Introduction to Translational Cardiovascular Research

Dennis V. Cokkinos
Editor

Introduction to Translational Cardiovascular Research

Springer

Editor
Dennis V. Cokkinos, MD, FESC
Biomedical Research Foundation
Academy of Athens
Athens
Greece

ISBN 978-3-319-08797-9 ISBN 978-3-319-08798-6 (eBook)
DOI 10.1007/978-3-319-08798-6
Springer Cham Heidelberg New York Dordrecht London

Library of Congress Control Number: 2014954073

Printed on acid-free paper

Springer is part of Springer Science+Business Media (www.springer.com)

All the authors dedicate this book to our families and our students. The editor (DVC) additionally dedicates it to his wife Vana, in translation

Foreword

It is with great pleasure that I write this foreword for two reasons:

First, the concept of this book emerged from two seminars held in our institution with the same title, *Introduction to Translational Cardiovascular Research*, with Professor Dennis V. Cokkinos, Director of the Heart and Vessel Department, who is also the Editor of this book as the course organizer, and Professor Evangelia Kranias, Director of Molecular Biology, Hanna Professor of Cardiology, Chair, Department of Pharmacology and Cell Biophysics, University of Cincinnati College of Medicine as co-organizer.

These courses were attended by young researchers either from a basic or a clinical background; many of them are students at or collaborating with our center.

Also, most of the instructors in this course, who have also authored the 31 chapters of the book, are either researchers or collaborators of our foundation.

Second, the Biomedical Research Foundation Academy of Athens, at its inception in 1992 and its inauguration in 2002, has been dedicated to the concept of translational research. This concept originated in the decade of 1990, and in essence, it concerns the successful implementation of laboratory findings in clinical care. When we refer to clinical care, we include the individual patient with his inalienable rights to health, quality of life, and well-being, but also the community and, finally, world health policies.

Although the value of basic research, which pertains to the quest of pure scientific knowledge, and clinical research, which includes mechanisms of human disease, therapeutic interventions, clinical trials, and the development of new technologies is well appreciated, there clearly exists a need for their integration, which defines translational research. This is not an easy task; meticulous planning, organizational expertise, and a generous budget allotment are essential. Our foundation strives to meet these challenges in collaboration with other institutes in Greece and abroad dedicated to these same meritorious goals.

I believe that this book, which represents a great effort by its Editor, Professor Dennis V. Cokkinos and all the participating authors, will further contribute to the awareness of the value of translational research.

I hope that it may prove successful and pursue a course productive to our application of research toward an improved quality of health services for our patients.

Professor-Academician
Gregory D. Skalkeas, MD
President, Biomedical Research Foundation Academy of Athens,
Athens, Greece

Preface

The term "translational research" has come to stay. It reflects today's integration of basic research ("bench") findings with the clinical practice of medicine and, in a wider scope, the application of results from the individual patient ("bedside") to entire populations for the improvement of public health.

In this book, we try to offer future researchers a stimulus in as many aspects of cardiovascular research as possible so as to promote their interest in future fields of cardiovascular disease, diagnosis, and treatment.

The idea for this book emerged from two series of seminars given at the Biomedical Research Foundation of the Academy of Athens under the title *Introduction to Translational Cardiovascular Research.*

Many presentations were added, deleted, or, more importantly, upregulated and transformed as the lessons progressed.

However, the constant "leitmotif" of the book is the interaction of basic and applied knowledge.

Another aspect that is constantly stressed by the editor by many cross-referrals is that the various processes described are very closely interrelated.

Inevitably, this book is incomplete and will be partially outdated by the time it appears, given the constant explosion of both knowledge and information.

As editor, I have tried to give a logical sequence to the chapters. Thus, fundamental and important aspects are discussed first: an introduction to the subject, translational research, cardiac development and regeneration, basis of cell excitability, and conduction. Next, I thought appropriate to describe the great axes such as the renin-angiotensin-aldosterone system, the beta adrenergic receptors, and the hypothalamic-pituitary-adrenal axis.

After this, the ubiquitous and constantly enlarging subject of genetic polymorphisms is discussed both generally and specifically as regards the vascular endothelium, which involves so many mechanisms regulating cardiac and vascular structure and function. MicroRNAs are another constantly expanding subject; they are practically involved in all processes affecting the cardiovascular system as well as the organism as a whole.

The next unit that is discussed concerns fundamental processes such as cardiac hypertrophy, calcium cycling, inflammation, stress proteins and the adaptive response, cell death, repair of the infarcted myocardium, and myocardial remodeling, together with the arrhythmic potential of the heart.

Animal models of cardiovascular disease are subsequently described together with the aspects of the assessment of cardiac function and imaging in vitro in animals and in man. Next are discussed two currently widely studied entities in which novel, both basic and clinical knowledge is constantly emerging: the cardiomyopathies and the cardiorenal syndrome.

The book finishes with therapeutic aspects strongly pertaining to the interaction of basic and clinical research: pre-, peri-, and postconditioning and gene and cell therapy.

As a final chapter, an article on the translational application of the results of the continuously expanding heart failure trials is included.

Inevitably, there is considerable overlap of the data presented in the various chapters. However, all the processes described have many common pathways and mechanisms of action.

When starting this endeavor, I was asked by Springer to whom this book was addressed. The answer came gradually through the comments of the students attending these seminars and their numerous enlivening questions. Thus, it can be proposed that this book pertains to young physicians, nurses, and other scientists engaged in the clinical cardiovascular field who want to add a research-oriented dimension to their efforts toward a better understanding and practice of medicine. It also aims to attract young basic researchers who want to develop a better comprehension of the organism as a whole, man or animal, which they are investigating.

I want to express my gratitude to all the authors of this book, who also are significant contributors in their respective fields. First as teachers, they gave their best efforts to educate the young translational investigators of the future. We should not forget the wise aphorism of Henry Brooks Adams:

> A teacher affects eternity. He can never tell where his influence stops.

The same teachers, often with the aid of other colleagues, expressed their thoughts in print with great diligence. Our collaboration has always been friendly, punctual, and rewarding. They are the protagonists of this book, together with our students, whose interest and curiosity prompted many outstanding considerations included in this volume.

If the current endeavor proves successful, an ongoing process of evolution will hopefully commence.

Acknowledgments and thanks are due to many:

I am indebted to all the contributors: teachers, authors, and students. Foremost, Professor Evangelia Kranias is my cochair of the course from which this book originated. She added her prestige, suggestions, and insight.

Theodora Tzanavari is a constant asset as course organizer. Additionally, her help in editing manuscripts and the work in print is invaluable.

My secretary Athinais Danou generously contributed her outstanding talents and painstaking conscientiousness throughout this effort. Tonia Kyriakoulakou and Konstantinia Karpouzi also contributed their valuable secretarial aid.

The Biomedical Research Foundation Academy of Athens, a center of international excellence, is strongly represented in this book both by faculty and students. This foundation, which, in essence, made this book possible by its organizational help, practical support, and creative environment, is the result of the vision and inspired leadership of Professor Academician Gregory D. Skalkeas, my mentor of 45 years, who contributes a foreword to the volume.

The initiation of this series and the support of the efforts toward the production of the book would not be possible without the generous financial support of the Onassis Foundation and its President Mr. Anthony Papadimitriou, a true and long-standing friend. Mr. Grant Weston of the Springer Publishing Company strongly encouraged me in planning, editing, and finishing this book.

Ms. Govindan Meena has been an outstanding project manager.

The Editor joins the faculty in dedicating this book to our families and to our students over the years, especially those who attended these seminars; they are all a constant inspiration.

I personally dedicate it additionally as a translation of my lifelong gratitude to my wife Vana.

I have tried to give due thanks to all my co-contributors for the possible success of this book. If this does not materialize as hoped, the responsibility rests solely with the Editor.

Dennis V. Cokkinos, MD, FESC
Professor Emeritus University of Athens,
Honorary Director Onassis Cardiac Surgery Center,
Heart and Vessel Department,
Biomedical Research Foundation of the Academy of Athens,
Athens, Greece

Contents

Contributors

Constantinos D. Anagnostopoulos, MD, PhD, FRCP, FRCR, FESC PET/CT Unit, Centre for Experimental Surgery, Clinical and Translational Research, Biomedical Research Foundation, Academy of Athens, Athens, Greece

Katherine Anagnostopoulou Cardiology Department, Onassis Cardiac Surgery Center, Kallithea, Greece

Nicholas P. Anagnou, MD, PhD Laboratory of Cell and Gene Therapy, Biomedical Research Foundation of the Academy of Athens (IIBEAA), Athens, Greece

Laboratory of Biology, University of Athens School of Medicine, Athens, Greece

Aris Anastasakis, MD, PhD Unit of Inherited Cardiovascular Diseases, 1st Department of Cardiology, University of Athens, Athens, Greece

Ioanna Andreadou Department of Pharmaceutical Chemistry, University of Athens School of Pharmacy, Athens, Greece

Emmanuel Androulakis 1st Cardiology Unit, Hippokration Hospital, Athens University Medical School, Athens, Greece

Antonis A. Armoundas, PhD Cardiology Division, Cardiovascular Research Center, Massachusetts General Hospital, Charlestown, Boston, USA

Feriel Azibani UMR-S 942 Inserm, University Paris Diderot, Paris, France

Dimitris Beis Developmental Biology, Biomedical Research Foundation, Academy of Athens, Athens, Greece

Dimitrios T Boumpas, MD, FACP 1st Department of Medicine, Attiko Hospital, Chaidari, Athens, Greece

Evangelia Charmandari, MD, MSc, PhD, MRCP(UK), CCST(UK) Division of Endocrinology and Metabolism, Clinical Research Center, Biomedical Research Foundation of the Academy of Athens, Athens, Greece

Division of Endocrinology, Metabolism and Diabetes, First Department of Pediatrics, University of Athens Medical School, "Aghia Sophia" Children's Hospital, Athens, Greece

Aristidis S. Charonis, MD, PhD Center of Clinical, Experimental Surgery and Translational Research, Biomedical Research Foundation of the Academy of Athens, Athens, Greece

George P. Chrousos, MD, MACP, MACE, FRCP (London) Division of Endocrinology and Metabolism, Clinical Research Center, Biomedical Research Foundation of the Academy of Athens, Athens, Greece

First Department of Pediatrics, University of Athens Medical School, "Aghia Sophia" Children's Hospital, Athens, Greece

Division of Endocrinology, Metabolism and Diabetes, UNESCO Chair on Adolescent Health Care, University of Athens Medical School, "Aghia Sophia" Children's Hospital, Athens, Greece

Distinguished Visiting Scientist, NICHD, NIH, Bethesda, MD, USA

Saudi Diabetes Study Research Group, King Fahd Medical Research Center, King Abdulaziz University, Jeddah, Saudi Arabia

Dennis V. Cokkinos Heart and Vessel Department, Biomedical Research Foundation Academy of Athens, Athens, Greece

Nikolaos Dagres Second Department of Cardiology, University of Athens Medical School, Attikon University Hospital, Athens, Greece

Claude Delcayre, PhD UMR-S 942 Inserm, University Paris Diderot, Paris, France

Inês Falcão-Pires, MSc, PhD Department of Physiology and Cardiothoracic Surgery, Faculty of Medicine, Universidade do Porto, Alameda Prof Hernâni Monteiro, Porto, Portugal

Loubina Fazal UMR-S 942 Inserm, University Paris Diderot, Paris, France

Gerasimos Filippatos, MD, FESC, FACC Department of Cardiology, Athens University Hospital Attikon, Athens, Greece

Nikolaos G Frangogiannis, MD Department of Medicine (Cardiology), The Wilf Family Cardiovascular Research Institute, Albert Einstein College of Medicine, Bronx, NY, USA

Charalampia V. Geladari, MD Division of Cardiology, Department of Medicine, Center for Life Sciences, Beth Israel Deaconess Medical Center, Boston, MA, USA

Department of Internal Medicine, Evangelismos State General Hospital, Athens, Greece

Eleni V. Geladari, MD Division of Cardiology, Department of Medicine, Center for Life Sciences, Beth Israel Deaconess Medical Center, Boston, MA, USA

4th Department of Internal Medicine, Evangelismos State General Hospital, Athens, Greece

Mihai Gheorghiade, MD Division of Cardiology, Department of Medicine, Center for Cardiovascular Innovation, Northwestern University Feinberg School of Medicine, Chicago, IL, USA

Kobra Haghighi Department of Pharmacology and Cell Biophysics, University of Cincinnati, College of Medicine, Cincinnati, OH, USA

E. Kevin Heist, MD, PhD Cardiology Division, Massachusetts General Hospital, Boston, MA, USA

Efstathios K. Iliodromitis Second Department of Cardiology, University of Athens Medical School, Attikon University Hospital, Athens, Greece

Stamatia Kalogirou Developmental Biology, Biomedical Research Foundation, Academy of Athens, Athens, Greece

Katia P. Karalis, MD, PhD Developmental Biology Lab, Center of Basic Research I, Biomedical Research Foundation of the Academy of Athens, Athens, Greece

Theodore Karatzas Second Department of Propaedeutic Surgery, Medical School, National and Kapodistrian University of Athens, Athens, Greece

Sadiya S. Khan, MD Division of Cardiology, Department of Medicine, Center for Cardiovascular Innovation, Northwestern University Feinberg School of Medicine, Chicago, IL, USA

Genovefa Kolovou Department of Cardiology, Onassis Cardiac Surgery Center, Kallithea, Greece

Maria Irene Kontaridis, PhD Division of Cardiology, Department of Medicine, Center for Life Sciences, Beth Israel Deaconess Medical Center, Boston, MA, USA

Department of Biological Chemistry and Molecular Pharmacology, Harvard Medical School, Boston, MA, USA

Michael Koutsilieris, MD, PhD Department of Experimental Physiology, Medical School, National and Kapodistrian University of Athens, Goudi-Athens, Greece

Elias Kouvelas Department of Physiology, University of Patras, Patras, Greece

Evangelia G. Kranias, PhD Department of Pharmacology and Cell Biophysics, University of Cincinnati, College of Medicine, Cincinnati, OH, USA

Academy of Athens Foundation of Biomedical Research, Athens, Greece

Dimitrios T. Kremastinos Second Department of Cardiology, University of Athens Medical School, Attikon University Hospital, Athens, Greece

Adelino F. Leite-Moreira, MD, PhD Department of Physiology and Cardiothoracic Surgery, Faculty of Medicine, Universidade do Porto, Alameda Prof Hernâni Monteiro, Porto, Portugal

André P. Lourenço, MD, PhD Department of Physiology and Cardiothoracic Surgery, Faculty of Medicine of University of Porto, Porto, Portugal

Konstantinos Makaritsis, MD Department of Medicine, University of Thessaly, School of Medicine, Larissa University Hospital, Larissa, Greece

Konstantinos Malliaras, MD 3rd Department of Cardiology, University of Athens, Athens, Greece

Maria Maridaki Department of Sports Medicine and Biology of Physical Activity, Faculty of Physical Education and Sport Science, National and Kapodistrian University of Athens, Athens, Greece

Manolis Mavroidis Cell Biology Division, Biomedical Research Foundation, Academy of Athens, Athens, Greece

Theofanie Mela, MD Cardiology Division, Massachusetts General Hospital, Boston, MA, USA

Faisal M. Merchant, MD Cardiology Division, Emory University School of Medicine, Atlanta, GA, USA

John Nanas, MD, PhD 3rd Department of Cardiology, University of Athens, Athens, Greece

Stephan G. Nekolla, PhD, FESC Multimodal Cardiac Imaging, NuklearmedizinischeKlinik und PoliklinikKlinikumrechts der Isar der Technischen Universitaet München, Munich, Germany

Nicolas C. Nicolaides, MD, PhD Division of Endocrinology and Metabolism, Clinical Research Center, Biomedical Research Foundation of the Academy of Athens, Athens, Greece

Petros Nihoyannopoulos, MD, FRCP, FESC, FACC, FAHA National Heart and Lung Institute, Imperial College London, London, UK

Hammersmith Hospital, London, UK

Eva D. Papadimitraki, MD Department of Cardiology, Laikon General Hospital, Athens, Greece

Eleni Papanikolaou Laboratory of Cell and Gene Therapy, Biomedical Research Foundation of the Academy of Athens (IIBEAA), Athens, Greece

Laboratory of Biology, University of Athens School of Medicine, Athens, Greece

Anna N. Paschali, MD, MSc, PhD Medical School and Centre for Clinical Research, University of Patras, Biomedical Research Foundation, Academy of Athens, Athens, Greece

Anastassios Philippou Department of Experimental Physiology, Medical School, National and Kapodistrian University of Athens, Goudi-Athens, Greece

Mathilde Prudhomme UMR-S 942 Inserm, University Paris Diderot, Paris, France

Dheeraj Puppala, MD Cardiology Division, Cardiovascular Research Center, Massachusetts General Hospital, Charlestown, Boston, USA

Helene Ragot UMR-S 942 Inserm, University Paris Diderot, Paris, France

Jane-Lise Samuel UMR-S 942 Inserm, University Paris Diderot, Paris, France

Despina Sanoudou Department of Pharmacology, Medical School, University of Athens and Biomedical Research Foundation of the Academy of Athens, Athens, Greece

Omid Sayadi, PhD Cardiology Division, Cardiovascular Research Center, Massachusetts General Hospital, Charlestown, Boston, USA

Jagmeet P. Singh, MD, PhD Cardiology Division, Massachusetts General Hospital, Boston, MA, USA

Irini Skaliora, PhD Neurophysiology Laboratory, Center for Basic Research, Biomedical Research Foundation of the Academy of Athens (BRFAA), Athens, Greece

Vasileios Sousonis, MD 3rd Department of Cardiology, University of Athens, Athens, Greece

Christodoulos Stefanadis 1st Cardiology Unit, Hippokration Hospital, Athens University Medical School, Athens, Greece

Bernard Swynghedauw, PhD, MD INSERM, U 942-INSERM Hôpital Lariboisière, Paris, France

John Terrovitis, MD 3rd Department of Cardiology, University of Athens, Athens, Greece

Dimitris Tousoulis, MD, PhD, FACC 1st Cardiology Unit, Department of Cardiology, Hippokration Hospital, Athens University Medical School, Athens, Greece

Filippos Triposkiadis, MD Department of Cardiology, University of Thessaly, School of Medicine, Larissa University Hospital, Larissa, Greece

Nikolaos Tsigkas Developmental Biology, Biomedical Research Foundation, Academy of Athens, Athens, Greece

Theodora Tzanavari, PhD Developmental Biology Lab, Center of Basic Research I, Biomedical Research Foundation of the Academy of Athens, Athens, Greece

Demetrios V. Vlahakos Renal Unit, B'Department of Medicine, Attikon University Hospital, Haidari, Athens, Greece

Junhong Wang Department of Medicine (Cardiology), The Wilf Family Cardiovascular Research Institute, Albert Einstein College of Medicine, Bronx, NY, USA

James S.M. Yeh, MBChB, MRCP, PhD National Heart and Lung Institute, Imperial College London, London, UK

Part I

General Aspects

Introduction: What Is Translational Research

1

Dennis V. Cokkinos

Abstract

There are many definitions of Research, Basic, Clinical and Translational Research. A very practical and short definition of Translational Research could be, the application of findings from Basic Research to patient, community and population care and to the advancement of the delivery of health services.

Usually three steps can be defined:

T1 (T for translation): is the transfer of new understanding of disease mechanisms gained in the laboratory into the development of new methods for diagnosis and therapy.

T2 is the translation of results from clinical studies into everyday clinical practice and health decision making.

T3 is the dissemination and implementation of research translation into practice/community/large populations.

Corresponding blocks or impediments are delineated to the successful employment of these steps. A newly introduced concept is the Valley of Death, separating research results from successful innovation-application.

To overcome these problems, the foundation and collaboration of centers able to conduct Translational Research, such as the National Institutes of Health and the National Clinical and Translational Science Award Consortium is important.

The teaching, training, and formation of translational researchers is difficult, varied and a matter of constant effort.

To overcome increasing costs the combination of "wet" –i.e. biological labs with "dry" or computational data is being increasingly employed.

Keywords

Research • Basic research • Valley of death • Translational Research

D.V. Cokkinos MD, FESC
Heart and Vessel Department, Biomedical Research Foundation, Academy of Athens, Athens, Greece
e-mail: dcokkinos@bioacademy.gr

D.V. Cokkinos (ed.), *Introduction to Translational Cardiovascular Research*,
DOI 10.1007/978-3-319-08798-6_1, © Springer International Publishing Switzerland 2015

Abbreviations

ACRT	Association for Clinical Research Training
AHCs	Academic Health Centers
BRFAA	Biomedical Research Foundation Academy of Athens
CTSA	Clinical and Translational Science Awards
GCRCs	General Clinical Research Centers
NCATS	National Center for Advancing Translating Services
NCI	Translational Research Institute
NIH	National Institutes of Health
TR	Translational Research

1.1 Definitions

The term "Translational Research" (TR) is being increasingly employed in the last 20 years. It has come to imply to some scientists a more advanced type of research. Before an attempt is made to define TR one should first try to define Research. According to the National Science Foundation [1]:

Research is planned search or critical investigation aimed at discovery of new knowledge with the hope that such knowledge will be useful in developing a new product or service or a new process or technique or in bringing about a significant improvement to a planned product process.

In the Oxford English Dictionary, Research is defined more simply as [2]: A search or investigation directed to the discovery of some fact by careful consideration or study of a subject; a course of critical or scientific inquiry.

K. Popper in 1972 discussed the philosophy of research. According to him [3] research should follow five steps:

1. Seek a problem,
2. Propose a solution
3. Formulate a testable hypothesis from that proposal
4. Attempt to refute the hypothesis by observations and experiments
5. Establish preference between competing theories.

According to Jan Illing [4], the following practical considerations apply when studying research: The area, the topic, and general, specific and data collection questions. She also points out that the important aspects of research are:

The aim, testing hypothesis, cause and effect, generalizability, adding to existing knowledge, and vigour, viability and reliability.

Before trying to define TR, which in very plain words is the link between Basic and Clinical Research, one should try to define its two components:

1.2 Basic Research

According to the National Science Foundation [1]: Basic Research is performed without practical ends. It results in general knowledge and an understanding of nature and its laws. This general knowledge provides the means of answering a large number of important practical problems, though it may not give a complete specific answer to any one of them.

In other words it is research for the acquisition of knowledge. This would take us to the early Greek philosophers, Thales and Empedocles among others.

However, even those thinkers in the eve of knowledge acquisition, must have had a problem in mind, i.e. some potential application towards improving the state of the world they were living in. The function of Applied Research (to be further defined) is to provide such complete answers [5].

According to Hecker and Birla [6], Basic Research is the planned systemic approach of new knowledge or understanding toward general application. According to the same authors, Applied Research is the acquisition of knowledge or understanding to meet a specific recognized need.

Please note that in neither of the definitions is the object of research explicitly mentioned.

Many of the early studies, i.e. of the pulse and the ECG can be in some way be considered basic, although undoubtedly Sir Thomas Lewis, Karel Frederic Wenckebach and Willem Einthoven had therapeutic goals in mind.

1.3 Clinical Research

Clinical Research is much more widely applied. Again one can use the NIH Directors Panel definition [7, 8]: It is tantamount to:
Patient-oriented research,
Epidemiologic and behavioral studies, and
Health services research.

Seely and Grinspoon point out [9] that from Clinical Research are excluded in vitro studies utilizing human tissues that cannot be linked to living individuals. They add that according to the National Institution of Health (NIH), under Patient-oriented Research can be included Research conducted with human subjects, or on material of human origin such as tissues, specimens and cognitive phenomena for which an investigator (or colleague) directly interacts with human subjects.

Obviously, no definition can be correct or complete in a waterproof manner. Thus, if one investigates or just studies "mechanisms of human disease", without interacting with the patient as an individual, he could well claim to be carrying-out Basic Research.

Clinical Research is currently much more widely practiced than the other two types of research described. It is widely divided into Retrospective and Prospective. Obviously the latter is considered more worthwhile. However, when a clinical question arises, it is easier and faster to look back at already existing data than start acquiring new ones. Of course, only prospective trials can be randomized, and placebo-controlled, thus requiring Ethics Committee approval and informed consent. Our era has seen the triumph of the multicenter randomized placebo-controlled megatrials. Some concerns about them still exist. Thus Robert M. Califf [10], one of the most experienced clinical trial researchers, points out that less than 15 % of major guidance recommendations are evidence-based. It should not be forgotten that since September 2004 it has been announced by the International Committee of Medical Journal Editors that registration of clinical trials is a prerequisite of publication.

However, description of this process is not the subject of this chapter, nor is ethics of research.

1.4 Translational Research

The term "Translational Research" (TR) or Science was first used in the 1990 decade and referred to efforts devoted to the discovery of the new antitumor genes [11].

It was soon extended to other disciplines and of course to Cardiology [12].

Very soon the term "from bench to bedside" was introduced. Other names had been previously employed, i.e., pre-clinical research, research targeted to the disease [13].

One of the pioneers in the endeavour of establishing the identity of TR, Steven H. Woolf gives these definitions [14]: Bench-to-bedside enterprise, harnessing basic science to produce new drugs, devices and treatment options for patients.

An Interface between basic science and clinical medicine.

Dische and Saunders [15] mention the definition given by Julie Denekamp: Translational Research is the application of scientific method to address a health need. Barry S. Coller has very simply defined [16] it as:

Successful implementation of a laboratory concept into a clinical protocol.

He also reiterates the older paradigm of the three-legged stool, in which Research is one of the three legs, together with patient care and education, and the newer paradigm in which Research is the cushion that covers a four legged stool – patient care, Education, Community service and Global health, being the four legs. He further points out that TR differs from scientific discovery in both its goals and processes. The latter pertains to adding to the store of human knowledge. The former springs from the motivation to improve human health, searching for the identification of discoveries that can fill this need [17].

Williams and Robertson [18] in the introduction to their excellent book "Clinical and Translational Science" state that TR originally used to describe the translation of animal studies to humans, but that more recently it has applied to a great variety of activities, from cell-based experiment results to whole organs and organisms, to epidemiologic data and the delivery of health or health services. The information provided by translating epidemiology data ultimately affects the delivery of health services.

The same authors [19], add the population-based study dimension.

For the academic community TR signifies the effort to close the gap between knowledge and practice, as well as the transfer of results of research studies to practice [20].

According to the TR Working Group of the National Cancer Institute (NCI): Translational Research transforms scientific discoveries arising from laboratory, clinical or population studies into clinical application to reduce cancer incidence, morbidity, and mortality [21].

If one interprets the Institute of Medicine Clinical Research Roundtable [22, 23]:

T1 (T for translation): is the transfer of new understanding of disease mechanisms gained in the laboratory into the development of new methods for diagnosis and therapy.

T2 is the translation of results from clinical studies into everyday clinical practice and health decision making. These authors, and Robertson and Williams, point out [19] that one more subgroup is commonly provided: T3, i.e. dissemination and implementation of research translation into practice/community/large populations.

According to Westfall et al. [24] T1 involves Basic Research.

T2 includes guideline development, meta-analyses, and systematic reviews, while T3 includes dissemination and implementation research. It is obvious that all these steps are essential if a fruitful transfer of research findings to improved public health is desired.

It is stressed that a continuum exists from Basic Science to Clinical Science- In essence this constitutes the bench to bedside process (T1).

Then comes the implementation of findings. From the bedside to practice, i.e., to the general population, Healthcare and Health Services (T2 and T3).

Malliaras et al. [25] very opportunely correlate these three stages to phase I, II, III trials

Waldman and Terzic [26] maintain that 6 T steps can be differentiated:

TO: Targets, Biomarkers, Genes, Pathways, Mechanisms

T1: First in Human phase I-II Trials. Proof of Concept

T2: Phase III Trials. Clinical Efficiency. Clinical Guidelines

T3: Dissemination. Community Engagement. Health Service Research.

Comparative Effectiveness.

T4: Public Health. Prevention. Population Health Impact. Behavioural

Modifications. Lifestyle Modifications

T5: Social Health Care. Political Security. Economic Opportunity. Access to Education. Access to Health Care.

Of course the problem with definitions and aphorisms is that they can get very pedantic.

According to Schteingart [8] and to Mc Gartland Rubio et al. [27] to improve community practice, T2 should cater to the development of new treatments and to the use of new tools to validate diagnosis and treatment. Other aspects to be addressed are comparative effectiveness, the use of bioinformatics to integrate large datasets, and the application of genomics to determine efficacy and safety of drugs. The same authors [27] describe how the members of the ACRT (Association for Clinical Research Training) developed this working definition of TR:

Translational Research fosters the multidirectional integration of Basic Research, patient-oriented research, and population-based research, with the long-term aim of improving the health of the public.

T1 research expedites the movement between Basic Research and patient-oriented research that leads to new or improved scientific understanding or standards of care.

T2 research facilitates the movement between patient-oriented research and population-based research but leads to better patient outcomes, the implementation of best practices, and improved health status in communities.

T3 research promotes interaction between laboratory-based research and population-based research to stimulate a robust scientific understanding of human health and disease.

They also mention that the NIH has followed another definition in directions about applying for Clinical and Translational Science Awards (CTSA) (http://grants.nih.gov/grants/guide/rfa-files/RFA-RM-07-007.html):

Translational Research includes two areas of translation. One is the process of applying discoveries generated during research in the laboratory, and in preclinical studies, to the development of trials and studies in humans. The second area of translation concerns research aimed at enhancing the adoption of best practices in the community. Cost-effectiveness of prevention and treatment strategies is also an important part of translational science.

Again, it is realized according to the NIH Roadmap for Clinical Research, that there are three TR models [8]:

In the unidirectional model, the laboratory findings are applied to the patient and then to the wider public. A good example is the development of a new drug. In the bidirectional model, population findings have to be tested back in the laboratory. The new hypothesis that statins are associated with increased prevalence of type 2 diabetes mellitus, emerging mostly from observational studies, can be studied in the laboratory.

A more realistic model is the multidirectional one in which Basic Research, patient oriented research and population-based research are interconnected [8].

In a very recent lecture Walter J. Koch [28] described the following process:

A clinical observation creates a design for its therapeutic application. Small and large animal models are then studied. The findings from these studies prompt the design of the appropriate clinical trials.

In another representation, after the "bench" results are applied to the "bedside", the time comes for clinical trials. The knowledge acquired from these is then applied to wide population implementation.

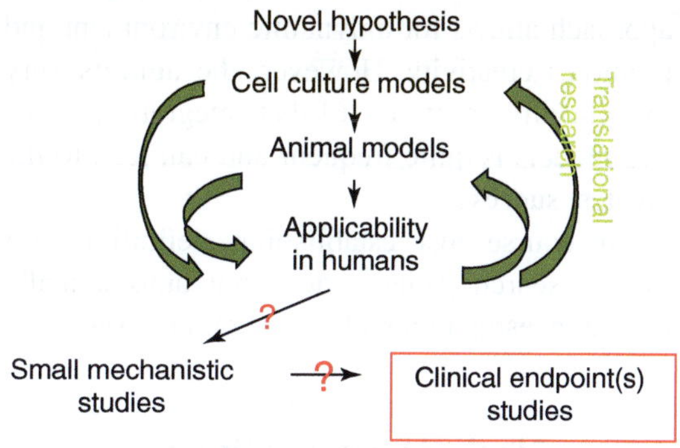

Fig. 1.1 Transferring knowledge from basic science to the clinical area (Reproduced from Antoniades [30] with permission)

Kieburtz and Olanow propose another approach [29], while describing The Experimental Translational Therapeutic Pathway:

From the in vitro experiments in which mechanisms and candidate interventions are defined, whole animal (in vivo) experiments are carried out to assess efficacy. Safety experiments and drug activity studies follow. Then comes FDA application in the US and to corresponding organizations elsewhere. After approval, one moves to phase I, II, and III studies. Very important is postmarketing surveillance which further determines both safety and efficacy.

Charalambos Antoniades [30] has proposed another roadmap in Fig. 1.1.

Again it must be pointed out that these are definitions given by experienced investigators which are similar among them, but differ somewhat according to their creators' backgrounds and research interests.

Hecker and Birla [6] stress that strategy in research consists of two differing directions: The more frequent, especially, I would think, in well organized departments in the academic setting, is the Top Down Strategy, in which a vision is set. To ensure successful implementation of this vision, one must set objectives to be attained, and research activities to be undertaken.

The same authors describe that in the bottom-up approach, the outcome of experimentation dictates the overall strategic research direction.

The finding by Murry et al. [31] of ischemic preconditioning is such an example. This latter approach allows for a dynamic environment and promotes creativity. However, the authors very thoughtfully point out [6] that integration of the two models is quite frequent and can lead to the greatest success.

Of course just establishing definitions for these research patterns does not automatically ensure investigational bliss and clinical success.

1.5 Blocks to Translational Research

Lauer and Scarlatos [23], reiterate the three translational blocks or obstacles identified by the Institute of Medicine Clinical Research Roundtable [22], pertaining to T1, T2 and T3.

Chautard et al. [32] have further defined the first block as this limiting translation of new knowledge into clinical practice and health decision making towards improved health. As components of the former they cite lack of willing participants, regulatory burdens, fragmented infrastructure, incompatible databases, and lack of qualified investigators. As components of the latter, they mention career disincentives, practice limitations, high research costs and lack of funding. A T3 block can be regarded as limitation of dissemination into practice, communities, and large populations.

Here it must be stressed that the NIH itself points out that funding between T1 and T2 is not evenly balanced, to some extent explaining the block between these stage.

Thus, according to some 2007 data the NIH allots 13 billion dollars to Basic Research but only 787 millions to Health Services Research. Researchers from the National Cancer Institute stresses another important point, that research dissemination and diffusion are costly by themselves [33].

Hecker and Birla [6] give two interesting additional definition pertaining to research.

Thus they propose two more entities:

(a) Development is the systematic use of the knowledge or understanding gained from research of practical experience directed toward the production or significant improvement of useful products.

(b) Applied Research is the acquisition of knowledge or understanding to meet a specific recognized need".

According to Vanovar Bush [5] the function of applied research is to give answers which Basic Research cannot provide.

Another goal of TR which the European Society of Cardiology specifically endorses is innovation, which should be the strong point of discovery.

Deborah Zucker [34] describes that innovation connotes something novel, original, visionary, and hopefully improved. It necessitates the generation of new ideas and hypotheses.

These newer notions signify the quest for the attainment of results and not just the acquisition of new data, which is becoming more pressing with time.

The question then arises, by what measures can TR be carried out and produce favorable results for the improvement of the care of the individual patient and the human populations?

1.6 Organizational Aspects

The evolution towards organizing TR in the United States is interesting and didactic, as presented by Robertson and Williams [19]. They describe how the General Clinical Research Centers (GCRCs) evolved to the Clinical and Translational Science Award (CTSA) program in 2005.

They give a draft of the conceptual framework of the National CTSA Consortium.

The CTSA consortium comprises numerous Academic Health Centers (AHCs) in various states.

From their Fig. 1.1 one can readily appreciate the complexity but also the scope of these clinical and Translational Research Institutes.

Recently, Gordon R Bernard [35] described the establishment of a new NIH center, the National Center for Advancing Translational Services (NCATS) with a budget of $576.5 millions, comprising the Clinical and Translational Science Award (CTSA) program, a consortium of 60 sites.

1.6.1 The Value of Collaborations-Paradigms

First, the necessity of collaborations must be realized and appreciated. Thus, Lauer and Scarlatos [23] point out in the Progenitor Cell Biology Consortium that collaborations among institutions are essential. They describe the path from discovery (presumably produced through Basic Research), as producing early (pilot) T1 studies and ancillary studies towards yielding clinical applications.

In the Basic Research component, this Consortium is the main vehicle. A large number of Research Units is coordinated by the Administrative Coordinating Center, which is the University of Maryland, Baltimore.

As regards clinical applications, the Cardiovascular Cell Therapy Research Network consists of important clinical departments: i.e. the Vanderbilt University, the University of Florida, the Cleveland Clinic and the Texas Heart Institute.

A similar paradigm is offered by the Pediatric Cardiovascular Translational Bench to Bassinet Program.

Again one can mark three stages:

Discovery is managed by the Cardiovascular Development Consortium, managed by four research Units (Gladstone, Harvard, Pittsburgh, Utah).

Early T1 is effected by the Pediatric Cardiac Genomics Consortium, comprising outstanding units (Boston, Columbia, Philadelphia, Mt. Sinai, Yale).

Finally the Clinical Application part is implemented by eight clinical sites which constitute the Pediatric Heart Network, a multicenter approach.

Bernard [35] also stresses the importance of collaboration to enable multi-site translational science.

This accent on collaboration brings into focus a consideration by Hecker and Birla [6]: They stress that many investigators or departments have a conception of territorial belonging or ownership of an idea. This narrow outlook is counter-productive and hampers collaboration.

1.6.2 Training Translational Research Scientists

This brings into focus the question: Can and should TR be taught? The answer to both is yes. Before considering how, let us outline the requirements of becoming a Translational Researcher.

In the aforementioned excellent and detailed book, K. E Hartman, E. Heitman, and N. Brown [36] devote a chapter on recommended knowledge bases for T1 and T2 Translational Research. Not surprisingly the requirements for the former discipline are simpler.

Thus, they describe that for T1, recommended knowledge base includes:

Human and molecular biology and pathophysiology, animal models, and laboratory techniques.

The TR translational science components include genomics, proteomics, imaging technology, biomarker development, biomedical informatics, dataset acquisition, and management.

Finally, core competences additionally include biostatistics, epidemiology, study design, research ethics, writing and communication.

For a T2 career, health care epidemiology and other care epidemiology methods are additionally required.

The authors point out that guidelines exist for the education in Clinical and Translational Research of students since 2008, and residents since 2007. They point out that although the mentored/apprentice research prototype still applies, participation into a core didactic curriculum is essential, as well as participation in formal career and leadership development activities. They also describe that some academic medical centers have established training programs in Clinical and early Translational Research, are their majority directed at MDs in post-doctoral training. These curricula vary widely. Moreover, for more advanced training a few programs offer PhDs in Clinical and TR per se.

Barry Coller according to David Schteintgart [8] proposes that the Basic and Clinical Researchers represent two separate cultures.

Similar specifications are proposed by many authors.

Thus, according to Williams and Robertson [37], a TR team should include:

- Laboratory-based investigators
- Clinical investigators
- Statisticians
- Data managers
- Research nurses and coordinators
- Research Pharmacists

The same authors, propose that the twenty first century human research laboratory should have the following picture (Fig. 1.2).

According to Schteingart [8] an appropriate collaborative model should encourage partnerships between researchers, practitioners and people skilled in translation.

A proposed concept of who is and who is not a translational investigator is given by Williams and Robertson [37] as adapted from Lee M Nadler, who gave some further thoughts on this subject in 2007 [38].

To produce such results many medical schools are proposing various teaching courses for producing this type of researchers.

However, it must be realized that there is no formal training to produce a translational researcher. David Schteingart [8] proposes how to train such scientists:

For those coming from a clinical background he proposes courses and seminars in genetics, molecular biology, computational biology, molecular imaging, epidemiology, and therapeutics.

From those coming from a basic laboratory, he proposes clinical immersion and to learn principles of clinical research. Furthermore, he recommends:

- Translational Research training principles
- Multidisciplinary training
- Training customized to an individual's background and skills
- Mentoring by mentoring committees with diverse areas of expertise
- Adaptation to working in multidisciplinary teams

The same author thoroughly accepts that many challenges remain:

- Translational Research training challenges
- Career paths uncertain

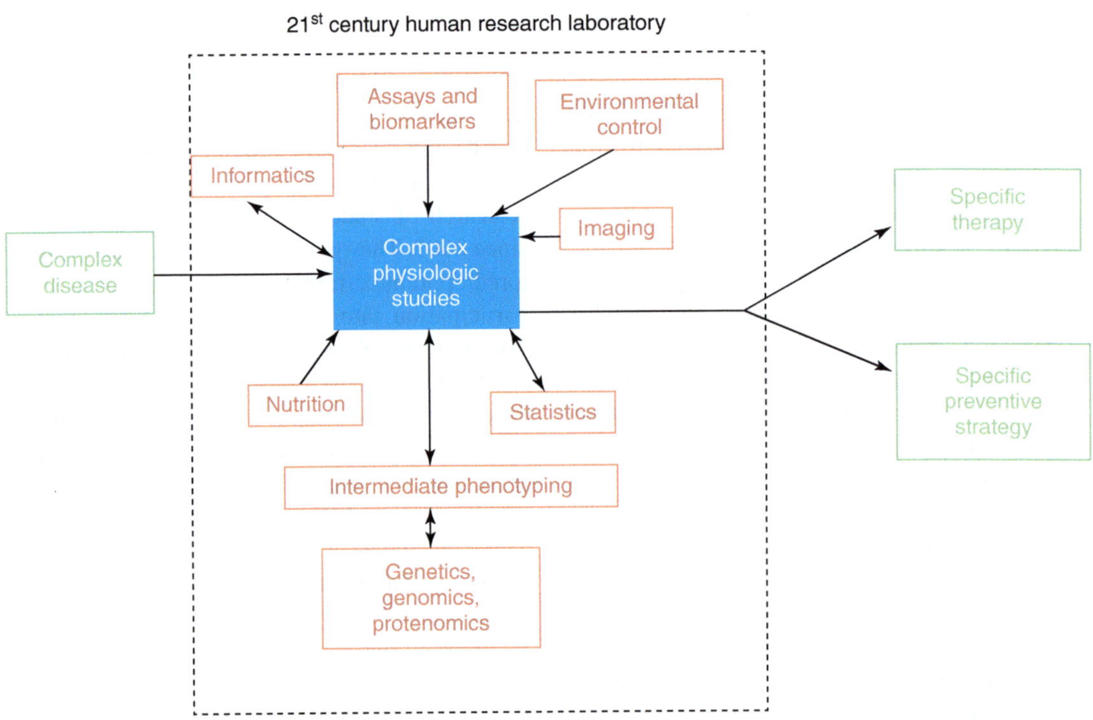

Fig. 1.2 The twenty-first century human translational investigator's laboratory (Reprinted from: Williams and Robertson [37], with permission of Elsevier)

- Limited number of well trained mentors
- Competences still being developed
- Unclear role in the academic research environment
- No specific evaluation criteria

McGartland Rubio et al. [27] discuss the implications for the design of training programs. They stress that since there exists a great diversity of educational background it may be necessary to design a separate curriculum for every individual trainee. They add that those with basic research background will need to acquire practice in clinical sciences and practice, while clinical background trainees will need additional exposure to basic science. They also stress the importance of mentoring, which will be further discussed. This aspect they consider demanding but highly rewarding.

Bernard [35] stresses the importance of educating and training scientists in clinical and translational research.

At the Biomedical Research Foundation of the Academy of Athens (BRFAA), we are conducting a yearly course, which actually gave the momentus for this book.

1.6.2.1 Leadership

It should be appreciated that, as in all fields of scientific endeavor, correct mentoring of the younger investigators is important and essential. The word "mentor" emerges from Homer's Odyssey. The Goddess Athena is disguised as Mentis or Mentor, a friend of Ulysses, who offers to guide his son Telemachus in a journey to gather news about his father.

A strategy in any department cannot be fruitful unless a sense of leadership is cultivated. Leadership develops leaders at all levels, with as a result exponential growth according to Hecker and Birla [6].

The same authors point out that success in scientific research can be determined by both tangible and, equally important, intangible factors, As tangible factors one can enumerate publications, impact factor, citations, Hirsch index, invited lectures and articles, positions in committees, grants, patents, and finally return on investment stock prices, etc.

Intangible rewards are to this and to many authors more important and long-lasting. Hecker and Birla [6] describe them as creating a positive work environment momentum and managing innovation. Additionally, these authors point out that leadership is different from management:

The latter term is impersonal and concerns resource allocation and accountability, while the former concerns the ability to work and connect with people and to convince them to implement change.

In this sense, in an inspiring article, Verkoeijen and Tabbers point out that good research requires productive theories and guidelines [39].

The PLoS Medicine Editors Tikki Pang and Robert F. Terry stress that in the twenty first century it seems astonishing that decisions on healthcare are still made without a solid grounding one research evidence [40].

1.6.3 The Blocks and Problems

Here, it should be stressed that the effort toward advancing T1 are well delineated and adequately stressed.

However, T2 is also gradually acquiring greater importance, because it is realized that many blocks in its implementation remain.

White et al. [41] and Green et al. [42] point out that the great majority of patients are treated in primary care centers.

Thus, we do not often get a real picture of everyday medicine if we only take into account the academic clinical centers, in which an "artificial" atmosphere may be said to exist.

To counteract this problem, has been created, which according to Westfall et al. [24], the NIH Roadmap tries to connect major academic laboratories to physicians and primary physician offices.

The authors further point out that since recommendations and guidelines are created from relatively small groups in selected tertiary centers their applicability may be limited and not reflect real world day –to-day practice.

Martin et al. [43] very recently point out that apart from the above mentioned factors, additional patient and trial barriers exist. Patient-specific factors were older age, out-of-state residence and female gender Trial specific barriers exist were intensive trial-related testing and long anticipation (>6 months).

The first item mentioned, which is essential to the success of clinical trials is simplicity, the principle of KISS (keep it simple and stupid), since intensive testing militates against adherence.

These considerations become more important currently because of the increasing cost and difficulty of conducting research; a main consideration is how to produce worthwhile results.

However, many researchers Dirk Brutsaert [44] being a distinguished example, question the future of clinical trials, in this instance in chronic heart failure. According to him, most single target-oriented clinical trials are doomed to fail. He advocates that we should incorporate Genome Wide Association Studies (GWAs), and research should be multiscaled- and multitarget-based and network medicine oriented. This is in contrast to the vast majority of multicenter clinical trials. Robert Calif [45] underlines the difficulties facing the planners of clinical trials. He points out that unintended biological targets are common (for example intracranial haemorrhage in thrombolysis for acute myocardial infarction), and that interactions among therapies and long-term effects are unpredictable. He points out to the necessity of embedding clinical trials within disease registries [46].

The Multicenter Research Group [47] realizing the shortcomings and mounting expenses of collaborative clinical trials have advanced many proposals. In accordance with the previous concerns about too much simplicity, they propose the evaluation of the effect of combing different therapies that target diverse pathways or mechanisms in complex medical disorders.

Very recently Sipido et al. [48] propose a clinical trial checklist:

1. Robust number of observations to ensure data care reliable.
2. Randomization and blinded observations.
3. Correct data processing.

In this aspect Kaul and Diamond [49] point out that research has many levels of importance. Thus, it may be (tough luck) both statistically insignificant and clinically unimportant.

It may be statistically significant but not clinically important; a $p<0.05$ may not mean anything as it may affect cardiac remodelling after an anterior myocardial infarction as regards end-diastolic volume. The best case scenario would be to have both clinically and statistically important results.

This brings again blocks T2 and T3. Balas and Boren [50] point out that it takes an estimated average of 17 years for only 14 % of new discoveries to reach clinical practice and patient care.

Contopoulos- Ioannidis et al. [51] examined the life of TR for medical interventions. Even for the most highly published and non refuted interventions for first use in human, they found a range of 0–28 years. They propose the following measures:

- Multidisciplinary collaboration involving both basic and clinical scientists.
- Large robust randomized clinical trials to provide proof of effectiveness.
- Effort at producing novel agents and new cutting-edge technologies.

Antoniades [31] notes that 95 % of hypotheses generated by basic science fail in the clinical arena. Translational research is able to filter these observations, and is the first priority of funding bodies: ERC/MRC/BHF/BRC, etc. Translational Research saves money! Negative findings in Translational Research are publishable, and may be more important than positive ones.

1.7 A New Concept: The Valley of Death

The difficulties described, or blocks T1, T2, T3 have in the last 5 year been given a new name referring to the Bible or Western films, The Valley of Death concept is the phase between research and successful innovation [52].

Declan Butler [53], describes this valley as an abyss in which neither basic researchers nor physicians busy with patient are keen to venture. According to this author lack of communication is the main problem.

1.7.1 Proposed Ways to Cross the Valley of Death

Roberts et al. [54] define the "death valley" as the gap between bench research and clinical application, and defined the varied barriers impending the crossing of this valley.

They point out that despite unprecedented US government funding of public research, the dramatic drop of new drugs and treatments reaching patient use should be of concern. They believe that a major factor is the increasing isolation of basic researchers from clinicians. They believe that clinician-scientists can built bridges across this valley. They point out that up to 2005 more funding goes to PhD than MD scientists.

Coller and Callif [55] again highlight the gap between finding a promising new agent and demonstrating its safety and efficacy. They also point out that basic scientists try to advance from the discovery to the development phase, but their institutions lack systems to support such research.

They propose six categories of questions in an effort to cross the valley of death.

1. Is it worth the effort?
2. Is there an adequate potential market?
3. What can be referred from human and animal data about likely safety and efficacy?
4. Can the agent be delivered to its target at an adequate concentration?
5. Is there an industry partner that can develop the agent effectively and efficiently?
6. Can a pivotal trial be designed and completed?

Bodi et al. [56] in a very recent article actually describe three death Valleys:
First: Transition to research in humans
Second: Preliminary validation in patients
Third: Use of the model in routine practice.

All these studies point out that barriers exist throughout the continuum of TR. Moses et al. [57] already in 2005 pointed out that the study of financial anatomy of biomedical research provides staggering facts. They quantify 10 year funding trends (from 1994 to 2004) in Basic, Translational and Clinical biomedical research. Funding increased from \$37.1 billions in 1994 to \$94.3 in 2003, doubling when adjusted for inflation. There was an increase from \$4.0 to \$14.2 billions for industry sponsorship of clinical trials, while proportions devoted to Basic and Applied Research were unchanged. These facts underlie the increasing trends for Clinical Research.

They urge more effective translation of Basic Research to clinical application, the very essence of TR.

1.7.2 New Concepts. The Dry Lab

The spiralling costs of research have highlighted another necessity. According to Quinn and Kohl [58] combining wet and dry research: experience with model development for cardiac mechano-electric structure function studies is important.

The wet lab, i.e. animal experimental work can be profitably complemented by the "dry" or computational model. In a very far reaching spotlight review they point out that this interactive combination of "wet" and "dry" experimentation can be very beneficial, through many processes:

The "wet" investigations (experimental and clinical) help develop experimental and/or clinical theoretical models.

On the other hand, the computational simulation results generate novel hypotheses and predictions. Wet lab studies are used to prove or disprove these model-created hypotheses.

Newly generated insight is employed to further advance computational models.

Another benefit of this wet/dry integration according to the authors is that computational modelling can help avoid a "fishing expedition". They also pertinently point out that an eventual mismatch between model prediction and experimental validation can identify directions for subsequent development. This integrative process further promotes translational medicine.

According to the Swedish Academy of Sciences [59] in a report on the occasion of the award of the Nobel Prize in Chemistry for 2013, experiments can be carried out in the laboratory but planned in the computer. The very recent concept of 3D organ printer, which is a transfer of the "dry" lab planning to the "wet" lab (organ production) is a very important paradigm.

Before concluding this chapter, it must still be mentioned that there is hope for the –even near – future. Hudson and Khazragui [52] point out that the "Valley of Death" can be crossed, even with profits. Even though they admit that co-operation between researchers from academia, the pharmaceutical-technical industry, government agencies and international funding bodies is still far from perfect, many countries are beginning to employ research as a tool for innovation and ultimately for expanding industrial and economic policy. The new HORIZON research project is such an example.

Curry [60] offers some thoughts on what expected from translational science over the next 10 years.

(i) A boost to biomarker research in the universities.
(ii) Transfer of early clinical testing work into academic control.
(iii) Create better opportunities for universities to commercialize their discoveries, and
(iv) Promote the regulation of the efficacy and quality of the process and its products.

To give some more concrete ideas on what can be expected from Translational Cardiovascular Research, E. Braunwald [61] describes the following aspects in which hopes exist for the next years from Translating Research into improved care:

Research in microRNAs, dilated cardiomyopathy, adaptive immunity in atherogenesis, cardiac hypertrophy and failure, gene therapy, regenerative therapy, sudden cardiac death, myocardial reperfusion injury, nitrosylation. Actually all of them are addressed in this book.

Finally, the deliberations of The Associations of Professors of Medicine should be taken into consideration: They specifically refer to the Translational of academic discovery into societal benefit which should be the final goal of TR [62].

Conclusions

The author has tried to give an overview on various modalities of Research, focusing on Translational Research.

The obstacles still existing in translation of laboratory findings to patient and population benefits through a multidirectional interactive model.

The need for educating translational Research and collaboration of large centers is evident. The integration of wet (animal) and dry (computational) laboratories for greater economy and efficacy is imperative.

References

1. NSF. Definition of research. National Science Foundation 2007. http://www.Nsf.gov/statistics/rand-def/business. cfm.
2. Oxford English Dictionary. www.oed.com.
3. Popper KR. Objective knowledge. 2nd ed. Oxford: Clarendon press; 1972. p. 191–205.
4. Illing J. Thinking about research: frameworkers, ethics and scholarships. Edinburgh: Association for the Study of Medical Education; 2007. p. 2–37.
5. Bush V. Science: the endless frontier; a report to the President by Vannevar Bush, Director of the Office of Scientific research and Development. Washington, DC: United states Government Printing Office; 1945. Accessed 13 Nov 2009. Section 3 (the importance of basic research), chapter 3 (science and the public welfare) http://nsf.gov/about/history/nsf50/vbush1945_content.jsp.
6. Hecker L, Birla RV. Intangible factors leading to success in research: strategy, innovation and leadership. J Cardiovasc Transl Res. 2008;1:85–92.
7. Glossary of themes for human subjects protection and inclusion issues based on the 1997 report of the NIH Director's Panel on clinical research, entry: "clinical research". http://grants.nih.gov/grants/peer/tree_glossary.pdf. Accessed 13 Nov 2009.
8. Schteingart DE. Introduction to principles of clinical and translational research. Athens: ESCI Core Course on Clinical Research; 2010.
9. Seely WE, Grinspoon S. Patient-oriented research: clinical pathophysiology and clinical therapeutics. In: Robertson D, Williams GH, editors. Clinical and translational science. 1st ed. London: Elsevier; 2009. p. 3–12.
10. Califf RM, Zarin DA, Kramer JM, Sherman RE, Aberle LH, Tasneem A. Characteristics of clinical trials registered in ClinicalTrials.gov, 2007–2010. JAMA. 2012;307:1838–47.
11. Karp JE, McCaffrey RP. New avenues of translational research in leukemia and lymphoma: outgrowth of a Leukemia Society of America-National Cancer Institute workshop. J Natl Cancer Inst. 1994;86:1196–201.
12. Feldman AM, Koch WJ, Force TL. Developing strategies to link basic cardiovascular sciences with clinical drug development: another opportunity for translational sciences. Clin Pharmacol Ther. 2007;81:887–92.
13. Littman BH, Di Mario L, Plebani M, Marincola FM. What's next in translational medicine? Clin Sci (Lond). 2007;112:217–27.
14. Woolf SH. The meaning of translational research and why it matters. JAMA. 2008;290:211–3.

15. Dische S, Saunders M. Translational research–a new entity? Acta Oncol. 2001;40:995–9.
16. Coller BS. Translational research: forging a new cultural identity. Mt Sinai J Med. 2008;75:478–87.
17. Coller BS. Translating from the rivers of Babylon to the coronary bloodstream. J Clin Invest. 2012;122: 4293–9.
18. Williams DR. Introduction to clinical research. In: Robertson D, Williams GH, editors. Clinical and translational science. 1st ed. London: Elsevier; 2009. p. xvii–xx.
19. Williams GH, Robertson D. Clinical and translational science in infrastructure. In: Robertson D, Williams GH, editors. Clinical and translational science. 1st ed. London: Elsevier; 2009. p. 171–81.
20. Davis D, Evans M, Jadad A, Perrier L, Rath D, Ryan D, et al. The case for knowledge translation: shortening the journey from evidence to effect. BMJ. 2003; 327(7405):33–5.
21. National Cancer Institute. Translational research working group definition of translational research. http://www.cancer.gov/trwg/TRWG-definition–ND-tr-continuum.
22. Sung NS, Crowley Jr WF, Genel M, Salber P, Sandy L, Sherwood LM, et al. Central challenges facing the national clinical research enterprise. JAMA. 2003;289:1278–87.
23. Lauer M, Scarlatos S. Translational research for cardiovascular diseases at the national heart lung and blood institute. Moving from bench to bedside and from bedside to community. Circulation. 2010;121:929–33.
24. Westfall JM, Mold J, Fagnan L. Practice-based research–"Blue Highways" on the NIH roadmap. JAMA. 2007;297:403–6.
25. Malliaras K, Kreke M, Marbán E. The stuttering progress of cell therapy for heart disease. Clin Pharmacol Ther. 2011;90:532–41.
26. Waldman SA, Terzic A. Clinical and translational science: from bench-bedside to global village. Clin Transl Sci. 2010;5:254–7.
27. Mc Garland Rubio D, Schoenbaum E, Lee S, Schteinggard DE, Marantz PR, Anderson KE, et al. Defining translational research: implications for training. Acad Med. 2010;85:470–5.
28. Koch WJ. Targeting the beta-adrenergic receptor kinase in heart failure. Lecture presented at the 1st international scientific conference on cardiovascular biotechnology: from cell to man. Biomedical Research Foundation of the Academy of Athens, 31 May 2013.
29. Kieburtz K, Olanow CW. Translational experimental therapeutics: the translation of laboratory-based discovery into disease-related therapy. Mt Sinai J Med. 2007;74:7–14.
30. Antoniades CH. Bridging the gap between basic science and clinical practice: the role of translational medicine. Lecture presented at the Biomedical Research Foundation Academy of Athens, 31 Oct 2012.
31. Murry CE, Jennings KA, Reimer KA. Preconditioning with ischemia: a delay of lethal cell injury in ischemic myocardium. Circulation. 1986;74:1124–36.
32. Chautard E, Thierry-Mieg N, Ricard-Blum S. Interaction networks: from protein functions to drug discovery. A review. Pathol Biol (Paris). 2009;57:324–33.
33. Kerner JF, Hall KL. Research dissemination and diffusion. Res Soc Work Practice 2009;19:519–30.
34. Zucker DR. What is needed to promote translational research and how do we get it? J Investig Med. 2009;57:468–70.
35. Bernard GR. Preparedness of the CTSA's structural and scientific assets to support the mission of the National Center for Advancing Translational Sciences (NCATS). Clin Transl Sci. 2012;5:121–9.
36. Hartmann KE, Heitman E, Brown NJ. Training basic, clinical and translational investigators. In: Robertson D, Williams GH, editors. Clinical and translational science. 1st ed. London: Elsevier; 2009. p. 191–9.
37. Williams GH, Robertson D. The future of clinical research. In: Robertson D, Williams GH, editors. Clinical and translational science. 1st ed. London: Elsevier; 2009. p. 565–70.
38. Nadler LM, Roberts WC. Lee Marshall Nadler, MD: a conversation with the editor. Proc Baylor Univ Med Cent. 2007;20:381–9.
39. Verkoeijen PPJL, Tabbers HK. Good research requires productive theories and guidelines. Med Educ. 2013; 47:858–65.
40. Pang T, Terry RF, The PLoS Medicine Editors WHO/PLoS Collection. No health without research: a call for papers. PLoS Med. 2011;8:4 e1001008.
41. White KL, Williams TF, Greenberg BG. The ecology of medical care. N Engl J Med. 1961;265:885–92.
42. Green LA, Fryer Jr GE, Yawn BP, Lanier D, Dovey SM. The ecology of medical care revisited. N Engl J Med. 2001;344:2021–5.
43. Martin SS, Ou FS, Newby LK, Sutton V, Adams P, Felker GM, Wang TY. Patient- and trial-specific barriers to participation in cardiovascular randomized clinical trials. J Am Coll Cardiol. 2013;61:762–9.
44. Brutsaert DL. Heart failure: Quo Vadis. Lecture presented at cardiovascular biotechnology: from cell to man. Biomedical Research Foundation Academy of Athens, 31 May–1 June 2013.
45. Califf RM. Clinical trials. In: Robertson D, Williams GH, editors. Clinical and translational science. 1st ed. London: Elsevier; 2009. p. 13–37.
46. Welke KF, Ferguson Jr TB, Cooms LP, Dokholygan RS, Murray CJ, Sehrader MI, et al. Validity of the society of thoracic surgeons national adult cardiac surgery database. Ann Thorac Surg. 2004;77: 1137–9.
47. Moss AJ, Francis CW, Rayan D. Collaborative clinical trials. N Engl J Med. 2011;364:789791.
48. Sipido KR, Casadei B, Holvoet P, Janssens S, Luttun A, Sampaolesi M. Bedside to bench: a look at experimental research with a clinical trial checklist. Cardiovasc Res. 2014;101:1–3.

49. Kaul S, Diamond GA. Trial and error. How to avoid commonly encountered limitations of published clinical trials. J Am Coll Cardiol. 2010;55:415–27.
50. Balas EA, Boren SA. In: Balas EA, editor. Yearbook of medical informatics: managing clinical knowledge for health care improvement. Stuttgart: Shattauer Verlagsgesellschaft mbH; 2000, p. 65–70.
51. Contopoulos-Ioannidis DG, Alexiou GA, Grouvias TC, Ioannidis JPA. Life circle of translational research for medical interventions. Science. 2008;321:1298–9.
52. Hudson J, Khazhragui HF. Into the valley of death; research to innovation. Drug Discov Today. 2012;18: 610–3.
53. Butler D. Translational research; crossing the valley of death. Nature. 2008;453:840–2.
54. Roberts SF, Fischhoff MA, Sakowski SA, Feldman EL. Perspective: transforming science into medicine: how clinician-scientists can build bridges across research's "valley of death". Acad Med. 2012;87:266–70.
55. Coller BS, Califf RM. Traversing the valley of death: a guide to assessing prospects for translational success. Sci Transl Med. 2009;1:10cm9. doi:10.1126/scitranslmed.3000265.
56. Bodi V, Marrachelli VG, Husser O, Chorro FJ, Viña JR, Monleon D. Metabolomics in the diagnosis of acute myocardial ischemia. J Cardiovasc Trans Res. 2013;6:808–15.
57. Moses 3rd H, Dorsey ER, Matheson DH, Their SO. Financial anatomy of biomedical research. JAMA. 2005;294:1333–42.
58. Quinn T, Kohl P. Combining wet and dry research: experience with model development for cardiac mechano-electric structure-function studies. Cardiovasc Res. 2013;97:601–11.
59. The Royal Swedish Academy of Science. press release: pressmeddecande, 9 october 2013. Nobel prize in Chemistry. 2013.
60. Curry SH. Translational science: past, present, and future. Bio Tech. 2008;44:Pii–vii.
61. Braunwald E. Cardiovascular science: opportunities for translating research into improved care. J Clin Invest. 2013;123:6–10.
62. Stamler JS, Taber RL, Califf RM. Translation of academic discovery into societal benefit: proposal for a balanced approach–part 1. Am J Med. 2003;115:596–9.

Insights into Heart Development and Regeneration

2

Dimitris Beis, Stamatia Kalogirou, and Nikolaos Tsigkas

Abstract

The heart is one of the first organs to form and function during the development of an organism. Cardiac development, morphology and transcriptional networks involved in cardiac patterning, across species, are reviewed. These genes are most commonly mutated in Congenital Heart Disease. In parallel, recent advances in understanding how the cardiac development program is recapitulated during cardiac regeneration are also presented. We discuss models of cardiac regeneration in zebrafish and newborn mice and how these could be utilized in the context of translational research.

Keywords

Heart development • Regeneration • Heart diseases • Animal models

Abbreviations

ANF	Atrial natriuretic factor
AVC	Atrioventricular canal
BMP	Bone morphogenetic protein
CMC	Cardiomyocytes
ECM	Extracellular cell matrix
EMT	Epithelial to mesenchymal transition
Eomes	Eomesodermin
FGF	Fibroblast growth factor
FHF	First heart field
FUCCI	Fluorescent ubiquitination-based cell cycle indicator
NGF	Nerve growth factor
OFT	Outflow tract
PDGF	Platelet-derived growth factor
REG	Regeneration
SHF	Second heart field
SRF	Serum response factor
TGF-β	Transforming growth factor beta

D. Beis (✉) • S. Kalogirou • N. Tsigkas
Developmental Biology, Biomedical Research Foundation, Academy of Athens, Athens, Greece
e-mail: dbeis@bioacademy.gr

2.1 Heart Development

The heart is one of the most elegant yet durable organs of an organism. It is designed to pump blood efficiently, throughout its lifetime at rates that vary from an average of 8 beats per minute (bpm) in the blue whale to 72 bpm in humans, 150 bpm in zebrafish and 600 bpm in mice.

D.V. Cokkinos (ed.), *Introduction to Translational Cardiovascular Research*,
DOI 10.1007/978-3-319-08798-6_2, © Springer International Publishing Switzerland 2015

The heart's life-long mission is to deliver oxygenated blood (or hemolymph in arthropods) to every part of the body. Hearts come in different shapes and size. They have evolved from a single peristaltic chamber in insects, to a two-chambered heart in fish and the complex four-chamber organ with septa and valves in mammals that can weigh up to 500 kg in whales. Despite the remarkable variation in shape and morphogenesis across species, it has become evident that conserved transcription factors and signaling pathways contribute to the making of the heart. Therefore, studying heart development in Drosophila, mice and more recently zebrafish are giving increasing insight on how the human heart forms and functions. In addition, a number of experimental animals such as the fruit fly, zebrafish, chicken, mice and rats are now being used to model a number of Heart Diseases (HD).

2.1.1 Embryonic Origin of the Heart

During gastrulation of the developing embryo, a single-layered blastula is re-organized into three germ layers: a dorsal ectodermal layer, a ventral endodermal layer and a mesodermal layer in between these two [1]. The heart tissue, which consists of myocardial, endocardial and epicardial cells, derives predominantly from the splanchnic mesoderm, a subpopulation of the mesodermal layer facing the endoderm, located on the ventral side, beneath the pharynx [2–4]. In addition, ectoderm-derived cardiac neural crest cells have been identified in the cushions of the outflow tract, through genetic tools that allow tracing of the cell lineage [5]. In mice, the prospective cardiogenic cells originate from the posterior epiblast cells, the precursors of mesodermal tissues [6]. In the chick embryos these cells are bilaterally distributed on both sides of the primitive streak, caudal to node [7] and in zebrafish they are located in the ventral marginal zone at the mid-late blastula stages [8]. Fate mapping studies in mouse and chicken embryos indicated that the fate of gastrulating cells is indicated by the time and location of cell ingression through the **primitive streak (PS)** in the blastula stage (Fig. 2.1) [9].

2.1.2 Cardiac Differentiation Is Induced by Signaling Cues from Adjacent Tissues

Mesoderm induction is conserved and regulated by numerous signaling pathways. Some of the key players are: Nodal (a member of the **transforming growth factor beta superfamily, TGF-β**); **bone morphogenetic protein (BMP)**; the **Wnt signaling pathway** and **fibroblast growth factors (FGF)** [1, 9]. Signaling anterior to endodermal cells positively regulate cardiac specification, whereas signaling from the neural plate, somatic and axial mesoderm represses heart formation [10]. Higher levels of Nodal favor cardiac mesoderm induction [11]. BMP function is not clear in the earliest stages of cardiac commitment, although inhibiting BMP signaling seems important to promote the emergence of the cardiac mesoderm [12]. BMP signaling is active in cardiac progenitor cells prior to their differentiation into cardiomyocytes (CMC), and it is continuously required during somitogenesis within the anterior lateral plate mesoderm (LPM) to induce myocardial differentiation in zebrafish. However, at later stages BMP signaling is actively repressed in the ventricle through Smad6a,[1] in order to allow for proper chamber differentiation [13]. BMPs seem to be important for expansion of cardiac progenitors, as genetic deletion of the BMP receptor in Mesp1-expressing mesoderm results in major defects in heart formation [14]. Mesp1 expression marks cardiogenic mesoderm (around E6.5 in mouse embryogenesis) and Mesp1$^{-/-}$; Mesp2$^{-/-}$ double knockout mice lack all mesodermal layer between endoderm and ectoderm [15]. BMP inhibitors noggin and chordin present in the dorsal neural tube and notochord restrict cardiac commitment through Wnt8, Wnt3a inhibition [16]. Wnt antagonists dickkopf1 (Dkk1) and Crescent, inhibit the induction of multiple cardiac foci in adjacent mesodermal cells [17, 18]. FGFs induces cardiac differentiation from the cardiac progenitor cells in early mesoderm [19, 20]. In

[1] Smads are cytoplasm-signaling proteins which regulate gene transcription in response to BMP and its receptors of the TGF-β superfamily.

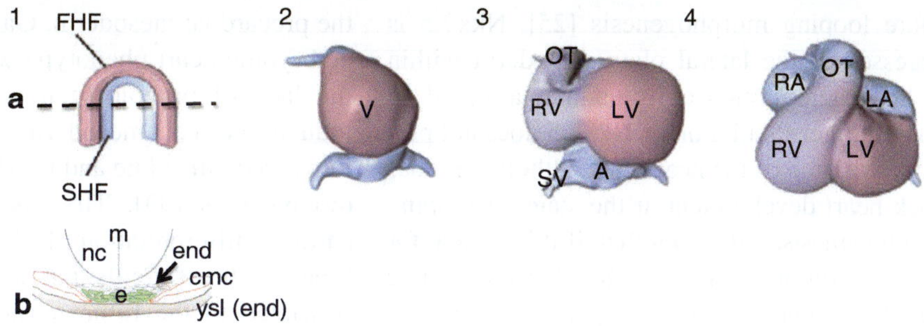

	(1) Cardiac crescent	(2) Linear heart tube	(3) Looped heart	(4) Mature heart
Zebrafish embryo (hours post fertilization, hpf)	18 hpf	24 hpf	36 hpf	120 hpf
Mouse embryo (day)	E 7.5	E 8.5	E 9.5	E 11.5
Human embryo (day)	Day 15	Day 20	Day 28	Day 32
Developmental milestones	Bilateral cardiac cell differentiation Migration to the midline	Heart tube forms First heartbeat	Looping to the right Chamber differentiation	Cushions, valve and septa Conduction system Trabeculation of the myocardium Epicardial enveloping
Representative signaling pathways and genes involved	BMPs, Wnt, FGFs, Eomes	Nkx2.5, Mef2C, eHAND, dHAND Tbx5, GATA4	Nodal, Lefty, Shh, Pitx2, Anf, Cx40, Cx43	NFATC, BMPs, HAS2, Wnt, ErbB2, Wt1, Tcf21

Fig. 2.1 (**a**) Early steps in heart development. Diagrams of heart development are shown in ventral views. At the earliest stages of heart formation (cardiac crescent), two pools of cardiac precursors exist. The first heart field (*FHF*) contributes to the left ventricle (*LV*), and the second heart field (*SHF*) contributes to the right ventricle (*RV*) and later to the outflow tract (*OT*), sinus venosus (*SV*), and left and right atria (*LA* and *RA*, respectively). *V* ventricle. In (**b**) a cross section at the level of the dotted line is depicted. Myocardial (cmc) and endocardial (e) progenitors migrate to the midline (m) to form the linear heart tube. They are flanked by endodermal cells (end) and the yolk syncytial layer (YSL) in zebrafish or the endoderm (that invaginates from where the YSL is depicted) in mouse and chick embryos. (An interactive version of the figure can be found at http://pie.med.utoronto.ca/HTBG/index.htm. Images courtesy of F. Yeung, University of Toronto, Canada)

zebrafish, $fgf8^{-/-}$ mutants fail to initiate proper gene expression of *nkx2.5* and *gata4* and exhibit severe heart malformations [21].

Specification of splanchnic mesoderm into cardiogenic mesoderm also requires the T-box transcription factor **Eomesodermin (Eomes)** [22]. In PS stage embryo, Eomes directly activates the basic helix-looped helix transcription factor mesoderm posterior 1 (Mesp1) [23].

T-box factors direct **serum response factor (SRF)** gene activity early in development and SRF is essential for cardiac regulation of the T-box factors during mesoderm specification [24]. Finally, **Tinman** (nkx2.5) is the first regulatory gene in any species that was described to be expressed in the precardiac mesoderm and to function in the differentiation of cardiac precursors. In *tinman* mutants, cardiogenesis is arrested before looping morphogenesis [25]. Nkx2.5 is expressed in the lateral plate mesoderm within the heart field in mouse, frog and avians [26]. In mouse, targeted ablation of Nkx2.5 does not prevent formation of the heart tube, although it does block heart development at the stage of looping morphogenesis, indicating that, if it is critical for the initiation of cardiac cell fate decisions, there must be redundant pathways [27]. The hematopoietic/erythroid cell fate is suppressed via Nkx2.5 during mesodermal fate determination, and that the Gata1 gene is one of the targets that are suppressed by Nkx2.5 [28]. In zebrafish, *nkx2.5* and *nkx2.7* are redundant during development [29]. Wnt signals from the neural tube normally act to block cardiogenesis in the adjacent anterior paraxial mesendoderm in chick embryos at HH8-9 stage [16].[2]

2.1.3 Cardiac Crescent Formation

The bilateral precursor pools unite in the midline, cranial to the stomatopharyngeal membrane, forming the cardiac crescent at 3 weeks of human development (E7.5 in mouse) when the embryo is a flat tri-laminar disc [5, 30]. The differentiation of the cardiac crescent into CMCs is dependent on signals derived from the adjacent endoderm. Multiple signals from the craniolateral endoderm are most likely required to induce myocardial specification, and these are balanced by inhibitory factors from other tissues. Candidates that promote specification of myocardial fate include members of the TGF-β, BMP, and FGF [31]. Downstream of these, are members of the MEF2 family expressed in the primary myocardium. In zebrafish, *mef2c* is expressed in the precardiac mesoderm, followed by *mef2A*, both apparently limited to the premyocardial and not pre-endocardial cells [32]. **GATA transcription factors** are also found in the precardiac mesoderm. Gata4$^{-/-}$ mice have an embryonic heart phenotype with more profound the lack of proepicardial cells while, GATA5 induction directs mesoderm-committed progenitors to a cardiac fate and the development of cardiomyocytes [33]. Tbx5 is also essential for cardiac differentiation. It is expressed in the bilateral heart fields but at later stages it is restricted to the future atria [34]. Mutation in human Tbx5 cause the **Holt-Oram syndrome**, which consists of heart defects and hand bone defects [35]. In zebrafish, *tbx5.1* is expressed in cells from the 15-somite stage and marks the bilateral (at both sides of the midline) migrating heart population [36]. Zac1 is strongly expressed in the heart from the cardiac crescent stages and in the looping heart show a chamber-restricted pattern. Zac1$^{-/-}$ mice exhibit ventricular and atrial septal defects, chamber abnormalities and defects in neural tube closure [37].

2.1.4 Linear Heart Tube Formation

At E8 in mouse, or 3 weeks in human gestation, the cardiac crescent fuses at the midline and gives rise to the **First Heart Field (FHF)** derived linear heart tube. This structure starts beating and subsequently undergoes rightward looping and rapid growth [38]. During the stages that follow, the heart tube expands and additional cells are recruited [5, 39]. Cells from the **Second Heart Field (SHF)** are added to the heart tube, with preference to the venous and arterial poles [40]. The SHF is located medially to the FHF in the cardiac crescent [5] and the anterior lateral plate mesoderm in zebrafish [41]. SHF cells contribute to the formation of the **outflow tract (OFT)**, the septa, right ventricle, and the inflow of atria [42–45]. SHF is required also in zebrafish for its arterial pole formation [46] and activates FGF signaling pathway [47]. Isl-1 (LIM homeodomain transcription factor) is a marker of SHF, dependent on the Wnt pathway [48]. Isl-1 is required for proliferation and survival of SHF cells as well as for the migration of cardiac progenitors [45]. BMP mediates TGF-β signaling and functions to induce SHF progenitors to differentiate into myocardium [49].

[2] Differences in nomenclature rules between species are indicated in the way orthologue genes and proteins are written: for example GATA4 refers to the human gene, Gata4 to the mouse and gata4 to the zebrafish orthologue. When referring to proteins GATA4 refers to the human or mouse while Gata4 to the zebrafish one.

The Notch signaling pathway, negatively regulates β-catenin and keeps progenitors in an undifferentiated state [49]. Loss of β-catenin leads to reduction of Islet-1 cells due to reduced proliferation of these cells. Canonical Wnt signaling[3] is involved in the differentiation of the right ventricle, the OFT and the atria [50]. Non canonical- wnt5a, wnt11 ligands are expressed in OFT and are essential for SHF progenitor development and act by restraining the canonical Wnt/β-catenin signaling [48].

2.1.5 Endocardium Development

Cardiac crescent contains both endocardial and myocardial progenitors. The endocardium contributes to the heart tube assembly by directing myocardial migration during heart tube fusion [51]. Studies in zebrafish and chicken embryos showed that endocardial progenitor cells are sequestered within the Heart field [52, 53]. In zebrafish studies, endocardial precursors are restricted in the most ventral zone of the heart field in the early blastula stage [52]. The **endocardium** of the primary heart tube forms directly from the ventral plexus of endothelial precursor cells, which are in close association with the anterior endoderm. Importantly, endocardial cells have a common origin with **myocardial cells**, as suggested in quail embryos [54]. QH-1, a quail endothelial marker was first detected in quail embryos at stage 7 [55]. Mouse studies suggested that mesodermal precursor cells in the cardiac crescent maintain fate plasticity and can give rise to both myocardium and endocardium or that the cardiogenic precursors are pre-specified when they migrate from the primitive streak to the cardiac crescent [56]. Endothelial progenitor cells from SHF contribute to the development of endocardium through OFT migration. There is heterogeneity in the origin of endocardium; a part of it derives from vascular endothelial cells [57]. Tal1 is a transcription factor required for endocardial cells migration. In *tal1*$^{-/-}$ zebrafish mutants morphogenesis the endocardial cells do not form a single cell layer lining the myocardium, and do not form atrial endocardium. Instead, endocardial cells aggregate at the arterial pole of the heart [58]. GATA5 is required for differentiation of cardiogenic precursors into endothelial endocardial cells [59]. Gata5 is expressed in the endocardium, early in mouse development (E12.5) in atrial endocardium and regulates smooth muscle cell transcription program. NFATC1 interacts with GATA5 to activate endocardial transcription factors [59]. Etv (Etsrp71) transcription factor is expressed in endocardium/endothelium at E8.5 stage and regulates tie2 expression [60]. The transcriptional network involved in endocardial specification is reviewed in [61].

2.1.6 Looping of the Heart

The Heart tube is the first organ that exhibits left-right (L-R) asymmetry. It becomes apparent in chicken embryos at stage HH9 [62] and in zebrafish embryos as cardiac jogging (leftward displacement of the heart cone) at 28 h post fertilization (hpf), and as s-loop at 36 hpf [8]. In humans, s-looping occurs at CS9-10 with the formation of an inner and an outer curvature that gives rise to the ventricles. There is proliferating and differentiating myocardium (secondary/chamber myocardium) from which arise the heart chambers [5]. In zebrafish, the cardiac cone rotates clockwise (venous pole left side, arterial pole midline). In this way, L-R polarity is converted to Dorsal-Ventral axis during heart tube formation, a process dependent on BMP signaling in the LPM, which also directs cardiac progenitor cells migration. For this rotation and migration (cardiac jogging) the Hyaluronan synthase 2 (Has2) expression in cardiac progenitors cells is required [63]. In zebrafish, *southpaw*, (*spaw*) a Nodal related gene, is expressed in the left LPM and activates Nodal at the onset of asymmetric morphogenesis in an *one eyed pinhead*, (*oep*)-dependent manner at 21-somite stage. Nodal acts in L-R asymmetry by regulating the speed and the direction of CMCs [64]. Nodal signaling directs asymmetric cardiac morphogenesis through establishing and reinforcing

[3] Wnt canonical signaling refers to the signaling mediated by the β-catenin.

laterality information over the course of cardiac development. Cardiac jogging is driven by an asymmetric atrial myocardial migration, influenced by the laterality of gene expression [65]. *bmpr1* and *bmpr2* are essential for L-R asymmetry in zebrafish, are upstream of *pitx2* and *spaw* and regulate *lefty1* [66]. Wnt-GATA4 signaling controls the asymmetric signal propagation from the LPM to the cardiac field. Wnt/β-catenin signaling negatively regulates Gata4 expression in the cardiac field, which subsequently modulates Lefty2 expression in the cardiac primodium. In contrast to the inductive role of Spaw, Wnt/β-catenin signaling imposes a permissive function on the cardiac field, allowing it to respond to asymmetric cues such as Spaw [67]. Sonic Hedgeghog (Shh) in mouse is expressed in the node (the source of mouse left-right asymmetry), the notochord and the gut endoderm [68]. Hedgehog controls L/R asymmetry by the induction of left-side determinants and is required for activation of Gdf1 (Tgf family, upstream of Nodal, lefty1/2, Pitx2) within the node [69].

2.1.7 Chamber Formation

The heart starts functioning and transitions from a linear tube to a looped structure with distinct differentiated chambers. During cardiac looping an inner and an outer curvature of the myocardium are being specified [6, 70]. The outer curvature gives rise to the future ventricles and in the dorsolateral side of the primary heart tube, two atrial appendices form [6]. The Atrial Natriuretic Factor (ANF) gene is expressed in the working myocardium in the outer curvature of ventricle and atrium of chicken stage HH9 [71]. In zebrafish embryos by 28hpf, sided by the heart tube, in regions supposed to become outer curvatures of ventricle and atrium [72]. The molecular signals in chamber formation are *Nppa* (*anf*), the gene encoding ANF and the transcription factors COUP-TFII, Hand1, Irx4 and Irx5, Nkx2-5, Gata4 and members of the T-box gene family. These, in turn, regulate a number of chamber specific genes such as those encoding the gap-junction proteins connexins [73] and as reviewed in [1].

2.1.8 Cardiac Valves and Septa

Cardiac valves originate from endocardial cells at specific positions along the anteroposterior axis of the heart after the heart starts beating. They serve throughout the lifespan of an organism to prevent retrograde blood flow. A number of processes, including **Epithelial to Mesenchymal Transition (EMT),** lead to the differentiation of valve progenitor cells at the **AtrioVentricular (AV) canal** from the endocardium [74]. In mice, this process initiates at day (E9.5–10.5) with the formation of cushions by the migration of these mesenchymal cells into the cardiac jelly secreted by the overlying myocardial cells. Highly regulated signaling pathways orchestrate their development. These pathways include Notch, BMP/TGF-β, Wnt/β-catenin, NFATc, VEGF, Erb2/4, has2, microRNAs and others, as reviewed in [75], [76] and chapter 9 of this book. In addition to the above-mentioned signaling pathways, cardiac valve morphogenesis is regulated by the heart function and intracardiac flow dynamics. Endocardial cells at the **AV canal** as well as the OFT of the heart, experience retrograde blood flow when the heart starts to function and before the valves are formed. Studies in zebrafish embryos, which can survive for several days and develop in the absence of a functional heart beat or blood circulation, revealed the importance of intracardiac flow dynamics in valve morphogenesis [77–80]. Valve cushion mesenchyme differentiates into the fibrous connective tissue of both inlet and outlet valvular leaflets. In addition, the tricuspid valves as well as the septa are partially myocardialized, due to the invasion of cushions by myocardial cells to give a muscular component to the terminally differentiated tissues. Thus, myocardialization appears to be a normal morphogenetic event occurring in most vertebrates, including humans, to give specific cushion structures their mature phenotype. The **extracellular cell matrix (ECM)** proteins fibrillin and fibulin as well as proteoglycans are thought to be involved in the remodeling of the cushions into valvuloseptal tissue. These molecules accumulate at the cell surface or pericellular matrix of the migrating cushion cells that secrete them and appear to play a role in the final positioning and spacing of cells within the differentiated tissue, reviewed in [74].

2.2 The Signaling Pathways Involved in Cardiac Development Are Responsible for Congenital Heart Diseases

It is no surprise that the above-described complexity of form and function of the heart, leads to an increased incidence of related diseases. A core of conserved transcription factors, including Nkx2.5, GATA4 and Tbx5 are critical in regulating the development of the heart. These transcription factors, as well as their regulatory network (upstream activators and downstream targets) represent a significant percentage of **congenital heart diseases** (CHD) in humans reviewed in [81]. GATA4 has multiple roles during development in the specification of the myocardium as well as in later stages in AV cushion morphogenesis. In addition, GATA4 is activated during pathologic hypertrophy. Both in the United States and Europe, heart disease (HD) is the leading cause of death and disability and the greatest public health problem. HD is the result of a genetic mutation, congenital diseases, as well as different types of insults in the adult heart, such as coronary artery disease, hypertension and chemotherapy [82]. Although these insults have a different pathophysiological mechanism of action, they all lead progressively to CMCs loss and consequently to the deterioration of heart function. For example, in myocardial infarction, after the initial deprivation of O_2 in the myocardium an ischemic cascade is activated with the end result being cell death and its replacement by a collagen rich scar tissue. Scar tissue deposition allows for the initial stabilization of the induced damage, but it is not contractile and thus compromises heart function in the long run. The loss of contractility elicits a hypertrophic response through the activation of signaling pathways like GATA4 but this does not result in an increased number of cardiomyocytes in mammals, that lack the regenerative response capable of replenishing the lost cardiomyocytes. A new research field has emerged, aiming to understand the mechanisms in animal models that maintain the ability to regenerate their hearts and how this could be activated in humans.

2.3 Regenerative Capacity

Regeneration (REG) is the replacement of cells after trauma and results in a partially or fully restored and functional organ. The renewal of the intestinal lining or the maintenance of skin, hair and bone of an organism, are examples of regenerative potential. This natural replacement of cells lost in day-to-day minor and physiological damage, is referred to as homeostatic REG, while the actual REG per se is a unique posttraumatic response. The first paradigm of REG was first observed and reported in Hellenic mythology through the myth of the Titan Prometheus. The myth describes that Prometheus was chained to a rock where each day an eagle devoured his liver, which was growing back. Hundreds of years had passed since the myth of Prometheus until 1768 when Spallanzani reported that amputated salamander limbs were capable to fully regenerate [83]. In the following centuries, more organisms were added to the list of organisms capable to regenerate, among them lizards, frogs and fish. These can regenerate not only their limbs but also different organs.

2.3.1 Heart Regeneration Across Different Species

In mammals, several organs retain their regenerative capacity during adult life. Skin and liver, for example, demonstrate robust examples of mammalian organ REG. Other organs, in the contrary, such as the nervous system and the heart lose their regenerative potential early after birth. However, when hearts of neonatal mice were amputated 1 day after birth, they demonstrated a robust regenerative response completely restoring the damaged ventricle [84]. In addition, neonatal mice retain a regeneration response up to 7 days after birth not only after ventricle amputation but also after coronary ligation, an experimental model closer to the pathophysiology of myocardial infarction [85]. Interestingly, contrary to the long-standing belief that adult human hearts lose their regenerating capacity, there is growing evidence of cardiomyocyte renewal during the lifespan of an adult human. Using the integration of radiocarbon 14C, cardiomyocytes were found to renew at a rate of ~1 % of the entire population per year in a person at the age of 25 years, but this rate drops progressively with the advancement of age [86]. Although the heart of higher adult vertebrates loses its ability to regenerate after an injury, the above studies reveal that regenerative potential is not an evolutionary advantage (Fig. 2.2).

2.3.2 Regeneration in Zebrafish

The urodeles (for example, salamanders) are the champions of heart REG. They can regenerate it even after a 50 % injury [87], by a mitotic response of the preexisting mature cardiomyocytes, which undergo successive cell divisions [88]. Lately, zebrafish has emerged as a novel model with remarkable regenerative capacity and with numerous additional advantages, such as the amenability to in vivo cell biological studies and to forward and reverse genetics approaches [89]. Zebrafish (Danio rerio) is a fish found in fresh water streams from South and East Asia. Zebrafish is a cyprinid and belongs to the greater family of teleosts. Organs such as the kidney, liver, pancreas, spinal cord, CNS, retina and fin can be regenerated in zebrafish after injury [90–92]. The ability of zebrafish to regenerate its heart, was first demonstrated in 2002 when part of the ventricle was amputated and it fully regenerated within 60 days [93]. This unique characteristic of the zebrafish heart it is not a transitory ability but it is preserved throughout its lifetime [94]. The technique of ventricular apex amputation creates initially a thrombus and subsequent activation of the regeneration response [93]. Since then, several techniques have been developed to study heart REG in zebrafish. In cryoinjury-induced damage, a probe that is precooled in liquid nitrogen is applied on the surface of the ventricle, resulting in massive cell death [95, 96]. This type of injury elicits initially an inflammatory response where inflammatory cells invade the injured tissue. In the following days, there is a gradual activation of different type of cells that migrate to the site of injury and initiate the reparative phase with collagen deposition. The cryoinjury method resembles the events that follow a myocardial infarction. In both methods of injury, fully replenished myocardial tissue is achieved after 60 days.

In addition to these surgical methods, genetic approaches have been developed, using transgenic zebrafish that express the bacterial nitroreductase specifically in the heart. Nitroreductase is an enzyme that catalyzes the reduction of the prodrug metronidazole in a cytotoxic product. When zebrafish are exposed to media with metronidazole, cell death is induced in a time and dose dependent manner [97]. Alternatively a heart specific tamoxifen inducible Cre recombinase line was created and crossed with a line capable of expressing diphtheria toxin under the promoter of β-actin upon recombination achieving more than 60 % cardiomyocyte specific death [98]. Finally, ventricular specific embryonic ablation during development showed that atrial cells can transdifferentiate to contribute to ventricular regeneration [99]. In conclusion, genetic methods allow a more global injury of the ventricle in respect to the focally located mechanical injury, thus allowing the study of acute and chronic heart failure mechanisms in regenerative models.

Chemical induction of hypoxia and hypoxia-induced injury is also used to study zebrafish heart REG. Hypoxia refers to the lack of oxygen in the blood and is the hallmark of the ischemia induced heart injury in higher mammals. Since the previously described methods lack the ability to generate an oxygen-deprived environment in the heart tissue, this methodology provides an alternative and a more reliable method to study ischemia induced rather than infarcted injuries [100]. Finally, exposure to aristolochic acid during early development causes a reduction of cardiomyocyte proliferation and heart failure at the

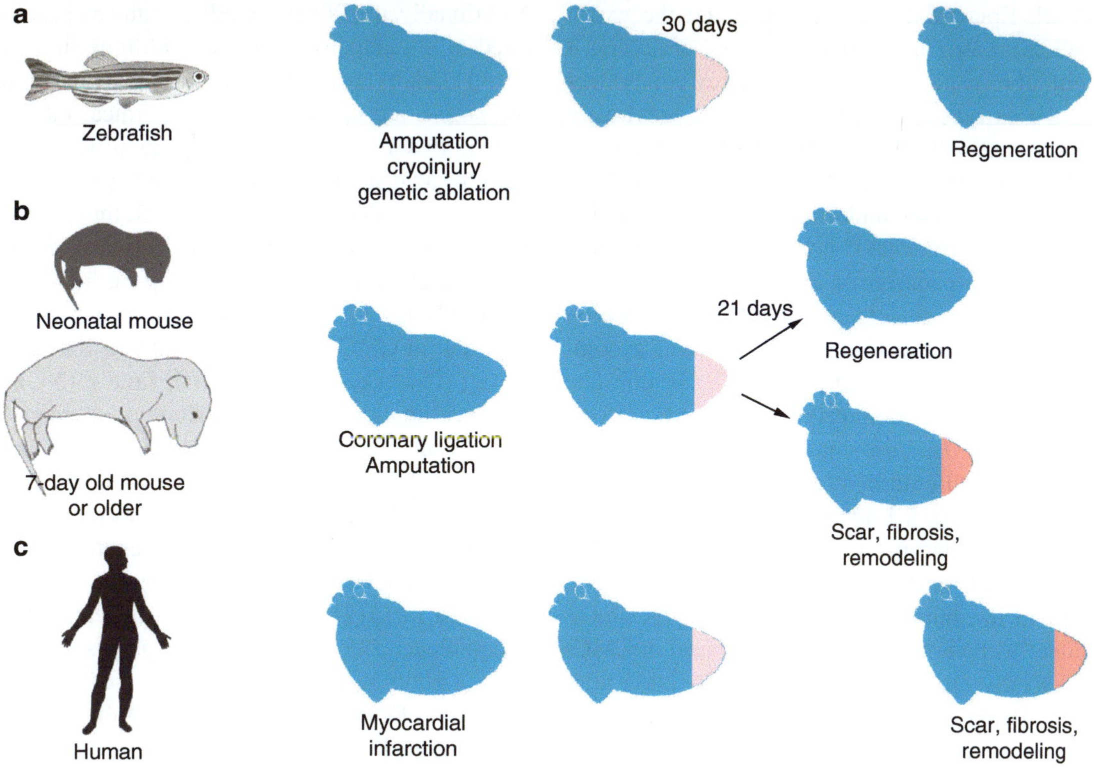

Fig. 2.2 Regenerative capacity is lost in the adult human heart but is maintained in neonatal mouse and zebrafish. (**a**) Zebrafish maintain their ability to fully regenerate their myocardium within a month after injury. Current experimental models include cryoinjury, ventricular amputation or genetic ablation of myocardial cells. Activated epicardium is necessary for the induction of myocardial proliferation. (**b**) In neonatal mice, upon ventricular amputation or coronary ligation the myocardium regenerates and is fully functional with no signs of fibrosis. However, this competence is lost after the first week of life. (**c**) In contrast, in humans upon myocardial injury, a collagenous scar is deposited compromising the myocardial function and initiating a remodeling transcriptional program

larval stage [101]. This model allows the study of progression to heart failure and heart regeneration at early stages, where zebrafish retains a plethora of advantages, including the ability to do large-scale chemical screens.

2.3.3 Epicardial Cells and Transcriptional Networks Involved in Heart Regeneration

Understanding the mechanisms that are activated during the regenerative response after injury is necessary to be able to re-activate them in humans. It is therefore important to elucidate both the sources of the different types of cells and the relevant signaling pathways. One of the first questions that were addressed was if the sources of the new cardiomyocytes were either undifferentiated progenitor cells or existing cardiomyocytes, which undergo dedifferentiation and proliferation. Amputation experiments in zebrafish showed that undifferentiated progenitor cells initiate REG, in addition to epicardial cells. The **activated epicardial cells** express FGF receptors and migrate to the site of injury playing a key role to the REG process. Blocking the FGF receptor by expressing negative dominant FGF receptor or treating with an FGFR inhibitor, arrests heart REG. Coronary neovascularization is impaired because the endocardial cells fail to undergo endothelial to mesenchymal transition

[102]. Epicardial cells also regulate the extracellular matrix at the injury site, by enriching it with fibronectin. Fibronectin is a key component of the extracellular matrix and it is previously associated with fibrosis after cardiac damage in adult mammals [103, 104]. A transgenic zebrafish that expresses under a heat-shock inducible promoter a truncated, not functional fibronectin after amputation of the ventricle was used to show that defects in fibronectin deposition are associated with impaired REG and accompanied by increased fibrosis [105]. Genetic fate mapping studies demonstrated that pre-existing cardiomyocytes are capable of dedifferentiation and proliferation after resection of zebrafish heart [106, 107]. Furthermore, not only de-differentiation and proliferation of existing CMCs is essential for heart REG but also their migration to the injury site. Pharmacological blocking of a chemokine receptor expressed in CMCs especially after injury arrests regeneration after amputation of the ventricle [108]. The Notch signaling pathway is highly conserved across species and plays a key role in cell-to-cell communication regulating cell fate decisions during embryogenesis [109]. In particular, Notch signaling is involved in the development both of the myocardium-ventricular morphogenesis-and the formation of the valves [110]. Interestingly, the Notch signaling pathway has also been implicated in the REG process after ventricular amputation of zebrafish heart [111]. In particular, different components of the Notch signaling pathway are upregulated before REG takes place, designating an activation of embryonic genetic program during injury.

Another study, using microarray technology to analyze genome expression during REG in heart zebrafish after amputation of the ventricle, identified that **platelet-derived growth factor (PDGF)** signaling is upregulated [109]. PDGF molecules and their receptors are growth factors found in the serum of mammals. PDGFs play a key role both in heart development and fibrosis after myocardial infarction. In cardiac fibrosis, different studies of gain or loss of function suggested the important role of PDFG signaling pathway in neovascularization and healing response [112]. Additionally, the PDGF signaling pathway is activated in inflammatory cells that infiltrate injured heart [113]. In amputated zebrafish hearts, *pdfg-a* and *pdgf-b* are upregulated and chemical inhibition of PDGF impairs heart regeneration [109]. Retinoic acid signaling pathway is a key regulator during heart development [114]. Retinoic acid also plays an important role in zebrafish heart REG. After injury, the activated epicardium and endocardium produce retinoic acid, which is required for CMC proliferation and thus for heart REG [115]. Also, **nerve growth factor (NGF)** has been implicated both in mice to promote cardiac repair after myocardial infarction [116] and in zebrafish to promote CMC proliferation and REG [101]. In addition, the thyroid hormone can induce cardiac repair and (or) regeneration by reactivating developmental gene programming, as reviewed in [117]. The concept that heart REG recapitulates the developmental programs has been applied in an elegant system to screen for induction of cardiomyocyte proliferation in vivo. A transgenic line where the cardiomyocyte proliferation can be monitored in vivo was generated using a myocardial specific promoter driving the **fluorescent ubiquitination-based cell cycle indicator (FUCCI)**. This technology allows the screening of small compound libraries that enhance myocardial proliferation during cardiac development. This approach, identified several compounds that when used in the resection model of cardiac injury, could enhance heart regeneration. These include compounds that act via the Hedgehog pathway, the Insulin-like growth factor or the TGF-β, signaling pathways [118]. These results highlight the importance of chemical genetic screens in zebrafish but also further support the notion that regeneration and development are highly analogous.

2.4 Conclusion

It is becoming apparent that modeling cardiac regeneration in fish and mice is a powerful approach to understand the mechanisms that need being activated after an ischemic injury in humans. During heart regeneration, several signaling pathways that have been identified as key regulators of heart development are recruited. It is thus important to decode the mechanisms of heart development, since this knowledge would enhance the ability to control heart regeneration.

References

1. Rana MS, Christoffels VM, Moorman AF. A molecular and genetic outline of cardiac morphogenesis. Acta Physiol (Oxf). 2013;207:588–615.
2. Srivastava D, Olson EN. A genetic blueprint for cardiac development. Nature. 2000;407:221–6.
3. Harvey RP. Patterning the vertebrate heart. Nat Rev Genet. 2002;3:544–56.
4. Abu-Issa R, Kirby ML. Heart field: from mesoderm to heart tube. Annu Rev Cell Dev Biol. 2007; 23:45–68.
5. Tam PP, Parameswaran M, Kinder SJ, Weinberger RP. The allocation of epiblast cells to the embryonic heart and other mesodermal lineages: the role of ingression and tissue movement during gastrulation. Development. 1997;124:1631–42.
6. Sylva M, van den Hoff MJ, Moorman AF. Development of the human heart. Am J Med Genet A. 2013. doi:10.1002/ajmg.a.35896.
7. López-Sánchez C, García-Martínez V. Molecular determinants of cardiac specification. Cardiovasc Res. 2011;91:185–95.
8. Stainier DY, Lee RK, Fishman MC. Cardiovascular development in the zebrafish. I. Myocardial fate map and heart tube formation. Development. 1993;119: 31–40.
9. Brade T, Pane LS, Moretti A, Chien KR, Laugwitz KL. Embryonic heart progenitors and cardiogenesis. Cold Spring Harb Perspect Med. 2013;3:a013847.
10. Abu-Issa R, Kirby ML. Patterning of the heart field in the chick. Dev Biol. 2008;319:223–33.
11. Brennan J, Lu CC, Norris DP, Rodriguez TA, Beddington RS, Robertson EJ. Nodal signalling in the epiblast patterns the early mouse embryo. Nature. 2001;411:965–9.
12. Yuasa S, Itabashi Y, Koshimizu U, Tanaka T, Sugimura K, Kinoshita M, et al. Transient inhibition of BMP signaling by Noggin induces cardiomyocyte differentiation of mouse embryonic stem cells. Nat Biotechnol. 2005;23:607–11.
13. de Pater E, Ciampricotti M, Priller F, Veerkamp J, Strate I, Smith K, et al. Bmp signaling exerts opposite effects on cardiac differentiation. Circ Res. 2012;110:578–87.
14. Klaus A, Saga Y, Taketo MM, Tzahor E, Birchmeier W. Distinct roles of Wnt/beta-catenin and Bmp signaling during early cardiogenesis. Proc Natl Acad Sci U S A. 2007;104:18531–6.
15. Kitajima S, Takagi A, Inoue T, Saga Y. MesP1 and MesP2 are essential for the development of cardiac mesoderm. Development. 2000;127:3215–26.
16. Tzahor E, Lassar AB. Wnt signals from the neural tube block ectopic cardiogenesis. Genes Dev. 2001;15:255–60.
17. Marvin MJ, Di Rocco G, Gardiner A, Bush SM, Lassar AB. Inhibition of Wnt activity induces heart formation from posterior mesoderm. Genes Dev. 2001;15:316–27.
18. Logan CY, Nusse R. The Wnt signaling pathway in development and disease. Annu Rev Cell Dev Biol. 2004;20:781–810.
19. Rossant J, Ciruna B, Partanen J. FGF signaling in mouse gastrulation and anteroposterior patterning. Cold Spring Harb Symp Quant Biol. 1997;62:127–33.
20. Zaffran S, Frasch M. Early signals in cardiac development. Circ Res. 2002;91:457–69.
21. Reifers F, Walsh EC, Léger S, Stainier DY, Brand M. Induction and differentiation of the zebrafish heart requires fibroblast growth factor 8 (fgf8/acerebellar). Development. 2000;127:225–35.
22. Arnold SJ, Huang GJ, Cheung AF, Era T, Nishikawa S, Bikoff EK, et al. The T-box transcription factor Eomes/Tbr2 regulates neurogenesis in the cortical subventricular zone. Genes Dev. 2008;22:2479–84.
23. Costello I, Pimeisl IM, Dräger S, Bikoff EK, Robertson EJ, Arnold SJ. The T-box transcription factor Eomesodermin acts upstream of Mespl to specify cardiac mesoderm during mouse gastrulation. Nat Cell Biol. 2011;13:1084–91.
24. Barron MR, Belaguli NS, Zhang SX, Trinh M, Iyer D, Merlo X, et al. Serum response factor, an enriched cardiac mesoderm obligatory factor, is a downstream gene target for Tbx genes. J Biol Chem. 2005;280: 11816–28.
25. Bodmer R. The gene tinman is required for specification of the heart and visceral muscles in Drosophila. Development. 1993;118:719–29.
26. Fishman MC, Chien KR. Fashioning the vertebrate heart: earliest embryonic decisions. Development. 1997;124:2099–117.
27. Lyons I, Parsons LM, Hartley L, Li R, Andrews JE, Robb L, et al. Myogenic and morphogenetic defects in the heart tubes of murine embryos lacking the homeo box gene Nkx2-5. Genes Dev. 1995;9:1654–66.
28. Caprioli A, Koyano-Nakagawa N, Iacovino M, Shi X, Ferdous A, Harvey RP, et al. Nkx2-5 represses Gata1 gene expression and modulates the cellular fate of cardiac progenitors during embryogenesis. Circulation. 2011;123:1633–41.
29. Tu CT, Yang TC, Tsai HJ. Nkx2.7 and Nkx2.5 function redundantly and are required for cardiac morphogenesis of zebrafish embryos. PLoS One. 2009;4:e4249.
30. Sizarov A, Ya J, de Boer BA, Lamers WH, Christoffels VM, Moorman AF. Formation of the building plan of the human heart: morphogenesis, growth, and differentiation. Circulation. 2011;123:1125–35.

31. Sugi Y, Lough J. Activin-A and FGF-2 mimic the inductive effects of anterior endoderm on terminal cardiac myogenesis in vitro. Dev Biol. 1995;168: 567–74.
32. Ticho BS, Stainier DY, Fishman MC, Breitbart RE. Three zebrafish MEF2 genes delineate somitic and cardiac muscle development in wild-type and mutant embryos. Mech Dev. 1996;59:205–18.
33. Turbendian HK, Gordillo M, Tsai SY, Lu J, Kang G, Liu TC, et al. GATA factors efficiently direct cardiac fate from embryonic stem cells. Development. 2013;140:1639–44.
34. Bruneau BG, Logan M, Davis N, Levi T, Tabin CJ, Seidman JG, et al. Chamber-specific cardiac expression of Tbx5 and heart defects in Holt-Oram syndrome. Dev Biol. 1999;211:100–8.
35. Basson CT, Bachinsky DR, Lin RC, Levi T, Elkins JA, Soults J, et al. Mutations in human TBX5 [corrected] cause limb and cardiac malformation in Holt-Oram syndrome. Nat Genet. 1997;15:30–5.
36. Begemann G, Ingham PW. Developmental regulation of Tbx5 in zebrafish embryogenesis. Mech Dev. 2000;90:299–304.
37. Yuasa S, Onizuka T, Shimoji K, Ohno Y, Kageyama T, Yoon SH, et al. Zac1 is an essential transcription factor for cardiac morphogenesis. Circ Res. 2010;106:1083–91.
38. Moorman A, Webb S, Brown NA, Lamers W, Anderson RH. Development of the heart: (1) formation of the cardiac chambers and arterial trunks. Heart. 2003;89:806–14.
39. van den Berg G, Abu-Issa R, de Boer BA, Hutson MR, de Boer PA, Soufan AT, et al. A caudal proliferating growth center contributes to both poles of the forming heart tube. Circ Res. 2009;104:179–88.
40. Buckingham M, Meilhac S, Zaffran S. Building the mammalian heart from two sources of myocardial cells. Nat Rev Genet. 2005;6:826–35.
41. Guner-Ataman B, Paffett-Lugassy N, Adams MS, Nevis KR, Jahangiri L, Obregon P, et al. Zebrafish second heart field development relies on progenitor specification in anterior lateral plate mesoderm and nkx2.5 function. Development. 2013;140:1353–63.
42. Mjaatvedt CH, Nakaoka T, Moreno-Rodriguez R, Norris RA, Kern MJ, Eisenberg CA, et al. The outflow tract of the heart is recruited from a novel heart-forming field. Dev Biol. 2001;238:97–109.
43. Waldo KL, Kumiski DH, Wallis KT, Stadt HA, Hutson MR, Platt DH, et al. Conotruncal myocardium arises from a secondary heart field. Development. 2001;128:3179–88.
44. Kelly RG, Brown NA, Buckingham ME. The arterial pole of the mouse heart forms from Fgf10-expressing cells in pharyngeal mesoderm. Dev Cell. 2001;1:435–40.
45. Cai CL, Liang X, Shi Y, Chu PH, Pfaff SL, Chen J, et al. Isl1 identifies a cardiac progenitor population that proliferates prior to differentiation and contributes a majority of cells to the heart. Dev Cell. 2003;5:877–89.
46. Hami D, Grimes AC, Tsai HJ, Kirby ML. Zebrafish cardiac development requires a conserved secondary heart field. Development. 2011;138:2389–98.
47. de Pater E, Clijsters L, Marques SR, Lin YF, Garavito-Aguilar ZV, Yelon D, et al. Distinct phases of cardiomyocyte differentiation regulate growth of the zebrafish heart. Development. 2009;136:1633–41.
48. Cohen ED, Miller MF, Wang Z, Moon RT, Morrisey EE. Wnt5a and Wnt11 are essential for second heart field progenitor development. Development. 2012;139:1931–40.
49. Dyer LA, Kirby ML. The role of secondary heart field in cardiac development. Dev Biol. 2009;336:137–44.
50. Cohen ED, Tian Y, Morrisey EE. Wnt signaling: an essential regulator of cardiovascular differentiation, morphogenesis and progenitor self-renewal. Development. 2008;135:789–98.
51. Holtzman NG, Schoenebeck JJ, Tsai HJ, Yelon D. Endocardium is necessary for cardiomyocyte movement during heart tube assembly. Development. 2007;134:2379–86.
52. Lee RK, Stainier DY, Weinstein BM, Fishman MC. Cardiovascular development in the zebrafish. II. Endocardial progenitors are sequestered within the heart field. Development. 1994;120:3361–6.
53. Cohen-Gould L, Mikawa T. The fate diversity of mesodermal cells within the heart field during chicken early embryogenesis. Dev Biol. 1996;177: 265–73.
54. Linask KK, Lash JW. Early heart development: dynamics of endocardial cell sorting suggests a common origin with cardiomyocytes. Dev Dyn. 1993;196:62–9.
55. Sugi Y, Markwald RR. Formation and early morphogenesis of endocardial endothelial precursor cells and the role of endoderm. Dev Biol. 1996;175:66–83.
56. Harris IS, Black BL. Development of the endocardium. Pediatr Cardiol. 2010;31:391–9.
57. Milgrom-Hoffman M, Harrelson Z, Ferrara N, Zelzer E, Evans SM, Tzahor E. The heart endocardium is derived from vascular endothelial progenitors. Development. 2011;138:4777–87.
58. Bussmann J, Bakkers J, Schulte-Merker S. Early endocardial morphogenesis requires Scl/Tal1. PLoS Genet. 2007;3:e140.
59. Nemer G, Nemer M. Cooperative interaction between GATA5 and NF-ATc regulates endothelial-endocardial differentiation of cardiogenic cells. Development. 2002;129:4045–55.
60. Ferdous A, Caprioli A, Iacovino M, Martin CM, Morris J, Richardson JA, et al. Nkx2-5 transactivates the Ets-related protein 71 gene and specifies an endothelial/endocardial fate in the developing embryo. Proc Natl Acad Sci U S A. 2009;106:814–9.
61. De Val S, Black BL. Transcriptional control of endothelial cell development. Dev Cell. 2009;16:180–95.
62. Männer J. Cardiac looping in the chick embryo: a morphological review with special reference to

terminological and biomechanical aspects of the looping process. Anat Rec. 2000;259:248–62.
63. Smith KA, Chocron S, von der Hardt S, de Pater E, Soufan A, Bussmann J, et al. Rotation and asymmetric development of the zebrafish heart requires directed migration of cardiac progenitor cells. Dev Cell. 2008;14:287–97.
64. de Campos-Baptista MI, Holtzman NG, Yelon D, Schier AF. Nodal signaling promotes the speed and directional movement of cardiomyocytes in zebrafish. Dev Dyn. 2008;237:3624–33.
65. Baker K, Holtzman NG, Burdine RD. Direct and indirect roles for Nodal signaling in two axis conversions during asymmetric morphogenesis of the zebrafish heart. Proc Natl Acad Sci U S A. 2008;105:13924–9.
66. Monteiro R, van Dinther M, Bakkers J, Wilkinson R, Patient R, ten Dijke P, et al. Two novel type II receptors mediate BMP signalling and are required to establish left-right asymmetry in zebrafish. Dev Biol. 2008;315:55–71.
67. Lin X, Xu X. Distinct functions of Wnt/beta-catenin signaling in KV development and cardiac asymmetry. Development. 2009;136:207–17.
68. Ramalho-Santos M, Melton DA, McMahon AP. Hedgehog signals regulate multiple aspects of gastrointestinal development. Development. 2000;127:2763–72.
69. Zhang XM, Ramalho-Santos M, McMahon AP. Smoothened mutants reveal redundant roles for Shh and Ihh signaling including regulation of L/R symmetry by the mouse node. Cell. 2001;106:781–92.
70. Moorman AF, Christoffels VM. Cardiac chamber formation: development, genes, and evolution. Physiol Rev. 2003;83:1223–67.
71. Houweling AC, Somi S, Van Den Hoff MJ, Moorman AF, Christoffels VM. Developmental pattern of ANF gene expression reveals a strict localization of cardiac chamber formation in chicken. Anat Rec. 2002;266:93–102.
72. Auman HJ, Coleman H, Riley HE, Olale F, Tsai HJ, Yelon D. Functional modulation of cardiac form through regionally confined cell shape changes. PLoS Biol. 2007;5:e53.
73. Christoffels VM, Hoogaars WM, Tessari A, Clout DE, Moorman AF, Campione M. T-box transcription factor Tbx2 represses differentiation and formation of the cardiac chambers. Dev Dyn. 2004;229:763–70.
74. Eisenberg LM, Markwald RR. Molecular regulation of atrioventricular valvuloseptal morphogenesis. Circ Res. 1995;77:1–6.
75. Armstrong EJ, Bischoff J. Heart valve development: endothelial cell signaling and differentiation. Circ Res. 2004;95:459–70.
76. Bakkers J. Zebrafish as a model to study cardiac development and human cardiac disease. Cardiovasc Res. 2011;91:279–88.
77. Hove JR, Köster RW, Forouhar AS, Acevedo-Bolton G, Fraser SE, Gharib M. Intracardiac fluid forces are an essential epigenetic factor for embryonic cardiogenesis. Nature. 2003;421:172–7.
78. Bartman T, Walsh EC, Wen KK, McKane M, Ren J, Alexander J, et al. Early myocardial function affects endocardial cushion development in zebrafish. PLoS Biol. 2004;2:E129.
79. Beis D, Bartman T, Jin SW, Scott IC, D'Amico LA, Ober EA, et al. Genetic and cellular analyses of zebrafish atrioventricular cushion and valve development. Development. 2005;132:4193–204.
80. Vermot J, Forouhar AS, Liebling M, Wu D, Plummer D, Gharib M, et al. Reversing blood flows act through klf2a to ensure normal valvulogenesis in the developing heart. PLoS Biol. 2009;7:e1000246.
81. McCulley DJ, Black BL. Transcription factor pathways and congenital heart disease. Curr Top Dev Biol. 2012;100:253–77.
82. Kelly BB, Narula J, Fuster V. Recognizing global burden of cardiovascular disease and related chronic diseases. Mt Sinai J Med. 2012;79:632–40.
83. Spallanzani L. An essay on animal reproductions. London: T. Becket and P.A. de Hondt; 1768.
84. Porrello ER, Mahmoud AI, Simpson E, Hill JA, Richardson JA, Olson EN, et al. Transient regenerative potential of the neonatal mouse heart. Science. 2011;331:1078–80.
85. Porrello ER, Mahmoud AI, Simpson E, Johnson BA, Grinsfelder D, Canseco D, et al. Regulation of neonatal and adult mammalian heart regeneration by the miR-15 family. Proc Natl Acad Sci U S A. 2013;110:187–92.
86. Kajstura J, Urbanek K, Perl S, Hosoda T, Zheng H, Ogorek B, et al. Cardiomyogenesis in the adult human heart. Circ Res. 2010;107:305–15.
87. Oberpriller JO, Oberpriller JC. Response of the adult newt ventricle to injury. J Exp Zool. 1974;187:249–53.
88. Bettencourt-Dias M, Mittnacht S, Brockes JP. Heterogeneous proliferative potential in regenerative adult newt cardiomyocytes. Cell Sci. 2003;116:4001–9.
89. Beis D, Stainier DY. In vivo cell biology: following the zebrafish trend. Trends Cell Biol. 2006;16:105–12.
90. Becker T, Wullimann MF, Becker CG, Bernhardt RR, Schachner M. Axonal regrowth after spinal cord transection in adult zebrafish. J Comp Neurol. 1997;377:577–95.
91. Moss JB, Koustubhan P, Greenman M, Parsons MJ, Walter I, Moss LG. Regeneration of the pancreas in adult zebrafish. Diabetes. 2009;58:1844–51.
92. Kyritsis N, Kizil C, Zocher S, Kroehne V, Kaslin J, Freudenreich D, et al. Acute inflammation initiates the regenerative response in the adult zebrafish brain. Science. 2012;338:1353–6.
93. Poss KD, Wilson LG, Keating MT. Heart regeneration in zebrafish. Science. 2002;298:2188–90.
94. Itou J, Kawakami H, Burgoyne T, Kawakami Y. Life-long preservation of the regenerative capacity in the fin and heart in zebrafish. Biol Open. 2012;1:739–46.
95. Gonzalez-Rosa JM, Mercader N. Cryoinjury as a myocardial infarction model for the study of cardiac

regeneration in the zebrafish. Nat Protoc. 2012;7: 782–8.
96. Chablais F, Veit J, Rainer G, Jazwinska A. The zebrafish heart regenerates after cryoinjury-induced myocardial infarction. BMC Dev Biol. 2011;11:21.
97. Curado S, Stainier DY, Anderson RM. Nitroreductase-mediated cell/tissue ablation in zebrafish: a spatially and temporally controlled ablation method with applications in developmental and regeneration studies. Nat Protoc. 2008;3:948–54.
98. Wang J, Panáková D, Kikuchi K, Holdway JE, Gemberling M, Burris JS, et al. The regenerative capacity of zebrafish reverses cardiac failure caused by genetic cardiomyocyte depletion. Development. 2011;138:3421–30.
99. Zhang R, Han P, Yang H, Ouyang K, Lee D, Lin YF, et al. In vivo cardiac reprogramming contributes to zebrafish heart regeneration. Nature. 2013;498: 497–501.
100. Jopling C, Sune G, Faucherre A, Fabregat C, Izpisua Belmonte JC. Hypoxia induces myocardial regeneration in zebrafish. Circulation. 2012;126:3017–27.
101. Lam NT, Currie PD, Lieschke GJ, Rosenthal NA, Kaye DM. Nerve growth factor stimulates cardiac regeneration via cardiomyocyte proliferation in experimental heart failure. PLoS One. 2012;7:e53210.
102. Lepilina A, Coon AN, Kikuchi K, Holdway JE, Roberts RW, Burns CG, et al. A dynamic epicardial injury response supports progenitor cell activity during zebrafish heart regeneration. Cell. 2006;127:607–19.
103. Knowlton AA, Connelly CM, Romo GM, Mamuya W, Apstein CS, Brecher P. Rapid expression of fibronectin in the rabbit heart after myocardial infarction with and without reperfusion. J Clin Invest. 1992;89: 1060–8.
104. Rysä J, Leskinen H, Ilves M, Ruskoaho H. Distinct upregulation of extracellular matrix genes in transition from hypertrophy to hypertensive heart failure. Hypertension. 2005;45:927–33.
105. Wang J, Karra R, Dickson AL, Poss KD. Fibronectin is deposited by injury-activated epicardial cells and is necessary for zebrafish heart regeneration. Dev Biol. 2013;382:427–35.
106. Jopling C, Sleep E, Raya M, Marti M, Raya A, Izpisua Belmonte JC. Zebrafish heart regeneration occurs by cardiomyocyte dedifferentiation and proliferation. Nature. 2010;464:606–9.
107. Kikuchi K, Holdway JE, Werdich AA, Anderson RM, Fang Y, Egnaczyk GF, et al. Primary contribution to zebrafish heart regeneration by gata4(+) cardiomyocytes. Nature. 2010;464:601–5.
108. Itou J, Oishi I, Kawakami H, Glass TJ, Richter J, Johnson A, et al. Migration of cardiomyocytes is essential for heart regeneration in zebrafish. Development. 2012;139:4133–42.
109. Lien C-L, Schebesta M, Makino S, Weber GJ, Keating MT. Gene expression analysis of zebrafish heart regeneration. PLoS Biol. 2006;4:e260.
110. Niessen K, Karsan A. Notch signaling in cardiac development. Circ Res. 2008;102:1169–81.
111. Raya A, Koth CM, Buscher D, Kawakami Y, Itoh T, Raya RM, et al. Activation of Notch signaling pathway precedes heart regeneration in zebrafish. Proc Natl Acad Sci U S A. 2003;100 Suppl 1:11889–95.
112. Andrae J, Gallini R, Betsholtz C. Role of platelet-derived growth factors in physiology and medicine. Genes Dev. 2008;22:1276–312.
113. Raines EW. PDGF and cardiovascular disease. Cytokine Growth Factor Rev. 2004;15:237–54.
114. Hoover LL, Burton EG, Brooks BA, Kubalak SW. The expanding role for retinoid signaling in heart development. Sci World J. 2008;8:194–211.
115. Kikuchi K, Holdway Jennifer E, Major Robert J, Blum N, Dahn Randall D, Begemann G, et al. Retinoic acid production by endocardium and epicardium is an injury response essential for zebrafish heart regeneration. Dev Cell. 2011;20:397–404.
116. Meloni M, Caporali A, Graiani G, Lagrasta C, Katare R, Van Linthout S, et al. Nerve growth factor promotes cardiac repair following myocardial infarction. Circ Res. 2010;106:1275–84.
117. Pantos C, Mourouzis I, Cokkinos DV. Thyroid hormone and cardiac repair/regeneration: from Prometheus myth to reality? Can J Physiol Pharmacol. 2012;90:977–87.
118. Choi WY, Gemberling M, Wang J, Holdway JE, Shen MC, Karlstrom RO, et al. In vivo monitoring of cardiomyocyte proliferation to identify chemical modifiers of heart regeneration. Development. 2013;140:660–6.

Basis of Cell Excitability and Cardiac Conduction System

3

Irini Skaliora, Manolis Mavroidis, and Elias Kouvelas

Abstract

In this chapter we review essential aspects of cellular electrical excitability, which apply to all excitable cells, including neurons and cardiac tissue. We present the concept of the equilibrium potential, describe the factors that create the resting potential, and discuss the channel activity that leads to the generation of the action potential. We subsequently focus specifically on the peculiarities of the cardiac conduction system. We discuss the types of action potentials present in myocardial cells, the anatomical and ionic basis of automaticity, the regulatory mechanisms of heart rate and several aspects of electrocardiography, as well as the different types of arrhythmias.

Keywords

Ion channels • Fast/slow response action potentials • Automaticity of the heart • Electrocardiography • Arrhythmias

Abbreviations

AN	Atrionodal
AP	Action potential
ATP	Adenosine triphosphate
ATPase	Adenosine triphosphatase
AV	Atrioventricular
AVN	Atrioventricular node
CCS	Cardiac conduction system
CFS	Central fibrous body
CN	Compact node
CS	Coronary sinus
E_{Na}	Sodium equilibrium potential
GABA	γ-Aminobutyric acid
GHK	Goldman-Hodgkin-Katz
G_{K}^{+}	Conductance for potassium
G_{Na}^{+}	Conductance for sodium
I_{Ki}	Inwardly rectifying K^+ current
LNB	Lower nodal bundle
N	Nodal
NH	Nodo-His
PNE	Posterior nodal extension

I. Skaliora, PhD (✉)
Neurophysiology Laboratory, Center for Basic Research, Biomedical Research Foundation of the Academy of Athens (BRFAA),
Soranou Efessiou 4, Athens 11527, Greece
e-mail: iskaliora@bioacademy.gr

M. Mavroidis
Cell Biology Division, Biomedical Research Foundation, Academy of Athens, Athens, Greece

E. Kouvelas
Department of Physiology, University of Patras, Patras, Greece

D.V. Cokkinos (ed.), *Introduction to Translational Cardiovascular Research*,
DOI 10.1007/978-3-319-08798-6_3, © Springer International Publishing Switzerland 2015

SA	Sinoatrial
TV	Tricuspid valve
Vm	Membrane potential

3.1 Introduction: Basis of Electrical Excitability of Cells

3.1.1 What Are Excitable Cells?

All living cells in very organism have a transmembrane potential, or in other words a voltage difference across their plasma membrane. But not all cells are electrically excitable. Excitable cells include neurons, muscle and heart cells, as well as fertilized eggs, glandular tissue and some plants. A cell is generally defined as 'excitable' if it manifests a *nonlinear* response to depolarization, causing an amplification and propagation of the depolarization, in the form of an action potential. Or, in other words, if it can generate an action potential, which can be transmitted along the membrane. In the fist part of this chapter, we present the concept of the equilibrium potential, which is crucial for understanding all electrical phenomena in cell membranes. We then describe the resting potential, which forms the basis of cell excitability and, finally, we discuss the voltage-gated ion channels present in excitable cells, whose activity results in the generation and propagation of the action potential (AP).

3.1.1.1 Equilibrium Potential

The plasma membrane of all cells is a lipid bilayer that acts as an electrical insulator, largely impermeable to charged species. It would require an enormous amount of energy to move an ion through the hydrophobic interior of the bilayer. Instead, the membrane permeability arises as a result of the presence of ion channels, which are specialized proteins that form aqueous pores across the membrane, and through which specific ions can flow. It is the flow of ions through membrane channels that is responsible for electrical signalling in excitable cells.

The flow rate of an ion across the membrane is determined by three factors: (1) the difference in concentration of that ion between the two sides of the membrane, i.e. the concentration gradient, which creates a force that compels the ion to move towards the side with the lowest concentration; (2) the difference in voltage across the plasma membrane, i.e. the electrical gradient, which creates a force that compels the ion to move towards the side with the fewer similarly charged ions; and (3) the conductance of the ion channel, i.e. the ease with which a specific ion can move (through the channels) across the plasma membrane.

Let us consider a simple membrane that separates two aqueous solutions (Fig. 3.1a). If positive charges (ions) are added to one side only, a condition of electrical and chemical imbalance, or un-equilibrium, is immediately created. Provided the membrane is permeable to the specific ions (i.e. provided it contains channels selective to that ion) then both the electrical and chemical gradients would force the X^+ ions to flow towards the other side until electrical and chemical equilibrium is reached (Fig. 3.1b).

If, instead, we also add an equal amount of negative ions (Y^-) to which the membrane is not permeable, then we do not disturb the electrical equilibrium (since the net charge on either side is zero), but we create a chemical un-equilibrium for both types of ions (Fig. 3.1c). In this case, the positive ions will cross the membrane, forced by their concentration gradient, as before. In contrast, the negative ions, in spite an identical concentration gradient, will be unable to move because the membrane does not contain Y^--selective channels. The result would be the creation of an electrostatic imbalance, which was not present before, because there are now more negative charges on the left side of the membrane (Fig. 3.1d). The final steady-state of this system is depicted in Fig. 3.1e, where some of the permeant ions have moved back to the left side, so that the electrical un-equilibrium counterbalances the chemical un-equilibrium to create a resting steady-state.

Hence, it becomes evident that there are always two forces acting on the ions, one generated by the difference in concentration and the other by the difference in electrical charges

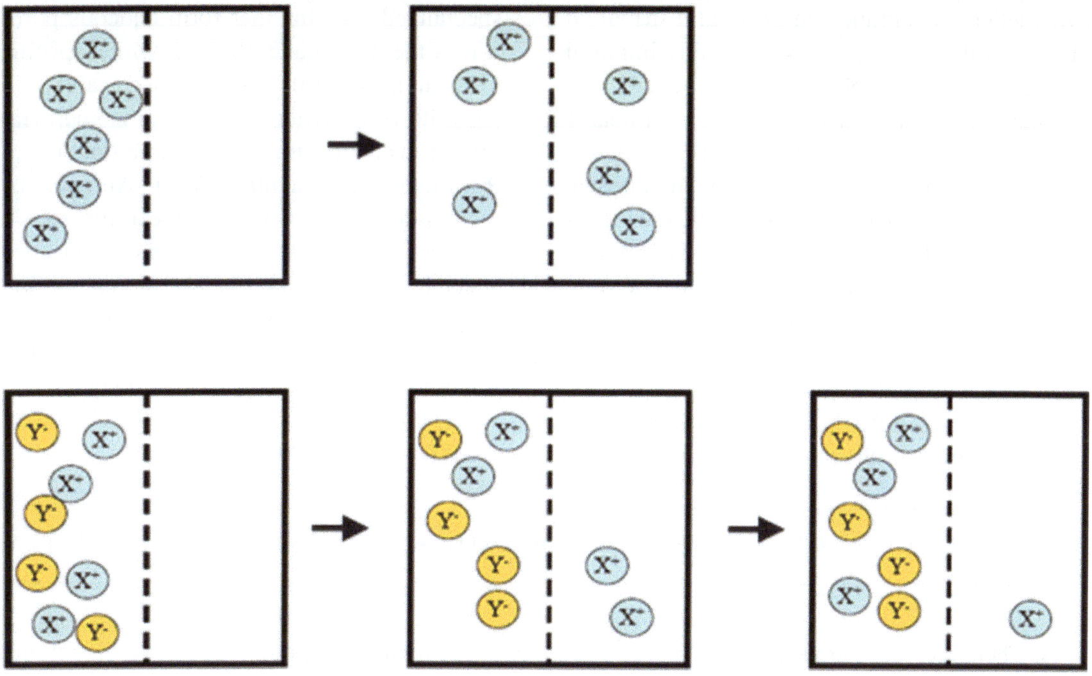

Fig. 3.1 Schematic illustration of the principles governing the movement of ions through membranes. The membrane separating the two sides of the container is permeable to ion X^+ but not to ion Y^-. In the *top row*, where there are no impermeant ions, the steady state is a state of chemical and electrical equilibrium (*as illustrated in the right panel*). In contrast, when impermeant ions are present, as in the examples depicted in the *bottom row*, the steady state (*as illustrated in the rightmost panel*) is the condition at which the electrical gradient counterbalances the chemical gradient

across the two sides of the membrane. The electrical gradient (voltage) required to counterbalance the chemical gradient (concentration difference) resulting in a net flow = 0, is called the equilibrium potential for that particular ion and is described by the famous Nernst equation:

$$E_X = RT / zF \log_e \left[X^+\right]_o / \left[X^+\right]_i \quad (3.1)$$

Where *R* is the gas constant, *T* is the temperature in degrees Kelvin, *z* is the charge of the ion, and *F* is the Faraday (the amount of charge in coulombs carried my a mole of monovalent ions). For monovalent ions at room temperature (~20 °C), the Nernst equation is reduced to:

$$E_X = 58 \log_{10} \left[X^+\right]_o / \left[X^+\right]_i \quad (3.2)$$

Hence, if we take the case of potassium ions (K^+) as an example and we measure the K^+ concentrations on both sides of the membrane, we can calculate that, for concentrations $[K^+]_o = 5$ and $[K^+]_i = 140$ nM, the equilibrium potential for K^+, will be: 58 $\log_{10}$ 5/140 = −84 mV. That means that if the membrane potential (Vm) is set at −84 mV (there are ways to do that experimentally, with the voltage-clamp method), there would be no *net* flow of K^+ across the membrane. Or, in other words, potassium ions would be at equilibrium.

3.1.2 Resting Potential

The principles just discussed regarding the two forces (electrostatic and chemical) acting on the ions also apply in real cells, except that in this case there are multiple ions present, and real membranes have different permeabilities for the various ions. In the previous example with the hypothetical membrane, the unequal distribution of ions on the two sides was artificially imposed for the purpose of explaining the principles, and the membrane was either completely permeable to one type of ions (as in X^+) or completely impermeable (as in Y^-). In real cells the unequal distribution is created primarily (1) by the differential permeability of cell membranes for different types of ions (including the presence of non-permeant ions inside the cell); and secondarily (2) by the presence of energy-consuming ion pumps, or transporters.

1. The differential permeability arises as a result of the presence of selective ion channels, i.e. specialized proteins that form aqueous pores across the membrane, through which specific ions can flow. Furthermore, as we shall see in the following section, the membrane permeability can change dramatically as a function of the membrane potential (Vm). At rest, the membrane exhibits high permeability to K^+, i.e. many potassium channels are in an open state. In contrast, membranes at rest exhibit very low permeability to Na^+ and Cl^-, as most sodium and chloride channels are closed. The relationship between membrane potential and ionic concentrations is given by the Goldman-Hodgkin-Katz (GHK) equation:

$$V_m = RT/zF\log_e\left[\left(K_o + [P_{Na}/P_K]Na_o + [P_{Cl}/P_K]Cl_i\right)/\left(K_i + [P_{Na}/P_K]Na_i + [P_{Cl}/P_K]Cl_o\right)\right] \quad (3.3)$$

Therefore, the permeabilities (*P*) for each ion, in combination with the intracellular and extracellular ionic concentrations determine the final value of the membrane potential. There are, of course, other ions present besides the three just described (Na^+, Cl^-, and K^+), but these are either present at very low concentrations, or there are no ion channels that permit them to cross the membrane. Hence, they contribute very little to the Vm and can be ignored for present purposes. Thus, when the Na^+ and Cl^- channels are closed, i.e. when P_{Na} and P_{Cl} are close to zero, and the membrane is permeable only to potassium, the GHK equation reverts to the Nernst equation, as discussed before (Eq. 3.1).

2. Besides the passive flow along electrochemical gradients through ion channels, the membranes also contain energy-driven pumps or transporters, which use the energy from adenosine triphosphate (ATP) to overcome the barrier imposed by the lipophilic nature of the plasma membrane. Such pumps or transporters are proteins that physically grab ions from one side of the membrane and transport them to the other. These pumps are essential for the establishment of concentration gradients of various inorganic ions across the plasma membrane. Many of them are electroneutral, but some are electrogenic, i.e. they contribute to the membrane potential, since their activity results in a net flow of ions across the membrane. One such pump is the sodium-potassium pump, or Na^+/K^+ adenosine triphosphatase (ATPase), which transports *three* sodium ions out of the cell for every *two* potassium ions pumped in (Fig. 3.2). Hence, this specific pump helps to maintain the negative levels of the membrane potential [1].

This unequal distribution of charged particles on the intracellular and extracellular sides of the plasma membrane creates the voltage difference know as the "resting potential". The resting potential, which in most cells is usually around −75 mV, can be viewed as a form of stored energy and lies at the basis of all cellular excitability. The resting potential is exactly large enough to balance the ion flow caused by the various permeant ions with their different concentration gradients and membrane permeabilities. At this voltage the net charge flow is zero and the membrane is at a resting steady-state, but not at equilibrium (Fig. 3.1e).

3.1.3 Action Potential

The plasma membrane of all excitable cells, including neurons and cardiac tissue, contains voltage-gated channels that are responsible for

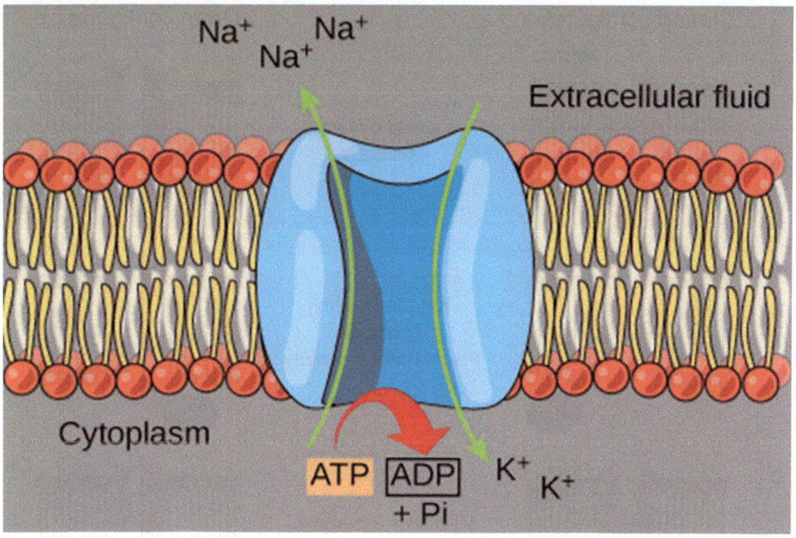

Fig. 3.2 Graphic illustration of the $Na^{\pm}$-$K^{\pm}$ pump. The protein spans the plasma membrane of all animal cells and is an antiporter enzyme that pumps sodium out of cells, while pumping potassium into cells, against their concentration gradient using ATP as an energy source. The protein is a sodium dependent ATPase. Because the transport ratio is 2 K^+ pumped in for 3Na^+ pumped out, the Na^+-K^+ pump is an electrogenic antiporter, as it contributes to maintaining the negativity of the resting potential. An antiporter is a cotransporter and integral membrane protein involved in secondary active transport of two or more different molecules or ions across a phospholipid membrane, in opposite directions (Illustration reproduced with permission from: OpenStax College. ATP: Adenosine Triphosphate [OpenStax-CNX Web site]. 28 Jan 2013. Available at: http://cnx.org/content/m44427/1.3/)

these cells' non-linear response to depolarization and the generation of the AP. These channels can be in a closed or an open state, and the transition between the two is regulated in different ways (Fig. 3.3): in some channels the probability of opening is determined by the voltage difference across the membrane (voltage-gated channels), in others by the binding of a specific molecule on the channel (ligand-gated channels), and some may be activated by conformational change of the membrane itself (stretch-activated channels).

The most important channels for the generation of the action potential are the voltage-gated channels, which open when the membrane potential reaches a certain value, and either remain open for as long as the voltage remains within a certain range, or close after a given time period (temporally regulated inactivation). All channels are selectively permeable to one or few types of ions and once open allow the specific ion(s) to move through it according to their electrochemical gradient, as described in the previous section.

To examine the sequence of events that leads to the generation of an AP we can refer to Fig. 3.4. At rest, the membrane potential is at a hyperpolarized level (−75 mV). This value may vary as it reflects the particular combination of ion channels present on the membrane, but is usually between −80 and −70 mV. When small hyperpolarizing stimuli are applied to the cell, the membrane potential becomes hyperpolarized to values below the resting potential (blue traces). When small depolarizing pulses are applied the membrane becomes depolarized accordingly (green traces). However, with a larger depolarizing pulse the membrane potential reaches the threshold level and a couple of action potentials are generated (red trace).

The upstroke of the action potential (indicated by circle-1 in Fig. 3.4) reflects the opening of the voltage-gated Na^+ channels, which were almost completely closed at rest. Once open, the conductance for sodium ions is dramatically increased and Na^+ rushes in, down its electrochemical

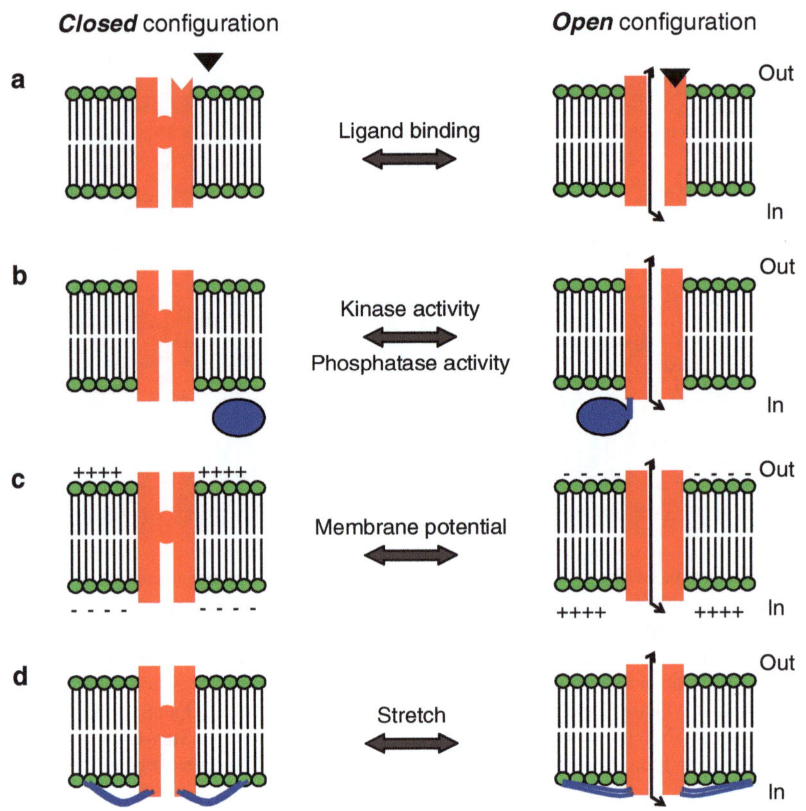

Fig. 3.3 Mechanisms of channel gating. (**a**) In ligand-gated channels, a molecule (*black triangle*) binds to the extracellular side of the channel protein and causes a conformational change that leads to channel opening. An example of a ligand-gated channel is the γ-aminobutyric acid $(GABA)_A$ receptor, where the binding of GABA on the channel leads to the opening of a Cl^- channel. (**b**) Channel gating can also occur by phosphorylation or dephosphorylation of the channel protein, caused by the activity of kinases or phosphatases, respectively. (**c**) Gating in voltage-gated channels occurs through local changes in membrane potential, which lead to conformational change in the channel protein. (**d**) There are also channels that are activated by physical stretching of the membrane. In these, the channel protein is linked to the cytoskeleton (*blue lines*) and the gating is mechanical (Illustration modified with permission from: http://employees.csbsju.edu/)

gradient. This will cause further depolarization of the membrane, which will exceed the zero value and will tend towards the equilibrium potential for sodium (E_{Na} = about +35 mV). The depolarization cannot exceed this level since at E_{Na}, sodium ions are at electrochemical equilibrium and the net flow across the membrane will be zero – even if all Na^+ channels were open. The reason that the depolarization does not quite reach the level of E_{Na} is two-fold: (1) On one hand the voltage-gated sodium channels are temporally regulated and will have started to become inactivated, causing the conductance for Na^+ to go back to resting levels and thus preventing further inflow. The inactivated state is different from the closed state, in that it is a state from which the channel cannot open. (2) At the same time K^+ channels, which are also voltage sensitive but with slower kinetics, will have started to open and K^+ will have started to move outwards along its concentration gradient, which is no longer counterbalanced by the electrical gradient as when the cell was at rest. The downstroke of the AP (indicated by circle-2 in Fig. 3.4) reflects the delayed opening of potassium channels and the outflow of K^+ along its electrochemical gradient. After the return to baseline (or even below baseline in cells that exhibit an afterhypolarization) the cell will enter a refractory period, which is determined by the rate of recovery from inactivation of the Na^+

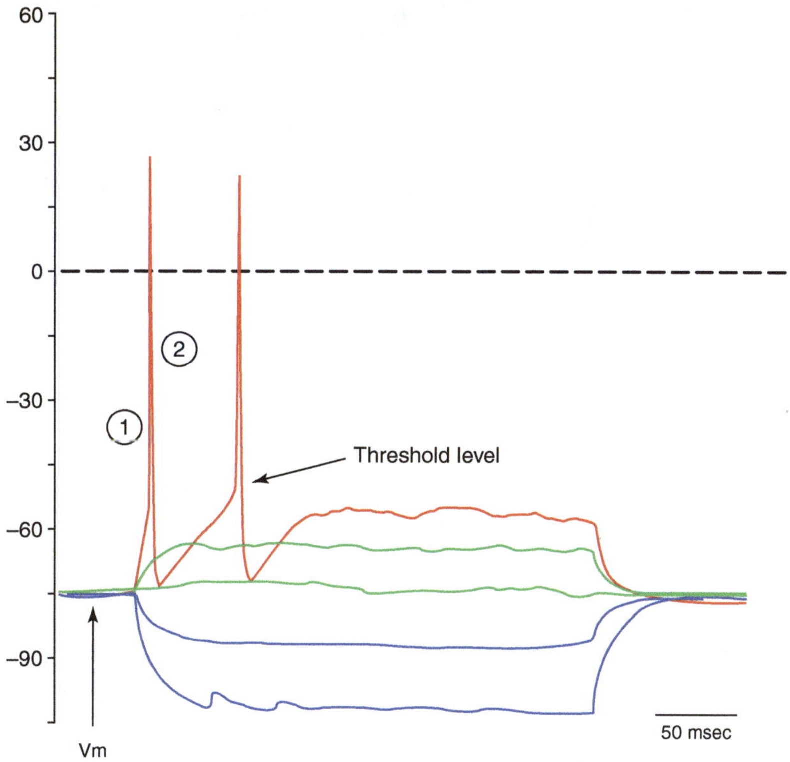

Fig. 3.4 Current-clamp whole cell recordings obtained from a cultured neuron. Three hundred millisecond-long hyperpolarizing and depolarizing current pulses are applied to the cell body and the change in membrane voltage is recorded. The resting potential is –75 mV

channels. Until the termination of the (absolute) refractory period, no AP can be generated. The time course of the sequence of events that underlie the AP, and thus the duration of an individual AP, varies between cells. In most neurons and axons the entire sequence of events is over in a few milliseconds. In other cells, as in certain cells of the pituitary gland, APs may last for tens of milliseconds, whereas in cardiac muscle they can be hundreds of milliseconds long, as described in the next section.

3.2 Cardiac Conduction System

3.2.1 Electrical Properties of the Heart

The cells of the heart, like neurons or striated muscle fibers, are excitable and generate APs. The cardiac tissue consists of two types of muscle cells: (1) cells that initiate and conduct impulses; and (2) cells that, in addition to conducting impulses, respond to stimuli by contracting. Figure 3.5 illustrates APs found in different types of cardiac cells. Two types of impulses occur in the heart: the fast response AP occurs in atrial and ventricular myocardial cells; while the slow response AP occurs in (i) the **sinoatrial (SA) node,** which is the natural pacemaker region of the heart, and (ii) the **atrioventricular (AV) node,** which is the specialized tissue that conducts the cardiac impulse from the atria to the ventricles, but can also act as a pacemaker [2].

As with most cells of the other tissues of the body (discussed in previous paragraphs), the intracellular K^+ concentration of myocardial cells ($[K^+]_i$) exceeds the concentration outside the cell ($[K^+]_o$). The reverse gradient exists for Na^+, Cl^-, and Ca^{2+}. Several types of potassium channels are present in cardiac muscle cell membranes [3], and the specific K^+ channel which is active (i.e. open)

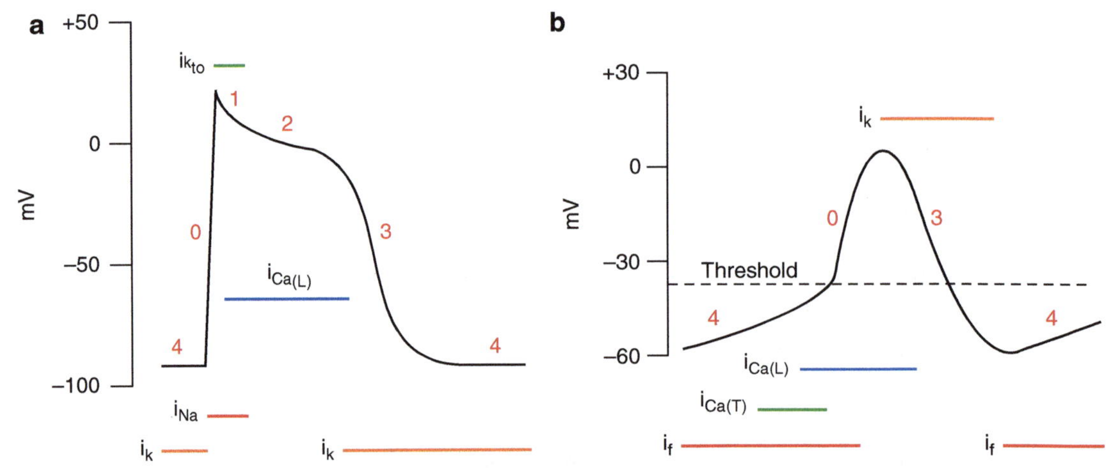

Fig. 3.5 (**a**) Fast response action potential, as found in ventricular myocytes. (**b**) Slow-response action potentials, as found in sinoatrial node cells (Illustration reproduced with permission from: www.cvphysiology.com)

at rest is the voltage-gated channel that conducts the **inwardly rectifying K⁺ current (IK_i).** Inwardly rectifying potassium channels are a specific subset of potassium-selective ion channels. A channel that is "inwardly rectifying" is one that passes current (in this case potassium ions) more easily in the inward direction (into the cell) than in the outward direction (out of the cell). These channels, by mediating a small depolarizing K^+ current at negative membrane potentials, help establish the resting membrane potential [4]. As for most cells, conductance for K^+ (g_K) in a resting myocardial cell is about 100 times higher than the conductance for Na^+ (g_{Na}).

3.2.1.1 Fast-Response Action Potentials

The characteristics of fast response APs are shown in Fig. 3.5a. When the cell is electrically stimulated (typically by a current from an adjacent cell), a sequence of events is set in motion, involving the influx and efflux of ions. When the resting membrane potential is depolarized to the threshold level of about −65 mV, the cell membrane properties change dramatically and Na^+ enters into the myocardial cells through specific **voltage-gated Na^+ channels** (upstroke, depolarization, **phase 0**). The Na^+ channels open very rapidly (in 0.1 msec), resulting in an abrupt increase of g_{Na}. Once open, the Na^+ channels inactivate and g_{Na} rapidly decreases. The Na^+ channels remain inactivated until the membrane begins to repolarize. Phase 0 is followed by a brief period of limited repolarization (**phase 1**) reflected in the notch between the end of the upstroke and the beginning of the plateau. This repolarization is the result of activation of a **transient outward current** carried mainly by potassium ions.

The plateau phase (**phase 2**) of the cardiac AP is sustained by a balance between inward movement of Ca^{2+} and outward movement of K^+. Ca^{2+} enters in the cell via voltage-gated **L-type Ca^{2+} channels**. These channels are activated when V_m reaches −20 mV and, like the sodium channels, inactivate slowly thus providing a long lasting Ca^{2+} inflow. Opening of Ca^{2+} channels results in an increase in Ca^{2+} conductance (g_{Ca}). Because [Ca^{2+}] inside the cells is much less than outside, the increase of g_{Ca} promotes the influx of Ca^{2+} throughout the plateau. During the peak of the upstroke g_K decreases (Fig. 3.5a), thus preventing the excessive loss of K^+ during the plateau.

The process of final repolarization (**phase 3**) starts at the end of the plateau phase, when efflux of K^+ from the myocardial cells begins to exceed Ca^{2+} influx, with several outward K^+ channels contributing to the repolarization of the myocardial cell [5–7].

Refractory Period

From the beginning of phase 0 until nearly the end of phase 2, the cell is in an **absolute refractory period,** during which it is impossible to evoke another AP. This is followed by a **relative refractory period** that lasts until phase 4, and during which a stronger stimulus is required to elicit another impulse. These two refractory periods are caused by changes in the state of sodium and potassium channels. As described in the first part of the chapter, sodium channels enter an 'inactivated' state at the end of phase 0 of the AP, from which they cannot progress to an 'open' state regardless of the membrane potential, thus leading to the absolute refractory period. Even after a sufficient number of sodium channels have transitioned back to their resting state, a fraction of potassium channels may remain open, making it more difficult for depolarization to occur, thereby leading to the relative refractory period. This has important functional consequences, as it prevents a sustained tetanic contraction of the cardiac muscle, which would interfere with the normal pumping function of the heart.

3.2.1.2 Slow-Response Action Potentials

A completely different type of impulse, the slow response AP, is exhibited by cells in SA and AV node (Fig. 3.5b). Here, the upstroke is much slower and the depolarizing current is carried into the cell primarily by relatively slow Ca^{2+} currents, instead of fast Na^+ channels. Also, the plateau is less prolonged and the transition to the repolarization is less distinct. The ionic basis of the slow-response APs underlies the automaticity of the heart and will be described in detail in the following paragraphs.

3.2.1.3 Automaticity

In heart physiology, automaticity is the ability of cardiac cells, contrary to skeletal muscles, to depolarize spontaneously without external stimulation from the nervous system. The ordered excitation of the heart occurs via the heart's conduction system (Fig. 3.6).

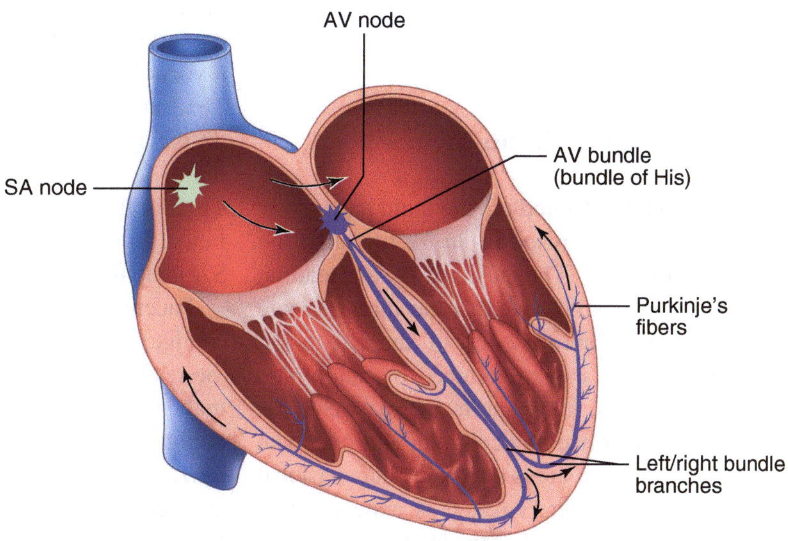

Fig. 3.6 The-conducting system of the heart (Illustration reproduced with permission from: medical-dictionary.thefreedictionary.com)

The cardiac conduction system (CCS) is a series of specialized tissues in the heart responsible for the initiation and co-ordination of the heartbeat. Each normal heartbeat is achieved by a wave of depolarizing impulses originating from a group of cells collectively called the ***sinus node***. The impulse spreads rapidly through the atria, activating the myocardium to contract, and is collected in the **atrioventricular node**. It is then slowed, before spreading rapidly through the histologically specialized and insulated fibers of the **atrioventricular bundle (bundle of His)** and its branches, to the finest ramifications of the peripheral ventricular conduction system, thus activating the ventricular myocardium to contract [8].

The major parts of the CCS were discovered in the nineteenth and early twentieth centuries. The Purkinje fibers were discovered in 1839 by Jan Purkinje, a Czech physiologist and anatomist; the bundle of His was discovered in 1893 by Wilhelm His, a Swiss cardiologist and anatomist; and the atrioventricular node was discovered in 1906 by a Japanese, Sunao Tawara, working in the laboratory of Ludwig Aschoff in Marburg in Germany. Finally, the sino-atrial node was discovered in 1907 by Sir Arthur Keith in a farmhouse in Kent together with a young medical student, Martin Flack [9].

3.2.2 Sinoatrial Node

The **sinoatrial (SA) node** is the main pacemaker of the heart, and is responsible for the initiation of the cardiac AP. The position of the leading pacemaker site is not fixed as the initiation site can shift in different zones of the SA node. Pacemaker shifts can be induced by autonomic regulatory inputs, temperature, atrial stretch, as well as by pharmacological interventions. The leading pacemaker site is situated wherever local automaticity is faster. Thus, it is expected that sympathetic input will shift the leading site where automaticity is most sensitive to adrenergic stimulation, while parasympathetic activity will shift pacemaking where automaticity is less inhibited by cholinergic transmitters [10]. In humans, the leading pacemaker site (i.e. the site where the cardiac AP is first initiated) can be anywhere from the superior vena cava to the inferior vena cava (and not just at the junction of the superior vena cava with the right atrium, as most textbooks would lead us to believe). This has been confirmed in normal human subjects [11] and it is also the case in rats and rabbits [12, 13]. The SA node contains two principal cell types: (1) small, round cells and (2) elongated cells that are intermediate in appearance between the round and the ordinary atrial myocardial cells. The round cells are the primary pacemaker site within the heart. In these cells the resting membrane potential is less negative (−55 to −65 mV) than the atrial or ventricular myocardial cells (−85 to −95 mV) because nodal cells lack the inward rectifying (IK_i) type K^+ channels.

The principal feature of a SA node cell that distinguishes it from an atrial or ventricular cell is that in the latter the resting membrane potential remains constant, whereas a pacemaker cell is characterized by slow diastolic depolarization throughout the resting membrane potential (Fig. 3.5b). Depolarization proceeds at a steady rate until a threshold is attained and an AP is triggered. It is believed that a common element in the formation of the conduction system is its failure to differentiate into mature working myocardium [14]. The T-box transcription factor Tbx3 and the homeodomain transcription factor Shox2 appear to be involved in the formation of the SA node region. Ectopic expression of Tbx3 in the adult atria of transgenic mice is sufficient to reactivate focal automaticity and some SA node markers [15, 16].

Pacemaker frequency may be varied by changes in (1) the rate of depolarization during the resting membrane potential, or (2) the maximal negativity during the resting membrane potential (Fig. 3.5b). When the rate of slow depolarization is increased, the threshold potential is attained earlier, and the heart rate increases. When the maximal negative potential is at more hyperpolarized values, a longer time is required to reach the threshold potential and the heart rate decreases.

3.2.2.1 Ionic Basis of Automaticity

Many studies have examined the ionic basis of cardiac automaticity [17–20]. At the end of repolarization of SA node cells, when the membrane potential is about −60 mV, ion channels open that conduct slow, inward Na^+ currents (Fig. 3.5b). These currents are called **"funny" currents** (I_f) and cause the resting membrane potential to begin to depolarize, thereby initiating **phase 4.** Since the discovery of a pacemaker current (I_f) in 1978, multiple studies have shown that rhythmic changes in membrane voltage (the "membrane voltage clock") underlie the mechanisms of automaticity. Recent studies, however, suggest that increased intracellular calcium $[Ca^{2+}]_i$ induced by spontaneous rhythmic sarcoplasmic reticulum calcium release (the "calcium clock") is also jointly responsible for the initiation of the heartbeat. Elevated $[Ca^{2+}]_i$ activates another ionic current (the sodium–calcium exchanger current or *I*NCX), leading to spontaneous phase 4 depolarization. Under normal conditions, both clocks are needed to initiate the heart beat. Malfunction of the clocks is associated with sinus node dysfunction in heart failure and atrial fibrillation. More studies are needed to determine how both clocks work together to initiate the heart beat under normal and disease conditions [21]. Ivabradine, a novel medication used for symptomatic management of stable angina pectoris, acts by reducing the heart rate via specific inhibition of the I_f channel, a mechanism different from beta blockers and calcium blockers, two commonly prescribed antianginal drugs [22, 23]. As the membrane potential reaches about −50 mV, another type of channel opens. This channel is called transient or **T-type Ca^{2+} channel.** As Ca^{2+} enters the cell through these channels down its electrochemical gradient, the inwardly directed Ca^{2+} currents cause further depolarization of the cell and when the membrane reaches about −40 mV, a second type of Ca^{2+} channel opens. These are the so-called long lasting or **L-type Ca^{2+} channels.** During phase 4 there is also a slow decline in the outward movement of K^+ as the K^+ channels responsible for phase 3 continue to close. This fall in K^+ conductance contributes to the depolarizing pacemaker potential. **Phase 0** depolarization is primarily caused by increased Ca^{2+} conductance through the L-type Ca^{2+} channels that began to open toward the end of phase 4. Repolarization occurs (**phase 3**) as K^+ channels open, thereby increasing the outwardly directed, hyperpolarizing K^+ currents. At the same time, the L-type Ca^{2+} channels become inactivated and close, which leads to a decrease in Ca^{2+} conductance and the inward depolarizing Ca^{2+} current (Fig. 3.5b).

3.2.3 Atrial Conduction

From the SA node the cardiac impulse spreads radially throughout the myocardium of the right and left atrium and eventually to the AV node along ordinary atrial myocardial fibers with a conduction velocity of about 0.5 m/s. However, conduction is somewhat more rapid in several small bundles of atrial muscle fibers, some of which pass directly from SA to AV node. Their distinct nature has not been definitely established.

3.2.4 Atrioventricular Conduction

The primary role of the AV node is to conduct the AP from the atria to the ventricles. In adult humans, the AV node is approximately 15 mm long, 10 mm wide and 3 mm thick. The conductive system is so organized that the cardiac impulses will do not travel unimpeded from the atria to the ventricles. The principal delay occurs in the AN and N regions (see below) of the AV node and accounts, in the electrocardiogram, for the delay between the P wave (the electrical manifestation of the atrial excitation) and the QRS complex (the electrical manifestation of ventricular excitation). This delay provides time for the atria to empty their contents into the ventricles before ventricular contraction begins. Although teleological explanations are avoided in science, the atrial "boost" just before ventricular contraction utilizes the starling law to provide optimal ventricular stroke volume. The AV node can also act as a backup pacemaker in the case of failure of the sinus node, and can hamper rapid atrial contractions as in atrial fibrillation, from being conducted into the ventricles. On the other hand, the AV node is part of the circuit underlying AV nodal re-entrant tachycardia (AVNRT). A debate still exists between morphologists and physiologists about which structures of the atrioventricular junction should be included in an ideal "true" AVN [24]. In this review, we will endorse the definition that includes all structures contributing to the atrial-His conduction interval. Anatomically, the AV node is located within the triangle of Koch, a region located at the base of the right atrium defined by the following landmarks: the coronary sinus (CS) ostium, the tendon of Todaro (tT), and the septal leaflet of the tricuspid valve (TV). Using the central fibrous body (CFB) as the demarcation between the His bundle and AV node as Tawara suggested, the AV node can be further divided morphologically into the lower nodal bundle (LNB) and the compact node (CN) [25]. In the LNB, the cells are longer and arranged more parallel to one another, whereas in the CN the cells are small and spindle-shaped with no clear orientation. Extending proximally from the LNB towards the coronary sinus (CS) is the inferior nodal extension, also known as the rightward nodal extension in humans [26].

The second nodal extension (or leftward nodal extension), present only in humans, extends from the CN towards the CS, and is usually shorter than the rightward extension. Functionally, the AV node area can be described as having two pathways – the slow pathway and the fast pathway. It has been shown that the anatomical substrate for the slow pathway involves structures embedded within an isthmus of myocardium located along the tricuspid annulus below the coronary sinus [27, 28]. Consequently, evidence exists involving the area of the LNB as the anatomical substrate of the slow pathway [29]. It is, however, still debated whether the slow pathway conduction also includes inferior transitional cells overlaying this nodal extension. The fast pathway is less well-defined from an anatomical and structural standpoint. The probable anatomical substrate of this pathway is the transitional cell layers located around the CN at the interface between the CN and transitional cells, which express Cx43 at levels similar to the interatrial septum [30]. The AP configuration and the expression of ion channels in the AVN are heterogeneous. Three types of AP waveforms have been identified in early studies: atrionodal (AN), nodal (N), and nodo-His (NH). The N-type AP is characterized by slow upstroke velocity and AP amplitude, while AN and NH APs have intermediate properties between nodal and atrial or His APs, respectively.

The location of the leading AVN pacemaker site has also been a matter of debate. Initiation of automaticity has been identified in the N-NH part of the node [25]. But the posterior (or inferior) nodal extension (PNE) of the AVN is also able to generate pacemaking and can effectively pace the atrioventricular junction. It is possible that, in vivo, both the PNE and NH-CS region can generate junctional automaticity. It would be interesting to test if pacemaker shift exists in the AVN. Indeed, it cannot be excluded that the dominant site can shift between the PNE and the NH-CS region depending on the physiological conditions. In clinical terms this explains the great diversity in the form of P waves found in so-called AVN or "junctional" ectopic beats or rhythms.

3.2.5 Ventricular Conduction

The bundle of His passes subendocardially down the right side of the interventricular septum for about 1 cm and then divides into the right and left bundle branches (Fig. 3.6). The right bundle branch is a direct continuation of the bundle of His, and proceeds down the right side of the interventricular septum. The left bundle branch proceeds on the subendocardial surface of the left side of the interventricular septum, and splits into a thin anterior division and a thick posterior division. The bundles of His ultimately subdivide into a network of conducting fibers, called Purkinje fibers, which spread out over the subendocardial surfaces of both ventricles. Purkinje fibers are the broadest cells of the heart [31]. Because of their large diameter, conduction velocity in these fibers exceeds that of any other fiber type within the heart. The conduction velocity varies along the cardiac tissue: the Purkinje fibers are the fastest with values at about 4 m/s, while the AV node are the slowest with velocities at about 0.05 m/s. Intermediate velocities are found in the atria (0.5 m/s) and in the bundle of His and its branches (2 m/s). The systematic differences in conduction velocity permit rapid activation of the entire endocardial surface of the ventricles. The APs of the Purkinje fibers resemble those of the ordinary ventricular myocardial fibers. Because of the long refractory period many premature excitations are blocked by the Purkinje fibers.

The first parts of the ventricles to be excited are the left and the right side of the interventricular septum and the papillary muscles. The early activation and contraction of the septum makes it more rigid and allows it to serve as an anchor for the contraction of the myocardium of the ventricles. Furthermore, early contraction of the papillary muscles prevents eversion of the AV valves into the atria during ventricular systole. Although the endocardial surfaces of both ventricles are excited rapidly, the wave of excitation spreads from the endocardium to the epicardium at a slower velocity. The epicardial surface of the right ventricle is activated earlier than that of the left ventricle because the right ventricular wall is thinner than the left. The apical and central regions of the epicardium of both ventricles are activated somewhat earlier than the respective basal regions. The last portions of the ventricles to be excited are the posterior basal epicardial regions and a small region in the basal portion of the interventricular septum.

3.3 Control of Excitation of the Heart

Due to its automaticity, the heart is able to beat even without the participation of external inputs. Nevertheless, adaptation of cardiac function to the changing needs of the organism is, to a large degree, dependent upon the cardiac nerves (Fig. 3.7), whose function can modify the following aspects of cardiac activity: (1) the frequency at which impulses are initiated in the pacemaker, and thus the heart rate (**chronotropism**); (2) the speed of conduction of excitation, especially in the AV node (**dromotropism**); (3) the force of contraction, i.e. the contractility of the heart (**inotropism**); (4) the excitability, via alterations in the threshold of excitation (**bathmotropism**). The efferent cardiac nerves via which the function of the heart can be influenced are the **parasympathetic** fibers of the **vagus nerve** (cholinergic) and the **sympathetic nerves**.

The average resting heart rate is about 70 beats/min in normal adults, and it is significantly greater in children. During sleep the heart rate decreases by 10–20 beats/min, while during emotional excitement or muscular activity it may accelerate to rates well above 100 beats/min. Both divisions of the autonomic nervous system tonically influence the cardiac pacemaker, normally the SA node. The sympathetic system enhances the heart rate, whereas the parasympathetic system inhibits it. Thus, the heart rate ordinarily increases as a result of the combined decrease in parasympathetic activity and increase in sympathetic activity, whereas it decreases with the opposite changes. Parasympathetic tone usually predominates in healthy, resting individuals.

3.3.1 Effects of the Parasympathetic System

The cardiac parasympathetic fibers originate in the medulla oblongata, in cells that lie in the dorsal motor nucleus of the vagus nerve or in the nucleus ambiguous. Centrifugal preganglionic parasympathetic fibers of the vagus nerve synapse with postganglionic vagal cells. These cells are located either in the epicardial surface or within the walls of the heart (Fig. 3.7). The right vagus nerve predominantly affects the SA node, whereas the left vagus nerve predominantly affects the AV node. This is why the right carotid sinus is preferentially "massaged" to produce SA cardiac slowing.

Acetylcholine (ACh) released quickly, binds to M2 (muscarinic) receptors and, via the $\beta\gamma$ subunit of a G protein, leads to the opening of a special set of potassium channels. The ensuing increase in potassium efflux hyperpolarizes the SA nodal fibers to a level as low as −65 to −75 mV, rather than the usual level of −55 to

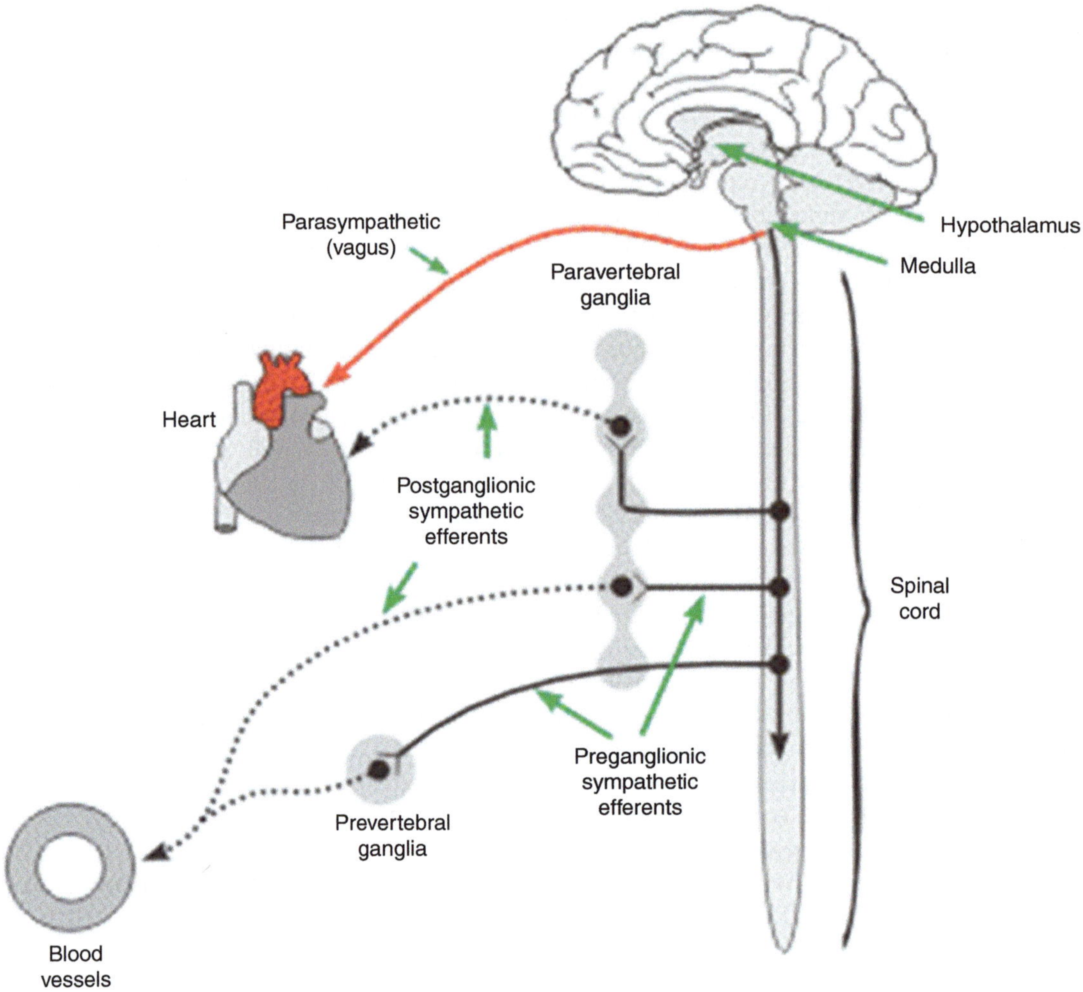

Fig. 3.7 Innervation of the heart by the autonomic nervous system (Illustration reproduced with permission from: www.cvpharmacology.com)

–60 mV. Therefore the upward drift of the resting membrane potential caused by the flow of sodium inside the cell requires much longer to reach the threshold potential for excitation. Obviously, this causes a large reduction in the rate of rhythmicity of these nodal cells and, consequently, of the heart (negative chronotropic effect). If the vagal stimulation is strong enough, the rhythmical self-excitation of this node may even completely stop. In the AV node, the state of hyperpolarization causes a delay in the conduction of the impulse (negative dromotropic effect). A strong stimulation, especially of the left vagus, may produce various degrees of AV block [2, 32].

3.3.2 Effects of the Sympathetic System

The cardiac sympathetic fibers originate in the intermediolateral columns of the upper five or six thoracic and lower one or two cervical segments of the spinal cord. These preganglionic fibers emerge from the spinal column through the white communicating branches and enter the paravertebral chains of ganglia. The postganglionic cardiac sympathetic fibers are distributed to the various chambers as an extensive epicardial plexus. They then penetrate the myocardium, usually accompanying the coronary vessels (Fig. 3.7). Sympathetic stimulation causes the opposite effects to those caused by vagal stimulation, as follows: First, it increases the rate of SA node discharge and hence the heart rate (positive chronotropic effect). Second, it increases the rate of conduction and excitability in all portions of the heart (positive dromotropic effect). Third, it increases the contractility of both the atrial and ventricular myocardia (positive inotropic effect). In short, the sympathetic system increases the overall activity of the heart and hence the cardiac output.

Stimulation of the sympathetic nerves leads to the release of norepinephrine at the sympathetic nerve terminals. The cardiac effects of the released norepinephrine are mediated by β adrenergic receptors (described elsewhere in this book) and the cyclic AMP (cAMP) second messenger system. The cAMP second messenger system is used for intracellular signal transduction, such as transferring into cells the effects of hormones or neurotransmitters like epinephrine and norepinephrine, which cannot pass through the plasma membrane. It is involved in the activation of protein kinases, causing them to phosphorylate ion channels of the cell membrane and thereby increasing their probability of activation [33]. Through this mechanism norepinephrine and epinephrine increase the activity of all ion channels involved in SA node automaticity. However, the slope of the resting potential in the SA and AV node increases because the augmentation of depolarizing channels I_f and I_{Ca} is greater than the increase of the repolarizing channels I_K. These changes result in increases of heart rate (positive chronotropic effect) and the conduction (positive dromotropic effect) of the impulses from the atria to the ventricles [2, 32].

3.3.3 Central Control of Heart Rate-Baroreceptor Reflex

The heart rate is regulated by the pontomedullary **cardiovascular centers** of the brain, which are located bilaterally in the reticular formation of the medulla and the lower part of the pons. Certain important areas of the cardiovascular center have been identified: **The pressure zone** of the centers is located in the anterolateral portions of the upper medulla and lower pons. The fibers of the neurons of this area are distributed throughout the spinal cord where they excite the sympathetic neurons, causing an increase of the heart rate (mainly) and vasoconstriction. The **depressure zone** of the centers is located in the anterolateral portion of the lower part of the medulla. The fibers of these neurons project to the pressure zone and inhibit its activity, thus causing a decrease of the heart rate and vasodilatation. A sensory area is located bilaterally in the **tractus solitarius.** The neurons of this area receive nerve signals mainly from the vagus and the glossopharyngeal nerves.

Stimulation of various brain regions can either excite or inhibit the cardiovascular centers, thereby causing significant effects on cardiac rate and contractility. Stimulation of the motor cortex, for instance, excites the pressure zone because of impulses transmitted downward to the hypothalamus and thence to the cardiovascular centers. Also, stimulation of the anterior temporal lobe, the orbital areas of the frontal cortex, the anterior part of the cingulate gyrus, the amygdala, the septum and the hippocampus can all either excite or inhibit the cardiovascular centers. Sudden changes in arterial blood pressure initiate a reflex that evokes an opposite change in heart rate (Fig. 3.8). Baroreceptors located in the aortic arch and carotid sinuses are responsible for this reflex. Baroreceptors are nerve endings and are extremely abundant in the wall of each internal carotid artery slightly above the carotid bifurcation, an area known as the carotid sinus, and in the wall of the aortic arch. A rise in pressure stretches the baroreceptors and causes them to transmit signals to the central nervous system. After the baroreceptor signals have entered the tractus solitarius of the medulla, secondary signals activate the depressor zone and the center and inhibit the pressor zone. The net effects are (1) decreased heart rate and reduced strength of heart contraction; and (2) vasodilatation throughout the peripheral circulatory system. Thus, excitation of the baroreceptors by pressure

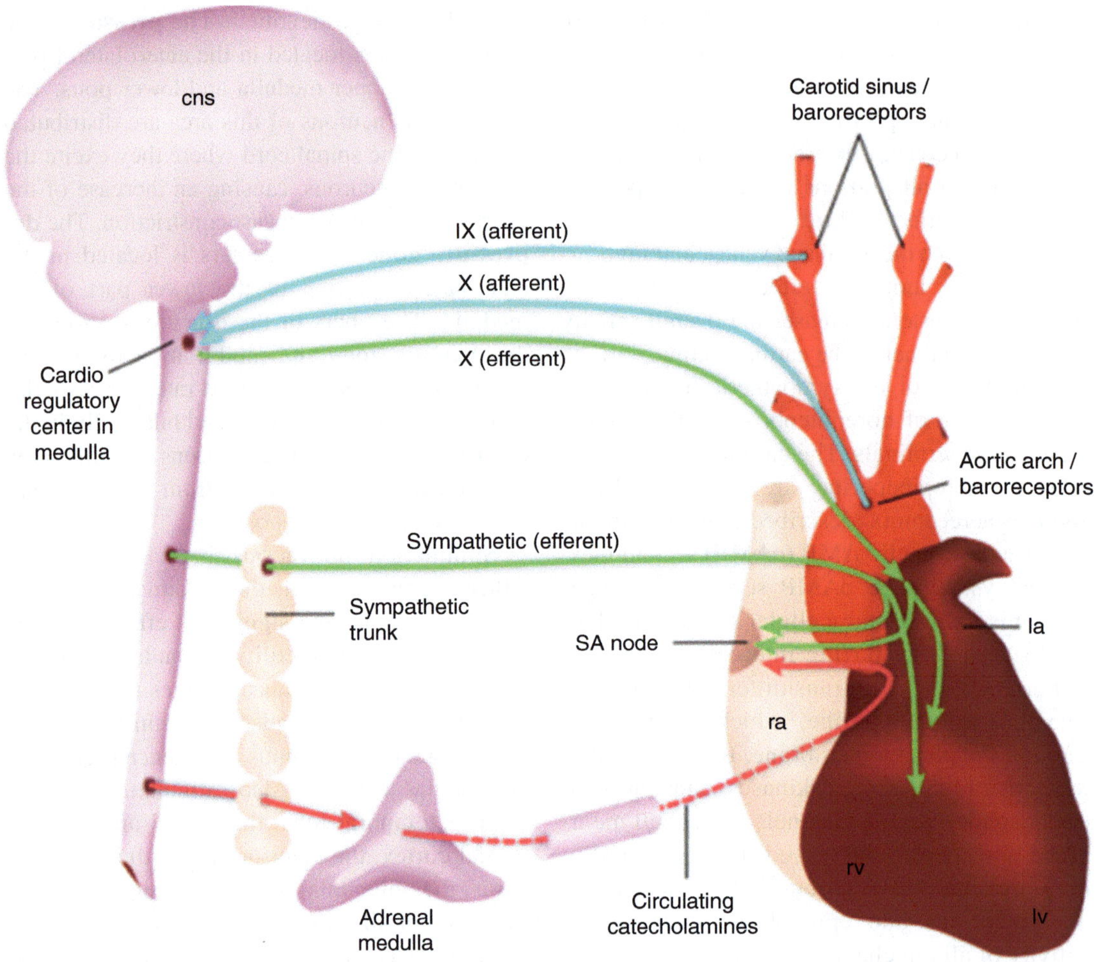

Fig. 3.8 Control of heart rate: baroreceptor reflex. Baroreceptors transmit afferent signals to the cardioregulatory center of medulla through the *IX* and *X* cranial nerves. Efferent signals are transmitted from the parasympathetic nuclei of the medulla through the *X* cranial nerve and from the sympathetic centers of the spinal cord through sympathetic efferent sympathetic fibers and the circulating catecholamines released from the adrenal medulla (Illustration reproduced with permission from BioMed Central, McNeill et al. Neural development 2010: http://www.neuraldevelopment.com/content/5/1/6)

in the arteries reflexly causes the arterial pressure to decrease because of reductions both in cardiac output and peripheral resistance. Conversely, low pressure has the opposite effect, reflexly causing the pressure to rise back toward normal levels. The baroreceptors respond extremely rapidly to changes in arterial pressure, in fact the rate of impulse firing increases during systole and decreases during diastole. Thus baroreceptors function as a buffer system, which does not permit extreme fluctuations of blood pressure during the cardiac cycle [2, 32].

Conclusions

We gave a concise view of cell excitability which governs the cardiac rhythm and the cardiac conduction system, and is involved in many pathological conditions these data provide a translational new integrating basic knowledge to cardiac structure and function.

References

1. Levitan IB, Kaczmarek LK. The neuron. 3rd ed. Oxford: Oxford University Press; 2002. p. 135–7.
2. Berne R, Levy M, Koeppen B, Stanton B. Physiology. Philadelphia: Elsevier/Mosby; 2008. p. 292–308.
3. Deal KK, England SK, Tamkun MM. Molecular physiology of cardiac potassium channels. Physiol Rev. 1996;76:49–67.
4. Nichols CG, Lopatin AN. Inward rectifier potassium channels. Annu Rev Physiol. 1997;59:171–91.
5. Gernot S, Pourrier M, Melnyk P, Nattel S. Differential distribution of cardiac ion channel expression as a basis for regional specialization in electrical function. Circ Res. 2002;90:939–50.
6. Klabunde RE. Conduction of action potentials within the heart. In: Cardiovascular physiology concepts. Baltimore/Philadelphia: Lippincott, Williams and Wilkins; 2011. p. 21–4.
7. Zaza A. Control of the cardiac action potential: the role of repolarization dynamics. J Mol Cell Cardiol. 2010;48:106–11.
8. Boyett MR. And the beat goes on. The cardiac conduction system: the wiring system of the heart. Exp Physiol. 2009;94:1035–49.
9. Silverman EM, Grove D, Upshaw BC. Why does the heart beat? The discovery of the electrical system of the heart. Circulation. 2006;113:2775–81.
10. Mackaay AJ, Op't Hof T, Bleeker WK, Jongsma HJ, Bouman LN. Interaction of adrenaline and acetylcholine on cardiac pacemaker function. Functional inhomogeneity of the rabbit sinus node. J Pharmacol Exp Ther. 1980;214:417–22.
11. Ramanathan C, Jia P, Ghanem R, Ryu K, Rudy Y. Activation and repolarization of the normal human heart under complete physiological conditions. Proc Natl Acad Sci U S A. 2006;103:6309–14.
12. Yamamoto M, Dobrzynski H, Tellez J, Niwa R, Billeter R, Honjo H, Kodama I, Boyett MR. Extended atrial conduction system characterised by the expression of the HCN4 channel and connexin45. Cardiovasc Res. 2006;72:271–81.
13. Fedorov VV, Hucker WJ, Dobrzynski H, Rosenshtraukh LV, Efimov IR. Postganglionic nerve stimulation induces temporal inhibition of excitability in the rabbit sinoatrial node. Am J Physiol Heart Circ Physiol. 2006;291:H612–23.
14. Magnoni M, Nargeot J. Genesis and regulation of the heart automaticity. Physiol Rev. 2008;88: 919–82.
15. Blaschke RJ, Hahurij ND, Kuijper S, Just S, Wisse LJ, Deissler K, et al. Targeted mutation reveals essential functions of the homeodomain transcription factor Shox2 in sinoatrial and pacemaking development. Circulation. 2007;115:1830–8.
16. Hoogaars WM, Engel A, Brons JF, Verkerk AO, de Lange FJ, Wong LY, et al. Tbx3 controls the sinoatrial node gene program and imposes pacemaker function on the atria. Genes Dev. 2007; 21:1098–112.
17. Hiraoka M, Furukawa T. Functional modulation of cardiac ATP-sensitive K^+ channels. News Physiol Sci. 1998;13:131–7.
18. Irisawa H, Brown HF, Giles W. Cardiac pacemaking in the sinoatrial node. Physiol Rev. 1993;73:197–227.
19. James TN. Structure and function of the sinus node, AV node and His bundle of the human heart: part I-structure. Prog Cardiovasc Dis. 2002;45:235–67.
20. Sangunetti MC, Keating MT. Role of delayed rectifier channels in cardiac repolarization and arrhythmias. News Physiol Sci. 1997;12:152–7.
21. Chen PS, Joung B, Shinohara T, Das M, Chen Z, Lin SF. The initiation of the heart beat. Circ J. 2010;74:221–5.
22. Tardiff JC, Ford I, Tendera M, Bourassa MG, Fox K. Efficacy of ivabradine a new selective I_f inhibitor, compared with atenolol in patients with chronic stable angina pectoris. Eur Heart J. 2005;26:2529–36.
23. Ruzyllo W, Tendera M, Ford I, Fox KM. Antianginal efficacy and safety of ivabradine compared with amlodipine in patients with stable effort angina pectoris: a 3 month randomised double-blind, multicentre, noninferiority trial. Drugs. 2007;67:393–405.
24. Efimov IR, Nikolski VP, Rothenberg F, Greener ID, Li J, Dobrzynski H, et al. Structure-function relationship in the AV junction. Anat Rec. 2004;280:952–65.
25. Meijler FL, Janse MJ. Morphology and electrophysiology of the mammalian atrioventricular node. Physiol Rev. 1998;68:608–47.
26. Inoue S, Becker AE. Posterior extensions of the human compact atrioventricular node: a neglected anatomic feature of potential clinical significance. Circulation. 1998;97:188–93.
27. Nikolski VP, Jones SA, Lancaster MK, Boyett MR, Efimov IR. Cx43 and dual-pathway electrophysiology of the atrioventricular node and atrioventricular nodal reentry. Circ Res. 2003;92:469–75.
28. Hucker WJ, Sharma V, Nikolski VP, Efimov IR. Atrioventricular conduction with and without AV nodal delay: two pathways to the bundle of His in the rabbit heart. Am J Physiol Heart Circ Physiol. 2007;293:H1122–30.
29. Medkour D, Becker AE, Khalife K, Billette J. Anatomic and functional characteristics of a slow posterior AV nodal pathway: role in dual-pathway physiology and reentry. Circulation. 1998;98:164–74.
30. Hucker WJ, McCain ML, Laughner JI, Iaizzo PA, Efimov IR. Connexin 43 expression delineates two discrete pathways in the human atrioventricular junction. Anat Rec (Hoboken). 2008;291:204–15.
31. Ryu S, Yamamoto S, Andersen CR, Nakazawa K, Miyake F, James TN. Intramural Purkinje cell network of sheep ventricles as the terminal pathway of conduction system. Anat Rec (Hoboken). 2009;292:12–22.
32. Guyton AC, Hall JE. Textbook of medical physiology. 12th ed. Philadelphia: Saunders Elsevier; 2011. p. 115–20.
33. Gray PC, Scott JD, Caterall WA. Regulation of ion channels by cAMP dependent protein kinase anchoring proteins. Curr Opin Neurobiol. 1998;59:171–91.

Part II

The Main Axes

4 The Renin-Angiotensin-Aldosterone System in Cardiovascular Diseases

Claude Delcayre, Loubina Fazal, Helene Ragot,
Mathilde Prudhomme, Feriel Azibani,
and Jane-Lise Samuel

Abstract

Angiotensin II and aldosterone have both beneficial and deleterious effects that affect the function of cardiovascular system (blood vessels and heart), the kidneys and other organs. The history of the discoveries of Angiotensin II and aldosterone, and of the molecules that inhibit their synthesis or antagonize their receptors, is an excellent example of translational research. Indeed, a series of experiments have been determinant to initiate clinical studies, and conversely, some unexpected secondary effects observed in treated patients have been understood by experimental research. This chapter will describe the functions of the renin-angiotensin-aldosterone system and the progression of ideas which have allowed to introduce some of the most successful drugs used in hypertension and heart failure.

Keywords

Blood pressure • Hypertension • Heart failure • Renin • Angiotensin II • Aldosterone • Angiotensin converting enzyme • Angiotensin converting enzyme inhibitors • Angiotensin receptor blockers • Mineralocorticoid receptor antagonists

C. Delcayre, PhD (✉) • L. Fazal • H. Ragot
M. Prudhomme • F. Azibani • J.-L. Samuel
UMR-S 942 Inserm, University Paris Diderot,
Paris, France
e-mail: claude.delcayre@inserm.fr

D.V. Cokkinos (ed.), *Introduction to Translational Cardiovascular Research*,
DOI 10.1007/978-3-319-08798-6_4,

Abbreviations

ACE	Angiotensin converting enzyme
ALD	Aldosterone
Ang I	Angiotensin
Ang II	Angiotensin II
ARB	Angiotensin receptor blockers
ARNi	Angiotensin Receptor-Neprilysin Inhibitors
CVD	Cardiovascular diseases
CTGF	Connective tissue growth factor
DRI	Direct Renin Inhibitors
EF	Ejection fraction
11β-HSD2	11-β-hydroxysteroid dehydrogenase type II
GR	Glucocorticoid receptor
HF	Heart failure
LV	Left ventricular
MI	Myocardial infarction
MR	Mineralocorticoid receptor
MRA	Mineralocorticoid receptor antagonists
PRA	Plasma renin activity
RAAS	Renin-angiotensin-aldosterone system
REM	Remodeling
SHR	Spontaneously hypertensive rats
VSMC	Vascular smooth muscle cell

4.1 Introduction

The renin-angiotensin-aldosterone system (RAAS) plays a key role in the regulation of blood pressure on the short and long term through renal and nonrenal mechanisms. The main hormones of this system are Angiotensin II (Ang II) and aldosterone (ALD); they have both beneficial and pathological effects that affect the function of blood vessels, heart, kidney, brain, and other organs. The RAAS functions as an endocrine system, but it also serves local paracrine and autocrine functions in organs and tissues.

Cardiovascular diseases (CVD) are an important health problem in the modern world and their incidence will increase with the aging of populations. The cardiovascular system is one of the first targets of hypertension, in which hypertrophy and fibrosis are evidenced in the arterial wall and in the myocardial interstitium. This remodeling (REM) secondary to hypertension is generally attributed to mechanical factors and to the hypertrophic, pro-inflammatory and pro-fibrotic effects of vasoactive hormones, namely Ang II, catecholamines, ALD, and endothelin [1]. Arterial hypertension induces long-term structural changes in several organs that are risk factors for myocardial infarction (MI) and heart failure (HF). Thus, the pharmacological treatment of hypertension, MI, and chronic HF, is mainly based on the combined inhibition of the vasoactive hormones that are chronically activated in these syndromes.

The history of the discoveries of Ang II and ALD, and of the molecules that inhibit their synthesis or antagonize their receptors, is an excellent example of translational research. Indeed, a series of experiments have been determinant to initiate clinical studies, and conversely, some unexpected secondary effects observed in treated patients have been understood by experimental research. This chapter will describe the progression of ideas which have introduced some of the most successful drugs used in hypertension, heart failure, coronary disease and diabetic nephropathy. It must be realized that the RAAS domain is very active as indicated by the number of Pubmed citations (Ang: 106,901; renin: 53,097; ALD: 35,404), and numerous reviews are available, especially related to cardiovascular diseases [2–10].

4.1.1 Overview of the Renin-Angiotensin-Aldosterone System

The effects of the activation of the RAAS include vasoconstriction, sodium and water retention, increased arterial blood pressure and increased myocardial contractility, which in combination increase the circulating volume. Any decrease in perfusion of the kidney triggers production of renin by juxtaglomerular cells. Conversely, an increase in perfusion of the juxtaglomerular apparatus inhibits the release of renin through a negative feedback mechanism. Renin is a protease

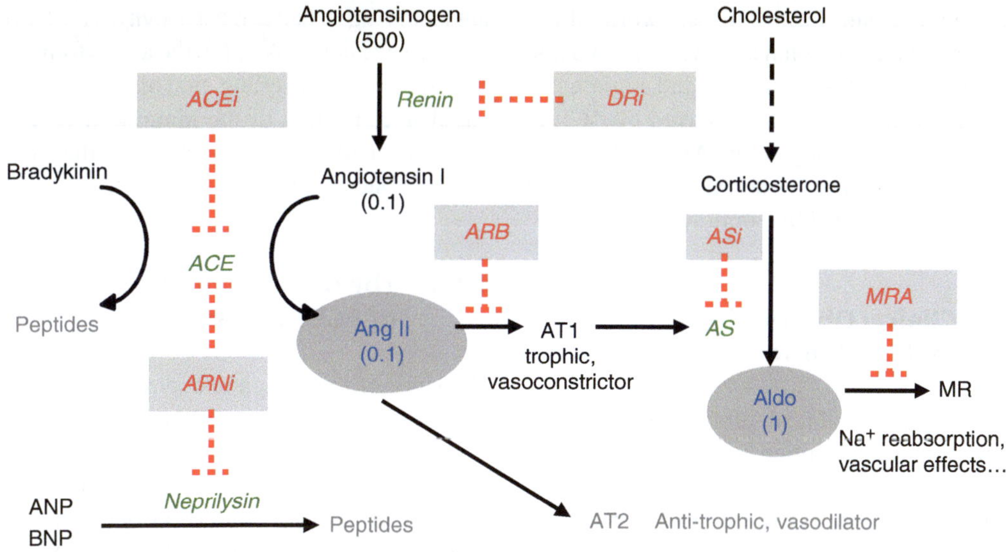

Fig. 4.1 Scheme of the RAAS and its inhibitors. Enzymes are in *green*, inhibitors are in *red*. Abbreviations: *ACE* angiotensin converting enzyme, *ACEi* ACE inhibitors, *Dri* direct renin inhibitors, *ARB* angiotensin receptor blockers, *Aldo* aldosterone, *AS* aldosterone synthase, *ASi* AS inhibitors, *MRA* mineralocorticoid receptor antagonists, *ARNi* angiotensin receptor-neprilysin inhibitors. Values in *brackets* are mean concentrations in nMol/L

of 40 kDa that regulates the initial and rate-limiting step of the RAAS by converting angiotensinogen to angiotensin I. Angiotensin I is a biologically inactive decapeptide, which requires further activation by the angiotensin converting enzyme (ACE), a dipeptidyl carboxypeptidase, to form the biologically active octapeptide Ang II. ACE is a membrane-bound zinc metalloprotease, mainly produced by the lungs. Angiotensin II binds to membrane receptors AT1 and AT2 to induce numerous cellular effects via kinases activation and calcium mobilization. Ang II modulates blood pressure by acutely regulating sodium and water homeostasis, and inducing vasoconstriction; it is one of the strongest known endogenous vasoconstrictors. Chronic stimulation of Ang II induces hyperplasia and hypertrophy of vascular smooth muscle cells, and cardiac hypertrophy and REM. Ang II acts on the adrenal cortex and causes the release of ALD, whose main role is to induce sodium reabsorption in epithelial tissues (namely kidney and colon), which triggers movements of water and electrolytes, and therefore increases plasma volume. Aldosterone binds to the intracellular mineralocorticoid receptor, a transcription factor that triggers transcription of genes mainly related to ionic movements (Fig. 4.1).

4.1.2 Angiotensin II

4.1.2.1 History (Table 4.1)

Early Discoveries

The story of the RAAS begins with the discovery that the injection of an extract of renal cortex from ischemic rabbits induced an increase of blood pressure in control rabbits [11]. However, it was not until 1934 that Goldblatt and other groups confirmed the pressor effects of ischemic kidney extracts, identified as a product of renin and called hypertensin or angiotonin [12]. Then, it was realized that the effect of renin was due to a peptide produced by the proteolytic enzyme renin [13, 14]. In 1952, an increased "hypertensin" activity was evidenced in arterial blood samples of hypertensive humans compared to normotensive subjects [15]. The protein substrate, a globulin mainly produced by the liver [31], was later named angiotensinogen and the peptide named angiotensin [32]. Further works have demonstrated that angiotensin existed in two distinct forms: angiotensin I (Ang I) and angiotensin II (Ang II), where Ang I was cleaved by ACE to generate the biologically active Ang II. The relationship between Ang II and ALD hypothesized by Gross [20] was rapidly confirmed [33].

4.1.3 Clinical Observations in Hypertension

In the 1960s, the clinical problem of essential hypertension was identified but there was no consensus on the interest to treat this disorder. It had previously been shown that ganglionic blockade improved cardiac output in dogs with experimentally induced hypertension [34]. In addition, clinical observations had already demonstrated that nitroglycerin provided immediate relief in patients with dyspnea. In the 1960s, several groups demonstrated increased sympathetically mediated vasoconstriction in HF patients [35]. These discoveries paved the way to the observations that nitroprusside or nitroglycerin given in patients within the first 24 h of acute MI improved congestive symptoms, left ventricular pressure, and cardiac output. Further studies demonstrated similar hemodynamic benefits of afterload reduction in patients with chronic HF using phentolamine or nitroprusside. Thus, the role of afterload reduction in the treatment of HF was firmly established in patients and the stage was set for the next series of clinical studies using RAAS blockade in patients with hypertensive HF [36].

Before 1970, it was well-appreciated that oversecretion of ALD and renin-angiotensin were responsible for end-organ damage in adrenal tumors and in malignant hypertension. In 1972, however, Brunner et al. were the first to report that high renin levels were associated with heart attack, stroke, and LV hypertrophy in patients with essential hypertension [23]. At the same time, striking reductions in blood pressure were observed in patients with renovascular hypertension using the angiotensin peptide analog, saralasin. Saralasin had to be administered intravenously and had a 2-min half-life. It bound to the Ang II receptor and prevented Ang-II binding but, in being structurally similar to Ang II, had agonist activity. The discovery of the conversion of Ang I to the active form Ang II by angiotensin-converting enzyme (ACE), and the full characterization of the kininase II ACE were determinant for the development of the first oral ACE inhibitor, captopril.

4.1.4 The Development of ACE Inhibitors

The story of the design and synthesis of the first inhibitors of ACE is one of the great success stories of modern medicinal chemistry. It has been described as one of the first examples of true 'rational drug design'. Several detailed reviews of this story have been published [37, 38]. In the 1960s, Sergio Ferreira prepared an extract of the venom of the Brazilian viper Bothrops jararaca and established that it potentiated the actions of bradykinin. The extract was tested on ACE and found to be a potent inhibitor thereof. A nonapeptide named teprotide, was isolated from the venom extract and tested intravenously in hypertensive patients by Dr John Laragh, a strong supporter of the ACE concept. The result was positive and this led to a top priority effort at Squibb pharmaceutical company to develop an orally active form of the drug, which company scientists (namely David Cushman and Miguel Ondetti) accomplished. Captopril (trade name Capoten) was approved by the FDA in the early 1980s and it opened a new approach for the treatment of this serious disease. When the adverse effects of Captopril (skin rash and loss of taste) became apparent new derivates were designed, first Enalaprilat and Lisinopril, then many others. Indeed, several major clinical trials using ACE inhibitors were initiated in the late 1970s, first in hypertension then in HF.

Most of the ACE inhibitors on the market today are non-selective towards the two active sites of ACE because their binding to the enzyme is based mostly on the strong interaction between the zinc atom in the enzyme and the chelating group on the inhibitor. Although N- and C-domain have comparable rates in vitro of ACE hydrolyzing, it seems like that in vivo the C-domain is mainly responsible for regulating blood pressure. Ang I is mainly hydrolyzed by the C-domain in vivo but bradykinin is hydrolyzed by both active sites. Apparently, the N-domain does not play a big role in controlling blood pressure but it seems to be the principal metabolizing enzyme for Acetyl-SDKP, a natural haemoregulatory hormone. Thus, C-domain selective inhibition could possibly result in specialized control of blood pressure with less vasodilator-related adverse effects.

4.1.5 The Development of AT1 Antagonists

The dipeptidyl carboxypeptidase ACE cleaves not only Ang I but also bradykinin, which generates enkephalins and substance P. These substrates are involved in bronchoconstriction and inflammation and their accumulation may contribute to cough or asthma-like symptoms or both. In addition, before the development of captopril, there was evidence for alternative pathways to ACE for formation of Ang II through chymase, trypsin, kallikrein, tissue plasminogen activator and cathepsin-G. The potential pathophysiological significance of alternative Ang II-forming pathways in human CVD remained obscure until Urata and Husain reported that a chymotrypsin-like serine protease accounted for 90 % of the Ang II-forming capacity in tissue extracts from human myocardium [39], suggesting that ACE was not the major Ang II-forming enzyme in the human left ventricle. To address the problems of ACE inhibitor-induced cough and alternative pathways for Ang II production, Saralasin was developed in the early 1970s. Saralasin was an octapeptide analogue of Ang II, in which three amino acids were different. Saralasin was not orally bioavailable, had a short duration of action and showed partial agonist activity and therefore it was not clinically suitable as a drug. Research investigators at Takeda company discovered in 1982 the weak nonpeptide Ang II antagonists S-8307 and S-8308 which had moderate potency and short duration of action, however they were selective AT1 receptor antagonists without partial agonist activity. Then, the pharmaceutical company DuPont modified the Takeda molecule and produced the first AT1 receptor antagonist, losartan (DuP-753) in 1989 [40]. A series of AT1 antagonists, called angiotensin receptor blockers (ARB), have been rapidly synthesized by several companies. The modifications on the molecule aimed to increase the bioavailability, elimination half-life, affinity for the AT1 receptor and activity, namely on blood pressure reduction. Telmisartan is the only ARB that can cross the blood–brain barrier and can therefore inhibit centrally mediated effects of Ang II, contributing to even better blood pressure control (Table 4.1).

Table 4.1 Chronology of discoveries and clinical observations in the RAAS

Authors/year	Discovery
Tigerstedt and Bergman 1898 [11]	Renal extracts contain a pressor substance
Goldblatt et al. 1934 [12]	Renal artery constriction produces hypertension in dogs
Braun-Menendez et al. 1940 [13]; Page and Helmer 1940 [14]	Renin is a peptidase producing angiotonin/hypertensin
Kahn et al. 1952 [15]	Increased "hypertensin" activity in blood of hypertensive humans
Simpson et al. 1953 [16]	Discovery of aldosterone
Skeggs et al. 1954 [17]	Identification of Ang I and Ang II
Skeggs et al. 1956 [18]	Identification of ACE
Liddle 1957 [19]	SC-5233 increased urinary excretion of Na in a patient with HF
Gross 1958 [20]	Ang II releases aldosterone
Kagawa et al. 1959 [21]	Isolation of spironolactone at Searle laboratories
Pals et al. 1971 [22]	Saralasin, the 1st Ang II peptide antagonist
Brunner et al. 1972 [23]	High renin levels associated with heart attack and stroke
Cushman et al. 1977 [24]	Synthesis of the 1st ACE inhibitor, captopril
Carini and Duncia 1988 [25]	Synthesis of 1st orally active nonpeptide ARB, losartan
Brilla et al. 1993 [26]	Cardiac fibrosis by aldosterone-salt, prevented by spironolactone
Pitt et al. 1997 [27]	ELITE I study, captopril: decreased mortality in HF
Pitt et al. 1999 [28]	RALES study, spironolactone decreases mortality in HF
Pitt et al. 2000 [29]	ELITE II study, losartan=captopril to decrease mortality in HF
Pitt et al. 2003 [30]	EPHESUS study, eplerenone decreases mortality in post-MI

4.2 Cellular Mechanisms

The ACE cleaves Ang I to give the octapeptide Ang II. In addition, several peptidases (chymase, chymotrypsin, ACE2 (a homolog of ACE) and aminopeptidase A) generate a number of bioactive peptides from angiotensin I and/or Ang II, such as Ang III, angiotensin IV and angiotensin (1–7). In the heart the majority of Ang I is converted by chymase [41]. The carboxypeptidase ACE2 cleaves one amino acid from either Ang I or Ang II, decreasing Ang II levels and increasing the metabolite Ang 1–7, which has vasodilator properties. Thus the balance between ACE and ACE2 is an important factor controlling Ang II levels. The main pathway of Ang II synthesis occurs in plasma, but so-called local RAASs have also been evidenced in the kidneys, heart, brain, adrenal glands, and possibly other tissues [42, 43]. The local RAASs operate in a paracrine or autocrine manner and it is generally considered that they work with the classical circulating RAAS in a complementary manner.

The receptor subtypes AT1 and AT2 are polypeptides containing seven trans-membrane domains [44]. Despite their similar affinities for Ang II, AT1 and AT2 receptors are functionally distinct, with a sequence homology of only 30 %. Composed of 359 amino acids, the AT1 receptor (40 kDa) belongs to the superfamily of G protein-coupled receptors. AT1 receptors bind Ang II with an affinity similar to its circulating concentration (0.1 nM) and they are regulated by their rates of biosynthesis and recycling (up- and down-regulation). Most known physiological effects of Ang II are mediated by AT1 receptors, which are widely distributed in all organs, including liver, adrenals, brain, lung, kidney, heart, and vasculature. AT2 receptors exert anti-proliferative and pro-apoptotic changes in vascular smooth muscle cells, mainly by antagonizing AT1 receptors via activation of tyrosine or serine/threonine phosphatases. AT2 receptor expression declines after birth, suggesting that it may play an important role in fetal development, and it is induced again in adult heart under pathological conditions.

4.2.1 Cardiovascular Effects of Ang II

Ang II, within seconds to minutes of binding to AT1 receptors, activates signaling pathways leading to vascular smooth muscle cell contraction, maintaining vascular tone. In addition to stimulating the synthesis and release of ALD and increasing renal Na^+ absorption, Ang II's actions on the central nervous system are critical in maintaining sympathetic outflow to the vasculature and in autoregulating cerebral blood flow. Ang II is extremely important in modulating minute to minute changes that occur in spatial adaptation. For example, when we stand up from a supine position, Ang II increases myocardial inotropy and chronotropy via an increase of inward Ca^{2+} current through L-type channels.

The binding of Ang II to AT1 receptor leads to the dissociation of subunits of a guanine-nucleotide-binding protein (Gq/11), which activates phospholipase C to generate diacylglycerol, and inositol trisphosphate which releases calcium from intracellular stores. Ang II also increases the entry of calcium into cells. Calcium and diacylglycerol activate various enzymes, such as protein kinase C and calcium-calmodulin kinases that catalyze the phosphorylation of proteins, and this ultimately regulates the cell functions affected by Ang II. These signal-transduction events are completed within seconds or minutes. However, they also initiate slower responses to Ang II including vascular growth and ventricular hypertrophy. The stimulation of growth by Ang II also involves other processes common to growth factors in general, such as the phosphorylation of tyrosine, and the activation of mitogen-activated protein kinase and Stat 91, proteins that affect the cell nucleus and activate DNA transcription. In vivo experiments in rats reported that AT1 receptor antagonists prevent Ang II-induced cardiac hypertrophy. The cellular responses depend on receptor biosynthesis, insertion into the membrane, internalization and degradation. The internalization of receptors is initiated by binding to hormone and is one mechanism by which target cells can become desensitized during prolonged exposure to agonists. RAAS blockade causes an increase in renin levels as a result of interference with a negative feedback loop between Ang II and renin release. This effect explains, at least in part, why Ang II and ALD breakthroughs occur. In addition to renin, the levels of its precursor, prorenin, might also increase during breakthroughs. Since the discovery of the prorenin receptor [45], which induces profibrotic effects in vitro in response to renin or prorenin binding, it has been proposed that increases in renin and prorenin levels will not only result in diminished RAAS suppression, but also in unwanted effects via the prorenin receptor stimulation.

4.2.2 Pathophysiological Role of Ang II in Cardiovascular Disorders

Experimental studies have demonstrated that abnormal elevation of Ang II and ALD levels in plasma induce structural and functional alterations in the heart, kidneys, and vessels with effects such as vascular inflammation and REM, cardiac fibrosis, nephrosclerosis, and disturbed fibrinolysis. This large spectrum of actions explains that dysregulation of the RAAS is a major factor in the development of cardiovascular pathologies including hypertension, MI, congestive HF and stroke, as well as renal disorders especially diabetic nephropathy. In atherosclerotic plaques, the local RAAS system is activated, with high levels of ACE, Ang II, and AT1 receptor. Ang II's cytokine-like effects usually occur with longer exposure, and promote cell growth and migration, extracellular matrix deposition, and vascular and electrical remodeling. It is important to underscore that the dramatic increase of salt (and fat) in the modern food will amplify the effects of the RAAS in cardiovascular pathologies. In other words, the primitive function of the RAAS is less and less adapted to the conditions of high salt intake, and this is a problem of increasing importance [46].

4.2.2.1 Experimental Models

The experimental models of hypertension or HF are detailed in another chapter of this book. To summarize, hypertension is experimentally obtained in rodents by either strain selection (spontaneously hypertensive rats, SHR), lower aorta or renal artery ligation, or genetic intervention (REN-2 rats, Ren-TgKC mice, etc.). Severe experimental hypertension evolves generally towards with time (this is also the case in humans, but their hypertensin is cured). Heart failure is produced in rats or mice by MI, aortic stenosis, aortic insufficiency, infusion of angiotensin, ALD-salt, isoproterenol or other hormones or drugs, generally infused by osmotic minipumps, and by numerous genetic models of gene overexpression or invalidation. Each of the RAAS genes has been eliminated by gene targeting in embryonic stem cells and blood pressure phenotypes have been established for each, see review in [47]. For example, the complete absence of angiotensinogen, ACE or AT-1a receptor cause a significant decrease in blood pressure. Specific knockout of the tissue-bound ACE that does not alter circulating ACE also causes a decrease in blood pressure, thus supporting the hypothesis that tissue-bound ACE is critical in the physiologic generation of Ang II. These studies are also in agreement with those showing a lack of correlation between the hypertensive effect of ACE inhibitors and circulating levels of ACE. The decrease in arterial pressure in the AT-1a (an AT1 receptor subtype only present in rodents) knockout is similar to the blood pressure observed in angiotensinogen and ACE knockout mice, in agreement with previous observations that most of the effects of Ang II on blood pressure are mediated by AT-1a receptors. Many transgenic models have used the insertion of human renin (hRen) and/or angiotensinogen (hAGT) genes in the mouse or rat genome in order to develop models emulating human hypertension. For example, overexpression of the renin gene in liver induces hypertension and renal alterations, with a relation between the severity of the symptoms and the number of gene copies inserted [48].

4.2.2.2 Ang II, Inflammation and Remodeling

In rats, Ang II infusion for 2-weeks leads to hypertension and vascular smooth muscle cell (VSMC) hypertrophy [49]. Shear stress from elevated blood pressure has been shown to upregulate Ang II receptors [50], linking hypertension to vascular REM. Independently from the mechanical effect of hypertension that stimulates cell growth, several in vitro and in vivo experiments have shown that Ang II is an important growth factor, causing cell proliferation, VSMC hypertrophy, cell differentiation, and apoptosis [51]. The main targets of Ang II are VSMC [52]. However, it has multiple effects on endothelial cells, such as producing reactive oxygen species, activating apoptotic signaling pathways, and promoting thrombosis. The increase in oxidative stress caused by Ang II leads to impaired endothelial relaxation and endothelial dysfunction. Ang II has been shown to stimulate the production of TNF-α, an important contributor to vascular inflammation in adult mammalian heart. Ang II also stimulates the production of matrix metalloproteinases, which are necessary for vascular REM. Ang II-induced EGFR- and MAPK-dependent pathways participate in the matrix formation and regulation. Ang II-mediated EGFR transactivation regulates fibronectin and TGF-β synthesis. Additionally, production of matrix metalloproteinases like MMP-2 and breakdown of collagen IV is also modulated by Ang II. Cardiac repair occurs in the infarcted myocardium and structural REM is developed in noninfarcted myocardium, which are accompanied by activated cardiac RAAS. The spatial and temporal sequence of cardiac expression of key-components of RAAS has been nicely described using autoradiography in sections of rat infarcted myocardium [53]. In these experiments, ACE and AT1 receptor expressions are enhanced in the infarcted myocardium within a few days post-MI and cells expressing ACE and AngII receptors are primarily macrophages in the early stage of repair. These observations suggest that locally produced AngII may regulate the function of macrophages in an autocrine manner.

4.2.3 Clinical Studies

Besides the successful classes of ACE inhibitors and AT1 blockers, other RAAS inhibitors have been developed, namely direct renin inhibitor (DRI), ALD antagonists or better termed mineralocorticoid receptor antagonists (MRA), and ALD synthesis inhibitors. All these classes of drugs have proven good efficiency in animal models of hypertension, HF and MI. But the endpoint being treatment of human diseases, it is necessary to verify that the promising results are confirmed in the "real life" of clinical practice. This is necessary for at least two reasons: first, patients with chronic, and often severe, CVD have treatments involving several drugs, and possible deleterious interactions between all these drugs (which are never tested in the laboratory for reasons of time and money) may only be evidenced in clinical studies enrolling hundreds to thousands of patients; secondly, approval for sale may be obtained only if the new drug brings a significant benefit over the standard of care. In this highly competitive field, several drugs have been eliminated on one of these criteria after large clinical studies.

It would be tedious here to analyze in detail the results of all clinical studies involving ACE inhibitors and ARBs. Numerous extensive and comprehensive reviews on this important topic have be published [5, 6, 8, 9].

4.2.3.1 Hypertension and Heart Failure

To summarize, ACE inhibitors have an established role as the first-line treatment for a number of cardiovascular and renal diseases. Their role in the management of hypertension is proven, and they have been shown to reduce mortality associated with both HF with reduced ejection fraction and left-ventricular dysfunction after MI. Furthermore, ACE inhibitors have been shown to reduce the rate of stroke, MI, and death in high-risk individuals without known HF. ACE inhibitors are indicated by the European Society of Cardiology in potentially all patients with symptomatic (NYHA functional class II– IV) systolic HF, with a Class of recommandation I and a Level of evidence A (together with beta blockers and mineralocorticoid receptor antagonists) [54]. In fact, there is consensus that a beta-blocker and an ACE inhibitor should both be started as soon as possible after diagnosis of HF with reduced left ventricular (LV) ejection fraction (EF). This is in part because ACE inhibitors have a modest effect on LV whereas beta-blockers often lead to a substantial improvement in EF. Furthermore, beta-blockers are anti-ischaemic and probably more effective in reducing the risk of sudden cardiac death, and lead to a striking and early reduction in overall mortality.

Angiotensin receptor blockers (ARBs) have been compared with other classes of drugs and namely ACE inhibitors in large clinical trials. The results show that ARBs remain an appropriate alternative in patients who are intolerant to ACEI. However, according to the Guidelines of the European Society of Cardiology, ARBs are no longer the first choice recommendation in patients with HF and an ejection ≤40 % who remain symptomatic despite optimal treatment with an ACE inhibitor and beta-blocker. This is because in the EMPHASIS-HF trial (discussed in the Aldosterone paragraph), eplerenone led to a larger reduction in morbidity-mortality than seen in the ARB 'add-on' trials, and because in both the RALES and EMPHASIS-HF studies, MR antagonists treatment reduced all-cause mortality, whereas ARB 'add-on' treatment did not [54]. Useful meta-analyses are often published, which help to keep a clear mind on the subtle conclusions of the large clinical trials. For example, a recent pooled analysis of 20 cardiovascular morbidity–mortality trials in hypertension, involving a total of around 160,000 patients, showed that use of ACE inhibitors was associated with a significant 10 % reduction in all-cause mortality, whereas no mortality reduction could be demonstrated with ARB treatment [55].

4.2.3.2 Combination Therapy of ACEI and ARB

The rationale of giving ACE inhibitors in combination with ARB is based on the evidence that standard doses of ACE inhibitors only offer a partial blockade of ACE. One proposed explanation was that Ang II may be generated from angiotensinogen and other peptide substrates, in a mode independent of ACE, by enzymes such as chymase or cathepsin G. Moreover, one would expect more specific Ang II blockade at AT1 receptors and theoretically unopposed AT2 receptor agonism. However, the results of several trials (CHARM-Added, VALIANT, ONTARGET) were somewhat conflicting and failed to find benefit for a combination treatment over a single drug use.

4.2.3.3 Other Pathologies

The pharmacological treatment of HF with preserved LV ejection fraction remains challenging, and effective treatment is urgently needed for this disease, which may be as common and lethal as HF with reduced LV ejection fraction. Activation of RAAS and other neurohormonal pathways occurs in HF with preserved LV ejection fraction; however, several studies of ACE inhibitors and ARBs in this disease have failed to show convincing benefit. On the other hand, several clinical trials have shown that the frequency of new onset of type 2 diabetes can be reduced by ACE inhibitors and ARBs (as opposed to beta-blockers and diuretics), thus supporting a role of RAAS in diabetes mellitus. However, the level of renin activity or Ang II in plasma of diabetic patients is generally normal and the mechanistic links remain to be determined.

4.2.3.4 Direct Renin Inhibitors (DRI)

Development of DRIs dates back to the 1980s, but the early DRIs had poor bioavailability (<2 %), a short half-life, lack of specificity, and low potency. Aliskiren is the first of a new class of nonpeptide-orally active DRIs, and further DRIs are in development. Aliskiren has limited bioavailability (2.7 %), but its half-life is 45 h, and it is therefore suitable as a once-daily medication. Aliskiren blocks the active site of renin and therefore can block the action of both renin and prorenin. It has the potential to block both circulating and tissue RAAS and has been shown to reduce renin activity. In a study of spontaneously hypertensive rats, aliskiren blocked RAAS more effectively than ACE inhibitors or ARBs.

Aliskiren is effective at reducing blood pressure and is approved for the treatment of hypertension. The role of DRIs in HF has not yet been well defined, with early trials suggesting that they may have a role in HF but subsequent studies failing to show a significant impact on mortality and hospital admissions, raising clear concerns about safety. We await the outcome of the ATMOSPHERE trial, designed to test the effect of aliskiren in systolic HF, for further clarification [5].

4.2.3.5 Angiotensin Receptor-Neprilysin Inhibitors (ARNi)

Neprilysin, like ACE, is a zinc metalloproteinase enzyme that is expressed, in the kidney, lung, endothelial cells, vascular smooth muscle cells, cardiac myocytes, fibroblasts, and neutrophils, with the highest concentrations being present in the renal proximal tubule. Neprilysin degrades biologically active natriuretic peptides, including atrial natriuretic peptide, BNP, cardiac natriuretic peptide, angiotensin I, bradykinin, and endothelin-1. By augmenting the active natriuretic peptides, neprilysin inhibition increases generation of myocardial cyclic guanosine 3′,5′-monophosphate, which improves myocardial relaxation and reduces hypertrophy. However, neprilysin also contributes to the breakdown of angiotensin, which is the rationale for dual-acting compounds that both inhibit this enzyme and block the action of angiotensin. Hence, drugs that inhibit both neprilysin and ACE were developed and were referred to as vasopeptidase inhibitors. These drugs decrease peripheral vascular resistance and improve both local blood flow and the sodium/water balance. However, in the OCTAVE trial, the frequency of angioedema was three to four times higher with the first vasopeptidase inhibitor to be developed, omapatrilat, than with enalapril. Novel approaches have been explored to avoid angioedema. One proposed concept was to combine neprilysin inhibition with ARBs, i.e., a dual-acting ARB-neprilysin inhibitor (ARNI), which would not directly affect ACE or aminopeptidase and may therefore be a safer approach to inhibiting the RAAS and increasing natriuretic peptide levels. LCZ696 is a first-in-class angiotensin receptor-neprilysin inhibitor that comprises the molecular moieties of the ARB valsartan and AHU377 (the prodrug of the neprilysin inhibitor) in a 1:1 molar ratio. AHU377 is metabolized by enzymatic cleavage to LBQ657, the active inhibitor of neprilysin. Preliminary data in hypertension and in HF are promising [5].

4.3 Aldosterone

The classic role of ALD is to adjust the hydro-mineral balance in the body, and thus to participate to the regulation of blood pressure. ALD has several modes of action. The best known involves activation of the cytoplasmic mineralocorticoid receptor (MR) by binding of ALD; the MR-aldosterone complex enters the nucleus and binds to a specific DNA sequence which initiates transcription of target genes (as subunits of the amiloride-sensitive sodium channel, Na^+K^+ -ATPase and others) which activates sodium reabsorption in the kidney and epithelial tissues. The MRAs prevent the binding of ALD to its receptor and thus prevent its action. As discussed below, these antagonists have been first marketed as diuretics, which is probably too restrictive in regard to their recently recognized efficacy in CVD. Like other steroid hormones, ALD may also cause ionic effects (activation of sodium currents) in a few minutes at the membrane level, without activation of the MR. A third mode of action has been evidenced more recently by which ALD can quickly activate kinases, through binding to the MR but without gene transcription [56]. The physiological role of this latter intermediate mode is still poorly defined.

4.3.1 History of Aldosterone Discovery (Table 4.1)

Aldosterone, the last A of RAAS, was isolated 60 years ago. A substance secreted by the cortex of adrenal glands and having the ability to retain salt has been evidenced in the 30s by the teams of Kendall and Reichstein (for a more detailed review on the discovery of aldosterone, see [57]). From the crystallization of glucocorticoids and mineralocorticoids, researchers have discovered that a fraction extracted from adrenals was not crystallized. This so-called "amorphous" fraction had an important mineralocorticoid activity, albeit different from that of deoxycorticosterone or other steroids. A potentially confounding issue was the fact that cortisol possessed effects both on carbohydrate metabolism and electrolyte secretion, leading to a widely held opinion that cortisol was the physiologically important mineralocorticoid hormone. Nevertheless, some researchers were convinced of the existence of a mineralocorticoid different from deoxycorticosterone. The isolation of electrocortin (subsequently termed aldosterone) relied on two important technical developments: the use of partition chromatography and the development of a specific radiolabeled bioassay (Na24/K42). Sylvia and James Tait, working in London, purified a very small quantity of ALD, carried out pilot studies and identified some chemical groupings. In 1952, they began a collaboration with Pr Tadeus Reichstein in Basel. The initial isolation of adequate quantities of ALD was carried out at Ciba AG, Basel, where material from 1,500 kg of pig adrenals yield 60 mg of amorphous pure ALD, which Reichstein crystallized in August 1953. The hormone was then better characterized under the name of ALD [57]. That this hormone was secreted by the adrenal gland was then evidenced by Tait's team, showing that the hormones extracted from beef or dog adrenal perfusate were identical.

4.3.2 Development of MR Antagonists

The development of spironolactone by the Searle laboratories in the 1950s was intended to provide a diuretic drug with a complementary mode of action to that of the diuretics currently used. When coadministered with a thiazide, it would cause an additional Na^+/water loss, but also reverse the hypokalemic effects of chronic thiazide therapy. Frank Sturtevant was working on experimental mineralocorticoid and renal hypertension while in the nearby labs Charlie Kagawa was examining the effects of a spirolactones series in blocking the activities of the sodium-retaining actions of DOCA and ALD. At lunchtime, they discussed their exploratory findings with the spirolactones and suggested that the compound SC-5233 be taken into clinical trials. Thus the first ALD antagonist was discovered serendipitously using compounds synthesized for very different reasons. In 1957, Grant Liddle at Vanderbilt University showed that SC-5233 increased the urinary excretion of sodium in a patient with congestive HF, as well as the sodium-retaining actions of DOCA in patients with Addison's disease [19]. Then, Liddle's group published the clinical effects of five analogs of SC-5233 in edematous patients. They concluded that a number of steroid 17-spirolactones have proved to be effective diuretic agents in man by antagonizing the renal tubular actions of ALD. One of the spirolactone analogs was SC-9420, which was subsequently named spironolactone. Spironolactone was marketed as a novel diuretic with additional antihypertensive effects [21]. While spironolactone has useful clinical effects, it has significant tolerability problems due to painful gynecomastia and menstrual disturbances in premenopausal women. These side effects are attributed to its androgenic and progesteronergic properties. The introduction of epoxy groups into the spironolactone molecule resulted in more potent and highly selective MR antagonists, of which epoxymexrenone (CGP30083) proved to be the optimal compound. This compound, now called eplerenone, was patented in 1984 and later taken into clinical trials [58].

4.3.3 Cellular Mechanisms

4.3.3.1 Biosynthesis of Aldosterone

Aldosterone is a steroid hormone synthesized from cholesterol in the zona glomerulosa of adrenal cortex. The first rate-limiting step involves a transport of cholesterol into mitochondria controlled by the steroidogenic acute regulatory protein (StAR). The last steps of its biosynthesis involve the mitochondrial P-450 aldosterone-synthase which catalyses the

11beta-hydroxylation of deoxycorticosterone to form corticosterone, then a 18-hydroxylation and 18-methyloxidation to yield ALD. This enzyme is encoded by the CYP11B2 gene and its activity is stimulated mainly by Ang II and potassium, and more weakly by ACTH and sodium. Inhibitors of aldosterone-synthase have been developed but, despite promising results in experimental HF [59], side-effects compromise their use in humans. Extra-adrenal sites of production of ALD have been also described, such as the brain, vessels and heart. The level of ALD synthesis in these organs is generally low in resting conditions, suggesting that the secreted hormone could have local autocrine or paracrine actions, if any. The relevance of ALD synthesis in heart is a matter of debate, but several observations have been made in pathological conditions where the well described stimulation of the intracardiac renin-angiotensin system could lead to an increased level of ALD within the cardiac tissue, with likely deleterious consequences. This has been observed in post-MI in rat, where the increased AngII and ALD cardiac production played a key role in the development of cardiac fibrosis [60]. Similarly, ALD production is activated in proportion to severity in failing ventricle in humans [61], and myocardial ALD and aldosterone synthase mRNA levels are elevated by 4- to 6-fold in humans with hypertrophic cardiomyopathy, and provoke expression of hypertrophic markers in rat cardiac myocytes and expression of collagens and transforming growth factor-beta1 in rat cardiac fibroblasts [62].

The Mineralocorticoid Receptor (MR)

The MR and glucocorticoid receptor (GR) belong to the nuclear hormone receptors superfamily, and they have a high sequence homology. Sequence evolution studies suggest that MR is the first receptor to have diverged within this subfamily [63]. Interestingly, primitive fishes living in salt water express the MR but not ALD, suggesting that this « orphan » MR is activated by glucocorticoids. Glucocorticoids (cortisol in humans and corticosterone in rats and mice) bind to GR and MR with a strong affinity. ALD binds to MR with strong affinity, while its affinity for GR is much lower. Since plasma ALD levels are three orders of magnitude lower than those of GR, the latter should occupy most of the MRs. However, this theoretical excess is around ten-fold decreased by the 97 % binding of GR to plasma transcortin, while the binding of ALD to albumin is lower (30 % of plasma ALD is free). In addition, transfection studies have shown that cortisol has a transactivation activity of MR ten-fold lower than that of ALD despite identical binding affinities, and the cortisol-MR complex is less stable than the ALD-MR complex due to differences in the conformation changes of MR induced by hormone binding. A first conclusion is that ALD seems disadvantaged compared to cortisol to bind to MR, but probably not as much as the ratio of plasma concentrations suggests. But in these conditions, how can ALD have a specific action?

The answer depends on the cell type. In epithelial cells and in endothelial and smooth muscle cells, which express the MR, the binding of ALD to the MR is made possible by the presence of the 11-β-hydroxysteroid dehydrogenase type II (11β-HSD2), which metabolizes cortisol and corticosterone in inactive metabolites [64]. In contrast, in cells such as cardiomyocytes which express the MR but not the 11-HSD2, the MR is probably mostly occupied by GR. But, as outlined above, there are possible other mechanisms that allow the binding of ALD on the MR, even in the absence of 11β-HSD2. The studies on isolated cardiomyocytes evidence effects of ALD on calcium or potassium currents, but these effects are observed using high concentrations of ALD in a milieu containing no GR. Transgenic mice overexpressing the MR in cardiomyocytes [65] or in other cell types are a powerful and elegant means to explore these mechanisms, this is discussed below. To conclude, a distinction must be made between inhibition of MR and antagonism of the effects of ALD. Indeed, the high concentration of GR in plasma, their close structural similarity to ALD, and of their receptors, the hormone-receptor affinities measured in vitro that conclude to the possible binding of GR on the MR (and vice-versa), complicate the understanding of the mode of action of aldosterone in the cardiovascular system.

4.3.3.2 Pathophysiological Role of Aldosterone in Cardiovascular Disorders

An increase of ALD concentration in plasma occurs in several clinical situations, as primary aldosteronism, acute MI, and HF. A major consequence of primary aldosteronism is sustained hypertension that can be explained by both sodium retention and vascular effects. Recent studies evidence that the incidence of primary aldosteronism in hypertensive patients has been largely underestimated in the past, and should be between 11 and 15 %. As to regards the major CVD, experimental studies have demonstrated that elevation of aldosterone induces structural and functional changes in the heart, kidneys and blood vessels that include fibrosis, inflammation, vascular remodeling, and impairment of fibrinolysis.

Aldosterone Induces Cardiac Fibrosis (…?)

Studies on cardiac fibrosis induced by ALD give an excellent example of translational, or "bench to bedside" research. The first observations of a deleterious effect of a mineralocorticoid on the heart were made by Bois and Selye who described periarteritis nodosa of the cardiac arteries and hyalinized nodules in myocardium of rats treated by deoxycorticosterone acetate for 20 days [66]. Twenty four years ago, a relationship has been established between the plasma level of ALD and mortality in patients with HF [67], or with left ventricle mass [68] which is a highly predictive index of morbidity and mortality. This was one of the first indications that ALD may have effects on myocardial function in clinical HF. In the same line, plasma cortisol and ALD levels have more recently been identified as complementary and incremental predictors of mortality [69]. In the early 1990s, the group of Karl Weber demonstrated in rats that high levels of infused ALD induced a severe cardiac fibrosis, and that spironolactone prevented this fibrosis [26]. Importantly, this fibrosis was independent of the ALD-induced hypertension, i.e. it was not induced by mechanical stretch of the cardiac tissue. These pioneering works were confirmed and extended by other laboratories [70, 71]. In all these early studies, salt (1 %) was added to the drinking water to amplify the cardiac damage. This is an important point discussed below in this paragraph. The high level of MR expression in heart and blood vessels provided an explanation for the observed effects of ALD in these tissues. Although far from clinical situations, the above-described experimental models have allowed to describe the determinants and the biochemical steps of cardiac fibrosis. It is important to underline that these effects were due to concentrations of ALD that were strongly and chronically elevated, and inadequate for the body salt requirements. These experiments have also shown that spironolactone prevented the aldosterone-induced cardiac fibrosis, which brought one argument for launching clinical studies using MRAs. The plasma levels of Ang II and of ALD are increased in HF, and decrease upon ACE inhibitor treatment. Unfortunately, the level of ALD increases again after several months in the plasma of patients with HF treated with ACE inhibitors [72]. The mechanisms of this escape (or breakthrough) of ALD under ACE inhibition are not clearly established. Nevertheless, the ALD escape was a second strong argument to selectively inhibit the actions of ALD in HF.

The pathways of ALD action leading to inflammation and cardiovascular fibrosis are partially established [2, 4, 52, 73, 74]. Induction of a perivascular inflammatory phenotype has been demonstrated in the heart of uninephrectomised rats treated with ALD-salt [75]. Increases in inflammation markers such as Cox-2 and MCP-1, and upregulation of plasminogen activator inhibitor-1 (PAI-1), have been seen from the first week on, making the proliferation of inflammatory cells around the coronary arteries among the first events leading to fibrosis. A causal role for oxidative stress is suggested by the observations that ALD stimulates expression of NADPH oxidase in macrophages, induces cardiac CaMKII oxidation and activation through ROS generated by NADPH oxidase in cultured cardiomyocytes [4] and that spironolactone and antioxidants prevent these changes independently in the coronary and peripheral arteries. Activated fibroblasts and myofibroblasts that produce and release TGF-ß 1 play an essential role in sustaining collagen synthesis [10]. Interestingly, an interaction between ALD and AngII was found in the release of free radicals that can damage arterial smooth muscle cells [52]. This interaction between ALD and Ang II is a major point further discussed below, and it is a strong argument for a combined blockade of both hormones in clinical situations.

In the experimental models used above, the level of ALD in plasma was strongly increased (four to five fold compared to normal level). By contrast, moderate ALD elevation through transgenic overexpression of cardiomyocyte-specific aldosterone synthase (CYP11B2) in mice leads to coronary vessel dysfunction [76] by decreasing the expression of the repolarizing calcium-activated potassium channel BKCa in coronary smooth muscle cells [77]. Importantly, no cardiac fibrosis was found in the hearts of these AS mice. This is apparently in contrast with what was observed in the ALD-salt or DOCA-salt models, and in post-MI, but the rather moderate increase of ALD in AS mice probably explains that the markers of oxidative stress and of inflammation were not upregulated in this model. Moreover, the elegant work of Edith Hummler using a transgenic model of ENac gene invalidation (resulting in a 6.3- fold increased plasma ALD!) has shown that this chronic robust hyperaldosteronism fails to induce cardiac REM and fibrosis under a normal-salt diet [78]. It may therefore be concluded that increased ALD induces cardiovascular REM only when it is combined with another stress-generating factor, such as salt or Ang II (which is increased in post-MI or HF). This is what has been observed in AS mice crossed with mice made hypertensive by genetic increased plasma Ang II. Hyperaldosteronism in these hypertensive mice was associated with increased macrophage infiltration (CD68+ cells) and enhanced expression of mRNA for MCP1, osteopontin and galectin-3 in the heart [79]. Eplerenone decreased CD68 and galectin-3 levels in these mice. Galectin-3 is a beta-galactoside-binding lectin expressed in fibroblasts, endothelial cells and macrophages that has been shown to participate in inflammation, fibrosis, and HF. Interestingly, similar results were observed in aldosterone-treated hypertensive rats that have vascular hypertrophy, inflammation, fibrosis, and increased aortic Gal-3 expression [80]. Spironolactone reversed this phenotype, and ALD had no pro-fibrotic actions in galectin-3 knock-out mice [80]. Together, these results indicate a key role of ALD in the stimulation of macrophages and of their synthesis of galectin-3. Moreover, the moderate ALD excess in AS hypertensive mice was associated with a decrease in BNP [79] and ANP [81] expression. The natriuretic peptides ANP and BNP are antifibrotic and antihypertrophic [82]. Thus, ALD appears to play a determinant role in a balance between pro-fibrotic (TGF-ß, galectin-3) and anti-fibrotic (BNP, ANP) factors (Fig. 4.2).

The adverse consequences of fibrous tissue are: (a) tissue heterogeneity, accentuated in the diseased heart because fibrillar collagen ensnares neighboring cardiomyocytes and, by doing so, reduces cardiomyocyte workload and therefore induces cardiomyocyte atrophy, (b) increased passive tissue stiffness, and (c) electrical REM and enhanced arrhythmogenicity. It is thus of primary importance to better understand the mechanisms leading to cardiac fibrosis, with the aim to reduce or prevent it. This is especially important since atrial fibrosis is considered to be a critical determinant of cardiac arrhythmogenicity. The role of ALD in the generation of atrial fibrillation has been established in patients since, for a same level of hypertension, a history of atrial fibrillation was diagnosed in 7.3 % of patients with primary aldosteronism and in only 0.6 % of patients with essential hypertension [83]. In the same way, conditional MR overexpression in the mouse heart leads to life-threatening arrhythmias [65]. Moreover ALD blockade can reduce ventricular arrhythmias [84], and decreases ventricular premature complexes, LV collagen and noradrenaline content and improve heart rate variability parameters (meanRR and sdRR) [85]. Further, addition of atenolol, a beta-blocker, enhanced spironolactone effects on all of these parameters in a rat model of MI [85]. It is thus clear that ALD blockade could be of interest in prevention of cardiac arrhythmias.

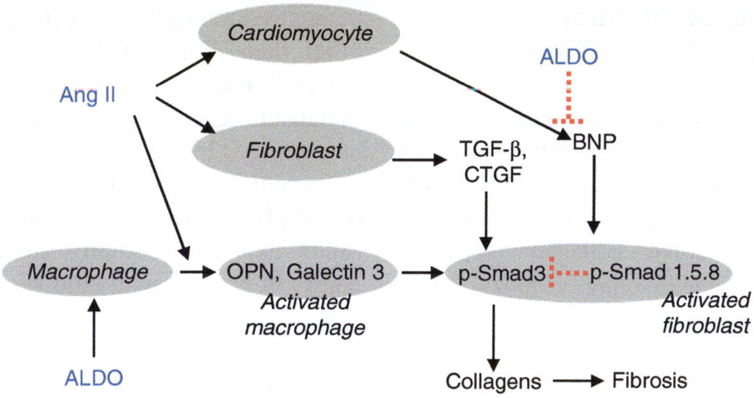

Fig. 4.2 The interaction of Ang II and aldosterone in cardiac fibrosis. Aldosterone amplifies the Ang II-induced fibrotic process by stimulating macrophages infiltration in the heart. Macrophages are activated by AngII and release osteopontin (OPN) and galectin-3 which strongly potentiate the action of TGFb and CTGF. Aldosterone also inhibits the the hypertension-induced BNP synthesis and release, this decreases the antifibrotic action of BNP (Redrawn with permission from Azibani et al. [79])

4.3.3.3 Activation of the MR Is Determinant in the Development of Cardiac Alterations

Perivascular fibrosis resulting from inflammation in the coronary arteries is a major step in the triggering of cardiac fibrosis by ALD. However, the question of the target cell of ALD in the heart remained unsolved. Several works have recently shed a brilliant light on the consequences of the activation of the ALD receptor in specific cell types on cardiac function and fibrosis, see review in [86]. It is now clear that imposition of stress (aortic stenosis, L-NAME/AngII, or aldosterone/salt) induces myocyte hypertrophy, oxidative stress and inflammation/fibrosis, thus predisposing to the development of HF. These effects are prevented by MR antagonists [87]. Studies using mice with cell type-selective deletion of the MR in cardiomyocytes [88], fibroblasts [88], macrophages [89], or myeloid cells that control macrophage polarization [90] demonstrated that fibrosis in hearts subjected to the above stresses was prevented only in the mice with macrophage-selective deletion of MR, although the recruitment of these cells to the stressed heart was not prevented. Interestingly, fibroblast-selective MR deletion did not affect the cardiac structural and functional alterations, whereas cardiomyocyte-elective MR deletion resulted in improved cardiac function. Macrophages are inflammatory cells that are present in the heart in very small numbers under normal conditions. However, stresses such as those mentioned above trigger the release of cytokines like MCP-1 which induce the infiltration of macrophages into the heart. These observations provide evidence that MR-mediated signaling in macrophages elicits the cardiac fibrosis associated with hemodynamic or hormonal challenges, even when plasma ALD is not elevated [91].

The question of which hormones bind to MR in the myocardium, ALD, or GR that bind efficiently to MR and whose plasma concentration is much higher than aldosterone, persists to this day [92]. A recent study using mice overexpressing MR in cardiomyocytes and treated with ALD, demonstrated that it specifically regulates the expression of 265 genes in cardiomyocytes despite the high concentration of GR in the plasma [93]. The connective tissue growth factor (CTGF) is one of the aldosterone-upregulated genes in cardiomyocytes, which seems pathologically relevant as the increase in CTGF observed in a model of HF (transverse aortic constriction) in rats was prevented by eplerenone [93].

4.4 From Experimental Observations to Clinics

The first study to show a beneficial cardiac effect in humans was published in 1995. The study found that spironolactone reduced cardiac sympathetic activity, ventricular arrhythmias, and markers of myocardial collagen [94]. The RALES study was the first large clinical study to evaluate the effects of adding a MRA to standard of care in 1,663 patients with severe HF [28]. Spironolactone was the only approved MRA at this time, and it was used despite the known side effects and the weak hope of financial return on it since it was already out of patent. But the results were very positive. The risk of death from all causes decreased by 30 %, and that of death of cardiac origin by 31 % using a mean dose of 26 mg/day of spironolactone in treated patients. There was also a reduction in hospital admissions for HF by 35 %. This unexpectedly excellent result has been an important step in the history of MRAs. A correlation between mortality and a reduction in cardiac fibrosis after spironolactone treatment has been observed in a subgroup of patients from the RALES study [95].

Eplerenone was tested in 6,642 patients with LV dysfunction (LV ejection fraction <40 %) after MI in the EPHESUS study [30]. Like in the RALES study, the results were positive. All-cause mortality decreased by 15 % in the eplerenone group, cardiovascular mortality was reduced by 17 %, and sudden cardiac death by 21 % when compared to placebo. Interestingly, a post hoc analysis of the EPHESUS trial showed a reduction of the risk of global mortality (−31 %), cardiovascular mortality (−32 %), and sudden death (−37 %) as early as 30 days after the onset of eplerenone treatment [96]. One of the main differences between the RALES and EPHESUS studies is the number of patients treated with beta-blockers, since the percentage was 11 % in RALES vs 75 % in EPHESUS. For this reason, the mortality benefit seen in the eplerenone group was primarily due to sudden cardiac death reduction. Importantly, plasma ALD and sodium levels in both RALES and EPHESUS studies trials were normal. This observation suggests pathophysiological MR activation by ligands other than ALD, likely by normal levels of cortisol, and provides clear evidence for the therapeutic utility of MR blockade in HF with normal ALD levels.

In contrast to the above described studies that tested MRAs in severe HF, the EMPHASIS-HF Study explored mortality and morbidity outcomes in patients with mild systolic HF and LV systolic dysfunction [95]. Eplerenone was used at a dose of up to 50 mg daily in addition to standard of care. This study enrolled 2,737 patients with NYHA class II HF and LV ejection fraction <35 %. The primary outcome was a composite of death from cardiovascular causes or hospitalization for HF. The trial was stopped prematurely, according to prespecified rules, after a median follow-up period of 21 months. Eplerenone, as compared with placebo, reduced both the risk of death and the risk of hospitalization among patients with systolic HF and mild symptoms. A multicentric randomized study to analyze the effect of MRAs in patients with HF and preserved LV ejection fraction has been recently completed. The TOPCAT study randomizes patients to spironolactone or placebo. This study begun in 2006 and results are expected in 2014.

These large clinical studies demonstrate that the inhibition of MR has very beneficial consequences in mild to severe HF, suggesting that an activation of the MR occurs over the course of the disease and plays an important role in the pathophysiology of HF. The European Society of Cardiology guidelines reflect these findings and now recommend MRAs in patients with LV ejection fraction <35 % and persisting NYHA class II–IV [54]. However, it seems that MRAs suffer from a somewhat “fuzzy” image in some physician’s mind: spironolactone has been initially viewed as a potassium-sparing diuretic among the pool of other drugs for HF treatment, such as diuretics, ACE inhibitors, and beta-blockers. The discovery in the 1980s that ALD had a range of extrarenal receptors and actions, especially in the heart and blood vessels, has certainly renewed interest in the field of ALD antagonists. Nevertheless, a clear understanding of the mechanisms of the MRAs that may fully explain

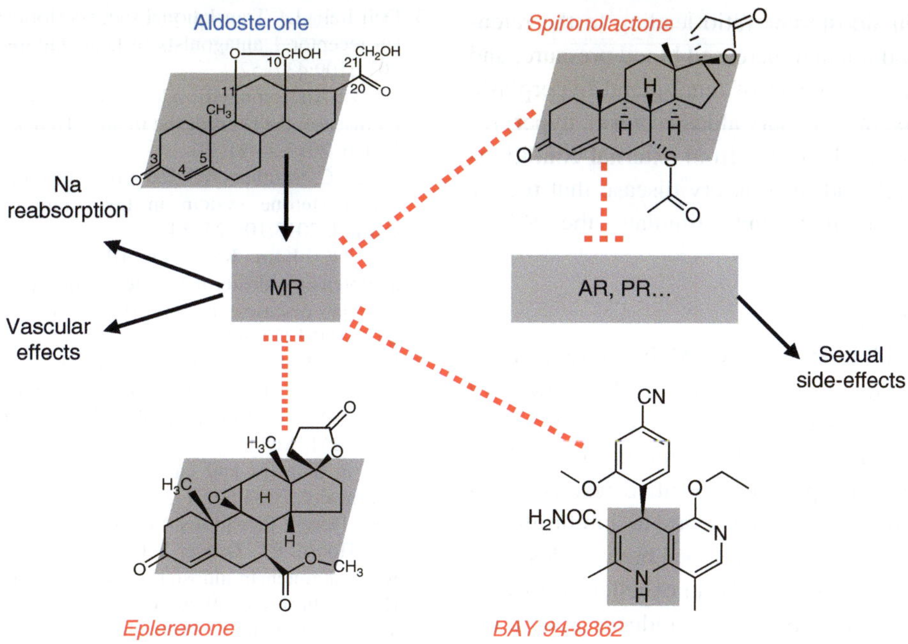

Fig. 4.3 The family of mineralocorticoid receptor antagonists. The "old" MR antagonists spironolactone and eplerenone are derived from aldosterone (the steroid core is shaded in *grey*). The new non steroidal BAY 94-8862 and its analogues to come are derived from the dihydropyridine molecule (shaded in *grey*). BAY 94-8862 combines the high affinity of spironolactone, and the selectivity of eplerenone, for the MR

their beneficial effects in HF is still lacking. Together, these reasons are probably determinants to the underuse of MRAs in HF [97, 98].

4.4.1 Future Developments

The properties of spironolactone (high affinity but low selectivity for the MR) and eplerenone (good selectivity but low affinity for MR) led several laboratories to develop nonsteroidal ARM. BAY 94–8862 from Bayer laboratories is a last generation nonsteroidal MRA. In pre-clinical studies, it has demonstrated a high selectivity and a higher affinity for MR that eplerenone. It is evaluated in the randomized ARTS phase II study comparing BAY 94–8862 to spironolactone [99]. This study is conducted in HF with mild to moderate renal impairment, mostly NYHA class II. At doses of 5 and 10 mg per day, BAY 94–8862 reduced the BNP, NT- proBNP and albuminuria in the same proportions as 25–50 mg of spironolactone, with a significantly lower risk of hyperkalemia than spironolactone. While concentrations of spironolactone observed are six times higher in the kidney compared to the heart, BAY 94–8862 was found similarly in heart and kidney. This suggests that the cardiac action will be observed even at low doses (Fig. 4.3).

4.4.2 Markers of RAAS Activity

As discussed above clinical symptoms of increased blood pressure or cardiac dysfunction are strong indications that the RAAS is activated. Obviously, this deserves to be verified and precised by assay of the plasma renin activity (PRA) and concentration, and Ang II (ELISA kits) and of aldosterone (ELISA kits, radio-immuno assay) in plasma. PRA is measured by generating Ang I from endogenous angiotensinogen, followed by measurement by RIA of the generated Ang I. Ang II and ALD are assayed using ELISA kits. Measurement of serum ALD in conjunction with plasma renin is used clinically to differentiate between primary and secondary aldosteronism. Primary aldosteronism is characterized by a very low renin:aldosterone ratio leading to the retention of sodium and increased blood pressure, and is typically the result of renal gland hyperplasia or tumors. In secondary aldosteronism, hyperproduction of ALD results from external conditions such as HF and renal artery disease that reduce renal blood flow and stimulate the RAAS mechanism.

Conclusion

The inhibition of the RAAS has a tremendous benefit in the management all CVD. The most successful interventions have been the use of ACE inhibitors and MRAs, both of which consistently produced positive results in trials. Alternative approaches to inhibiting the RAAS have been developed but with less success. ARBs are clearly an excellent substitute in cases of ACE inhibitor-induced cough, but they may have no other role in HF. DRIs have also been developed with some success, but recent results have raised concerns about their side-effect profile, meaning that more data are required to determine whether recent adverse effects are just chance occurrences. One exciting new possibility is the use of ARNis, for which the very preliminary data look encouraging. At present, the RAAS-modulating strategy recommended for HF is a combination of ACE inhibitors and MRAs. It will therefore be difficult for renin inhibitors to replace ACE/ARB and MRAs because these have proven efficacy.

Acknowledgements This work was supported by CNRS, Inserm, Université Paris-Diderot, the Fondation de France, Interface grant Inserm-APHP and the Société Française d'Hypertension Artérielle (SFHTA).

Disclosures The authors declare that they have no disclosures to declare.

References

1. Swynghedauw B. Molecular mechanisms of myocardial remodeling. Physiol Rev. 1999;79:215–62.
2. Brown NJ. Contribution of aldosterone to cardiovascular and renal inflammation and fibrosis. Nat Rev Nephrol. 2013;9:459–69.
3. Dell'Italia LJ. Translational success stories: angiotensin receptor 1 antagonists in heart failure. Circ Res. 2011;109:437–52.
4. He BJ, Anderson ME. Aldosterone and cardiovascular disease: the heart of the matter. Trends Endocrinol Metab. 2013;24:21–30.
5. Lang CC, Struthers AD. Targeting the renin-angiotensin-aldosterone system in heart failure. Nat Rev Cardiol. 2013;10:125–34.
6. Ma TK, Kam KK, Yan BP, Lam YY. Renin-angiotensin-aldosterone system blockade for cardiovascular diseases: current status. Br J Pharmacol. 2010;160:1273–92.
7. Messaoudi S, Azibani F, Delcayre C, Jaisser F. Aldosterone, mineralocorticoid receptor, and heart failure. Mol Cell Endocrinol. 2012;350:266–72.
8. Patel BM, Mehta AA. Aldosterone and angiotensin: role in diabetes and cardiovascular diseases. Eur J Pharmacol. 2012;697:1–12.
9. Seva Pessoa B, van der Lubbe N, Verdonk K, Roks AJ, Hoorn EJ, Danser AH. Key developments in renin-angiotensin-aldosterone system inhibition. Nat Rev Nephrol. 2013;9:26–36.
10. Weber KT, Sun Y, Bhattacharya SK, Ahokas RA, Gerling IC. Myofibroblast-mediated mechanisms of pathological remodelling of the heart. Nat Rev Cardiol. 2013;10:15–26.
11. Tigerstedt R, Bergman PG. Niere und Kreislauf. Skand Arch Physiol. 1898;8:223–7.
12. Goldblatt H, Lynch J, Hanzal RF, Summerville WW. Studies on experimental hypertension I. The production of persistent elevation of systolic blood pressure by means of renal ischemia. J Exp Med. 1934;59: 347–79.
13. Braun-Menendez E, Fasciolo JC, Leloir LF, Munoz JM. The substance causing renal hypertension. J Physiol. 1940;98:283–98.
14. Page IH, Helmer OM. A crystalline pressor substance (angiotonin) resulting from the reaction between renin and renin-activator. J Exp Med. 1940;71:29–42.
15. Kahn JR, Skeggs Jr LT, Shumway NP, Wisenbaugh PE. The assay of hypertensin from the arterial blood of normotensive and hypertensive human beings. J Exp Med. 1952;95:523–9.
16. Simpson SA, Tait JF, Wettstein A, Neher R, Von Euw J, Reichstein T. [Isolation from the adrenals of a new crystalline hormone with especially high effectiveness on mineral metabolism]. Experientia. 1953;9:333–5.
17. Skeggs Jr LT, Marsh WH, Kahn JR, Shumway NP. The existence of two forms of hypertensin. J Exp Med. 1954;99:275–82.
18. Skeggs Jr LT, Kahn JR, Shumway NP. The preparation and function of the hypertensin-converting enzyme. J Exp Med. 1956;103:295–9.
19. Liddle GW. Sodium diuresis induced by steroidal antagonists of aldosterone. Science. 1957;126:1016–8.
20. Gross F. Renin and hypertension, physiological or pathological agents? Klin Wochenschr. 1958;36: 693–706.
21. Kagawa CM, Sturtevant FM, Van Arman CG. Pharmacology of a new steroid that blocks salt activity

of aldosterone and desoxycorticosterone. J Pharmacol Exp Ther. 1959;126:123–30.
22. Pals DT, Masucci FD, Sipas F, Denning Jr GS. A specific competitive antagonist of the vascular action of angiotensin II. Circ Res. 1971;29:664–72.
23. Brunner HR, Laragh JH, Baer L, Newton MA, Goodwin FT, Krakoff LR, et al. Essential hypertension: renin and aldosterone, heart attack and stroke. N Engl J Med. 1972;286:441–9.
24. Cushman DW, Cheung HS, Sabo EF, Ondetti MA. Design of potent competitive inhibitors of angiotensin-converting enzyme. Biochemistry. 1977;16:5484–91.
25. Carini DJ, Christ DD, Duncia JV, Pierce ME. The discovery and development of angiotensin II antagonists. Pharm Biotechnol. 1998;11:29–56.
26. Brilla CG, Matsubara LS, Weber KT. Anti-aldosterone treatment and the prevention of myocardial fibrosis in primary and secondary hyperaldosteronism. J Mol Cell Cardiol. 1993;25:563–75.
27. Pitt B, Segal R, Martinez FA, Meurers G, Cowley AJ, Thomas I, Deedwania PC, Ney DE, Snavely DB, Chang PI. Randomized trial of losartan versus captopril in patients over 65 with heart failure (Evaluation of Losartan in Elderly Study, ELITE). Lancet. 1997;349:747–52.
28. Pitt B, Zannad F, Remme WJ, Cody R, Castaigne A, Perez A, et al. The effect of spironolactone on morbidity and mortality in patients with severe heart failure. Randomized Aldactone Evaluation Study Investigators. N Engl J Med. 1999;341:709–17.
29. Pitt B, Poole-Wilson PA, Segal R, Martinez FA, Dickstein K, Camm AJ, Konstam MA, Riegger G, Klinger GH, Neaton J, Sharma D, Thiyagarajan B. Effect of losartan compared with captopril on mortality in patients with symptomatic heart failure: randomised trial–the Losartan Heart Failure Survival Study ELITE II. Lancet. 2000;355(9215):1582–7.
30. Pitt B, Reichek N, Willenbrock R, Zannad F, Phillips RA, Roniker B, et al. Effects of eplerenone, enalapril and eplerenone/enalapril in patients with essential hypertension and left ventricular hypertrophy: the 4E-left ventricular hypertrophy study. Circulation. 2003;108:1831–8.
31. Menard J, Bouhnik J, Clauser E, Richoux JP, Corvol P. Biochemistry and regulation of angiotensinogen. Clin Exp Hypertens A. 1983;5:1005–19.
32. Braun-Menendez E, Page IH. Suggested revision of nomenclature–angiotensin. Science. 1958;127:242.
33. Yankopoulos NA, Davis JO, Kliman B, Peterson RE, Casper A. Evidence that a humoral agent stimulates the adrenal cortex to secrete aldosterone in experimental secondary hyperaldosteronism. J Clin Invest. 1959;38:1278–89.
34. Sarnoff SJ, Berglund E. Neurohemodynamics of pulmonary edema. IV. Effect of systemic vasoconstriction and subsequent vasodilation on flow and pressures in systemic and pulmonary vascular beds. Am J Physiol. 1952;170:588–600.
35. Zelis R, Mason DT. Compensatory mechanisms in congestive heart failure–the role of the peripheral resistance vessels. N Engl J Med. 1970;282:962–4.
36. Cohn JN. Vasodilator therapy for heart failure. The influence of impedance on left ventricular performance. Circulation. 1973;48:5–8.
37. Acharya KR, Sturrock ED, Riordan JF, Ehlers MR. Ace revisited: a new target for structure-based drug design. Nat Rev Drug Discov. 2003;2:891–902.
38. Cushman DW, Ondetti MA. History of the design of captopril and related inhibitors of angiotensin converting enzyme. Hypertension. 1991;17:589–92.
39. Urata H, Kinoshita A, Misono KS, Bumpus FM, Husain A. Identification of a highly specific chymase as the major angiotensin II-forming enzyme in the human heart. J Biol Chem. 1990;265:22348–57.
40. Duncia JV, Chiu AT, Carini DJ, Gregory GB, Johnson AL, Price WA, et al. The discovery of potent nonpeptide angiotensin II receptor antagonists: a new class of potent antihypertensives. J Med Chem. 1990;33:1312–29.
41. Wolny A, Clozel JP, Rein J, Mory P, Vogt P, Turino M, et al. Functional and biochemical analysis of angiotensin II-forming pathways in the human heart. Circ Res. 1997;80:219–27.
42. Kumar R, Thomas CM, Yong QC, Chen W, Baker KM. The intracrine renin-angiotensin system. Clin Sci (Lond). 2012;123:273–84.
43. Paul M, Poyan Mehr A, Kreutz R. Physiology of local renin-angiotensin systems. Physiol Rev. 2006;86:747–803.
44. Griendling KK, Lassègue B, Alexander RW. Angiotensin receptors and their therapeutic implications. Annu Rev Pharmacol Toxicol. 1996;36:281–306.
45. Nguyen G. Renin, (pro)renin and receptor: an update. Clin Sci (Lond). 2011;120:169–78.
46. Swynghedauw B, Delcayre C, Samuel JL, Mebazaa A, Cohen-Solal A. Molecular mechanisms in evolutionary cardiology failure. Ann N Y Acad Sci. 2010;1188:58–67.
47. Lavoie JL, Bianco RA, Sakai K, Keen HL, Ryan MJ, Sigmund CD. Transgenic mice for studies of the renin-angiotensin system in hypertension. Acta Physiol Scand. 2004;181:571–7.
48. Caron KM, James LR, Kim HS, Morham SG, Sequeira Lopez ML, Gomez RA, et al. A genetically clamped renin transgene for the induction of hypertension. Proc Natl Acad Sci U S A. 2002;99:8248–52.
49. Lombardi D, Gordon KL, Polinsky P, Suga S, Schwartz SM, Johnson RJ. Salt-sensitive hypertension develops after short-term exposure to Angiotensin II. Hypertension. 1999;33:1013–9.
50. Ruiz-Ortega M, Lorenzo O, Ruperez M, Esteban V, Suzuki Y, Mezzano S, et al. Role of the renin-angiotensin system in vascular diseases: expanding the field. Hypertension. 2001;38:1382–7.
51. Dzau VJ. Tissue angiotensin and pathobiology of vascular disease: a unifying hypothesis. Hypertension. 2001;37:1047–52.
52. Rautureau Y, Paradis P, Schiffrin EL. Cross-talk between aldosterone and angiotensin signaling in vascular smooth muscle cells. Steroids. 2011;76:834–9.

53. Sun Y, Zhang J, Lu L, Bedigian MP, Robinson AD, Weber KT. Tissue angiotensin II in the regulation of inflammatory and fibrogenic components of repair in the rat heart. J Lab Clin Med. 2004;143:41–51.
54. McMurray JJ, Califf RM, Bethel AM, Haffner SM, Holman RR. Comparative effectiveness of angiotensin-converting enzyme inhibitors and angiotensin receptor blockers for hypertension on clinical end points: a cohort study. J Clin Hypertens. 2012;14:731.
55. van Vark LC, Bertrand M, Akkerhuis KM, Brugts JJ, Fox K, Mourad JJ, et al. Angiotensin-converting enzyme inhibitors reduce mortality in hypertension: a meta-analysis of randomized clinical trials of renin-angiotensin-aldosterone system inhibitors involving 158,998 patients. Eur Heart J. 2012;33:2088–97.
56. Grossmann C, Benesic A, Krug AW, Freudinger R, Mildenberger S, Gassner B, et al. Human mineralocorticoid receptor expression renders cells responsive for nongenotropic aldosterone actions. Mol Endocrinol. 2005;19:1697–710.
57. Tait SA, Tait JF, Coghlan JP. The discovery, isolation and identification of aldosterone: reflections on emerging regulation and function. Mol Cell Endocrinol. 2004;217:1–21.
58. Menard J. The 45-year story of the development of an anti-aldosterone more specific than spironolactone. Mol Cell Endocrinol. 2004;217:45–52.
59. Mulder P, Mellin V, Favre J, Vercauteren M, Remy-Jouet I, Monteil C, et al. Aldosterone synthase inhibition improves cardiovascular function and structure in rats with heart failure: a comparison with spironolactone. Eur Heart J. 2008;29:2171–9.
60. Silvestre JS, Heymes C, Oubenaissa A, Robert V, Aupetit-Faisant B, Carayon A, et al. Activation of cardiac aldosterone production in rat myocardial infarction: effect of angiotensin II receptor blockade and role in cardiac fibrosis. Circulation. 1999;99:2694–701.
61. Mizuno Y, Yoshimura M, Yasue H, Sakamoto T, Ogawa H, Kugiyama K, et al. Aldosterone production is activated in failing ventricle in humans. Circulation. 2001;103:72–7.
62. Tsybouleva N, Zhang L, Chen S, Patel R, Lutucuta S, Nemoto S, et al. Aldosterone, through novel signaling proteins, is a fundamental molecular bridge between the genetic defect and the cardiac phenotype of hypertrophic cardiomyopathy. Circulation. 2004;109:1284–91.
63. Baker ME, Funder JW, Kattoula SR. Evolution of hormone selectivity in glucocorticoid and mineralocorticoid receptors. J Steroid Biochem Mol Biol. 2013;137:57–70.
64. Funder JW, Krozowski Z, Myles K, Sato A, Sheppard KE, Young M. Mineralocorticoid receptors, salt, and hypertension. Recent Prog Horm Res. 1997;52:247–60; discussion 61–2.
65. Ouvrard-Pascaud A, Sainte-Marie Y, Benitah JP, Perrier R, Soukaseum C, Nguyen Dinh Cat A, et al. Conditional mineralocorticoid receptor expression in the heart leads to life-threatening arrhythmias. Circulation. 2005;111:3025–33.
66. Bois P, Selye H. 2-Methyl-9(alpha)-chlorocortisol, a new synthetic mineralocorticoid with unusually intense nephrotoxic actions. Can Med Assoc J. 1956;75:720–4.
67. Swedberg K, Eneroth P, Kjekshus J, Wilhelmsen L. Hormones regulating cardiovascular function in patients with severe congestive heart failure and their relation to mortality. CONSENSUS Trial Study Group. Circulation. 1990;82:1730–6.
68. Rossi GP, Sacchetto A, Pavan E, Palatini P, Graniero GR, Canali C, et al. Remodeling of the left ventricle in primary aldosteronism due to Conn's adenoma. Circulation. 1997;95:1471–8.
69. Güder G, Bauersachs J, Frantz S, Weismann D, Allolio B, Ertl G, et al. Complementary and incremental mortality risk prediction by cortisol and aldosterone in chronic heart failure. Circulation. 2007;115:1754–61.
70. Robert V, Silvestre JS, Charlemagne D, Sabri A, Trouvé P, Wassef M, et al. Biological determinants of aldosterone-induced cardiac fibrosis in rats. Hypertension. 1995;26:971–8.
71. Young M, Fullerton M, Dilley R, Funder J. Mineralocorticoids, hypertension, and cardiac fibrosis. J Clin Invest. 1994;93:2578–83.
72. Pitt B. "Escape" of aldosterone production in patients with left ventricular dysfunction treated with an angiotensin converting enzyme inhibitor: implications for therapy. Cardiovasc Drugs Ther. 1995;9:145–9.
73. Azibani F, Fazal L, Chatziantoniou C, Samuel JL, Delcayre C. Aldosterone mediates cardiac fibrosis in the setting of hypertension. Curr Hypertens Rep. 2013;15:395–400.
74. Weber KT, Brilla CG, Campbell SE, Guarda E, Zhou G, Sriram K. Myocardial fibrosis: a role of angiotensin II and aldosterone. Basic Res Cardiol. 1993;88(Suppl1):107–24.
75. Gerling IC, Sun Y, Ahokas RA, Wodi LA, Bhattacharya SK, Warrington KJ, et al. Aldosteronism: an immunostimulatory state precedes proinflammatory/fibrogenic cardiac phenotype. Am J Physiol Heart Circ Physiol. 2003;285:H813–21.
76. Garnier A, Bendall JK, Fuchs S, Escoubet B, Rochais F, Hoerter J, et al. Cardiac specific increase in aldosterone production induces coronary dysfunction in aldosterone synthase-transgenic mice. Circulation. 2004;110:1819–25.
77. Ambroisine ML, Favre J, Oliviero P, Rodriguez C, Gao J, Thuillez C, et al. Aldosterone-induced coronary dysfunction in transgenic mice involves the calcium-activated potassium (BKCa) channels of vascular smooth muscle cells. Circulation. 2007;116:2435–43.
78. Wang Q, Clement S, Gabbiani G, Horisberger JD, Burnier M, Rossier BC, et al. Chronic hyperaldosteronism in a transgenic mouse model fails to induce cardiac remodeling and fibrosis under a normal-salt diet. Am J Physiol Renal Physiol. 2004;286:F1178–84.

79. Azibani F, Benard L, Schlossarek S, Merval R, Tournoux F, Fazal L, et al. Aldosterone inhibits antifibrotic factors in mouse hypertensive heart. Hypertension. 2012;59:1179–87.
80. Calvier L, Miana M, Reboul P, Cachofeiro V, Martinez-Martinez E, de Boer RA, et al. Galectin-3 mediates aldosterone-induced vascular fibrosis. Arterioscler Thromb Vasc Biol. 2013;33:67–75.
81. Azibani F, Devaux Y, Coutance G, Schlossarek S, Polidano E, Fazal L, et al. Aldosterone inhibits the fetal program and increases hypertrophy in the heart of hypertensive mice. PLoS One. 2012;7:e38197.
82. Calvieri C, Rubattu S, Volpe M. Molecular mechanisms underlying cardiac antihypertrophic and antifibrotic effects of natriuretic peptides. J Mol Med (Berl). 2012;90:5–13.
83. Milliez P, Girerd X, Plouin PF, Blacher J, Safar ME, Mourad JJ. Evidence for an increased rate of cardiovascular events in patients with primary aldosteronism. J Am Coll Cardiol. 2005;45:1243–8.
84. Shah NC, Pringle SD, Donnan PT, Struthers AD. Spironolactone has antiarrhythmic activity in ischaemic cardiac patients without cardiac failure. J Hypertens. 2007;25:2345–51.
85. Milliez P, Gomes S, Champ-Rigot L, Callebert J, Samuel JL, Delcayre C. Effects of spironolactone alone and in addition to a beta-blocker on myocardial histological and electrical remodeling in chronic severe failing rat hearts. J Cardiovasc Pharmacol. 2012;60:315–21.
86. Jaisser F, Swynghedauw B, Delcayre C. The mineralocorticoid receptor in heart: different effects in different cells. Hypertension. 2011;57:679–80.
87. Kuster GM, Kotlyar E, Rude MK, Siwik DA, Liao R, Colucci WS, et al. Mineralocorticoid receptor inhibition ameliorates the transition to myocardial failure and decreases oxidative stress and inflammation in mice with chronic pressure overload. Circulation. 2005;111:420–7.
88. Lother A, Berger S, Gilsbrach R, Rösner S, Ecke A, Barreto F, et al. Ablation of mineralocorticoid receptors in myocytes but not in fibroblasts preserves cardiac function. Hypertension. 2011;57:746–54.
89. Rickard AJ, Morgan J, Tesch G, Funder JW, Fuller PJ, Young MJ. Deletion of mineralocorticoid receptors from macrophages protects against deoxycorticosterone/salt-induced cardiac fibrosis and increased blood pressure. Hypertension. 2009;54:537–43.
90. Usher MG, Duan SZ, Ivaschenko CY, Frieler RA, Berger S, Schütz G, et al. Myeloid mineralocorticoid receptor controls macrophage polarization and cardiovascular hypertrophy and remodeling in mice. J Clin Invest. 2010;120:3350–64.
91. Bienvenu LA, Morgan J, Rickard AJ, Tesch GH, Cranston GA, Fletcher EK, et al. Macrophage mineralocorticoid receptor signaling plays a key role in aldosterone-independent cardiac fibrosis. Endocrinology. 2012;153:3416–25.
92. Funder JW. Aldosterone and mineralocorticoid receptors: a personal reflection. Mol Cell Endocrinol. 2012;350:146–50.
93. Messaoudi S, Gravez B, Tarjus A, Pelloux V, Ouvrard-Pascaud A, Delcayre C, et al. Aldosterone-specific activation of cardiomyocyte mineralocorticoid receptor in vivo. Hypertension. 2013;61:361–7.
94. MacFadyen RJ, Barr CS, Struthers AD. Aldosterone blockade reduces vascular collagen turnover, improves heart rate variability and reduces early morning rise in heart rate in heart failure patients. Cardiovasc Res. 1997;35:30–4.
95. Zannad F, McMurray JJ, Krum H, van Veldhuisen DJ, Swedberg K, Shi H, et al. Eplerenone in patients with systolic heart failure and mild symptoms. N Engl J Med. 2011;364:11–21.
96. Pitt B, White H, Nicolau J, Martinez F, Gheorghiades M, Aschermann M, et al. Eplerenone reduces mortality 30 days after randomization following acute myocardial infarction in patients with left ventricular systolic dysfunction and heart failure. J Am Coll Cardiol. 2005;46:425–31.
97. Albert NM, Yancy CW, Liang L, Zhao X, Hernandez AF, Peterson ED, et al. Use of aldosterone antagonists in heart failure. JAMA. 2009;302:1658–65.
98. Samuel JL, Delcayre C. Heart failure: aldosterone antagonists are underused by clinicians. Nat Rev Cardiol. 2010;7:125–7.
99. Pitt B, Kober L, Ponikowski P, Gheorghiade M, Filippatos G, Krum H, et al. Safety and tolerability of the novel non-steroidal mineralocorticoid receptor antagonist BAY 94–8862 in patients with chronic heart failure and mild or moderate chronic kidney disease: a randomized, double-blind trial. Eur Heart J. 2013;34:2453–63.

Beta Adrenergic Receptors

5

Konstantinos Makaritsis and Filippos Triposkiadis

Abstract

β-Adrenergic receptors (β-ARs) have a key position not in to the overall regulation of cardiac function and have been shown to play an important role in various cardiac diseases and heart failure in particular. Beta adrenergic receptors (β-ARs) belong to the G protein-coupled receptor (GPCR) superfamily with widespread expression and cardiovascular functions. Three β-AR subtypes (β_1-AR, β_2-AR, and β_3-AR) are expressed in cardiomyocytes. The positive inotropic effect of β-AR stimulation is one of the most effective measures for maintaining cardiac output. The β-AR stimulation induces protein kinase A (PK-A) activation through G protein, adenylyl cyclase (AC) and cyclic adenosine monophosphate (cAMP). PK-A mediated phosphorylation of many calcium-handling molecules enhances ventricular wall motion. However, long term stimulation of these receptors can lead to the deterioration of cardiac function. In addition, the prognosis of heart failure patients improves with β-AR blocking therapy. Prospective, randomized, placebo-controlled outcome trials of β-blockers in heart failure have demonstrated sustained improvements in left ventricular remodeling and significant reductions in mortality and hospitalizations. The clinical evidence for the long-term benefit of β -blocker therapy is so strong that it is now recommended therapy in all patients with Class II or III heart failure symptoms who do not have specific contraindications. Cardiac G protein–coupled receptor kinases are tightly related to the status of β-AR function in the heart and they have lately emerged not only as a potential therapeutic target in HF but also as a biomarker of HF status and response to treatment, potentially useful in HF clinical practice.

K. Makaritsis, MD (✉)
Department of Medicine, University of Thessaly, School of Medicine, Larissa University Hospital, Box 1425, Larissa 41110, Greece
e-mail: makarits@med.uth.gr

F. Triposkiadis, MD
Department of Cardiology, University of Thessaly, School of Medicine, Larissa University Hospital, Box 1425, Larissa 41110, Greece

D.V. Cokkinos (ed.), *Introduction to Translational Cardiovascular Research*,
DOI 10.1007/978-3-319-08798-6_5, © Springer International Publishing Switzerland 2015

Keywords
Beta adrenergic receptors • G protein-coupled receptors • Beta blockers • Heart failure • G protein–coupled receptor kinases

Abbreviations

ANS	Autonomous nervous system
APO	Apoptosis
ATP	Adenosine triphosphate
βARKct	$G_{\beta\gamma}$ protein sequestering peptide
BBs	β-blockers
CVD	Cardiovascular diseases
β-ARs	Beta adrenergic receptors
cAMP	cyclic Adenosine Monophosphate
eNOS	Endothelial Nitric Oxide Synthase
ISA	Intrinsic sympathomimetic activity
GPCR	G protein-coupled receptor
GRKs	G protein–coupled receptor kinases
LVEF	Left Ventricular Ejection Fraction
MI	Myocardial infarction
NE	Norepinephrine
RAAS	Renin-Angiotensin-Aldosterone System

5.1 Introduction- History

In the early 1900s John Newport Langley first proposed that there were specific receptors which bind certain medications resulting in specific biological effects within the cell itself [1]. Paul Ehrlich, who received the Nobel Prize for Medicine in 1908, suggested that these receptors were selective [2]. In 1897, John Jacob Abel successfully isolated epinephrine and in 1933, W. B. Cannon, while studying the sympathetic nervous system concluded that there were two chemical transmitters that he called sympathins [3]. However, it was not until 1948, where Raymond Ahlquist described the actions of epinephrine on two distinct receptors called alpha and beta [4]. After the discovery of the beta receptors the first β-blockers were synthesized and later on Sir James W. Black was the first to use propranolol for the management of angina pectoris [5]. His contribution was considered to be one of the most important to clinical medicine and as such he received the Nobel Prize for his work. β -Blockers became very popular for their cardiac clinical uses in angina pectoris, post myocardial infarction, hypertension, and arrhythmias. The first study which tested the use of β -blockers for the treatment of heart failure (HF) was published in 1975 [6] and afterwards many randomized controlled clinical trials in the 1980s and 1990s established the use of β -blockers in the treatment of HF.

5.2 Beta Adrenergic Receptors Physiology

Beta adrenergic receptors (β-ARs) are members of the G protein-coupled receptor (GPCR) superfamily with widespread expression and cardiovascular functions. Three subtypes of β-ARs have been cloned, the β_1-, β_2- and β_3-AR [7–9]. A fourth subtype has been suggested based on pharmacologic studies, but it has not yet been cloned and could represent a particular state of one of the known subtypes [10]. Traditionally, β-ARs can be distinguished according to their affinity to epinephrine and norepinephrine. The endogenous norepinephrine is ten-fold more selective for the β_1- compared to the β_2-AR subtype, while β_2-and β_3-AR subtypes have higher affinity to epinephrine. Under physiologic conditions the human heart expresses both β_1-and β_2-ARs and their stimulation increases cardiac contractility (positive inotropic effect), frequency (positive chronotropic effect), and rate of relaxation (lusitropic effect) as well as impulse conduction through the atrioventricular node (positive dromotropic effect). In fact, about 70–80 % of the expressed receptors are of the β_1-AR subtype and approximately 20–30 % of the β_2-AR subtype [11, 12]. Cardiac contractility is primarily regulated by the predominant cardiomyocyte β_1-AR subtype. The vasodilatory β_2-AR subtype contributes to blood pressure control and pathways activated by cardiomyocyte β_2-ARs provide inotropic support. The β_3-AR subtype is mainly related to noncardiac metabolic actions in adipose tissue and the gastrointestinal tract. However, direct cardiac actions of cardiomyocyte β_3-AR subtype have been also identified, indicating that unlike β_1-and β_2-AR subtypes, β_3-AR subtype activation may result in inhibition of myocardial contractility mediated by the nitric oxide synthase pathway [13, 14].

5.2.1 β-AR Activation

Agonist-induced activation of β-ARs catalyzes the exchange of guanosine triphosphate for guanosine diphosphate on the Gα-subunit and causes a conformational change in the receptor protein resulting in the dissociation of the heterotrimeric G protein into its active subunit components, $G\alpha_s$ and Gβγ [15]. The heterogeneity of G-protein α subunit, of which there are more than 20 subtypes (Gs, Gi, Gq, Go, and so on), is the central basis of GPCR signaling. In the human heart, activation of β_1- and β_2-ARs is the most powerful physiologic mechanism to acutely increase cardiac performance. β_1-ARs activate Gs proteins whereas β_2-ARs use both Gi and Gs proteins. Gs signaling acts as a "receptor-accelerator," while Gi signaling as a "receptor-brake" [16]. Gs signaling results in stimulation of adenylyl cyclases leading to dissociation of adenosine triphosphate (ATP) into the second messenger adenosine cyclic monophosphate (cAMP), which in turn binds to the regulatory subunits of protein kinase A (PK-A), causing the release of active catalytic PK-A subunits. PK-A phosphorylates serine and threonine residues on a number of proteins thereby affecting a spectrum of cellular processes and multiple gene expression patterns. Important PK-A-induced phosphorylation targets include: (1) the L-type calcium channels and ryanodine receptors, both leading to an increase in Ca^{2+} entry into the cell [17]; (2) the hyperpolarization-activated cyclic nucleotide-gated channels, which generate the hyperpolarization-activated cation inward current (I_f) affecting the initiation and modulation of rhythmic activity in cardiac pacemaker cells [18]; (3) phospholamban, a modulator of the sarcoplasmic reticulum associated ATP dependent calcium pump, which accelerates Ca^{2+} reuptake by the sarcoplasmic reticulum accelerating cardiac relaxation [19]; (4) troponin I and myosin binding protein-C, which reduce myofilament sensitivity to Ca^{2+} accelerating the relaxation of myofilaments [19]; (5) phospholemman, a subunit of Na^+/K^+-ATPase, relieving its inhibitory influence and resulting in the stimulation of the sodium pump [20]; and (6) the sarcoplasmic reticular Ca^{2+}/ATPase inhibitory protein (Fig. 5.1).

Furthermore, PK-A phosphorylates protein β-ARs themselves, resulting in partial uncoupling and desensitization of the receptor to further agonist stimulation [21]. As mentioned above, the β_1- and β_2-AR signaling pathways are both coupled to stimulation adenylyl cyclases. However, there is a marked difference between the two receptor subtypes. It seems that in human ventricular myocardium, stimulation of the β_2 -AR is much more efficiently coupled to the production of cAMP than is the β_1-AR [12, 22]. Myocardial contractility appears to be better associated with total β-AR density and β_2-ARs do not appear to stimulate contractility more efficiently than β_1-ARs [23].

Stimulation of β-ARs can also lead to the activation of MAP kinase members in a sub-selective way [24, 25], e.g. jun kinase and p38 kinase families [26]. These findings indicate that β-AR signaling pathways have significant mitogenic and proapoptotic actions. In particular, it has become clear that the β_1- and β_2-AR signaling pathways can be quite distinct [27]. For example, the β_1-AR appears to be coupled primarily to the Gs/adenylyl cyclase/PK-A pathway and to modulation of L-type Ca^{++} channels and phospholamban. On the contrary, the β_2-AR is not only coupled to Gs/adenylyl cyclase/PK-A, but also to the Gi pathway, and to "G protein-independent" functions such as regulation of the Na^+/H^+ exchanger.

As previously stated, cardiac function is mainly controlled by β-ARs and signaling and expression are tightly controlled by G protein–coupled receptor kinases (GRKs), which induce GPCR internalization and signal termination through phosphorylation. The GRKs are a family of cytosolic serine/threonine kinases consisting of seven isoforms that share structural and functional similarities [28]. The GRKs are classified into three subfamilies: (1) the rhodopsin kinase GRK1 and visual pigment kinase GRK7, (2) the β-AR kinases (or GRK2 and 3), and (3) the GRK4 group (GRK4–6). GRK2, GRK3, GRK5, and GRK6

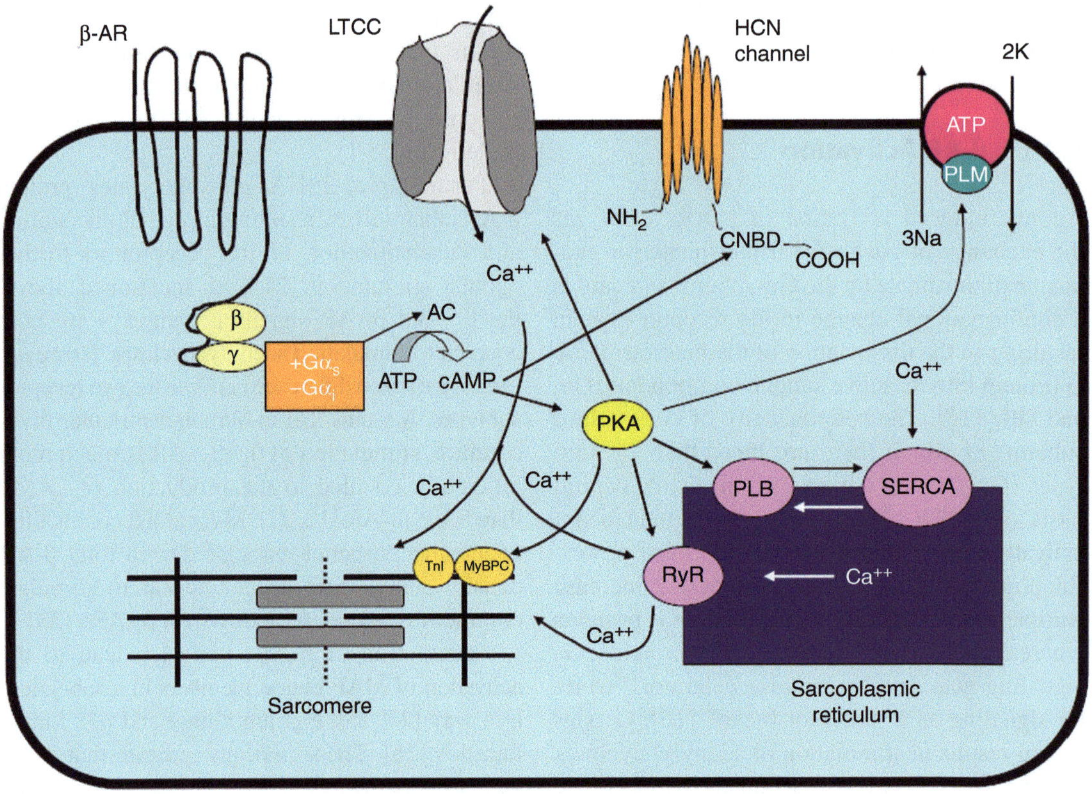

Fig. 5.1 β-AR signaling. The major intracellular effect of the sympathetic transmitters norepinephrine and epinephrine is mediated by formation of 3', 5'-cyclic monophosphate (*cAMP*), which increases the activity of the cAMP-dependent protein kinase A (*PKA*). PKA mediates a series of phosphorylations in diverse intracellular substrates, including the L-type Ca^{++} channels (*LTTC*), hyperpolarization-activated cyclic nucleotide-gated (*HCN*) channels, sarcoplasmic ryanodine receptors (*RyR*), phospholamban (*PLN*), myofibrillar proteins troponin I (*TnI*), cardiac myosin-binding protein C (*MyBPC*), and phospholemman (*PLM*). *AC* adenylyl cyclase, *AR* adrenergic receptor, *ATP* adenosine triphosphate, *CNBD* cyclic nucleotide-binding domain, $G_{alpha-i}$ and $G_{alpha-s}$ G protein alpha-subunit subtypes, *SERCA* sarcoendoplasmic reticulum (Adapted by permission from Triposkiadis et al. [21])

are expressed in a wide variety of tissues, whereas other GRKs display a more restricted expression pattern. GRK2, initially identified as βARK1 (βAR kinase-1), and GRK5 are the most abundant GRKs expressed in the heart [29].

Cardiac contractility is mainly controlled by catecholamines that are either locally released from sympathetic neurons or by circulating catecholamines that are released from the adrenal gland. When catecholamine levels are increased, there is an acute physiologic stimulation of cardiac β-ARs resulting in an adaptive increase in cardiac output, which ultimately activates a negative feedback loop to suppress further catecholamine release. β-AR desensitization and signal cessation is mediated by GRKs via agonist-receptor interactions. GRKs phosphorylate β-ARs in an agonist-occupancy dependent manner. When β-ARs are stimulated, the dissociated G protein βγ subunits interact with GRKs, bringing the kinases within close proximity of the transmembrane β-ARs. The resultant phosphorylation of β-ARs by GRKs reduces the affinity of the receptor for the stimulatory G protein, Gs, and consequently increases the affinity of interaction for the inhibitory G protein, Gi [30]. Furthermore, phosphorylation leads to the interaction of β-ARs with β-arrestin adaptor proteins which facilitate the internalization of receptors into endosomic vesicles. These processes are involved in receptor resensitization/reexpression and in receptor downregulation.

5.3 β-ARs and Cardiovascular Diseases

Reduced β-AR density and activity associated with elevated cardiac GRK expression and activity have been described in various cardiovascular diseases (CVD). Clinical and experimental studies suggest that this GRK-mediated receptor desensitization is initially an adaptive/protective mechanism because chronic β-AR stimulation can be deleterious to the heart. In the failing heart, diminishing cardiac output triggers a vicious cycle of persistent sympathetic activation, resulting in further β-AR desensitization and maladaptive signaling due in large part to GRK-mediated receptor phosphorylation and loss of responsiveness to sympathetic stimulation. GRKs are upregulated in HF and thus contribute to the decrease in β-AR signal transduction [31]. Desensitization of the β-AR has been associated with upregulation of GRK2 both at the mRNA and at the protein level.

Failing hearts have been shown to have desensitized β-adrenergic receptor signaling and this adaptive mechanism may help maintain cardiac function in HF [32]. Norepinephrine stimulates all β-AR (β_1-, β_2- and β_3-AR) subtypes and induces apoptosis (APO) in cardiomyocytes. Several mechanisms of β-AR stimulation-induced APO have been reported [33] (Fig. 5.2). However, not all subtypes of β-AR-mediated signaling induce cardiomyocyte APO. It is thought that the β_1-AR-mediated pathway mainly contributes to this cell death process [34]. Although all three subtypes are coupled to Gsα, β_2-AR and β_3-AR are also linked to the Gi protein. The β_2-AR exerts antiapoptotic effects through Gi βγ, phosphatidyl inositol-3 kinase (PI3K), and Akt (also known as protein kinase B) activation [35]. The β_3-AR expression is upregulated in the failing heart [36]. It is reported, that unlike β_1- and β_2-AR stimulation by catecholamines, β_3-AR negatively modulates ventricular contractility by activating endothelial nitric oxide synthase (eNOS). Catecholamines activate both positively inotropic and negatively inotropic path-

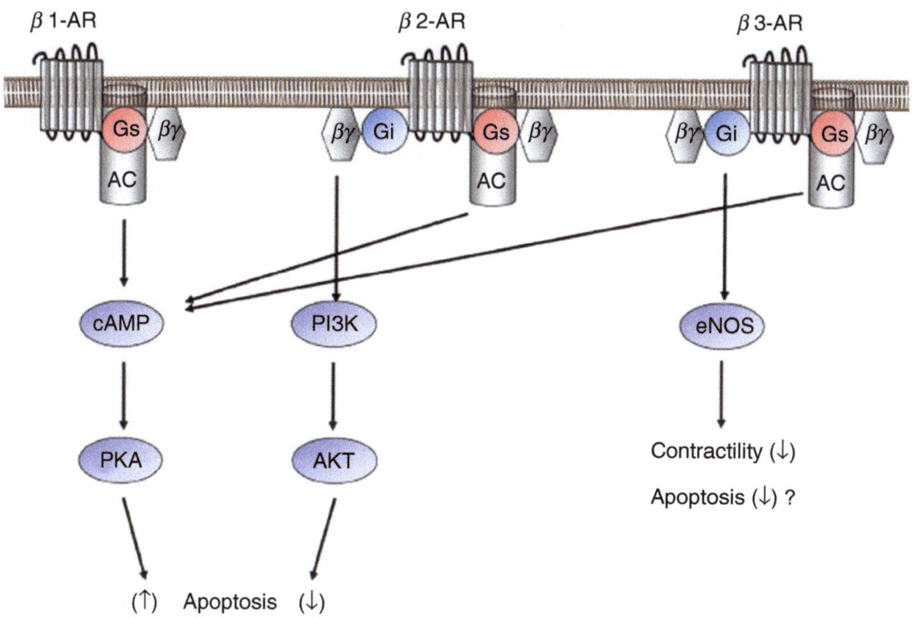

Fig. 5.2 The β-adrenergic receptor (β-AR) receptor-mediated signaling pathway for apoptosis. Three β-AR subtypes (β_1-AR, β_2-AR, and β_3-AR) are expressed in cardiomyocytes. Although all 3 subtypes are coupled to Gs, β_2-AR and β_3-AR are also linked to the Gi protein. β_1-AR is thought to be mainly involved in the apoptosis of cardiomyocytes. β_2-AR exerts antiapoptotic effects through Giβγ, PI3K, and Akt activation. β_3-AR negatively modulates ventricular contractility through endothelial nitric oxide synthase (eNOS) activation and might also be involved in the apoptosis of cardiomyocytes (Modified by permission from Fujita and Ishikawa [33])

ways in human cardiomyocytes, with β_1- and β_2-AR mediating the positive inotropic effect, while β_3-AR mediate a negative inotropic effect through eNOS overexpression [14]. Although the role of β_3-AR-mediated signaling in cardiomyocyte APO is still unknown, it is possible that β_3-AR exerts anti-apoptotic effects through nitric oxide as well [37].

The observation that stimulation of the β_1-AR (Gsα coupling) appears to promote APO in cardiomyocytes whereas stimulation of the β_2-AR (Gi $\beta\gamma$ coupling) induces antiapoptotic effects [38] has been confirmed in animal models. In rats with myocardial infarction, treatment for 2 weeks with β_2-AR agonists preserved cardiac contractility and reduced the number of apoptotic cardiomyocytes [39]. It has been shown that cardiac overexpression of the human β_2-AR in a transgenic mouse [40] produced a significant increase in cardiac contractility while overexpression of a mini-peptide inhibitor of βARK produced a hyperdynamic mouse with no apparent histopathology [41]. In contrast, a transgenic mouse overexpressing the human β_1-AR in ventricular myocardium [42, 43], unlike the β_2-AR overexpressing mouse, demonstrated a time dependent reduction in myocardial contractility as well as marked myocyte hypertrophy, myofibrillar disarray and replacement fibrosis. In addition, the β_1-AR transgenic mouse demonstrated upregulation of proapoptotic proteins and increased APO of cardiomyocytes. Thus regarding APO, the β_1-AR mouse is more similar to transgenic mice overexpressing the stimulatory G protein, Gαs [44], than it is to the β_2-AR mouse. It has been also shown that β-AR blockade in Gαs overexpressing mice can prevent the myocardial damage seen in this transgenic mouse model [45]. Therefore, attenuation of Gαs signaling, and presumably β_1-AR signaling by β-blockade, strengthens the positive clinical data of the use of β-blockade in HF treatment.

5.4 Beta Adrenergic Receptors and Heart Failure

HF is associated to dramatic changes in neurohormonal balance. To compensate for the reduced effective arterial volume because of the diminished cardiac output, the autonomous nervous system (ANS) and the Renin-Angiotensin-Aldosterone System (RAAS) are highly activated. As a consequence of ANS hyperactivity, norepinephrine (NE) and epinephrine plasma levels increase, due to adrenal gland secretion and adrenergic terminal spillover, thus leading to chronic sympathetic stimulation of the heart. Such stimulation of cardiac β-ARs increases oxygen demand and myocardial work, thus contributing to cardiac muscle stress. Chronic ANS activation is also responsible for the selective down-regulation of β_1-AR and for the functional uncoupling of both β_1- and β_2-ARs from their intracellular coupling mechanisms. These events are determined by activation of GRKs, particularly GRK2. Indeed, it has been demonstrated that, in chronic HF, GRK2 is up-regulated in cardiomyocytes, thus leading to a reduced responsiveness of the cardiac muscle to catecholamine stimulation [29]. GRK2-induced AR uncoupling and down-regulation also occur in the adrenal gland, where the inhibitory feedback on catecholamine release mediated by inhibitory α_2-ARs is reduced, thus determining an increase of circulating epinephrine [46].

In the failing human heart, the β_1-AR undergoes subtype selective downregulation at both the levels of mRNA and protein such that the β_1:β_2-AR subtype proportions become approximately equal [32]. Although there are some differences based on the etiology of HF, the extent of β_1-AR downregulation correlates well with the severity of heart disease. The expression of myocardial β_1-ARs also correlates well with systemic or coronary sinus plasma NE concentrations. A striking feature of HF is a characteristic set of molecular alterations in the components of the β-AR signaling pathway, including a decrease in β_1-AR density and messenger ribonucleic acid, uncoupling of β_1-AR from Gs, increased Gi protein and messenger ribonucleic acid, and impaired compartmentalization of cAMP/protein kinase A signaling [47–49]. β_1-AR abnormalities have been attributed to the recruitment of both β-AR kinase-1 and phosphoinositide 3-kinase to the ligand-activated receptor complex [50, 51]. In addition, the levels of both Gi signaling proteins and the G-protein receptor kinases are increased. It seems that β-AR desensitization is a predominantly protective adaptation, which follows the increase in NE plasma levels that keeps intracellular cAMP concentration constant [52]. As mentioned above, this is further supported by the fact that overexpression of human β_1-ARs in transgenic mice initially augments cardiac function but eventually leads to pathologic hypertrophy and HF [43, 53]. Many of the changes to the β-AR pathways associated with HF are also produced by the normal process of aging and there is also a good correlation between β_1-AR density and age; the older the individual, the lower the β_1-AR density [54].

Aging, like HF, does not appear to have a significant effect on β_2-AR density. The role of β_2-ARs in HF has not been delineated clearly [21]. In the failing human heart the β_2-AR may be uncoupled from its signaling pathway but it is not downregulated. There are a number of potential explanations for this. First, the endogenous catecholamine, NE, is approximately 10–30-fold more selective for the β_1- than the β_2-AR. Second, the β_1-AR appears to be localized to the synaptic cleft, thus it is more than likely exposed to higher concentrations of NE. Studies in transgenic animals have demonstrated that, in contrast to the early cardiomyopathy resulting from low-level (approx. 5-fold) cardiac overexpression of β_1-ARs, even a 100-fold overexpression of β_2-ARs in the mouse heart significantly increases cardiac contractile force without any cardiomyopathic consequences; extremely higher levels of overexpression (up to 350-fold) are needed to induce pathological changes [55]. Moreover, because β_2-AR signaling contributes to an increase in the levels of Gi, it has been suggested that this may activate a protective antiapoptotic pathway in the setting of catecholamine excess. Indeed, in an experimental study, selective inhibition of Gi signaling in response to myocardial ischemia was associated with a marked enhancement of myocardial infarct size and apoptotic signaling [56]. Because of the relative preservation of β_2-AR expression in the failing human heart, it has been the focus of therapeutic interest both for the development of β_2-AR-selective pharmacological agents, both agonist and antagonist, and for a gene-therapy approach of increased cardiac contractility [57].

β_3-AR mRNA is expressed in the human heart, but a corresponding receptor protein has not yet consistently been demonstrated. Furthermore, their physiological role remains highly controversial. For example, in human atria these receptors apparently do not promote cAMP formation and β_3-AR have no effect on atrial contraction but, as stated above, in human ventricles β_3-AR stimulation may exhibit negative inotropic effects [14]. However, more evidence is required that these effects indeed occur via β_3-AR [58]. The role of β_3-ARs in HF has not been fully elucidated. However, it has been proposed that in HF there is an excess of beta3-AR signaling, which exerts a negative inotropic effect potentially involving *Pertussis* toxin-sensitive G-proteins and activation of a NO synthase [36, 59].

In HF, sympathetic drive is selectively activated in several organ systems including the kidney, skeletal muscle and the heart. Increases in cardiac adrenergic activity result in marked increases in interstitial concentrations of NE within the failing human heart [60]. As discussed above, one consequence of the exposure of cardiomyocytes to high concentrations of NE is an alteration in cardiac adrenergic receptor pharmacology [48]. These changes decrease the sensitivity of cardiomyocytes to both endogenous and exogenous catecholamines. For example, there is a downward and rightward shift in dobutamine dose response curves in patients with heart failure compared to subjects with normal left ventricular function [61]. Maximal exercise workload as measured by peak VO_2 also falls in proportion to the loss of cardiac β-receptors [62].

Cardiomyocyte growth is modulated in part by β_1-, β_2- and α_1-ARs. Increases in signal transduction through these receptor pathways in the failing heart can contribute to pathological remodeling. Activation of these three receptors also results in increases in inotropic and chronotropic response. Myocardial energetics are adversely affected by these changes. Additionally, cardiac AR activation may promote arrhythmias. Another consequence of increased exposure of cardiomyocytes to increased concentrations of NE is myocyte toxicity. In tissue culture systems there is both a time- and concentration-dependent relationship between

NE exposure and cardiomyocyte death [63]. The toxic effects of NE incubation can be partially blocked with the addition of a β-AR antagonist and completely prevented with the addition of both a β- and α-blocker to the culture media. Apoptosis of cardiomyocytes can be induced in tissue culture by NE. This effect appears to be mediated primarily through the β_1-AR. Clinical examples of toxic effects of increased cardiac adrenergic drive include the observation of significant left ventricular dysfunction after catastrophic brain injury. However, the most compelling clinical support for the cardiotoxic role of cardiac NE are the beneficial effects that occur with the use of β-AR antagonists in patients with HF.

5.4.1 Beta Adrenergic Receptor Antagonists in Heart Failure

Beta adrenergic receptor antagonists (or β-blockers-BBs) are a wide and heterogeneous group of molecules acting as competitive and reversible antagonists of β-ARs. In addition to their ability to block β-AR-signaling, BBs show a variety of adjunctive actions that are often used as criteria for their classification. BBs can be classified according to β_1-AR selectivity, α-AR antagonism and vasodilation, intrinsic sympathomimetic activity (ISA), pharmacokinetics and other properties like metabolic effects. BBs can be also classified into generations: (1) *first generation*, which are nonselective and competitively block both the β_1- and β_2-AR (propranolol, nadolol, timolol); (2) *second generation*, with much higher affinity for the β_1- than for the β_2-AR (atenolol, metoprolol, bisoprolol); and (3) *third generation*, which may be selective (celiprolol, nebivolol) or nonselective (bucindolol, carvedilol, labetalol) but all cause peripheral vasodilation mediated via α_1-AR blockade (bucindolol, carvedilol, labetalol), β_2-AR agonism (celiprolol), or nitric oxide synthesis (nebivolol) [64]. Cardioselectivity of β-blockers is dose-dependent and decreases with larger doses. Both selective and nonselective agents have negative chronotropic and inotropic effects. Selective agents have a less inhibitory effect on the β_2- receptors and are less likely to cause peripheral vasoconstriction [65] and bronchial spasm. Exercise performance may be impaired to a lesser extent by β_1-selective agents, partially because β_2-blockade tends to blunt the exercise-induced increase in skeletal muscle blood flow. Finally, there are BBs that at low concentrations antagonize the cardiostimulant effects of catecholamines but at high concentrations cause cardiostimulation. These cardiostimulant BBs (e.g., pindolol, alprenolol, oxprenolol), widely known as nonconventional partial agonists, antagonize the effects of catecholamines through a high-affinity site (β_{1H}-AR), but cause cardiostimulation mainly through a low-affinity site (β_{1L}-AR) of the myocardial β_1-AR [66]. Nonconventional partial agonists are considered potentially arrhythmogenic and should not be used for HF treatment.

The majority of BBs are partially or totally metabolized by CYP2D6, whose gene has more than 90 different variants [67]. Individuals homozygous for nonfunctional alleles are considered poor metabolizers. Several inconsistencies have been reported regarding the genotype phenotype correlations for intermediate or extensive metabolizers [68]. Poor metabolizers treated with metoprolol have a five-fold higher risk for adverse effects [69], whereas the adverse effects of carvedilol and bisoprolol are less influenced by the genetic background [70, 71]. Various protective mechanisms have been attributed to BBs, namely: (1) inhibition of catecholamine cardiotoxic effects; (2) β_1-AR up-regulation (carvedilol is an exception); (3) attenuation of neurohumoral vasoconstrictive, growth-promoting, and pro-apoptotic systems (renin-angiotensin-aldosterone system, endothelin); (4) subendocardial coronary flow enhancement (as a result of diastolic prolongation); (5) restoration of the reflex control on the heart and circulation; and (6) improved myocardial performance by reducing heart rate and oxygen demand [72]. Among all BBs, bisoprolol, carvedilol, metoprolol and nebivolol are almost universally approved for the treatment of chronic HF [21]. Chronic BB therapy improves left ventricular performance and reverses left ventricular remodeling, reduces risk of hospitalization, and improves survival as will be further described.

5.4.1.1 Effects of β-Blocker Therapy in Heart Failure

Therapy of chronic HF with β-AR blockers has distinct acute (pharmacologic) and chronic (biologic) effects. The pharmacologic effects are the consequence of the acute changes in function that occur with withdrawal of sympathetic agonism and include a decrease in heart rate and contractile state. These detrimental effects can be tolerated only by initiating therapy with very low doses of β-blocker and slow up-titration of the dose over several weeks. There is significant variation in the severity of myocardial depression with different generations of BBs. Nonselective BBs such as propranolol reduce the contractile state and increase systemic resistance which profoundly decreases cardiac output [73]. As a consequence, the intolerance to initiation of propranolol is high (>20 %) and these agents have not been successfully used in long-term placebo-controlled trials. The initiation of β_1-AR-selective β-blockers such as metoprolol and bisoprolol is much better tolerated by HF patients. This appears to occur because unblocked β_2-ARs can support cardiac function either directly or indirectly (by β_2-AR-mediated facilitation of sympathetic norepinephrine release). In addition, peripheral β_2-ARs can mediate vasodilation. Thus, the overall detrimental effect upon organ perfusion is less severe than that observed with first generation compounds. β_1-AR-selective BBs have been utilized successfully in prospective trials in HF with a tolerability >80 %. The third generation BBs possess vasodilator properties which counteract the negative properties of adrenergic withdrawal. This permits a more comprehensive blockade of cardiac adrenergic pathways with high tolerability (≥90 % in clinical trials of carvedilol and bucindolol).

5.4.1.2 β-Blockers Clinical Trials in Heart Failure

BB treatment in HF results in improvements in right heart hemodynamics, reversal of ventricular remodeling (as evidenced by reductions in left ventricular volumes, increases in right and left ventricular ejection fraction (LVEF), decreases in left ventricular mass and favorable effects upon left ventricular geometry), and improvements in HF symptoms [74]. To date, four specific BBs have been shown to be effective in the treatment of HF: metoprolol, bisoprolol, carvedilol and nebivolol [75]. (1) The Metoprolol in Dilated Cardiomyopathy trial, studied metoprolol tartrate (100–150 mg daily) which showed a trend toward a reduction in morbidity of patients with idiopathic dilated cardiomyopathy [76]. (2) The Metoprolol CR/XL Randomized Intervention Trial in Congestive Heart Failure (MERIT-HF) used a more effective formula with metoprolol succinate and showed a significant relative risk reduction in mortality in patients with New York Heart Association (NYHA) functional class II–IV [77, 78]. (3) The Cardiac Insufficiency Bisoprolol Study II (CIBIS-II) demonstrated bisoprolol improved all-cause mortality by 32 %, sudden cardiac death by 45 % and reduced HF hospitalization by 30 % [79]. (4) The Australian New Zealand Heart Failure Research Collaborative Group (ANZ-HeFT) demonstrated significant improvement in left ventricular function and a significant reduction of left ventricular end diastolic volume index in a carvedilol group at 12 months in patients with NYHA class II or III [80]. Similarly, the Carvedilol Prospective Randomized Cumulative Survival (COPERNICUS) trial showed benefit in patients with NYHA class IV and an ejection fraction of <25 % with 38 % mortality risk reduction at 12 months [81]. The CAPRICORN trial focused on post myocardial infarction (MI) patients with LV dysfunction with ejection fraction of <40 % and incorporated current recommended therapy with the treatment of ACE inhibitors. The study demonstrated a 23 % further reduction of mortality with patients also receiving carvedilol 25 mg twice daily [82]. Long-term survival was good, particularly in patients with a nonischemic etiology for their dilated cardiomyopathy [83]. Finally, the SENIORS trial focused on elderly patients (>70 years old) with HF (ejection fraction <35 %) which demonstrated that nebivolol is an effective and well-tolerated treatment in this selected patient group [84].

5.4.1.3 Comparison Between β-Blockers

As previously mentioned, results from clinical trials demonstrated that blockade of β-AR signaling has beneficial effects in HF, both reducing mortality and improving symptoms of impaired cardiac function. Such protection has been demonstrated for different molecules belonging to BB class, and the degree of the beneficial effects was quite similar for any of the chosen drug. Thus, the idea existed that BB efficacy in HF was due to a "class effect." On the other hand, many researchers have pointed out that specific pharmacodynamics and/or pharmacokinetic properties (β_1-AR-selectivity, vasodilating actions, anti-oxidant activity, "pleiotropic effects", adequate bioavailability and low drug-drug interaction risk) could represent valuable characteristics for preferring a specific β-blocker over others in the treatment of HF. To verify this hypothesis, a specific head-to-head clinical trial was conducted in 2003. The Carvedilol or Metoprolol European Trial (COMET) study aimed to compare the mortality risk-reducing effects in 3,029 patients with HF randomized to receive either carvedilol 25 mg twice daily or metoprolol tartrate 50 mg twice daily, after a mean follow-up of 58 months. The results demonstrated that carvedilol decreased mortality by 17 % with respect to metoprolol [85]. However, subsequent analyses showed that the degree of β-blockade reached with the formulation of metoprolol used in the study (metoprolol tartrate) was not adequate, and probably not similar to that of the carvedilol arm. Basically, metoprolol tartrate should have been titrated up in the COMET study [86]. An answer to this issue has been also pursued by several meta analyses, most of which have been focused on carvedilol, possibly because of its unique pharmacodynamics profile. Nevertheless, results from these studies seem to be conflicting. In a systematic review of 11 randomized controlled trials in 5,207 patients, it was found that carvedilol reduced all-cause mortality in patients with HF significantly more when compared to other β-blockers such as atenolol, bisoprolol and metoprolol. The superiority of carvedilol over other β-blockers could be attributed to the special properties of carvedilol, such as: antiarrhythmic effect (and consequent reduction in the risk of sudden death), a more sustained increase in LVEF when compared to other β-blockers, blockade of up-regulated β_2-AR and vasodilation [87]. By contrast, in another meta-analysis of 21 trials including 23,122 HF patients, no significant differences were found in mortality outcome among the β-blockers considered (atenolol, bisoprolol, bucindolol, carvedilol, metoprolol, and nebivolol), thus concluding that the beneficial of β-blockers were due to a "class effect." Nonetheless, carvedilol showed the lowest cardiac mortality among all β-blockers tested, although this was not statistically significant [88]. Lack of clear data from clinical trials regarding the superiority of a given BB is reflected in the 2012 ESC guidelines for the management of HF, in which the use of a particular BB over the others is not recommended [75].

5.4.1.4 Pharmacogenomics and Therapeutic Impact of β-AR Polymorphisms

As for many other pharmacological treatments, variability in clinical and functional outcomes exists also for BB administration in HF patients. Actually, BB treatment fails to improve LVEF in a variable proportion of subjects, while a minority of patients experience worsening of HF symptoms during BB titration [89]. Such differences could be explained, at least in part, by genetic variation influencing BB pharmacodynamics and/or pharmacokinetics. To date, polymorphisms in β_1-AR, β_2-AR, GRK-5, CYP2C6, NET and UGT1A1 have been associated to variability in BB response.

Many studies have examined the impact of the aforementioned polymorphisms in response to β-blockade among HF patients. Preliminary studies in patients treated with various BBs have demonstrated a survival benefit [90] and a significant reduction in left ventricular end diastolic diameter [91] for those who carried the Gly49 allele as compared to the Ser49 homozygous patients. A similar reversal of the remodeling process has been reported for Arg389-homozygous HF patients treated with carvedilol as compared with

Gly389-homozygous [92] and Arg389Gly-heterozygous patients [93]. However, neutral results have also been reported. For example, no survival benefit was observed for the Ser49Gly or the Arg389Gly patients treated with carvedilol [94, 95], bisoprolol [94], or metoprolol [95], and for the Arg389-homozygous or Gly389 patients treated with metoprolol CR/XL [96]. Finally, a dose-dependent response to beta-blockade has been reported, whereby low doses in patients carrying the Gly49 allele portend worse outcomes than in Ser49-homozygous patients, whereas in higher doses, genotype dependent differences are not observed [97]. More recent data, however, suggest improvement in the therapeutic effect of bucindolol by pharmacogenetic targeting. In the deoxyribonucleic acid substudy of the Beta Blocker Evaluation of Survival Trial (BEST) [98], patients carrying the Arg389 genotype had a greater agonist promoted ventricular contractility along with improved age-, sex-, and race-adjusted survival than the Gly389 carriers [99].

Taken together, these results, although suggestive of the possibility to select BB according to a particular genotype, are not conclusive, thus requiring large prospective clinical trials. In this respect, the use of genetic polymorphisms as potential tools to guide therapeutic strategies seems a promising new approach. The subject of genetic polymorphisms is described in Chap. 7.

5.4.1.5 GRK2 as a Potential Target in Heart Failure Treatment

As mentioned above, the up-regulation of GRK2 (and also probably GRK5) caused by SNS activation acts as a "brake" for cardiac β-AR signaling and this is a partial reason why BBs have beneficial effects in HF as they can block the noxious effects of catecholamines on the cardiomyocyte. However, increased GRK2 activity has proven to be maladaptive in HF and its inhibition has emerged as a therapeutic target [100]. Interestingly, chronic BB use in HF models has been shown to decrease GRK2 expression levels, which could contribute to BBs' therapeutic effects [101, 102].

It has been shown that lowering GRK2 expression or activity in the injured, stressed or failing heart can prevent or reverse ventricular dysfunction at the functional and morphological level [103]. This has been shown using a peptide inhibitor known as the βARKct ($G_{\beta\gamma}$ protein sequestering peptide) and also in GRK2 knockout (KO) mice. First, cardiac-specific βARKct transgenic mice were created showing increased inotropic reserve [104] and these mice have been used to prevent HF in several genetic mouse models [105–107]. In addition, viral-mediated βARKct delivery to rats, rabbits, and pigs have shown significant beneficial effects including improved cardiac function and reverse ventricular remodeling [102, 108–111]. Similar findings were noted by induced KO of GRK2 in mice, after HF was evident, and this is consistent with βARKct-mediated inhibition of GRK2 [112]. Although there are some minor differences between GRK2 inhibition with βARKct and GRK2 KO, the data is overwhelming in supporting GRK2 inhibition as beneficial in the failing heart [112–114]. Importantly, a large animal HF study has been done that demonstrates the clinical potential of βARKct-mediated gene therapy [111]. This study used adeno-associated virus serotype-6 (AAV6) to deliver βARKct to a post-ischemic HF model in the pig [111, 115]. It was found that AAV6-βARKct delivery ameliorated LV function, and suppressed adverse cardiac remodeling and fetal gene expression in this model [111]. Of note, this study in pigs had similar results found with AAV6-βARKct delivery to a rat model of HF where it was also shown that βARKct worked significantly better that β-blockade alone and the two were complementary together [102]. Of importance, both of these studies showed that chronic GRK2 inhibition results in significant lowering of catecholamines and aldosterone demonstrating feedback to decrease the neurohormonal outflow associated with negative prognosis in HF [102, 111]. These two studies in particular are important as they show reversal of the disease process and the pig study closely reflect human pathophysiology and is a pre-requisite for future clinical trials.

Gene therapy for HF is now becoming a reality and AAV6-βARKct trials are in the planning stages; GRK2 inhibition by small pharmacological agents would offer many advantages to the HF patients [116]. Interestingly, several recent molecules have been developed and described that have GRK2 inhibitory properties. Two decades ago, heparin and related compounds were shown to block GRK2 activity but the direct access to GRK2, the high concentration and the intrinsic cytotoxicity made them not useful for *in vivo* administration [116]. RNA molecules such as aptamers have been also investigated as a new approach to efficiently block GRK2 activity and the RNA-aptamer C13, was shown to be able to bind to GRK2 with a high affinity and inhibit GRK2-catalyzed rhodopsin phosphorylation [117]. Molecules that target the GRK2-Gβγ protein-protein interaction and thus, have mechanisms identical to the βARKct have recently emerged. Gallein is a related molecule that blocks GRK2-Gβγ and it has also shown positive results *in vivo* [118]. However, these compounds are not true pharmacological agents and have severe limitations that preclude human use [119].

Recently, it was found that an existing FDA-approved drug has significant GRK2 inhibitory properties and potentially this off-target effect may be seen in humans. The serotonin reuptake inhibitor (SSRI), paroxetine has affinity for GRK2 and has significant GRK2 inhibitory properties *in vitro* and *in vivo* [120]. Paroxetine binds in the active site of GRK2 and stabilizes the kinase domain in a novel conformation in which a unique regulatory loop forms part of the ligand binding site [120]. Pretreatment *in vivo* of mice with paroxetine before isoproterenol administration significantly increases left ventricular inotropic reserve with no significant effect on heart rate [120]. This agent used for clinical depression probably is not viable for use as a specific GRK2 inhibitor but is a promising starting point for chemistry to develop novel GRK2 inhibitors that can be used eventually for cardiovascular disorders.

Conclusions

β-ARs are the most important GPCR class expressed in the human heart and represent the most powerful means to increase the pumping function of the heart. In particular, β-ARs are the prime modulators of heart rate and myocardial contractility in response to catecholamines originating from the SNS. From the discovery and characterization to their manipulation in clinical practices, β-ARs have been shown to play an important role in cardiac disease, and heart failure in particular. Their alterations lead to pathways desensitization and most importantly result in harmful effects upon the myocardium that lead to pathologic ventricular remodeling and heart failure progression.

Many large multicenter trials have shown that therapy with β_1-selective and third-generation BBs results in significant improvements in cardiac function and clinical outcomes. BBs use is strongly recommended in all current guidelines for patient with symptomatic HF and impaired systolic function, unless there is a contraindication. Although wide, randomized, controlled clinical trials have investigated efficacy of four molecules, thus driving to the registration of carvedilol, metoprolol, bisoprolol and nebivolol for the treatment of HF, it appears reasonable to suppose that BBs' efficacy lies in their ability to counteract adrenergic overactivation, more than in additional, molecule-related properties. Such consideration is supported by different meta-analyses suggesting that BBs efficacy should be considered as a class effect. However, certain actions of distinct BBs (i.e., vasodilation, NO release, antioxidant activity, anti-proliferation effect on vascular smooth muscle cells) might represent additional and useful tools for HF therapy and increase treatment tolerability, mainly in selected groups of patients. For instance, molecules such as carvedilol, which have been demonstrated to ameliorate insulin sensitivity, could be useful in patients with concomitant diabetes. Moreover, analysis of genetic polymorphisms in β-ARs and metabolic enzymes, might also contribute to find "the best drug to the best patient." BBs are currently a cornerstone in HF therapy, and their use should be extended also to groups of patients commonly undertreated, such as the elderly or patients with comorbidities.

References

1. Langley JN. Preliminary notice of experiments on the physiological action of jaborandi. Br Med J. 1875;1:241–2.
2. Limbird LE. The receptor concept: a continuing evolution. Mol Interv. 2004;4:326–36.
3. von Euler US. Hormones of the sympathetic nervous system and the adrenal medulla. Br Med J. 1951; 1:105–8.
4. Ahlquist RP. A study of the adrenotropic receptors. Am J Physiol. 1948;153:586–600.
5. Stapleton MP. Sir James Black and propranolol: the role of the basic sciences in the history of cardiovascular pharmacology. Tex Heart Inst J. 1997;24:336–42.
6. Waagstein F, Hjalmarson A, Varnauskas E, Wallentin I. Effect of chronic beta-adrenergic receptor blockade in congestive cardiomyopathy. Br Heart J. 1975;37:1022–36.
7. Frielle T, Collins S, Daniel KW, Caron MG, Lefkowitz RJ, Kobilka BK. Cloning of the cDNA for the human beta 1-adrenergic receptor. Proc Natl Acad Sci U S A. 1987;84:7920–4.
8. Kobilka BK, Dixon RA, Frielle T, Dohlman HG, Bolanowski MA, Sigal IS, et al. cDNA for the human beta 2-adrenergic receptor: a protein with multiple membrane-spanning domains and encoded by a gene whose chromosomal location is shared with that of the receptor for platelet-derived growth factor. Proc Natl Acad Sci U S A. 1987;84:46–50.
9. Emorine LJ, Marullo S, Briend-Sutren MM, Patey G, Tate K, Delavier-Klutchko C, et al. Molecular characterization of the human beta 3-adrenergic receptor. Science. 1989;245:1118–21.
10. Granneman JG. The putative beta 4-adrenergic receptor is a novel state of the beta1-adrenergic receptor. Am J Physiol Endocrinol Metab. 2001; 280:E199–202.
11. Bristow MR, Ginsburg R, Umans V, Fowler M, Minobe W, Rasmussen R, et al. Beta 1- and beta 2-adrenergic-receptor subpopulations in nonfailing and failing human ventricular myocardium: coupling of both receptor subtypes to muscle contraction and selective beta 1-receptor down-regulation in heart failure. Circ Res. 1986;59:297–309.
12. Bristow MR, Anderson FL, Port JD, Skerl L, Hershberger RE, Larrabee P, et al. Differences in beta-adrenergic neuroeffector mechanisms in ischemic versus idiopathic dilated cardiomyopathy. Circulation. 1991;84:1024–39.
13. Gauthier C, Tavernier G, Charpentier F, Langin D, Le Marec H. Functional beta3- adrenoceptor in the human heart. J Clin Invest. 1996;98:556–62.
14. Gauthier C, Leblais V, Kobzik L, Trochu JN, Khandoudi N, Bril A, et al. The negative inotropic effect of beta3-adrenoceptor stimulation is mediated by activation of a nitric oxide synthase pathway in human ventricle. J Clin Invest. 1998;102:1377–84.
15. Lohse MJ, Engelhardt S, Eschenhagen T. What is the role of beta-adrenergic signaling in heart failure? Circ Res. 2003;93:896–906.
16. Feldman DS, Carnes CA, Abraham WT, Bristow MR. Mechanisms of disease: beta-adrenergic receptors—alterations in signal transduction and pharmacogenomics in heart failure. Nat Clin Pract Cardiovasc Med. 2005;2:475–83.
17. Zhao XL, Gutierrez LM, Chang CF, Hosey MM. The alpha 1-subunit of skeletal muscle L-type Ca channels is the key target for regulation by A-kinase and protein phosphatase-1C. Biochem Biophys Res Commun. 1994;198:166–73.
18. Ludwig A, Zong X, Jeglitsch M, Hofmann F, Biel M. A family of hyperpolarization-activated mammalian cation channels. Nature. 1998;393:587–91.
19. Sulakhe PV, Vo XT. Regulation of phospholamban and troponin-I phosphorylation in the intact rat cardiomyocytes by adrenergic and cholinergic stimuli: roles of cyclic nucleotides, calcium, protein kinases and phosphatases and depolarization. Mol Cell Biochem. 1995;149:103–26.
20. Despa S, Bossuyt J, Han F, Ginsburg KS, Jia LG, Kutchai H, et al. Phospholemman-phosphorylation mediates the beta-adrenergic effects on Na/K pump function in cardiac myocytes. Circ Res. 2005;97:252–9.
21. Triposkiadis F, Karayannis G, Giamouzis G, Skoularigis J, Louridas G, Butler J. The sympathetic nervous system in heart failure physiology, pathophysiology, and clinical implications. J Am Coll Cardiol. 2009;54:1747–62.
22. Levy FO, Zhu X, Kaumann AJ, Birnbaumer L. Efficacy of beta 1-adrenergic receptors is lower than that of beta 2-adrenergic receptors. Proc Natl Acad Sci U S A. 1993;90:10798–802.
23. Zhou YY, Cheng H, Bogdanov KY, Hohl C, Altschuld R, Lakatta EG, et al. Localized cAMP-dependent signaling mediates beta 2-adrenergic modulation of cardiac excitation-contraction coupling. Am J Physiol. 1997;273:H1611–8.
24. Bogoyevitch MA, Andersson MB, Gillespie-Brown J, Clerk A, Glennon PE, Fuller SJ, et al. Adrenergic receptor stimulation of the mitogen-activated protein kinase cascade and cardiac hypertrophy. Biochem J. 1996;314:115–21.
25. Luttrell LM, Ferguson SS, Daaka Y, Miller WE, Maudsley S, Della Rocca GJ, et al. Beta-arrestin-dependent formation of beta 2 adrenergic receptor-Src protein kinase complexes. Science. 1999;283:655–61.
26. Williams NG, Zhong H, Minneman KP. Differential coupling of alpha1-, alpha2-, and beta-adrenergic receptors to mitogen-activated protein kinase pathways and differentiation in transfected PC12 cells. J Biol Chem. 1998;273:24624–32.
27. Steinberg SF. The molecular basis for distinct beta-adrenergic receptor subtype actions in cardiomyocytes. Circ Res. 1999;85:1101–11.

28. Penela P, Ribas C, Mayor Jr F. Mechanisms of regulation of the expression and function of G protein-coupled receptor kinases. Cell Signal. 2003;15:973–81.
29. Rengo G, Perrone-Filardi P, Femminella GD, Liccardo D, Zincarelli C, de Lucia C, et al. Targeting the β-adrenergic receptor system through G-protein-coupled receptor kinase 2: a new paradigm for therapy and prognostic evaluation in heart failure: from bench to bedside. Circ Heart Fail. 2012;5:385–91.
30. Daaka Y, Luttrell LM, Lefkowitz RJ. Switching of the coupling of the beta2-adrenergic receptor to different G proteins by protein kinase A. Nature. 1997;390:88–91.
31. Ungerer M, Bohm M, Elce JS, Erdmann E, Lohse MJ. Altered expression of beta-adrenergic receptor kinase and beta 1-adrenergic receptors in the failing human heart. Circulation. 1993;87:454–63.
32. Bristow MR, Hershberger RE, Port JD, Gilbert EM, Sandoval A, Rasmussen R, et al. Beta-adrenergic pathways in nonfailing and failing human ventricular myocardium. Circulation. 1990;82 Suppl 2:I12–25.
33. Fujita T, Ishikawa Y. Apoptosis in heart failure. The role of the β-adrenergic receptor-mediated signaling pathway and p53-mediated signaling pathway in the apoptosis of cardiomyocytes. Circ J. 2011; 75:1811–8.
34. Zaugg M, Xu W, Lucchinetti E, Shafiq SA, Jamali NZ, Siddiqui MA. Beta-adrenergic receptor subtypes differentially affect apoptosis in adult rat ventricular myocytes. Circulation. 2000;102:344–50.
35. Zhu WZ, Zheng M, Koch WJ, Lefkowitz RJ, Kobilka BK, Xiao RP. Dual modulation of cell survival and cell death by beta(2)-adrenergic signaling in adult mouse cardiac myocytes. Proc Natl Acad Sci U S A. 2001;98:1607–12.
36. Moniotte S, Kobzik L, Feron O, Trochu JN, Gauthier C, Balligand JL. Upregulation of beta(3)-adrenoceptors and altered contractile response to inotropic amines in human failing myocardium. Circulation. 2001;103:1649–55.
37. Stefanelli C, Pignatti C, Tantini B, Stanic I, Bonavita F, Muscari C, et al. Nitric oxide can function as either a killer molecule or an antiapoptotic effector in cardiomyocytes. Biochim Biophys Acta. 1999;1450:406–13.
38. Communal C, Singh K, Sawyer DB, Colucci WS. Opposing effects of beta(1)- and beta(2)-adrenergic receptors on cardiac myocyte apoptosis: role of a pertussis toxin-sensitive G protein. Circulation. 1999; 100:2210–2.
39. Ahmet I, Krawczyk M, Heller P, Moon C, Lakatta EG, Talan MI. Beneficial effects of chronic pharmacological manipulation of beta adrenoreceptor subtype signaling in rodent dilated ischemic cardiomyopathy. Circulation. 2004;110:1083–90.
40. Milano CA, Allen LF, Rockman HA, Dolber PC, McMinn TR, Chien KR, et al. Enhanced myocardial function in transgenic mice overexpressing the beta 2-adrenergic receptor. Science. 1994;264:582–6.
41. Koch WJ, Rockman HA, Samama P, Hamilton RA, Bond RA, Milano CA, et al. Cardiac function in mice overexpressing the beta-adrenergic receptor kinase or a beta ARK inhibitor. Science. 1995;268:1350–3.
42. Bisognano JD, Weinberger HD, Bohlmeyer TJ, Pende A, Raynolds MV, Sastravaha A, et al. Myocardial-directed overexpression of the human beta(1)-adrenergic receptor in transgenic mice. J Mol Cell Cardiol. 2000;32:817–30.
43. Engelhardt S, Hein L, Wiesmann F, Lohse MJ. Progressive hypertrophy and heart failure in beta1-adrenergic receptor transgenic mice. Proc Natl Acad Sci U S A. 1999;96:7059–64.
44. Iwase M, Uechi M, Vatner DE, Asai K, Shannon RP, Kudej RK, et al. Cardiomyopathy induced by cardiac Gs alpha overexpression. Am J Physiol. 1997;272:H585–9.
45. Asai K, Yang GP, Geng YJ, Takagi G, Bishop S, Ishikawa Y, et al. Beta-adrenergic receptor blockade arrests myocyte damage and preserves cardiac function in the transgenic G(salpha) mouse. J Clin Invest. 1999;104:551–8.
46. Lymperopoulos A, Rengo G, Koch WJ. Adrenal adrenoceptors in heart failure: fine-tuning cardiac stimulation. Trends Mol Med. 2007;13:503–11.
47. Dodge-Kafka KL, Soughayer J, Pare GC, Carlisle Michel JJ, Langeberg LK, Kapiloff MS, et al. The protein kinase A anchoring protein mAKAP coordinates two integrated cAMP effector pathways. Nature. 2005;437:574–8.
48. Bristow MR, Ginsburg R, Minobe W, Cubicciotti RS, Sageman WS, Lurie K, et al. Decreased catecholamine sensitivity and beta-adrenergic-receptor density in failing human hearts. N Engl J Med. 1982;307:205–11.
49. Engelhardt S, Bohm M, Erdmann E, Lohse MJ. Analysis of beta-adrenergic receptor mRNA levels in human ventricular biopsy specimens by quantitative polymerase chain reactions: progressive reduction of beta 1-adrenergic receptor mRNA in heart failure. J Am Coll Cardiol. 1996;27:146–54.
50. Perrino C, Naga Prasad SV, Patel M, Wolf MJ, Rockman HA. Targeted inhibition of beta-adrenergic receptor kinase-1-associated phosphoinositide-3 kinase activity preserves beta-adrenergic receptor signaling and prolongs survival in heart failure induced by calsequestrin overexpression. J Am Coll Cardiol. 2005;45:1862–70.
51. Noma T, Lemaire A, Naga Prasad SV, Barki-Harrington L, Tilley DG, Chen J, et al. Beta-arrestin-mediated beta1-adrenergic receptor transactivation of the EGFR confers cardioprotection. J Clin Invest. 2007;117:2445–58.
52. Eschenhagen T. Beta-adrenergic signaling in heart failure-adapt or die. Nat Med. 2008;14:485–7.
53. Böhm M, Ettelbrück S, Flesch M, van Gilst WH, Knorr A, Maack C, et al. Beta-adrenergic signal transduction following carvedilol treatment in hypertensive cardiac hypertrophy. Cardiovasc Res. 1998;40:146–55.

54. White M, Roden R, Minobe W, Khan MF, Larrabee P, Wollmering M, et al. Age related changes in beta-adrenergic neuroeffector systems in the human heart. Circulation. 1994;90:1225–38.
55. Liggett SB, Tepe NM, Lorenz JN, Canning AM, Jantz TD, Mitarai S, et al. Early and delayed consequences of beta(2)-adrenergic receptor overexpression in mouse hearts: critical role for expression level. Circulation. 2000;101:1707–14.
56. DeGeorge Jr BR, Gao E, Boucher M, Vinge LE, Martini JS, Raake PW, et al. Targeted inhibition of cardiomyocyte Gi signaling enhances susceptibility to apoptotic cell death in response to ischemic stress. Circulation. 2008;117:1378–87.
57. Drazner MH, Peppel KC, Dyer S, Grant AO, Koch WJ, Lefkowitz RJ. Potentiation of beta adrenergic signaling by adenoviral-mediated gene transfer in adult rabbit ventricular myocytes. J Clin Invest. 1997;99:288–96.
58. Michel MC, Harding SE, Bond RA. Are there functional β_3-adrenoceptors in the human heart? Br J Pharmacol. 2011;162:817–22.
59. Morimoto A, Hasegawa H, Cheng HJ, Little WC, Cheng CP. Endogenous beta3-adrenoreceptor activation contributes to left ventricular and cardiomyocyte dysfunction in heart failure. Am J Physiol Heart Circ Physiol. 2004;286:H2425–33.
60. Joseph J, Gilbert EM. The sympathetic nervous system in chronic heart failure. Prog Cardiovasc Dis. 1998;41:9–16.
61. Fowler MB, Laser JA, Hopkins GL, Minobe W, Bristow MR. Assessment of the beta-adrenergic receptor pathway in the intact failing human heart. progressive receptor down-regulation and subsensitivity to agonist response. Circulation. 1986;74:1290–302.
62. White M, Yanowitz F, Gilbert EM, Larrabee P, O'Connell JB, Anderson JL, et al. Role of beta-adrenergic receptor downregulation in the peak exercise response in patients with heart failure due to idiopathic dilated cardiomyopathy. Am J Cardiol. 1995;76:1271–6.
63. Mann DL, Kent RL, Parsons B, Cooper GT. Adrenergic effects on the biology of the adult mammalian cardiocyte. Circulation. 1992;85:790–804.
64. López-Sendón J, Swedberg K, McMurray J, Tamargo J, Maggioni AP, Dargie H, et al. Expert consensus document on beta-adrenergic receptor blockers. Eur Heart J. 2004;25:1341–62.
65. Triposkiadis F, Giamouzis G, Kelepeshis G, Sitafidis G, Skoularigis J, Demopoulos V. Acute hemodynamic effects of moderate doses of nebivolol versus metoprolol in patients with systolic heart failure. Int J Clin Pharmacol Ther. 2007;45:71–7.
66. Kaumann AJ, Molenaar P. The low-affinity site of the beta1-adrenoceptor and its relevance to cardiovascular pharmacology. Pharmacol Ther. 2008; 118:303–36.
67. Sistonen J, Sajantila A, Lao O, Corander J, Barbujani G, Fuselli S. CYP2D6 worldwide genetic variation shows high frequency of altered activity variants and no continental structure. Pharmacogenet Genomics. 2007;17:93–101.
68. Ingelman-Sundberg M, Sim SC, Gomez A, Rodriguez-Antona C. Influence of cytochrome P450 polymorphisms on drug therapies: pharmacogenetic, pharmacoepigenetic and clinical aspects. Pharmacol Ther. 2007;116:496–526.
69. Wuttke H, Rau T, Heide R, Bergmann K, Böhm M, Weil J, et al. Increased frequency of cytochrome P450 2D6 poor metabolizers among patients with metoprolol associated adverse effects. Clin Pharmacol Ther. 2002;72:429–37.
70. Fujimaki M. Oxidation of R(+)- and S(−)-carvedilol by rat liver microsomes. Evidence for stereoselective oxidation and characterization of the cytochrome P450 isozymes involved. Drug Metab Dispos. 1994;22:700–8.
71. Horikiri Y, Suzuki T, Mizobe M. Pharmacokinetics and metabolism of bisoprolol enantiomers in humans. J Pharm Sci. 1998;87:289–94.
72. Adamson PB, Gilbert EM. Reducing the risk of sudden death in heart failure with beta-blockers. J Card Fail. 2006;12:734–46.
73. Talwar KK, Bhargava B, Upasani PT, Verma S, Kamlakar T, Chopra P. Hemodynamic predictors of early intolerance and long-term effects of propranolol in dilated cardiomyopathy. J Card Fail. 1996;2:273–7.
74. Lombardi WL, Gilbert EM. Carvedilol in the failing heart. Clin Cardiol. 2001;24:757–66.
75. McMurray JJ, Adamopoulos S, Anker SD, Auricchio A, Böhm M, Dickstein K, et al. ESC guidelines for the diagnosis and treatment of acute and chronic heart failure 2012: The Task Force for the Diagnosis and Treatment of Acute and Chronic Heart Failure 2012 of the European Society of Cardiology. Developed in collaboration with the Heart Failure Association (HFA) of the ESC. Eur J Heart Fail. 2012;14:803–69.
76. Waagstein F, Bristow MR, Swedberg K, Camerini F, Fowler MB, Silver MA, et al. Beneficial effects of metoprolol in idiopathic dilated cardiomyopathy. Metoprolol in Dilated Cardiomyopathy (MDC) Trial Study Group. Lancet. 1993;342:1441–6.
77. Effect of metoprolol CR/XL in chronic heart failure: Metoprolol CR/XL Randomised Intervention Trial in Congestive Heart Failure (MERIT-HF). Lancet. 1999;353:2001–7.
78. Wikstrand J, Hjalmarson A, Waagstein F, Fagerberg B, Goldstein S, Kjekshus J, et al. Dose of metoprolol CR/XL and clinical outcomes in patients with heart failure: analysis of the experience in metoprolol CR/XL randomized intervention trial in chronic heart failure (MERIT-HF). J Am Coll Cardiol. 2002;40:491–8.
79. The Cardiac Insufficiency Bisoprolol Study II (CIBIS-II): a randomised trial. Lancet. 1999;353:9–13.
80. Australia/New Zealand Heart Failure Research Collaborative Group. Randomised, placebo-controlled trial of carvedilol in patients with congestive heart failure due to ischaemic heart disease. Lancet. 1997;349:375–80.
81. Wollert KC, Drexler H. Carvedilol prospective randomized cumulative survival (COPERNICUS) trial:

carvedilol as the sun and center of the beta-blocker world? Circulation. 2002;106:2164–6.
82. Dargie HJ. Effect of carvedilol on outcome after myocardial infarction in patients with left-ventricular dysfunction: the CAPRICORN randomised trial. Lancet. 2001;357:1385–90.
83. MacGregor JF, Wachter SB, Munger M, Stoddard G, Bristow MR, Gilbert EM. Carvedilol produces sustained long-term benefits: follow-up at 12 years. Congest Heart Fail. 2009;15:5–8.
84. Flather MD, Shibata MC, Coats AJ, Van Veldhuisen DJ, Parkhomenko A, Borbola J, et al. Randomized trial to determine the effect of nebivolol on mortality and cardiovascular hospital admission in elderly patients with heart failure (SENIORS). Eur Heart J. 2005;26:215–25.
85. Poole-Wilson PA, Swedberg K, Cleland JG, Di Lenarda A, Hanrath P, Komajda M, et al. Comparison of carvedilol and metoprolol on clinical outcomes in patients with chronic heart failure in the Carvedilol or Metoprolol European Trial (COMET): randomized controlled trial. Lancet. 2003;362:7–13.
86. Talber RL. Pharmacokinetics and pharmacodynamics of beta blockers in heart failure. Heart Fail Rev. 2004;9:131–7.
87. DiNicolantonio JJ, Lavie CJ, Fares H, Menezes AR, O'Keefe JH. Meta-analysis of carvedilol versus beta 1 selective beta-blockers (atenolol, bisoprolol, metoprolol, and nebivolol). Am J Cardiol. 2013;111:765–9.
88. Chatterjee S, Biondi-Zoccai G, Abbate A, D'Ascenzo F, Castagno D, Van Tassell B, et al. Benefits of β blockers in patients with heart failure and reduced ejection fraction: network meta-analysis. BMJ. 2013;346:f55.
89. Talameh JA, McLeod HL, Adams Jr KF, Patterson JH. Genetic tailoring of pharmacotherapy in heart failure: optimize the old, while we wait for something new. J Card Fail. 2012;18:338–49.
90. Borjesson M, Magnusson Y, Hjalmarson A, Andersson B. A novel polymorphism in the gene coding for the beta(1)-adrenergic receptor associated with survival in patients with heart failure. Eur Heart J. 2000;21:1853–8.
91. Terra SG, Hamilton KK, Pauly DF, Lee CR, Patterson JH, Adams KF, et al. Beta1-adrenergic receptor polymorphisms and left ventricular remodeling changes in response to beta-blocker therapy. Pharmacogenet Genomics. 2005;15:227–34.
92. Mialet Perez J, Rathz DA, Petrashevskaya NN, Hahn HS, Wagoner LE, Schwartz A, et al. Beta 1-adrenergic receptor polymorphisms confer differential function and predisposition to heart failure. Nat Med. 2003;9:1300–5.
93. Chen L, Meyers D, Javorsky G, Burstow D, Lolekha P, Lucas M, et al. Arg389Gly-beta1-adrenergic receptors determine improvement in left ventricular systolic function in nonischemic cardiomyopathy patients with heart failure after chronic treatment with carvedilol. Pharmacogenet Genomics. 2007;17:941–9.
94. de Groote P, Helbecque N, Lamblin N, Hermant X, Mc Fadden E, Foucher-Hossein C, et al. Association between beta-1 and beta-2 adrenergic receptor gene polymorphisms and the response to beta-blockade in patients with stable congestive heart failure. Pharmacogenet Genomics. 2005;15:137–42.
95. Sehnert AJ, Daniels SE, Elashoff M, Wingrove JA, Burrow CR, Horne B, et al. Lack of association between adrenergic receptor genotypes and survival in heart failure patients treated with carvedilol or metoprolol. J Am Coll Cardiol. 2008;52:644–51.
96. White HL, de Boer RA, Maqbool A, Greenwood D, van Veldhuisen DJ, Cuthbert R, et al. An evaluation of the beta-1 adrenergic receptor Arg389Gly polymorphism in individuals with heart failure: a MERIT-HF sub-study. Eur J Heart Fail. 2003;5:463–8.
97. Magnusson Y, Levin MC, Eggertsen R, Nyström E, Mobini R, Schaufelberger M, et al. Ser49Gly of beta1-adrenergic receptor is associated with effective beta-blocker dose in dilated cardiomyopathy. Clin Pharmacol Ther. 2005;78:221–31.
98. Beta-Blocker Evaluation of Survival Trial Investigators. A trial of the beta-blocker bucindolol in patients with advanced chronic heart failure. N Engl J Med. 2001;344:1659–67.
99. Liggett SB, Mialet-Perez J, Thaneemit-Chen S, Weber SA, Greene SM, Hodne D, et al. A polymorphism within a conserved beta(1)-adrenergic receptor motif alters cardiac function and beta-blocker response in human heart failure. Proc Natl Acad Sci U S A. 2006;103:11288–93.
100. Lymperopoulos A, Rengo G, Koch WJ. GRK2 inhibition in heart failure: something old, something new. Curr Pharm Des. 2012;18:186–91.
101. Iaccarino G, Tomhave ED, Lefkowitz RJ, Koch WJ. Reciprocal *in vivo* regulation of myocardial G protein-coupled receptor kinase expression by beta-adrenergic receptor stimulation and blockade. Circulation. 1998;98:1783–9.
102. Rengo G, Lymperopoulos A, Zincarelli C, Donniacuo M, Soltys S, Rabinowitz JE, et al. Myocardial adeno-associated virus serotype 6-betaARKct gene therapy improves cardiac function and normalizes the neurohormonal axis in chronic heart failure. Circulation. 2009;119:89–98.
103. Huang ZM, Gold JI, Koch WJ. G protein-coupled receptor kinases in normal and failing myocardium. Front Biosci. 2011;16:3047–60.
104. Koch WJ, Inglese J, Stone WC, Lefkowitz RJ. The binding site for the beta gamma subunits of heterotrimeric G proteins on the beta-adrenergic receptor kinase. J Biol Chem. 1993;268:8256–60.
105. Rockman HA, Chien KR, Choi DJ, Iaccarino G, Hunter JJ, Ross Jr J, et al. Expression of a beta-adrenergic receptor kinase 1 inhibitor prevents the development of myocardial failure in gene-targeted mice. Proc Natl Acad Sci U S A. 1998;95:7000–5.
106. Freeman K, Lerman I, Kranias EG, Bohlmeyer T, Bristow MR, Lefkowitz RJ, et al. Alterations in cardiac adrenergic signaling and calcium cycling

differentially affect the progression of cardiomyopathy. J Clin Invest. 2001;107:967–74.

107. Harding V, Jones L, Lefkowitz RJ, Koch WJ, Rockman HA. Cardiac βARK1 inhibition prolongs survival and augments β blocker therapy in a mouse model of severe heart failure. Proc Natl Acad Sci U S A. 2001;98:5809–14.
108. White DC, Hata JA, Shah AS, Glower DD, Lefkowitz RJ, Koch WJ. Preservation of myocardial beta-adrenergic receptor signaling delays the development of heart failure after myocardial infarction. Proc Natl Acad Sci U S A. 2000;97:5428–33.
109. Shah AS, White DC, Emani S, Kypson AP, Lilly RE, Wilson K, et al. *In vivo* ventricular gene delivery of a β-adrenergic receptor kinase inhibitor to the failing heart reverses cardiac dysfunction. Circulation. 2001;103:1311–6.
110. Tevaearai HT, Eckhart AD, Shotwell KF, Wilson K, Koch WJ. Ventricular dysfunction following cardioplegic arrest is improved after myocardial gene transfer of a β-adrenergic receptor kinase inhibitor. Circulation. 2001;104:2069–74.
111. Raake PW, Schlegel P, Ksienzyk J, Reinkober J, Barthelmes J, Schinkel S, et al. AAV6.βARKct cardiac gene therapy ameliorates cardiac function and normalizes the catecholaminergic axis in a clinically relevant large animal heart failure model. Eur Heart J. 2013;34:1437–47.
112. Raake PW, Vinge LE, Gao E, Boucher M, Rengo G, Chen X, et al. G protein-coupled receptor kinase 2 ablation in cardiac myocytes before or after myocardial infarction prevents heart failure. Circ Res. 2008;103:413–22.
113. Matkovic SJ, Diwan A, Klanke JL, Hammer DJ, Marreez Y, Odley AM, et al. Cardiac-specific ablation of G-protein receptor kinase 2 redefines its roles in heart development and beta-adrenergic signaling. Circ Res. 2006;99:996–1003.
114. Völkers M, Weidenhammer C, Herzog N, Qiu G, Spaich K, von Wegner F, et al. The inotropic peptide βARKct improves βAR responsiveness in normal and failing cardiomyocytes through G(βγ)-mediated L-type calcium current disinhibition. Circ Res. 2011;108:27–39.
115. Pleger ST, Shan C, Kszienyk J, Bekeredjian R, Boekstegers P, Hinkel R, et al. Cardiac AAV9-S100A1 gene therapy rescues post-ischemic heart failure in a preclinical large animal model. Sci Transl Med. 2011;3:92ra64.
116. Cannavo A, Liccardo D, Koch WJ. Targeting cardiac β-adrenergic signaling via GRK2 inhibition for heart failure therapy. Front Physiol. 2013;4:264.
117. Mayer G, Wulffen B, Huber C, Brockmann J, Flicke B, Neumann L, et al. An RNA molecule that specifically inhibits G-protein-coupled receptor kinase 2 *in vitro*. RNA. 2008;14:524–34.
118. Piao L, Fang YH, Parikh KS, Ryan JJ, D'Souza KM, Theccanat T, et al. GRK2-mediated inhibition of adrenergic and dopaminergic signaling in right ventricular hypertrophy: therapeutic implications in pulmonary hypertension. Circulation. 2012; 126:2859–69.
119. Casey LM, Pistner AR, Belmonte SL, Migdalovich D, Stolpnik O, Nwakanma FE, et al. Small molecule disruption of G beta gamma signaling inhibits the progression of heart failure. Circ Res. 2010;107:532–9.
120. Thal DM, Homan KT, Chen J, Wu EK, Hinkle PM, Huang ZM, et al. Paroxetine is a direct inhibitor of g protein-coupled receptor kinase 2 and increases myocardial contractility. ACS Chem Biol. 2012;7: 1830–9.

6

The Hypothalamic-Pituitary-Adrenal Axis in Human Health and Disease

Nicolas C. Nicolaides, Evangelia Charmandari, and George P. Chrousos

Abstract

The hypothalamic-pituitary-adrenal (HPA) axis plays a fundamental role in the maintenance of basal and stress-related homeostasis. This neuroendocrine axis consists of three distinct components located in the hypothalamus, the pituitary gland and the adrenal cortex. Glucocorticoids, the end-products of the HPA axis, exert their diverse actions in virtually all tissues through their ubiquitously expressed glucocorticoid receptor. A broad spectrum of pathologic conditions affecting any of the three anatomical parts results in hypo- or hyper-activation of the HPA axis and subsequent clinical manifestations of glucocorticoid deficiency or excess, respectively. Moreover, our ever-increasing understanding of

N.C. Nicolaides, MD, PhD (✉)
Division of Endocrinology and Metabolism, Clinical Research Center, Biomedical Research Foundation of the Academy of Athens, 4 Soranou tou Efessiou Street, Athens 11527, Greece
e-mail: nnicolaides@bioacademy.gr

E. Charmandari, MD, MSc, PhD, MRCP(UK), CCST(UK)
Division of Endocrinology and Metabolism, Clinical Research Center, Biomedical Research Foundation of the Academy of Athens, 4 Soranou tou Efessiou Street, Athens 11527, Greece

Division of Endocrinology, Metabolism and Diabetes, First Department of Pediatrics, University of Athens Medical School, "Aghia Sophia" Children's Hospital, Thivon and Papadiamantopoulou Street, Athens 11527, Greece
e-mail: evangelia.charmandari@googlemail.com

G.P. Chrousos, MD, MACP, MACE, FRCP (London)
Division of Endocrinology and Metabolism, Clinical Research Center, Biomedical Research Foundation of the Academy of Athens, 4 Soranou tou Efessiou Street, Athens 11527, Greece

First Department of Pediatrics, University of Athens Medical School, "Aghia Sophia" Children's Hospital, Thivon and Papadiamantopoulou Street, Athens 11527, Greece

Division of Endocrinology, Metabolism and Diabetes, UNESCO Chair on Adolescent Health Care, University of Athens Medical School, "Aghia Sophia" Children's Hospital, Thivon and Papadiamantopoulou Street, Athens 11527, Greece

Distinguished Visiting Scientist, NICHD, NIH, Bethesda 20892, MD, USA

Saudi Diabetes Study Research Group, King Fahd Medical Research Center, King Abdulaziz University, Jeddah, Saudi Arabia
e-mail: chrousge@med.uoa.gr; chrousog@mail.nih.gov

D.V. Cokkinos (ed.), *Introduction to Translational Cardiovascular Research*,
DOI 10.1007/978-3-319-08798-6_6, © Springer International Publishing Switzerland 2015

glucocorticoid receptor signaling has allowed us to approach diagnostically and therapeutically these endocrine diseases in a more integrated way. However, the pathophysiology, differential diagnosis and therapy of some of these disorders still remain challenging. In this chapter, we describe the physiologic and endocrine aspects of the HPA axis, and we present the clinical manifestations and therapeutic management of its most common disorders.

Keywords
Adrenal cortex • Glucocorticoid receptor • Glucocorticoids • Hypothalamus • Pituitary gland

Abbreviations

ACTH	Adrenocorticotropic hormone
AP-1	Activator protein 1
AV	Arginine vasopressin
CBP	p300/CREB-binding protein
CLOCK	Circadian locomotor output cycle kaput
CNS	Central nervous system
CRH	Corticotropin-releasing hormone
DRIP/TRAP	Vitamin D receptor-interacting protein/thyroid hormone receptor-associated protein
eNOS	Endothelial nitric oxide synthase
GR	Glucocorticoid receptor
GREs	Glucocorticoid response elements
HPA Axis	hypothalamic-pituitary-adrenal axis
NF-κB	Nuclear factor κB
NL	Nuclear localization signal
p/CAF	p300/CBP-associated factor
POMC	Pro-opiomelanocortin
PVN	Paraventricular nucleus
SCN	Suprachiasmatic nucleus
STAT	Signal transducer and activator of transcription

6.1 Introduction

All living organisms maintain a complex dynamic equilibrium, called *homeostasis*, which may be threatened, or perceived as threatened, by a wide variety of extrinsic or intrinsic adverse challenges or forces, the *stressors* [1, 2]. To cope with these stressful stimuli, living organisms have developed a highly complex regulatory system, the *stress system*, which, upon activation, leads to a programmed repertoire of physiologic and behavioral central nervous system (CNS) and peripheral adaptive responses [1–3]. If the *stress response* is either inadequate or excessive or prolonged, it may adversely influence personality development and behavior, and may impair fundamental physiologic functions, such as growth, development, metabolism, reproduction, circulation and the immune response [3]. The hypothalamic-pituitary-adrenal (HPA) axis is one of the two major arms of the stress system, which acts synergistically with the locus caeruleus/norepinephrine-autonomic nervous systems to adjust homeostasis. This neuroendocrine axis consists of three components: the paraventricular nuclei (PVN) located in the hypothalamus, the corticotrope cells located in the pituitary gland and the *zona fasciculata* residing in the adrenal cortices. Glucocorticoids, the end-products of the HPA axis, are cholesterol-derived molecules that exert their pleiotropic actions through the glucocorticoid receptor (GR), which acts as an intracellular ligand-induced transcription factor, influencing the transcription rate of many thousands of genes in a positive or negative way [4]. Consequently, the dysfunction of the HPA axis at any of the above levels may represent the main pathogenetic mechanism underlying several pathologic conditions, which may strongly influence human health and quality of life. In this chapter, we describe the functional components of the HPA axis, we provide an overview of the endocrine effects of glucocorticoids through their cognate receptor, and we finally present the most common diseases associated with dysfunction of this axis.

6.1.1 Historical Development of the Stress and the HPA Axis

> ...he who knows things from their beginning and origins understands them better... (Aristotle, 4th Century BCE).

The concepts of stress go back to Greek antiquity [1, 2]. Pythagoras was the first to use the term *harmony* to describe the equilibrium of the human organism or the balance of the entire universe (*The harmony of the Cosmos*). This *harmony* is constantly challenged by disturbing forces, while other counteracting forces help *harmony* to be reestablished. Shortly afterwards, Alcmaeon of Croton used the term *isonomia* to describe the balance of opposing forces. Empedocles of Argigentum proposed that all matter consisted of four basic elements (= rhizomata or roots), the earth, the water, the air and the fire, which were in a dynamic opposition to one another, and that balance was a necessary prerequisite for the health of living organisms [2, 5]. The Empedoclean doctrine seems to be the precursor of the Hippocratic humoral system. Hippocrates, the father of medicine, equated health to a harmonious equilibrium of the four humors: blood, phlegm, black and yellow bile, corresponding to the heart, the brain, the liver and the spleen, respectively. The balance of the humors is termed *eucrasia*, whereas their imbalance or *dyscrasia* causes disease [2]. Hippocrates also suggested that the disturbing forces that produced *dyscrasia* and the counteracting forces that reestablish *eucrasia* both derived from nature. He, therefore, introduced the concept that "Nature is the healer of disease" [2]. Many years later, Epicurus suggested that the mind could be one of these healing forces and wrote that *ataraxia*, or "imperturbability of mind" and *aponia* (no pain) represented most desirable states [2].

In the years of Renaissance, Thomas Sydenham proposed that an individual's adaptive response to the disturbing forces that lead to systematic disharmony could result in pathologic changes. Two hundred years later, Claude Bernard, one of the world's greatest physiologists, pointed out that cells are surrounded by an internal medium, the *milieu intérieur*, which provides a steady state. He wrote that "it is the fixity of the *milieu intérieur*, which is the condition of free and independent life" [6]. Fifty years later, Walter Bradford Cannon coined the term *homeostasis* (from the Greek *homoios*, or similar, and *stasis*, or position) for all the physiologic processes that maintain the steady state of the organism [2, 6]. He published the concept of *homeostasis* in his book entitled "Wisdom of the Body" in 1932. Cannon also described an animal's response to threat. The concept of "*fight or flight reaction*" suggests that the adaptive response to stress is associated with catecholamine secretion due to activation of the sympathetic nervous system, priming the animal for fight against the threat or fleeing to save its life [2, 6]. This response was considered to be the first stage (acute stress response) of the general adaptation syndrome (GAS) suggested later by Hans Selye.

Hans Hugo Bruno Selye, the father of the concept of stress, observed that patients with different diseases manifested many of the same 'nonspecific' symptoms as a common response to stressors. Selye, and before him Cannon, borrowed the term "*stress*" from physics and defined it as the mutual actions of forces that happen across any section of body [2, 6]. He postulated that the presence of stereotypic psychological and physiological manifestations occurring in seriously ill patients represented the consequences of severe long-lasting adaptational responses. He named this condition the "*General Adaptation or Stress Syndrome*" and redefined Sydenham's concept in the "diseases of adaptation". In addition to clearly defining stress, Selye coined the term *heterostasis* (from the Greek *heteros*, or other), later named as *allostasis*, initially meaning "stability through change" [2, 6].

In parallel with the evolution of stress concepts, numerous advances in neuroendocrinology uncovered the physiologic biochemical effectors of the stress response and the central loci responsible for the regulation of their production and release. The locus caeruleus/autonomic nervous system and the HPA axis represent the major arms of the stress system. Coined by the physiologist John Newport Langley in 1898, the autonomic nervous system was shown to play an important role in the fight or flight reaction and the maintenance of homeostasis, especially in the cardiovascular system [6]. On the other hand, our understanding of the HPA axis has improved significantly in the last century. The pituitary gland had long been considered to be an autonomous regulator of many endocrine glands, such as the thyroid, the gonads and the adrenal cortex. However, experiments by Geoffrey Harris and William Rowan and others led to an acceptance of the novel concept that the pituitary gland functions under the control of the CNS. Evidence supporting the neurohumoral hypothesis of anterior pituitary control came from the pituitary stalk section and pituitary grafting experiments of Geoffrey Harris and Dora Jacobsohn, from the characterization of some of the neurohormonal molecules by Andrew Schally and Roger Guillemin, and from the proof that these neurohormones were directly secreted into hypophyseal portal veins [6]. Corticoctropin-releasing factor (CRF), a 41-amino acid peptide that controls the production and secretion of adrenocorticotropic hormone (ACTH), was isolated and sequenced by Wylie Vale and associates in 1981 [6]. Finally, glucocorticoids, the effector molecules of the HPA axis, were isolated and synthesized by Edward Kendall and Tadeus Reichstein [6]. Philip Hench was the first who tested cortisone, a synthetic pre-glucocorticoid, in patients with rheumatoid arthritis, and showed the anti-inflammatory effect of this compound [6]. Kendall, Hench, and Reichstein were jointly awarded the Nobel Prize for physiology and medicine in 1950. Despite the isolation and synthesis of glucocorticoids in the middle of the twentieth century, their mechanisms of pleiotropic actions were – and still remain – an enigma. In 1985, the human glucocorticoid receptor (hGR) cDNA was isolated by expression cloning, predicting two protein forms, of 777 (alpha) and 742 (beta) amino acids, which differ at their carboxyl termini [7]. Since then, the GR-mediated anti-inflammatory and immunosuppressive effects have been elucidated and accumulating evidence from *in vitro* and *in vivo* studies supports the stochastic (randomly determined) nature of glucocorticoid signaling [8].

6.1.2 The HPA Axis

The HPA axis consists of the paraventricular nuclei (PVN) located in the hypothalamus, the pituitary gland and the adrenal cortices. A broad spectrum of internal and external signals from various organs of the human body are detected and subsequently integrated by the CNS, which transduces this information to the PVN and other brain loci, such as the hypothalamic suprachiasmatic nucleus (SCN), the amygdala and the raphe nuclei of the brain stem, and controls the activity of the PVN [9]. The SCN functions also as a central circadian rhythm center (master CLOCK), under the control of light/dark changes during the 24 h day, and generates the circadian rhythmicity of the HPA axis through synaptic connections with the PVN, leading to the diurnal fluctuation of circulating concentrations of glucocorticoids [10]. Neurons of the PVN produce and release corticotropin-releasing hormone (CRH) and arginine vasopressin (AVP) into the hypophyseal portal system [9, 11]. Subsequently, CRH and, to a lesser degree, AVP trigger the synthesis and secretion of ACTH by the corticotrope cells of the anterior pituitary gland [12, 13] (Fig. 6.1). CRH is the strongest and probably the most important stimulator of ACTH secretion. AVP, although a potent synergistic factor of CRH, has little ACTH secretagogue activity on its own. ACTH is synthesized as part of a large precursor molecule of 214 amino acids, pro-opiomelanocortin (POMC). Depending on the cleavage enzymes, which are expressed in a tissue-specific fashion, ACTH and several other peptides, e.g. NH2-terminal peptide, joining peptide, β- or γ-lipotropins, β-endorphin,

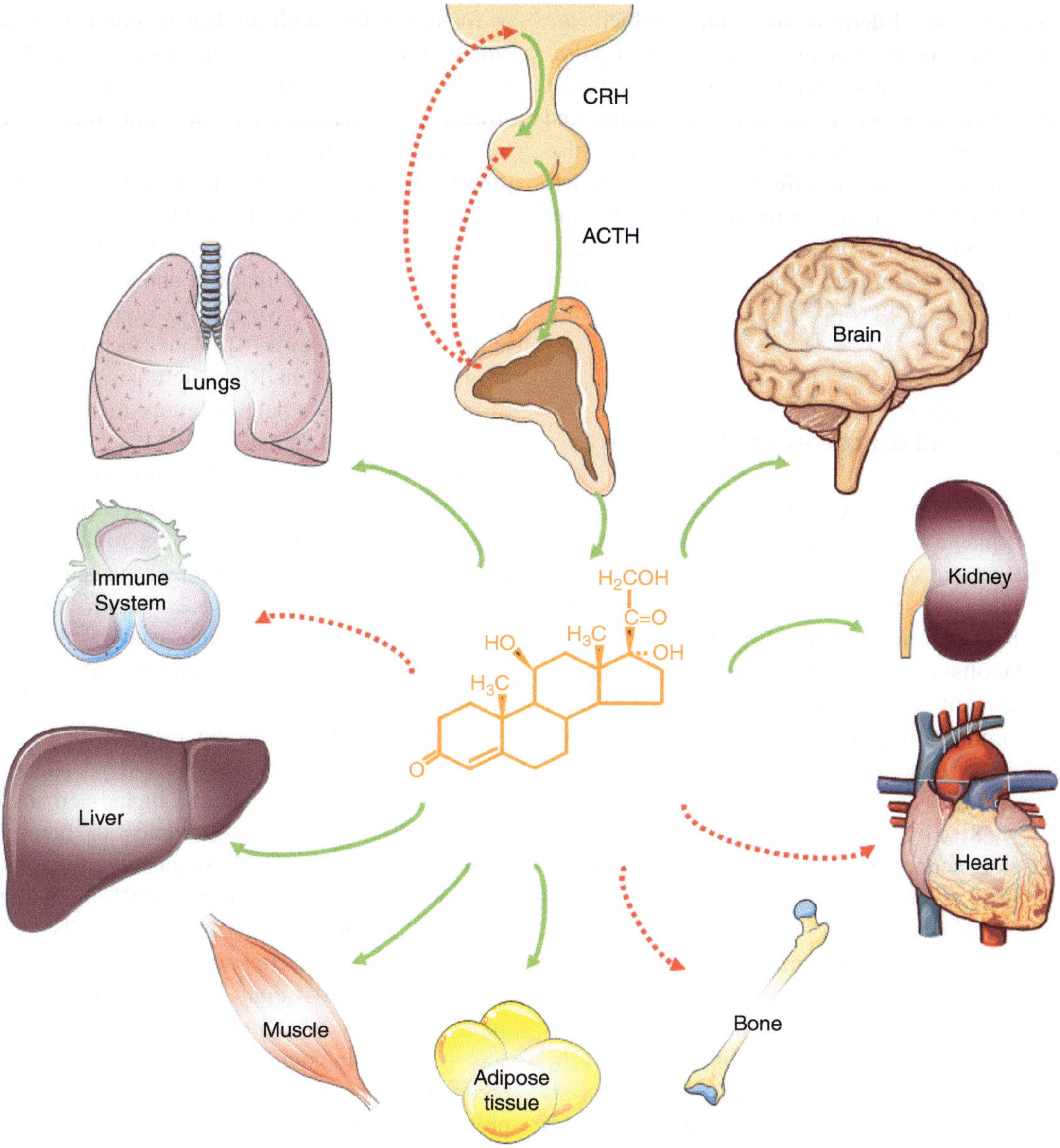

Fig. 6.1 The HPA axis and systemic actions of glucocorticoids. *CRH* corticotropin-releasing hormone, *ACTH* adrenocorticotropic hormone (Figure 6.1 was prepared using image vectors from Servier Medical Art (www.ervier.com), licensed under the Creative Commons Attribution 3.0 Unported License (http://creativecommons.org/license/by/3.0/))

α-melanocyte-stimulating hormone (MSH) and corticotropin-like intermediate peptide (CLIP), are produced [14]. ACTH is secreted in regular pulses of variable amplitude over 24 h, with peak concentrations attained in the early morning hours (04:00–08:00 h), thus forming the basis of the circadian pattern of ACTH and cortisol secretion. Upon binding to its cognate transmembrane G-protein-coupled receptor of the adrenocortical cells of the *zona fasciculata* of the adrenal cortex, ACTH induces the activity of proteins and the expression of genes implicated in the biosynthetic pathway of glucocorticoids (cortisol in humans, corticosterone in rodents) [15] Glucocorticoids are cholesterol-derived molecules, which are released into the systemic circulation in a pulsatile, circadian and stress-related fashion, and exert their numerous actions in almost all tissues and organs. However, these steroid hormones also have negative feedback effects on both PVN CRH and AVP synthesis and secretion, and inhibit pituitary synthesis of POMC, as well as ACTH secretion, forming a closed, tightly regulated, negative feedback loop [9] (Fig. 6.1).

6.1.3 Glucocorticoids and Glucocorticoid Receptor

Glucocorticoids, the end-products of the HPA axis, play a fundamental role in the maintenance of basal and stress-related homeostasis, and regulate a broad spectrum of physiologic functions, such as the cardiovascular tone, the intermediary metabolism primarily through catabolic actions, the quantity and the quality of the inflammatory and immune response and many other functions, by altering the transcription rate of a significant percentage of genes in a positive or negative way [3, 4, 8] (Fig. 6.1). Glucocorticoids exert their diverse actions through an intracellular, ubiquitously expressed protein, the human glucocorticoid receptor (hGR), which belongs to the nuclear receptor superfamily of transcription factors [16].

The *hGR* gene is located on the short arm of chromosome 5 and consists of 10 exons [16]. The alternative use of two distinct exons, 9α and 9β, generates two main isoforms, the hGRα and the hGRβ [17]. The hGRα is a 777-amino acid protein and represents the classic isoform, which binds endogenous and synthetic glucocorticoids, and mediates all genomic effects of these hormones in almost every cell type in the human organism [17]. On the other hand, the hGRβ contains 742 amino acids, does not bind glucocorticoids, and acts as a dominant negative regulator on the hGRα-mediated transcriptional activity through several mechanisms, such as heterodimerization and competition with hGRα for binding to glucocorticoid response elements (GREs) in the promoter regions of target genes, or for interacting with nuclear receptor coregulators (coactivators, corepressors) [17–21]. Furthermore, the hGRα mRNA was demonstrated to be translated from eight alternative initiation sites into functionally distinct hGRα protein isoforms by ribosomal leaky scanning or ribosomal shunting [22]. Given that hGRβ mRNA translation is initiated by the same 5′ termini, it is possible that the above translation mechanisms could give rise to eight different hGRβ proteins as well [8]. Thus, the 16 amino terminal hGRα and hGRβ protein isoforms may form 256 homo- or hetero-dimers to transduce the glucocorticoid signal.

At the cellular level, hGRα is primarily localized in the cytoplasm of the target cell in the absence of a ligand, as part of a multiprotein complex consisting of heat shock proteins and immunophilins [16] (Fig. 6.2). Upon ligand-binding, hGRα undergoes conformational change, dissociates from the rest of proteins, and translocates into the nucleus through the nuclear pore, via an active ATP-dependent process mediated by its nuclear localization signal (NL)-1 and −2 [19]. Within the nucleus, the ligand-activated GR directly interacts as a homo- or hetero-dimer with specific DNA sequences, the glucocorticoid response elements (GREs), in the promoter regions of target genes [19]. The GR contains two transactivation domains, activation function (AF)-1 and −2, located at its NTD and LBD, respectively, through which it interacts with protein complexes, such as the nuclear receptor coactivators p160, p300/CREB-binding protein (CBP) and p300/CBP-associated factor (p/CAF) complexes and the SWI/SNF and vitamin D receptor-interacting protein/thyroid hormone receptor-associated protein (DRIP/TRAP) chromatin-remodeling complexes; it influences the activity of the RNA polymerase II and its ancillary factors, thereby modulating the transcription rates of glucocorticoid-responsive genes [16] (Fig. 6.2).

Alternatively, hGRα may modulate gene expression independently of its DNA binding, by interacting with and altering the functions of other known transcription factors, such as NF-κB, STAT-5, and AP-1, possibly as monomer

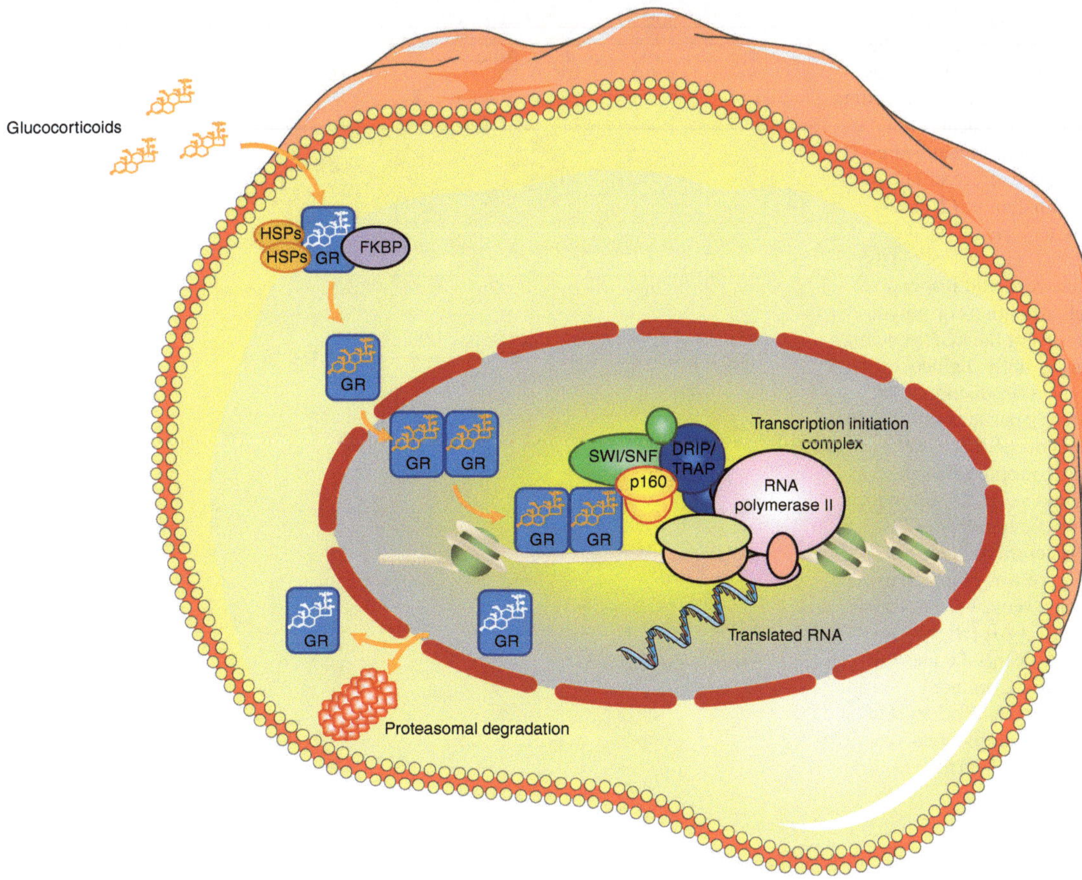

Fig. 6.2 Glucocorticoid signaling pathway. *GR* glucocorticoid receptor, *HSP* heat shock proteins, *FKBP* immunophilins, *p160* nuclear receptor coactivators p160, *SWI/SNF* switching/sucrose non-fermenting complex, *DRIP/TRAP* vitamin D receptor-interacting protein/thyroid hormone receptor-associated protein complex (Figure 6.2 was prepared using image vectors from Servier Medical Art (www.servier.com), licensed under the Creative Commons Attribution 3.0 Unported License (http://creativecommons.org/license/by/3.0/))

[16]. These interacting factors, in turn, may alter the actions of the glucocorticoid receptor acting on positive or negative GREs.

6.1.4 Disorders of the HPA Axis

The disorders of the HPA axis can be categorized according to the anatomical component(s) that is/are primarily affected: (1) the hypothalamus, (2) the pituitary gland, (3) the adrenal glands and (4) other tissues and organs, including alterations of glucocorticoid availability or action at target tissues (Fig. 6.3). These disorders may result in either elevated or reduced concentrations or effects of circulating glucocorticoids; thus, symptoms and signs are associated with increased or decreased actions of these hormones in the responsive tissues, (Table 6.1).

Indeed, chronic glucocorticoid excess results in central obesity, buffalo hump, purple striae of the skin, hypertension, osteoporosis, glucose intolerance/overt diabetes mellitus, dyslipidemia and leukocytosis, all of which are referred to as the "Cushing phenotype" [23]. Patients with pathologically increased concentrations of cortisol are at great risk of severe cardiovascular complications, such as ischemic heart/cerebral disease [23]. Moreover, they are more susceptible to infections secondary to any pathogens, since cortisol suppresses strongly the activity of the immune system.

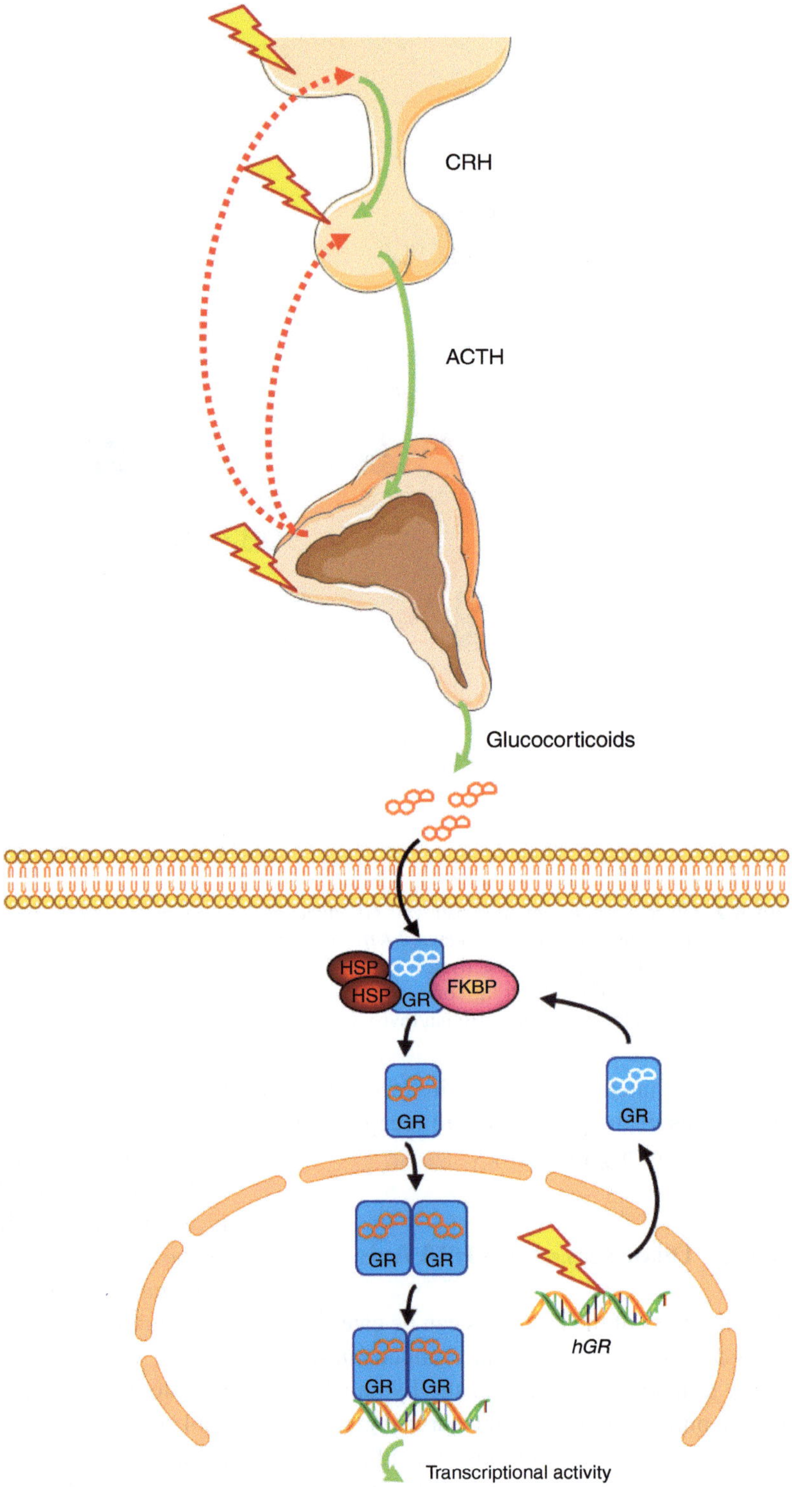

Fig. 6.3 The HPA axis and associated disorders. The disorders of the HPA axis can be categorized according to the anatomical component(s) that is/are primarily affected: (1) the hypothalamus, (2) the pituitary gland, (3) the adrenal glands and (4) the glucocorticoid-responsive cell. Mutations or polymorphisms of the *hGR* gene may impair normal glucocorticoid signal transduction, thus altering tissue sensitivity to glucocorticoids. *CRH* corticotropin-releasing hormone, *ACTH* adrenocorticotropic hormone, *GR* glucocorticoid receptor (Figure was prepared using image vectors from Servier Medical Art (www.servier.com), licensed under the Creative Commons Attribution 3.0 Unported License (http://creativecommons.org/license/by/3.0/))

Table 6.1 Expected clinical manifestations in tissue-specific glucocorticoid excess or hypersensitivity and deficiency or resistance

Target tissue	Glucocorticoid hypersensitivity =Glucocorticoid excess	Glucocorticoid resistance =Glucocorticoid deficiency
Central nervous system	Insomnia, anxiety, depression, defective cognition	Fatigue, somnolence, malaise, defective cognition
Liver	+ Gluconeogenesis, + lipogenesis	Hypoglycemia, resistance to diabetes mellitus
Fat	Accumulation of visceral fat (metabolic syndrome)	Loss of weight, resistance to weight gain
Blood vessels	Hypertension	Hypotension
Bone	Stunted growth, osteoporosis	
Inflammation/immunity	Immune suppression, anti-inflammation, vulnerability to certain infections and tumors	+ Inflammation,+ autoimmunity, + allergy

Modified from Ref. [8]

On the other hand, patients with isolated glucocorticoid deficiency or adrenal insufficiency including aldosterone deficiency may present with fatigue, vomiting, nausea, hypotension, hypoglycemia, hyponatremia, hyperkalemia in the absence of aldosterone secretion and eosinophilia [23]. The decreased concentrations of cortisol lead to compensatory elevations in plasma ACTH concentrations, which result in hyperpigmentation of the skin and buccal mucosa in these patients.

6.1.4.1 Hypothalamic Disorders Associated with Alterations in the HPA Axis

Many space-occupying lesions of the hypothalamus, including craniopharyngioma, Rathke's pouch cysts, head trauma, inflammatory or infiltrative diseases (encephalitis, meningitis, sarcoidosis, histiocytosis X) and brain malignant tumors (primary or metastatic) lead to destruction of the PVN neurons producing CRH or to dissection of the pituitary stalk that transfers CRH from the hypothalamus to the pituitary gland, thus causing decreased function of the HPA axis [24]. These conditions are often associated with dysfunction of other endocrine axes, such as the hypothalamic-pituitary-gonadal or thyroid axes and the growth hormone/insulin-like growth factor-I axis.

Prader-Willi syndrome is a rare genetic disorder, which is characterized by symptoms associated with hypothalamic dysfunction, such as hyperphagia, obesity, sleep disorders, hypogonadism, hypocortisolism, learning disabilities/borderline intellectual functioning and hypotonia [25].

Patients with the melancholic type of major depression show hyperactivity of the HPA axis and have increased cerebrospinal fluid CRH and norepinephrine, plasma ACTH and serum cortisol concentrations [26, 27]. This sustained hyperfunction of the HPA axis leads to central obesity, hypertension, impaired glucose tolerance, decreased libido and osteoporosis, all of which result in impaired quality of life.

One of the major eating disorders, anorexia nervosa, is also characterized by elevated cortisol concentrations via activation of the HPA axis caused by strict and prolonged energy restriction, as well as by mental stress [28]. Patients with anorexia nervosa demonstrate increased concentrations of CRH in their cerebrospinal fluid [28]. However, in contradistinction to depressed patients, they do not show any clinical manifestations suggestive of glucocorticoid excess. Indeed, they present with symptoms and signs associated with reduced action of glucocorticoids in target tissues, possibly due to lack of food substrate and changes of proteins that may influence the actions of glucocorticoids through the hGR, such as the AMP-activated protein kinase (AMPK) [29].

Any conditions associated with uncoupling of the cortisol circadian rhythm that is under the influence of the SCN CLOCK system, and the circadian peripheral tissue sensitivity to glucocorticoids, under the control of the peripheral CLOCK, may cause the development of components of the metabolic syndrome and its detrimental cardiovascular complications [10, 30]. Night-shift workers and people frequently exposed to jet lag are at an increased risk for developing symptoms and signs of chronic hypercortisolemia, such as central obesity, insulin resistance, dyslipidemia and hypertension, which represent the cardinal clinical manifestation of metabolic syndrome. These pathologic conditions were recently explained at the molecular and cellular level, when it was convincingly shown that the transcription factor "circadian locomotor output cycle kaput" (CLOCK) physically interacts with GR, and catalyzes enzymatically the acetylation of a lysine cluster, located in the hinge region of the receptor and leading to decreased sensitivity to glucocorticoids [10, 30, 31]. This effect of CLOCK on GR can lead to "functional" tissue hypersensitivity to glucocorticoids via uncoupling of circadian cortisol concentrations and peripheral tissue responsiveness to these hormones [10, 30, 31].

6.2 Pituitary Disorders Associated with Alterations in the HPA Axis

6.2.1 Cushing Disease (and Syndrome)

Cushing disease is part of Cushing syndrome, which is characterized by elevated concentrations of circulating cortisol and symptoms and signs of glucocorticoid excess. This disease is caused by semi-autonomous neoplasia or hyperplasia of corticotropes that result in oversecretion of ACTH from the pituitary gland. In contrast, Cushing syndrome indicates a disorder that derives from the adrenal glands, caused by either an adrenocortical adenoma or carcinoma, or from an ectopic site secreting CRH or ACTH (~15 % of ACTH-dependent forms of Cushing disease). Ectopic secretion of ACTH from non-pituitary tissues includes small cell carcinoma of the lung and lung carcinoids, pancreatic or adrenomedullary tumors, as well as other neoplasias [32].

The first manifestation of Cushing disease may be the loss of the diurnal rhythm in ACTH and cortisol secretion. Patients with either Cushing disease or syndrome present with "Cushingoid features", including moon facies, "buffalo hump", central obesity, purple skin striae, hypertension, insulin resistance/overt diabetes mellitus, mood changes, menstrual irregularity and osteoporosis [33]. The diagnosis should be made after careful medical history and physical examination, and confirmed by endocrinologic evaluation and imaging studies. Cushing disease is mostly caused by pituitary adenomas. They are usually microadenomas with a diameter less than 1 cm, and are sometimes quite difficult to detect even in the MRI scan with contrast material [34]. Bilateral inferior petrosal sinus sampling with CRH stimulation is helpful in some cases to localize pituitary adenomas in the pituitary including the site of the tumor inside the pituitary gland. The therapeutic approach of patients with Cushing disease starts with resection of the ACTH-secreting pituitary adenoma by transsphenoidal surgery [35]. However, 10–15 % of patients with remission may recur in the future. Bilateral adrenalectomy may be performed in difficult cases in which tumors cannot be successfully resected [35]. Radiation may also be applied to the pituitary gland in combination with medical therapy, usually with mitotane or ketoconazol.

6.2.2 Pituitary Disorders That Result in Hypofunction of the HPA Axis

Any space-occupying lesions in the pituitary gland may lead to hypofunction of the HPA axis and secondary adrenal insufficiency [24]. Pituitary adenomas, cysts, craniopharyngiomas, ependymomas, meningiomas and rarely carcinomas may interfere with ACTH secretion. In addition to these lesions, infections or infiltrative processes, including lymphocytic hypophysitis, haemochromatosis, tuberculosis, meningitis, sarcoidosis, actinomycosis, histiocytosis X and Wegener's granulomatosis can result in low ACTH release

[24]. Sheehan's syndrome is caused by pituitary apoplexy after labor and consequent pan-hypopituitarism, and used to be a major cause of secondary adrenal insufficiency. However, its incidence has been dramatically reduced because of the improved maternal care in developed countries.

Mutations in genes encoding crucial transcription factors and molecules essential for corticotrope survival and function can cause developmental defects and/or dysfunction in these cells leading to hypofunction of the HPA axis. So far, pathologic mutations have been identified in the genes expressing the transcription factors HESX homolog 1 (HESX1), orthodenticle homeobox 2 (OTX2), LIM homeobox 4 (LHX4), SRY (sex-determining region Y)-box 2 and 3 (SOX2 and SOX3), PROP paired-like homeobox 1 (PROP1) and T-box 19 (TBX19) [36]. Patients harboring these mutations may present with short stature, metabolic disorders, craniofacial abnormalities and learning difficulties/mental retardation associated with abnormalities in the CNS. The onset of adrenal insufficiency occurs generally early in life, although cases owing to PROP1 mutations usually manifest in adolescence.

Congenital pro-opiomelanocortin deficiency is another cause of secondary adrenal insufficiency. The molecular basis of this genetic condition has been ascribed to inactivating mutations in the pro-opiomelanocortin (POMC) gene. Patients develop a characteristic syndrome of hypocortisolism, early onset morbid obesity, and alterations in skin and hair pigmentation [37].

Achalasia-Adrenal Insufficiency-Alacrima syndrome or Allgrove Syndrome, also known as Triple-A syndrome, is a rare autosomal recessive disorder characterized by ACTH-resistant adrenal insufficiency, alacrima (absence of tear secretion), achalasia (dilatation of thoracic esophagus), autonomic dysfunction, and neurodegeneration. This syndrome is caused by mutations in the *AAAS* gene, which encodes the nuclear pore protein ALADIN with as yet unknown functions [38]. Adrenal insufficiency develops gradually within the first 10 years of life but sometimes becomes evident much later. It may present in some cases as an adrenal crisis with hypoglycemia and seizures.

6.3 Adrenal Disorders Associated with Alterations in the HPA Axis

6.3.1 Cushing Syndrome

Cushing syndrome can be caused by both benign and malignant lesions, such as glucocorticoid-producing adenomas, micro-nodular dysplasia, ACTH-independent macro-nodular hyperplasia or adenocarcinoma of the adrenal cortex [23, 33]. Patients with this syndrome appear with "Cushingoid features", as described above; however, their clinical manifestations depend on the severity and duration of cortisol excess. Cushing syndrome caused by adenocarcinoma is characterized by large tumors of more than 5 cm in diameter, and are usually rapidly progressing, whereas adenomas are usually small (less than 3 cm) and have generally an insidious onset and chronic course [39]. First choice treatment for Cushing syndrome remains the surgical removal of the tumor. Laparoscopic surgery is currently the approach of choice for the treatment of Cushing syndrome caused by adenomas [40]. In case of failure of resection of the entire mass, usually adenocarcinomas, or those with metastatic lesions, mitotane is used for suppressing both tumor growth and production of steroids [41]. This compound inhibits the cholesterol side-chain cleavage (SCC) enzyme (the human p450 CYP, cholesterol desmolase, or 20, 22 desmolase) and the 11β-hydroxylase (p450 11β or CYP11B1) [41]. Adrenal enzyme inhibitors, such as ketoconazole, metyrapone and etomidate, are also used in clinical practice for patients with surgical failure who remain hypercortisolemic [32].

6.3.2 Adrenal Disorders That Result in Hypofunction of the HPA Axis

Adrenal insufficiency is a disorder first described by Thomas Addison in 1855, which is characterized by deficient production or action of glucocorticoids and/or mineralocorticoids and adrenal androgens [24]. Any pathologic condition associated with destruction of the adrenal cortex can cause primary adrenal insufficiency. The etiology of primary adrenal insufficiency has changed over time. Prior to 1920, the most common cause of primary adrenal insufficiency was tuberculosis, while since 1950, the majority of cases (80–90 %) have been ascribed to autoimmune adrenalitis, which can be isolated (40 %) or in the context of an autoimmune polyendocrinopathy syndrome (60 %) [24]. The clinical symptoms of adrenal insufficiency include weakness, fatigue, anorexia, abdominal pain, weight loss, orthostatic hypotension, salt craving, and characteristic hyperpigmentation of the skin. Regardless of etiology, adrenal insufficiency was an invariably fatal disorder, until the synthesis of cortisone by Kendall and Reichstein in 1949, and the introduction of substitution therapy with life-saving synthetic glucocorticoids. Today, patients with primary adrenal insufficiency are treated with hydrocortisone or cortisone acetate if hydrocortisone is not available, and fludrocortisone to prevent intravascular volume depletion, hyponatremia and hyperkalemia [24]. One of the most important aspects of the management of chronic primary adrenal insufficiency is patient and family education. Patients should understand the reason for life-long replacement therapy, the need to increase the dose of glucocorticoids during minor or major stress and to inject hydrocortisone or methylprednisolone in emergencies.

6.4 Other Disorders Associated with Changes in the HPA Axis

6.4.1 Generalized Glucocorticoid Resistance Syndrome (Chrousos Syndrome)

Primary generalized glucocorticoid resistance (Chrousos syndrome) is a rare, familial or sporadic condition, which is characterized by generalized partial end-organ insensitivity to glucocorticoids [42, 43]. Affected patients have compensatory elevation in circulating cortisol and ACTH concentrations, which maintain circadian rhythmicity and appropriate responsiveness to stressors, and resistance of the HPA axis to dexamethasone suppression, but no clinical manifestations suggestive of Cushing syndrome. The clinical spectrum of this condition is broad, ranging from completely asymptomatic cases, displaying biochemical alterations only, to severe forms of mineralocorticoid and/or androgen excess [44]. The molecular basis of Chrousos syndrome has been ascribed to inactivating mutations in the *hGR* gene [16, 42–45]. Most of these mutations are located in the GR LBD, which alter functions of this subdomain, such as ligand-binding, activation of transcription and nuclear translocation. So far only two mutations have been reported in the DBD of GR: R477H and V423A [46]. All reported pathologic mutations causing familial or sporadic Chrousos syndrome are depicted in Fig. 6.4. Recently, a heterozygous mutation causing glucocorticoid hypersensitivity, ie the mirror image of glucocorticoid resistance, was described [47]. In this patient, Cushingoid features such as obesity and metabolic syndrome were associated with low normal cortisol levels.

6.4.2 hGR Polymorphisms

Inter-individual variations in tissue sensitivity to glucocorticoids have been described within the normal population and have been partly attributed to polymorphisms in the *hGR* gene [16]. A heterozygous polymorphism replacing aspartic acid to serine at amino acid 363 that mildly increases the transcriptional activity of the affected receptor *in vitro* is associated with glucocorticoid hypersensitivity, weakly correlating with the development of central obesity and, thus, influencing the metabolic profile and the longevity of humans in a negative fashion [48, 49].

The polymorphism in the GR gene that causes arginine to lysine replacement at amino acid 23 (ER22/23EK: GAG AGG to GA<u>A</u> A<u>A</u>G) is associated with relative glucocorticoid resistance by altering the expression levels of GR translational isoforms [50]. This polymorphism increases muscle mass in males and reduces waist to hip ratio in females [51], and is associated with greater insulin sensitivity, and lower total and low-density lipoprotein cholesterol levels [52], indicating

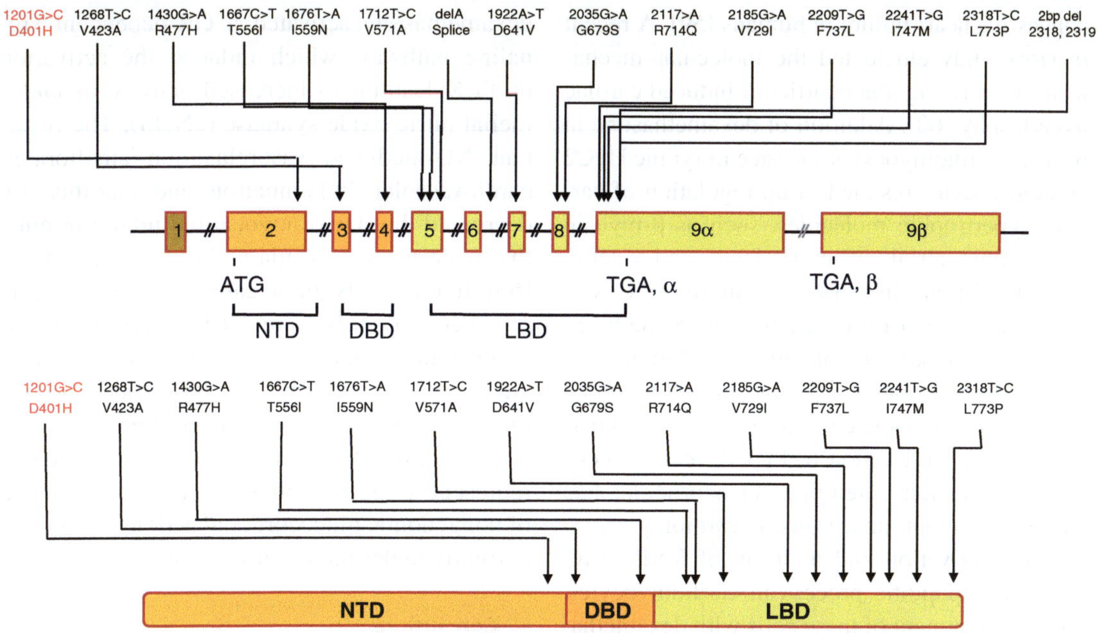

Fig. 6.4 Location of the identified mutations in the *hGR* gene causing Chrousos syndrome. A mutation that causes glucocorticoid hypersensitivity is included in *red color. NTD* N-terminal domain, *DBD* DNA-binding domain, *LBD* ligand-binding domain, *ATG* translation initiation codon, *TGA* stop codon, 1-8, 9α, 9β Exons 1-8, 9α, 9β (Modified from Ref. [43])

that this polymorphism has a beneficial effect on longevity by reducing glucocorticoid action.

6.4.3 Ectopic Tumors Producing ACTH or CRH

Ectopic ACTH producing tumors account for ~15 % of ACTH-dependent Cushing syndrome [53]. Most of them are malignant and occur more frequently in men than in women. These tumors usually derive from neuroendocrine cells, but adenocarcinoma and squamous cell carcinoma may also cause the syndrome [53]. Approximately half of the cases are due to small cell carcinoma of the lung. Carcinoids originating from the thymus, bronchi and other organs, pancreatic islet tumors, pheochromocytomas and ovarian adenocarcinomas may also be associated with this syndrome [54]. Patients with this condition have elevated concentrations of cortisol and ACTH, while concentrations of other POMC-related peptides and bioactive molecules, such as other pituitary hormones, calcitonin, somatostatin are sometimes increased because of their concurrent ectopic production by the tumors [54]. Hypokalemia occurs in most cases with this syndrome. Manifestations are of sudden onset and their progression is usually rapid and sometimes not responsive to treatment.

6.4.4 The Cardiomyocyte as a Glucocorticoid Target Cell

In addition to common cardiovascular manifestations, such as hypertension and metabolic syndrome, often observed in several pathologic conditions associated with alterations in the activity of the HPA axis, accumulating evidence suggests that glucocorticoids exert direct effects on cardiomyocytes. Indeed, glucocorticoids stimulate cardiomyocyte contraction by influencing calcium homeostasis [55–57]. Moreover, mice overexpressing GR in their cardiomyocytes exhibit atrioventricular block [58]. Furthermore, glucocorticoids may cause cardiac hypertrophy, a condition that represents a severe cause of congestive heart failure in humans [59]. A recent *in vitro* study elucidated the molecular mechanisms underlying glucocorticoid-induced cardiac hypertrophy [60]. Addition of dexamethasone in primary cardiomyocytes and rat embryonic H9C2 cardiomyocytes resulted in up-regulation of cardiac hypertrophic molecules, such as β-myosin heavy chain, atrial natriuretic factor and α-actin, resulting in an increased cardiomyocyte size [60]. These glucocorticoid effects were mediated by the GR, as exposure of cells to the GR antagonist RU 486 or addition of GR shRNA inhibited dexamethasone-induced cardiomyocyte hypertrophy [60]. In addition to hypertrophic effects, this study demonstrated that glucocorticoids had strong anti-apoptotic actions on cardiomyocytes. Serum deprivation and addition of TNFα triggered the apoptotic process in cardiomyocytes, whereas treatment of these cells with dexamethasone caused significant up-regulation of the key anti-apoptotic molecule *Bcl-xL* and concurrent down-regulation of *Gas2*, a known target of caspases-3 and −7 [60]. Importantly, these anti-apoptotic glucocorticoid actions may prevent cardiomyocyte death in severe pathologic conditions, such as ischemia/reperfusion injury.

6.4.5 Beneficial Nongenomic Glucocorticoid Effects in Cardiac Ischemia/ Reperfusion Injury

In the past, glucocorticoids were used in acute myocardial ischemia due to their cardioprotective effects. Indeed, the acute administration of glucocorticoids decreased myocardial ischemic injury in animal models [61, 62] and increased the critical short-term survival of patients after acute myocardial infarction [63]. However, synthetic glucocorticoids are not used in the current treatment of acute myocardial ischemia because of their severe side effects, such as cardiac rupture [64]. An interesting study shed light on the acute cardioprotective effects of glucocorticoids both in *in vitro* experiments and in cardiac ischemia /reperfusion injury animal models [65]. Acute administration of high doses of dexamethasone activated a GR-dependent signaling pathway, which induced the activation of PI_3K leading to increased activity of endothelial nitric oxide synthase (eNOS). The resultant NO-mediated vasorelaxation ameliorated cardiovascular inflammation and significantly decreased the size of myocardial infarct in mice that underwent ischemia and reperfusion injury [65]. Interestingly, these cardioprotective effects of glucocorticoids were GRE-independent and nongenomic, since the dexamethasone-bound GR activated acutely the synthesis of NO through non-transcriptional mechanisms. The acute cardioprotective effects of glucocorticoids represent a strong evidence for the importance of nongenomic glucocorticoid actions, which are currently under intense investigation.

Conclusions

The HPA axis plays a fundamental role in the maintenance of basal and stress-related homeostasis; dysfunction of hypothalamic nuclei, pituitary or adrenal glands may cause symptoms and signs associated with glucocorticoid excess or deficiency. Accordingly, the aim of treatment is to correct both the primary cause and the associated hormonal abnormality. During the last several decades, despite the well-recognized significant progress in the clinical care of patients with disorders of the HPA axis, there are still numerous challenges regarding the diagnosis and treatment of these conditions. Indeed, the ubiquitous presence and actions of glucocorticoids, the rapid advances in our general knowledge of the human genome and our ever-increasing understanding of cell signaling allow us to view the actions and functions of the HPA axis and its involvement in human health and disease in a more integrated fashion.

References

1. Chrousos GP. Stress and disorders of the stress system. Nat Rev Endocrinol. 2009;5:374–81.
2. Chrousos GP, Gold PW. The concepts of stress and stress system disorders: overview of physical and behavioral homeostasis. JAMA. 1992;267:1244–52.

3. Charmandari E, Tsigos C, Chrousos GP. Endocrinology of the stress response. Annu Rev Physiol. 2005;67:259–84.
4. Chrousos GP, Kino T. Glucocorticoid action networks and complex psychiatric and/or somatic disorders. Stress. 2007;10:213–9.
5. Kontopoulou TD, Marketos SG. Homeostasis. The ancient Greek origin of a modern scientific principle. Hormones. 2002;1:124–5.
6. Fink G. Stress: definition and history. In: Squire LR, editor. Encyclopedia of neuroscience, vol. 9. Oxford: Academic; 2009. p. 549–55.
7. Weinberger C, Hollenberg SM, Ong ES, Harmon JM, Brower ST, Cidlowski J, et al. Identification of human glucocorticoid receptor complementary DNA clones by epitope selection. Science. 1985;228(4700):740–2.
8. Chrousos GP, Kino T. Intracellular glucocorticoid signaling: a formerly simple system turns stochastic. Sci STKE. 2005;(304):e48.
9. Chrousos GP. The hypothalamic-pituitary-adrenal axis and immune-mediated inflammation. N Engl J Med. 1995;332:1351–62.
10. Nader N, Chrousos GP, Kino T. Interactions of the circadian CLOCK system and the HPA axis. Trends Endocrinol Metab. 2010;21:277–86.
11. Chrousos GP, Calabrese JR, Avgerinos P, Kling MA, Rubinow D, Oldfield EH, et al. Corticotropin releasing factor: basic studies and clinical applications. Prog Neuropsychopharmacol Biol Psychiatry. 1985;9:349–59.
12. Calogero AE, Bernardini R, Gold PW, Chrousos GP. Regulation of rat hypothalamic corticotropin-releasing hormone secretion in vitro: potential clinical implications. Adv Exp Med Biol. 1988;245:167–81.
13. Smith MA, Kling MA, Whitfield HJ, Brandt HA, Demitrack MA, Geracioti TD, Chrousos GP, Gold PW. Corticotropin-releasing hormone: from endocrinology to psychobiology. Horm Res. 1989;31:66–71.
14. Stevens A, White A. ACTH: cellular peptide hormone synthesis and secretory pathways. Results Probl Cell Differ. 2010;50:63–84.
15. Bornstein SR, Chrousos GP. Clinical review 104: Adrenocorticotropin (ACTH)- and non-ACTH-mediated regulation of the adrenal cortex: neural and immune inputs. J Clin Endocrinol Metab. 1999;84:1729–36.
16. Nicolaides NC, Galata Z, Kino T, Chrousos GP, Charmandari E. The human glucocorticoid receptor: molecular basis of biologic function. Steroids. 2010;75:1–12.
17. Kino T, Chrousos GP. Glucocorticoid and mineralocorticoid receptors and associated diseases. Essays Biochem. 2004;40:137–55.
18. Bamberger CM, Bamberger AM, de Castro M, Chrousos GP. Glucocorticoid receptor β, a potential endogenous inhibitor of glucocorticoid action in humans. J Clin Invest. 1995;95:2435–41.
19. Kino T, De Martino MU, Charmandari E, Mirani M, Chrousos GP. Tissue glucocorticoid resistance/hypersensitivity syndromes. J Steroid Biochem Mol Biol. 2003;85:457–67.
20. Charmandari E, Chrousos GP, Ichijo T, Bhattacharyya N, Vottero A, Souvatzoglou E, et al. The human glucocorticoid receptor (hGR) β isoform suppresses the transcriptional activity of hGRα by interfering with formation of active coactivator complexes. Mol Endocrinol. 2005;19:52–64.
21. Yudt MR, Jewell CM, Bienstock RJ, Cidlowski JA. Molecular origins for the dominant negative function of human glucocorticoid receptor β. Mol Cell Biol. 2003;23:4319–30.
22. Lu NZ, Cidlowski JA. Translational regulatory mechanisms generate N-terminal glucocorticoid receptor isoforms with unique transcriptional target genes. Mol Cell. 2005;18:331–42.
23. Chrousos GP. Glucocorticoid therapy. In: Felig P, Frohman LA, editors. Endocrinology & metabolism. 4th ed. New York: McGraw-Hill; 2001. p. 609–32.
24. Charmandari E, Nicolaides NC, Chrousos GP. Adrenal insufficiency. Lancet. 2014;383:2152–67.
25. de Lind van Wijngaarden RF, Otten BJ, Festen DA, Joosten KF, de Jong FH, Sweep FC, et al. High prevalence of central adrenal insufficiency in patients with Prader-Willi syndrome. J Clin Endocrinol Metab. 2008;93:1649–54.
26. Gold PW, Chrousos GP. The endocrinology of melancholic and atypical depression: relation to neurocircuitry and somatic consequences. Proc Assoc Am Physicians. 1999;111:22–34.
27. Gold PW, Goodwin FK, Chrousos GP. Clinical and biochemical manifestations of depression. Relation to the neurobiology of stress (2). N Engl J Med. 1988;319:413–20.
28. Kaye WH, Gwirtsman HE, George DT, Ebert MH, Jimerson DC, Tomai TP, et al. Elevated cerebrospinal fluid levels of immunoreactive corticotropin-releasing hormone in anorexia nervosa: relation to state of nutrition, adrenal function, and intensity of depression. J Clin Endocrinol Metab. 1987;64:203–8.
29. Nader N, Ng SS, Lambrou GI, Pervanidou P, Wang Y, Chrousos GP, et al. AMPK regulates metabolic actions of glucocorticoids by phosphorylating the glucocorticoid receptor through p38 MAPK. Mol Endocrinol. 2010;24:1748–64.
30. Kino T, Chrousos GP. Circadian CLOCK-mediated regulation of target-tissue sensitivity to glucocorticoids: implications for cardiometabolic diseases. Endocr Dev. 2011;20:116–26.
31. Nader N, Chrousos GP, Kino T. Circadian rhythm transcription factor CLOCK regulates the transcriptional activity of the glucocorticoid receptor by acetylating its hinge region lysine cluster: potential physiological implications. FASEB J. 2009;23:1572–83.
32. Veytsman I, Nieman L, Fojo T. Management of endocrine manifestations and the use of mitotane as a chemotherapeutic agent for adrenocortical carcinoma. J Clin Oncol. 2009;27:4619–29.
33. Orth DN, Kovacs WJ, DeBold CR. The adrenal cortex. In: Wilson JD, Foster DW, Kronenberg HM, Larsen R, editors. Textbook of endocrinology. 9th ed. Philadelphia: W.B. Saunders Co; 1998. p. 517–664.

34. Tsigos C, Chrousos GP. Differential diagnosis and management of Cushing's syndrome. Annu Rev Med. 1996;47:443–61.
35. Aghi MK. Management of recurrent and refractory Cushing disease. Nat Clin Pract Endocrinol Metab. 2008;4:560–8.
36. Kelberman D, Dattani MT. Hypopituitarism oddities: congenital causes. Horm Res. 2007;68 Suppl 5:138–44.
37. Krude H, Biebermann H, Luck W, Horn R, Brabant G, Gruters A. Severe early-onset obesity, adrenal insufficiency and red hair pigmentation caused by POMC mutations in humans. Nat Genet. 1998;19:155–7.
38. Cronshaw JM, Matunis MJ. The nuclear pore complex: disease associations and functional correlations. Trends Endocrinol Metab. 2004;15:34–9.
39. Patalano A, Brancato V, Mantero F. Adrenocortical cancer treatment. Horm Res. 2009;71 Suppl 1:99–104.
40. Porterfield JR, Thompson GB, Young Jr WF, Chow JT, Fryrear RS, van Heerden JA, et al. Surgery for Cushing's syndrome: an historical review and recent ten-year experience. World J Surg. 2008;32:659–77.
41. Terzolo M, Angeli A, Fassnacht M, Daffara F, Tauchmanova L, Conton PA, et al. Adjuvant mitotane treatment for adrenocortical carcinoma. N Engl J Med. 2007;356:2372–80.
42. Charmandari E. Primary generalized glucocorticoid resistance and hypersensitivity. Horm Res Paediatr. 2011;76:145–55.
43. Charmandari E, Kino T. Chrousos syndrome: a seminal report, a phylogenetic enigma and the clinical implications of glucocorticoid signalling changes. Eur J Clin Invest. 2010;40:932–42.
44. Charmandari E. Primary generalized glucocorticoid resistance and hypersensitivity: the end-organ involvement in the stress response. Sci Signal. 2012;5(244):pt5.
45. Charmandari E, Kino T, Ichijo T, Chrousos GP. Generalized glucocorticoid resistance: clinical aspects, molecular mechanisms, and implications of a rare genetic disorder. J Clin Endocrinol Metab. 2008;93(5):1563–72.
46. Roberts ML, Kino T, Nicolaides NC, Hurt DE, Katsantoni E, Sertedaki A, et al. A novel point mutation in the DNA-binding domain (DBD) of the human glucocorticoid receptor causes primary generalized glucocorticoid resistance by disrupting the hydrophobic structure of its DBD. J Clin Endocrinol Metab. 2013;98:E790–5.
47. Charmandari E, Ichijo T, Jubiz W, Baid S, Zachman K, Chrousos GP, et al. A novel point mutation in the amino terminal domain of the human glucocorticoid receptor (hGR) gene enhancing hGR-mediated gene expression. J Clin Endocrinol Metab. 2008;93:4963–8.
48. Huizenga NA, Koper JW, De Lange P, Pols HA, Stolk RP, Burger H, et al. A polymorphism in the glucocorticoid receptor gene may be associated with and increased sensitivity to glucocorticoids in vivo. J Clin Endocrinol Metab. 1998;83:144–51.
49. Dobson MG, Redfern CP, Unwin N, Weaver JU. The N363S polymorphism of the glucocorticoid receptor: potential contribution to central obesity in men and lack of association with other risk factors for coronary heart disease and diabetes mellitus. J Clin Endocrinol Metab. 2001;86:2270–4.
50. Russcher H, van Rossum EF, de Jong FH, Brinkmann AO, Lamberts SW, Koper JW. Increased expression of the glucocorticoid receptor-A translational isoform as a result of the ER22/23EK polymorphism. Mol Endocrinol. 2005;19:1687–96.
51. van Rossum EF, Voorhoeve PG, te Velde SJ, Koper JW, Delemarre-van de Waal HA, Kemper HC, et al. The ER22/23EK polymorphism in the glucocorticoid receptor gene is associated with a beneficial body composition and muscle strength in young adults. J Clin Endocrinol Metab. 2004;89:4004–9.
52. van Rossum EF, Koper JW, Huizenga NA, Uitterlinden AG, Janssen JA, Brinkmann AO, et al. A polymorphism in the glucocorticoid receptor gene, which decreases sensitivity to glucocorticoids in vivo, is associated with low insulin and cholesterol levels. Diabetes. 2002;51:3128–34.
53. Nieman LK, Ilias I. Evaluation and treatment of Cushing's syndrome. Am J Med. 2005;118:1340–6.
54. Isidori AM, Kaltsas GA, Pozza C, Frajese V, Newell-Price J, Reznek RH, et al. The ectopic adrenocorticotropin syndrome: clinical features, diagnosis, management, and long-term follow-up. J Clin Endocrinol Metab. 2006;91:371–7.
55. Whitehurst Jr RM, Zhang M, Bhattacharjee A, Li M. Dexamethasone-induced hypertrophy in rat neonatal cardiac myocytes involves an elevated L-type Ca(2+)current. J Mol Cell Cardiol. 1999;31:1551–8.
56. Hadoke PW, Iqbal J, Walker BR. Therapeutic manipulation of glucocorticoid metabolism in cardiovascular disease. Br J Pharmacol. 2009;156:689–712.
57. Wang L, Feng ZP, Duff HJ. Glucocorticoid regulation of cardiac K^+ currents and L-type Ca^{2+} current in neonatala mice. Circ Res. 1999;85:168–73.
58. Sainte-Marie Y, Nguyen Dinh Cat A, Perrier R, Mangin L, Soukaseum C, Peuchmaur M, et al. Conditional glucocorticoid receptor expression in the heart induces atrio-ventricular block. FASEB J. 2007;21:3133–41.
59. Lister K, Autelitano DJ, Jenkins A, Hannan RD, Sheppard KE. Cross talk between corticosteroids and alpha-adrenergic signaling augments cardiomyocyte hypertrophy: a possible role for SGK1. Cardiovasc Res. 2006;70:555–65.
60. Ren R, Oakley RH, Cruz-Topete D, Cidlowski JA. Dual role for glucocorticoids in cardiomyocyte hypertrophy and apoptosis. Endocrinology. 2012;153:5346–60.
61. Libby P, Maroko PR, Bloor CM, Sobel BE, Braunwald E. Reduction of experimental myocardial infarct size by corticosteroid administration. J Clin Invest. 1973;52:599–607.

62. Spath Jr JA, Lane DL, Lefer AM. Protective action of methylprednisolone on the myocardium during experimental myocardial ischemia in the cat. Circ Res. 1974;35:44–51.
63. Barzilai D, Plavnick J, Hazani A, Einath R, Kleinhaus N, et al. Use of hydrocortisone in the treatment of acute myocardial infarction. Summary of a clinical trial in 446 patients. Chest. 1972;61:488–91.
64. Hammerman H, Schoen FJ, Braunwald E, Kloner RA. Drug-induced expansion of infarct: morphologic and functional correlations. Circulation. 1984;69:611–7.
65. Hafezi-Moghadam A, Simoncini T, Yang Z, Limbourg FP, Plumier JC, et al. Acute cardiovascular protective effects of corticosteroids are mediated by non-transcriptional activation of endothelial nitric oxide synthase. Nat Med. 2002;8:473–9.

Part III

Fundamental Aspects and Processes

7 Genetic Polymorphisms

Katherine Anagnostopoulou and Genovefa Kolovou

Abstract

Human genetics has evolved rapidly during the past years. It is widely accepted that human diseases have a genetic component and can be characterized either as monogenic or polygenic (also known as complex or multifactorial) such as diabetes mellitus, obesity, cardiovascular disease, dyslipidemia, hypertension, psychiatric diseases, cancer and others. Polygenic diseases are more common and widely variable, and thus, very complex to be studied as they are influenced by both gene-to-gene and gene-to-environment interactions. Two randomly chosen individuals differ in about 0.1 % of their genomes while the rest 99.9 % is identical. This small genetic variability seems to be responsible for all the phenotypic differences among people. As cardiovascular management has shifted from acute intervention to prediction and prevention, genetic studies (linkage analysis, association studies, genome-wide association studies) are focused on identifying susceptibility loci on the DNA. Genetic science, after the completion of the Human Genome Project (the complete sequence of the human genome), has moved to the post-genomic era and with the remarkable growth of Bioinformatics, new technologies have been evolved which enabled the creation of numerous databases and the relevant tools for their analysis. Moreover, recent advances in molecular biology techniques have allowed parallel genotyping, using microarray technology, and genome sequencing, by massive next-generation sequencing in a cost- and time-effective way. These technological tools have led to a better understanding of the genetic structure of the human genome. This chapter describes in detail the different types of genetic variability and focuses on how this variation has contributed to identify candidate susceptibility genes that could predict cardiovascular disease risk.

K. Anagnostopoulou (✉) • G. Kolovou
Department of Cardiology, Onassis Cardiac Surgery Center, Kallithea, Greece
e-mail: kat_anag@yahoo.com; genovefa@kolovou.com

D.V. Cokkinos (ed.), *Introduction to Translational Cardiovascular Research*,
DOI 10.1007/978-3-319-08798-6_7, © Springer International Publishing Switzerland 2015

Keywords
Complex disease • Genetic polymorphisms • Genetic studies • Human genome project • Mutations

Abbreviations

ABCA1	ATP-Binding Cassette, sub-family A, member 1
ABCG5	ATP-Binding Cassette, sub-family G, member 5
ABCG8	ATP-Binding Cassette, sub-family G, member 8
ACE	Angiotensin Converting Enzyme
APOA5	Apolipoprotein A5
APOB	Apolipoprotein B
APOCII	Apolipoprotein CII
ARH	Low Density Lipoprotein Receptor Adaptor Protein 1
Array CGH	Comparative Genomic Hybridization
ATP	Adenosine Triphosphate
CAD	Coronary Artery Disease
CEPH	Centre d'Etude du Polymorphism Humain
CFTR	Cystic Fibrosis Transmembrane Conductance Regulator
CHD	Coronary Heart Disease
CNVs	Copy-Number Variations
CVD	Cardiovascular Disease
CYP7A1	Cytochrome P450, family 7, subfamily A, polypeptide 1
DNA	Deoxyribonucleic acid
GCK	Glucokinase (hexokinase 4)
GPIHBP1	Glycosylphosphatidylinositol-anchored High density lipoprotein-Binding Protein 1
GWAS	Genome-Wide Association Studies
HNF4A	Hepatocyte Nuclear Factor 4, Alpha
Indels	Insertions/deletions
IPF1/PDX1	Insulin Promoter Factor 1/ Pancreatic and Duodenal homeobox 1
LDL	Low-Density Lipoprotein
LDLR	LDL Receptor
LFM1	Lipase Maturation Factor 1
LPL	Lipoprotein Lipase
MI	Myocardial Infarction
mtDNA	Mitochondrial DNA
NGS	Next-Generation Sequencing
ORs	Odds Ratios
PCR	Polymerase Chain Reaction
PCSK9	Proprotein Convertase Subtilisin/Kexin type 9
RFLP	Restriction Fragment Length Polymorphism
rRNA	Ribosomal RNA
SCN5A	Sodium Channel α-subunit
SNPs	Single Nucleotide Polymorphisms
STRs	Short Tandem Repeats
TCF1/HNF1A	Transcription Factor 1/Hepatocyte Nuclear Factor 1 Alpha
TCF2/HNF1B	Transcription Factor 2/ Hepatocyte Nuclear Factor 1 homeobox B
tRNA	Transfer RNA
VNTRs	Variable Number of Tandem Repeats

7.1 Introduction

7.1.1 Genetics Basics

The term "Genetics" comes from Ancient Greek and means "genesis" (i.e. origin). The science of genetics studies the mechanisms related to heredity and biodiversity. Genetic science can be subdivided into five main fields: classical genetics (mode of inheritance), molecular genetics (gene function and expression), cytogenetics (study of chromosomes), microbial genetics (genetics of microorganisms) and population genetics (allele frequency distribution and change under the influence of natural selection, genetic drift, mutation and gene flow).

In humans, the genetic material, deoxyribonucleic acid (DNA) is located in the nucleus of every cell. It is a double-stranded molecule 3.3×10^9 base pairs that is organized in 46 chromosomes [22 pairs of autosomes (numbered 1–22) and 1 pair of sex chromosomes (X and Y)] in somatic cells and half the amount [23 chromosomes (1–22 autosomes and 1 sex chromosome, either X or Y)] in gametes. Thus each of the parents transmits 23 chromosomes to their offspring. DNA is composed of four nucleotide bases, abbreviated A, T, C and G, that stand for adenine, thymine, cytosine and guanine, respectively. The linear sequence of these bases specifies the genetic information (genetic code). Unlike germ cells, which are haploid, in a somatic cell (i.e. diploid), each chromosome appears twice (with the exception of sex chromosomes in men, XY) and these identical chromosomes are called homologues. Therefore, there are two copies of each gene, one on each homologue. An allele is one of a pair of genes that appear at a particular location on a chromosome and control the same characteristic [1]. A set of alleles at nearby loci located on the same chromosomal strand is called a haplotype. In the absence of recombination between homologous chromosomes at the time of gamete formation, loci located on the same chromosome are transmitted together as a haplotype [2].

Mitochondria have also a small amount of DNA (mitochondrial DNA, mtDNA), which codes for only 37 genes essential for normal mitochondrial function and consists of only about 16,600 base pairs. Human mtDNA is inherited solely from the mother. Thirteen of these genes encode enzymes involved in production of adenosine triphosphate by oxidative phosphorylation which takes place in the mitochondrion. The remaining genes encode transfer RNA (tRNA) and ribosomal RNA (rRNA) molecules. The disorders associated with mitochondrial genes include Leber hereditary optic neuropathy, Leigh syndrome, maternally inherited diabetes and deafness, mitochondrial encephalomyopathy, lactic acidosis, and stroke-like episodes, myoclonic epilepsy with ragged-red fibers, neuropathy-ataxia-retinitis pigmentosa, nonsyndromic deafness, palmoplantar keratoderma with deafness and progressive external ophthalmoplegia [3].

Genetic science has evolved rapidly through the twentieth century. In nineteenth century, Gregor Mendel, known as the founder of genetics, who was not aware of DNA existence, observed that certain traits in pea plants follow particular patterns of inheritance, now referred to as the laws of Mendel [4]. In 1911, Thomas Hunt Morgan revealed that genetic material is located on chromosomes [5]. In 1953, James D. Watson and Francis Crick [1] elucidated the structure of the DNA as double-helix and 9 years later, in 1962, they shared the Nobel Prize for solving one of the most important of all biological riddles. In 1983, Kary Mullis developed the polymerase chain reaction (PCR) an indispensable technique in medical and biological research and diagnosis [6]. In 1989, the gene CFTR (cystic fibrosis transmembrane conductance regulator), in which mutations are responsible for cystic fibrosis was the first gene whose sequence was determined [7] and in 1995, the genome of the bacteria *Haemophilus influenzae* was the first complete genome sequenced [8].

In 1990, the largest collaborative biological project "The Human Genome Project" was initiated aimed to determine the human DNA sequence and to identify and map the total number of genes in the human genome. An initial rough draft of the human genome was available in June 2000 and The Human Genome Project was declared complete on April 14, 2003. According to the report, 99 % of the human genome was sequenced with 99.99 % specificity [9]. The Human Genome Project revealed that human DNA consists of ~3 billion base pairs and ~25,000 haploid protein-coding genes. Paradoxically, only about 1.5 % of the genome codes for proteins, while the rest consists of noncoding RNA genes, regulatory sequences, introns and noncoding DNA (known as "junk DNA").

Humans have on average only three times the protein-coding genes compared to the fly or worm. However, the same gene can produce different protein products by a process known as "alternative splicing". Additionally, the DNA between two different individuals is 99.9 % similar and differs only in 0.1 % [10]. This small percentage, though, seems enough to account for all the observed interindividual differences in disease genetic predisposition and in therapeutic drug response.

As we have now proceeded to the post-genomic era, a new task for geneticists has emerged: the successful translation of this knowledge into clinical benefit. Consequently, genetic research has two main goals. Firstly, the prognosis of individuals at risk for disease by identifying and mapping disease-causing genes and secondly, to elucidate the biochemical pathways of pathogenesis. The latter is of high significance, since the identification of such pathways will make the development of new therapeutic targets feasible.

7.2 Evidence of Genetic Susceptibility for Cardiovascular Disease

Cardiovascular disease (CVD) has attracted geneticists' interest as it is the leading cause of death worldwide, causing 7,249,000 deaths in 2008, and 12.7 % of global mortality, which has not changed up to date. Since the 1970s, cardiovascular mortality rates have declined in many affluent countries but at the same time, morbidity and mortality have developed at a fast rate in low- and middle-income countries [11, 12]. Coronary heart disease (CHD) alone caused ≈ 1 of every 6 deaths in the United States in 2009. Approximately every 34 s, 1 American has a coronary event, and approximately every 1 min, an American will die of one [12]. The major risk factors for the development of CHD are male gender, increasing age, elevated levels of plasma low-density lipoprotein (LDL) cholesterol, elevated blood pressure, obesity and life style factors such as smoking, a high fat diet and lack of exercise. High plasma LDL cholesterol concentration promotes the formation of coronary atherosclerotic plaques. Vulnerable plaques can rupture, leading to vessel occlusion and ischemic events [13, 14].

The genetic predisposition for CVD has been widely accepted. CHD phenotype usually follows a heritable mode within families. An individual's family history is the most direct and cost-effective information to evaluate genetic susceptibility to CHD. According to the Framingham risk algorithm, a positive family history of premature CHD or stroke is associated with 2.4 fold higher risk in men and 2.2 fold higher risk in women for a future event [15]. Further studies in the past have shown that even after adjustment for age, sex, total cholesterol, high density lipoprotein cholesterol, hypertension, diabetes, cigarette smoking and body mass index, family history remains a highly significant predictor of future coronary artery disease (CAD) [16]. Moreover, the risk of myocardial infarction (MI) in men increases with decreasing age of parental MI. Paternal history of MI has been related to increased risk of coronary artery surgery and in general, a history of MI in either parent has been associated with an increased risk of CAD among men [17]. The INTERHEART study showed that after adjustment for age, sex, smoking and geographic region, a positive family history for MI increases significantly the CAD risk (odds ratio 1.54) [18].

Twin studies also support a genetic basis for CHD. Among 21,004 Swedish twins followed for 26 years, the relative hazard of death from CHD when one's twin died of CHD before the age of 55 years, as compared with the hazard when one's twin did not die before 55, was 8.1 for male monozygotic twins and 3.8 for male dizygotic twins. Among the women, when one's twin died of CHD before the age of 65 years, the relative hazard was 15.0 for monozygotic twins and 2.6 for dizygotic twins. These findings suggest that the younger the age of the CAD event, the stronger the genetic component which implies that the genetic effect decreases with increasing age [19]. Heritability estimates in 36-year follow-up of 20,966 Swedish twins were 0.57 and 0.38 among males and females, respectively [20].

7.2.1 Monogenic and Polygenic Heart Diseases

7.2.1.1 Lipid Disorders

Genetic diseases can be characterized either as monogenic or polygenic (also known as common or complex). In monogenic diseases, a single gene is responsible for the clinical phenotype. Monogenic disorders follow a Mendelian pattern of inheritance (autosomal dominant/recessive, X-linked, Y-linked or holandric). Familial hypercholesterolemia is characterized by considerably increased levels of total and LDL cholesterol, early incidence of MI and cutaneous lipid deposition (xanthomata and xanthelasmata). Familial hypercholesterolemia is known to occur due to mutations in either of six genes encoding proteins involved in the uptake of LDL cholesterol from the plasma. These genes are LDLR (LDL receptor), APOB (apolipoprotein B), PCSK9 (proprotein convertase subtilisin/kexin type 9), ARH (low density lipoprotein receptor adaptor protein 1), CYP7A1 (cytochrome P450, family 7, subfamily A, polypeptide 1), ABCG5 (ATP-binding cassette, sub-family G, member 5) or ABCG8 (ATP-binding cassette, sub-family G, member 8), and follow an autosomal dominant or recessive pattern of inheritance [14, 21–23]. Currently, more than 1,200 different LDLR mutations have been reported by Usifo et al. [24] but only one common in APOB (c.10580G>A, p.Arg3527Gln) and one in PCSK9 (c.1120G>T, p.Asp374Tyr) [25, 26]. Familial chylomicronemia is a rare autosomal recessive disorder (also called Hyperlipoproteinemia type I) caused by mutations in LPL (lipoprotein lipase) or APOCII (apolipoprotein CII) genes resulting in lipoprotein lipase or apolipoprotein C-II deficiency. It is characterized by marked elevation of chylomicron and triglyceride levels (>1,000 mg/dl), resulting in lipemic plasma and recurrent attacks of acute pancreatitis, eruptive xanthoma, hepatosplenomegaly, and lipemia retinalis [27]. Additional genes involved in monogenic early-onset familial hypertriglyceridemia with a typical Mendelian recessive inheritance include LPL, APOCII, LFM1 (lipase maturation factor 1), GPIHBP1 (glycosylphosphatidylinositol-anchored high density lipoprotein-binding protein 1), APOA5 (apolipoprotein A5) [28, 29].

Tangier disease is also a rare autosomal recessive disease caused by mutations in ABCA1 (ATP-binding cassette, sub-family A, member 1) gene, encoding ABCA1 protein. This and similar proteins, present in all species, are integral membrane proteins and use ATP as a source of energy to transport a wide assortment of molecules, such as ions, sugars, vitamins, lipids, amino acids, peptides, proteins and a large number of hydrophobic compounds and metabolites across intracellular and plasma membranes. The transmembrane domains form a pathway across the membrane through which substrates pass. Upon ATP binding and hydrolysis, ABC transporters undergo conformational change altering the affinity and orientation of the substrate binding sites. In patients with Tangier disease, the plasma lipid profile is very characteristic, with nearly zero high density lipoprotein cholesterol, very low LDL cholesterol and normal or increased triglyceride levels [30].

7.2.1.2 Channelopathies

Channelopaties such as long QT Syndrome, and the Brugada Syndrome, can also derive from mutations in single genes. Congenital long QT syndrome is a genetic condition characterized by a prolonged QT interval registered by electrocardiography and it is associated with the history of syncope and ventricular tachyarrhythmias, the evidence of T-wave abnormalities, and the high risk of a sudden cardiac death. The mode of inheritance varies, based on the subtype of the disease and can be either autosomal dominant or recessive. Mutations of KCNQ1, HERG and SCN5A genes account for the 95 % of the cases [31]. The Brugada syndrome is characterized by the presence of an abnormal electrocardiography with right bundle branch block pattern and coved-type ST elevation over the right precordial leads. This disease shows an increased risk of sudden cardiac death in patients with structurally normal hearts [32]. Patients with the syndrome can be asymptomatic for many years and the first clinical presentation is often sudden death [33]. The syndrome is inherited with an autosomal dominant pattern. It shows genetic heterogeneity and the first mutation linked to the syndrome was identified in the SCN5A (sodium channel α-subunit) gene [31].

7.2.1.3 Complex Forms

However, the most common disorders and major concern of public health, are complex and result from the combination of multiple genes and non-genetic factors (age, gender, cigarette smoking, alcohol consumption, nutritional status, exercise and others). Many complex diseases, like CVD, are thought to be inherited as they tend to run in families. Unlike monogenic, complex diseases do not follow a typical mendelian pattern of inheritance. These non-mendelian diseases are determined by more than one susceptibility loci and environmental influence. Their complexity lies on the following facts: Firstly, they constitute a multistage process, in which several genetic and environmental factors affect each stage, secondly, there are interindividual variations in response to environmental factors due to genetic heterogeneity of populations and thirdly, under certain environmental, physiological (pregnancy), or pathological (diabetes, cancer) conditions some alleles may no longer remain neutral [34]. Complex diseases are difficult to be studied since it is not feasible to control all these variables in a cohort. Moreover, the multifactorial nature of most traits obstructs the identification of each individual factor influencing them, because each factor may obscure or confound other factors' effects [35]. However, up to date, biological pathways have been elucidated through the elucidation of monogenic diseases, which in turn have helped in understanding some of the disease components. Monogenic diseases are characterized by rare genetic alterations with a severe phenotype (called mutations), while complex diseases may also derive from genetic alterations in the same genes as monogenic, but are much more frequent and have a lower effect size (polymorphisms). For instance, maturity-onset diabetes of the young (OMIM #606391), an autosomal dominant form of diabetes, is quite similar phenotypically to type 2 diabetes mellitus. Mutations in several genes have been implicated for the dominant form, namely HNF4A (hepatocyte nuclear factor 4, alpha), GCK [glucokinase (hexokinase 4)], TCF1/HNF1A (transcription factor 1/hepatocyte nuclear factor 1 alpha), IPF1/PDX1 (Insulin Promoter Factor 1/ Pancreatic and Duodenal homeobox 1) and TCF2/HNF1B (transcription factor 2/hepatocyte nuclear factor 1 homeobox B). Interestingly, polymorphisms (common variants) in the same genes have been associated with the common form type 2 diabetes mellitus [36].

7.3 Types of Human Genetic Variation

Analysis of whole genomes has revealed an unexpected amount of variability among humans and other primate species. These differences in the genome are known as genetic variations. DNA variations have a great contribution in medical and forensic science and have been widely used in studies of genes responsible for various diseases and in screening tumors for chromosomal abnormalities. The fraction of these genetic variations with a frequency equal or greater to 1 % in the general population, is classified as genetic polymorphisms [37]. A polymorphism arises as a result of mutation since errors may occur during DNA replication. Although most of these errors are repaired with no consequences, a mutation may persist and, if it affects the germ line, is transmitted from generation to generation. These genetic changes can be advantageous, deleterious or neutral. Polymorphism may often erroneously be referred as mutation. Both are derived from changes in genetic material, however polymorphism is not deleterious and thus it is unable by itself to cause disease, as mutation does. Polymorphism succeeds in spreading through a significant proportion of the population since it is not under negative selection. For that reason, polymorphism and mutation differ in frequency in the general population where alleles with frequencies less than 1 % are referred to as mutants [2].

Human DNA is highly polymorphic with a frequency of 1 change in every 1,000 bases. Genetic variation may occur within or outside genes which account for less than 5 % of the human genome [2, 38]. A polymorphism may have no effect (i.e. silent) or it may be considered functional, for example, if it affects an enzyme's catalytic activity, a protein's stability or levels of expression. Therefore, functional polymorphisms usually occur within or near coding regions. The different types of polymorphism correspond to the type of the mutation that created them [35]. There are five types of genetic variations and they can be divided into single nucleotide polymorphisms (SNPs), insertions/deletions (indels), short tandem repeats (STRs or microsatellites), variable number of tandem repeats (VNTRs or minisatellites) and copy-number variations (CNVs) [37]. These variations (also known as markers) have been used in genetic studies, such as linkage analysis, in order to identify genes responsible for hereditary diseases. Furthermore, they have helped in the construction of SNP maps and, along with SNP array platforms, they are used for genome-wide association studies aiming in the identification of genetic loci susceptible to common diseases or associated to drug response.

7.3.1 Single Nucleotide Polymorphisms

SNPs are the most common type of DNA variation and result from a single base change which substitutes one nucleotide for another. In the past, such variation was referred to by the method used to detect it, namely restriction fragment length polymorphism (RFLP). SNPs were originally determined based on the property of restriction enzymes to identify and digest a specific nucleotide sequence. A single base change could result in the loss or gain of a restriction site recognizable by the enzyme. Digestion of an amount of DNA containing a restriction site by the appropriate enzyme, yielded different fragment sizes. The different variants could be revealed based on the resulting fragment sizes via electrophoresis [35]. Most SNPs are biallelic, though triallelic and tetraallelic SNPs have been described. Human genome contains more than 10 million SNPs. Biallelic SNPs have a less frequent allele (minor allele) and a more frequent one (major allele), the frequency of which must sum up to 1 or 100 % (if working with percentages). Rare variants are observed at a frequency between 1 and 5 %, while common variants occur at a frequency >5 % [38, 39]. SNPs can be located within (intragenic) or outside of genes (intergenic). Intragenic SNPs may be in coding (exonic) or in non-coding region (intronic). Exonic SNPs can be synonymous or silent (no aminoacid change) or non-synonymous (aminoacid change). Non-synonymous SNPs are more likely to be functional. Functional SNPs usually are lying in exons, splicing sites and promoters [2]. Differences in allele frequencies can be observed among different populations and this has been attributed to the time passed of a SNP's first turn up in a specific population [40]. In the last decade, research was oriented towards identifying millions of SNP markers covering the entire genome and constructing a high-density SNP (haplotype) map. This map has been successfully used to conduct genetic association studies for complex traits.

7.3.2 Indels

Other types of genetic polymorphism result from the insertion or deletion of a section of DNA ranging from 1 to 10,000 base pairs in length. Despite the fact that small indels are highly abundant in human genomes, less attention has been drawn in identifying and studying indels compared to SNPs and other structural variations. Indels are likely to represent between 16 and 25 % of all sequence polymorphisms. Human populations are expected to collectively harbor at least 1.6–2.5 million indel polymorphisms. Several classes of indels have been identified including repeat expansions, transposon insertions and random sequences [41]. A large portion of small indels has been produced by mobile genetic elements such as Alu (named according to the restriction enzyme used to detect them, AluI), SVA and L1. Alu elements cause new insertions of about 300 base pairs, while SVA and L1 elements cause insertions that range from tens of base pairs up to 3 and 6 kilo bases in length, respectively. Many of these new insertions that occur in functionally important regions may affect gene function [42]. In general, indels can cause a substantial amount of genetic variation which can alter human traits and can cause human disease. For example, one of the most common genetic causes of cystic fibrosis is an indel variation, namely a 3 base pair deletion (i.e. elimination of a single amino acid), within exon 10 of the CFTR gene. DNA insertions within the promoter region of the FMR1 gene cause Fragile X syndrome. There is a critical nucleotide triplet repeat expansion that determines pathogenicity, > 200 repeats, and when this threshold size is exceeded, the promoter methylation pattern is altered leading to changes in gene expression [42]. However, most 3 base pair indels in human genomes do not cause disease. Mills et al. [41] reported that 61.1 % of coding indels identified in healthy individuals are multiples of 3 base pairs which maintain the open reading frames of proteins. One of the most common known indel polymorphism in the research for the cardiovascular susceptibility is that of angiotensin converting enzyme (ACE) insertion/deletion (I/D). The I allele is characterized by a 287 base pair inserted fragment in intron 16 of the gene encoding ACE. This polymorphism has been shown to affect enzyme's serum concentration and the D allele was associated with MI [43]. Interestingly, Yoshida et al. [44] showed that the insertion fragment has a sequence very similar to a silencer sequence which may explain why D/D individuals (who lack the silencer sequence) have higher serum ACE levels. Comprehensive variation maps, which include both SNPs and indels, will be more effective than SNP maps alone for identifying variants that underlie specific human phenotypes and diseases.

7.3.3 Short Tandem Repeats or Microsatellites

Microsatellite markers were first described by Weber and May in 1989 [45]. They are short segments of 2–9 base pairs repeated tandemly in tracts and are present at > 100,000 regions spanning the whole genome [37]. It is expected that the STR frequency within genome is one every 3–10 kilobase pairs. STR polymorphisms often result in many alleles (with different repeat sizes) and thus are considered highly polymorphic. Variation between different alleles is caused by a difference in the number of repeat units that results in alleles that are of different lengths. Hence, tandem repeat polymorphisms are also known as length POL. Based on such high level of heterozygosity, the probability that two unrelated individuals will have the same number of repeats can be quite low. For that reason, STRs have been used in paternity tests and in forensic science since they can distinguish individuals' alleles with high probability and in linkage analysis for indentifying disease loci, as well [35].

7.3.4 Various Number of Tandem Repeats or Minisatellites

Minisatellites were first reported by Nakamura et al. in 1987 [37]. The general structure of VNTRs and STRs is the same, with only the repeat size changing. VNTRs are repeated base patterns that range in size from 10 to 100 base pairs. They are highly polymorphic, like STRs, and show high heterozygosity due to wide variety of the copy number of tandem repeat DNA sequences within human genome. VNTRs are currently used in forensic science and also in clinics to monitor recipients of bone marrow transplants [37, 46].

7.3.5 Copy-Number Variations

Sequencing of the human genome helped in the discovery of CNVs and quite recently, it was shown that CNVs are widespread in the genomes of phenotypically normal humans [47, 48]. Initially, large duplications and deletions have been known to be present within human genome from cytogenetic only observations. CNVs are DNA segments that are duplicated or deleted in genomes and which range in length from

1 kilobase pair to 5 megabases. DNA changes larger than 5 megabases can be visualized microscopically at cytogenetic level (karyotype). Currently, more than 6,000 CNV regions have been reported in the human genome, covering about 12 % of the genome [49]. The mechanisms responsible for CNV creation include non-allelic homologous recombination, non-homologous end joining, replication slippage and retrotransposition [50]. Such type of variation is considered to affect more base pairs than other forms of variation. Between two individuals, structural differences in the form of CNVs are expected to be greater than the sum of all SNPs [51]. Polymorphisms at cytogenetic level (>5 magabases) also exist such as inversion 9 and some balanced translocations [52]. Variations such as CNVs, inversions and translocations, which change the structure of the genome, are classified as forms of genome structural variation.

Single copy genes can be duplicated or deleted in any individual, but deletions tend to be under stronger selection because deletions in coding sequences seem to be more deleterious than duplications. Additionally, selection is stronger against large CNVs, presumably due to higher probability of affecting functional DNA [50]. Functional CNVs may affect gene expression, chromatin organization and influence the regulation of nearby genes leading to differences in susceptibility to complex diseases and evolutionary adaptations. Approximately 23 % of known CNVs are intragenic, while intergenic CNVs are believed to have a potential influence on gene expression by affecting gene regulatory elements [49]. CNVs have been linked with interindividual differences in expression of immunological and environmental sensor genes and there is a strong possibility that CNVs play a role in common diseases such as diabetes, heart disease and cancer [53]. CNVs mainly contribute to human diversity. Increasing CNV number is being associated with complex human disease, dietary adaptation [49] but mostly with neurodevelopmental and neurodegenerative disorders [54]. CNVs can be found in different databases such as DECIPHER (https://decipher.sanger.ac.uk/) and in the Database of Genomic Variants (https://dgv.tcag.ca/). Efforts are underway for CNV research to establish a comprehensive atlas of CNVs in the human genome.

7.4 Molecular Technological Advances for the Study of Genetic Disease

Genetic studies aiming at exploring CVD heredity using DNA markers have been carried out for more than 30 years. Technology has rapidly evolved and allowed researchers to perform large-scale studies. In the pre-genomic era (1970s), microscopic cytogenetic analysis identifying chromosomal abnormalities was the only genetic test available. At the same time, many serological markers were studied in the place of DNA. For example, ABO blood groups or human leukocyte antigen classes were often used to test for disease association. In fact, these serological markers represent, in an indirect way, SNPs within genes on chromosomes 9 and 6, respectively. In the pre-genomic era, investigation between cases of MI and healthy individuals was based on measurements of clinical and laboratory features such as weight, blood pressure, blood glucose and lipids. In 1980, Botstein et al. [55] introduced a direct way of studying DNA variation through RFLP analysis and a new molecular technique was developed, Southern blotting [55]. RFLPs helped in mapping and identification of disease genes such as Huntington's disease, cystic fibrosis and familial breast cancer. The shift from protein-serological markers to DNA variants introduced the beginning of the genomic era [39].

In the mid-1980s, PCR replaced Southern blot analysis and upgraded genetic analysis allowing the multiplication of specific DNA fragments producing billion copies in a test tube and reducing time and cost. PCR is still a fundamental method in all laboratories in the fields of research and diagnosis. In 2000, the simultaneous genotyping of millions of SNPs across the genome in a single experiment was achieved by the development of microarray technology known as SNP chip [39]. Except for SNP genotyping, another category of microarrays is known as comparative genomic hybridization array (CGH) which examines insertions and deletions (CNVs) compared to a reference DNA sequence [2]. Microarray technology switched genetic research from locus-specific studies to genome-wide analyses of genetic variation. Advantages of array-based approaches include cost effectiveness and rapid screening of a large number of individuals. Similarly, Sanger sequencing, which is used to "read" the sequence of a gene, may take months and is usually quite expensive (depending on gene length), has evolved to Next-Generation Sequencing (NGS) which may read all coding sequence of the genome (Exome sequencing) or even full genome (whole-genome sequencing) in few days and cheaply. This new technology is able to identify novel genes associated with rare and common diseases. Both of these sophisticated technologies (microarray and NGS) along with the completion of the Human Genome Project launched genetic association studies and marked the beginning of the post-genomic era.

7.5 Genetic Studies

7.5.1 Linkage Analysis

For more than 30 years, linkage analysis has been the most commonly used approach to identify genes influencing disease traits. Botstein et al. [55] indicated that pedigrees in which inherited traits are known to be segregating could be analyzed, for mapping the gene(s) responsible for the trait, using DNA marker loci, without requiring direct access to a specified gene's DNA. In other words, linkage analysis assesses the transmission and co-segregation of marker loci with putative disease alleles. Genetic linkage studies require the availability of an appropriate number of families and family members with a certain disease trait. The fundamental basis of linkage analysis is the hypothesis that for a few generations, chromosomal segments harboring disease alleles will also carry genes at nearby loci that were on the ancestral chromosome harboring the disease-predisposing allele [35]. Evidence of existence of co-segregation between a disease trait and a locus leads to the examination of more DNA markers in that location to minimize the suspected disease region until an actual disease locus is identified. This procedure is referred as positional cloning. Linkage analysis using polymorphic DNA markers in families with genetic diseases of any inheritance pattern, has been a powerful tool to discover genes without a prior knowledge of the biochemical/biological mechanisms of the disease, an approach known as the "reverse genetics" method [37]. Exploiting the plethora of polymorphic DNA markers available in research, genetic linkage maps of all chromosomes have been constructed and are available to scientists [56]. Linkage mapping led to the discovery of many genes responsible for monogenic diseases such as familial polyposis coli, neurofibromatosis type 1 and others. Although this method was powerful in unraveling the genetics of monogenic traits, it was not ideal for studying complex diseases such as CVD. One of the reasons is that linkage analysis cannot tract genes with moderate or low effect on a multifactorial disease phenotype since such trait is the result of multiple genetic and non-genetic factors and the collection of thousands families would be required. Additionally, the lack of genetically informative families, particularly in late-onset diseases or in conditions with high infant mortality hampers linkage analysis experiments. Lastly, a single phenotype may be caused by any one of a multiple number of different genes (locus heterogeneity) [35, 57].

7.5.2 Association Studies

Association studies are the most popular assays for discovering susceptibility loci in common diseases. These studies investigate whether a genetic polymorphism occurs more frequently in individuals with a disease (cases) than in disease-free controls (case–control studies). If the allele is more commonly observed in cases, is defined as the risk allele. A positive association result means that the polymorphism is either in the susceptibility locus or in close proximity with the susceptibility locus (i.e. in linkage disequilibrium).

Linkage disequilibrium is the non-random association of alleles at two or more loci with limited recombination between them that descend from a single ancestral chromosome. Selection of a population is crucial and both groups should be matched according to variables that could influence the result, such as age, sex, medication, ethnicity and additional disorders that may affect biochemical measurement such as cancer and hypothyroidism. Another main concern of association studies is population stratification, which refers to the presence of subgroups differing in their genetic structure (e.g. different ethnic populations), which may lead to spurious results. For example it would be totally incorrect for a study to use Caucasians as cases and Africans as controls [2]. Association studies may involve families (case-parent trios, sib-pair analysis, transmission disequilibrium test) or unrelated individuals and rely on candidate gene methods. Candidate gene approach includes polymorphic alleles in genes with a known biological role that is relevant to the disease under investigation. Unlike linkage analysis where there is a connection between a trait and a chromosomal region, association studies are more specific and a connection between a trait and an allele is established. For that reason, these studies are sensitive to allelic heterogeneity a single phenotype may be caused by any one of a multiple number of different alleles in the same gene.

Association studies were used with enthusiasm in the effort to predict acute coronary syndromes, MI, blood pressure, lipid levels, sudden death from arrhythmias and the response to CVD medications. ACE I/D polymorphism was one of the first variations that involved in CVD association studies in relation to idiopathic cardiomyopathy, MI and left ventricular hypertrophy [58]. Association studies can also examine quantitative traits such as blood pressure, circulating lipid concentrations, postprandial triglyceride values or QT interval length. The study population is divided into genotype categories, for example homozygotes for either allele and heterozygotes, in case of a biallelic variant. Then, the mean value of the quantitative trait under investigation, is compared among the three genotype groups [39]. Many candidate gene associations have been tested regarding CVD and its risk factors are presented in Table 7.1.

Unfortunately, the results of many candidate gene studies have been inconsistent and were not replicated under further scrutiny. Some reported “positive” associations are the result of false findings and “negative” publication bias.

Table 7.1 CVD-associated candidate gene loc associated with CVD and its risk factors

Locus	Gene	Trait	Reference
1p32.3	PCSK9	LDL cholesterol	[59]
2p24.1	APOB	Total and LDL cholesterol	[60]
3p25	PPARG	HDL cholesterol	[61]
5q31	SEPP1	Insulin resistance	[62]
6q25.3	LPA	Lipoprotein(a)	[63]
8p21.3	LPL	HDL cholesterol	[61]
9q31.1	ABCA1	HDL cholesterol, Triglycerides	[64, 65]
11q23	APOA1/C3/A5	HDL cholesterol, Triglycerides	[66]
11q23	APOA5	Triglycerides, Metabolic syndrome	[67]
12q24.31	SCARB1	CAD, ischemic stroke	[68]
16q21	CETP	Coronary artery stenosis severity, Postprandial lipemia	[69–71]
16q22.1	LCAT	HDL cholesterol	[72]
19q13.32	APOE	Total and LDL cholesterol, Age of CAD onset	[73, 74]
20q13.12	PLTP	HDL cholesterol	[75]

Abbreviations
CAD coronary artery disease, *CVD* cardiovascular disease, *HDL* high-density lipoprotein cholesterol, *LDL* low-density lipoprotein cholesterol

A combination of small variant effect and a low sample size could lead to type 2 error which is the probability of a false negative result due to low statistical power. The probability of detecting association by chance (false positive) leads to type 1 error. Positive results are easier to publish, while negative studies, even if better-designed, may not reach criteria for publication and the significance of positive associations may be overestimated. The cardiovascular literature is enriched with positive genetic association studies, though few have true clinical value and have been helpful to clinical practice. Among the reasons for failing to replicate findings are incorrect SNP selection, variable definitions for cases and controls in different studies, important differences in enrolled cases due to variations in investigators' clinical skills, failure to control confounding variables, lack of sufficient power (insufficient number of participants) and genetic and phenotypic heterogeneity. Phenotypic definition is of great importance when stratifying cases and controls. For example, in association studies for CAD, MI should be separated from other angiographic coronary disease phenotypes, since different genes may be involved in each process [58, 76].

7.5.3 Genome Maps

The effort of mapping and pinpointing susceptibility genes was facilitated by the construction and availability of genetic maps bearing known DNA markers [77]. In 1980, a map of RFLPs was initially proposed and this first map contained 403 polymorphic loci including 393 RFLPs [55]. It was estimated that the linkage map was detectably linked to at least 95 % of the DNA in the human genome [78]. In 1990s, microsatellite markers were also included in maps due to their high level of polymorphism [35]. A great collaborative effort to map more DNA markers, initiated in 1990 by the Centre d'Etude du Polymorphism Humain (CEPH) in which 63 research laboratories from United States, Canada, Europe, South Africa, Japan and Australia participated [79, 80]. The present version of the database (V10.0 – November 2004) contains genotypes for 32,356 genetic markers including 21,480 biallelic markers and >9,900 microsatellite markers. The mean observed heterozygote frequency of all the loci is 0.438 and for identifiable microsatellite loci 0.698, of which 56 % are highly polymorphic (observed heterozygote frequency $\geq$ 0.70). The CEPH database now manages 6,081,570 genotypes [81].

In October 2002, another great step was made towards a high-density SNP map (or haplotype map) construction covering the entire genome. The International Hapmap Project (http://www.hapmap.org/) was initiated for establishing a SNP database for populations with ancestry from parts of Africa, Asia and Europe. The aims of the International HapMap Project was to determine the common patterns of DNA sequence variation in the human genome and to make this information freely available in the public domain. Exploiting such information, The HapMap was intended to assist in the discovery of sequence variants that affect common disease, to facilitate development of diagnostic tools, and to enhance our ability to choose targets for therapeutic intervention [82]. In stage I (completed in 2005), more than one million SNPs were genotyped in 269 DNA samples from four populations: the Yoruba in Ibadan, Nigeria (YRI), Utah, USA, from the CEPH collection (CEU), Han Chinese in Beijing, China (CHB) and Tokyo, Japan (JPT). These data documented the generality of recombination hotspots, a block-like structure of linkage disequilibrium and low haplotype diversity, leading to substantial correlations of SNPs with many of their neighbors (tag SNPs) [83]. Tag SNPs are covering the whole genome and are able to represent neighboring SNPs with high accuracy, without the need for genotyping them directly. This is known as genotype imputation (i.e. genotype guessing) [2]. In stage II (completed in 2007), over 3.1 million human SNPs were genotyped in 270 individuals from the same population. The resulting HapMap database yielded a SNP density of approximately 1 SNP per 1 kilobase and is estimated to contain approximately 25–35 % of all the 9–10 million common SNPs (minor allele frequency $\geq$0.05) in the assembled human genome [84].

7.5.4 Genome-Wide Association Studies

The information available from the completion of The Hapmap Project along with the development of large-scale genotyping SNP chips (microarrays) shifted research for common diseases, like CVD, from single/few gene associations to genome-wide association studies (GWAS). GWAS, also known as whole-genome association studies, involve the examination of genetic variation across a given genome using hundreds of thousands of SNPs (500,000–1 million) on DNA arrays. The SNPs throughout the genome are printed in large series of disease cases and disease-free controls [57]. There are two main companies offering high-throughput genome-wide scanning, Affymetrix and Illumina and the cost is decreasing with time. In contrast to candidate approach, in GWAS no a priori biological hypothesis is needed and previously unsuspected genes can be identified. GWAS are based on the concept of "common disease – common variant hypothesis" where common polymorphisms (minor allele frequency > 5 %) are believed to influence, in part (low effect size), genetic susceptibility to common diseases. As a consequence, very large sample sizes (>100,000 subjects) are needed to achieve statistical power to detect more variants associated with the disease under investigation. However, in GWAS the likelihood of false positive associations is high and thus stringent criteria are applied in order to declare true positive associations. Bonferroni correction adjusts the threshold of significance by dividing $P = 0.05$ with the number of tests and thus the P-value is often $P < 10^{-8}$ which is known as the "genome-wide significance" [14, 39]. Even though applying such stringent statistical methods, positive results should always be replicated by independent cohorts. Regarding reproduction, increased sample size and meta-analysis could result in the identification of associations missed by individual GWAS. In GWAS, odds ratios (ORs) provide an estimate of the risk conferred by an allele in a given SNP. An allele with OR > 1.0 is associated with increased probability of disease in carriers of this allele and thus it is considered as a risk allele [39]. It is important to note that GWAS do not test directly SNPs that alter structure or function and induce pathogenicity. Instead, they test tag SNPs, in other words SNPs that are linked to functional variants through linkage disequilibrium. The gene closest to an association signal that makes biological sense is nominated as the candidate one.

The expected outcomes of GWAS concerning CVD are the following: (1) the identified SNPs could lead to genomic regions carrying genes that influence new molecular mechanisms and pathways and, (2) SNP results could help to diagnose and treat specific patients which may lead to personalize treatment strategies [39]. GWAS have successfully confirmed already established loci and identified novel ones for CAD and its risk factors (diabetes mellitus, blood pressure, dyslipidemias) and are listed in Table 7.2. Although the responsible gene is clear in some studies, most genomic regions possess multiple candidate

Table 7.2 Results of GWAS analysis of CVD and its risk factors

Disease or trait	Gene	Reference
HDL cholesterol	SLC39A8	[85]
HDL cholesterol and Triglycerides	LPL	[86]
LDL cholesterol	MYLIP/GMPR	[85]
LDL cholesterol	PPP1R3B	[85]
Triglycerides	AFF1	[85]
Triglycerides	APOA5	[87]
Ischemic stroke	AGTRL1	[88]
Ischemic stroke	HDAC9	[89]
Ischemic stroke	PRKCH	[90]
Ischemic stroke	ARHGEF10	[91]
Ischemic stroke	ABO	[92]
Myocardial infarction	LTA	[93]
Myocardial infarction	LGALS2	[94]
Myocardial infarction	PSMA6	[95]
Myocardial infarction	MIAT	[96]
Myocardial infarction	ITIH3	[97]
Coronary artery disease	LIPA	[98]
Type 2 diabetes	TPMRSS6	[99]
Type 2 diabetes	BCL2	[100]

Abbreviations
CVD cardiovascular disease, *GWAS* genome-wide association studies, *LDL* low-density lipoprotein cholesterol, *HDL* high-density lipoprotein cholesterol

genes and therefore, further research is needed in order to filter out irrelevant variants. Additionally, GWAS have resulted in some novel loci bearing genes with either an unknown function or without a clear connection with CAD-related mechanisms. An example of this is the chr9p21.3 locus which appears to be GWAS hotspot and for many years it remains the strongest and most significant determinant of the risk for CAD and other CVD phenotypes (type 2 diabetes, abdominal aortic aneurysm and intracranial aneurysm) [14]. However, the exact mechanism whereby the chr9p21.3 variation increases CVD risk remains unidentified. The nearest protein coding genes, in relation to tag SNPs, are CDKN2A (150 kilobases) and CDKN2B (118 kilobases) and are known to control cellular proliferation and apoptosis [14]. Functional studies concerning the chr9p21.3 locus have shown that this region seems to have regulatory role on the activity of primary aortic smooth muscle cells. Deletion of the region in mouse models leads to increased expression of CDKN2A and CDKN2B genes and high proliferation of aortic smooth muscle cells [14, 101, 102].

Based on the polygenic model of CVD, most variants when considered alone have a very low impact on phenotype. In order to obtain meaningful information for clinical practice, the estimation of "genetic scores" has been recently introduced by combining data from as many as possible variants related with a given phenotype. Twenty SNP variations with additive effect on LDL cholesterol explain 14 % of this lipoprotein's variance in healthy men and women [103]. Furthermore, 116 independent blood pressure-related SNPs explain approximately 2.2 % of the variance observed in systolic and diastolic blood pressure measurements [104].

Unfortunately GWAS, based on common variation, have explained only a small portion of the expected heritability of CVD risk as previously reported by twin studies. This "missing heritability", is currently believed, might be explained by rare variants based on the alternative concept of "common disease – rare variant" hypothesis. Next-generation applications such as exome sequencing or whole genome sequencing will enable the identification of rare variants which may provide considerable clues in missing heritability [39].

GWAS are also expected to elucidate our knowledge in the fields of pharmacogenetics and pharmacogenomics. The two terms are often confused and used as one but actually they are quite different. Pharmacogenetics refers to the study of inherited differences (variation) in drug metabolism and response, while pharmacogenomics refers to the general study of the many different genes that determine drug behavior [105]. The information produced by these studies will help predicting the effectiveness, the risk of adverse reactions and the appropriate dose of drugs for each patient leading to personalized medicine [37]. Genetic tests for variations in CYP2C9 and VKORC1 genes are already established, prior to warfarin usage predicting slow metabolizers [106, 107]. Interestingly, two single-blind, randomized trials comparing a genotype-guided (based on CYP2C9 and VKORC1 variations) dosing of acenocoumarol or phenprocoumon did not reveal any improvement on the percentage of time in the therapeutic INR [108]. Concerning lipids, SLCO1B1 is a future biomarker candidate for simvastatin use influencing statin-induced myopathy [109]. Moreover, GATM is considered to be associated with cholesterol homeostatis and it has been recently identified to be associated with differences is susceptibility to statin-induced myopathy [110].

Conclusions

Technological advances have considerably contributed to our better understanding of the human genome structure. Genetic variability seems to account for most common diseases, such as CVD, as well as for drug response and adverse drug reactions. Genetic variability exists in many forms including SNPs, indels, STRs, VNTRs and CNVs. Most common diseases are complex, influenced by multiple genetic and non-genetic factors, and constitute a major concern of public health. GWAS are currently flourishing producing a massive amount of genetic data and have pointed out previously unsuspected candidate genes. Although GWAS have helped to illuminate previously unknown biological and metabolic pathways, clinical significance in predicting future risk of disease is still low. The study of genetics and its involvement in various disease entities offers an excellent paradigm of Translational Research, since basic research findings eventually find their way to the treatment of the individual patient but also to application in populations. An important issue raised by unraveling the genetic basis of complex traits in humans and yielding so much genetic information at individual level, is the management of this information. Genetic information should be handled with an ethical and confidential way avoiding genetic discrimination. And as Nakamura [37] has said "*although we are all different, we should have equal rights and should respect each other's differences*".

References

1. Watson JD, Crick FH. Molecular structure of nucleic acids; a structure for deoxyribose nucleic acid. Nature. 1953;171:737–8.
2. Bochud M. Genetics for clinicians: from candidate genes to whole genome scans (technological advances). Best Pract Res Clin Endocrinol Metab. 2012;26:119–732.
3. Genetics home reference, mitochondrial DNA. 2013. http://ghr.nlm.nih.gov/mitochondrial-dna. Accessed 2 Dec 2013.
4. Mendel GJ. Versuche uber Pflanzen-Hybriden. Verh Naturforsch Ver Brunn. 1866;4:215–22.
5. Morgan TH. Chromosomes and associative inheritance. Science. 1911;34:636–8.
6. Mullis KB. The unusual origin of the polymerase chain reaction. Sci Am. 1990;262:56–61.
7. Riordan JR, Rommens JM, Kerem B, Alon N, Rozmahel R, Grzelczak Z, et al. Identification of the cystic fibrosis gene: cloning and characterization of complementary DNA. Science. 1989;245:1066–73.
8. Fleischmann RD, Adams MD, White O, Clayton RA, Kirkness EF, Kerlavage AR, et al. Whole-genome random sequencing and assembly of Haemophilus influenzae Rd. Science. 1995;269:496–512.
9. Collins FS, Morgan M, Patrinos A. The Human Genome Project: lessons from large-scale biology. Science. 2003;300:286–90.
10. International Human Genome Sequencing Consortium. Initial sequencing and analysis of the human genome. Nature. 2001;409:860–921.
11. Finegold JA, Asaria P, Francis DP. Mortality from ischaemic heart disease by country, region, and age: statistics from World Health Organisation and United Nations. Int J Cardiol. 2013;168:934–45.
12. Go AS, Mozaffarian D, Roger VL, Benjamin EJ, Berry JD, Borden WB, et al. American Heart Association Statistics Committee and Stroke Statistics Subcommittee. Executive summary: heart disease and stroke statistics–2013 update: a report from the American Heart Association. Circulation. 2013;127:143–52.
13. Lloyd-Jones DM, Larson MG, Beiser A, Levy D. Lifetime risk of developing coronary heart disease. Lancet. 1999;353:89–92.
14. Swerdlow DI, Holmes MV, Harrison S, Humphries SE. The genetics of coronary heart disease. Br Med Bull. 2012;102:59–77.
15. Schildkraut JM, Myers RH, Cupples LA, Kiely DK, Kannel WB. Coronary risk associated with age and sex of parental heart disease in the Framingham Study. Am J Cardiol. 1989;64:555–9.
16. Hopkins PN, Williams RR, Kuida H, Stults BM, Hunt SC, Barlow GK, et al. Family history as an independent risk factor for incident coronary artery disease in a high-risk cohort in Utah. Am J Cardiol. 1988;62:703–7.
17. Colditz GA, Rimm EB, Giovannucci E, Stampfer MJ, Rosner B, Willett WC. A prospective study of parental history of myocardial infarction and coronary artery disease in men. Am J Cardiol. 1991;67:933–8.
18. Chow CK, Islam S, Bautista L, Rumboldt Z, Yusufali A, Xie C, et al. Parental history and myocardial infarction risk across the world: the INTERHEART Study. J Am Coll Cardiol. 2011;57:619–27.
19. Marenberg ME, Risch N, Berkman LF, Floderus B, de Faire U. Genetic susceptibility to death from coronary heart disease in a study of twins. N Engl J Med. 1994;330:1041–6.
20. Zdravkovic S, Wienke A, Pedersen NL, Marenberg ME, Yashin AI, De Faire U. Heritability of death from coronary heart disease: a 36-year follow-up of 20 966 Swedish twins. J Intern Med. 2002;252:247–54.
21. Kolovou G, Voudris V, Drogari E, Palatianos G, Cokkinos DV. Coronary bypass grafts in a young girl with sitosterolemia. Eur Heart J. 1996;17:965–6.
22. Pullinger CR, Kane JP, Malloy MJ. Primary hypercholesterolemia: genetic causes and treatment of five monogenic disorders. Expert Rev Cardiovasc Ther. 2003;1:107–19.
23. Rader DJ, Cohen J, Hobbs HH. Monogenic hypercholesterolemia: new insights into pathogenesis and treatment. J Clin Invest. 2003;111:1795–803.
24. Usifo E, Leigh SE, Whittall RA, Lench N, Taylor A, Yeats C, et al. Low-density lipoprotein receptor gene familial hypercholesterolemia variant database: update and pathological assessment. Ann Hum Genet. 2012;76:387–401.
25. Humphries SE, Cranston T, Allen M, Middleton-Price H, Fernandez MC, Senior V, et al. Mutational analysis in UK patients with a clinical diagnosis of familial hypercholesterolaemia: relationship with plasma lipid traits, heart disease risk and utility in relative tracing. J Mol Med (Berl). 2006;84:203–14.
26. Futema M, Whittall RA, Kiley A, Steel LK, Cooper JA, Badmus E, et al. Analysis of the frequency and

spectrum of mutations recognised to cause familial hypercholesterolaemia in routine clinical practice in a UK specialist hospital lipid clinic. Atherosclerosis. 2013;229:161–8.

27. Sugandhan S, Khandpur S, Sharma VK. Familial chylomicronemia syndrome. Pediatr Dermatol. 2007;24:323–5.
28. Johansen CT, Hegele RA. Genetic bases of hypertriglyceridemic phenotypes. Curr Opin Lipidol. 2011;22:247–53.
29. Surendran RP, Visser ME, Heemelaar S, Wang J, Peter J, Defesche JC, et al. Mutations in LPL, APOC2, APOA5, GPIHBP1 and LMF1 in patients with severe hypertriglyceridaemia. J Intern Med. 2012;272:185–96.
30. Kolovou G, Daskalova D, Anagnostopoulou K, Hoursalas I, Voudris V, Mikhailidis DP, et al. Postprandial hypertriglyceridaemia in patients with Tangier disease. J Clin Pathol. 2003;56:937–41.
31. Romano R, Parisi V, Pastore F, Riccio A, Petraglia L, Allocca E, et al. Genetic test for the channelopaties: useful or less than useful for patients? (part II). Transl Med UniSa. 2013;6:35–40.
32. Brugada P, Brugada J. Right bundle branch block, persistent ST segment elevation and sudden cardiac death: a distinct clinical and electrocardiographic syndrome. A multicenter report. J Am Coll Cardiol. 1992;20:1391–6.
33. Antzelevitch C, Brugada P, Borggrefe M, Brugada J, Brugada R, Corrado D, et al. Brugada syndrome: report of the second consensus conference: endorsed by the Heart Rhythm Society and the European Heart Rhythm Association. Circulation. 2005;111:659–70.
34. Gambaro G, Anglani F, D'Angelo A. Association studies of genetic polymorphisms and complex disease. Lancet. 2000;355:308–11.
35. Schork NJ, Fallin D, Lanchbury JS. Single nucleotide polymorphisms and the future of genetic epidemiology. Clin Genet. 2000;58:250–64.
36. Fajans SS, Bell GI, Polonsky KS. Molecular mechanisms and clinical pathophysiology of maturity-onset diabetes of the young. N Engl J Med. 2001;345:971–80.
37. Nakamura Y. DNA variations in human and medical genetics: 25 years of my experience. J Hum Genet. 2009;54:1–8.
38. Abecasis GR, Altshuler D, Auton A, Brooks LD, Durbin RM, Gibbs RA, et al. 1000 Genomes Project Consortium. A map of human genome variation from population-scale sequencing. Nature. 2010;467:1061–73.
39. Dubé JB, Hegele RA. Genetics 100 for cardiologists: basics of genome-wide association studies. Can J Cardiol. 2013;29:10–7.
40. Salisbury BA, Pungliya M, Choi JY, Jiang R, Sun XJ, Stephens JC. SNP and haplotype variation in the human genome. Mutat Res. 2003;526:53–61.
41. Mills RE, Luttig CT, Larkins CE, Beauchamp A, Tsui C, Pittard WS, et al. An initial map of insertion and deletion (INDEL) variation in the human genome. Genome Res. 2006;16:1182–90.
42. Mullaney JM, Mills RE, Pittard WS, Devine SE. Small insertions and deletions (INDELs) in human genomes. Hum Mol Genet. 2010;19 Suppl 2:131–6.
43. Cambien F, Poirier O, Lecerf L, Evans A, Cambou JP, Arveiler D, et al. Deletion polymorphism in the gene for angiotensin-converting enzyme is a potent risk factor for myocardial infarction. Nature. 1992;359:641–4.
44. Yoshida H, Mitarai T, Kawamura T. Functional significance of ACE I/D locus for controlling the ace gene. J Am Soc Nephrol. 1997;8:633A.
45. Weber JL, May PE. Abundant class of human DNA polymorphisms which can be typed using the polymerase chain reaction. Am J Hum Genet. 1989;44:388–96.
46. Gatti RA, Nakamura Y, Nussmeier M, Susi E, Shan W, Grody WW. Informativeness of VNTR genetic markers for detecting chimerism after bone marrow transplantation. Dis Markers. 1989;7:105–12.
47. Iafrate AJ, Feuk L, Rivera MN, Listewnik ML, Donahoe PK, Qi Y, et al. Detection of large-scale variation in the human genome. Nat Genet. 2004;36:949–51.
48. Sebat J, Lakshmi B, Troge J, Alexander J, Young J, Lundin P, et al. Large-scale copy number polymorphism in the human genome. Science. 2004;305:525–8.
49. Gökçümen O, Lee C. Copy number variants (CNVs) in primate species using array-based comparative genomic hybridization. Methods. 2009;49:18–25.
50. Schrider DR, Hahn MW. Gene copy-number polymorphism in nature. Proc Biol Sci. 2010;277:3213–21.
51. Kidd JM, Cooper GM, Donahue WF, Hayden HS, Sampas N, Graves T, et al. Mapping and sequencing of structural variation from eight human genomes. Nature. 2008;453:56–64.
52. de la Chapelle A, Schröder J, Stenstrand K, Fellman J, Herva R, Saarni M, et al. Pericentric inversions of human chromosomes 9 and 10. Am J Hum Genet. 1974;26:746–66.
53. Freeman JL, Perry GH, Feuk L, Redon R, McCarroll SA, Altshuler DM, et al. Copy number variation: new insights in genome diversity. Genome Res. 2006;16:949–61.
54. Stankiewicz P, Lupski JR. Structural variation in the human genome and its role in disease. Annu Rev Med. 2010;61:437–55.
55. Botstein D, White RL, Skolnick M, Davis RW. Construction of a genetic linkage map in man using restriction fragment length polymorphisms. Am J Hum Genet. 1980;32:314–31.
56. Nakamura Y, Lathrop M, Bragg T, Leppert M, O'Connell P, Jones C, et al. An extended genetic linkage map of markers for human chromosome 10. Genomics. 1988;3:389–92.
57. Singleton AB, Hardy J, Traynor BJ, Houlden H. Towards a complete resolution of the genetic architecture of disease. Trends Genet. 2010;26:438–42.

58. Ginsburg GS, Shah SH, McCarthy JJ. Taking cardiovascular genetic association studies to the next level. J Am Coll Cardiol. 2007;50:930–2.
59. Davignon J, Dubuc G, Seidah NG. The influence of PCSK9 polymorphisms on serum low-density lipoprotein cholesterol and risk of atherosclerosis. Curr Atheroscler Rep. 2010;12:308–15.
60. Delghandi M, Thangarajah R, Nilsen M, Grimsgaard S, Bønaa KH, Tonstad S, et al. DNA polymorphisms of the apolipoprotein B gene (XbaI, EcoRI, and MspI RFLPs) in Norwegians at risk of atherosclerosis and healthy controls. Acta Cardiol. 1999;54:215–25.
61. Bozina T, Simić I, Lovrić J, Pećin I, Jelaković B, Sertić J, et al. Effects of lipoprotein lipase and peroxisome proliferator-activated receptor-gamma gene variants on metabolic syndrome traits. Coll Antropol. 2013;37:801–8.
62. Hellwege JN, Palmer ND, Ziegler JT, Langefeld CD, Lorenzo C, Norris JM, et al. Genetic variants in selenoprotein P plasma 1 gene (SEPP1) are associated with fasting insulin and first phase insulin response in Hispanics. Gene. 2014;534:33–9.
63. Danik JS, Buring JE, Chasman DI, Zee RY, Ridker PM, Glynn RJ. Lipoprotein(a), polymorphisms in the LPA gene, and incident venous thromboembolism among 21483 women. J Thromb Haemost. 2013;11:205–8.
64. Kolovou V, Kolovou G, Marvaki A, Karakosta A, Vasilopoulos G, Kalogiani A, et al. ATP-binding cassette transporter A1 gene polymorphisms and serum lipid levels in young Greek nurses. Lipids Health Dis. 2011;10:56.
65. Ma XY, Liu JP, Song ZY. Associations of the ATP-binding cassette transporter A1 R219K polymorphism with HDL-C level and coronary artery disease risk: a meta-analysis. Atherosclerosis. 2011;215:428–34.
66. Yin RX, Li YY, Lai CQ. Apolipoprotein A1/C3/A5 haplotypes and serum lipid levels. Lipids Health Dis. 2011;10:140.
67. Zaki M, Amr K. Apolipoprotein A5 T-1131C variant and risk for metabolic syndrome in obese adolescents. Gene. 2014;534:44–7.
68. Wu Y, Marvelle AF, Li J, Croteau-Chonka DC, Feranil AB, Kuzawa CW, et al. Genetic association with lipids in Filipinos: waist circumference modifies an APOA5 effect on triglyceride levels. J Lipid Res. 2013;54:3198–205.
69. Kolovou GD, Anagnostopoulou KK, Karyofillis P, Salpea KD, Yiannakouris N, Zarkalis D, et al. Cholesteryl ester transfer protein gene polymorphisms and severity of coronary stenosis. Clin Invest Med. 2006;29:14–9.
70. Anagnostopoulou KK, Kolovou GD, Kostakou PM, Mihas C, Hatzigeorgiou G, Marvaki C, et al. Sex-associated effect of CETP and LPL polymorphisms on postprandial lipids in familial hypercholesterolaemia. Lipids Health Dis. 2009;8:24.
71. Kolovou GD, Anagnostopoulou KK, Kostakou PM, Mikhailidis DP. Cholesterol ester transfer protein (CETP), postprandial lipemia and hypolipidemic drugs. Curr Med Chem. 2009;16:4345–60.
72. Agirbasli D, Cirakoglu B, Eren F, Sumerkan M, Aksoy S, Aral C, et al. Effects of lecithin: cholesterol acyltransferase genotypes, enzyme levels, and activity on high-density lipoprotein levels. J Clin Lipidol. 2011;5:152–8.
73. Kolovou GD, Anagnostopoulou KK, Mikhailidis DP, Panagiotakos DB, Pilatis ND, Cariolou MA, et al. Association of apolipoprotein E genotype with early onset of coronary heart disease in Greek men. Angiology. 2005;56:663–70.
74. Zende PD, Bankar MP, Kamble PS, Momin AA. Apolipoprotein E gene polymorphism and its effect on plasma lipids in arteriosclerosis. J Clin Diagn Res. 2013;7:2149–52.
75. Aouizerat BE, Engler MB, Natanzon Y, Kulkarni M, Song J, Eng C, et al. Genetic variation of PLTP modulates lipoprotein profiles in hypoalphalipoproteinemia. J Lipid Res. 2006;47:787–93.
76. Chowdhury TA. Association studies of genetic polymorphisms and complex disease. Lancet. 2000;355:1277–8.
77. Lander ES, Weinberg RA. Genomics: journey to the center of biology. Science. 2000;287:1777–82.
78. Donis-Keller H, Green P, Helms C, Cartinhour S, Weiffenbach B, Stephens K, et al. A genetic linkage map of the human genome. Cell. 1987;51:319–37.
79. Dausset J, Cann H, Cohen D, Lathrop M, Lalouel JM, White R. Centre d'etude du polymorphisme humain (CEPH): collaborative genetic mapping of the human genome. Genomics. 1990;6:575–7.
80. Murray JC, Buetow KH, Weber JL, Ludwigsen S, Scherpbier-Heddema T, Manion F, et al. A comprehensive human linkage map with centimorgan density. Cooperative Human Linkage Center (CHLC). Science. 1994;265:2049–54.
81. The Foundation Jean Dausset-Centre d'Etude du Polymorphisme Humain (CEPH). 2008. http://www.cephb.fr/en/cephdb/. Accessed 2 Dec 2013.
82. International HapMap Consortium. The International HapMap Project. Nature. 2003;426:789–96.
83. International HapMap Consortium. A haplotype map of the human genome. Nature. 2005;437:1299–320.
84. International HapMap Consortium. A second generation human haplotype map of over 3.1 million SNPs. Nature. 2007;449:851–61.
85. Waterworth DM, Ricketts SL, Song K, Chen L, Zhao JH, Ripatti S, et al. Genetic variants influencing circulating lipid levels and risk of coronary artery disease. Arterioscler Thromb Vasc Biol. 2010;30:2264–76.
86. Kathiresan S, Manning AK, Demissie S, D'Agostino RB, Surti A, Guiducci C, et al. A genome-wide association study for blood lipid phenotypes in the Framingham Heart Study. BMC Med Genet. 2007;8 Suppl 1:S17.
87. Wu DF, Yin RX, Cao XL, Chen WX, Aung LH, Wang W, et al. Scavenger receptor class B type 1 gene rs5888 single nucleotide polymorphism and the

risk of coronary artery disease and ischemic stroke: a case–control study. Int J Med Sci. 2013;10:1771–7.
88. Hata J, Matsuda K, Ninomiya T, Yonemoto K, Matsushita T, Ohnishi Y, et al. Functional SNP in an Sp1-binding site of AGTRL1 gene is associated with susceptibility to brain infarction. Hum Mol Genet. 2007;16:630–9.
89. International Stroke Genetics Consortium (ISGC); Wellcome Trust Case Control Consortium 2 (WTCCC2), Bellenguez C, Bevan S, Gschwendtner A, et al. Genome-wide association study identifies a variant in HDAC9 associated with large vessel ischemic stroke. Nat Genet. 2012;44:328–33.
90. Kubo M, Hata J, Ninomiya T, Matsuda K, Yonemoto K, Nakano T, et al. A nonsynonymous SNP in PRKCH (protein kinase C eta) increases the risk of cerebral infarction. Nat Genet. 2007;39:212–7.
91. Matsushita T, Ashikawa K, Yonemoto K, Hirakawa Y, Hata J, Amitani H, et al. Functional SNP of ARHGEF10 confers risk of atherothrombotic stroke. Hum Mol Genet. 2010;19:1137–46.
92. Williams FM, Carter AM, Hysi PG, Surdulescu G, Hodgkiss D, Soranzo N, et al. Ischemic stroke is associated with the ABO locus: the EuroCLOT study. Ann Neurol. 2013;73:16–31.
93. Ozaki K, Ohnishi Y, Iida A, Sekine A, Yamada R, Tsunoda T, et al. Functional SNPs in the lymphotoxin-alpha gene that are associated with susceptibility to myocardial infarction. Nat Genet. 2002;32:650–4.
94. Ozaki K, Inoue K, Sato H, Iida A, Ohnishi Y, Sekine A, et al. Functional variation in LGALS2 confers risk of myocardial infarction and regulates lymphotoxin-alpha secretion in vitro. Nature. 2004;429:72–5.
95. Ozaki K, Sato H, Iida A, Mizuno H, Nakamura T, Miyamoto Y, et al. A functional SNP in PSMA6 confers risk of myocardial infarction in the Japanese population. Nat Genet. 2006;38:921–5.
96. Ishii N, Ozaki K, Sato H, Mizuno H, Saito S, Takahashi A, et al. Identification of a novel non-coding RNA, MIAT, that confers risk of myocardial infarction. J Hum Genet. 2006;51:1087–99.
97. Ebana Y, Ozaki K, Inoue K, Sato H, Iida A, Lwin H, et al. A functional SNP in ITIH3 is associated with susceptibility to myocardial infarction. J Hum Genet. 2007;52:220–9.
98. Wild PS, Zeller T, Schillert A, Szymczak S, Sinning CR, Deiseroth A, et al. A genome-wide association study identifies LIPA as a susceptibility gene for coronary artery disease. Circ Cardiovasc Genet. 2011;4:403–12.
99. He M, Workalemahu T, Manson JE, Hu FB, Qi L. Genetic determinants for body iron store and type 2 diabetes risk in US men and women. PLoS One. 2012;7:e40919.
100. Saxena R, Elbers CC, Guo Y, Peter I, Gaunt TR, Mega JL, et al. Large-scale gene-centric meta-analysis across 39 studies identifies type 2 diabetes loci. Am J Hum Genet. 2012;90:410–25.
101. Jarinova O, Stewart AF, Roberts R, Wells G, Lau P, Naing T, et al. Functional analysis of the chromosome 9p21.3 coronary artery disease risk locus. Arterioscler Thromb Vasc Biol. 2009;29:1671–7.
102. Visel A, Zhu Y, May D, Afzal V, Gong E, Attanasio C, et al. Targeted deletion of the 9p21 non-coding coronary artery disease risk interval in mice. Nature. 2010;464:409–12.
103. Talmud PJ, Drenos F, Shah S, Shah T, Palmen J, Verzilli C, et al. Gene-centric association signals for lipids and apolipoproteins identified via the HumanCVD BeadChip. Am J Hum Genet. 2009;85: 628–42.
104. International Consortium for Blood Pressure Genome-Wide Association Studies, Ehret GB, Munroe PB, Rice KM, Bochud M, Johnson AD, et al. Genetic variants in novel pathways influence blood pressure and cardiovascular disease risk. Nature. 2011;478:103–9.
105. Ito RK, Demers LM. Pharmacogenomics and pharmacogenetics: future role of molecular diagnostics in the clinical diagnostic laboratory. Clin Chem. 2004;50:1526–7.
106. D'Andrea G, D'Ambrosio RL, Di Perna P, Chetta M, Santacroce R, Brancaccio V, et al. A polymorphism in the VKORC1 gene is associated with an interindividual variability in the dose-anticoagulant effect of warfarin. Blood. 2005;105:645–9.
107. Anderson JL, Horne BD, Stevens SM, Grove AS, Barton S, Nicholas ZP, et al.; Couma-Gen Investigators. Randomized trial of genotype-guided versus standard warfarin dosing in patients initiating oral anticoagulation. Circulation. 2007;116: 2563–70.
108. Verhoef TI, Ragia G, de Boer A, Barallon R, Kolovou G, Kolovou V, et al. A randomized trial of genotype-guided dosing of acenocoumarol and phenprocoumon. N Engl J Med. 2013;369:2304–12.
109. SEARCH Collaborative Group, Link E, Parish S, Armitage J, Bowman L, Heath S, et al. SLCO1B1 variants and statin-induced myopath- genomewide study. N Engl J Med. 2008;359:789–99.
110. Mangravite LM, Engelhardt BE, Medina MW, Smith JD, Brown CD, Chasman DI, et al. A statin-dependent QTL for GATM expression is associated with statin-induced myopathy. Nature. 2013;502: 377–80.

Genetic Polymorphisms and the Vascular Endothelium

8

Emmanuel Androulakis, Christodoulos Stefanadis, and Dimitris Tousoulis

Abstract

The healthy vascular endothelium exerts atheroprotective actions through vasoactive mediators such as nitric oxide and prostacyclin. It should be noted that inflammation and genetics are both prominent mechanisms in the pathogenesis of endothelial dysfunction and atherosclerosis. Currently, a growing body of evidence has emerged regarding genetic component and its role in the aim of assessing vascular endothelium. Of note, genetic variation within the population seems to determine endothelial responses and potential modify both atherogenesis and individual's responses to risk factors. It has been estimated that only 10–20 % of the variation in endothelial function may be accounted for by genes. Moreover, several studies have explored the association of vascular disease with gene polymorphisms of candidate genes, such as of endothelial nitric oxide synthase, cytokines, chemokines and of other proinflammatory molecules. Although their results are preliminary and to a certain extent conflicting, current data provide some evidence that alterations in the genetics, especially of the inflammatory cascade, may modify vascular disease.

Keywords

Vascular endothelium • Endothelial dysfunction • Genetic polymorphisms

Abbreviations

ACE II	Angiotensin Converting Enzyme Gene
ACS	Acute Coronary Syndromes
ADMA	Asymmetrical dimethylarginine
AGT	Angiotensinogen Gene
AngII	Angiotensin-II
ATH	Atherosclerosis
BH4	Tetrahydrobiopterin

E. Androulakis • C. Stefanadis
D. Tousoulis, MD, PhD, FACC (✉)
1st Cardiology Unit, Hippokration Hospital,
Athens University Medical School,
Athens, Greece
e-mail: drtousoulis@hotmail.com

D.V. Cokkinos (ed.), *Introduction to Translational Cardiovascular Research*,
DOI 10.1007/978-3-319-08798-6_8,

CAMs	Cell Adhesion Molecules
CD 40L	CD40 ligand
CPR	C-reactive protein
CVDs	Cardiovascular Diseases
eNos	Endothelial Nitric Oxide Synthase
EPCs	Endothelial Progenitors Cells
ET-1	Endothelin −1
FMD	Flow Mediated Dilation
ICAM-1	Intercellular Adhesion molecule −1
IL-1	Interleukin-1
IMT	Carotid Intima Media Thickness
iNos	Inducible Nitric Oxide Synthase
MCP-1	Monocyte Chemotactic Protein −1
NADPH	Nicotinamide Adenine Dinucleotide Phosphate Oxidase
NO	Nitric Oxide
Ox LDL	Oxidized Low-density Lipoprotein
PAI-1	Plasminogen Activator inhibitor-1
PGI 2	Prostacyclin
ROS	Reactive Oxygen Species
SMCs	Smooth Muscle Cells
TNF-a	Tumor Necrosis Factor-a
TXA2	Thromboxane
VSMC	Vascular Smooth Muscle Cells
vWF	Von Willebrand Factor
XO	Xanthine Oxidase

8.1 Introduction

The vascular endothelium is nowadays considered as a paracrine organ which secretes several mediators exerting anti-atherogenic effects. Endothelial damage is also crucial for the development of atherosclerosis and risk factors such as hyperlipidemia, hypertension, smoking, diabetes mellitus and genetics represent important factors predisposing to endothelial dysfunction (ED), by triggering underlying processes such as thrombosis and inflammation [1–3].

Moreover, nitric oxide (NO) is the key molecule managing the vascular homeostasis, while decreased bioavailability of NO due to reduced synthesis and increased scavenging by reactive oxygen species (ROS), plays a crucial role in developing ED. Importantly, ED plays pivotal role in disease initiation and progression of atherosclerosis(ATH); it seems to precede atherosclerotic lesions in coronary vessels, and even occur in offspring with a history for cardiovascular diseases (CVDs) [4, 5].

Recently, growing data have focused on detection and monitoring of biomarkers, which may increase the ability to predict vascular disease. Circulating inflammatory markers are implicated in the pathogenesis of ED and ATH. It also seems rational that molecules, such as C-reactive protein (CRP), interleukin-1 (IL-1) and intercellular adhesion molecule-1 (ICAM-1) could be used as diagnostic objectives in that state [6–8]. Of note, many studies have assessed the effects of a range of candidate genes on ED, the results of which could provide useful insights into genetic influences on atherothrombotic disease and others CVDs [9, 10].

In the present review we highlight findings regarding the pathophysiology of vascular disease and will discuss the role of genetic polymorphisms in that state.

8.2 Physiology of Vascular Endothelium

Vascular endothelium has emerged as a paracrine organ responsible for the secretion of several beneficial substances with anti-atherogenic effects; thus its structural and functional integrity are fundamental. It consists of a thin semipermeable layer of cells covering the internal surface of vessels and develops a border between the vessel and circulation, exerting significant autocrine, paracrine and endocrine actions and influencing smooth muscle cells (SMCs), platelets and peripheral leucocytes [2, 11].

More specifically, circulating molecules across the endothelial cells (ECs) to the subendothelial space are transported via several mechanisms to meet the metabolic demands of the surrounding tissue cells. Also, tight junctions between ECs create a selective barrier to the egress of molecules from the circulation [12]. Notably, there exists a phenotypic deviation between ECs in various parts of the vascular system, expressing different surface antigens and receptors and generating different responses to the same stimuli [2].

Principally, vascular endothelium participates in the regulation of vascular tone, producing several vasoactive mediators, such as NO, prostacyclin (PGI2) and endothelin-1 (ET-1) which arc powerful vasoactive substances released in response to both hormonal and mechanical stimuli and affecting both the function and structure of the underlying vascular smooth muscle cells (VSMC). NO is a profound vasodilator, produced by both endothelial nitric oxide synthase (eNOS) and inducible nitric oxide synthase (iNOS) which catalyze the conversion of L-arginine to NO and maintain the vasculature in a state of vasodilation. On the other hand, ET is a powerful vasoconstrictor which is also produced by ECs, with marked effects on vascular tone [13, 14]. NO bioavailability is recognised to exert various actions on vascular endothelium and more specifically, it is capable of reversing constrictive effects of acetylcholine leading to vasorelaxation and maintaining the balance against various endothelium-derived contracting factors, such as ET-1 and thromboxane A2 (TXA2). Furthermore, decreased NO bioavailability critically participates in atherothrombosis, given its antithrombotic, antiapoptotic, antiinflammatory and antioxidant effects [15, 16].

In particular, the endothelium secretes the tissue-type plasminogen activator (t-PA), along with the von Willebrand factor (vWF), the plasminogen activator inhibitor-1 (PAI-1), and the platelet activating factor. Thus, it seems to play a key role in the regulation of coagulation in response to vascular injury, inflammation, or other stimuli such as oxidized low-density lipoprotein (oxLDL), tumor necrosis factor-α (TNF-a) and IL-1 [17, 18]. In addition, ECs can produce a variety of principal molecules including cytokines and growth factors, such as IL-1, IL-6, IL-8, insulin growth factor, transforming growth factor and colony stimulating factor in response to stimulation with bacterial products, inflammation, hypoxemia and other mediators [19, 20].

8.2.1 Pathophysiology of Endothelial Dysfunction

Endothelial dysfunction is now considered an important early event in the pathogenesis of ATH, contributing to plaque initiation and progression [21]. Generally, it is characterised by a shift of the aforementioned actions of the endothelium toward reduced vasodilation and toward a proinflammatory and prothrombotic state. This process is the consequence of high prevalence of both traditional risk factors (smoking, increased cholesterol levels, hypertension) and non-traditional risk factors (inflammation, oxidative stress, hyperhomocysteinemia etc.) [1] (Fig. 8.1). Also, ED has been repeatedly associated with low NO bioavailability as a result of impaired NO production by the endothelium and/or increased NO inhibition by ROS [1].

The withdrawal of NO-mediated beneficial effects on vascular function and to the formation of free radicals with proatherogenic properties. In particular, the term "oxidative stress" describes conditions involving increased ROS levels, produced by enzymes within vascular tissue, such as nicotinamide adenine dinucleotide phosphate oxidase (NADPH), and xanthine oxidase [22]. Also, tetrahydrobiopterin, an essential cofactor for NO synthases, has been recently suggested as a critical determinant for eNOS activity. Moreover, significant data have demonstrated that vascular but not plasma tetrahydrobiopterin (BH4) is a central factor of eNOS coupling, endothelium-dependent vasodilation, and superoxide production in human vessels, whereas plasma biopterins are associated with systemic inflammation [23, 24].

NO is essential to vascular homeostasis, while disturbance of the eNOS ability to produce NO is a major contributor to the pathogenesis of vascular disease. It has been shown by *in vivo* studies that expression of eNOS is vital for endothelial function and that this enzyme is subjected to significant degrees of regulation by numerous physiological and pathophysiological stimuli via mechanisms that alter steady-state eNOS mRNA levels. Such stimuli include shear stress, transforming growth factors, cell growth, hydrogen peroxide (H_2O_2), hypoxia and oxLDL [25–27]. Moreover, it is well-known that oxidative stress is implicated in all stages of inflammation, including hypertrophy, apoptosis, migration, fibrosis, angiogenesis and ED participating in complex processes leading in vascular remodeling. It stimulates inflammatory processes, via multiple intracellular proteins, enzymes and transcription

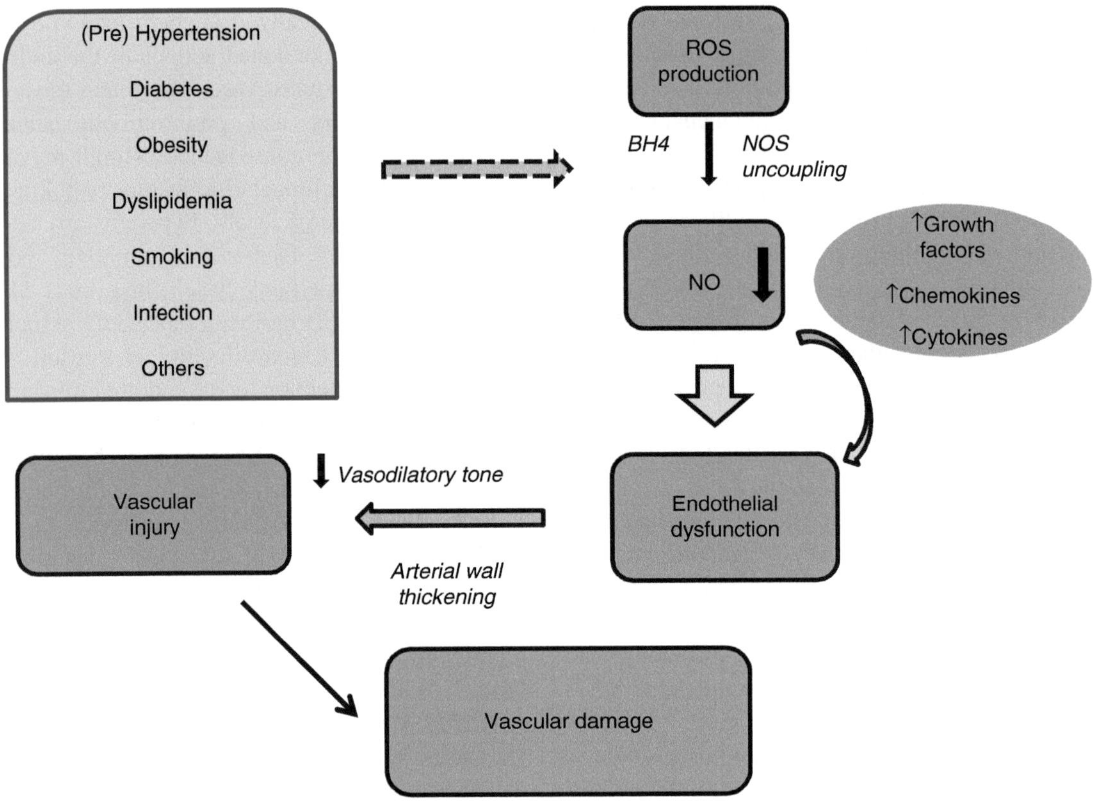

Fig. 8.1 Pathophysiological mechanisms contributing to vascular disease

factors activated by ROS [28, 29]. Importantly, angiotensin-II (Ang II) plays a pivotal role in cascades leading in expression of proinflammatory mediators and extracellular matrix modification. Accordingly, vascular NADPH oxidase is activated, and the produced ROS stimulate redox-sensitive inflammatory genes, such as those encoding monocyte chemotactic protein-1 (MCP-1) and IL-6 [29, 30].

8.2.2 Biomarkers in Vascular Disease

Comprehension of mechanisms which are implicated in the development of ED is vital for establishing biomarkers as potential diagnostic tools and designing prevention or treatment strategies. This approach could be equally attractive in both preclinical and clinical ATH and accordingly, in CVDs [31]. According to recent studies, selected biomarkers may be associated with ED and scientific interest has focused on detection and monitoring of them (Table 8.1).

8.2.2.1 C-Reactive Protein (CRP)

The most exploited circulating inflammatory marker in plasma is CRP. In addition to its role as a marker, it can exert modulatory effects through its well-demonstrated presence in atherosclerotic plaques [32]. CRP is an acute-phase protein produced in the liver and has a homopentameric structure, each with 206 amino acids that are combined in a three-dimensional structure, and Ca^{2+}-binding specificity for phosphocholine [33]. Besides being a sensitive marker for the detection of subclinical inflammation, CRP has been suggested to participate in the pathophysiology of ATH. Moreover, it stimulates the secretion of proinflammatory cytokines and tissue factor and may contribute to vascular remodeling via its effects on eNOS [34].

Table 8.1 Biomarkers associated with endothelial dysfunction

Category	Biomarker (plasma)
Acute phase protein	CRP
Adhesion molecules	ICAM-1
	VCAM-1
Cytokines/chemokines	IL-1, IL-6
	TNF-a
	MCP-1
Pro-coagulant and thrombotic markers	PAI-1
	Fibrinogen
	vWF
Other biomarkers	EPCs
	Soluble CD40 ligand
	Selectins (E-Selectin)
	Tetrahydrobiopterin

Abbreviations: *CRP* C-reactive protein, *ICAM* intercellular cell adhesion molecules, *VCAM-1* vascular cell adhesion molecule-1, *MCP-1* monocyte chemoattractant protein-1, *IL* interleukin, *TNF-a* tumor necrosis factor-alpha, *PAI-1* tissue plasminogen activator inhibitor-1, *vWF* von Wilebrand factor, *EPCs* endothelial progenitor cells

A growing body of literature has demonstrated that CRP levels may be correlated with ED. Moreover, it may stimulate expression of various biomarkers, such as ICAM, vascular cell adhesion molecule 1 (VCAM-1) and E-selectin [35]. Moreover, according to experimental data CRP may also induce a significant impairment of endothelial-dependent vasorelaxation in various conditions which could lead to an increased cardiovascular risk profile [36]. In line with this evidence, Venugopal et al. [37] have demonstrated that CRP decreased eNOS mRNA, protein abundance, and enzyme activity in cultured human aortic ECs. Furthermore, increased CRP plasma levels across the coronary circulation have been associated with impairment in coronary endothelial-dependent function, even though its relationship with the severity and extent of coronary atherosclerosis is not clear [38].

8.2.2.2 Other Biomarkers in ED

Impaired endothelium dependent vasodilation along with alterations in the expression of adhesion molecules and proinflammatory molecules are present in state of ED. More specifically, increased IL-6, TNF-a, and especially ICAM-1, VCAM-1, and E-selectin are associated with ED. These molecules may also participate in ECs stimulation to promote an atherogenic phenotype [39]. In addition, other chemotactic factors could be expressed such as MCP-1, macrophage colony-stimulating factor, and TNF-β which contribute to the development of inflammation within the arterial wall related with the pathogenesis of atherosclerosis [40]. As aforementioned, vascular endothelium produces various other molecules that affect blood fluidity and thrombosis, such as plasminogen activator inhibitor-1 (PAI-1), tissue factor and vWF. These in turn, are regulated by the production of NO, prostacyclin, tissue plasminogen activator and thrombomodulin [41]. Moreover, CD40 ligand (CD40L) is expressed on monocyte/macrophages, ECs, smooth muscle cells and platelets, and as a consequence of CD40L binding to CD40, several inflammatory processes are initiated by the release of cytokines and the expression of adhesion molecules. In particular, the link between CD40/CD40L and CVDs has been established in numerous studies [41]. The pathophysiological substrate is still under investigation however, evidence suggests that initially, CD40L has an unfavorable effect on the vascular redox state [41].

Accordingly, it has been suggested that circulating markers of oxidative stress, including F2 isoprostanes and antibodies against oxLDL, are increased in humans with diabetes [42]. Notably, given that there is oxidative degradation of BH4 by ROS in ED, BH4 plasma levels along with levels in the vascular wall could reflect vascular endothelial health [43]. Moreover, clinical data have suggested that hyperhomocysteinemia may be associated with impaired renal function, potentially through affecting endothelial function. Thus, plasma homocysteine levels may be considered as an intermediate factor between ED and renal function [44]. Also, asymmetrical dimethylarginine (ADMA) as an endogenous eNOS inhibitor has been associated with ED in several CVDs, such as hypercholesterolemia and coronary artery disease [45]. It is worth mentioning, endothelial progenitor cells (EPCs) are currently considered to participate in vascular repair and maintain endothelial integrity thus, they may exhibit a role as prognostic biomarker in CVD. EPC number and function may be used as biomarkers and more specifically, reduced circulating numbers and functional capacity may predict future cardiovascular events, independently of other cardiovascular risk factors [46].

8.3 Genetic Contribution in Vascular Endothelium: The Role of Polymorphisms

Currently, a growing body of evidence has emerged regarding genetic component and its role in the aim of assessing vascular endothelium. Of note, genetic variation within the population seems to determine endothelial responses and potential modify both atherogenesis and an individual's responses to risk factors. It has been estimated that only 10–20 % of the variation in endothelial function may be accounted for by genes [47].

8.3.1 eNOS

The eNOS gene includes 26 exons, 25 introns and it is located at 7q35–7q36 of chromosome 7, while the protein consists of 1,203 amino acids and has a molecular weight of 133 kDA [48]. It has been the focus of intensive research to identify potentially functional polymorphisms influencing ED, as more than 100 polymorphisms have been identified in the eNOS gene (Table 8.2). Some of them (e.g. T–786C promoter polymorphism) are situated in the eNOS promoter and might influence mRNA transcription reducing gene expression [53]. More spe-

Table 8.2 Most important single nucleotide polymorphisms of eNOS gene and their relationship with endothelial dysfunction

SNPs	Participants	Examined parameters	Comments
G894T [49]	104 patients with CAD	Endothelium-dependent vasorelaxations	It is associated with impaired NO-mediated endothelial vasomotor function
G894T [50]	248 healthy subjects	FMD/GTN-induced dilation	It is associated with differences in endothelial responses to both smoking and n-3 FA in healthy young subjects
G894T [51]	Human endothelial cells	Subcellular localization and interaction of eNOS with modulatory proteins	It does not have a major effect in modulating eNOS activity *in vivo*
G894T [52]	56 patients with a history of premature MI	Forearm blood flow	It is associated with impaired endothelial function and higher levels of von Willebrand factor
T786C [53]	11 patients with CAD and 9 controls	Endothelial NO synthesis and coronary spasm	It is associated with reduced endothelial NO synthesis and predisposes to coronary spasm
T786C [54]	Endothelial cells cultures (154 patients with CAD and 174 non-CAD subjects)	NO-dependent relaxation was examined in segments of saphenous vein Shear stress-induced NOS-3 mRNA and protein expression	It is associated with blocking shear stress-dependent maintenance of NOS-3 expression
ecNOS4a/b [55]	549 subjects with, and 153 without CAD	Distribution of polymorphism in CAD in relation to smoking	It is associated with predisposition to endothelial dysfunction
A922G [53]	11 patients with CAD and 9 controls	Endothelial NO synthesis and coronary spasm	It is associated with coronary spasm
T1468A [53]	11 patients with CAD and 9 controls	Endothelial NO synthesis and coronary spasm	It is associated with coronary spasm

Abbreviations: *CAD* coronary artery disease, *NO* nitric oxide, *FMD* flow mediated dilation, *GTN* glyceryl trinitrate, *eNOS* endothelial nitric oxide synthase, *FA* fatty acid, *MI* myocardial infarction cifically, Nakayama et al. [53] have demonstrated the existence of three linked mutations in the 5′-flanking region of the eNOS gene (T-786C, A-922G, and T-1468A) which are more prevalent in patients with coronary spasm than in the control group. Also, the T-786C mutation resulted in a significant reduction in eNOS gene promoter activity, whereas neither the A-922G nor the T-1468A mutation had any affect, suggesting that this single nucleotide polymorphism (SNP) may reduce endothelial NO synthesis and predispose to coronary spasm.

One of the most studied NOS polymorphisms is the polymorphism in exon 7 of NOS3, a G-T transition at position 894 that results in a Glu to Asp amino acid substitution for codon 298 (894GT) within exon 7. It is the only common polymorphism identified thus far that encodes an amino acid substitution. Significant data have shown that eNOS Asp298 is subjected to selective proteolytic cleavage in ECs and vascular tissues that might account for reduced vascular NO generation, even though it has been elsewhere suggested that eNOS Asp298 could be a marker for another possibly functional variant [51, 56, 57]. Moreover, given a novel method to accurately determine molar quantities of each variant of G894T polymorphism (expressing them as green fluorescent protein fusion proteins and using recombinant adenoviruses to facilitate transient infection of human microvascular ECs), the Asp substitution at 298 does not seem to have a major effect in modulating eNOS activity *in vivo* [51]. In turn, Guzik et al. [49] have investigated the relationships between NO-mediated endothelial function with the presence of the eNOS Glu298Asp variant via endothelium-dependent vasorelaxation to different agonists which were determined in human saphenous veins of coronary artery disease (CAD) patients. NO-mediated endothelial vasorelaxation was highly variable between patients, and reduced values were associated with increased number of clinical risk factors for ATH. This variant was not associated with any differences in contractions to phenylephrine, NO-mediated vasorelaxations to acetylcholine, bradykinin or calcium ionophore, nor relaxations to the NO donor sodium nitroprusside, suggesting that this polymorphism may not have a major direct functional effect on vascular eNOS activity in human ATH [49].

More recently however, a study by Antoniades et al. [52] has provided new evidence about its potential association with endothelial function and with markers of ECs injury and activation. The study population consisted of 56 patients with a history of premature myocardial infarction, while the forearm blood flow was measured using strain-gauge plethysmography. Of note, the presence of 894 T allele on eNOS gene is associated with impaired endothelial function and higher levels of von Willebrand factor in relatively young patients with myocardial infarction. Subsequently, the same investigators have attempted to explore the determinants of GCH1 gene expression, which codes for a rate-limiting enzyme in the biosynthesis of BH4, an eNOS cofactor important for maintaining enzymatic coupling. They have demonstrated that GCH1 gene expression modulated by a particular GCH1 haplotype, is a major determinant of BH4 bioavailability both in plasma and in the vascular wall thus, this genetic variation may be a determinant of eNOS coupling, vascular redox state, and endothelial function in human vascular disease [58].

8.3.1.1 CRP Gene Variation

Its role has already been discussed in Sect. 8.2.2. It has been suggested to participate in several related processes, such as the binding of LDL-cholesterol from macrophages to form foam cells and the development of vulnerable plaques, while it stimulates the secretion of pro-inflammatory cytokines and tissue factor, thus contributing to vascular remodeling [59, 60]. Moreover, CRP levels have been inversely correlated with ED and with the prediction of future or recurrent cardiovascular events [61]. The CRP gene is located on chromosome 1 in the region 1q21–q23. It consists of two exons encoding the CRP monomer of 206 amino acids, with an intervening intron, while the circulating protein is a symmetric, noncovalently associated pentamer with a central pore [62]. Due to the fact that circulating levels of CRP are widely used to determine inflammatory response, it is not surprising that CRP gene variation has been studied in relation to inflammatory disorders. More specifically, it seems that CRP SNPs may be associated with the risk of developing inflammatory disease and also with its severity [63]. Furthermore, multiple CRP gene polymorphisms have been shown to associate with circulating CRP, and in turn with CVD. According to Lawlor et al. [64], however, according to data derived from five large trials (a total of 18,637 individuals) rs1130864 (on the 3′ untranslated region of CRP) was associated with serum CRP, and serum CRP was associated with coronary heart disease, though there was no a direct association between the SNP and disease.

8.3.1.2 Cytokines

Most of the cytokines are glycoproteins with a monomeric molecular mass of 15–25 kDa. IL-6 and TNF-a are some of the main cytokines participating in atherogenesis and as regards their structure, IL-6 is a four helix bundle, while TNF-a is a trimeric protein [1]. Notably, genetic variants of interleukin genes have been associated with their plasma concentrations and with the risk of CVDs [65, 66]. Moreover, according to experimental studies which examined the functional effect of four polymorphisms in the IL-6 promoter (G-597A, G-572GC, −373A(n)T(n), G-174GC), more than one of the polymorphic sites is functional and they may influence IL-6 transcription not by a simple additive mechanism but rather through complex interactions determined by the haplotype [67]. Also, Stoica et al. [68] have recently evaluated the association between IL-6 (G-174 T, nt565 G/A) and IL-10 (G-1082A, C819T, C-592A) gene polymorphisms with the short-term risk of postoperative cardiovascular events and with endothelial function in patients with peripheral artery disease (Table 8.3). They

Table 8.3 Most important single nucleotide polymorphisms associated with endothelial dysfunction

Study	SNPs	Genes	Comments
Antoniades et al. [52]	G894T	eNOS	Association with impaired endothelial function and higher levels of von Willebrand factor
Nakayama et al. [53]	T786C	eNOS	Association with reduced endothelial NO synthesis and predisposition to coronary spasm
Wang et al. [55]	ecNOS4a/b	eNOS	Association with predisposition to endothelial dysfunction
Nakayama et al. [53]	A922G	eNOS	Association with coronary spasm
Nakayama et al. [53]	T1468A	eNOS	Association with coronary spasm
Stoica et al. [68]	G-174 T	IL-6	Association with ED
Stoica et al. [68]	nt565 G/A	IL-6	Association with ED
Stoica et al. [68]	G-1082A C819T C-592A	IL-10	Association with ED (ATA haplotypes)
Ponthieux et al. [69]	G/R241	ICAM-1	Association with serum ICAM-1 levels
Motawi et al. [70]	K469E	ICAM-1	Association with vascular disease
Motawi et al. [70]	Ser128Arg	E-selectin	Association with vascular disease
Yoshida et al. [71]	Thr715Pro	E-selectin	Association with predisposition to atherosclerosis
Vadapalli et al. [72]	3A/4A Lys198Asn	ET-1	Association with more pronounced ED
Ezzidi et al. [73]	4G/5G G-844A	PAI-1	Association with PAI-1 levels and microvascular disease
Robinson et al. [74]	C-7351T T20 099C T27445A	tPA	No association with endothelial function and microvascular disease

Abbreviations: *NO* nitric oxide, *eNOS* endothelial nitric oxide synthase, *BH4* tetrahydrobiopterin, *CRP* C-reactive protein, *IL* interleukins, *ED* endothelial dysfunction, *GCH1* GTP-cyclohydrolase I is encoded by GCH1, *ICAM-1* intercellular adhesion molecule 1, *PAI-1* plasminogen activator inhibitor-1, *ET-1* endothelin-1, *tPA* tissue plasminogen activator have shown that IL-6 -174CC and nt565AA genotypes, as well as IL-10 ATA haplotypes are correlated with ED in these patients, as indicated by decreased values of flow mediated dilation (FMD), and with a high short-term risk of acute postoperative cardiovascular events. Moreover, in the setting of non-ST-elevation acute coronary syndromes (ACS), genetic variation at the IL-1 gene locus contributes to the changes in soluble endothelial activation markers (vWF and E-selectin) [75]. It is also worth-noting that according to preliminary data, there is a significant and independent association between the IL-6 G-572C gene polymorphism (presence of C allele) and adolescents with a family history of premature ATH [76].

8.3.1.3 Adhesion Molecules-Chemokines

Cell adhesion molecules (CAMs) are transmembrane glycoproteins consisting of an extracellular component with a hydrophobic transmembrane component and an intracytoplasmic component. Integrins, the immunoglobulin superfamily and the selectins are the three families of CAMs. Also, chemokines are members of a group of structurally related and secretable, chemotactic cytokines divided into four families (CC, CXC, CX3C, XC) and can be located in different vascular cell types, such as ECs but also inflammatory cells [77, 78]. ICAM-1 is thought to be associated with non-ECs inflammation, while VCAM-1 is expressed more locally within the vascular system. It has been assessed the effect of a single-base polymorphism at codon 241 in exon 4 of ICAM-1 gene on serum ICAM-1 (sICAM-1) concentration in a large healthy population, taking into account other biological determinants of sICAM-1 level. The R241 allele was significantly associated with lower sICAM-1 levels and explained 3.4 and 1.9 % of the sICAM-1 variability in children and adults, respectively, probably due to the impairment in binding of ICAM-1 to leukocyte integrin Mac-1 protein [69].

Notably, it has been recently hypothesized that several candidate genes may be associated with markers of systemic inflammation and ED in an aging population. Blood samples were analyzed for 202 SNPs in 25 candidate genes, while the relationship between markers of systemic inflammation and ED and these SNPs was evaluated in order to identify novel candidate genes which may elucidate the etiology and pathogenesis of CVD. It has been suggested that candidate genes potentially influence levels of serum markers of inflammation and ED, such as ICAM-1, VCAM-1, CRP and fibrinogen via several novel SNP associations which have not previously been associated with CVDs [79]. It is also worth mentioning that there are genotype-specific associations between circulating soluble cellular adhesion molecules and preclinical ATH in community residents. It has been suggested that sVCAM-1 is independently associated with carotid intima media thickness (IMT) in subjects with the angiotensin converting enzyme gene (ACE II) genotype or apolipoprotein E gene (apoE4) genotype. Similarly, the plasma level of sICAM-1 was independently associated with carotid IMT in angiotensinogen gene (AGT) M carriers. These findings suggest that genetic background could be involved in the association between plasma CAMs and ATH [80]. Of note, the investigation of the association of both ICAM-1 and endothelial cell adhesion molecule (E-selectin) polymorphisms as well as their role in the pathogenesis of ATH have recently been attempted. Particularly, Ser 128Arg of E-selectin and the K469E of ICAM-1 polymorphisms may be involved in predisposition to ATH. More specifically, the frequency of the mutant AC genotype of E-selectin in peripheral, cerebral and cardiovascular atherosclerotic patients was significantly higher than in control subjects. Also, the frequency of the mutant EE homozygotes of ICAM-1 in peripheral, cerebral and cardiovascular atherosclerotic patients was significantly higher compared to controls, while the frequency of EK of ICAM-1 showed no significant difference between atherosclerotic patients and the control group. The frequency of the mutant E allele of ICAM-1 was significantly higher in peripheral, cerebral and cardiovascular patients compared to controls [70].

On the other hand, selectins are a family of cell adhesion molecules which include a single-chain transmembrane glycoprotein. According to previous data, the heritability of circulating P-selectin levels has been estimated between 45 and 70 %. Specifically, the Thr715Pro polymorphism (rs6136) of the P-selectin gene (SELP) has been associated with lower soluble P-selectin levels, accounting for approximately 10–20 % of the variation in healthy European-American populations, while other SELP polymorphisms, such as Val599Leu (rs6133), appear to account for some of the residual variance in soluble P-selectin among these populations [81, 82]. Of note, it has been demonstrated by Yoshida et al. [71] that the E-selectin Ser128Arg polymorphism was significantly associated with rolling and adhesion of neutrophils and mononuclear cells as well as phosphorylation of extracellular signal regulated kinase 1 and 2 and p38 mitogen-activated protein kinase, suggesting that an altered endothelial signaling pathway is associated with this polymorphism. Moreover, according to data derived from the population-based CARDIA study which assessed relationship of 25 P-selectin SNPs with atherosclerotic risk, common SELP polymorphisms were associated with soluble P-selectin and carotid IMT in young adults, even though the patterns of association differed between European-Americans and African-American, supporting the role of P-selectin in the preclinical stages of atherosclerosis [83]. In line with this evidence, it had been previously suggested in a large cohort of patients with documented CAD an association between P-selectin gene polymorphisms (C-2123G, A-1969G, and Thr715Pro) and serum P-selectin levels which altogether explained 7.3 and 18.6 % of the P-selectin variability in patients and controls, respectively. Also, it has been revealed a complex age-dependent relation between soluble P-selectin levels and CAD, which suggests that this molecule might have different roles in the atherothrombotic process [82]. Moreover, according to Volcic et al. [84] who examined the association of the P-selectin Thr715Pro polymorphism with the incident of coronary heart disease (CHD) and ischemic stroke among 14,595 participants, genotypes carrying the P-selectin Pro715 variant allele were associated with decreased P-selectin levels compared to the homozygous wild-type genotype, even though this polymorphism was not associated with incident CHD or ischemic stroke.

8.3.1.4 Other Endothelium-Derived Mediators

In addition, it is well-established that ET-1 is an endothelium-derived peptide with multiple functions affecting cardiovascular system, given its role as a powerful vasoconstrictor with mitogenic activity on vascular smooth muscle and fibroblasts. Also, vascular endothelium produces a variety of other molecules that affect blood fluidity and thrombosis, such as PAI-1, tissue factor, and vWF which are regulated by the production of NO, prostacyclin, tPA, and thrombomodulin. Furthermore, the CD40L protein is a type II membrane protein, the extracellular region of which belongs to the TNF superfamily. The B cells are the main cell type expressing CD40; however, a variety of cells involved in ATH, such as ECs, SMCs, macrophages, T lymphocytes and platelets, also express both CD40 and CD40L. As a consequence of CD40L binding to its receptor, several inflammatory processes are initiated. Noticeably, both are molecules with a dual prothrombotic and proinflammatory role [1, 85].

ET-1 is produced as a 212 amino acid preproendothelin and is processed to a relatively inactive 39 amino acid molecule, which is then converted by the membrane-bound endothelin converting enzyme-1 to a 21 amino acid functional peptide. Genetic variants of the ET-1 gene (3A/4A, Lys198Asn) have been suggested to alter its expression and play a role in endothelial function. More specifically, according to a recent study which evaluated their contribution to endothelial function in patients with idiopathic pulmonary hypertension, ED was more pronounced in the individuals with ET-1 variants, and they were shown to play a significant role in susceptibility to the disease and its clinical progression [72].

Furthermore, mutations in the PAI-1 gene, along with altered PAI-1 and tPA levels, have been implicated in vascular disease. In 856 type 2 diabetes patients PAI-1 4G/5G and -844G/A genotyping was investigated in regards to microvascular damage. Alterations in PAI-1 levels have been identified, while genetic variations at the PAI-1 locus have been revealed as risk factors for diabetic retinopathy [73]. In addition, our insight into the regulation of the synthesis and release of t-PA has extended markedly in the last decade, however mechanisms underlying acute release of t-PA from the endothelium are still under investigation. Therefore, Robinson et al. [74] have evaluated whether polymorphisms of the t-PA gene (C-7351T, T20 099C, T27445A) could influence endothelial function, as evaluated from forearm blood flow in response to intra-brachial infusion of substance P and sodium nitroprusside, and acute endogenous t-PA release in 96 patients with CAD. However, they have found no effect of the polymorphisms on two complementary aspects of endothelial function, or a major influence on acute t-PA release in this population. Moreover, it is unknown whether genetic variations in CD40/CD40L genes contribute to atherogenesis and the development of vascular disease. It is worth noting that genetic polymorphisms related to plasma CD40L levels could be used to examine whether this molecule constitutes a causal factor. Accordingly, it has been evaluated the role of genetic variation in CD40 and CD40L genes in subclinical ATH assessed by coronary artery calcification and IMT in subjects from families in the Diabetes Heart Study. The results of the study showed that the two SNPs in the CD40 gene (rs1535045 and rs3765459) were significantly associated with decreased coronary artery calcification in this population. However, they were not associated with other parameters of the study [85, 86].

Conclusions

It is widely accepted that atherosclerosis is a disease which for the most part is characterised by endothelial dysfunction and vascular inflammation. Moreover, vascular disease is a multi-factorial disorder with many environmental and genetic factors involved, while its genetic predisposition has been studied with respect to several candidate genes. The genes encoding components of the inflammatory cascade, including cytokines, adhesion molecules and other biomarkers have been the most studied as candidate ones for that state, as well as related disorders. However, results have not always been consistent and data were limited to single studies, therefore it has been difficult to draw firm conclusions about these genes. Some of these uncertainties could be resolved by systematic reviews and meta-analyses of the relevant genotype–disease association studies and undoubtedly, further large-scale studies are required in the aim of defining genes that regulate vascular function.

References

1. Tousoulis D, Kampoli AM, Papageorgiou N, Androulakis E, Antoniades C, Toutouzas K, et al. Pathophysiology of atherosclerosis: the role of inflammation. Curr Pharm Des. 2011;17:4089–110.
2. Galley HF, Webster NR. Physiology of the endothelium. Br J Anaesth. 2004;93:105–13.
3. Glasser S, Selwyn A, Ganz P. Atherosclerosis: risk factors and the vascular endothelium. Am Heart J. 1996;131:379–84.
4. Libby P, Theroux P. Pathophysiology of coronary artery disease. Circulation. 2005;111:3481–8.
5. Tousoulis D, Briasoulis A, Papageorgiou N, Tsioufis C, Tsiamis E, Toutouzas K, et al. Oxidative stress and endothelial function: therapeutic interventions. Recent Pat Cardiovasc Drug Discov. 2011;6:103–14.
6. Tousoulis D. Biomarkers in cardiovascular disease. Curr Med Chem. 2012;19:2483–4.
7. Tousoulis D, Antoniades C, Koumallos N, Stefanadis C. Pro-inflammatory cytokines in acute coronary syndromes: from bench to bedside. Cytokine Growth Factor Rev. 2006;17:225–33.
8. Damas JK, Aukrust P. Systemic markers of inflammation – are they useful predictive tools in coronary artery disease? Scand Cardiovasc J. 2006;40:262–6.
9. Jones LC, Hingorani AD. Genetic regulation of endothelial function. Heart. 2005;91:1275–7.
10. Vallance P, Chan N. Endothelial function and nitric oxide: clinical relevance. Heart. 2001;85:342–50.
11. Gallagher G, Sumpio BE. Vascular endothelial cells. In: Sumpio BE, Sidawy AS, editors. Basic science of vascular disease. Mt Kisco: Futura Publishing Co; 1997. p. 151–86.
12. Rubanyi GM. The role of endothelium in cardiovascular homeostasis and diseases. J Cardiovasc Pharmacol. 1993;22 Suppl 4:S1–14.

13. Inoue A, Yanagisawa M, Kimura S, Kasuya Y, Miyauchi T, Goto K, et al. The human endothelin family: three structurally and pharmacologically distinct isopeptides predicted by three separate genes. Proc Natl Acad Sci U S A. 1989;86:2863–7.
14. Gardiner SM, Kemp PA, March JE, Bennett T, Davenport AP, Edvinsson L. Effects of an ET1-receptor antagonist, FR139317, on regional haemodynamic responses to endothelin-1 and [Ala11,15] Ac-endothelin-1 (6–21) in conscious rats. Br J Pharmacol. 1994;112:477–86.
15. Esper RJ, Nordaby RA, Vilariño JO, Paragano A, Cacharrón JL, Machado RA. Endothelial dysfunction: a comprehensive appraisal. Cardiovasc Diabetol. 2006;5:4. doi:10.1186/1475-2840-5-4.
16. Wennmalm A. Endothelial nitric oxide and cardiovascular disease. J Intern Med. 1994;235:317–27.
17. Stehouwer CD, Lambert J, Donker AJ, van Hinsbergh VW. Endothelial dysfunction and pathogenesis of diabetic angiopathy. Cardiovasc Res. 1997;34:55–68.
18. Erickson LA, Hekman CM, Loskutoff DJ. The primary plasminogen-activator inhibitors in endothelial cells, platelets, serum, and plasma are immunologically related. Proc Natl Acad Sci U S A. 1985;82:8710–4.
19. Tousoulis D, Charakida M, Stefanadis C. Endothelial function and inflammation in coronary artery disease. Heart. 2006;92:441–4.
20. Harrison DG. Cellular and molecular mechanisms of endothelial cell dysfunction. J Clin Invest. 1997;100:2153–7.
21. Hirata Y, Nagata D, Suzuki E, Nishimatsu H, Suzuki J, Nagai R. Diagnosis and treatment of endothelial dysfunction in cardiovascular disease. A Review. Int Heart J. 2010;51:1–6.
22. Hansson GK. Inflammation, atherosclerosis, and coronary artery disease. N Engl J Med. 2005;352:1685–95.
23. Schmidt TS, Alp NJ. Mechanisms for the role of tetrahydrobiopterin in endothelial function and vascular disease. Clin Sci (Lond). 2007;113:47–63.
24. Antoniades C, Shirodaria C, Crabtree M, Rinze R, Alp N, Cunnington C, et al. Altered plasma versus vascular biopterins in human atherosclerosis reveal relationships between endothelial nitric oxide synthase coupling, endothelial function, and inflammation. Circulation. 2007;116:2851–9.
25. Wilcox JN, Subramanian JNR, Sundellet CL, Tracey WR, Pollock JS, Harrison DG, et al. Expression of multiple isoforms of nitric oxide synthase in normal and atherosclerotic vessels. Arterioscler Thromb Vasc Biol. 1997;17:2479–88.
26. Stuehr DJ. Mammalian nitric oxide synthases. Biochim Biophys Acta. 1999;1411:217–30.
27. Dimmeler S, Fleming I, Fisslthaler B, Hermann C, Busse R, Zeiher AM. Activation of nitric oxide synthase in endothelial cells by Akt-dependent phosphorylation. Nature. 1999;399:601–5.
28. Touyz RM, Briones AM. Reactive oxygen species and vascular biology: implications in human hypertension. Hypertens Res. 2011;34:5–14.
29. Bautista LE. Inflammation, endothelial dysfunction, and the risk of high blood pressure: epidemiologic and biological evidence. J Hum Hypertens. 2003;17:223–30.
30. Chiarugi P, Cirri P. Redox regulation of protein tyrocine phosphatases during receptor tyrocine kinase signal transduction. Trends Biochem Sci. 2003;28:509–14.
31. Briasoulis A, Tousoulis D, Androulakis ES, Papageorgiou N, Latsios G, Stefanadis C. Endothelial dysfunction and atherosclerosis: focus on novel therapeutic approaches. Recent Pat Cardiovasc Drug Discov. 2012;7:21–32.
32. Tousoulis D, Hatzis G, Papageorgiou N, Androulakis E, Bouras G, Giolis A, et al. Assessment of acute coronary syndromes: focus on novel biomarkers. Curr Med Chem. 2012;19:2572–87.
33. Srinivasan N, White HE, Emsley J, Wood SP, Pepys MB, Blundell TL. Comparative analyses of pentraxins: implications for protomer assembly and ligand binding. Structure. 1994;2:1017–27.
34. Hein TW, Singh U, Vasquez-Vivar J, Devaraj S, Kuo L, Jialal I. Human C-reactive protein induces endothelial dysfunction and uncoupling of eNOS in vivo. Atherosclerosis. 2009;206:61–8.
35. Kampoli AM, Tousoulis D, Antoniades C, Siasos G, Stefanadis C. Biomarkers of premature atherosclerosis. Trends Mol Med. 2009;15:323–32.
36. Ikeda U, Takahashi M, Shimada K. C-reactive protein directly inhibits nitric oxide production by cytokine-stimulated vascular smooth muscle cells. J Cardiovasc Pharmacol. 2003;42:607–11.
37. Venugopal SK, Devaraj S, Yuhanna I, Shaul P, Jialal I. Demonstration that C-reactive protein decreases eNOS expression and bioactivity in human aortic endothelial cells. Circulation. 2002;106:1439–41.
38. Tousoulis D, Papageorgiou N, Latsios G, Siasos G, Antoniades C, Stefanadis C. C-reactive protein and endothelial dysfunction: gazing at the coronaries. Int J Cardiol. 2011;152:1–3.
39. Kampoli AM, Tousoulis D, Briasoulis A, Latsios G, Papageorgiou N, Stefanadis C. Potential pathogenic inflammatory mechanisms of endothelial dysfunction induced by type 2 diabetes mellitus. Curr Pharm Des. 2011;17:4147–58.
40. Tabit CE, Chung WB, Hamburg NM, Vita JA. Endothelial dysfunction in diabetes mellitus: molecular mechanisms and clinical implications. Rev Endocr Metab Disord. 2010;11:61–74.
41. Tousoulis D, Androulakis E, Papageorgiou N, Briasoulis A, Siasos G, Antoniades C, et al. From atherosclerosis to acute coronary syndromes: the role of soluble CD40 ligand. Trends Cardiovasc Med. 2010;20:153–64.
42. Meigs JB, Larson MG, Fox CS, Keaney Jr JF, Vasan RS, Benjamin EJ. Association of oxidative stress, insulin resistance, and diabetes risk phenotypes: the Framingham Offspring Study. Diabetes Care. 2007;30:2529–35.
43. Cunnington C, Van Assche T, Shirodaria C, Kylintireas I, Lindsay AC, Lee JM, et al. Systemic

and vascular oxidation limits the efficacy of oral tetrahydrobiopterin treatment in patients with coronary artery disease. Circulation. 2012;125:1356–66.
44. Stam F, van Guldener C, Schalkwijk CG, ter Wee PM, Donker AJ, Stehouwer CD. Impaired renal function is associated with markers of endothelial dysfunction and increased inflammatory activity. Nephrol Dial Transplant. 2003;18:892–8.
45. Das UN, Repossi G, Dain A, Eynard AR. L-arginine, NO and asymmetrical dimethylarginine in hypertension and type 2 diabetes. Front Biosci. 2011;16:13–20.
46. Bakogiannis C, Tousoulis D, Androulakis E, Briasoulis A, Papageorgiou N, Vogiatzi G, et al. Circulating endothelial progenitor cells as biomarkers for prediction of cardiovascular outcomes. Curr Med Chem. 2012;19:2597–604.
47. Tousoulis D, Androulakis E, Papageorgiou N, Siasos G, Latsios G, Charakida M, et al. Novel biomarkers assessing endothelial dysfunction: role of microRNAs. Curr Top Med Chem. 2013;13:1518–26.
48. Marsden PA, Schappert KT, Chen HS, Flowers M, Sundell CL, Wilcox JN, et al. Molecular cloning and characterization of human endothelial nitric oxide synthase. FEBS Lett. 1992;307:287–93.
49. Guzik TJ, Black E, West NE, McDonald D, Ratnatunga C, Pillai R, et al. Relationship between the G894T polymorphism (Glu298Asp variant) in endothelial nitric oxide synthase and nitric oxide-mediated endothelial function in human atherosclerosis. Am J Med Genet. 2001;100:130–7.
50. Leeson CP, Hingorani AD, Mullen MJ, Jeerooburkhan N, Kattenhorn M, Cole TJ, et al. Glu298Asp endothelial nitric oxide synthase gene polymorphism interacts with environmental and dietary factors to influence endothelial function. Circ Res. 2002;90:1153–8.
51. McDonald DM, Alp NJ, Channon KM. Functional comparison of the endothelial nitric oxide synthase Glu298Asp polymorphic variants in human endothelial cells. Pharmacogenetics. 2004;14:831–9.
52. Antoniades C, Tousoulis D, Vasiliadou C, Pitsavos C, Toutouza M, Tentolouris C, et al. Genetic polymorphisms G894T on the eNOS gene is associated with endothelial function and vWF levels in premature myocardial infarction survivors. Int J Cardiol. 2006;107:95–100.
53. Nakayama M, Yasue H, Yoshimura M, Shimasaki Y, Kugiyama K, Ogawa H, et al. T-786—>C mutation in the 5′-flanking region of the endothelial nitric oxide synthase gene is associated with coronary spasm. Circulation. 1999;99:2864–70.
54. Cattaruzza M, Guzik TJ, Słodowski W, Pelvan A, Becker J, Halle M, et al. Shear stress insensitivity of endothelial nitric oxide synthase expression as a genetic risk factor for coronary heart disease. Circ Res. 2004;95:841–7.
55. Wang XL, Sim AS, Badenhop RF, McCredie RM, Wilcken DE. A smoking-dependent risk of coronary artery disease associated with a polymorphism of the endothelial nitric oxide synthase gene. Nat Med. 1996;2:41–5.
56. Hingorani AD. Endothelial nitric oxide synthase polymorphisms and hypertension. Curr Hypertens Rep. 2003;5:19–25.
57. Persu A, Stoenoiu MS, Messiaen T, Davila S, Robino C, El-Khattabi O, et al. Modifier effect of ENOS in autosomal dominant polycystic kidney disease. Hum Mol Genet. 2002;11:229–41.
58. Antoniades C, Shirodaria C, Van Assche T, Cunnington C, Tegeder I, Lötsch J, et al. GCH1 haplotype determines vascular and plasma biopterin availability in coronary artery disease effects on vascular superoxide production and endothelial function. J Am Coll Cardiol. 2008;52:158–65.
59. Wilson AM, Ryan MC, Boyle AJ. The novel role of C-reactive protein in cardiovascular disease: risk marker or pathogen. Int J Cardiol. 2006;106:291–7.
60. Singh U, Devaraj S, Vasquez-Vivar J, Jialal I. C-reactive protein decreases endothelial nitric oxide synthase activity via uncoupling. J Mol Cell Cardiol. 2007;43:780–91.
61. Fichtlscherer SG, Rosenberger DH, Walter S, Breuer S, Dimmeler S, Zeiher AM. Elevated C-reactive protein levels and impaired endothelial vasoreactivity in patients with coronary artery disease. Circulation. 2000;102:1000–6.
62. Hage FG, Szalai AJ. The role of C-reactive protein polymorphisms in inflammation and cardiovascular risk. Curr Atheroscler Rep. 2009;11:124–30.
63. Hage FG, Szalai AJ. C-reactive protein gene polymorphisms, C-reactive protein blood levels, and cardiovascular disease risk. J Am Coll Cardiol. 2007;50:1115–22.
64. Lawlor DA, Harbord RM, Timpson NJ, et al. The association of C-reactive protein and CRP genotype with coronary heart disease: findings from five studies with 4,610 cases amongst 18,637 participants. PLoS One. 2008;3:e3011.
65. Brull DJ, Montgomery HE, Sanders J, Dhamrait S, Luong L, Rumley A, et al. Interleukin-6 gene – 174 G>C and – 572 G>C promoter polymorphism are strong predictors of plasma interleukin-6 levels after coronary artery by-pass surgery. Arterioscler Thromb Vasc Biol. 2001;21:1458–63.
66. Humphries S, Luong L, Ogg MS, Hawe E, Miller GJ. The interelukin-6, −174G/C promoter polymorphism is associated with risk of coronary heart disease and systolic blood pressure in healthy men. Eur Heart J. 2001;22:2243–52.
67. Terry CF, Loukaci V, Green FR. Cooperative influence of genetic polymorphisms on interleukin-6 transcriptional regulation. J Biol Chem. 2000;275:18138–44.
68. Stoica AL, Stoica E, Constantinescu I, Uscatescu V, Ginghina C. Interleukin-6 and interleukin-10 gene polymorphism, endothelial dysfunction, and postoperative prognosis in patients with peripheral arterial disease. J Vasc Surg. 2010;52:103–9.
69. Ponthieux A, Lambert D, Herbeth B, Droesch S, Pfister M, Visvikis S. Association between Gly241Arg ICAM-1 gene polymorphism and serum sICAM-1 concentration in the Stanislas cohort. Eur J Hum Genet. 2003;11:679–86.

70. Motawi T, Shaker O, Taha N, Abdel Raheem M. Genetic variations in E-selectin and ICAM-1: relation to atherosclerosis. Med Sci Monit. 2012;18:CR381–9.
71. Yoshida M, Takano Y, Sasaoka T, Izumi T, Kimura A. E-selectin polymorphism associated with myocardial infarction causes enhanced leukocyte-endothelial interactions under flow conditions. Arterioscler Thromb Vasc Biol. 2003;23:783–8.
72. Vadapalli S, Rani HS, Sastry B, Nallari P. Endothelin-1 and endothelial nitric oxide polymorphisms in idiopathic pulmonary arterial hypertension. Int J Mol Epidemiol Genet. 2010;1:208–13.
73. Ezzidi I, Mtiraoui N, Chaieb M, Kacem M, Mahjoub T, Almawi WY. Diabetic retinopathy, PAI-1 4G/5G and -844G/A polymorphisms, and changes in circulating PAI-1 levels in Tunisian type 2 diabetes patients. Diabetes Metab. 2009;35:214–9.
74. Robinson SD, Ludlam CA, Boon NA, Newby DE. Tissue plasminogen activator genetic polymorphisms do not influence tissue plasminogen activator release in patients with coronary heart disease. J Thromb Haemost. 2006;4:2262–9.
75. Ray KK, Camp NJ, Bennett CE, Francis SE, Crossman DC. Genetic variation at the interleukin-1 locus is a determinant of changes in soluble endothelial factors in patients with acute coronary syndromes. Clin Sci (Lond). 2002;103:303–10.
76. Çelik A, Özçetin M, Ates O, et al. Association between C-reactive protein, endothelial nitric oxide synthase, and interleukin-6 gene polymorphisms in adolescents with a family history of premature atherosclerosis. J Am Coll Cardiol. 2013;62(18_S2):C125–6.
77. Price DT, Loscalzo J. Cellular adhesion molecules and atherogenesis. Am J Med. 1999;107:85–97.
78. Braunersreuther V, Mach F, Steffens S. The specific role of chemokines in atherosclerosis. Thromb Haemost. 2007;97:714–21.
79. Wilker EH, Alexeeff SE, Poon A, Litonjua AA, Sparrow D, Vokonas PS, et al. Candidate genes for respiratory disease associated with markers of inflammation and endothelial dysfunction in elderly men. Atherosclerosis. 2009;206:480–5.
80. Kohara K, Tabara Y, Yamamoto Y, Igase M, Nakura J, Miki T. Genotype-specific association between circulating soluble cellular adhesion molecules and carotid intima-media thickness in community residents: J-SHIPP study. Shimanami Health Promoting Program. Hypertens Res. 2002;25:31–9.
81. Hixson JE, Blangero J. Genomic searches for genes that influence atherosclerosis and its risk factors. Ann N Y Acad Sci. 2000;902:1–7.
82. Barbaux SC, Blankenberg S, Rupprecht HJ, Francomme C, Bickel C, Hafner G, et al. Association between P-selectin gene polymorphisms and soluble P-selectin levels and their relation to coronary artery disease. Arterioscler Thromb Vasc Biol. 2001;21:1668–73.
83. Reiner AP, Carlson CS, Thyagarajan B, Rieder MJ, Polak JF, Siscovick DS, et al. Soluble P-selectin, SELP polymorphisms, and atherosclerotic risk in European-American and African-African young adults: the Coronary Artery Risk Development in Young Adults (CARDIA) Study. Arterioscler Thromb Vasc Biol. 2008;28:1549–55.
84. Volcik KA, Ballantyne CM, Coresh J, Folsom AR, Wu KK, Boerwinkle E. P-selectin Thr715Pro polymorphism predicts P-selectin levels but not risk of incident coronary heart disease or ischemic stroke in a cohort of 14595 participants: the Atherosclerosis Risk in Communities Study. Atherosclerosis. 2006; 186:74–9.
85. Antoniades C, Bakogiannis C, Tousoulis D, Antonopoulos AS, Stefanadis C. The CD40/CD40 ligand system: linking inflammation with atherothrombosis. J Am Coll Cardiol. 2009;54:669–77.
86. Burdon KP, Langefeld CD, Beck SR, Wagenknecht LE, Carr JJ, Rich SS, et al. Variants of the CD40 gene but not of the CD40L gene are associated with coronary artery calcification in the Diabetes Heart Study (DHS). Am Heart J. 2006;151:706–11.

The Role of microRNAs in Cardiovascular Disease

9

Despina Sanoudou, Dimitris Tousoulis,
and Dennis V. Cokkinos

Abstract

MicroRNAs were discovered approximately two decades ago, and have dramatically changed our understanding of physiological and pathological functions since. These small (≈22 nucleotides in length) non-coding RNAs, have the ability to silence the expression of various genes either through mRNA degradation or prevention of mRNA translation to proteins.

They have been associated with cardiac development, structure and function but also with every aspect of cardiovascular disease. They can be detected in organs but also in the circulation. A constantly expanding number is shown to have diagnostic or prognostic value. Finally, they are already serving as novel therapeutic targets and/or tools, through a broad range of approaches.

Keywords

microRNAs, miRs • Cardiovascular disease • Non-coding RNAs • Nucleotides

Abbreviations

AMI	Acute myocardial infarction
APO	Apoptosis
CAD	Coronary artery disease
CD	Cell death
CLOCK	Circadian locomotor output cycles Kaput
CV	Cardiovascular development
DNA	Regions
EC	Endothelial cell
ECM	Extracellular matrix
ECs	Endothelial cells
eNOS	Oxide synthase

D. Sanoudou
Department of Pharmacology, Medical School, University of Athens and Biomedical Research Foundation of the Academy of Athens, Athens, Greece
e-mail: dsanoudou@bioacademy.gr

D. Tousoulis
1st Cardiology Unit, Department of Cardiology, 'Hippokration' Hospital, University of Athens Medical School, Athens, Greece
e-mail: drtousoulis@hotmail.com

D.V. Cokkinos, MD, FESC (✉)
Heart and Vessel Department, Biomedical Research Foundation Academy of Athens, Athens, Greece
e-mail: dcokkinos@bioacademy.gr

D.V. Cokkinos (ed.), *Introduction to Translational Cardiovascular Research*,
DOI 10.1007/978-3-319-08798-6_9, © Springer International Publishing Switzerland 2015

HYP	Hypertrophy
MiRs	MicroRNAs
MS	Metabolic syndrome
N	Necrosis
PAD	Peripheral artery disease
REM	Remodelling
ROS	Reactive oxygen species
SENSC	Senescence
TAC	Transverse aortic constriction
UTRs	3′ untranslated regions
VEGF	Vascular endothelial growth factor
VSMC	Vascular smooth muscle cell

9.1 Introduction – General Knowledge

9.1.1 What are microRNAs?

MicroRNAs (miRs) are small non-coding RNA molecules (approximately 18–25 nucleotides in size), which can bind to mRNA molecules and interfere with their stability. Specifically, mirRs are complementary to regions of the mRNA molecules, which allow their binding and can consequently affect their translation through mechanisms such as translational repression, mRNA cleavage and deadenylation. Lee et al. [1], were the first to describe this new class of molecules in 1993, in the nematode caenorhabditis elegans regulating its transition through the lower stages (miRNA lin-4). So far 2,042 miRs processed from 1,600 precursors have been reported in humans (miR base, www.Mitbase.org/index.shtml). According to Poller et al. [2], there are 1,424 separate miRNA genes in humans, while 1 % of genes are estimated to contain miRs they belong to the class of small RNAs, together with ncRNAs.

Thousands of publications have become available describing the involvement of miRs in physiological and pathological processes; large public databases have been created to store the related information and numerous bioinformatical tools have been developed to complement and expedite in vitro and in vivo research (e.g. miRBase, microRNA.org, miRWalk, TarBase, miRTarBase, miR2disease, PhenomiR, miRNA-bodymap, and more).

9.1.2 How Are microRNAs Produced? (Biogenesis)

MiRs are transcribed from a variety of DNA regions (intergenic, intronic or polycistronic) but are not translated into proteins. For example, in many cases they reside in intronic regions of mRNA-coding genes, and share their regulatory elements, whereas in some cases they are coded by independent DNA regions with their own promoters. MiRs are transcribed by RNA polymerase II. The primary transcripts of miRs, pri- miRNAs, are hairpin-shaped molecules bearing a 5′ cap and a poly (A) adenosine tail on the 3′ edge [3, 4]. While still in the cell nucleus the pri-miRNAs are processed by the microprocessor complex, which consists of Dorsha (an RNAse III enzyme) and Pasha/DGCR8 (a double-stranded-RNA-binding protein) [5, 6]. This process gives rise to the 70-nucleotide long pre-miRNA molecules. These are initially folded into imperfect stem-loop structures, and then form heterotrimers together with exportin 5 and the Ran-GTPase, which enables their export to the cytoplasm through the nuclear pores [7]. Characteristically, they do not contain introns. In the cytoplasm, the RNase III enzyme Dicer interacts with the 3′ end of the hairpin and cleaves the loop joining the 3′ and 5′ ends, leading to an imperfect miRNA duplex of approximately 22 nucleotides in length. The more unstable (thermodynamic instability and weaker base-pairing) of these two strands is then incorporated into the RNA-induced silencing complex (RISC), and called “guide strand”. The remaining strand, referred to as “passenger strand” is degraded. The RISC complex contains Dicer and many associated proteins, including members of the Argonaute protein family, which are key to RISK function [8, 9] Argonaute proteins contain conserved RNA binding domains that enable their direct interaction with the “guide strand”, and once this is integrated in the RISC complex, they orient it for interaction with a target mRNA. A number of miRs are expressed in clusters, signifying that two or three miRs are derived from a common parent mRNA. The miRs are highly conserved among species.

9.1.3 What is the Function of microRNAs?

MiRs exert their regulatory effects by binding to imperfect complementary sites within the 3′ untranslated regions (UTRs) of their mRNA targets. The formation of the double-stranded RNA, resulting from the binding of the miR, leads to gene silencing, either through the direct action of specific Argonaute proteins or through the recruitment of additional proteins. Gene silencing can be achieved either through mRNA degradation or through prevention of mRNA translation to protein. The eventual course of this process depends on the extent of complementarity between the miR and the target mRNA. Consequently, in cases of complete complementarity the mRNA molecules are degraded, whereas incomplete complementarity leads to translational repression. It should be noted, that even in the scenario of incomplete complementarity, a "seed region" of approximately 2–7 nucleotides of the miR molecule, need to be perfectly complementary to its mRNA target. Once bound to each other, translation repression can be achieved either through the inhibition of mRNA translation to protein or through the faster deadenylation of the mRNA molecules, leading to their early degradation [10]. Incomplete complementarity is the primary mode of miRs function in animals.

Less frequent functions of miRs include histone modification and DNA methylation of promoter sites which affected the expression of the target genes, as well as activation of gene expression [11, 12].

On average according to Da Costa Marins and de Windt [13], a single miRNA can affect more than 100–200 target mRNA sites by degradation or translational inhibition or deadenylation [14, 15]. It is estimated that in mammals over 1/3 of the genes are regulated by miRs.

9.2 MicroRNAs in Cardiovascular Disease

It is becoming increasingly clear that miRNAs are involved in practically every aspect of cardiovascular (CV) development and pathophysiology. Latronico et al. [16] give a very detailed review of the miRs in cardiovascular biology, which will be referred to in many points of this chapter.

9.2.1 MicroRNA Role in Cardiac Development, Differentiation and Proliferation

A number of miRs have been implicated in cardiogenesis, including: miR-1, -133, -126α, -30c, -26α, -208, -30c, –264 and let-7. miR-1-1 is first expressed in the atria, while miR-1-2 is prevalent in the ventricles. Its overexpression in transgenic mice results in thin-walled ventricles.

The miR-133 family promotes proliferation and inhibits differentiation of myoblasts, an action opposite to miR-1. However both increase in expression with cardiac development, which suggests that they may derive from a common miRNA polycistron. Lagendijk et al. [17] have found that miR-23 restricts cardiac valve and specifically endocardial cushion formation in zebra fish and mice, through inhibiting hyaluronic acid synthase.

Porello et al. [18] point out that up-regulation of the miR-15 family, especially miR-195, was 5-fold higher in the ventricles at 10 days of age as compared to day 1, in mice. These family members are upregulated postnatally in the heart, thus causing myocyte cell cycle arrest. More specifically, overexpression of miR-195 (a member of the miR-15 family) is upregulated in ventricular septal defects and cardiac myocyte hypoplasia.

Another aspect of miR function probably belonging in this entity is the regulation of the mitochondrial genome in the heart; miRs regulate the expression of ≈30 % of nuclear genome in the heart, as well as mitochondrial gene expression function and ROS generation. This can be effected by their translocation from the nucleus to the mitochondria [19].

Suárez and Sessa [20] point out that miRs are also involved in angiogenesis. They stress the importance of Dicer, the rate-limiting enzyme involved in miR maturation. Its loss leads to developmental defects which vary according to the difference status of development in

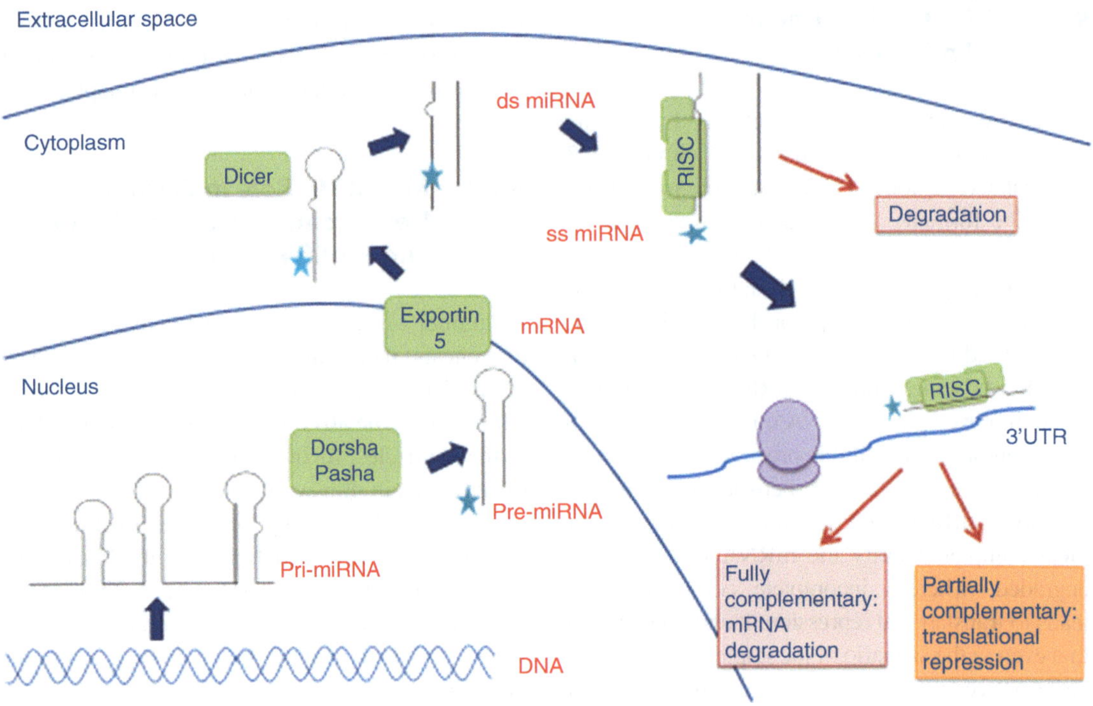

Fig. 9.1 MiR formation (From Sanoudou and Kalozoumi [24] by permission)

which Dicer is depleted. Latronico et al. [16] further point out that at angiogenesis highly co-ordinated multistep processes are required, and that Dicer K/O mice were characterized by embryonic lethality and disorganized blood vessels. According to Poliseno et al. [21] 15 highly expressed miRs have angiogenic properties in HUVECs, with miR-221 and -222 being most prominent. The interaction between miR-222 and c-Kit, the receptor of the angiogenic stem cell factor controls the ability of endothelial cells (ECS) to form new capillaries. However, they also include the following: miR-126,-130α, -210, -15 and −16, 37β, the 17–92 cluster, -296, -135. Boon [22] further describes the influence of miRNAs on the control of vascular endothelial formation through the vascular endothelial growth factor (VEGF) signalling.

Cordes and Sristava [23] also describe that miRs-1 and -133 which are derived from a common precursor transcript (bicistronic) are involved in the function of the cardiac conduction system: miR-1-2 mutant mice experienced sudden death and a spectrum of cardiac arrhythmias. They also exhibited a short PR and a prolonged QRS. In post-infarct rats, miR-1 overexpression increased arrhythmias while miR-133 represses the K + ion channels KCNQ1 and KCNH2.

The influence of miRNAs on cardiac development and specifically their involvement in the "fetal gene expression program" is described by Kalozoumi and Sanoudou [24] who differentiate between pro-and anti-hypertrophic miRs, as will be further described.

These data will be further discussed in 9.4.4. They also give a very comprehensive picture of miR action (Fig. 9.1).

9.2.2 MicroRNAs in Cardiac Hypertrophy

Numerous studies have assessed the involvement of miRs in cardiac hypertrophy (HYP). For example, van Rooj et al. [25] report the overexpression of miRs 23a and b, 24, 195, 199a and 214, and the underexpression of 150 and 181b in hypertrophic hearts. miR-208 has been shown to regulate β-MHC as a response to stress, but not during normal development. Furthermore, Cheng et al. [26] found that approximately 50 miRs were up- and 52 downregulated following TAC. According to van Roooiij et al. [27] miR-208 knockout mice had blunted HYP and fibrosis in response to transverse aortic constriction (TAC), while αMHC was increased, as well as the thyroid hormone receptor associated protein 1, together with absence of hypertrophy or fibrosis. Yang et al. [28] describe that Angiotensin II- induces hypertrophy (HYP) through miR-98/let-7 upregulation. They also point out that cyclin D2 which enhances postnatal growth is downregulated in this process.

Kalozoumi and Sanoudou (24) consider the following to be pro-hypertophic: -195, -23a, 23b, 24, 214, 211, 129, 212, 199a and b, 27b, 208a, 499, while 1 and 133 are antihypertrophic. It is interesting that 199b and 27b affect both HYP and heart failure, while 208a and 499 both HYP and arrhythmias, (also see Latronixo et al. [16]). Influences are signalled by diverse and multiple pathways enumeration of which lies outside the scope of this review.

Significant miR changes related to cardiac HYP, can also be detected in blood circulation. For example, Roncarati et al. [29] showed that in patients with hypertrophic cardiomyopathy 12 miRs were increased in the plasma; however, only miRs 199a-5p, 27a, and 29a were correlated with left ventricular (LV) hypertrophy, while only the latter was associated with both HYP and fibrosis.

9.2.3 MicroRNAs in Atherosclerosis

Extensive work has unveiled a major role of miRNAs in atherosclerosis (ATH). A brief outline on the findings relating to peripheral artery (PAD) and coronary artery disease (CAD) are presented herein.

As Papageorgiou et al. [12] and Tousoulis et al. [30] point out, miRs influence atherosclerosis through many different molecular mechanisms, including angiogenesis, vascular smooth muscle cell (VSMC) proliferation, inflammation, and apoptosis (APO), which characterize vascular plaque vulnerability.

For example, miR-92a is an endogenous repressor of the endothelial cell (EC) angiogenic program along with miR-21, 17, 221, 222 and 24. Meanwhile many miRs have been reported to affect VSMC growth and proliferation, such as the inhibitor miR-33. Inhibition of miR-26 promotes SMC differentiation miR-21 is induced by shear stress and decreases apoptosis (APO) by upregulation of endothelial nitric oxide synthase (eNOS) [12]. As regards their influence on the phenotype of VSMCs, miRs 143 and 145 are critical for maintaining their contractile phenotype. They are downregulated in "synthetic" VSMCs.

MiRs 143 and 145 can prevent vascular remodeling and restenosis. Overexpression of miR-145 leads to reduced neointima formation in balloon-injured arteries; miR-221, 222 and 21 are upregulated in neointimal lessions. Knockdown of miR-221 and 222 suppresses VSMC proliferation and neointimal lesion formation after carotid angioplasty in rats. The same is seen after downregulation of overexpressed miR-21.

Another aspect by which miRs are involved in ATH is their influence on inflammation. MiR-126 decreases VCAM-1 expression and leukocyte adhesion to EC. Consistently with these reports, miR-126 is considered a master regulator of endothelial function; it is highly enriched and actually expressed only in ECs. Its targeted deletion causes vessel leakage and hemorrhages, while its expression preserves vascular integrity by inhibiting inflammatory mediation such as VCAM-1. It also upgrades modulation of stromal cell-derived factor-1, which promotes the recruitment and mobilization of progenitor cell to the ischemic region. It has long been known that fatty meals cause an exaggerated postprandial increase of triglycerides (TGL) which is atherogenic. Sun et al. [31] describe that increased TGL and expression of the VCAM-1 receptor which promotes monocyte adherence to the endothelium, is mediated through increased miR-126 activity. Furthermore, miR-31 and miR-17-3p exert an anti-inflammatory action by regulating the TNFα induced expression of E-selectin and intercellular adhesion molecule-1 (ICAM-1) in EC [32].

The multi-faced nature of the atherosclerotic vascular involvement is further stressed by Zampetaki and Mayr [33], who point out that the metabolic derangements leading to ATH and coronary artery disease CAD are associated with miRs related to increased cholesterol synthesis but also reduced cellular cholesterol export. For example, miR-122 inhibition reduces total cholesterol (by decreasing its synthesis) and increases hepatic fatty acid oxidation; miR-122 is regulated by miR-370. Chen and Juo [34] note that it is the most abundant miR in the liver (75 % of total miR expression). Its deficiency in various strains of transgenic mice results in a $\approx$30 % reduction of total cholesterol and TGL levels. Its inhibition leads to a reduction of fatty acid liver content and synthesis.

Chen et al. [32] describe the miR-33 involvement in atherosclerosis; its inhibition increases HDL levels in African green monkeys; miR-33 also reduces fatty acid oxidation, increases intracellular TGL levels and promotes hepatic TGL synthesis. Its overexpression increases the level of hepatic bile acids. It also reduces the production of IL-1β and TNF-α, serving as an anti-inflammatory agent in macrophages. It also inhibits the activation of downstream insulin-signaling pathways. Torella et al. [35] point out that while miR-1 vascular levels are negligible, miR-133 is robustly expressed in VSMCs and has protective actions. Actually, miR-133 reduces but anti miR 133 exacerbates VSCM proliferation and migration.

Norata et al. [36] reviewed the relationship of miRs and lipoproteins. They describe that miR-33, and 122, 106, 758, 26, 370, 378, let-7, 27, 103, 107, 34α, 143, and 335 finely regulate lipid metabolism and progression and regression of ATH.

They further note that miR-33b is not conserved in rodents, which may explain some of the differences between rodent models of ATH and humans. They repeat that its inhibition leads to an increase of plasma HDL and regression of ATH, while it also increases the degradation of VLDL. Overexpression of miR-33 significantly inhibits insulin signaling. Thus, anti-miR-33 therapies may be an attractive therapeutic approach.

Importantly, circulating miRs may not act only as markers but also as effectors: LDL and HDL have been shown to transport miRs [37]. Affecting their bioavailability, and probably their contribution to immunity. In this context Wang et al. [38] have shown that repression of miR-10b promotes reverse macrophage cholesterol transport in mice.

Ma et al. [39] studied miR-155, a multifunctional miRNA that is expressed in the ECs, where it suppresses the expression of Angiotensin II type 1 receptor, a modulator of expression of inflammation. Interestingly, miR-155 is also expressed in the macrophages and atherosclerotic plaques, where it is induced by oxidized LDL. Furthermore, it seems to negatively modulate inflammation, and confer protective effects in VSMCs.

One can only marvel at this huge array of molecular players and realize the complexity of attempting atherosclerotic treatment through miRNA manipulation.

9.2.4 Action of microRNAs on Platelets

Stakos et al. [37] have written a pertinent review on this role of miRs, pointing out that human platelets express high levels of megakaryocyte-derived miRs. They mention that in 2008 it was first reported that the platelets of patients with polycythemia vera and essential thrombocythemia had a higher expression of miR26-b in their platelets. The authors further describe in detail how miRs regulate platelet function: The P2Y12 receptor plays a central role in platelet activation; miR-223 represses its gene expression; miR-200b may keep platelets in a hyporeactive state. MiR-107 targets and reduces the mRNA of the circadian locomotor output cycles Kaput (CLOCK) which regulate circadian rhythm in many species. It may be associated together with increased plasma von Willebrand factor levels with a pro-thrombotic state.

Further associations include: Platelet coagulation and wound healing are impeded by miR-17 overexpression due to fibronectin inhibition; miR-29 is associated with a decrease in fibrogen production; miR-96 decreases platelet reactivity; while miR-495 is associated with platelet hypo-reactivity to epinephrine. The angio-miRs-126, -21 and -210 appear to have a very interesting role as well. MiR-126 which is endothelial specific is also proangiogenic miRNA, which is also abundant in platelets, suggesting that platelets may communicate with ECs. miR-200b prevents platelet activation by suppressing CAMP-dependent protein kinase II-β regulation subunit gene expression in the megakaryocytes.

Zampetaki and Mayr [33] stress that platelets contain abundant quantities of small miRs, resulting into a higher miR/mRNA ratio as compared to nucleated cells. They cite miRs 223, 123, 103, let-7, 21, 107, 24 and 222.

Tousoulis et al. [30] provide a detailed list of miRs involved in the atherosclerotic process which in many ways affect various processes:

Platelet activation (17, 24, 191, 197, 223)

Nitric oxide (21, 155, 222/222, 214, 217), apoptosis (21)

Angiogenesis (28b, 130, 217, 222/222, 378)

VSCM proliferation (21, 143/145, 222/222)

Inflammation (125a/b, 221/222) adhesion molecules (17–30, 31), and

Collagen formation (133), among others.

9.3 MicroRNAs in Diabetes Mellitus

MiRNAs have been implicated in diabetes through multiple mechanisms: they contribute to insulin resistance, impaired angiogenesis, and diabetic cardiomyopathy. Shantikumar et al. [40] studied the role of miRs in diabetes and its cardiovascular complications through a variety of diabetic animal models i.e. rats, mice, rabbits, as well as humans, and in various tissues, such as skeletal and cardiac muscles, liver, adipose tissue, omentum, subcutaneous fat, ECs and retina. The following miRs were found to be upregulated: 29 family (a/b/c), 103, 125a,b, 195, 27a, 221, 222, 181a, 147, 197, 320, 503, 1, 206, 206b, 146, 155, 131, 21, 133. In contrast the following were found to be downregulated: 24,10b, 17-5p, 132, 134, 27a, 30e, 140, 155, 210, 133a, 200b.

Mortuza and Chakrabarti [41] recently also investigated the role of miRs in diabetes. They found that miR133a downregulation in chronically diabetic rat hearts was associated with SGK1 and IGF1 upregulation which induce HYP. MiR-133 however, has been described as either increased or decreased across different studies, which could be only partly explained by the diversity of conditions examined. Some points should be stressed: miR-133 is downregulated in the myocardium according to some authors but upregulated according to others. This upregulation caused a reduction of the G protein levels with resultant QT prolongation. It can also be the cause of hypertrophy in diabetic cardiomyopathy [42].

Baseler et al. [43] studied the myocardium of mice rendered diabetic after streptozotocin treatment and identified 26 upregulated miRs, notably miR-205, -141, 208b, and 200c. They comment on the role of miR-141 as a regulator of the production of ATP for the inner mitochondrial membrane.

According to Zampetaki and Mayr [33], multiple miRs are also involved in glucose homeostasis. For example, miR-375 suppresses insulin secretion, while miRs -9, -96 and -124a fine-tune insulin release. Importantly, while miR 124 promotes insulin secretion under basal conditions, it attenuates it in response to glucose stimulation. MiRs-34a and -146 induce b-cell APO, while miRs-103 and -107 are negative regulators of insulin sensitivity. The let-7 family of miRs, when blocked, promotes an insulin-sensitized state.

These authors also describe the role of miRs in glucose homeostasis. They point out that knockdown of miRNAs-24, 26, 182 and 148 in cultured b-cells or in isolated primary islets suppresses insulin promoter activity and insulin mRNA levels. Furthermore, miR-37 suppresses insulin secretion, while miRNAs-103 and -107 are negative regulators of insulin sensitivity, while miR-34α and -146 induce b-cell APO. According to the authors miR-9 is mandatory for optional secretory capacity of b-cells, while miR-96 increases granuphilin which enhances basal but inhibits K1- induced insulin secretion miRs in the metabolic syndrome (MS):

Pulakat et al. [44] focused on cardiac insulin resistance, and described how miR-143 inhibits insulin-stimulated Akt activation, while miR-122 dampens insulin signaling, consistently with aforementioned studies.

Feng et al. [45] found that let-79 and miR-221 were higher in the MS prominently in females.

9.3.1 Obesity

Obesity is a condition closely associated with diabetes. Jordan et al. [46] have shown that in this state, overexpression of miR-143 inhibits insulin-mediated Akt activation and impairs glucose metabolism. Of note, Wang et al. [47] found that let-7 and miR-221 were increased in patients with the metabolic syndrome and particularly in women.

Blumensalt et al. [48] found that Activin A which is released from epicardial adipose tissue inhibits insulin action on cardiomyocytes through the induction of miR-143 which inhibits the Akt pathway.

9.3.2 Senescence

Another aspect of ATH is endothelial senescence (SENSC). Menghini et al. [49] mention the following miRs involved in SENSC: mIR-34, -217, and -146: miR-34 is abundantly expressed in EC and increases with SENSC.

MiR-217 is preferentially expressed in aged but not in young cells.

These 2 miRs directly inhibit Sir T1 which plays a protective role in the endothelium, with eNOS as one of its main targets. SirT1 activity is also essential for maintenance of TIMP3 expression, which antagonizes MMPs. As already stated, miR-126 inhibits expression of inflammatory mediators such as VCAM1; miR-92α is an endogenous repressor of the angiogenic program in EC; its inhibition improves functional recovery in hindlimb ischemia and acute myocardial infarction. MR-21 is a negative regulator of angiogenesis miR-146α decreases with SENSC. It results into an increase of NOX4 protein, which induces the reduction of molecular oxygen to ROS in the vessel walls, further promoting SENSC.

The authors describe that on the whole miRs34a, 217 and 92a promote while miRs126 and 146a inhibit SENSC and ATH.

Dimmeler and Nicotera [50] note an age induced increase in vascular miR-29, 34α, 146, 217. They also note that in cardiac tissue miR-21 is increased, together with 22 and 24, and 18 and 19 are decreased in age-induced fibrosis.

Finally, Olivieri et al. [51] describe that circulating inflammatory miRs in age-related diseases are related to diabetes mellitus, cardiovascular disease and Alzheimer's disease.

9.4 Coronary Artery Disease

Tousoulis et al. [30] and Papageorgiou et al. [52] give an account of miRs involved in stable coronary artery disease (CAD). They point out that miR-126, -17, 92a and 155 (which is associated with inflammation) are downregulated in CAD. MiR-126 was found to be intensely related to LDL cholesterol by Sun et al. [53] who however did not find differences in its levels between patients with CAD and controls.

Fichtlscherer et al. [54] in a small group of eight patients with stable CAD versus 8 controls found 46 significantly downregulated and 20 upregulated miRs. They further analyze their findings in a larger numbers of patients. The circulating levels of endothelial-expressed miRs 126, 92a and 17 were significantly reduced, as well as the vascular smooth muscle enriched miR-145 and the inflammatory miR-155. A trend towards an increase of cardiac-muscle enriched miR-208a and -133a was seen.

Van Aelst and Heymans [55] cite the following miRs as biomarkers for asymptomatic CAD, as regards the serum levels:

<u>Increased:</u> 133a, 135a. 134. 370, 140, 140-3p, 182, 92a,b.

<u>Decreased</u>: 126, 17. 92a, 199a, 155, 145, 24, 21, 206, 15a, 191, 197, 223, 320, 486.

They remark that miR1 and 133a are abundantly expressed cardiac miRs as well as miR208a/b which are derived from the introns of a- and β-MHC. Further associations are beyond the scope of this review.

Zhu and Fan [56] point out that the reduced concentration of circulating vascular miRs detected in patients with CAD may seem paradoximal but it could be due to an increased uptake of circulating miRs into the widely disturbed atherosclerotic lessons.

Concerning the prognostic role of microRNAs we cannot conclude as the prospective studies are limited. Zampetaki et al. [57] based on the Brunech cohort of 820 participants followed up for 10 years concluded that 3 miRNAs were consistently and significantly related to incident myocardial infarction: miR-126 showed a positive association, whereas miR-223 and miR-197 were inversely associated with disease risk [pmid 22813605].

9.4.1 Acute Myocardial Infarction (AMI)

The main and most dramatic manifestation of CAD is the emergence of a severe acute myocardial infarction (AMI). A large number of miRs have been associated with AMI during the last year.

Fiedler and Thum [58] in a very recent review point out the following in rat models:

miR-1 is overexpressed in ischemic myocardium. Its role in heart failure (HF) will be discussed later.

miR-15 is upregulated in the infarct and border zone in rat and porcine models of AMI.

miR-24 is increased in EC at hypoxia and cardiac ischemia; this miR is also pro-apoptotic.

miR-29 is highly abundant in fibroblasts. Its role in post-AMI cardiac remodelling (REM) will be discussed later.

miR-29a is increased in hindlimb ischemic and AMI, and is antiangiogenic.

miR-101 is chronically downregulated in this peri-infarct zone,

miR-126 is involved in endothelial function and integrity.

miR-214 is upregulated in HF.

As the aforementioned authors imply, most of these miRs can constitute therapeutic targets in AMI.

9.4.1.1 Circulating microRNAs in AMI

An important role has also been described for circulating miRs, which could serve as novel biomarker in acute coronary syndromes (ACS). For example, Pleister et al. in a detailed review [59] site the increased miRs: 1,133, 133a, 208a and b, 499-5p, 499, 122, 126, as well as the decreased: 122, 375, 663b, and 1291. It is postulated that these miRs originate mainly from the injured myocardium.

In the already mentioned review of Van Aelst and Heymans [55], the following miRs are cited in acute coronary syndromes (ACS):

Increased: miR1, 133a and b, 499-5p, 208b, 328, 21.

Decreased: miR122, 375, 126.

Nabialek et al. [60] studied three miRs (425-5p, 208a and 1) in AMI and stable CAD. They found an early (<6 h) increase of miR-423-p, normalizing at 6 h.

In stable CAD pts there were no differences.

Several studies have also aimed at identifying circulating miRs that could serve as biomarkers of AMI. Among the different miRs that have been proposed as promising in that respect are miR-1, -133a, -208a, -208b, -499 and -499-5p, which appear significantly changed predominantly during the first few hours post AMI [61]. Serum levels of miR-1 have been associated with infarct size.

Also, Olivieri et al. [62] found that miR-499-5p increased 80-fold in non-ST elevation myocardial infarction; its diagnostic value was higher than hs and classical cTnT.

Importantly miR-208a which is encoded by an intron of the aMHC gene is the only heart-specific miR, while miR-499,1 and 133 are also expressed in skeletal muscle.

Presumably the same miR profile could emerge in myocardial injury after a precutaneous coronary intervention (PCI). However, few studies on this subject exist. Recently Yu et al. [63] found that miR-126 after PCI was associated with a worse prognosis in patients under dual antiplatelet treatment, up to 1 year. D' Alessandra et al. [64] gave a detailed review. In patients with coronary reperfusion after PCI they found increases in miR1, 133a and b, 499-5p, while miR-122 and 375 were decreased. Their patients with thrombolysis were too few for meaningful comments.

Jaguszewski et al. [65] very recently found that a unique signature comprising miR-1, -16, -26a and 133a differentiated Takotsubo cardiomyopathy from healthy subjects and from patients with AMI.

They also found a correlation with pressure and duration of balloon inflation and consider it as a new target of presentation and treatment of endothelial dysfunction. Polimeni et al. [66] give a recent review in this subject. They describe how miRs regulate VSMCs and ECs after vascular injury. The former are responsible for in-stent restenosis. They describe many miRs affecting VSMC regulating either the pro-contractile (1, 133a, 143, 145), and the pro-synthetic phenotype (26a, 31, 146a, 221, 24 222). MiR21 can be either pro-contractile or prosynthetic. They also describe miRs implicated in various ways in EC function, including 126, 217, 17-as, 17–50, 18a, 19a, 20a, 92a, 221/222 and 663. All these can be the target of future therapeutic interventions.

Lu et al. [67] comment on another aspect: they observed that miR-1 overexpression in ischemic myocardium was reversed by propranolol which also had beneficial cardiac effects. This was likely achieved through the inhibition of the β-adrenoreceptor-CANP-protein, kinase A signaling pathway by propranolol, which could regulate miR-1 expression.

9.4.1.2 Prognostic Value of microRNAs After an Acute Myocardial Infarction

Eitel et al. [68] assessed the relation between miR-133a myocardial damage by CMR and prognosis at 6 months, in 216 consecutive patients. They found a significant correlation of infarct size, microvascular obstruction, and myocardial salvage index with miR133a, however its concentrations could not independently predict clinical events.

Matsumoto et al. [69] attempted to identify circulating miRs as predictors of CHF in post-MI patients. They collected sera ~18 days after MI onset, in 21 patients followed for 1 year. The levels of 3 miRs which are p53 responsive miRs, 192, 194 and 349 were upregulated.

In a similar context, miR146a was upregulated and miR-150 and -155 were downregulated in post-MI ventricular rupture; these miRs are involved in innate immunity [70].

Further considerations on these associations will be given when heart failure is discussed.

9.4.2 MicroRNAs in Cell Death

The work of Matsumoto et al. [69] has been already mentioned.

The tumor suppressor p53 is an inducer of the APO pathways, partly through the co-ordinated induction of multiple miRs expression.

According to Hullinger et al. [71], the miR-15 family is increased in the heart within 24 h after I/R. Its inhibition reduced cardiomyocyte cell death and improved mitochondrial function, since this family targets Bcl-2 and the mitochondrial protective protein ADP-ribosylation factor like 2.

Inhibition of the pro-apoptotic miR-34 family, which targets SIRT1, had the same effects.

According to Aurora et al. [72] miR-214 protects the mouse heart from I/R injury by controlling Ca^{2+} overload by repression of the mRNA encoding the sodium/calcium exchanger 1, a key regulator of Ca^{2+} influx.

Orogo and Gustafsson [73] describe the following associations between miRs and cell death (CD): miR-21, 199α, 210 and 494 promote cardiomyocyte survival during ischemia. miR-1 reduces the anti-apoptotic Bcl-2, while miR-214 deletion increases apoptosis after I/R.

In cell loss, miR-1 and miR-133 have opposing roles, the former promoting it through increased APO through HSP60 and 70 suppression, which the latter decreased APO by decreasing caspase-9 protein levels and activity.

Ruan et al. [74] suggest that miR-23α may be involved in TNF-α induced EC APO through the caspase -7 and 3 pathway activation.

Li et al. [75] have found that miR-150 aggravates H_2O_2 induced apoptosis in cultured rat cardiomyopathies.

Fu et al. [76] found that let-7 is involved doxorubicin induced myocardial injury.

Also acute doxorubicin apoptosis was associated with miR-146α induced inhibition of the neuregulin-ErbB pathway [77].

9.4.3 Heart Failure and microRNAs

Many miRs have been investigated in CHF. One of the main causes of heart failure is post-MI remodelling (REM) which has already been discussed.

van Rooij et al. [78] stress that miR-92α increases early after AMI; its inhibition increases capillary density and improves cardiac function. miR-24 has intriguing actions; it inhibits angiogenesis but it also attenuates infarct size. miRr-29 which is repressed after aortic banding and reduced after AMI since it is antifibrotic, its downregulation in the border zone would promote fibrosis. miR-21 blocking by antagonists prevents cardiac fibrosis. However, it also has an antiapoptotic action and decreases infarct size. miR-101 is profibrotic; It is downregulated after MI. Its forced overexpression inhibited proliferation of cardiac fibroblast and reduced collagen production [79].

Zile et al. [80] first reported that miR29a early post-MI was associated with left ventricular end-diastolic volume at 3 months.

Many additional studies have been devoted to the subject. Devaux et al. [81] noted that miR-150 is a marker for REM.

Divakaran and Mann [82] also describe in depth the role of miRs in REM. They point out an important fact which will explain many of the data to be referred to, that miR-1, let7, miR26a, 30c, 126-3p and 133 are the more highly expressed in the human heart.

They further describe the following associations as regards.

9.4.3.1 Myocyte Hypertrophy

The subject has already been described in Sect. 9.2.2.

Reduced expression of miR-1 and 133 has been found in hypertrophic hearts [24]. The authors comment on the controversial findings as regards miR-21: this miR is upregulated post transverse aortic banding, and increased by the well-known hypertrophy induce, Angiotensin II and phenylephrine; however they also refer to studies in which antisense knock down of miR-21 actually provoked hypertrophy and increased fetal gene expression.

As regards the occurrence of CHF which is the eventual outcome of REM, it is –as already stated in Chaps. 16, 17 of this book, characterized by cardiomyocyte loss mostly through Apoptosis (APO) and Necrosis (N), and changes in the composition of the extracellular matrix (ECM).

An important step in the process towards REM is the inability of angiogenesis to cope with the ensuing hypertrophy. A number of pro- and anti-angiogenic miRs have been found. As already stated, miR-126 knockdown resulted in loss of vascular integrity; this miR also enhances the pro-angiogenic actions of VEGF and FGF [56]. Importantly however, the authors point out that miR126 is increased in the failing human hearts.

As regards to the increase in fibrotic tissue through ECM proliferation, van Rooij et al. pointed out that miR-208 is required for cardiac fibrosis [78].

Topkara and Mann [83], analyzing the role of miRs in cardiac REM and CHF also point out the role of miR-1 as a negative regulator of hypertrophy; miR-133 is down-regulated in many hypertrophy models, while its adenoviral overexpression attenuates hypertrophic growth. However, they point out that transient versus long-term suppression of its expression may have different effects. They also try to elucidate the role of miR-21, repeating that it is up-regulated in the failing myocardium, while its role in cardiac hypertrophy is not convincingly proven, while its antiapoptotic and pro-survival activity is discussed. The authors also describe the role of miR-199a in inducing hypertrophy, while its downregulation leads to hypoxic cell death through up-regulation of the hypoxia inducible factor 1-a (HIF-1a) which stabilizes the pro-apoptotic factor p53.

MiR-320 leads to APO-induced CD, while its knockdown by an antagonist leads to reduction of I/R injury. As regards the upregulation of fibrosis, the authors stress the role of miR-21, which increases fibroblast survival and fibrosis; it is upregulated in the border zone of post-Mi hearts, which is characterized by increased fibrosis compared to the remote region.

miR-29 is also downregulated in the border zone, thus promoting collagen deposition. They also point out the already discussed anti fibrotic effect of miR-133a.

miR-208a is also necessary for the development of fibrosis. A detailed review was given 2 years ago by Zhu and Fan [56].

They connect to a large extent the protection against I/R injury to the size of the infarct, which as stressed elsewhere in this book, determines to a large extent the course towards cardiac REM.

They stress the results of many investigations, mainly in rodent I/R models, and the increase of miR-133a at I/R in the rat, while in the human they are both down-regulated.

According to these authors miR-21 has controversial effects on REM; the same holds true for miR-29 and -24, while miR-126, -210, -494 and -499 have protective effects.

They additionally describe the protective effects of the following miRs:

miR-126 as a pro-angiogenic factor; It also upregulates the homing ability of endothelial progenitor cells and to promote myocardial regeneration. Its upregulation decreases REM.

miR-210 is also pro-angiogenic, and anti-apoptotic; as will be discussed further, it mediates ischemic pre-conditioning.

Hu et al. [84] showed that it directly increases myocyte survival and decreases REM.

The most recent detailed review on cardiac REM and HF is given by Kumarswamy and Thum [85].

They underline that the following miRs contribute to $\approx 90\ \%$ of total cardiac miRs in order of abundance: 1/206, let 7/98, 30, 29, 26, 378, 143, 24, 133 etc.

These authors also provide a list of "good" and "bad" cardiac-influencing miRs, as follows:

Protective miRs: 1, 101, 133, 142, 144/41, 145, 17, 18, 19, 210, 214, 30, 494, 9.

Detrimental miRs: 132/212, 141. 199b, 208, 21, 22, 221, 23, 24. 34, 350, 98/let-7.

They Provide the Following Data on Cardiac Hypertrophy, HF and REM

miR-208 is important for cardiac hypertrophy; specifically miR-208a is sufficient to induce cardiac REM and β-MHC expression. They cite the work of Sayed et al. [86], who found miR-1 downregulation in pressure-overload cardiac hypertrophy. This miR probably plays a protective role against HF emergence; It is also restored after adenoviral SERCA-2 gene therapy [87].

miR-1 also targets the Na^{+} –Ca^{2+} exchanger. miR-214 protects against I/R injury through the repression of this exchanger.

The action of miR-499 are somewhat contradictory and at this stage beyond the scope of this review.

The authors also describe the important action of non-cardiomyocyte specific miRs. As already noted in the Chap. 17 on cardiac REM in this book, fibrosis is a hallmark of REM. In this context, miR-21 promotes, and its antagonism inhibits, fibrosis.

Importantly, transforming growth factor-β which is profibrotic, upregulates miR-21.

miR-12b is highly abundant in EC already described. Its loss may be construed to limit neovascularization in HF. Conversely, it suppresses angiogenesis. Also, miR-24 induces EC apoptosis and inhibits capillary network formation. MiR-23α is prohypertrophic and is actually transactivated by the prohypertrophic NFATC 3; this also transactivates miR-199b which is upregulated in HF. Moreover, deletion of miR-22 accelerates the progression to cardiac dysfunction through a reduction of SERCA2a transporting activity.

A very interesting finding was recently reported in an uncommon but serious cause of HF, peripartum cardiomyopathy. Haghikia et al. [88] found an increase of serum levels of cathepsin-D, an enzyme induced by oxidative stress with proapoptotic properties which generates 16 k Da Prolactin whose target, miR-146α, is also increased in the serum. This is an antiangiogenic miR located in EC; after its release it is absorbed by cardiomyocytes, where it changes their metabolic profile.

Its increase in the serum as a result of an increase of endothelial microparticles. The upregulation of 146a has been discussed.

Papageorgiou et al. [12] describe the utility of miRs in the diagnosis and classification of the HF. Thus, Schipper et al. [89] studied 17 consecutive patients with end-stage heart failure. They found a decrease in miRs-1, 133α 133β, 208; LVAD support led to partial restoration of this expression.

In another paradigm of HF, doxorubicin cardiotoxicity, Vacchi-Suzzi et al. [90] found that it upregulates miRs 208b, 216b, 215, 34c and 367 in rat hearts in their course towards REM.

9.4.4 MicroRNAs in Arrhythmias-Conduction Defects

The work of Cordes and Srivastava [23] has already been discussed in 9.2.1.

The more frequent arrhythmia is Atrial Fibrillation (AF).

Wang et al. [91] discuss in a detailed review that miR-133a/b/c, -26a/b -let 7a/b/c/f/g, -24, -125 a/b, -27a/b, -126, -23a/b, -29 a/b, -12, -21, -92, and -100, are the more abundantly expressed in the myocardium. They then describe that AF has a multifunctional causative etiology: Ionic remodelling, structural remodelling, abnormalities of intracellular Ca^{2+} homeostasis, and enhanced spontaneous activity – which implicate multiple miRNAs at multiple levels.

<u>miR-1</u> has arrhythmogenic potential.

<u>miR-26</u> upregulates I_{K1}; it is downregulated in AF. An increase in I_{K1}(inward rectifier K^+ current) leads to a shortening of atrial action potential (APD) duration creating the substrate for AF.

<u>miR-328</u> is upregulated in AF. It enhances vulnerability to AF, diminishes I Cal (L-type Ca^{2+} currents) in the left atrium and this shortens atrial APD.

<u>miR-133</u> is upregulated in diabetic hearts and is associated with QT prolongation. It depresses Ikr. It prolongs APD. Its downregulation in AF would be expected to shorten APD.

9.4.4.1 Influence on Apoptosis and Fibrosis in the Genesis of Atrial Fibrillation

Down-regulation of the antifibrotic miR-133 and miR-590 also favors AF through production of atrial structural remodeling. Interestingly they are also downregulated by nicotine [91]. These authors also postulated that other miRs may have a potential role, through their action on fibrogenesis. Thus, miR-208 and -21 are characterized as pro- and miR-29, -30 (and-133, -590, as already mentioned) as anti-fibrotic. In this sense they may affect vulnerability to AF.

Another mechanism is induction of apoptotic cell death, the pro-apoptotic miR-1 and the anti-apoptotic miR-133 could be direct contributors to this pathogenetic phase.

Also, miR-29, -320 are considered to be pro- and -21 and -199α anti-apoptotic. However, Wang et al. [91] stress that the role of these miRs in AF is not proven.

Liu et al. [92] have examined the levels of various miRs in the plasma in AF. They found reduced levels or miR150, which interestingly had an inverse relationship with CRP.

Kim [93] gives a review on the role of miRs in arrhythmias and cardiac conduction;

He shows the action of various miRs on the APD. He cites the work of Zhao et al. [94] who showed that deletion of miR-1-2 caused conduction blocks in mice. Also they note that an increase in miR-1 in ischemic hearts was accompanied by arrhythmogenesis.

Overexpression of this miR resulted in QRS prolongation. QT prolongation is associated with increased miR-133 and miR-1.

Atrioventricular conduction slowing is seen in miR-208α knockdown mice; this miR is required for Connexin 40 expression; miR-1 reduces Connexin 43 protein levels.

miR-1 enhances cardiac excitation-contraction coupling by selectively increasing the L-type Ry R2 channels and is associated with development of arrhythmia [95].

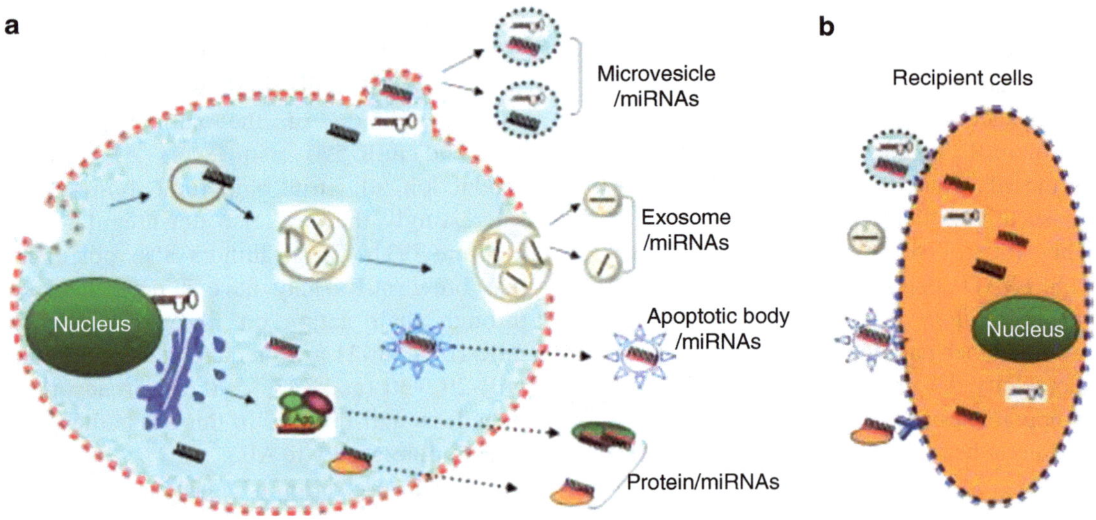

Fig. 9.2 Cellular releases (**a**) and uptake (**b**) of miRNAs. (**a**) Extracellular miRNAs may be contained within vesicles, including microvesicles, exosomes, and apoptotic bodies, as well as within proteins such as Ago2, HDL, and other RNA-binding proteins. (**b**) Extracellular miRNAs may potentially interact with recipient cells via direct fusion, internalization, receptor-mediated interactions and other possible mechanisms (From Zhu and Fan [56] by permission)

9.4.5 MicroRNAs in the Blood Circulation

A constantly expanding subject is the number of miRs detected in the periphery with new miRs being added every month. Many authors have provided lists of miRs to be found either in plasma, serum, peripheral mononuclear cells, and whole blood. Their content in the platelets has already been described [37]. Four recent reviews are very inclusive [56, 96–98]

According to Kinet et al. [96] miRs are unexpectedly stable, since naked RNA is readily targeted by exonucleases expressed in various body fluids. To achieve this protection, miRs are packaged in microparticles, such as exosomes microvesicles, and apoptotic bodies. They are also protected through their association with RNA binding proteins such as Argonaute 2 or nucleophosmin and also are bound by HDL. Microvesicles are produced from many cells including epithelial endothelial and tumour cells. They are also called microparticles or ectosomes.

These are shown in Fig. 9.2

They are also expressed in urine, milk, saliva, and sperm.

According to Zhu and Fan [56] released miRs by exosomes do not reflect their abundance in the cell of organ. Their assumption and that of Stakos et al. [37] should not be overlooked: That low levels of some miRs in the circulation may reflect their increased uptake into vascular lesions. Moreover, they point out that whether miRs are actively secreted outside cardiomyopathies remains obscure.

Exosomes are small exfoliated membrane microvesicles 40–120 nm, released from multivesicular bodies, produced by many and diverse cells.

Microvesicles are shed from budding of vesicles from the plasma membrane of many cells, 0.1–1 μm in size. Presumably, they may be formed by an apoptotic process as are the Apoptotic bodies or blebs already described in the Chap. 15 on Cell Death. Interestingly, endothelial cell-derived apoptotic bodies not only do not trigger innate immunity but actually may, through miR-126 limit atherosclerosis. Their size is 1–5 μm or 0.5–2 μm and their shape heterogenous average size of 8–12 μm [96].

As already stated, miRs are also joined to RNA proteins (nucleophosmin) to protect them from degradation and to proteins of the Argonaute family, and lipoprotein (mostly HDL) complexes.

Importantly when miRs become extracellular, they can effect extracellular cell-to-cell

Table 9.1 Circulating miRs in various conditions

Condition	miRNAs involved Increased	Decreased
Acute myocardial infarction	1,133a, 208a, 126, 30a, 409,499-5p, 145, 30c, 195, let 7-b, 328, 21, 155 (indication for AICD placement)	92, 122, 375, 126
Atherosclerosis[a]	130a, 27b, 210, 135a	155 (?) 147
Stable coronary artery disease	133, 135a, 134, 370, 92a,b 140-3p, 370, 92a,b, 208a, 140, 182,135, 499, 21, 146	126, 92a, 155, 145, 147, 17, 199a, 24, 21, 206, 15a, 191, 197,223, 320, 486
Heart failure	423-5p18b, 129-5p, 622, 654-3p, 499, 122, 126, 124-5p (DCM)	142-3p DCM
Diastolic dysfunction	1,246	454, 500
Stroke	210, 215, 324, -3p, 422, 451, 134	
Hypertension	296-5p, let-7e	
Diabetes mellitus	28-3p	126, 15a, 29b, 223, 21, 24, 20b, 15a, 191, 197, 223, 320, 486
Peripartum cardiomyopathy	146a	
HOCM	229, 27a, 199a-5p	
Atrial fibrillation		150
Metabolic syndrome	let 7, 221	

Circulating microRNAs in various pathological conditions
Compiled from References: [25, 30, 31, 34, 35, 39, 40, 47, 51, 53–65, 87, 88, 92, 96–98]
[a]Findings in this entity overlap with those in coronary artery disease and diabetes mellitus

communication. As Kinet et al. [96] point out, three paradigms of cell-to-cell communication are effected by miRs:

Shear-stress induces the expression of miR143/145 from endothelial cells and through vesicles they gather into smooth muscle cells to induce an atheroprotective phenotype.

It should be realized that the majority of miRs detectable in serum are concentrated in the exosomes.

In both reviews, miRs are described as mediators of cell to cell RNA communication.

Creemers et al. [97] point out the prospect that miRs are secreted from one cell and taken up by a distant cell to regulate its gene expression. They also describe various ways in which miRs are released from the cells; according to their intracellular level, selectively retained, or selectively released.

The latter is true for pre-miRs. These mechanisms are described in Fig. 9.2.

The exact percentage of miRs circulating in a free or bound form is discussed by Creemers et al. [97] who stress the importance of miR binding with the Argonaute proteins. Further description of the ways in which miRs accomplish cell-to-cell communication are beyond the scope of this chapter, especially as it is a constantly expanding field. A compilation of many studies is given in Table 9.1. As many authors have pointed out it should be taken into account, that there may be differences in plasma with EDTA and serum.

9.5 Cardiovascular Therapeutics and microRNAs

As early as 2008 van Rooij et al. [99] discussed this aspect.

They point out that miR modulation as a therapeutic approach can be affected by two distinct processes:

1. Reduction of the levels of pathogenic or aberrantly expressed miRs, with activation of a gene expression as a result.
2. miR mimics can elevate miR levels, with resultant gene expression suppression.

They also cite some early results:

(a) miR-122 inhibition led to serum cholesterol reduction.
(b) Cardiac miR-133 inhibition induced cardiac hypertrophy with fetal gene expression. This would not be expected to be beneficial.
(c) miR-29 inhibition was antifibrotic.

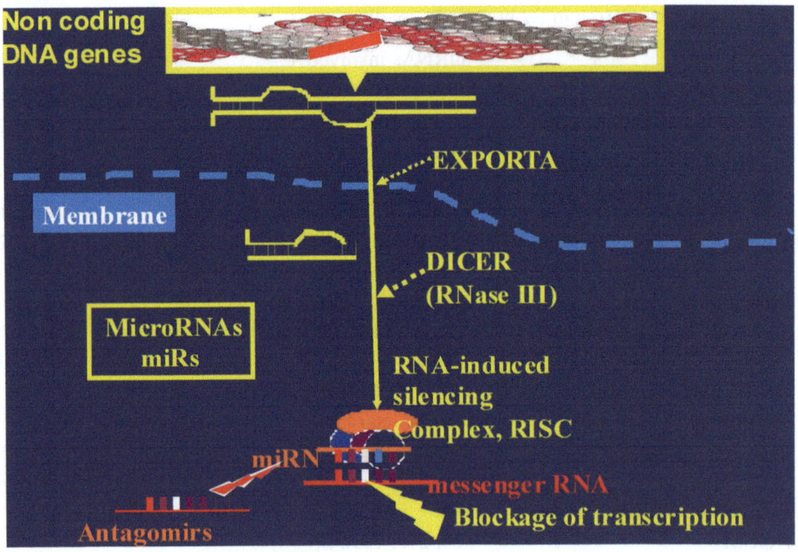

Fig. 9.3 Blocking of miR action by Antagomirs (Courtesy of Bernard Swynghedauw)

Very detailed reviews have been given by Chistiakov et al. [100] and Caroli et al. [101].

9.5.1 Antisense Oligonucleotides

As already stated they are considered for diseases caused by an upregulated miRNA.

These are small synthetic RNAs which are complementary to the specific miR target.

To increase stability and efficiency an antisense oligonucleotide can be modified by many approaches, such as modification with the 2-0-methyl-group (OMe antagomiRs) or with 2-0- methyloxyethyl groups; (MOE); the latter have stronger affinity and specificity to RNAs; characteristically cholesterol constructs are linked to an antagomir to enhance cellular uptake. Also longer antagomirs exhibit more profound miR repression. Stakos et al. [37] describe how HDL and LDL lipoproteins transport miRs in the human blood. This mechanism is presented in Fig. 9.3.

Another type of molecules is the locked nucleic acids, which have greater stability and affinity for binding to target miRs. They are resistant to degradation when given systemically and thus longer half-lines according to Topkara and Mann [83].

Another technique which is gaining ground is the use of miRNA "sponges" or "decoys". "Sponges" are constructed with inserted miR binding sites. The sponge technique can better inhibit functional classes of miRs than the antagomirs [100, 101].

Also miR decoy constructs have been generated, causing miR degradation.

Van Rooij et al. [99], Chistiakov et al. [100] and Caroli et al. [101] enumerate some of the preclinical and clinical applications of miRs, offering the following examples from mouse model studies:

Treatment of cholesterol (miR-122).

Increase of HDL, decrease of VLDL triglycerides (miR33a/b).

Increase of macrophage cholesterol efflux (miR-758).

Decrease of cardiac hypertrophy (miR-133).

Improvement of cardiac function, reduction of fibrosis (miR-21, miR-199b). Increase of angiogenesis (miR-92α, miR-24).

Reduction in infarct size (miR-320).

Abrogation of atrial fibrillation (miR-328).

Prevention of aortic dilatation (miR-29).

Caroli et al. [101] describe the therapeutic possibilities of miRs in ischemic heart disease. They consider a potential therapeutic advantage of miRs, that they target multiple genes involved in the same pathway. The problems that this may generate are evident. However, they also state that miRs have a specific and defined target on the disease mechanisms, and the effects of interventions on miRs are long-lasting.

However, multiple gene affection may have unexpected effects.

Apart from the effects described by Chistiakov et al. [100], the authors describe some additional actions:

Thus, miR-101 has antifibrotic action, miR-599 increases cardiomyocyte proliferation.

Hinkel et al. [102] have recently (LNA-transfer) reported that miR92α inhibition protected against experimental I/R in pigs.

Halkein et al. [103] showed that miR146α inhibition with LNA or antagomirs attenuated peripartum cardiomyopathy in mice.

Also very recently, Wahlquinst et al. [104] showed that inhibition of miR-25 by an antagomir markedly halted established HF in a mouse model; mir-25 delays calcium uptake kinetics in cardiomyocytes by interacting with SERCA 2α and is upregulated in HF.

Quatrocelli et al. [105] found that adeno-associated viral intraventricular delivery of miR-669α alleviated chronic DCM in dystrophic mice.

9.5.2 MicroRNA Mimics

They are to be used in conditions where a decreased miR is the cause of a disease or with the purpose of antagonizing the function of adversely upregulated miRs. Increases of miR levels can be effected by employing a synthetic RNA duplex in which one strand is identical to the native double –stranded mature miRs.

A main consideration is that, as mentioned in the beginning of this chapter miRs have numerous targets and one single miR can affect many processes.

9.5.2.1 Delivery Techniques

According to van Rooij et al. [99] and Chistiakov et al. [100] the following are some of the delivery techniques:

Viral-based using mostly adenoviral or lentiviral-based vectors.

Nanocarriers Nanoparticles of sub-100-nm scale achieve highly effective delivery.

Aptamers are molecules that bind to specific molecules: Exosomes/microvesicles and apoptotic bodies. This is not yet achievable technically.

Lipid nanoparticles have been developed to decrease the effective needed dose of oligonucleotides. These novel techniques are considered to be 30–100 times more efficient than typical lipid-based delivery carriers [100]. Novel developments include encapsulating nucleic acids in lipid-forming vesicles ranging from 50 to 500 nm in size.

One major problem of miR therapy is the method of delivery, so that the oligonucleotides can enter the cells. Up to now, as van Rooij et al. [98] point out efficient delivery has been shown to be achieved only in the liver.

Efficient delivery to the heart still remains a problem.

9.5.3 Non-microRNA Therapy Affecting miR Levels

Caroli et al. [101] also described that non-miR therapeutic interventions can affect miRs:

Thus, bone marrow mononuclear cell therapy in AMI blocks cardiomyocyte apoptosis through a paracrine regulation of miR-34α according to Iekushi et al. [106].

A parallel finding has been reported by Kumarswamy et al. [87] who found that SERCA-2 gene therapy restored miR-1 in HF.

Also the hypolipidemic drug ezetimibe inhibits monocyte to macrophage differentiation through downregulation of miRs-155, -233, -424 and -503. These actions should be assessed further [107].

The action of propranolol on miR-1 has already been discussed [67].

Another example of a drug regulating miR activation is given by Ye et al. [108] who found that pioglitazone, a PPAR-γ agonist diminishes miR 29a/c levels in rat hearts, while both pioglitazone and rosiglitazone did the same in Hg, 2 cells. Down regulation of miR-29 by an antistase inhibitor or PIO protected H9 c2.

Another non-pharmacologic therapeutic intervention is exercise Ntanasis-Stathopoulos et al. [109] gave a recent review.

They report that in the plasma miR-21 and -221 are altered by exhaustive exercises, miR-20α, by sustained aerobic exercise training, and miR-146α and -222 by both types of exercise. Also, miR 126 increases after endurance exercise.

Also, very recently, Mooren et al. [110] measured circulating miRs in the plasm of 14 individuals after a marathon run. The strongest increase was that of miR206; miRs 1-333, 206, 499 and 208β were increased. Interestingly miR-1, 133α and 206 correlated to aerobic performance parameters. Also, none of these miRs correlated with troponins and NT-proBNP.

9.5.4 Ischemic Preconditioning

A phenomenon which protects against various types of cardiac injury is preconditioning its association with various miRs has been studied.

Yin et al. [111] have shown that in the late preconditioning (PC) miR-1, -21 and -24 were significantly increased together with an increase in eNOS, both mRNA and protein. Additionally, these researchers injected miRs derived from preconditioning hearts with a protective phenotype as a result.

Rane et al. [112] found that miR-199α is acutely downregulated in cardiac myocytes during hypoxia. This decline is required according to the authors for the upregulation of the hypoxia-inducible factor –H1F1α, which stabilizes PI3. Knockdown of miR-199α, induces upregulation of Hif-1α and Sirtuin 1, reproducing PC.

Cheng et al. [113] found that ischemic IPC upregulates miR-21 which acts against APO.

Salloum et al. [114] found that miR-1, miR-133, miR-21, miR-126, miR-320, miR-92a, and miR-199a, are regulated after PC. These miRs also drive the synthesis of heat shock protein (HSP)-70, eNOs, inducible nitric oxide synthase, HSP-20, Sirt1, and hypoxia-inducible factor 1a.

9.5.5 Stem Cell Therapy

Another cardioreparative intervention is stem cell therapy: Seeger et al. [115] very recently demonstrated that many miRs influence the fate of these cells.

Specifically, improvement of cell survival and function is effected by miR-123; this miR is also released acting in a paracrine manner, together with miR-296, demonstrating a pro-angiogenic action. Conversely miR-34α which is increased by aging, adversely affects functional capacity and survival of cells. It has also been found that a "cocktail" of miRs-21, -24 and -221 improved cell engraftment and survival.

Also, many miRs affected in the migration of cells miR-150 and 146 enhance homing of cells into ischemic tissues. In contrast, miR-15α -16 inhibit the migratory potential of proangiogenic cells.

Seeger et al. [115] differentiate into the following miRs actions involved in the post-infarct myocardium.

Cell death	: miR15, 24, 34, 24
Fibrosis	: miR21, 29, 101
CMC Proliferation	: miR-15.195, 199, 510
Angiogenesis	: miR-15, 24, 12a
Cardiac reprogramming	: miR-1, 208, 499

Throhatou et al. [116] found that miR-21 inhibited Sox-2 expression in mesenchymal stem cells, reducing their clonogenic and proliferative potential and arresting cell cycle.

Finally, miR-1 increases cardiac differentiation of embryonic stem cells.

Apart from their action on "stem cells" many miRs are involved in endogenous cardiac regeneration; miR-15 family members induce postnatal mitotic arrest of cardiac cells, and inhibit their proliferation, while miR-590 and 199α promotes it. miRs can also influence cardiac reprograming.

Jayawardena et al. [117] found that a combination of miR-1, -133, -208, and -499 increased reprogramming of cardiac fibroblasts into cardiomyocytes.

Poller et al. [2] give a very recent review of therapeutic possibilities of ncRNAs, which amount to tens of thousands.

As already stated, they stress that there exist 1,424 separate miR genes in humans. They describe the mechanisms of RNA interference (RNAi), which are used to silence protein-coding genes. They underline that it is directed toward many targets: Heart, myocytes, atheroscrerotic plaques, stem cells, cardiac allografts and towards imaging.

They also stress potential side effects, which may arise from immune system stimulation Thus the question of safety will keep continuously emerging [87].

They also mention Braveheart, an Icn RNA required for cardiovascular linage Commitment for the identification of IncRNAs of potential clinical relevance.

Finally Porrello [118] approaches the association of miRs and the very important aspect of cardiac regeneration focusing in the mR-15 family and miR-133.

In their already mentioned review Kumarswamy and Thum [85] give a long list of genetically modified animal models for miRNA research in the heart. Four models involve Dicer, 2 miR1, one 126, 2, 133, 4 the 133 family, 3 the 208, 2 the -22 family, 3 the 328 and 2 the 499 family. In this sense Matkovich et al. [119] recently stress another important point, that indirect miRNa modulatory effects of miRs greatly outnumber direct target suppressions. In more hearts generated to overexpress miRs-143, 378, and 499, the last 2 indirectly regulated hundreds of cardiac miRNAs and 15–30 Cardiac miRs.

Conclusions

MicroRNAs have emerged in the last years as an important aspect of cardiovascular disease, both from a diagnostic but also a therapeutic standpoint. New miRs are constantly found and their role elucidated, since one miR can influence many functions. Despite technical problems, the therapeutic application of miRs is an emerging and constantly expanding field with a very important potential. The point of safety, should not be neglected, exactly due to the fact that miRs may have off-target effects.

References

1. Lee RC, Feinbaum RL, Ambros V. The C. elegans heterochronic gene lin-4 encodes small RNAs with antisense complementarity to lin-14. Cell. 1993;75:843–54.
2. Poller W, Tank J, Skurk C, Gast M. Cardiovascular RNA interference therapy: the broadening tool and target spectrum. Circ Res. 2013;113:588–602.
3. Smalheiser NR. EST analyses predict the existence of a population of chimeric microRNA precursor-mRNA transcripts expressed in normal human and mouse tissues. Genome Biol. 2003;4:403.
4. Cai X, Hagedorn CH, Cullen BR. Human microRNAs are processed from capped, polyadenylated transcripts that can also function as mRNAs. RNA. 2004;10:1957–66.
5. Han J, Lee Y, Yeom KH, Kim YK, Jin H, Kim VN. The Drosha-DGCR8 complex in primary microRNA processing. Genes Dev. 2004;18:3016–27.
6. Denli AM, Tops BB, Plasterk RH, Ketting RF, Hannon GJ. Processing of primary microRNAs by the Microprocessor complex. Nature. 2004;432: 231–5.
7. Lund E, Güttinger S, Calado A, Dahlberg JE, Kutay U. Nuclear export of microRNA precursors. Science. 2004;303:95–8.
8. Pratt AJ, MacRae IJ. The RNA-induced silencing complex: a versatile gene-silencing machine. J Biol Chem. 2009;284:17897–901.
9. Rana TM. Illuminating the silence: understanding the structure and function of small RNAs. Nat Rev Mol Cell Biol. 2007;8:23–36.
10. Filipowicz W, Jaskiewicz L, Kolb FA, Pillai RS. Post-transcriptional gene silencing by siRNAs and miRNAs. Curr Opin Struct Biol. 2005;15:331–41.
11. Tan Y, Zhang B, Wu T, Skogerbø G, Zhu X, Guo X, He S, et al. Transcriptional inhibition of Hoxd4 expression by miRNA-10a in human breast cancer cells. BMC Mol Biol. 2009;10:12.
12. Papageorgiou N, Tousoulis D, Androulakis E, Siasos G, Briasoulis A, Vogiatzi G, et al. The role of microRNAs in cardiovascular disease. Curr Med Chem. 2012;19:2605–10.
13. Da Costa Martins PA, De Windt LJ. Targeting microRNA targets. Circ Res. 2012;111:506–8.
14. Callis TE, Chen JF, Wang DZ. MicroRNAs in skeletal and cardiac muscle development. DNA Cell Biol. 2007;26:219–25.
15. Sandberg K, Samson WK, Ji H. Decoding noncoding RNA: da Vinci redux? Circ Res. 2013;113:240–1.
16. Latronico MV, Catalucci D, Condorelli G. Emerging role of microRNAs in cardiovascular biology. Circ Res. 2007;101:1225–36.
17. Lagendijk AK, Goumans MJ, Burkhard SB, Bakkers J. MicroRNA-23 restricts cardiac valve formation by inhibiting Has2 and extracellular hyaluronic acid production. Circ Res. 2011;109:649–57.
18. Porrello ER, Johnson BA, Aurora AB, Simpson E, Nam YJ, Matkovich SJ, et al. MiR-15 family regulates

postnatal mitotic arrest of cardiomyocytes. Circ Res. 2011;109:670–9.
19. Das S, Ferlito M, Kent OA, Fox-Talbot K, Wang R, Liu D, et al. Nuclear miRNA regulates the mitochondrial genome in the heart. Circ Res. 2012;110:1596–603.
20. Suárez Y, Sessa WC. MicroRNAs as novel regulators of angiogenesis. Circ Res. 2009;104:442–54.
21. Poliseno L, Tuccoli A, Mariani L, Evangelista M, Citti L, Woods K, et al. MicroRNAs modulate the angiogenic properties HUVECs. Blood. 2006;108:3068–71.
22. Boon RA. MicroRNAs control vascular endothelial growth factor signalling. Circ Res. 2012;11:1388–90.
23. Cordes KR, Srivastava D. MicroRNA regulation of cardiovascular development. Circ Res. 2009;104:724–32.
24. Sanoudou D, Kalozoumi G. Micro-RNAs: new biomarkers and novel applications for heart disease prevention and treatment. Hosp Chron. 2012;7:9–15.
25. van Rooij E, Sutherland LB, Liu N, Williams AH, McAnally J, Gerard RD, et al. A signature pattern of stress-responsive microRNAs that can evoke cardiac hypertrophy and heart failure. Proc Natl Acad Sci U S A. 2006;103:18255–60.
26. Cheng Y, Ji R, Yue J, Yang J, Liu X, Chen H, et al. MicroRNAs are aberrantly expressed in hypertrophic heart: do they play a role in cardiac hypertrophy? Am J Pathol. 2007;170:1831–40.
27. van Rooij E, Sutherland LB, Qi X, Richardson JA, Hill J, Olson EN. Control of stress-dependent cardiac growth and gene expression by a microRNA. Science. 2007;316:575–9.
28. Yang Y, Ago T, Zhai P, Abdellatif M, Sadoshima J. Thioredoxin 1 negatively regulates angiotensin II-induced cardiac hypertrophy through upregulation of miR-98/let-7. Circ Res. 2011;108:305–13.
29. Roncarati R, Anselmi CV, Losi MA, Papa L, Cavarretta E, Costa Martins PD, et al. Circulating miR-29a, among other upregulated microRNAs, is the only biomarker for both hypertrophy and fibrosis in patients with hypertrophic cardiomyopathy. J Am Coll Cardiol. 2013;pii: S0735-1097(13)05589-7.
30. Tousoulis D, Papageorgiou N, Charakida M, Briasoulis A, Androulakis E, Tentolouris C, et al. Prognostic role of miRNAs in coronary artery disease. Curr Top Med Chem. 2013;13:1540–7.
31. Sun C, Alkhoury K, Wang YI, Foster GA, Radecke CE, Tam K, et al. IRF-1 and miRNA126 modulate VCAM-1 expression in response to a high-fat meal. Circ Res. 2012;111:1054–64.
32. Chen WJ, Zhang M, Zhao GJ, Fu Y, Zhang DW, Zhu HB, et al. MicroRNA-33 in atherosclerosis etiology and pathophysiology. Atherosclerosis. 2013;227:201–8.
33. Zampetaki A, Mayr M. MicroRNAs in vascular and metabolic disease. Circ Res. 2012;110:508–22.
34. Chen KC, Juo SH. MicroRNAs in atherosclerosis. Kaohsiung J Med Sci. 2012;28:631–40.
35. Torella D, Iaconetti C, Catalucci D, Ellison GM, Leone A, Waring CD, et al. MicroRNA-133 controls vascular smooth muscle cell phenotype switch in vitro and vascular remodeling in vivo. Circ Res. 2011;109:880–93.
36. Norata GD, Sala F, Catapano AL, Fernández-Hernando C. MicroRNAs and lipoproteins: a connection beyond atherosclerosis? Atherosclerosis. 2013;227:209–15.
37. Stakos DA, Gatsiou A, Stamatelopoulos K, Tselepis AD, Stellos K. Platelet microRNAs: from platelet biology to possible disease biomarkers and therapeutic targets. Platelets. 2013;24:579–89.
38. Wang D, Xia M, Yan X, Li D, Wang L, Xu Y, et al. Gut microbiota metabolism of anthocyanin promotes reverse cholesterol transport in mice via repressing miRNA-10b. Circ Res. 2012;111:967–81.
39. Ma X, Ma C, Zheng X. MicroRNA-155 in the pathogenesis of atherosclerosis: a conflicting role? Heart Lung Circ. 2013;22:811–8.
40. Shantikumar S, Caporali A, Emanueli C. Role of microRNAs in diabetes and its cardiovascular complications. Cardiovasc Res. 2012;93:583–93.
41. Mortuza R, Chakrabarti S. Glucose-induced cell signaling in the pathogenesis of diabetic cardiomyopathy. Heart Fail Rev. 2014;19:75–86.
42. Xiao J, Luo X, Lin H, Zhang Y, Lu Y, Wang N, et al. MicroRNA miR-133 represses HERG K+channel expression contributing to QT prolongation in diabetic hearts. J Biol Chem. 2007;282:12363–7.
43. Baseler WA, Thapa D, Jagannathan R, Dabkowski ER, Croston TL, Hollander JM. miR-141 as a regulator of the mitochondrial phosphate carrier (Slc25a3) in the type 1 diabetic heart. Am J Physiol Cell Physiol. 2012;303:C1244–51.
44. Pulakat L, Aroor AR, Gul R, Sowers JR. Cardiac insulin resistance and microRNA modulators. Exp Diabetes Res. 2012;2012:654904.
45. Feng B, Chen S, McArthur K, Wu Y, Sen S, Ding Q, et al. miR-146a-mediated extracellular matrix protein production in chronic diabetes complications. Diabetes. 2011;60:2975–84.
46. Jordan SD, Krüger M, Willmes DM, Redemann N, Wunderlich FT, Brönneke HS, et al. Obesity-induced overexpression of miRNA-143 inhibits insulin-stimulated AKT activation and impairs glucose metabolism. Nat Cell Biol. 2011;13:434–46.
47. Wang YT, Tsai PC, Liao YC, Hsu CY, Juo SH. Circulating microRNAs have a sex-specific association with metabolic syndrome. J Biomed Sci. 2013;20:72.
48. Blumensatt M, Greulich S, Herzfeld de Wiza D, Mueller H, Maxhera B, Rabelink MJ, et al. Activin A impairs insulin action in cardiomyocytes via up-regulation of miR-143. Cardiovasc Res. 2013;100:201–10.
49. Menghini R, Casagrande V, Federici M. MicroRNAs in endothelial senescence and atherosclerosis. J Cardiovasc Transl Res. 2013;6:924–30.
50. Dimmeler S, Nicotera P. MicroRNAs in age-related diseases. EMBO Mol Med. 2013;5:180–90.
51. Olivieri F, Rippo MR, Procopio AD, Fazioli F. Circulating inflamma-miRs in aging and age-related diseases. Front Genet. 2013;4(121):1–9.

52. Papageorgiou N, Tousoulis D, Charakida M, Briasoulis A, Androulakis E, Tentolouris C, et al. Prognostic role of miRNAs in coronary artery disease. Curr Top Med Chem. 2013;13:1540–7.
53. Sun X, Zhang M, Sanagawa A, Mori C, Ito S, Iwaki S, et al. Circulating microRNA-126 in patients with coronary artery disease: correlation with LDL cholesterol. Thromb J. 2012;10:16.
54. Fichtlscherer S, De Rosa S, Fox H, Schwietz T, Fischer A, Liebetrau C, et al. Circulating microRNAs in patients with coronary artery disease. Circ Res. 2010;107:677–84.
55. Van Aelst LN, Heymans S. MicroRNAs as biomarkers for ischemic heart disease. J Cardiovasc Transl Res. 2013;6:458–70.
56. Zhu H, Fan GC. Extracellular/circulating microRNAs and their potential role in cardiovascular disease. Am J Cardiovasc Dis. 2011;1:138–49.
57. Zampetaki A, Willeit P, Tilling L, Drozdov I, Prokopi M, Renard JM, et al. Prospective study on circulating MicroRNAs and risk of myocardial infarction. J Am Coll Cardiol. 2012;60:290–9.
58. Fiedler J, Thum T. MicroRNAs in myocardial infarction. Arterioscler Thromb Vasc Biol. 2013;33:201–5.
59. Pleister A, Selemon H, Elton SM, Elton TS. Circulating miRNAs: novel biomarkers of acute coronary syndrome? Biomark Med. 2013;7:287–305.
60. Nabiałek E, Wańha W, Kula D, Jadczyk T, Krajewska M, Kowalówka A, et al. Circulating microRNAs (miR-423-5p, miR-208a and miR-1) in acute myocardial infarction and stable coronary heart disease. Minerva Cardioangiol. 2013;61:627–37.
61. Wang GK, Zhu JQ, Zhang JT, Li Q, Li Y, He J, et al. Circulating microRNA: a novel potential biomarker for early diagnosis of acute myocardial infarction in humans. Eur Heart J. 2010;31:659–66.
62. Olivieri F, Antonicelli R, Spazzafumo L, Santini G, Rippo MR, Galeazzi R, et al. Admission levels of circulating miR-499-5p and risk of death in elderly patients after acute non-ST elevation myocardial infarction. Int J Cardiol. 2014;pii: S0167-5273(14)00063-1.
63. Yu XY, Chen JY, Zheng ZW, Wu H, Li LW, Zhang ZW, et al. Plasma miR-126 as a potential marker predicting major adverse cardiac events in dual antiplatelet-treated patients after percutaneous coronary intervention. EuroIntervention. 2013;9:546–54.
64. D'Alessandra Y, Devanna P, Limana F, Straino S, Di Carlo A, Brambilla PG, et al. Circulating microRNAs are new and sensitive biomarkers of myocardial infarction. Eur Heart J. 2010;31:2765–73.
65. Jaguszewski M, Osipova J, Ghadri JR, Napp LC, Widera C, Franke J, et al. A signature of circulating microRNAs differentiates takotsubo cardiomyopathy from acute myocardial infarction. Eur Heart J. 2014;35:999–1006.
66. Polimeni A, De Rosa S, Indolfi C. Vascular miRNAs after balloon angioplasty. Trends Cardiovasc Med. 2013;23:9–14.
67. Lu Y, Zhang Y, Shan H, Pan Z, Li X, Li B, et al. MicroRNA-1 downregulation by propranolol in a rat model of myocardial infarction: a new mechanism for ischaemic cardioprotection. Cardiovasc Res. 2009;84:434–41.
68. Eitel I, Adams V, Dieterich P, Fuernau G, de Waha S, Desch S, et al. Relation of circulating MicroRNA-133a concentrations with myocardial damage and clinical prognosis in ST-elevation myocardial infarction. Am Heart J. 2012;164:706–14.
69. Matsumoto S, Sakata Y, Suna S, Nakatani D, Usami M, Hara M, et al. Circulating p53-responsive microRNAs are predictive indicators of heart failure after acute myocardial infarction. Circ Res. 2013;113:322–6.
70. Zidar N, Boštjančič E, Glavač D, Stajer D, et al. MicroRNAs, innate immunity and ventricular rupture in human myocardial infarction. Dis Markers. 2011;31:259–65.
71. Hullinger TG, Montgomery RL, Seto AG, Dickinson BA, Semus HM, Lynch JM, et al. Inhibition of miR-15 protects against cardiac ischemic injury. Circ Res. 2012;110:71–81.
72. Aurora AB, Mahmoud AI, Luo X, Johnson BA, van Rooij E, Matsuzaki S, et al. MicroRNA-214 protects the mouse heart from ischemic injury by controlling Ca^{2+} overload and cell death. J Clin Invest. 2012;122:1222–32.
73. Orogo AM, Gustafsson ÅB. Cell death in the myocardium: my heart won't go on. IUBMB Life. 2013;65:651–6.
74. Ruan W, Xu JM, Li SB, Yuan LQ, Dai RP. Effects of down-regulation of microRNA-23a on TNF-α-induced endothelial cell apoptosis through caspase-dependent pathways. Cardiovasc Res. 2012;93:623–32.
75. Li X, Kong M, Jiang D, Qian J, Duan Q, Dong A. MicroRNA-150 aggravates H2O2-induced cardiac myocyte injury by down-regulating c-myb gene. Acta Biochim Biophys Sin (Shanghai). 2013;45:734–41.
76. Fu J, Peng C, Wang W, Jin H, Tang Q, Wei X. Let-7 g is involved in doxorubicin induced myocardial injury. Environ Toxicol Pharmacol. 2012;33:312–7.
77. Horie T, Ono K, Nishi H, Nagao K, Kinoshita M, Watanabe S. Acute doxorubicin cardiotoxicity is associated with miR-146a-induced inhibition of the neuregulin-ErbB pathway. Cardiovasc Res. 2010;87:656–64.
78. van Rooij E, Sutherland LB, Thatcher JE, DiMaio JM, Naseem RH, et al. Dysregulation of microRNAs after myocardial infarction reveals a role of miR-29 in cardiac fibrosis. Proc Natl Acad Sci U S A. 2008;105:13027–32.
79. Pan Z, Sun X, Shan H, Wang N, Wang J, Ren J, et al. MicroRNA-101 inhibited postinfarct cardiac fibrosis and improved left ventricular compliance via the FBJ osteosarcoma oncogene/transforming growth factor-β1 pathway. Circulation. 2012;126:840–50.
80. Zile MR, Mehurg SM, Arroyo JE, Stroud RE, DeSantis SM, Spinale FG, et al. Relationship between the temporal profile of plasma microRNA and left ventricular remodeling in patients after myocardial infarction. Circ Cardiovasc Genet. 2011;4:614–9.
81. Devaux Y, Vausort M, McCann GP, Zangrando J, Kelly D, Razvi N, et al. MicroRNA-150: a novel marker of

left ventricular remodeling after acute myocardial infarction. Circ Cardiovasc Genet. 2013;6:290–8.
82. Divakaran V, Mann DL. The emerging role of microRNAs in cardiac remodeling and heart failure. Circ Res. 2008;103:1072–83.
83. Topkara VK, Mann DL. Role of microRNAs in cardiac remodeling and heart failure. Cardiovasc Drugs Ther. 2011;25:171–82.
84. Hu S, Huang M, Li Z, Jia F, Ghosh Z, Lijkwan MA, et al. MicroRNA-210 as a novel therapy for treatment of ischemic heart disease. Circulation. 2010;122:S124–31.
85. Kumarswamy R, Thum T. Non-coding RNAs in cardiac remodeling and heart failure. Circ Res. 2013;113:676–89.
86. Sayed D, Hong C, Chen IY, Lypowy J, Abdellatif M. MicroRNAs play an essential role in the development of cardiac hypertrophy. Circ Res. 2007;100:416–24.
87. Kumarswamy R, Lyon AR, Volkmann I, Mills AM, Bretthauer J, Pahuja A, et al. SERCA2a gene therapy restores microRNA-1 expression in heart failure via an Akt/FoxO3A-dependent pathway. Eur Heart J. 2012;33:1067–75.
88. Haghikia A, Podewski E, Libhaber E, Labidi S, Fischer D, Roentgen P, et al. Phenotyping and outcome on contemporary management in a German cohort of patients with peripartum cardiomyopathy. Basic Res Cardiol. 2013;108:366.
89. Schipper MEI, van Kuik J, de Jonge N, Dullens HFJ, deWeger RA. Changes in regulatory microRNA expression in myocardium of heart failure patients in left ventricular assist device support. J Heart Lung Transplant. 2008;27:1282–5.
90. Vacchi-Suzzi C, Bauer Y, Berridge BR, Bongiovanni S, Gerrish K, Hamadeh HK, et al. Perturbation of microRNAs in rat heart during chronic doxorubicin treatment. PLoS One. 2012;7(7):e40395.
91. Wang Z, Lu Y, Yang B. MicroRNAs and atrial fibrillation: new fundamentals. Cardiovasc Res. 2011;89:710–21.
92. Liu Z, Zhou C, Liu Y, Wang S, Ye P, Miao X¨, et al. The expression levels of plasma micoRNAs in atrial fibrillation patients. PLoS One. 2012;7:e44906.
93. Kim GH. MicroRNA regulation of cardiac conduction and arrhythmias. Transl Res. 2013;161:381–92.
94. Zhao Y, Ransom JF, Li A, Vedantham V, von Drehle M, Muth AN, et al. Dysregulation of cardiogenesis, cardiac conduction, and cell cycle in mice lacking miRNA-1-2. Cell. 2007;129:303–17.
95. Terentyev D, Belevych AE, Terentyeva R, Martin MM, Malana GE, Kuhn DE, et al. miR-1 overexpression enhances Ca(2+) release and promotes cardiac arrhythmogenesis by targeting PP2A regulatory subunit B56alpha and causing CaMKII-dependent hyperphosphorylation of RyR2. Circ Res. 2009;104:514–21.
96. Kinet V, Halkein J, Dirkx E, Windt LJ. Cardiovascular extracellular microRNAs: emerging diagnostic markers and mechanisms of cell-to-cell RNA communication. Front Genet. 2013;4:214.
97. Creemers EE, Tijsen AJ, Pinto YM. Circulating microRNAs: novel biomarkers and extracellular communicators in cardiovascular disease? Circ Res. 2012;110:483–95.
98. De Rosa S, Curcio A, Indolfi C. Emerging role of microRNAs in cardiovascular diseases. Circ J. 2014;78:567–75.
99. van Rooij E, Marshall WS, Olson EN. Toward microRNA-based therapeutics for heart disease: the sense in antisense. Circ Res. 2008;103:919–28.
100. Chistiakov DA, Sobenin IA, Orekhov AN. Strategies to deliver microRNAs as potential therapeutics in the treatment of cardiovascular pathology. Drug Deliv. 2012;19:392–405.
101. Caroli A, Cardillo MT, Galea R, Biasucci LM. Potential therapeutic role of microRNAs in ischemic heart disease. J Cardiol. 2013;61:315–20.
102. Hinkel R, Penzkofer D, Zühlke S, Fischer A, Husada W, Xu QF, et al. Inhibition of microRNA-92a protects against ischemia/reperfusion injury in a large-animal model. Circulation. 2013;128:1066–75.
103. Halkein J, Tabruyn SP, Ricke-Hoch M, Haghikia A, Nguyen NQ, Scherr M, et al. MicroRNA-146a is a therapeutic target and biomarker for peripartum cardiomyopathy. J Clin Invest. 2013;123:2143–54.
104. Wahlquist C, Jeong D, Rojas-Muñoz A, Kho C, Lee A, Mitsuyama S, et al. Inhibition of miR-25 improves cardiac contractility in the failing heart. Nature. 2014. doi:10.1038/nature13073.
105. Quattrocelli M, Crippa S, Montecchiani C, Camps J, Cornaglia AI, Boldrin L, et al. Long-term miR-669a therapy alleviates chronic dilated cardiomyopathy in dystrophic mice. J Am Heart Assoc. 2013;2(4):e000284. doi:10.1161/JAHA.113.000284.
106. Iekushi K, Seeger F, Assmus B, Zeiher AM, Dimmeler S. Regulation of cardiac microRNAs by bone marrow mononuclear cell therapy in myocardial infarction. Circulation. 2012;125:1765–73. S1–7.
107. Muñoz-Pacheco P, Ortega-Hernández A, Miana M, Cachofeiro V, Fernández-Cruz A, Gómez-Garre D. Ezetimibe inhibits PMA-induced monocyte/macrophage differentiation by altering microRNA expression: a novel anti-atherosclerotic mechanism. Pharmacol Res. 2012;66:536–43.
108. Ye Y, Hu Z, Lin Y, Zhang C, Perez-Polo JR. Downregulation of microRNA-29 by antisense inhibitors and a PPAR-gamma agonist protects against myocardial ischaemia-reperfusion injury. Cardiovasc Res. 2010;87:535–44.
109. Ntanasis-Stathopoulos J, Tzanninis JG, Philippou A, Koutsilieris M. Epigenetic regulation on gene expression induced by physical exercise. J Musculoskelet Neuronal Interact. 2013;13:133–46.
110. Mooren FC, Viereck J, Krüger K, Thum T. Circulating microRNAs as potential biomarkers of aerobic exercise capacity. Am J Physiol Heart Circ Physiol. 2014;306:H557–63. doi:10.1152/ajpheart.00711.2013. Epub 2013 Dec 20.
111. Yin C, Salloum FN, Kukreja RC. A novel role of microRNA in late preconditioning: upregulation of

endothelial nitric oxide synthase and heat shock protein 70. Circ Res. 2009;104:572–5.
112. Rane S, He M, Sayed D, Vashistha H, Malhotra A, Sadoshima J, et al. Downregulation of miR-199a derepresses hypoxia-inducible factor-1alpha and Sirtuin 1 and recapitulates hypoxia preconditioning in cardiac myocytes. Circ Res. 2009;104:879–86.
113. Cheng Y, Zhu P, Yang J, Liu X, Dong S, Wang X, et al. Ischaemic preconditioning-regulated miR-21 protects heart against ischaemia/reperfusion injury via anti-apoptosis through its target PDCD4. Cardiovasc Res. 2010;87:431–9.
114. Salloum FN, Yin C, Kukreja RC. Role of microRNAs in cardiac preconditioning. J Cardiovasc Pharmacol. 2010;56:581–8.
115. Seeger FH, Zeiher AM, Dimmeler S. MicroRNAs in stem cell function and regenerative therapy of the heart. Arterioscler Thromb Vasc Biol. 2013;33:1739–46.
116. Trohatou O, Zagoura D, Bitsika V, Pappa KI, Antsaklis A, Anagnou NP, et al. Sox2 suppression by miR-21 governs human mesenchymal stem cell properties. Stem Cells Transl Med. 2014;3:54–68.
117. Jayawardena TM, Egemnazarov B, Finch EA, Zhang L, Payne JA, Pandya K, et al. MicroRNA-mediated in vitro and in vivo direct reprogramming of cardiac fibroblasts to cardiomyocytes. Circ Res. 2012;110:1465–73.
118. Porrello ER. microRNAs in cardiac development and regeneration. Clin Sci (Lond). 2013;125:151–66.
119. Matkovich SJ, Hu Y, Dorn 2nd GW. Regulation of cardiac microRNAs by cardiac microRNAs. Circ Res. 2013;113:62–71.

Pathways to Myocardial Hypertrophy

10

Maria Irene Kontaridis, Eleni V. Geladari, and Charalampia V. Geladari

Abstract
Pathological cardiac hypertrophy occurs as a consequence of adaptive responses to pressure or volume overload, mutations in sarcomeric (or other) proteins, or loss of contractile mass from prior infarction. While initially compensatory, over time when the heart can no longer meet with the increased metabolic demands of the mechanical work load imposed on the heart, dilation and heart failure ensue. Several signaling pathways are critically important in mediating myocardial hypertrophy, including the G-protein coupled receptor, the calcineurin/NFAT, MAPK, and the PI3K/AKT/mTOR signaling pathways. Importantly, these signaling pathways also control molecular processes, such as cell proliferation, differentiation, survival, migration and other functions of the cell. In addition, the heart is comprised of several cell lineages make up the heart, including cardiomyocytes, fibroblasts, endothelial cells, and vascular smooth muscle cells, each integrally involved in modulating the signaling events that promote the

M.I. Kontaridis, PhD (✉)
Department of Biological Chemistry and Molecular Pharmacology, Harvard Medical School, Boston, MA, USA

Division of Cardiology, Department of Medicine, Center for Life Sciences, Beth Israel Deaconess Medical Center,
Room 908, 3 Blackfan Circle, Boston, MA, USA
e-mail: mkontari@bidmc.harvard.edu

E.V. Geladari, MD
Division of Cardiology, Department of Medicine, Center for Life Sciences,
Beth Israel Deaconess Medical Center,
Room 908, 3 Blackfan Circle, Boston, MA, USA

Department of Internal Medicine, Evangelismos State General Hospital, Athens, Greece

C.V. Geladari, MD
4th Department of Internal Medicine, Evangelismos State General Hospital, Athens, Greece

Division of Cardiology, Department of Medicine, Center for Life Sciences, Beth Israel Deaconess Medical Center,
Room 908, 3 Blackfan Circle, Boston, MA, USA

D.V. Cokkinos (ed.), *Introduction to Translational Cardiovascular Research*,
DOI 10.1007/978-3-319-08798-6_10, © Springer International Publishing Switzerland 2015

hypertrophic growth of the heart. In this chapter we discuss these molecular pathways and how the aberrant regulation of initially compensatory responses becomes pathological. We will also discuss potential therapeutic targets for hypertrophic cardiomyopathy and heart failure, with a focus on treating this devastating worldwide disease.

Keywords
Hypertrophy • Cardiomyocytes • Heart failure • Cardiomyopathy • Signaling • GPCR • MAPK • PI3K • AKT • Calcineurin • NFAT • Neurohumoral • Fibroblasts • HCM

Abbreviations

ACEIs	Angiotensin-converting-enzyme inhibitors
AngII	Angiotensin II
ATP	Adenosine triphosphate
ATR	Angiotensin receptor
b-FGF	basic fibroblast growth factor
C	Adenylyl cyclase
CaMKII	Ca^{2+}/calmodulin-dependent protein kinase II
cAMP	Cyclic adenosine 3′ 5′ monophosphate
CICR	Calcium-induced Calcium Release
CMs	Cardiomyocytes
CsA	Cyclosporine A
ECM	Extracellular matrix
ECs	Endothelial cells
ERK	Extracellular regulated kinase
G protein	Guanosine triphosphate binding protein
G-protein	GTP-binding protein
GSK3β	Glycogen synthase kinase 3-β
HCM	Hypertrophic Cardiomyopathy
HDACs	Histone deacetylases
HF	Heart Failure
IGF-1	Insulin-like growth factor-1
JNK	Jun N-terminal kinase
LTCC	Long-type Calcium Channel
LV	Left ventricular
MAPK	Mitogen activated protein kinase
MI	Myocardial infarction
mTOR	Mammalian target of Rapamycin
Na^+	Sodium irons
NFAT	Nuclear factor for activation of T cells
NO	Nitric Oxide
PI3K	xPhosphatidylinositol 3′ kinase
PKC	Protein kinase C
PLN	Phospholamban
PTEN	Phosphatase and tensin homolog deleted on chromosome ten
RAS	Renin–angiotensin system
RyR	Ryanodone receptor
SR	Sarcoplasmic reticulum
STAT	Signal transducer and activators of transcription
TGFβ	Transforming growth factor-β
T-tubule	Transverse tubule2
VEGF	Vascular endothelial growth factor
VSMCs	Vascular smooth muscle cells
α-AR	Alpha adrenergic receptor
β1AR	Beta 1adrenergic receptor
βAR	Beta adrenergic receptor
βMHC	Beta myosin heavy chain

10.1 Cardiomyocyte Function and Regulation

The heart's primary function in the body is to maintain proper oxygenation and pump blood to the lungs and body through contraction. Cardiomyocytes (CMs), cells regulating the contractile motion of the heart, are critical for this process. Initiation of contraction is mediated through a process called excitation contraction [1]. The action potential (AP) in CMs stems from the entry of sodium (Na+) ions across the sarcolemma. As the muscle impulse spreads from the sarcolemma to the transverse tubule (T-tubule), calcium ions (Ca^{2+}) are released into the sarcoplasm. In addition, an inward flux of extracellular Ca^{2+} enters the cell through voltage-gated long (L)-type calcium channels (LTCCs) to sustain the depolarization and to maximize the duration of contraction [2]. Then, through a mechanism of calcium-induced calcium release (CICR), additional Ca^{2+} is released into the sarcoplasm from the sarcoplasmic reticulum (SR), increasing intracellular Ca^{2+} levels. This increase in calcium flux inside the cell mediates Ca^{2+} binding to the protein troponin on the actin filament, allowing it undergo a conformational change that exposes the binding sites for myosin on actin filaments [3]. Once myosin is bound to actin, it initiates "cross-bridge cycling," a process which regulates the normal, rhythmic contraction of cardiac muscle cells [3, 4] (Fig. 10.1).

10.2 Cardiac Hypertrophy

Hypertrophic growth of the heart is considered an adaptive response to pressure or volume overload, mutations of sarcomeric (or other) proteins, or loss of contractile mass from myocardial infarction. However, over time, the heart loses its ability to keep up with the chronic metabolic demands of increased mechanical workload, and dilation and heart failure (HF) ensue [5]. For this reason, myocardial hypertrophy is considered to be the interface between a normal and failing heart.

There are two types of hypertrophy: concentric and eccentric. Chronic left ventricular (LV) pressure overload (afterload) results in a concentric type of hypertrophy, where new sarcomeres are added in parallel to existing sarcomeres, and consequently, the wall thickness becomes increased [6]. Concentric Hypertrophy typically occurs in cases of aortic stenosis and hypertension and is believed to function by

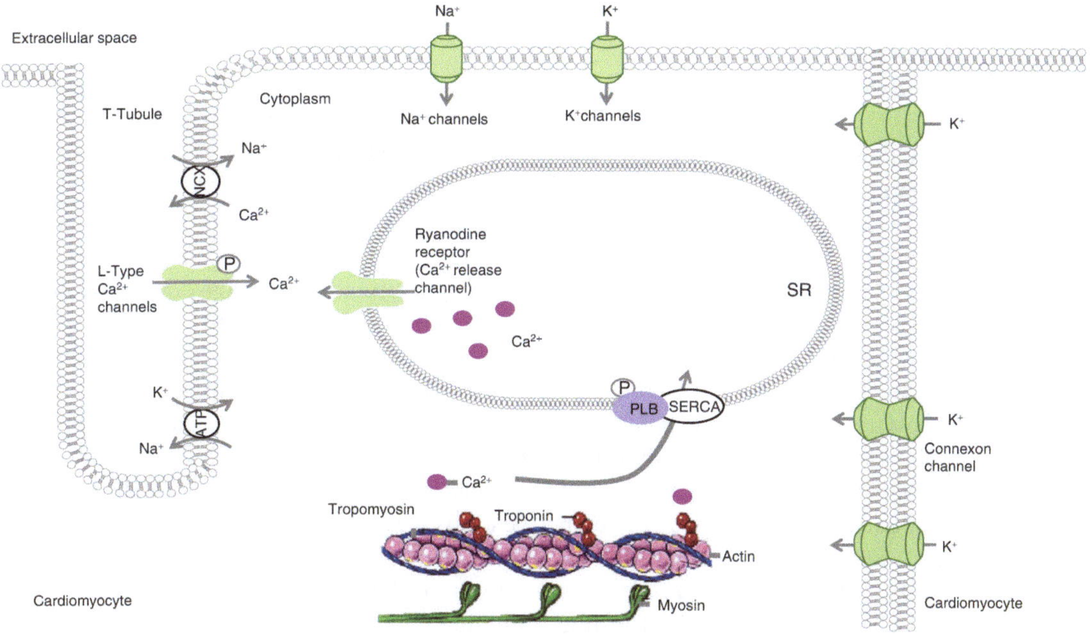

Fig. 10.1 Excitation-contraction coupling in cardiac muscle. The initial event in the cardiac muscle contraction is membrane depolarization, which occurs with ion entry through connexon channels from a neighboring cardiomyocyte, followed by opening of voltage-gated Na^+ channels and Na^+ entry. The resultant rapid depolarization of the membrane inactivates Na^+ channels and opens both K^+ channels and Ca^{2+} channels. Entry of Ca^{2+} into the cell triggers the release of Ca^{2+} from the sarcoplasmic reticulum through the ryanodine channel. Ca^{2+} then binds to the troponin complex and activates the contractile apparatus. Cellular relaxation occurs on removal of Ca^{2+} from the cytosol by the Ca^{2+}-uptake pumps of the sarcoplasmic reticulum and by Na^+/Ca^{2+} exchange with the extracellular fluid

diminishing wall stress and oxygen consumption [7]. It is characterized by normal peak systolic and end diastolic wall stresses, with little or no change in chamber volume, but with increased h (wall thickness)/R (radius) ratio [8]. In contrast, eccentric hypertrophy, which increases the number of sarcomeric units in series, occurs in response to chronic LV volume overload (preload) and is typically characterized by an enlarged LV chamber [6]. Eccentric hypertrophy is typically observed in patients with aortic or mitral valve insufficiency. It induces an increased end diastolic wall stress, normalizes h/R ratio, and in general, presents with normal peak systolic wall stress, thereby increasing the shortening capacity of the myocyte and preserving LV function [8]. However, despite this, eccentric hypertrophy with elongation of myocytes can be a hallmark of end-stage pressure overload hypertrophy as well. Therefore, it is important to distinguish between adaptive elongation of the cardiomyocyte and elongation associated with failure [9].

10.2.1 Hypertrophic Cardiomyopathy

The principal anatomical feature of pathological growth of the heart is referred to as hypertrophic cardiomyopathy (HCM), an abnormal, asymmetric LV thickening of the heart [4]. Specifically, pathological hypertrophy is defined as an increase in the overall size of cardiac cells, with increased myocardial fibrosis that is distributed throughout the interstitium and in discrete foci [10]. Data suggest a remarkable and characteristic cardiac histopathology in HCM; hearts have misaligned myocytes with enlarged nuclei and expanded interstitial matrix, combined with both increased perivascular and interstitial fibrosis [11]. Interestingly, HCM usually affects the interventricular septum more than the LV–free wall [11].

Cardiac hypertrophy can also occur as a consequence of genetic alterations. Specific, autosomal dominant sarcomeric mutations can cause HCM, with over 400 mutations in at least 13 different sarcomeric proteins identified thus far [12]. Mutations in β-myosin heavy chain myosin (βMHC) were the first to be identified in HCM and cause ~30 % of all cases [13]. Mutations in α-cardiac actin, tropomyosin, and troponin have also been associated with cardiomyopathy [11].

Cardiac hypertrophy can also be caused by ischemic disease, hypertension, HF, and valvular disease [10]. When an increased work load is chronically imposed on the myocardium, such as by external stimuli and/or pathological stress such as hypertension, heart muscle injury (myocardial infarction), or neurohumoral stimulation, there is increased adenosine triphosphate (ATP) utilization by cardiac cells, increasing energy consumption of the heart and reducing inotropic reserves [6]. However, over time, this increased signaling induces pathological remodeling of the heart, causing the heart to become abnormally thickened or hypertrophic [12]. When the heart can no longer keep up with this excess demand, it decompensates, transitioning to dilation and, ultimately causing end-stage HF [12], a serious life-threatening condition and one of the most common causes of death worldwide [4].

10.2.2 Pathological Signaling Pathways

Several types of pathological conditions induce cardiac hypertrophy by activating a variety of membrane receptors to engage downstream intracellular signaling pathways, including the G-protein coupled receptor (GPCR), receptor tyrosine kinase (RTK), cytokine, and calcium-modulated pathways [14]. Acutely, the purpose for the activation of these pathways is to enhance excitation-contraction coupling, to allow for the heart to compensate for the excess demand [2, 3] (Fig. 10.1). Chronically, however, constitutive activation of these signaling pathways leads to sustained hypertrophic responses that induce maladaptive remodeling of the heart.

Interestingly, there is significant cross-talk between the proteins within these various signaling cascades, allowing for specific and directed responses to downstream effectors [15]. For example, stimulation of the mitogen activated protein kinase (MAPK) cascade by each of the three family members, the extracellular regulated kinases (ERK1/2, ERK5), p38 and the c-Jun N-terminal kinase (JNK), culminates in the activation of nuclear transcription factors that drive hypertrophic responses within the cell [16]. Increases in intracellular Ca2+, which leads to the activation of calmodulin-dependent protein kinase II (CaMKII) and/or calcineurin, induces activation of the nuclear factor for activation of T cells (NFAT), enhancing cardiac hypertrophy [17]. In addition, increased CaMKII activity modulates hypertrophic gene transcription by controlling nuclear shuttling of class II histone deacetylases (HDACs) [18]. Therefore, it is the concomitant increase in multiple signaling cascades that ultimately leads to the panoply of responses that drive enhanced (and chronic) hypertrophic gene transcription [19].

10.2.2.1 G-Protein Coupled Receptor Signaling

GPCRs are the largest class of cell surface receptors, with nearly 800 family members identified to date [20]. The GPCR consists of a cytosolic region, a ligand-binding extracellular region and seven transmembrane domains. Intracellularly, GPCRs are associated with heterotrimeric GTP-binding proteins (G-proteins) consisting of multiple isoforms of distinct Gα, β and γ subunits [21]. There are four sub-classes of G-proteins: Gαs and Gαi, which either stimulate or inhibit adenylyl cyclase (AC), respectively; Gαq/11, which activates phospholipase C (PLC); and Gα12/13, which activates the Rho family of G proteins [22]. Because the signal transducing properties of the various possible βγ combinations do not appear to radically differ from one another, these classes are defined principally according to the isoform of their α-subunit; however, βγ dimers are important in that they are involved in enhancing the complexity of possible interactions between G proteins and their targets [23].

In the absence of signal, the GPCR-associated heterotrimeric G protein is bound to guanosine diphosphate (GDP) and is inactive. However, upon binding of the agonist to the GPCR, a conformational change takes place which enables the receptor to act as its own guanine nucleotide exchange factor (GEF), activating the associated G-protein by exchanging its bound GDP for guanosine triphosphate (GTP) [24]. The G-protein's α subunit then, together with the bound GTP, dissociates from the βγ subunit to further affect intracellular signaling proteins or target functional proteins directly dependent on the α subunit type [22]. GPCR activation drives downstream signaling cascades controlled by ACs, phospholipases and ion channels, as well as by various RTK cascades (ERK, JNK, p38, ERK5) and the phosphatidylinositol 3′ kinase (PI3K/Akt) pathway. In fact, GPCR signaling controls most important and vital molecular processes, such as cell proliferation, differentiation, survival, migration and other functions; however, chronic activation can also lead to the development of cardiovascular disease and HF [25].

10.2.2.2 Gαs and Gαi Signaling

β-1 adrenergic receptors (B1AR), β-2 adrenergic receptors (B2AR), dopamine-1 receptors, histamine-2 receptors, and vasopressin-2 receptors are examples of Gαs protein-coupled receptors [26]. Upon agonist binding, dissociated Gαs ("s" for stimulatory) leads to stimulation of AC and increased generation of cyclic adenosine 3′ 5′ monophosphate (cAMP), a key second messenger that mediates excitation-contraction coupling of the heart [27, 28]. The cAMP subsequently mediates activation of the serine/threonine-specific protein kinase A (PKA), which is ultimately required to modulate cardiac contractility via intracellular Ca2+ movements [26] (Fig. 10.2).

Once activated, the catalytic subunit of PKA phosphorylates a range of substrates within the cardiomyocyte, including cardiac troponin I (cTnI), the ryanodine receptor (RyR), the LTCCs, and phospholamban (PLB), all of which are required to enhance cardiomyocyte contractility through modulation of Ca^{2+} transients released from the SR [26] (Fig. 10.2). In addition, PKA activity is regulated by A-kinase anchoring proteins (AKAPs) and phosphodiesterases (PDEs) to similarly modulate cardiomyocyte contractility and function [29].

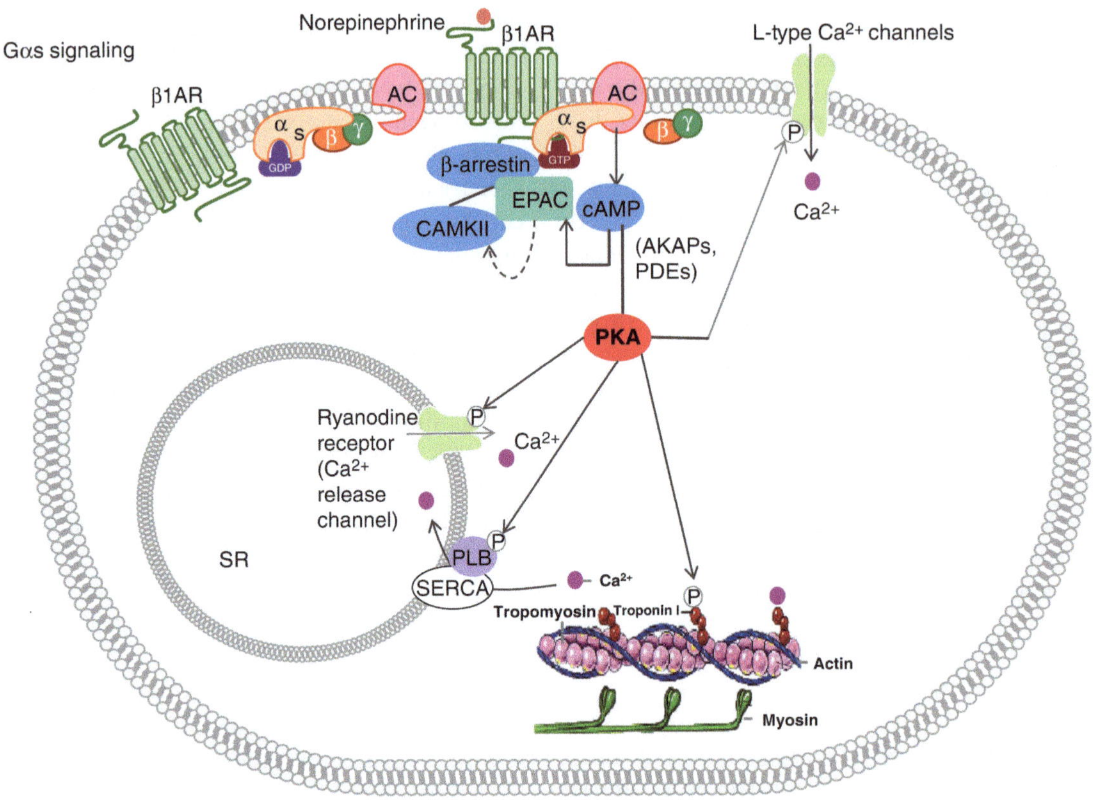

Fig. 10.2 Gαs signaling. When no signal molecule is present, the G protein binds to the GDP and is inactive. However, upon binding of a signal protein to the ligand-binding site, a conformational change of the receptor takes place. This enables the receptor to interact with the α subunit of the associated G protein, which then exchanges its bound GDP to GTP. This activates the G protein and causes βγ subunit to dissociate, thus enabling it to relay the signal by regulating the activity of additional intracellular signaling proteins. When norepinephrine (NE) binds to the β1AR, the G protein becomes activated and adenylate cyclase becomes stimulated. Cyclic AMP increases and phosphorylation events inside the cell take place, leading thus to increased cellular contraction. A β arrestin dependent scaffold including CAMKII and EPAC can be recruited to β1AR on stimulation, allowing cAMP-EPAC-mediated activation of CAMKII and regulation of contractility

AC activity is inhibited by stimulation of the Gαi-coupled muscarinic acetylcholine receptor-2 (mAchR2) as well as by stimulation of the sphingosine-1 phosphate receptor-1 (S1PR). In addition, Gβγ subunits, when released from the Gα subunits, function to open muscarinic K^+ channels (K_{ach}) and promote membrane hyperpolarization of the cardiomyocyte. Reduction of the action potential duration follows, and chronotropy and inotropy are decreased [30] (Fig. 10.3).

10.2.2.3 Gαq/11 Signaling

Angiotensin receptors (ATRs), endothelin receptors (ETRs), serotonin receptors and α-adrenergic receptors (αARs) are coupled to Gαq/11 signaling proteins [31]. Angiotensin I (AngI), Angiotensin II (AngII), and endothelin-1 (ET1) are examples of pro-hypertrophic hormones that bind these receptors during mechanical and/or pathological stress (i.e. stretch due to pressure or volume overload) [32]. Mechanistically, stimulation of Gαq/11-coupled receptors leads to activation of phospholipase C-β (PLCβ) and subsequent cleavage of membrane-bound phosphatidylinositol 4,5-biphosphate (PIP2) into the second messengers inositol (1,4,5) trisphosphate (IP3) and diacylglycerol (DAG) [33]. IP3 induces the IP3 receptor-mediated release of Ca^{2+} from the SR and is required to activate the downstream effectors CaMKII and calcineurin, whereas DAG

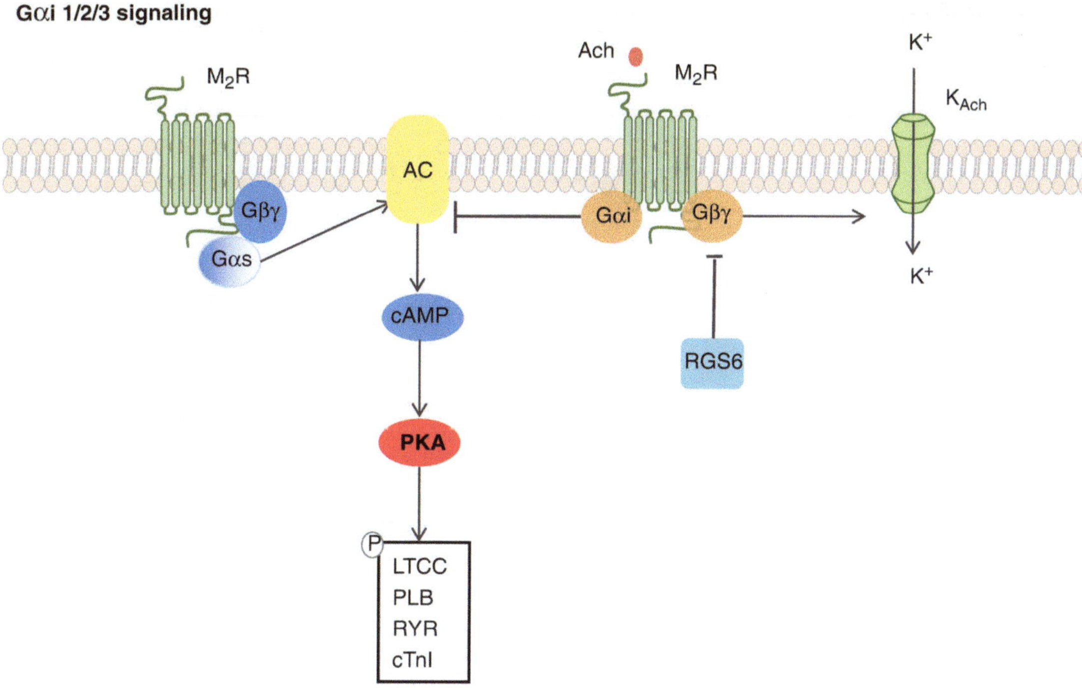

Fig. 10.3 Gαi 1/2/3 signaling. The muscarinic acetylcholine receptor 2 is Gαi coupled, and upon its stimulation, AC activity is decreased. Moreover, the Gβγ subunit is released and stimulates the muscarinic K+ channels to open. Hyperpolarization of the cardiomyocyte follows, dampening the contractile response. This is antagonized by RGS6

diffuses along the plasma membrane and activates membrane bound forms of the serine/threonine protein kinase C (PKC) and/or protein kinase D, which in turn drive the downstream activation of ERK1/2 [33] (Fig. 10.4).

Importantly, while all Gαq/11-coupled receptors function to control hypertrophy in response to cardiac stress, they each have additional important functional properties: α1-adrenergic receptor signaling is required to modulate Na^+-H^+ exchange transporter regulation; angiotensin receptor signaling controls Ca^{2+} signaling and collagen synthesis/deposition, and endothelin-1 mediates cardiac rhythm and collagen expression [34]. In addition, cardiac hypertrophy associated with Gαq signaling mediates the reactivation of embryonic genes, such as atrial natriuretic factor (ANF), skeletal α-actin, and βMHC [34].

Taken together, activation of Gαq signaling leads to an increase in transcriptional regulation of genes that control cardiomyocyte cell size and protein content, which over time, ultimately leads to hypertrophy and cardiac failure [35]. Indeed, transient overexpression of a constitutively active mutant of Gαq in transgenic mice consistently results in cardiac hypertrophy and dilatation with progressive heart failure and death [36]. Specifically, the transgenic overexpression of the angiotensin-1 (AT1R) receptor develops significant cardiac hypertrophy, with increased expression of atrial natriuretic factor (ANF) and interstitial collagen deposition, and the mice die prematurely of heart failure [37]. In contrast, mice carrying inactivating mutations of Gαq or Gα11 exhibit embryonic cardiomyocyte hypoplasia, suggesting that Gαq/Gα11-mediated signaling not only regulates myocardial growth during embryogenesis, but likely plays a critical role in pathological processes leading to cardiac hypertrophy and failure as well [38]. Importantly, moderate levels of Gαq signaling induce myocardial hypertrophy, while chronic and sustained activation caused cardiomyocyte death and HF through downstream activation of p38-MAPK

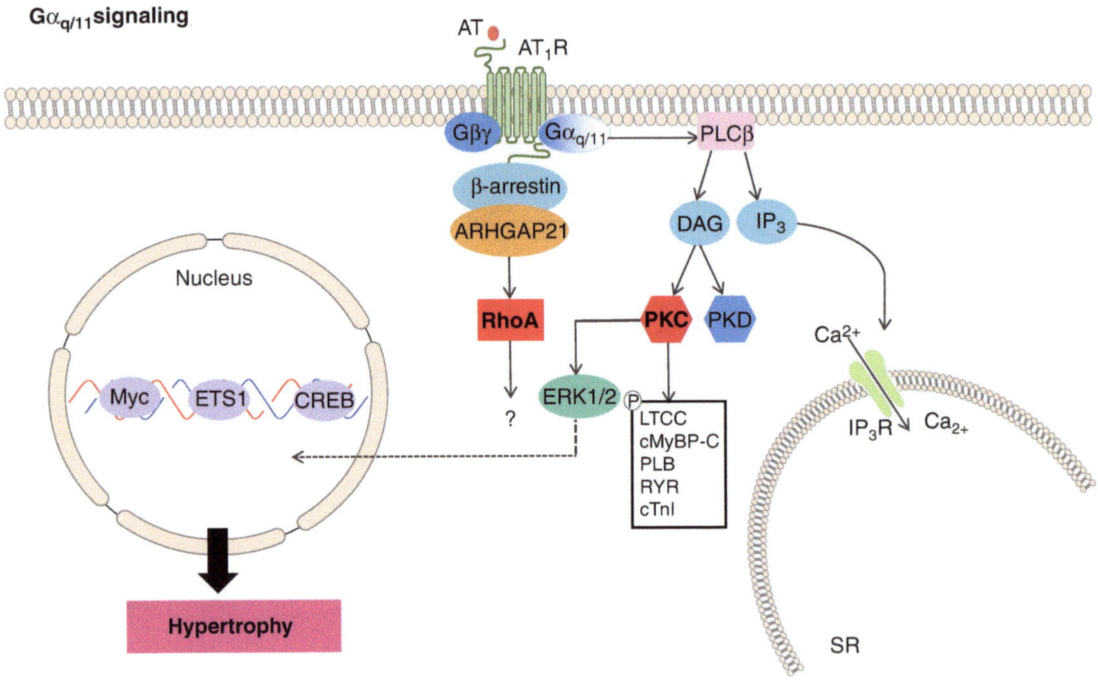

Fig. 10.4 Gαq/11 signaling. The AT1R is Gαq/11 coupled. Upon AT1R stimulation, PLCβ mediated generation of DAG and IP3 follows. IP3 induces IP3 receptor-mediated release of Ca^{2+} from the SR and is required to activate the downstream effectors CaMKII and calcineurin to drive hypertrophic transcription and induce cardiac contractility. DAG activates PKC and PKD. PKC leads to phosphorylation of LTCCs, cardiac myosin binding protein C, phospholamban, ryanodine receptor and cardiac troponin T, increasing cardiomyocyte contractility. In addition, increased ERK1/2 activity, leads to increased cellular transcription and cardiac hypertrophy results

and Janus kinases/signal transducer and activators of transcription (JAK/STAT) signaling pathways [39].

Therapeutically, it has been demonstrated that angiotensin-converting-enzyme inhibitors (ACEIs) are beneficial in hypertensive patients, as well as in patients with acute myocardial infarction (MI), chronic systolic HF, stroke and diabetic renal disease, specifically by targeting GPCR signaling [40]. Patients treated with ramipril, an ACEI, have improved clinical outcomes, with diminished left ventricular dysfunction, and reduced rates of death, myocardial infarction, and stroke [41]. Importantly, these data demonstrate a role for Ang II-mediated Gαq signaling in the development of cardiac hypertrophy and failure; however, the data also imply that the potential for targeted therapeutic interventions also exists, likely through specific inhibition of the Gαq downstream signaling effectors.

10.2.2.4 Gα12/13 Signaling

The most recently identified class of heterotrimeric G proteins is the Gα12/13 family. Gα13 was first identified as an oncogene, and overexpression of GTPase-deficient Gα12 or Gα13 altered cell shape, gene expression, and cell growth [42]. It is now clear that these responses resulted, at least in part, from activation of the small G protein Rho [43, 44] .

The Rho family of small G proteins includes more than 18 members, the best characterized of which are RhoA, Rac1, and Cdc42. A molecular link between the Gα12/13 family and RhoA was recently identified through work demonstrating that p115RhoGEF binds Gα12/13 proteins and is activated by Gα13 [43, 44] (Fig. 10.5). Similar interactions were shown for other GEFs, e.g., PDZRhoGEF and LARG, and Gα13 [42]. Interestingly, there is also evidence to suggest that signaling via AT1R-Gα12/13-mediated

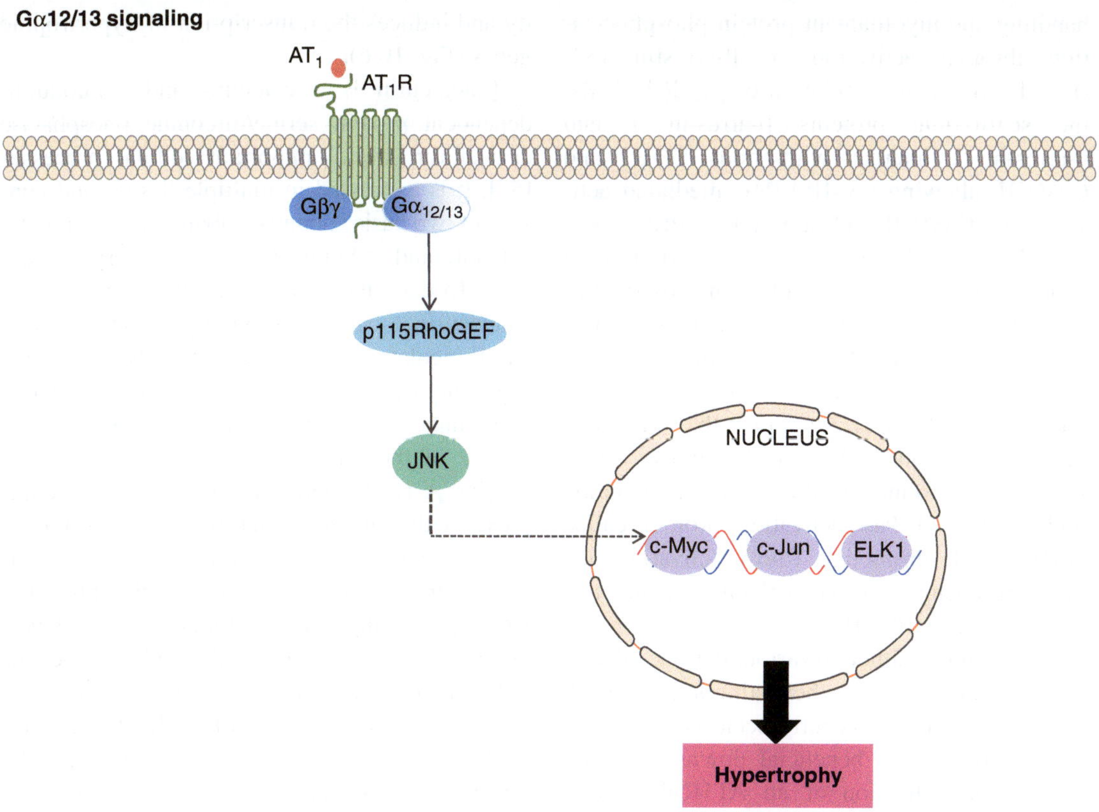

Fig. 10.5 Gα12/13 signaling. Stimulation of Gα12/13-coupled AT1R leads to p115RhoGEF mediated activation of JNK, which subsequently binds to nuclear transcription factors, increasing the expression of several hypertrophic genes, leading to cardiac muscle hypertrophy

p115RhoGEF contributes specifically to activation of JNK-MAPK in response to both phenylephrine (PE) [45] and ET1 [46] (Fig. 10.5). Interestingly, GPCRs that couple to Gα12/13 also couple to (and signal through) other sub-classes, often Gαq/11.

10.2.2.5 β-Arrestins and Desensitization Signaling

Normally, the cell has mechanisms in place to turn GPCR signaling off. This inactivation can occur by one of two ways: The first is vesicular translocation, where the GPCR is engulfed by a clathrin-coated vesicle, removed from the membrane, disassembled from its agonist, and then is either recycled or degraded [47]. The second consequence is β-arrestin linking; here, the GPCR becomes phosphorylated by a G protein-coupled receptor kinase (GRK), recruiting β-arrestin and blocking further communication between the G protein and the GPCR agonist [48] (Figs. 10.2 and 10.4). This latter mechanism is termed desensitization [49]. In many cases, binding of β-arrestin to the receptor is a prerequisite for translocation. For example, β-arrestin bound to β2-ARS acts as an adaptor for binding with clathrin and with the beta-subunit of AP2 (clathrin adaptor molecules); thus, the arrestin here acts as a scaffold assembling the components needed for clathrin-mediated endocytosis of β2-adrenoreceptors [50].

Activity of GRKs and subcellular targeting is tightly regulated by interaction with receptor domains, G protein subunits, lipids, anchoring proteins and calcium-sensitive proteins [51]. In the myocardium, the β-adrenergic signaling exchange protein activated by cAMP (EPAC) plays a critical role in regulating cardiomyocyte handling and myofilament protein phosphorylation through activation of β-arrestin [52] (Fig. 10.2). Upon stimulation of β1AR in CMs, the scaffolding proteins β-arrestin 1 and β-arrestin 2 interact with both EPAC and CaMKII, allowing cAMP-EPAC-mediated activation of CaMKII and subsequent PLB phosphorylation and regulation of heart muscle contraction [30] . In addition, β-arrestin-dependent β1AR-mediated epidermal growth factor receptor (EGFR) transactivation decreases cardiac apoptosis, possibly via internalization of a β1AR-EGFR-ERK1/2 complex that directs an unknown cytosolic cell survival response. AT1R stimulation also induces β-arrestin-1 association with a Rho GTPase-activating protein called ARHGAP21, promoting RhoA activation and inducing changes in cytoskeletal structure and cell shape [53] (Fig. 10.4).

Interestingly, although various cardiac GPCRs have negative effects when stimulated chronically, β-arrestin has recently been recognized to mediate potentially beneficial downstream signaling. Internalization of an AT1R-β-arrestin-ERK1/2 complex has been shown to increase MAP kinase-interacting kinase-1 activation, enhancing eukaryotic translation of initiation factor-4E-mediated mRNA translation and contributing to the compensatory increase in cell size and protein content in response to hypertrophic stimuli. In addition, AT1R-β-arrestin-ERK1/2-mediated activation of ribosomal S6 kinase (rS6K) inhibits BAD-induced apoptosis, which could contribute to increased cardiomyocyte cell survival [30].

10.2.2.6 Calcineurin/NFAT Signaling

There is a clear correlation between force production and perturbation of Ca^{2+} regulation, alterations of which might directly induce pathological, anatomical, and functional alterations that lead to HF. Importantly, GPCR signaling leads to activation of PLC, inducing Ca^{2+} release from the sarcoplasmic reticulum (SR) which activates calmodulin, phosphorylates calcineurin, and, ultimately, modulates sarcomeric contractility and induces the transcription of hypertrophic genes (Fig. 10.6).

Calcineurin is a calcium- and calmodulin-dependent protein serine/threonine phosphatase critical for several important cellular processes [54]. It is expressed in multiple tissues and consists of two basic subunits: subunit A, the catalytic subunit; and subunit B, the regulatory subunit [54]. To date, there have been three mammalian calcineurin A catalytic subunit genes (a, b, c) and two B regulatory subunit genes (B1, B2) identified [55]. Importantly, calcineurin is uniquely activated by sustained elevations in intracellular Ca^{2+} [56].

Use of the immunosuppressive drugs cyclosporine A (CsA) and FK506, which form complexes with immunophilin protein and thus inhibit calcineurin catalytic activity, essentially have elucidated the physiological role for this phosphatase. Specifically, when cytoplasmic Ca^{2+} levels increase inside the cell, calmodulin associates with calcineurin, thereby activating the enzyme [17]. Consequently, cytosolic NFAT becomes dephosphorylated, allowing it to translocate to the nucleus where it can participate in mediating calcium-inducible gene expression [57] (Fig. 10.6).

To help modulate the signal, kinases such as ERK1/2, JNK, p38, glycogen synthase kinase-3β (GSK3β) and casein kinase I (CKI), casein kinase II (CKII), and PKA phosphorylate NFAT family members, antagonizing nuclear translocation [58]. In addition, many of the same kinases also participate in re-phosphorylating NFAT within the nucleus, aiding in extrusion of NFAT back into the cytosol [58]. Indeed, transgenic mice that overexpresses activated forms of calcineurin or NFAT3 in the heart develop cardiac hypertrophy that progresses rapidly to dilation, with interstitial fibrosis, congestive HF, and sudden death [59]. However, use of CsA and FK 506 block the ability of cultured CMs to undergo hypertrophy in response to AngII and PE stimulation [59]. Furthermore, CsA administration prevents cardiac hypertrophy and the associated pathology in calcineurin transgenic mice, suggesting calcineurin activation exacerbates hypertrophic signals and expedites the transition to dilation.

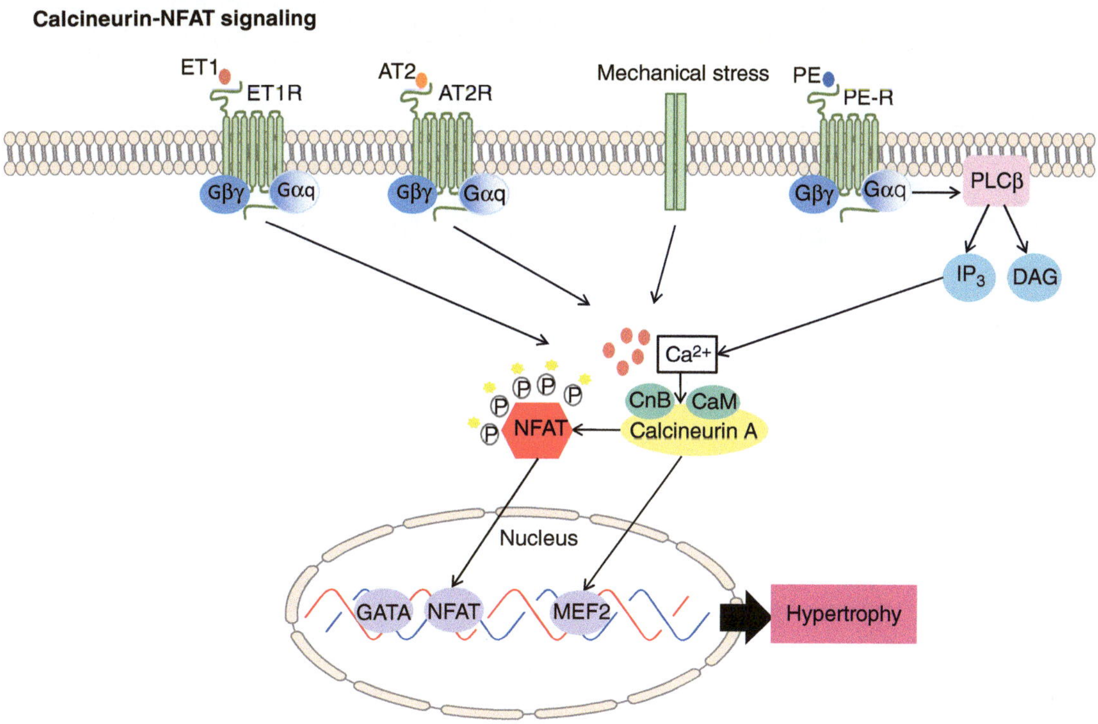

Fig. 10.6 Calcineurin/NFAT signaling. Upon stimulation of Gαq coupled receptors (i.e., ET1R, AT2R, or PE) or mechanical stress, the levels of intracellular calcium increase. Calcium then binds to calmodulin, thereby activating calcineurin through sustained elevations in intracellular calcium. This leads to nuclear localization of NFAT transcription factors as well as direct activation of nuclear MEF2 factors. Subsequent cardiac muscle hypertrophy follows

Together, these results define a novel signaling pathway that couples hypertrophic signals at the cell membrane to changes in cardiac gene expression and suggests possible opportunities for pharmacologic intervention to prevent cardiac hypertrophy and HF [17].

Several endogenous calcineurin inhibitors exist, including AKAP79, Cabin/Cain-1, and DSCR/MCIP [60, 61]. Specifically, AKAP79 interacts with calcineurin, PKA, and PKC to serve as a scaffold that integrates these signaling pathways [62]. Cain/Cabin-1 is a 230-kDa protein highly expressed in the brain that contains a potent noncompetitive calcineurin inhibitory domain in its C terminus [60, 61]. The fact that neither AKAP79 nor Cain is expressed at significant levels in the heart suggests that they are not physiologic regulators of cardiac calcineurin activity [63]. On the other hand, MCIP1 and MCIP2 (DSCR1 and ZAKI-4) were recently identified calcineurin inhibitory genes shown to be highly expressed in the myocardium, potentially representing physiologic regulators of calcineurin activity in cardiac muscle [14].

10.2.2.7 MAPK Signaling

Nearly all MAPK signaling components (upstream and downstream) are activated in end-stage human HF and are subdivided into three main branches consisting of p38 kinases, JNKs, and ERK1/2 and ERK5 [15]. The MAPK signaling cascade is classically initiated by activation of small G proteins in response to both RTK-mediated and GPCR-mediated activation. However, the functional outcome of specific MAPK activation can be modulated and altered by scaffolds in a specific spatiotemporal pattern [64] (Fig. 10.7). This complexity leads to different phenotypes ranging from "physiological" compensated hypertrophy and cardioprotection to

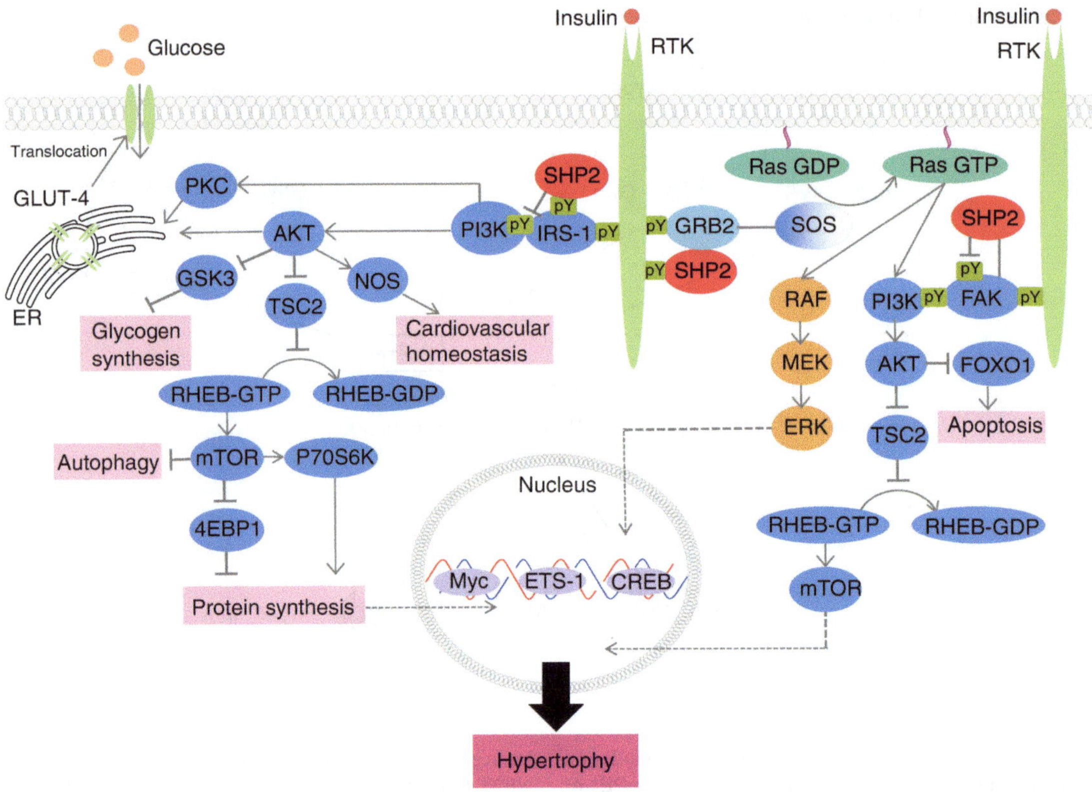

Fig. 10.7 Signaling pathways leading to SHP2-dependent signaling pathways leading to hypertrophy. When an RTK, such as insulin, binds to the receptor, both ERK/MAPK and PI3K/AKT signaling ensues. Importantly, ERK/MAPK translocates to the nucleus where it binds to transcription factors necessary to induce cardiac hypertrophy. The PI3K/AKT pathway will lead to the downstream activation of glycogen synthesis, autophagy and protein synthesis, culminating in mechanisms that can lead to cardiac hypertrophy. The PI3K pathway is also important in regulating the metabolic effects of insulin signaling. Stimulation of PKC and AKT by PI3K leads to translocation of GLUT-4 from the endoplasmic reticulum to the plasma membrane to mediate glucose metabolism in the cardiomyocyte

pathological HCM and cardiac remodeling, determined by the level, duration, mode, and timing of induction involving different isoforms and upstream/downstream pathways [64].

Pharmacologic inhibition of MAPK-signaling has demonstrated a necessary role for p38, JNK and ERK1/2 signaling in mediating hypertrophic growth of cultured CMs [65, 66]. In mice, constitutive activation of ERK1/2 signaling in the heart through expression of activated MEK1 causes a concentric type of hypertrophy [67]. In contrast, cardiac-specific inhibition of ERK1/2, through either a constitutively active ERK1/2-dual-specificity phosphatase or combinatorial deletion of ERK1 and ERK2, induces cardiac dilation [15]. Interestingly, and in contrast to ERK1/2, the related MEK5-ERK5 branch of the MAPK cascade preferentially induces eccentric hypertrophy [15]. Transgenic mice with cardiomyocyte-specific overexpression of MEK5, which induces downstream ERK5 activation, develop cardiac dilation and decompensation with loss of contractile function [68].

The JNK and p38 MAPK kinases, are activated by MEK4/7 and MEK3/6, respectively. These MAPKs generally serve as more specialized transducers of stress or injury responses, hence their classification as stress-activated protein kinases. Overexpression of MKK6 (p38 activation) or MKK7 (JNK activation) in hearts of transgenic mice show severe cardiac dilation and HF [65, 66].

10.2.2.8 PI3K/AKT Signaling

Phosphatidylinositol kinases are phospho-lipids tethered at cellular membranes that contribute to the recruitment and activation of multiple signaling components. They play a particularly key role in cell survival pathways, in the regulation of gene expression and cell metabolism, as well as in the process of cell growth and differentiation [69]. PI3K activation via protein kinase C-dependent or cAMP-dependent pathways are essential for the hypertrophic growth of adult CMs [70] (Fig. 10.7). RTK stimulation by growth factors, such as the insulin-like growth factor-1 (IGF-1) and the platelet derived growth factor (PDGF), lead to activation of the PI3K signaling cascade [70]. In addition, GPCR activation of both α-adrenergic and β-adrenergic signaling can also activate this pathway [70, 71].

Akt is the major downstream effector of PI3K signaling, mediating many processes important to cardiac adaptation including protein synthesis, inhibition of apoptosis, and metabolism. For example, cardiomyocyte-specific overexpression of the constitutively active catalytic subunit of PI3K, p110α, induces physiological, not pathological, H [72]. Conversely, dominant negative p110α overexpression in the heart induces a non-pathological atrophy, even in the presence of Insulin-like growth factor 1 receptor (IGFR) overexpression and exercise training [72]. Cardiac-restricted loss of the lipid phosphatase, phosphatase and tensin homolog deleted on chromosome ten (PTEN), which increases phosphorylation of Akt and GSK-3β, also promotes heart growth and prevents the development of maladaptive ventricular remodeling, with preservation of angiogenesis and metabolic gene expression in response to pressure overload [73].

Akt1-null mice, however, display growth retardation and are refractory to physiological cardiac hypertrophy when subjected to exercise training. Similarly, overexpression of dominant negative Akt1 prevents hypertrophic growth of the heart [74]. Importantly, while acute cardiomyocyte-specific expression of a constitutively active Akt1 initially promotes a physiological type of hypertrophy, its prolonged activation is ultimately pathological [74, 75]. Taken together, these results indicate that acute Akt activation promotes an adaptive cellular growth program in the heart, but that sustained Akt signaling leads to pathological hypertrophy and heart failure [76]. Indeed, the mediators of PI3K/Akt-induced hypertrophy are two well-defined direct downstream targets: GSK3β and the mammalian target of rapamycin (mTOR) [14].

10.2.2.9 GSK3 Signaling

GSK3, of which there are two isoforms, GSK3α and GSK3β, was originally characterized in the context of regulation of glycogen metabolism, though it is now known to regulate many other cellular processes and thus, is an emerging important therapeutic target in a variety of pathologies. In the heart, emphasis has been placed particularly on GSK3β rather than GSK3α; catalytically-active GSK3β has been directly implicated in anti-hypertrophic signaling. Conversely, inhibition of GSK3 alters the transcriptional and translational machinery in the heart, inducing hypertrophic responses.

GSK-3β is unphosphorylated and constitutively active in the healthy heart; phosphorylation of GSK-3β by AKT inactivates it, inducing hypertrophy [77] (Fig. 10.7). In mouse models, overexpression of activated GSK-3β causes a reduction in heart size and decreases hypertrophy in response to pathological stimuli. Moreover, in genetic models of HCM with mutations in sarcomeric proteins, GSK-3β is inactivated, consistent with hypertrophy in these models and demonstrated downstream alterations in AKT.

10.2.2.10 mTOR Signaling

The second downstream effector of PI3K/Akt activation in hypertrophy is mTOR, a key serine/threonine kinase that functions as both a positive regulator of cell growth and protein synthesis and negative regulator of a process called autophagy [78]. Rapamycin is an immunosuppressive drug that binds to its intracellular receptor FKBP12 and forms a complex which subsequently inhibits mTOR activity. Inhibition of mTOR results in impaired protein synthesis and decreased cell size via inhibition of its downstream effectors, p70S6 kinase and 4EBP1/eIF4E [79] (Fig. 10.7).

In addition, rapamycin also attenuates cardiac hypertrophy that is secondary to constitutive activation of Akt, completely blocking the increase in cardiomyocyte size that normally results as a consequence of oxidative stress, treatment with PE or AngII, or fetal calf serum [14, 74, 80].

10.2.2.11 Autophagy

CMs are intricately involved in autophagy, the catabolic process of regulating the synthesis, degradation and recycling of a cell's own components through lysosomal machinery [81]. While autophagy is a normal process that occurs in cells, it can be further induced by cellular stress, such as nutrient deprivation [82]. The PI3K signaling pathway, through its activation of mTOR, is a key negative regulator of this process [83] (Fig. 10.7).

Autolysosomal degradation of membrane lipids and proteins through autophagy generates fatty acids (Fas) and amino acids, which are reused by the cell to maintain mitochondrial ATP production and protein synthesis, thereby promoting cell survival [82]. Interestingly, autophagy also promotes programmed cell death in some circumstances, although the mechanism for this dual-functionality in the heart remains unclear [84].

Autophagy plays a dual role in cardiac function as well. Increased autophagy is observed in acute and chronic ischemia, end-stage HF, and aging hearts [85]. Acute activation of autophagy under a wide range of pathological conditions appears initially compensatory and critical for proper maintenance of cardiac metabolism and cellular homeostasis [86]. However, in response to chronic stress, when autophagy is excessive, HF ensues, likely due to the decline in both number and function of mitochondria, and a perturbation in cardiomyocyte metabolic flux [86]. Additional work is needed to fully define the profit and loss conferred by autophagy in cardiac hypertrophy and failure [86].

10.2.3 Diabetes and Obesity: Role of Leptin Signaling

Recent studies suggest that obesity, hypertension, and diabetes confer increased risk for structural heart disease. Leptin, the obesity gene product, is a 16 kDa protein monomer produced mainly by adipocytes but also other sources as well, including the heart [87]. Leptin suppresses appetite via central mechanisms and plays a key role in the regulation of body weight and metabolism. Recent evidence has shown that leptin exerts a negative inotropic effect in isolated CMs [88]. Interestingly, leptin causes hypertrophy in cultured neonatal rat ventricular myocytes [89]. Still, other studies have demonstrated that infusion of leptin has antihypertrophic effects in mice [90]. MAPK [91], JAK/STAT [92], and nitric oxide (NO) [93] signaling pathways have each been implicated in mediating some of the biological actions of leptin on heart disease (Fig. 10.7).

Like stretch, binding of leptin to its receptor activates downstream signaling pathways that result in activation of ERK1/2 and subsequent activation of both the angiotensin and endothelin systems. The hypertrophic response occurs as a consequence of transcriptional activation of genes mediated by AngII or ET-1 stimulation of AT1 or ET1 receptors, respectively, and the subsequent ERK1/2 activation that ensues. Use of the AT1R antagonist, losartan, or the endothelin-A (ETA) receptor antagonist, BQ123, blocks hypertrophy. Similarly, by preventing Ang II or endothelin-1 synthesis with an ACE inhibitor such as captopril, or with an endothelin converting enzyme (ECE) inhibitor such as PPRD, hypertrophy is also abrogated [94].

10.3 Role of Non-cardiomyocyte Cells in Myocardial Hypertroply

10.3.1 Cardiac Fibroblasts

Cardiac fibroblasts (CFs), together with their activated form as myofibroblasts, are the most abundant cell type in the myocardium. They have multiple functional roles, in both cardiac development and disease, a function through regulation of structural, paracrine, and electrical interactions with CMs [95].

The primary function of fibroblasts is to produce structural extracellular matrix (ECM) proteins, with a particularly critical focus on wound healing. As such, they play a key role in modulating myocardial hypertrophy and HF; in mice, they have a demonstrated role in regulating hypertrophic myocardial responses to pressure overload [96]. "Cardiac fibroblasts produce a variety of pro-hypertrophic paracrine factors such as cytokines, such as TNF, IL-6, IL1, and growth factors, including PDGF and IGF-1" [97].

10.3.1.1 Extracellular Matrix

As mentioned above, the primary function of cardiac fibroblasts is to produce the ECM, which is a network structure that provides structural and functional integrity to the heart. ECM is mainly comprised of fibrillar collagen types I and III, as well as less abundant collagen types IV, V and VI. ECM also includes fibronectin, laminin, elastin and fibrillin, proteoglycans and glycoproteins. CFs are the primary source of all of these ECM proteins.

ECM plays a critical role in mediating the mechanical connection among the CMs, CFs, and the blood vessels within the heart. It is through ECM that extracellular mechanical signals are transmitted to the CMs [98]. A number of growth factors such as PDGF, basic fibroblast growth factor (b-FGF) and transforming growth factor-β (TGFβ), can induce ECM proteins during cardiac development and disease [99].

The increased numbers of non-myocyte cells and extracellular matrix proteins contribute to cardiac fibrosis and progressive HF [100]. Numerous studies have demonstrated that both systemic and myocardial TGF-β levels are increased in patients with many forms of myocardial involvement. Specifically, increased TGF-β levels are observed in fibrotic hearts [85]. Patients with idiopathic HCM also have upregulated TGF-β in their hearts [101]. The latter is also observed in patients with aortic stenosis [102], with increased TGF-β1 levels associated with higher transvalvular gradients and worse hypertrophy [103]. Recently, it was shown that increased serum TGF-β1 levels are correlated with increased left ventricular mass in subjects with increased blood pressure [104], suggesting this may be a useful disease prognostic for the severity of myocardial hypertrophy in patients.

Full significance of TGF-β signaling in human cardiac hypertrophy and fibrosis remains to be elucidated. Evolving evidence suggests that TGF-β is critically involved in cardiac injury, repair and remodeling. TGF-β1 heterozygous mutant mice exhibit less age-associated myocardial fibrosis and diastolic disease than normal mice, with ameliorated age-associated myocardial fibrosis and improved LV compliance [105].

The renin–angiotensin system is a key mediator in the development of cardiac hypertrophy and HF [106]. Importantly, TGF-β1 acts downstream of Ang II to promote CM growth [104]. Ang II induces the expression of TGF-β1 in cardiac myocytes and fibroblasts [107], activating fibroblasts and enhancing production and deposition of ECM proteins between CMs. Autocrine/paracrine mechanisms play a critical role in this process [108].

10.3.2 Endothelial Cells

Cardiac endothelial cells (ECs) play a key role in regulating and maintaining cardiac function in the endocardium. In the myocardial capillaries, ECs directly interact with adjacent CMs. This interaction is a prerequisite for normal cardiac development and growth and is governed by molecular mechanisms and cellular signals, such as neuregulin, vascular endothelial growth factor (VEGF), and angiopoietin, that continue to maintain the phenotype and survival of CMs in the adult heart [109].

NO, ET1, prostaglandin I2, and AngII, directly influence cardiac metabolism, growth, contractile performance, and rhythmicity of the adult heart. These autocrine and paracrine agents are expressed and released by cardiac ECs [110]. ET-1 is a vasoconstrictor secreted primarily by ECs and also by macrophages, fibroblasts and CMs in response to mechanical and chemical stimuli [111]. Vascular ECS can release these agents as well. It has been showed that peripheral endothelial dysfunction is an early finding in the progression of HF [112].

10.3.3 Vascular Smooth Muscle Cells

Both contractile and synthetic functions can be performed by vascular smooth muscle cells (VSMCs), which are associated with and characterized by changes in morphology, proliferation and migration rates, and the expression of different marker proteins. By contraction and relaxation, they alter their luminal diameter, and enable blood vessels to maintain an appropriate blood pressure [113].

10.4 Future Directions

The incidence and prevalence of heart failure is still increasing, underscoring the need for agents that act earlier, target more specifically, or are more effective. Pathological signaling pathways discussed here fit a central theme of emerging pathways causing and/or potentiating cardiac hypertrophy, including the G-protein coupled, the calcineurin/NFAT, MAPK, and the PI3K/AKT/mTOR signaling pathways. Importantly, these signaling pathways control vital molecular processes, such as cell proliferation, differentiation, survival, migration and other functions. Understanding the regulatory and functional mechanisms of these pathways in the heart will allow us to better understand ways to design more specific and targeted therapies to cardiac disease and end-stage heart failure.

References

1. Rapila R, Korhonen T, Tavi P. Excitation-contraction coupling of the mouse embryonic cardiomyocyte. J Gen Physiol. 2008;132:397–405.
2. Bootman MD, Higazi DR, Coombes S, Roderick HL. Calcium signalling during excitation-contraction coupling in mammalian atrial myocytes. J Cell Sci. 2006;119:3915–25.
3. McDowell SA, McCall E, Matter WF, Estridge TB, Vlahos CJ. Phosphoinositide 3-kinase regulates excitation-contraction coupling in neonatal cardiomyocytes. Am J Physiol Heart Circ Physiol. 2004;286:H796–805.
4. Kontaridis MI, Geladari EV, Geladari CV. Role of the shp2 protein tyrosine phosphatase in cardiac metabolism. In: Bence KK, editor. Protein tyrosine phosphatase control of metabolism. London: Springer; 2013. p. 147–67.
5. Levy D, Labib SB, Anderson KM, Christiansen JC, Kannel WB, Castelli WP. Determinants of sensitivity and specificity of electrocardiographic criteria for left ventricular hypertrophy. Circulation. 1990; 81:815–20.
6. Badeer HS. Biological significance of cardiac hypertrophy. Am J Cardiol. 1964;14:133–8.
7. Mihl C, Dassen WR, Kuipers H. Cardiac remodelling: concentric versus eccentric hypertrophy in strength and endurance athletes. Neth Heart J. 2008;16:129–33.
8. Grossman W, Jones D, McLaurin LP. Wall stress and patterns of hypertrophy in the human left ventricle. J Clin Invest. 1975;56:56–64.
9. van Nierop BJ, van Assen HC, van Deel ED, Niesen LB, Duncker DJ, Strijkers GJ, et al. Phenotyping of left and right ventricular function in mouse models of compensated hypertrophy and heart failure with cardiac MRI. PLoS One. 2013;8:e55424.
10. Hunter JJ, Chien KR. Signaling pathways for cardiac hypertrophy and failure. N Engl J Med. 1999;341: 1276–83.
11. Harvey PA, Leinwand LA. The cell biology of disease: cellular mechanisms of cardiomyopathy. J Cell Biol. 2011;194:355–65.
12. Maron BJ. Hypertrophic cardiomyopathy: a systematic review. JAMA. 2002;287:1308–20.
13. Arad M, Penas-Lado M, Monserrat L, Maron BJ, Sherrid M, Ho CY, et al. Gene mutations in apical hypertrophic cardiomyopathy. Circulation. 2005; 112:2805–11.
14. Frey N, Olson EN. Cardiac hypertrophy: the good, the bad, and the ugly. Annu Rev Physiol. 2003; 65:45–79.
15. van Berlo JH, Maillet M, Molkentin JD. Signaling effectors underlying pathologic growth and remodeling of the heart. J Clin Invest. 2013;123:37–45.
16. Muslin AJ. MAPK signalling in cardiovascular health and disease: molecular mechanisms and therapeutic targets. Clin Sci (Lond). 2008;115:203–18.
17. Wilkins BJ, Molkentin JD. Calcineurin and cardiac hypertrophy: where have we been? where are we going? J Physiol. 2002;541:1–8.
18. Anderson ME, Brown JH, Bers DM. CaMKII in myocardial hypertrophy and heart failure. J Mol Cell Cardiol. 2011;51:468–73.
19. Ashrafian H, Redwood C, Blair E, Watkins H. Hypertrophic cardiomyopathy: a paradigm for myocardial energy depletion. Trends Genet. 2003; 19:263–8.
20. Bjarnadottir TK, Gloriam DE, Hellstrand SH, Kristiansson H, Fredriksson R, Schioth HB. Comprehensive repertoire and phylogenetic analysis of the g protein-coupled receptors in human and mouse. Genomics. 2006;88:263–73.

21. Wettschureck N, Offermanns S. Mammalian g proteins and their cell type specific functions. Physiol Rev. 2005;85:1159–204.
22. Hamm HE. The many faces of g protein signaling. J Biol Chem. 1998;273:669–72.
23. Clapham DE, Neer EJ. New roles for g-protein beta gamma-dimers in transmembrane signalling. Nature. 1993;365:403–6.
24. Kobilka BK. G protein coupled receptor structure and activation. Biochim Biophys Acta. 2007;1768: 794–807.
25. Salazar NC, Chen J, Rockman HA. Cardiac gpcrs: Gpcr signaling in healthy and failing hearts. Biochim Biophys Acta. 2007;1768:1006–18.
26. Madamanchi A. Beta-adrenergic receptor signaling in cardiac function and heart failure. McGill J Med. 2007;10:99–104.
27. Rockman HA, Koch WJ, Lefkowitz RJ. Seven-transmembrane-spanning receptors and heart function. Nature. 2002;415:206–12.
28. Xiang Y, Kobilka BK. Myocyte adrenoceptor signaling pathways. Science. 2003;300:1530–2.
29. Mauban JR, O'Donnell M, Warrier S, Manni S, Bond M. Akap-scaffolding proteins and regulation of cardiac physiology. Physiology (Bethesda). 2009;24:78–87.
30. Tilley DG. G protein-dependent and g protein-independent signaling pathways and their impact on cardiac function. Circ Res. 2011;109:217–30.
31. Yoshida H, Kakuchi J, Yoshikawa N, Saruta T, Inagami T, Phillips 3rd JA, Ichikawa I. Angiotensin ii type 1 receptor gene abnormality in a patient with Bartter's syndrome. Kidney Int. 1994;46:1505–9.
32. Sadoshima J, Xu Y, Slayter HS, Izumo S. Autocrine release of angiotensin ii mediates stretch-induced hypertrophy of cardiac myocytes in vitro. Cell. 1993;75:977–84.
33. Nicol RL, Frey N, Olson EN. From the sarcomere to the nucleus: role of genetics and signaling in structural heart disease. Annu Rev Genomics Hum Genet. 2000;1:179–223.
34. Feuerstein GZ, Rozanski D. G proteins and heart failure: is galphaq a novel target for heart failure? Circ Res. 2000;87:1085–6.
35. Mishra S, Ling H, Grimm M, Zhang T, Bers DM, Brown JH. Cardiac hypertrophy and heart failure development through gq and cam kinase ii signaling. J Cardiovasc Pharmacol. 2010;56:598–603.
36. D'Angelo DD, Sakata Y, Lorenz JN, Boivin GP, Walsh RA, Liggett SB, Dorn 2nd GW. Transgenic galphaq overexpression induces cardiac contractile failure in mice. Proc Natl Acad Sci U S A. 1997;94:8121–6.
37. Paradis P, Dali-Youcef N, Paradis FW, Thibault G, Nemer M. Overexpression of angiotensin ii type i receptor in cardiomyocytes induces cardiac hypertrophy and remodeling. Proc Natl Acad Sci U S A. 2000;97:931–6.
38. Offermanns S, Zhao LP, Gohla A, Sarosi I, Simon MI, Wilkie TM. Embryonic cardiomyocyte hypoplasia and craniofacial defects in g alpha q/g alpha 11-mutant mice. EMBO J. 1998;17:4304–12.
39. Adams JW, Sakata Y, Davis MG, Sah VP, Wang Y, Liggett SB, et al. Enhanced galphaq signaling: a common pathway mediates cardiac hypertrophy and apoptotic heart failure. Proc Natl Acad Sci U S A. 1998;95:10140–5.
40. Chrysant SG. Current status of dual renin angiotensin aldosterone system blockade for the treatment of cardiovascular diseases. Am J Cardiol. 2010;105: 849–52.
41. Yusuf S, Sleight P, Pogue J, Bosch J, Davies R, Dagenais G. Effects of an angiotensin-converting-enzyme inhibitor, ramipril, on cardiovascular events in high-risk patients. The Heart Outcomes Prevention Evaluation Study Investigators. N Engl J Med. 2000;342:145–53.
42. Radeff-Huang J, Seasholtz TM, Matteo RG, Brown JH. G protein mediated signaling pathways in lysophospholipid induced cell proliferation and survival. J Cell Biochem. 2004;92:949–66.
43. Hart MJ, Jiang X, Kozasa T, Roscoe W, Singer WD, Gilman AG, et al. Direct stimulation of the guanine nucleotide exchange activity of p115 rhogef by galpha13. Science. 1998;280:2112–4.
44. Kozasa T, Jiang X, Hart MJ, Sternweis PM, Singer WD, Gilman AG, et al. P115 rhogef, a gtpase activating protein for galpha12 and galpha13. Science. 1998;280:2109–11.
45. Maruyama Y, Nishida M, Sugimoto Y, Tanabe S, Turner JH, Kozasa T, et al. Galpha(12/13) mediates alpha(1)-adrenergic receptor-induced cardiac hypertrophy. Circ Res. 2002;91:961–9.
46. Arai K, Maruyama Y, Nishida M, Tanabe S, Takagahara S, Kozasa T, et al. Differential requirement of g alpha12, g alpha13, g alphaq, and g beta gamma for endothelin-1-induced c-jun nh2-terminal kinase and extracellular signal-regulated kinase activation. Mol Pharmacol. 2003;63:478–88.
47. Krueger KM, Daaka Y, Pitcher JA, Lefkowitz RJ. The role of sequestration in g protein-coupled receptor resensitization. Regulation of beta2-adrenergic receptor dephosphorylation by vesicular acidification. J Biol Chem. 1997;272:5–8.
48. Penela P, Murga C, Ribas C, Tutor AS, Peregrin S, Mayor Jr F. Mechanisms of regulation of g protein-coupled receptor kinases (grks) and cardiovascular disease. Cardiovasc Res. 2006;69:46–56.
49. Oakley RH, Laporte SA, Holt JA, Barak LS, Caron MG. Association of beta-arrestin with g protein-coupled receptors during clathrin-mediated endocytosis dictates the profile of receptor resensitization. J Biol Chem. 1999;274:32248–57.
50. Laporte SA, Oakley RH, Holt JA, Barak LS, Caron MG. The interaction of beta-arrestin with the ap-2 adaptor is required for the clustering of beta 2-adrenergic receptor into clathrin-coated pits. J Biol Chem. 2000;275:23120–6.
51. Penela P, Ribas C, Mayor Jr F. Mechanisms of regulation of the expression and function of g protein-

coupled receptor kinases. Cell Signal. 2003;15:973–81.
52. Metrich M, Berthouze M, Morel E, Crozatier B, Gomez AM, Lezoualc'h F. Role of the camp-binding protein epac in cardiovascular physiology and pathophysiology. Pflugers Arch. 2010;459:535–46.
53. Anthony DF, Sin YY, Vadrevu S, Advant N, Day JP, Byrne AM, et al. Beta-arrestin 1 inhibits the gtpase-activating protein function of arhgap21, promoting activation of rhoa following angiotensin ii type 1a receptor stimulation. Mol Cell Biol. 2011;31:1066–75.
54. Kissinger CR, Parge HE, Knighton DR, Lewis CT, Pelletier LA, Tempczyk A, et al. Crystal structures of human calcineurin and the human fkbp12-fk506-calcineurin complex. Nature. 1995;378:641–4.
55. Olson EN, Williams RS. Calcineurin signaling and muscle remodeling. Cell. 2000;101:689–92.
56. Crabtree GR. Generic signals and specific outcomes: signaling through Ca^{2+}, calcineurin, and NF-AT. Cell. 1999;96:611–4.
57. Wilkins BJ, Dai YS, Bueno OF, Parsons SA, Xu J, Plank DM, et al. Calcineurin/nfat coupling participates in pathological, but not physiological, cardiac hypertrophy. Circ Res. 2004;94:110–8.
58. Molkentin JD. Calcineurin-nfat signaling regulates the cardiac hypertrophic response in coordination with the mapks. Cardiovasc Res. 2004;63:467–75.
59. Yamazaki T, Yazaki Y. Is there major involvement of the renin-angiotensin system in cardiac hypertrophy? Circ Res. 1997;81:639–42.
60. Lai MM, Burnett PE, Wolosker H, Blackshaw S, Snyder SH. Cain, a novel physiologic protein inhibitor of calcineurin. J Biol Chem. 1998;273:18325–31.
61. Sun L, Youn HD, Loh C, Stolow M, He W, Liu JO. Cabin 1, a negative regulator for calcineurin signaling in T lymphocytes. Immunity. 1998;8:703–11.
62. Coghlan VM, Perrino BA, Howard M, Langeberg LK, Hicks JB, Gallatin WM, Scott JD. Association of protein kinase A and protein phosphatase 2b with a common anchoring protein. Science. 1995;267:108–11.
63. De Windt LJ, Lim HW, Bueno OF, Liang Q, Delling U, Braz JC, et al. Targeted inhibition of calcineurin attenuates cardiac hypertrophy in vivo. Proc Natl Acad Sci U S A. 2001;98:3322–7.
64. Rose BA, Force T, Wang Y. Mitogen-activated protein kinase signaling in the heart: Angels versus demons in a heart-breaking tale. Physiol Rev. 2010;90:1507–46.
65. Liao P, Georgakopoulos D, Kovacs A, Zheng M, Lerner D, Pu H, et al. The in vivo role of p38 map kinases in cardiac remodeling and restrictive cardiomyopathy. Proc Natl Acad Sci U S A. 2001;98:12283–8.
66. Wang Y, Su B, Sah VP, Brown JH, Han J, Chien KR. Cardiac hypertrophy induced by mitogen-activated protein kinase kinase 7, a specific activator for c-jun nh_2-terminal kinase in ventricular muscle cells. J Biol Chem. 1998;273:5423–6.
67. Bueno OF, De Windt LJ, Tymitz KM, Witt SA, Kimball TR, Klevitsky R, et al. The mek1-erk1/2 signaling pathway promotes compensated cardiac hypertrophy in transgenic mice. EMBO J. 2000;19:6341–50.
68. Nicol RL, Frey N, Pearson G, Cobb M, Richardson J, Olson EN. Activated MEK5 induces serial assembly of sarcomeres and eccentric cardiac hypertrophy. EMBO J. 2001;20:2757–67.
69. Cantley LC. The phosphoinositide 3-kinase pathway. Science. 2002;296:1655–7.
70. Schluter KD, Goldberg Y, Taimor G, Schafer M, Piper HM. Role of phosphatidylinositol 3-kinase activation in the hypertrophic growth of adult ventricular cardiomyocytes. Cardiovasc Res. 1998;40:174–81.
71. Chesley A, Lundberg MS, Asai T, Xiao RP, Ohtani S, Lakatta EG, Crow MT. The beta(2)-adrenergic receptor delivers an antiapoptotic signal to cardiac myocytes through g(i)-dependent coupling to phosphatidylinositol 3′-kinase. Circ Res. 2000;87:1172–9.
72. Shioi T, Kang PM, Douglas PS, Hampe J, Yballe CM, Lawitts J, et al. The conserved phosphoinositide 3-kinase pathway determines heart size in mice. EMBO J. 2000;19:2537–48.
73. Oudit GY, Kassiri Z, Zhou J, Liu QC, Liu PP, Backx PH, et al. Loss of pten attenuates the development of pathological hypertrophy and heart failure in response to biomechanical stress. Cardiovasc Res. 2008;78:505–14.
74. Shioi T, McMullen JR, Kang PM, Douglas PS, Obata T, Franke TF, et al. Akt/protein kinase b promotes organ growth in transgenic mice. Mol Cell Biol. 2002;22:2799–809.
75. Shiojima I, Sato K, Izumiya Y, Schiekofer S, Ito M, Liao R, et al. Disruption of coordinated cardiac hypertrophy and angiogenesis contributes to the transition to heart failure. J Clin Invest. 2005;115:2108–18.
76. Maillet M, van Berlo JH, Molkentin JD. Molecular basis of physiological heart growth: fundamental concepts and new players. Nat Rev Mol Cell Biol. 2013;14:38–48.
77. Sugden PH, Fuller SJ, Weiss SC, Clerk A. Glycogen synthase kinase 3 (gsk3) in the heart: a point of integration in hypertrophic signalling and a therapeutic target? A critical analysis. Br J Pharmacol. 2008;153 Suppl 1:S137–53.
78. Wullschleger S, Loewith R, Hall MN. Tor signaling in growth and metabolism. Cell. 2006;124:471–84.
79. Fingar DC, Salama S, Tsou C, Harlow E, Blenis J. Mammalian cell size is controlled by mtor and its downstream targets S6K1 and 4EBP1/eif4e. Genes Dev. 2002;16:1472–87.
80. Sadoshima J, Izumo S. Rapamycin selectively inhibits angiotensin ii-induced increase in protein synthesis in cardiac myocytes in vitro. Potential role of

70-kd s6 kinase in angiotensin ii-induced cardiac hypertrophy. Circ Res. 1995;77:1040–52.
81. Levine B, Klionsky DJ. Development by self-digestion: molecular mechanisms and biological functions of autophagy. Dev Cell. 2004;6:463–77.
82. Lum JJ, DeBerardinis RJ, Thompson CB. Autophagy in metazoans: cell survival in the land of plenty. Nat Rev Mol Cell Biol. 2005;6:439–48.
83. Ravikumar B, Vacher C, Berger Z, Davies JE, Luo S, Oroz LG, et al. Inhibition of mtor induces autophagy and reduces toxicity of polyglutamine expansions in fly and mouse models of Huntington disease. Nat Genet. 2004;36:585–95.
84. Matsui Y, Takagi H, Qu X, Abdellatif M, Sakoda H, Asano T, et al. Distinct roles of autophagy in the heart during ischemia and reperfusion: roles of AMP-activated protein kinase and Beclin 1 in mediating autophagy. Circ Res. 2007;100:914–22.
85. Hein S, Arnon E, Kostin S, Schonburg M, Elsasser A, Polyakova V, et al. Progression from compensated hypertrophy to failure in the pressure-overloaded human heart: structural deterioration and compensatory mechanisms. Circulation. 2003;107:984–91.
86. Wang ZV, Ferdous A, Hill JA. Cardiomyocyte autophagy: metabolic profit and loss. Heart Fail Rev. 2013;18:585–94.
87. Purdham DM, Zou MX, Rajapurohitam V, Karmazyn M. Rat heart is a site of leptin production and action. Am J Physiol Heart Circ Physiol. 2004;287: H2877–84.
88. Nickola MW, Wold LE, Colligan PB, Wang GJ, Samson WK, Ren J. Leptin attenuates cardiac contraction in rat ventricular myocytes. Role of NO. Hypertension. 2000;36:501–5.
89. Rajapurohitam V, Gan XT, Kirshenbaum LA, Karmazyn M. The obesity-associated peptide leptin induces hypertrophy in neonatal rat ventricular myocytes. Circ Res. 2003;93:277–9.
90. Tritos NA, Manning WJ, Danias PG. Role of leptin in the development of cardiac hypertrophy in experimental animals and humans. Circulation. 2004; 109:e67; author reply e67.
91. Banks AS, Davis SM, Bates SH, Myers Jr MG. Activation of downstream signals by the long form of the leptin receptor. J Biol Chem. 2000; 275:14563–72.
92. Ghilardi N, Skoda RC. The leptin receptor activates janus kinase 2 and signals for proliferation in a factor-dependent cell line. Mol Endocrinol. 1997;11:393–9.
93. Vecchione C, Maffei A, Colella S, Aretini A, Poulet R, Frati G, et al. Leptin effect on endothelial nitric oxide is mediated through Akt-endothelial nitric oxide synthase phosphorylation pathway. Diabetes. 2002;51:168–73.
94. Zeidan A, Purdham DM, Rajapurohitam V, Javadov S, Chakrabarti S, Karmazyn M. Leptin induces vascular smooth muscle cell hypertrophy through angiotensin II- and endothelin-1-dependent mechanisms and mediates stretch-induced hypertrophy. J Pharmacol Exp Ther. 2005;315:1075–84.
95. Ieda M, Tsuchihashi T, Ivey KN, Ross RS, Hong TT, Shaw RM, Srivastava D. Cardiac fibroblasts regulate myocardial proliferation through beta1 integrin signaling. Dev Cell. 2009;16:233–44.
96. Takeda N, Manabe I, Uchino Y, Eguchi K, Matsumoto S, Nishimura S, et al. Cardiac fibroblasts are essential for the adaptive response of the murine heart to pressure overload. J Clin Invest. 2010;120:254–65.
97. Vivar R, Humeres C, Varela M, Ayala P, Guzman N, Olmedo I, et al. Cardiac fibroblast death by ischemia/reperfusion is partially inhibited by IGF-1 through both PI3K/Akt and MEK-ERK pathways. Exp Mol Pathol. 2012;93:1–7.
98. Eghbali M. Cardiac fibroblasts: function, regulation of gene expression, and phenotypic modulation. Basic Res Cardiol. 1992;87 Suppl 2:183–9.
99. Fan D, Takawale A, Lee J, Kassiri Z. Cardiac fibroblasts, fibrosis and extracellular matrix remodeling in heart disease. Fibrogenesis Tissue Repair. 2012;5:15.
100. Basso C, Maron BJ, Corrado D, Thiene G. Clinical profile of congenital coronary artery anomalies with origin from the wrong aortic sinus leading to sudden death in young competitive athletes. J Am Coll Cardiol. 2000;35:1493–501.
101. Li RK, Li G, Mickle DA, Weisel RD, Merante F, Luss H, et al. Overexpression of transforming growth factor-beta1 and insulin-like growth factor-i in patients with idiopathic hypertrophic cardiomyopathy. Circulation. 1997;96:874–81.
102. Fielitz J, Hein S, Mitrovic V, Pregla R, Zurbrugg HR, Warnecke C, et al. Activation of the cardiac renin-angiotensin system and increased myocardial collagen expression in human aortic valve disease. J Am Coll Cardiol. 2001;37:1443–9.
103. Villar AV, Cobo M, Llano M, Montalvo C, Gonzalez-Vilchez F, Martin-Duran R, et al. Plasma levels of transforming growth factor-beta1 reflect left ventricular remodeling in aortic stenosis. PLoS One. 2009;4:e8476.
104. Dobaczewski M, Chen W, Frangogiannis NG. Transforming growth factor (tgf)-beta signaling in cardiac remodeling. J Mol Cell Cardiol. 2011;51: 600–6.
105. Brooks WW, Conrad CH. Myocardial fibrosis in transforming growth factor beta(1)heterozygous mice. J Mol Cell Cardiol. 2000;32:187–95.
106. Schnee JM, Hsueh WA. Angiotensin II, adhesion, and cardiac fibrosis. Cardiovasc Res. 2000;46: 264–8.
107. Campbell SE, Katwa LC. Angiotensin ii stimulated expression of transforming growth factor-beta1 in cardiac fibroblasts and myofibroblasts. J Mol Cell Cardiol. 1997;29:1947–58.
108. Rosenkranz S. TGF-beta1 and angiotensin networking in cardiac remodeling. Cardiovasc Res. 2004;63: 423–32.

109. Murphy JF, Fitzgerald DJ. Vascular endothelial growth factor induces cyclooxygenase-dependent proliferation of endothelial cells via the VEGF-2 receptor. FASEB J. 2001;15:1667–9.
110. Brutsaert DL. Cardiac endothelial-myocardial signaling: Its role in cardiac growth, contractile performance, and rhythmicity. Physiol Rev. 2003;83:59–115.
111. Yamazaki T, Komuro I, Kudoh S, Zou Y, Shiojima I, Hiroi Y, et al. Endothelin-1 is involved in mechanical stress-induced cardiomyocyte hypertrophy. J Biol Chem. 1996;271:3221–8.
112. Bank AJ, Lee PC, Kubo SH. Endothelial dysfunction in patients with heart failure: relationship to disease severity. J Card Fail. 2000;6:29–36.
113. Rensen SS, Doevendans PA, van Eys GJ. Regulation and characteristics of vascular smooth muscle cell phenotypic diversity. Neth Heart J. 2007;15:100–8.

The Multiple Actions of the Insulin-Like Growth Factor-I Signaling in the Myocardium

11

Anastassios Philippou, Maria Maridaki, Theodore Karatzas, and Michael Koutsilieris

Abstract

The insulin-like growth factor-I (IGF-I) is an important growth factor which regulates a variety of cellular responses and has important roles in multiple biological systems. IGF-I is produced by many tissues including the myocardium, indicating that a significant component of its action is due to an autocrine and paracrine mode of function. Multiple transcripts of the *Igf1* gene code for several precursor polypeptides (isoforms). IGF-I actions are mediated through its binding to several cell-membrane receptors, inducing cell proliferation, differentiation, migration and survival, and implicating this growth factor in mitogenic, myogenic and anti-apoptotic processes in cardiac muscle. In this chapter, focus has been driven on the signaling pathways that IGF-I triggers in the regulation of physiological and pathophysiological processes during cardiac hypertrophy, regeneration and remodeling. The concept of a potentially differential bioactivity and signaling of the different IGF-I peptides in the myocardium is also discussed.

Keywords

Myocardial cell survival • Cardiac hypertrophy • Cardiac function • Cardiac remodeling • Cardiac regeneration • IGF-I bioregulation system • IGF-I peptides • IGF-I signaling • IGF-I splice variants

A. Philippou • M. Koutsilieris, MD, PhD (✉)
Department of Experimental Physiology, Medical School, National and Kapodistrian University of Athens, 75 Micras Asias, Goudi-Athens, 115 27, Greece
e-mail: mkoutsil@med.uoa.gr

M. Maridaki
Department of Sports Medicine and Biology of Physical Activity, Faculty of Physical Education and Sport Science, National and Kapodistrian University of Athens, Athens, Greece

T. Karatzas
Second Department of Propaedeutic Surgery, Medical School, National and Kapodistrian University of Athens, Athens, Greece

D.V. Cokkinos (ed.), *Introduction to Translational Cardiovascular Research*,
DOI 10.1007/978-3-319-08798-6_11, © Springer International Publishing Switzerland 2015

Abbreviations

Akt	Protein kinase B
ALS	Acid-labile subunit
AMPK	AMP-activated protein kinase
APO	Apoptosis
ERKs	Extracellular signal-regulated kinases
GH	Growth hormone
GPCRs	G-protein coupled receptors
Grb2	Growth receptor binding protein 2
HGF	Hepatocyte growth factor
HSP60	Heat shock protein 60
IGFBPs	IGF binding proteins
IGF-I	Insulin-like growth factor-I
IGF-IEa	IGF-IEa isoform
IGF-IEb	IGF-IEb isoform
IGF-IIR	Type 2 IGF receptor
IGF-IR	Type 1 IGF receptor
IR	Insulin receptor
IRS	Insulin receptor substrate proteins
JNK1	c-Jun N-terminal kinase 1
MAPKs	Mitogen-activated protein kinases
MGF	Mechano-growth factor
MSCs	Mesenchymal stem cells
mTOR	Mammalian target of rapamycin
PDK1	Phosphoinositide-dependent kinase-1
PI3-K	Phosphatidylinositol 3-kinase
REG	Regeneration
SGK1	Serum/glucocorticoid regulated kinase 1
SH2	Src homology 2
Shc	Src homology/collagen
siRNA	Small interfering RNA
SirT1	Sirtuin 1
Sos	Son of Sevenless
TGF-β_1	Transforming growth factor beta 1
uPA	Urokinase-type plasminogen activator

11.1 Introduction

The insulin-like growth factor-I (IGF-I) is a cellular and secreted growth factor which is critical for normal body growth, development and maintenance and has important roles in various biological systems [1, 2]. IGF-I is produced by many tissues including skeletal and cardiac muscle, spleen, kidney and brain, indicating that a significant component of IGF-I action is due to an autocrine and paracrine mode of function, although it also acts as a classical circulating hormone [2–4]. Hormonal actions of circulating IGF-I, which is derived mainly from the liver but also from skeletal muscle [5], mediate the growth-promoting effects of pituitary growth hormone (GH) [6]. Both in plasma and tissue, IGF-I is mostly bound to high affinity IGF binding proteins, which protect it from degradation and modulate its interaction with the IGF-I receptors [1, 7]. IGF-I mediate its actions through the binding and activation of several receptors, inducing cellular responses such as proliferation, differentiation, migration and survival [7–9]. Thus, this growth factor is implicated in the mitogenic, myogenic and anti-apoptotic processes during myocardial development, regeneration and hypertrophy [3, 10–12].

The IGF-I domain which is responsible for the receptor binding and the activation of its downstream signaling pathways is the biologically active mature peptide. It is the common part of several IGF-I precursor proteins (isoforms) derived after their post-translational cleavage and the removal of their carboxy-terminal extension peptides, or E-peptides [13], (Fig. 11.1). Interestingly, it has been proposed that the E-peptides of the IGF-I isoforms also possess bioactivity that is distinct from that of mature IGF-I [14, 15] and particularly in cardiomyocytes [16–18]. In this chapter, focus has been driven on the signaling pathways that IGF-I triggers in the regulation of physiological and pathophysiological processes during cardiac growth/hypertrophy, regeneration and remodeling, while the concept of a potentially differential bioactivity and signaling of the IGF-I peptides in the myocardium is also discussed.

11.2 The IGF-I Bioregulation System

The IGF-I system consists of IGF-I, which produces three isoforms in humans, the type 1 (IGF-IR) and type 2 (IGF-IIR) IGF receptors, insulin receptor (IR), and several atypical receptors, such as the hybrid IGF-IR/IR [19], as well as of the IGF binding proteins (IGFBPs) [20, 21].

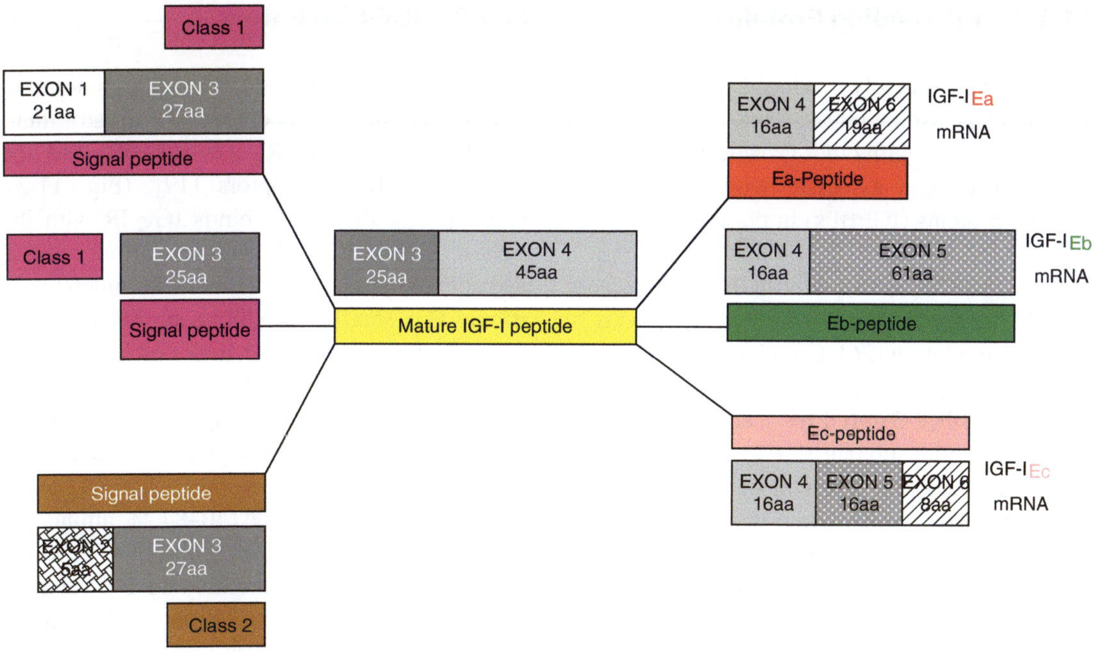

Fig. 11.1 Human *Igf1* gene alternative splicing. Different leader sequences of the *Igf1* gene result in two different classes of mRNA variants; class 1 transcripts use exon 1 as leader exon, whereas class 2 transcripts have the leader sequences on exon 2. All possible combinations between signal peptide sequences and terminal exon (5 or 6) can occur in different IGF-I mRNA isoforms. The mature IGF-I peptide is coded by exons 3 and 4. It is a common part of the IGF-I precursor polypeptides and it is derived from post-translational processing of each of the multiple IGF-I precursors, by which the signal peptides and the E-peptides (Ea, Eb, Ec) are removed. The different E-peptides are encoded by three mRNA variants produced by alternative splicing of the 3′ end of the pre-IGF-I mRNA. The first 16 amino acids of the amino-terminal portion of each of the IGF-I E peptides are coded by exon 4, while exons 5 and 6 encode distinct portions of the E-peptides with alternative carboxy-terminal sequences

11.2.1 IGF-I Alternative Splicing/Isoforms

The *Igf1* gene is a highly conserved sequence in mammals and primates. It contains six exons and as a result of its alternative splicing, different IGF-I mRNA transcripts are produced, encoding for several IGF-I precursor proteins [4]. Specifically, class 1 or class 2 mRNA transcripts are produced by differential splicing of exons 1 or 2, respectively, to the common exon 3. Alternative splicing of exon 5 results also in different mRNA variants containing exon 5, (class B, or IGF-IEb variant), or containing exon 6 (and excluding exon 5) defined as class A (or IGF-IEa variant). A third transcript variant, the IGF-IEc, which corresponds to IGF-IEb in rodents, is also generated by alternative splicing in the human *Igf1* gene and contains both exon 5 and 6. All possible combinations between leader exon (1 or 2) and terminal exon (5 or 6) can occur in different IGF-I transcripts [13]. Thus, the corresponding IGF-I protein isoforms, namely the IGF-IEa, IGF-IEb and IGF-IEc in humans, differ by the structure of their E-peptides, on the carboxy-terminal end, and by the length of their amino-terminal signal peptides, however they share the same mature peptide [13, 14], (Fig. 11.1).

Recent studies have shown that the IGF-I splice variants are differentially transcribed in response to varying conditions and pathologies, such as exercise-induced muscle damage [22], myocardial infarction [17, 18], endometriosis [23], and cancer [24, 25]. The differential expression/regulation of the IGF-I splice variants in various pathologies could indicate distinct biological roles of the different IGF-I isoforms, however their particular functions remain, as yet, unclear.

11.2.2 IGF Binding Proteins

IGF-I is constitutively produced from many tissues and can also be released into the circulation [19]. In contrast with other growth factors, IGF-I (and IGF-II) can associate with specific IGF binding proteins (IGFBPs) in plasma and tissues [3]. At least six IGFBPs modulate the biological actions of IGF-I, as they bind IGF-I and increase its half-life both in the extracellular environment and the circulation [26]. Circulating IGF-I exists predominantly as a ternary complex, consisting of IGF-I, IGFBP-3 or IGFBP-5 and the glycoprotein acid-labile subunit (ALS). This complex retains a circulating reservoir of IGF-I and protects it from proteolytic degradation [21]. Moreover, in a ternary complex IGF-I is inactive, because in this form it is unable to cross capillary membranes or activate the receptor(s) [11, 19]. Hence, IGFBPs are expected to modulate the extent of IGF-dependent cellular effects, both in the circulation and in the extracellular matrix, via regulation of free IGF-I concentration and its local bioavailability in the tissue [20, 26]. Under stress conditions (e.g., trauma) the affinity of IGFBPs, and particularly of IGFBP-3, for IGFs is reduced by proteolytic clipping of IGFBP-3 and, thus, IGF-I can re-associate with lower molecular weight binding proteins in binary complexes, which enables it to cross capillary membranes and target the peripheral tissues [11]. On the other hand, IGFBPs compete with IGF-IR, as they normally have higher affinity to IGF-I than IGF-IR. Therefore, binding of IGFBPs to IGF-I prevents the ligand to interact with the receptor, thus suppressing IGF-I actions. The ratio between free IGF-I and IGFBP-IGF-I bound, as well as the tissue-specific distribution of particular IGFBPs control the IGF-I-inhibitory or stimulatory activities of IGFBPs [7, 27].

Further, it appears that the IGFBPs have also independent activity in modulating mitogenesis, cell survival and apoptosis [27, 28], while there is also a subgroup of binding proteins, known as IGFBP-related proteins, that exhibit low binding affinity to IGFs and their functions regarding the IGFs actions are yet unclear [11, 29].

11.2.3 IGF-I Receptors

IGF-I actions are mediated through its binding to specific cell surface receptors (R) already mentioned, i.e., the IGF-IR, IGF-IIR, IR, and the hybrid IGF-IR/IR receptors [19], (Fig. 11.2). More specifically, IGF-I binds IGF-IR with the highest affinity, IGF-IIR with low affinity and is also able to interact with IR, but with much lower affinity [1]. The IGF-I exhibits significant structural similarity to insulin and both can cross-activate IGF-IR and IR, while the IGF-IR signaling pathways share multiple intracellular mediators with the insulin signaling cascade [13]. Moreover, various domains in the IGF-IR have a high degree of similarity (40–84 % aminoacid sequence homology) to IR [3, 30], both of which are comprised of 2 α-subunits and 2 β-subunits linked by disulfide bonds. However, the affinity of insulin for the IGF-IR is about 100-fold less than that of IGF-I and, thus, high concentrations of insulin are needed to cause IGF-IR activation. Nevertheless, and despite the similarities in their intracellular signaling cascades, the IGF-IR and the IR elicit different responses, probably due to differences in their subcellular localization and in the structure within the kinase containing β-subunit, as well as due to ligand specificity and, thus, the different conformational changes conferred by the α-subunits (reviewed in Suleiman et al. [11]).

IGF-IR/IR hybrid receptors are present in many mammalian tissues including the heart. They are heterologous IGF-IR and IR α–β hemi-receptors that maintain autophosphorylation activity upon ligand binding. The IGF-IR/IR hybrid receptor binds both insulin and IGF-I, however is thought to function predominantly as an IGF-I receptor, since its binding affinity for IGF-I is higher than that for insulin [21, 31]. The functional importance of IGF-IR/IR hybrid receptors remains poorly understood, however there is evidence that they may play an important role in both IGF-I and insulin-mediated cardiac growth (reviewed in DeBosch and Muslin [6]).

IGF-I acts primarily through the binding and activation of the IGF-IR. This is a transmembrane, ligand-activated receptor tyrosine kinase consisting

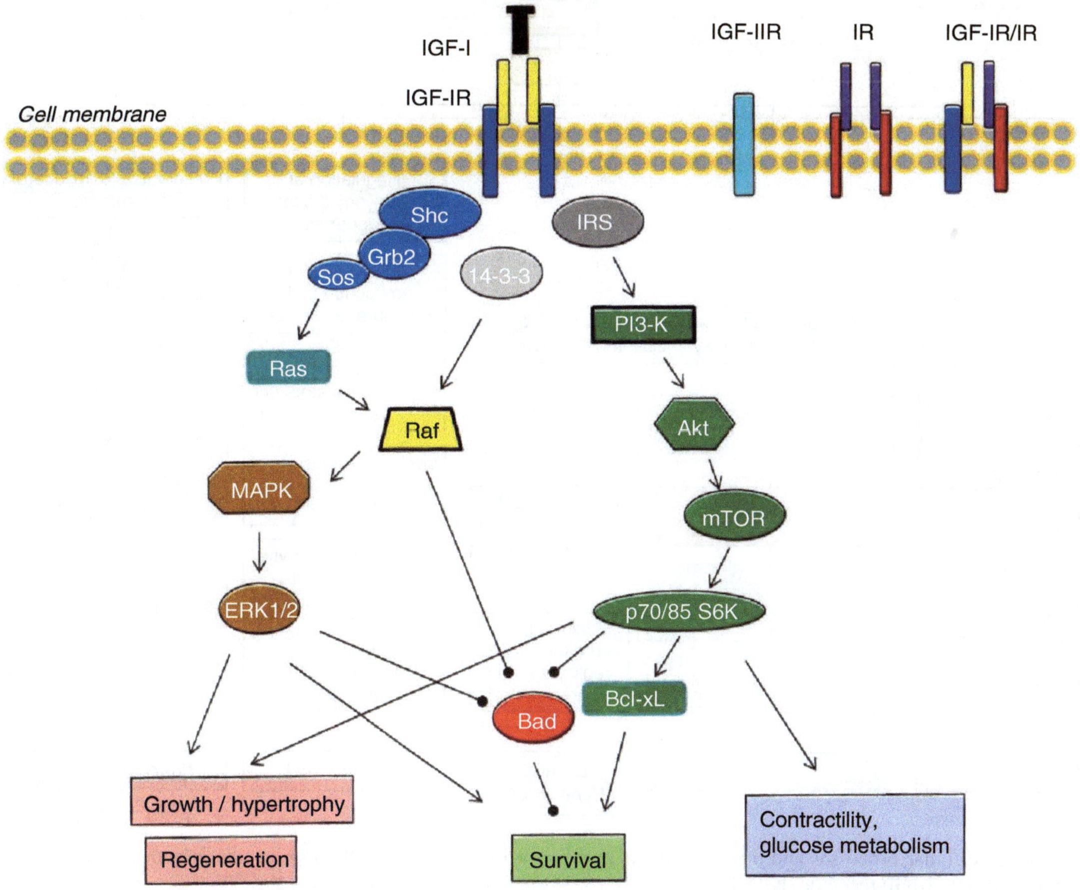

Fig. 11.2 Schematic representation of the insulin-like growth factor I (IGF-I) receptors, and IGF-I signaling pathways downstream of IGF-IR that result in specific biologic effects in myocardial cells

of two extracellular α-subunits, which contain the cysteine-rich ligand binding site, and two transmembrane β-subunits which have a cluster of three tyrosine residues that undergo phosphorylation and thus activation upon IGF-I binding [1, 30, 32], (Fig. 11.2). Ligand binding to the IGF-IR causes a structural rearrangement in the transmembrane β-subunits of the receptor, resulting in trans-autophosphorylation of the tyrosine residues as one kinase domain phosphorylates the other, and thus destabilizing the auto-inhibitory conformation within the kinase domain of the receptor [33]. The IGF-IR activation leads to a trend in protein substrates in favor of the catalytic site, thus recruiting and phosphorylating specific cytoplasmic molecules and adaptor proteins, including Src homology/collagen (Shc) and insulin receptor substrate (IRS) proteins [2], (Fig. 11.2). IRS-1 and IRS-2 do not have an intrinsic kinase activity and act to recruit other enzymes, in order to elicit a variety of responses through specific intracellular signaling pathways. The IGF-IR, after its ligand-induced activation, is usually down-regulated by endocytic internalization [11].

11.3 IGF-I/IGF-IR Signaling and Biological Actions on the Myocardium

There is a growing interest in recent years regarding the role of IGF-I in cardiac physiology, largely within the context of cardiac repair and stem cell research, and numerous studies have implicated

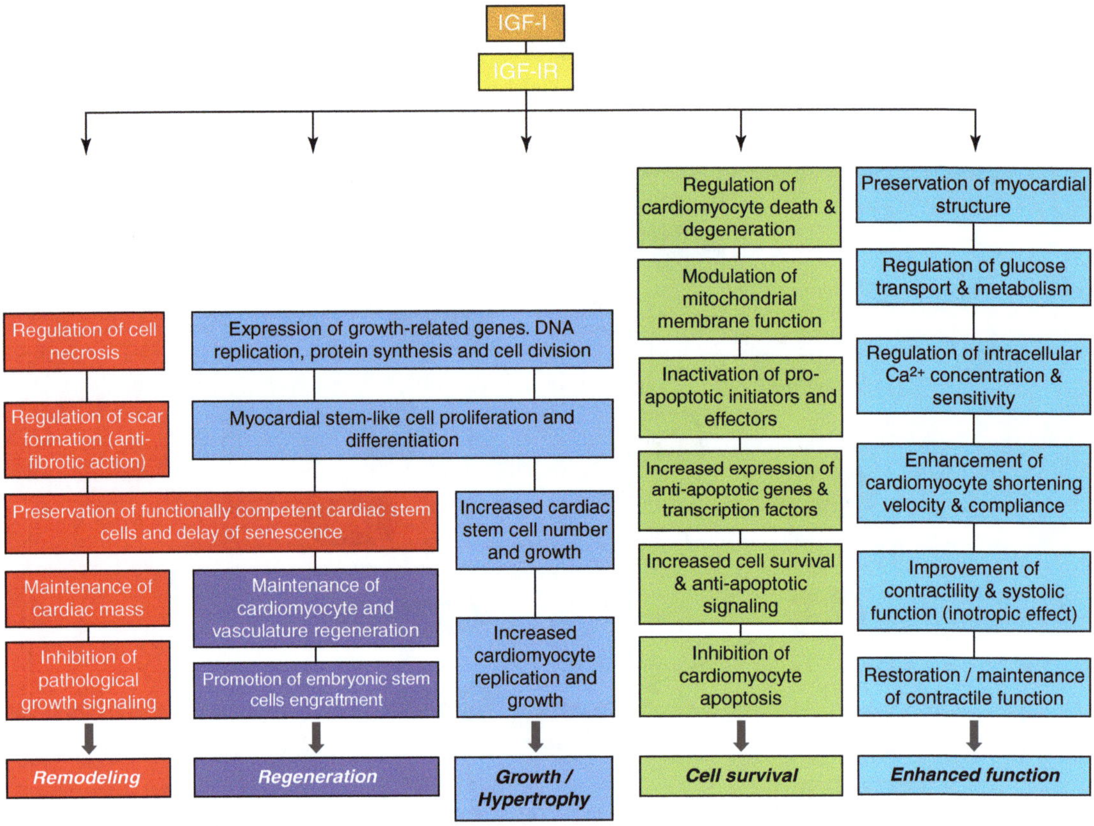

Fig. 11.3 Cellular processes and biologic effects in myocardium induced by the insulin-like growth factor I (IGF-I) binding to type 1 IGF receptor (IGF-IR)

IGF signaling in the regulation of cardiac growth, homeostasis, viability and regeneration [3, 11, 34].

It is widely recognized that most of the observed IGF-I biological effects on cell proliferation, differentiation and survival depend on the activation of IGF-IR [7, 11]. Ligation of IGF-IR phosphorylates specific molecules and initiates intracellular signaling cascades involved in mitogenic, myogenic and cell-survival/anti-apoptotic activities [11, 34], (Fig. 11.2). IGF-I is produced locally in the heart and IGF-IR is also present in cardiac muscle [3]. Thus, based on the well known IGF-IR cellular signaling, IGF-I actions on cardiomyocytes are expected to include an increase in cell size, prevention of apoptosis, regulation of glucose metabolism and intracellular Ca^{2+}, and direct effects on cardiac muscle contractile function [11, 35]. A variety of biological effects is regulated by the IGF-IR-induced stimulation of several phosphorylation cascades. Site-directed mutagenesis has been used to map specific signaling pathways, functions, and phenotypes associated with IGF-IR signaling, and receptor domain-dependent functions were identified for protection from apoptosis, anchorage-independent growth (i.e., cells grow in suspension or soft media where they float instead of growing on a solid substratum), and DNA synthesis (reviewed in Kurmasheva and Houghton [9]). Specific IGF-I/IGF-IR-dependent signaling and biological actions in myocardium are discussed in the next sections, (Figs. 11.2 and 11.3).

11.3.1 IGF-I Signaling in Cardiac Development and Growth/Hypertrophy

Heart growth is often referred to as cardiac hypertrophy (H) and can be defined as physiological or pathological; physiological H includes heart growth during postnatal development (sometimes also called eutrophy) and in response to exercise training (as occurs in elite aerobic exercise athletes) and is associated with preserved or enhanced cardiac function. Pathological cardiac H occurs in disease settings such as myocardial infarction, hypertension and valve disease, and is typically associated with histopathology and depressed cardiac function. The activation of distinct signaling transducers causes the different phenotypes of cardiac hypertrophy [36, 37].

That the IGF system plays an important role in the development and growth of the heart [11], GH/IGF-I axis may influence myocardial growth [38], and GH/IGF-I deficiency may lead to cardiac atrophy and impaired cardiac function [39]. More specifically, IGF-I appears to be crucial for the embryonic growth with age of the myocardium and it has an important role in its response [3]. Physiological cardiac hypertrophy in athletes is also associated with increased cardiac IGF-I production. This growth factor has been shown to have specific cardiac effects, stimulating DNA and protein synthesis, cardiomyocyte proliferation, differentiation and H [37, 40], and has been associated with the induction of expression of contractile proteins in neonatal rat cardiomyocytes [40], for review see [3], (Fig. 11.3).

Although substantial data suggest that IGF-I is a potent cardiomyocyte growth factor, nevertheless the research data regarding the IGF-I-induced myocardial hypertrophy appear controversial [11]. Specifically, IGF-I overexpression in mice increased cardiac stem cell number and growth [41], while myocardium-specific overexpression of IGF-I resulted in increased number of cardiomyocytes and total heart weight [42]. Moreover, it has been reported that overexpression of IGF-I in the hearts of transgenic mice induced a hypertrophic phenotype [43], in other studies transgenic mice overexpressing IGF-IR in the heart exhibited increased cardiomyocyte size, enhanced contractile function and no evidence of histopathology [44, 45]. However, other studies failed to find cellular hypertrophy in cardiomyocytes *in vitro*, or in individual muscle fibers in the hearts of IGF-I overexpressing mice, or of mice overexpressing IGF-I specifically in the heart [42, 46], reviewed in Suleiman et al. [11].

The cardiac growth/hypertrophy-promoting actions of IGF-I are mediated through various IGF-IR signaling components, involving extracellular signal-regulated kinases (ERKs), IRS-1 and phosphatidylinositol 3-kinase (PI3-K) [2, 34, 37], (Fig. 11.2). Specifically, mitogenic IGF-I signaling cascades are activated through the phosphorylation of Shc, which connects IGF-IR tyrosine kinases to mitogen-activated protein kinases (MAPK) through the Ras-Raf-MEK-ERK signaling pathway. Shc binds to phosphorylated tyrosines on activated IGF-IR and its subsequent phosphorylation generates a binding site for the growth receptor binding protein 2 (Grb2) and subsequently a Shc/Grb2/Son of Sevenless (Sos) complex. Sos activates the small G protein Ras, which is located at the plasma membrane and in its turn associates with and activates protein serine kinase Raf [3, 13, 34], (Fig. 11.2). The activation of Ras/Raf signals to MKKs (specifically MEK1/2) and these kinases phosphorylate on specific sites (Thr-Glu-Tyr) and activate ERKs (ERK1/2), which then can activate by phosphorylation other protein kinases and several transcription factors [34].

Although the Ras-Raf-MEK-ERK signaling pathway appears to regulate certain intracellular hypertrophic responses, however the importance of this pathway in the regulation of cardiac H has been disputed [34, 47]. Specifically, both *in vivo* and *in vitro* studies have shown that acute exposure of rat adult ventricular cardiomyocytes and the cardiomyoblast cell line H9C2 to IGF-I resulted in the activation of the IGF-IR, followed by the sequential activation of the Ras-Raf-MEK-ERK cascade, which is required for the anabolic effects of IGF-I [11]. In addition, it was demonstrated that ERK signaling is necessary for phenylephrine-induced cardiomyocyte H in culture [48], and that ERKs are required for sarcomeric organization induced by hypertrophic agonists, suggesting a more specialized role in cardiomyocyte H [49]. Moreover, agonist stimulation or cell stretching resulted in the activation of ERK1/2 in cultured cardiomyocytes [50], implicating ERK1/2 signaling proteins as regulators of a hypertrophic response.

Nevertheless, there are also studies suggesting a minimal role for ERKs in cardiac hypertrophy [51]. Overall, although the necessity of ERK signaling as a hypertrophic mediator is disputed, it appears that ERKs are implicated as downstream effectors of the hypertrophic response in the myocardium [34].

Other signaling molecules that appear to regulate the physiological hypertrophy phenotype in the myocardium are the components of the IGF-I/PI3-K/Akt pathway [35–37]. In particular, the regulatory subunit of PI3-K contains a src homology 2 (SH2) domain which interacts with IRS-1, resulting in PI3-K activation [36]. PI3-K then leads to the activation of Akt (protein kinase B) as well as p70S6K and p85S6K, which affect diverse intracellular processes such as translational regulation, cardiac cell growth/hypertrophy and survival (discussed in the next section), [34, 35, 52]. IGF-I receptor tyrosine kinases activate the PI3-K(p110-alpha) pathway leading to physiological H, whereas pathological H involves the activation of PI3-K(p110-gamma) pathway induced by G-protein coupled receptors (GPCRs) [12, 53]. Cardiac-specific overexpression of a constitutively active PI3-K catalytic subunit (p110) in mice resulted in cardiac H, which was associated with a comparable increase in myocyte size, while the changes in heart size were correlated with PI3-K activity. Moreover, transgenic overexpression of a dominant negative PI3-K resulted in smaller hearts and myocytes [54].

One of the most comprehensively studied signaling molecules in the regulation of cardiac growth and function is Akt kinase [12, 55]. Akt is downstream of the IGF-I/PI3-K/Akt physiological H pathway and it regulates a range of downstream targets involved in the modulation of local responses. It also regulates processes such as cell growth, differentiation and survival, as well as cell metabolism and contractile function [12, 55], (Fig. 11.2). Studies utilizing various Akt mutant mouse models suggest that the subcellular distribution of Akt activity is a determinant for the resulting cardiac phenotype. Moreover, short-term activation of Akt induces physiological H, whereas its prolonged activation results in pathological H, indicating that, depending on the timing and extent of stimulation, the IGF-I/Akt pathway may sustain either physiological or pathological hypertrophy [12, 56]. Indeed, Akt is critical both at baseline and for hypertrophic adaptation and the activation of the IGF-I/PI3-K/Akt pathway plays an important role in the mechanism of physiological cardiac H, by promoting a coordinated angiogenic program. Overall, physiological H is associated with the activation of the IGF-I/PI3-K/Akt pathway, which is critical in modulating cardiac growth and vasculogenesis (reviewed in Catalucci et al. [12], see also next Sect. 11.3.3).

In addition, there is evidence that the IGF-I/PI3-K/Akt signaling pathway downstream effectors, p70S6K and p85S6K, may also play a role in regulating physiologic cardiac H. Ventricular pressure overloading resulted in the activation of both p70S6K and p85S6K [52], while selective inhibition of p70S6K blocked the augmentation of agonist-induced protein synthesis and the subsequent hypertrophic response of cultured cardiomyocytes [34, 57].

11.3.2 IGF-I Signaling in Cardiac Cell Survival/Inhibition of Apoptosis

Programmed cell death apoptosis (APO) is a key contributor to myocyte loss that accompanies many forms of myocardial disease, such as acute myocyte death after ischemic injury. APO in cardiomyocytes contributes to the development of heart failure [58], while it may also occur even during normal aging. It has been demonstrated that the constitutively expressed biochemical apoptotic machine in cultured cardiomyocytes can be suppressed by the anti-apoptotic signals of IGF-I in the serum [59].

IGF-I has been well characterised as an anti-apoptotic factor and in many respects it appears to be a more potent survival than mitogenic factor. The identity of all the signaling proteins and interactions that mediate the IGF-I survival effect remains to be fully elucidated, however many components have been identified [11]. Thus, IGF-I is a potent cardiomyocyte survival factor and may affect the cardiac muscle mass by preventing APO and cardiomyocyte loss [11, 60]. Indeed, IGF-I has protective effects on the heart, as cardiac-specific IGF-I overexpression is anti-apoptotic [41] and results in reduced reperfusion injury and less cardiomyocyte death and fibrosis in chronic coronary artery disease [60], (Fig. 11.3). On the other hand, IGF-I-deficient mice have been shown to exhibit increased APO after myocardial infarction [61]. Moreover, IGF-I can decrease myocyte APO and prolong cell survival in cultured cardiomyocytes, and the anti-apoptotic effects of IGF-I on cardiac muscle cells can occur at physiological concentrations [59, 62]. Short-term administration of IGF-I in animals has been reported to counteract APO and improve cardiac contractility, however clinical trials in which IGF-I was administered chronically have shown conflicting results [3, 12, 44].

Several signaling pathways have been suggested to mediate the anti-apoptotic effects of IGF-I [63]. Specifically, three different pathways, originating from different domains of the IGF-IR, are involved in cell survival: the IRS-1/PI3-K/Akt/p70S6K pathway, acting through the tyrosine kinase domain; the Shc/MAPK pathway, acting preponderantly through the Y950 domain; and a third pathway which is dependent on the serine cluster motif (S1280–1283) of the IGF-IR and acts in cooperation with 14-3-3 proteins. The latter pathway results in the translocation of Raf-1 to mitochondria where it can phosphorylate, and so inactivate, the pro-apoptotic protein Bad, a member of the Bcl-2 family of proteins, (Fig. 11.2). Indeed, IGF-I acts as a survival factor via the stimulation of the Bcl-2 proteins [8], as IGF-I-mediated inhibition of APO has been shown to be associated with increased expression of an anti-apoptotic member (Bcl-xL) of the Bcl-2 family of proteins [64]. Mitochondria appear to have an important role in the apoptotic death and IGF-I has been shown to modulate mitochondrial membrane function through activation of PI3-K/Akt pathway [65]. The operation of any two of the above three pathways is sufficient to protect cells from APO, while inactivation of Bad appears to be a target for each pathway [9, 13], (Fig. 11.2).

The most frequently implicated pathways in IGF-induced survival signaling are MAPK and PI3-K pathways. IGF-IR signaling via IRS-1, Akt or MAPK regulates positively the expression of anti-apoptotic genes and transcription factors that themselves regulate anti-apoptotic programs, and negatively regulates the expression of pro-apoptotic genes. The requirement of PI3-K or ERK1/2 in mediating IGF-survival appears to be depended on the model system and the stress stimulus used. Inhibition of PI3-K or MAPK ablates the survival effect of IGF-I and under serum starvation conditions activation of both PI3-K and ERK1/2 is required, indicating that both are vital components of the anti-apoptotic effects of IGF-I [9, 11, 63]. In the absence of IRS proteins, sustained activation of ERK1/2 appears largely dependent on the Y950 domain, although the relationship between IGF-I-mediated survival and activation of ERKs is not absolute [9].

The primary cell survival pathway activated by IGF-I is the PI3-K/Akt signaling pathway (Fig. 11.2), which is activated in the presence of IRS-1 [9]. Tyrosine kinase-phosphorylated IRS-1 and IRS-2 interacts with specific cytoplasmic proteins, leading to the transduction of downstream cell survival and anti-apoptotic signals [33]. IRS proteins may play differential roles in the anti-apoptotic effects of IGF-I with IRS-1 being predominant. IRS-1 appears to be important in mediating IGF-I protection from APO under serum-starved conditions, as PI3-K activity and Akt phosphorylation were found to be reduced in IRS-1 deficient cells [9]. Phosphorylation of PI3-K activates the Akt pathway which inhibits activation of pro-apoptotic initiators, such as Bad, and effectors, e.g., caspases [8, 11, 36], while inhibition of PI3-K signaling would prevent the completion of the cell cycle, leading potentially to cell APO or differentiation. Moreover, it has been shown that the PI3-kinase/Akt pathway protects cells from reperfusion injury and promotes cardiomyocyte viability both *in vitro* and *in vivo* [66], and Akt appears to be a critical component of the survival pathway, regulating the activities of apoptotic factors [9, 59, 67]. Overall, IGF-I/PI3-K pathway provides cardiac protection and the mechanisms responsible for this protection include its anti-apoptotic and anti-fibrotic properties, inhibition of signaling cascades that lead to pathological growth, and maintenance of contractile function in a disease setting and the regeneration (reviewed in McMullen [36]), (Figs. 11.2 and 11.3).

11.3.3 IGF-I Signaling in Cardiac Regeneration/Remodeling

There is increasing evidence for new myocyte formation in the adult heart and a growing interest in the extent and mechanisms of cardiomyocyte regeneration (REG) [68–70]. A large number of cardiomyocytes in mitosis and a high frequency of cardiomyocyte replication in normal hearts have been observed both in response to increased work load and in acute or chronic cardiac failure of ischemic and non-ischemic origin, both in animals and humans. These findings indicate that cardiomyocyte REG is an important contributor to the maintenance of cardiac mass in physiological and pathological conditions [68–70]. Myocyte death and REG are part of the normal homeostasis of the heart and the generation of new cardiomyocytes predominates over cell death and contributes significantly to the normal growth of the heart into adulthood [53]. Thus, although the adult heart is mainly composed of terminally differentiated cells, it should not be considered as a post-mitotic organ, since it exhibits a significant capacity for myocyte REG that is markedly enhanced in acute and chronic heart failure. In human end-stage ischemic hearts and in idiopathic dilated cardiomyopathy, a high increase in the number of mitotic cells has been reported compared to control hearts [68]. Nevertheless, human and animal studies have provided evidence that in the failing adult heart the magnitude of cardiomyocyte replication and REG is far below the extent of the myocyte death [62].

The cardiac regenerative capacity is supported by a subpopulation of cycling, myocardial stem-like cells which possess the potential of regenerating the muscle cells and the coronary vasculature of the myocardium [70, 71]. Whether the origin of the cardiac stem cells permanently resides in the myocardium or they are taken up from the circulation/bone marrow is not clear [71].

IGF-I appears not only to protect myocardial cells from death and degeneration, but also to be an important stimulant for the REG of the adult heart, by promoting the expression of growth-related genes, DNA replication and cell division [10], (Fig. 11.3). Specifically, IGF-I has been shown to promote myocyte renewal and myocardial REG in experimental protocols of ischaemic cardiac injury [72, 73]. In addition, intracoronary injections of IGF-I and hepatocyte growth factor (HGF) were capable of activating cardiac stem cells and subsequently regenerating new myocytes and vasculature lost after myocardial infarction in pigs. This myocardial REG was accompanied by improved cardiomyocyte survival and ventricular function [73], while an increase in cell number in IGF-I transgenic animals has been also observed, suggesting that IGF-I may play a role in the REG of the myocardium [36]. Moreover, cardiac stem cell division in IGF-I transgenic mice has been shown to be induced via the IGF-IR, and it was accompanied by preservation of a reservoir of functionally competent cardiac stem cells and delayed senescence [41], (Fig. 11.3).

The REG capacity of IGF-I has been particularly explored in transgenic mice overexpressing a class 1 IGF-IEa isoform (see previous Sect. 11.2.1), implicating it as a powerful mediator of the REG response [72]. In particular, this isoform has been reported to have regenerative properties and to promote cell survival and renewal and its expression in cardiac myocytes induced a hypertrophic response [74]. The IGF-IEa transgene was reported to induce repair of the injured tissue, by promoting regenerative properties in damaged heart tissue with minimal scar formation and restoring of cardiac function through increased anti-apoptotic signaling [72, 74].

In conditions such as myocardial infarction, ischemia/reperfusion injury and heart failure, there is often myocyte loss, although a later increase in myocardial mass may occur through compensatory myocyte hypertrophy/remodeling and/or increased collagen deposition (fibrosis) [58]. Thus, after the segmental loss of myocardium due to ischemic heart disease, myocyte REG and H processes are activated contributing together to the development of new cardiac muscle mass. However, both processes are restricted to the remaining viable myocardium and the border zone of the infarct, while a scar formation occurs in the healed infarcted area [70]. The urokinase-type plasminogen activator (uPA)/transforming growth factor beta 1 (TGF-β_1) bioregulation system appears to have an important role as a main regulator of the myocardial collagen accumulation and fibrosis, and the extracellular matrix remodeling [12, 75, 76].

Interestingly, intracoronary injections of IGF-I/HGF have been proven effective to reduce the pathological cardiac remodeling (REM) and fibrosis after myocardial infarction [53]. In addition, the influence of IGF-I on myocardial remodeling involves also an adaptation of the coronary vasculature [11]. Thus, increased expression of IGF-I has been observed in rat aortas following balloon injury [77]. Moreover, in a variety of disorders such as hypertrophic cardiomyopathy, "hypertensive" heart disease and "ischaemic" cardiomyopathy, there is an initial up-regulation of IGF-I and IGF-IR, which has been suggested to be involved in a cardiac remodeling response [3, 11], (Fig. 11.3). Besides, higher serum IGF-I levels immediately after the onset of acute myocardial infarction have been associated with less myocardial remodeling and improved ventricular function [78], (see discussion in the next section).

11.3.4 IGF-I Signaling and Cardiac Function

IGF-I affects cardiac functional changes by improving cardiac contractility, stroke volume, cardiac output and ejection fraction [3], although enhanced cardiac contractility and elevated blood pressure have been reported in IGF-I-deficient mice, indicating that IGF-I deficiency can selectively modulate blood pressure and left ventricular function, yet normal IGF-I levels are not required for adaptive myocardial hypertrophy in response to sustained hemodynamic load [79]. Chronic heart failure (HF) leads to the appearance of cardiac cachexia in the late stages of the disease [80], which is accompanied by increased rate of APO and reduced local expression of IGF-I. There is strong evidence that a low IGF-I level increases the risk of HF. In patients with HF, IGF-I levels are low and have been correlated with left ventricular mass and ventricular systolic dysfunction [39]; GH/IGF-I deficiency may lead to cardiac atrophy and impaired cardiac function [3, 39]. Moreover, it has been shown that serum IGF-I concentrations at the time of cardiac infarction in humans can be used to predict later development of HF [62, 78]. In addition, in elderly people without a previous myocardial infarction, serum IGF-I levels were found to be inversely related to the risk for congestive HF [81], while the relative risk of coronary artery disease mortality has been associated with decreased levels of circulating IGF-I [82]. Besides, IGF-I can decrease systemic vascular resistance resulting potentially in indirect effects on the heart [83], while intravascular infusion of IGF-I resulted in significant increase in regional forearm blood flow when administered to humans [84], implying that IGF-I may be involved in the regulation of vasodilatation [11].

It has been suggested that IGF-I administration could benefit the cachectic heart, since this growth factor increases cardiac stem cell numbers and growth and leads to an increase in myocyte turnover and function [11, 41]. Indeed, intracoronary administration of IGF-I has been shown to significantly improve myocardial function during the early phase of myocardial infarction in pigs, and this functional improvement was associated with the preservation of myocardial structure [85]. Nevertheless, chronic infusion of IGF-I has been shown to result in mild cardiac hypertrophy in rats [86], and sustained overproduction of IGF-I may lead to hypertrophic cardiomyopathy [3]. In addition, local IGF-I overexpression in skeletal and cardiac muscle has been shown to initially induce first physiological and later pathological cardiac H in transgenic mice [43]. Collectively, it has been suggested that both extreme IGF-I overproduction and deficiency may lead to deterioration of cardiac function [62], (see also discussion below).

In rat models of acute cardiac injury or ischemic cardiomyopathy, it has been demonstrated that IGF-I is an important mediator in promoting cell engraftment at the site of injury and functional improvement after transferring embryonic stem cells for myocardial restoration [87]. Besides, cardiac muscle specific overexpression of IGF-I resulted in cardiomegaly and it was associated with enhanced cardiomyocyte shortening velocity and cellular compliance [46]. Moreover, the specific overexpression of IGF-IR in cardiac myocytes results in increased heart size and enhanced systolic function [44]; (Fig. 11.3).

Notably, while in both ischemic and hypertrophic cardiomyopathy there is an increased expression of IGF-I receptors, a reduction in the concentration and an increased ubiquitination of the IGF-IR have been shown in cardiac muscle of diabetic animals. Moreover, this down-regulation of IGF-IR in the myocardium was accompanied by concurrent reduction of heat shock protein HSP60 [88]. It was suggested that the anti-apoptotic action of HSP60 in cardiomyocytes observed in ischemia/reperfusion injuries may involve the augmentation of IGF-IR signaling, while the down-regulation of HSP60 in the diabetic heart may be a fundamental mechanism contributing to impaired IGF-IR signaling in diabetic cardiomyopathy [62, 88]. The reduction in IGF-IR signaling could potentially lead to increased myocardial vulnerability during myocardial stress and, thus, play an important role in the development of diabetic cardiomyopathy [62].

IGF-IR has been shown to be essential for myocardial performance through the PI3-K/Akt pathway, which mediates functional effects of IGF-I on the target cells, such as enhanced glucose transport and cardiomyocyte contractility [11, 12, 55, 89], (Figs. 11.2 and 11.3). Mice with cardiac muscle-specific deficiency in phosphoinositide-dependent kinase-1 (PDK1), a PI3-K-dependent kinase, exhibit severe systolic dysfunction, decreased cardiomyocyte volume and decreased cardiac mass [90]. Furthermore, the IGF-I/PI3-K/Akt pathway appears to be critical in modulating myocardial growth, cardiac inotropic function and vasculogenesis while, particularly, IGF-IR/PI3-K(p110α and γ) signaling is critical for physiological and pathological heart growth, respectively [53]. Various cardiac phenotypes, ranged from no H associated with protection from myocardial ischaemic injury, to substantial H associated with a pathological phenotype and premature death, have been attributed to different degrees of Akt activation, a well characterised target of PI3-K activity [12, 53], (see also previous Sect. 11.3.1). Moreover, acute activation of Akt has been shown to reduce both infarction size and dysfunction after ischemia/reperfusion injury, while its chronic activation resulted in decreased functional recovery and increased injury by inducing feedback inhibition of PI3-K activity [56]. Thus, it was suggested that PI3-K-dependent but Akt-independent signaling intermediates are required for rescuing function and reducing injury after ischemia/reperfusion injury of the heart [56].

An inotropic effect of acute exposure of the heart to IGF-I has been demonstrated in isolated perfused rat hearts, while the addition of IGF-I to canine cardiac myocytes and to human cardiomyocytes from end-stage failing hearts caused an increase in their contractility (reviewed in Suleiman et al. [11]). More specifically, IGF-IR activation is associated with regulation of intracellular Ca^{2+} concentration and glucose metabolism [35], and IGF-I has been shown to enhance myocardial contraction and intracellular Ca^{+2} sensitivity by regulatory proteins on the contractile machinery [11, 89, 91], (Fig. 11.3). Besides, PI3-K appears to be critical for the maintenance of contractile function in a disease setting, as expression of PI3-K (p110a) prevented the fall in sarcoplasmic reticulum Ca^{2+}-ATPase that usually occurs in models of heart failure [45]. In addition, IGF-IR-mediated activation of Akt increases inotropism through the functional regulation of critical Ca^{2+}-handling proteins [35]. It is noted, however, that Akt activation in cardiomyocytes inhibits AMP-activated protein kinase (AMPK) phosphorylation and function [92], which is a key regulator of energy metabolism and has the potential to increase energy production in the heart.

11.3.5 Evidence for IGF-I Peptide-specific Actions and Novel Signaling in Myocardium

By general consensus, the bioactive IGF-IR ligand is the mature IGF-I peptide derived from each of the IGF-I protein isoforms after the removal of the (isoform-specific) E-peptides (see previous Sect. 11.2.1 and Fig. 11.1). However, differential biological activities have been reported for the different IGF-I isoforms, or for their E-peptides, in various *in vivo* and *in vitro* models [14–16], implying that IGF-I peptides, other than the IGF-IR ligand, also possess bioactivity, or supporting the bioactivity of the pro-IGF-I forms [93]. In particular, there has been growing interest in the potential of differential IGF-I isoforms actions through IGF-I peptides-specific signaling in skeletal [22, 94] and cardiac myoblasts [17, 18], or in cardiac-specific IGF-I transgenic models [72, 95, 96].

Specifically, an increased endogenous expression of both rodent IGF-I isoforms, i.e., IGF-IEa and IGF-IEb (also named mechano-growth factor, MGF), was found in rat and mice myocardium during the post-infarction period after artery ligation–induced infarction, indicating the implication of the IGF-I isoforms in the myocardial repair/remodeling process [17, 18]. Moreover, overexpression of the IGF-IEa propeptide specifically in cardiac muscle of transgenic mice induced restoration of cardiac function post-infarction, by modulating the inflammatory response, decreasing scar formation, and increasing proliferative activity and anti-apoptotic signaling [72]. In addition, constitutively overexpression of this specific isoform was shown to increase a cardiogenic differentiation program [96] and protect the heart from oxidative stress via Sirtuin 1 (SirT1) / c-Jun N-terminal kinase 1 (JNK1) activity while, conversely, circulating (mature) IGF-I triggered oxidative stress in the heart and did not affect SirT1 activity [95, 97]. Interestingly, although both, mature IGF-I and IGF-IEa propeptide, triggered the phosphorylation of the same receptor (IGF-IR), however the canonical PI3-K/Akt/mTOR signaling pathway was not induced in the IGF-IEa overexpressing transgenic mice [72]. Instead, the IGF-IEa activated alternate signaling intermediates, such as PDK1 and serum/glucocorticoid regulated kinase 1 (SGK1), as well as SirT1. Thus, it was suggested that this downstream of IGF-IR signaling activated by IGF-IEa employs novel pathways and that the divergent signaling mechanisms between the mature IGF-I and IGF-IEa propeptide may account for their opposing effects in heart tissue [72, 96, 97].

Considering particularly the bioactivity of the E-peptides in cardiac cells, both *in vitro* and *in vivo* studies have suggested that the E domain of the human IGF-IEc isoform may act as independent growth factor [16–18]. Thus, exogenous administration of a synthetic peptide corresponding to the E domain of the IGF-IEc isoform has been reported to reduce post-infarction APO in the peri-infarct zone of sheep myocardium and to protect myocardium against ischaemia, ultimately improving cardiac function [16]. In addition, the administration of a similar synthetic 24-amino acid peptide analog at the time of myocardial infarction in mice has been reported to ameliorate the decline in function and result in significant preservation of cardiac contractility 2 weeks post-infarction. These changes were accompanied by inhibition of pathologic H and significantly fewer apoptotic nuclei in the viable myocardium [18].

Our group has characterized the synthetic E peptide bioactivity and its respective signaling in H9C2 myocardial-like cells [17], by utilizing a synthetic peptide corresponding to the last 24 aminoacids of the E domain of the human IGF-IEc isoform [98]. It was demonstrated that this synthetic peptide stimulated the proliferation of H9C2 cells as mature IGF-I did, however in contrast with the mature IGF-I, the proliferative action of the synthetic E peptide on H9C2 cells was not blocked by an anti–IGF-IR neutralizing antibody, suggesting that synthetic E peptide action may be mediated by an IGF-IR–independent mechanism [17]. Moreover, exogenous administration of mature IGF-I produced a time-dependent increase of ERK1/2 and Akt phosphorylation in H9C2 cells; however, the synthetic E peptide activated only ERK1/2 without affecting Akt phosphorylation, reinforcing the notion that biologic actions and signaling of the synthetic E peptide in H9C2 cells are possibly mediated via an IGF-IR–independent mechanism. Further evidence that the synthetic analog of the human Ec peptide possesses distinct signaling and independent bioactivity, compared with the (mature) IGF-I ligand, has been provided by our group [22, 24, 99] and others, showing the selective activation of only ERK1/2 and not Akt canonical pathway downstream of IGF-IR, and also a bioactivity of this synthetic peptide in IGF-IR and IR siRNA knock-out models, in various human cell lines [23–25].

Accordingly, treatment of H9C2 cells with a similar synthetic peptide analog indicated a rapid cellular uptake mechanism that did not involve IGF-IR activation but resulted in a nuclear localization and inhibition of the intrinsic apoptotic pathway in H9C2 cells [18]. Similarly, it has been reported that a similar peptide analog of the human Ec domain aminoacid sequence caused a significant increase in the migration of human mesenchymal stem cells (MSCs), which was greater than that induced by the mature IGF-I polypeptide while, in contrast with the mature IGF-I, the synthetic peptide had no effect on proliferation of MSCs [100]. It was suggested that regions of the IGF propeptides may act differentially, or in a combinatorial manner, to benefit cardiac tissue recovery after injury [100].

11.4 Clinical Implications and Future Perspectives

IGF-I appears to be a pluripotent factor that promotes mitogenic, myogenic and anti-apoptotic processes during cardiac muscle growth and development, REG and remodeling. This growth factor can improve cardiac function and opens new approaches for both prevention and treatment of cardiac diseases. Thus, its ability to activate/recruit cardiac stem cells to the site of myocardial infarction and to promote the engraftment and functional improvement of embryonic stem cells transplanted into myocardium could be an interesting therapeutic perspective for enhancing myocardial regeneration within the context of cardiac cell therapy. Besides, given the IGF-I-induced protection of myocardium against apoptotic cell death, the regulation of IGF-I production in the myocardium might become a promising intervention to repair diseased myocardium and prevent myocardial dysfunction. In addition, IGF-I administration could have a protective effect on the heart during surgical settings that involve its isolation from the body. New strategies, however, are needed to tailor the delivery of IGF-I to the heart in a systemic IGF-I administration, allowing for heightened levels of IGF-I where it is needed and avoiding any systemic risks and side effects of its administration.

New insights into the interactions between IGF-I and other factors in cardiac muscle cells could further define the IGF-IR intracellular pathways that regulate signaling in the normal and diseased heart. Furthermore, a mechanistic understanding of how IGF-I signaling modulates cardiac physiological responses may help in the development of feasible, non-invasive molecular therapeutic strategies in cardiac diseases, targeting basic mechanisms of cardiomyocyte growth, regeneration, survival and function. In this context, further verification and characterization of the intrinsic IGF-I isoform-specific actions and signaling in myocardial cells is a particularly interesting aspect of the role of IGF-I in myocardial physiology.

References

1. Laviola L, Natalicchio A, Giorgino F. The igf-i signaling pathway. Curr Pharm Des. 2007;13:663–9.
2. Le Roith D. Seminars in medicine of the beth Israel deaconess medical center. Insulin-like growth factors. N Engl J Med. 1997;336:633–40.
3. Ren J, Samson WK, Sowers JR. Insulin-like growth factor i as a cardiac hormone: physiological and pathophysiological implications in heart disease. J Mol Cell Cardiol. 1999;31:2049–61.
4. Philippou A, Maridaki M, Halapas A, Koutsilieris M. The role of the insulin-like growth factor 1 (igf-1) in skeletal muscle physiology. In Vivo. 2007;21:45–54.
5. Barton ER, Park S, James JK, Makarewich CA, Philippou A, Eletto D, et al. Deletion of muscle grp94

impairs both muscle and body growth by inhibiting local igf production. FASEB J. 2012;26:3691–702.
6. DeBosch BJ, Muslin AJ. Insulin signaling pathways and cardiac growth. J Mol Cell Cardiol. 2008; 44:855–64.
7. Jones JI, Clemmons DR. Insulin-like growth factors and their binding proteins: biological actions. Endocr Rev. 1995;16:3–34.
8. Kooijman R. Regulation of apoptosis by insulin-like growth factor (igf)-i. Cytokine Growth Factor Rev. 2006;17:305–23.
9. Kurmasheva RT, Houghton PJ. Igf-i mediated survival pathways in normal and malignant cells. Biochim Biophys Acta. 2006;1766:1–22.
10. Anversa P, Nadal-Ginard B. Myocyte renewal and ventricular remodelling. Nature. 2002;415:240–3.
11. Suleiman MS, Singh RJ, Stewart CE. Apoptosis and the cardiac action of insulin-like growth factor i. Pharmacol Ther. 2007;114:278–94.
12. Catalucci D, Latronico MV, Ellingsen O, Condorelli G. Physiological myocardial hypertrophy: how and why? Front Biosci. 2008;13:312–24.
13. Philippou A, Armakolas A, Koutsilieris M. Evidence for the possible biological significance of the igf-1 gene alternative splicing in prostate cancer. Front Endocrinol (Lausanne). 2013;4:31.
14. Siegfried JM, Kasprzyk PG, Treston AM, Mulshine JL, Quinn KA, Cuttitta F. A mitogenic peptide amide encoded within the e peptide domain of the insulin-like growth factor ib prohormone. Proc Natl Acad Sci U S A. 1992;89:8107–11.
15. Kuo YH, Chen TT. Novel activities of pro-igf-i e peptides: regulation of morphological differentiation and anchorage-independent growth in human neuroblastoma cells. Exp Cell Res. 2002;280:75–89.
16. Carpenter V, Matthews K, Devlin G, Stuart S, Jensen J, Conaglen J, et al. Mechano-growth factor reduces loss of cardiac function in acute myocardial infarction. Heart Lung Circ. 2008;17:33–9.
17. Stavropoulou A, Halapas A, Sourla A, Philippou A, Papageorgiou E, Papalois A, et al. Igf-1 expression in infarcted myocardium and mgf e peptide actions in rat cardiomyocytes in vitro. Mol Med. 2009;15:127–35.
18. Mavrommatis E, Shioura KM, Los T, Goldspink PH. The E-domain region of mechano-growth factor inhibits cellular apoptosis and preserves cardiac function during myocardial infarction. Mol Cell Biochem. 2013;381:69–83.
19. Le Roith D, Bondy C, Yakar S, Liu JL, Butler A. The somatomedin hypothesis: 2001. Endocr Rev. 2001;22:53–74.
20. Baxter RC, Martin JL. Binding proteins for the insulin-like growth factors: structure, regulation and function. Prog Growth Factor Res. 1989;1:49–68.
21. Yu H, Rohan T. Role of the insulin-like growth factor family in cancer development and progression. J Natl Cancer Inst. 2000;92:1472–89.
22. Philippou A, Papageorgiou E, Bogdanis G, Halapas A, Sourla A, Maridaki M, et al. Expression of igf-1 isoforms after exercise-induced muscle damage in humans: characterization of the mgf e peptide actions in vitro. In Vivo. 2009;23:567–75.
23. Milingos DS, Philippou A, Armakolas A, Papageorgiou E, Sourla A, Protopapas A, et al. Insulinlike growth factor-1ec (mgf) expression in eutopic and ectopic endometrium: characterization of the mgf e-peptide actions in vitro. Mol Med. 2010;17:21–8.
24. Armakolas A, Philippou A, Panteleakou Z, Nezos A, Sourla A, Petraki C, et al. Preferential expression of igf-1ec (mgf) transcript in cancerous tissues of human prostate: evidence for a novel and autonomous growth factor activity of mgf e peptide in human prostate cancer cells. Prostate. 2010;70:1233–42.
25. Philippou A, Armakolas A, Panteleakou Z, Pissimissis N, Nezos A, Theos A, et al. Igf1ec expression in mg-63 human osteoblast-like osteosarcoma cells. Anticancer Res. 2011;31:4259–65.
26. Baxter RC. Insulin-like growth factor (igf)-binding proteins: interactions with igfs and intrinsic bioactivities. Am J Physiol Endocrinol Metab. 2000;278: E967–76.
27. Werner H, Bruchim I. The insulin-like growth factor-i receptor as an oncogene. Arch Physiol Biochem. 2009;115:58–71.
28. Oh Y. Igf-independent regulation of breast cancer growth by igf binding proteins. Breast Cancer Res Treat. 1998;47:283–93.
29. Hwa V, Oh Y, Rosenfeld RG. The insulin-like growth factor-binding protein (igfbp) superfamily. Endocr Rev. 1999;20:761–87.
30. De Meyts P, Whittaker J. Structural biology of insulin and igf1 receptors: implications for drug design. Nat Rev Drug Discov. 2002;1:769–83.
31. Kristensen C, Wiberg FC, Andersen AS. Specificity of insulin and insulin-like growth factor i receptors investigated using chimeric mini-receptors. Role of c-terminal of receptor alpha subunit. J Biol Chem. 1999;274:37351–6.
32. Philippou A, Halapas A, Maridaki M, Koutsilieris M. Type i insulin-like growth factor receptor signaling in skeletal muscle regeneration and hypertrophy. J Musculoskelet Neuronal Interact. 2007;7:208–18.
33. LeRoith D, Werner H, Beitner-Johnson D, Roberts CT. Molecular and cellular aspects of the insulin-like growth factor i receptor. Endocr Rev. 1995;16: 143–63.
34. Molkentin JD, Dorn GW. Cytoplasmic signaling pathways that regulate cardiac hypertrophy. Annu Rev Physiol. 2001;63:391–426.
35. Latronico MV, Costinean S, Lavitrano ML, Peschle C, Condorelli G. Regulation of cell size and contractile function by akt in cardiomyocytes. Ann N Y Acad Sci. 2004;1015:250–60.
36. McMullen JR. Role of insulin-like growth factor 1 and phosphoinositide 3-kinase in a setting of heart disease. Clin Exp Pharmacol Physiol. 2008;35:349–54.
37. Rohini A, Agrawal N, Koyani CN, Singh R. Molecular targets and regulators of cardiac hypertrophy. Pharmacol Res. 2010;61:269–80.

38. Fazio S, Palmieri EA, Biondi B, Cittadini A, Sacca L. The role of the gh-igf-i axis in the regulation of myocardial growth: from experimental models to human evidence. Eur J Endocrinol. 2000;142:211–6.
39. Shahi M, Beshyah SA, Hackett D, Sharp PS, Johnston DG, Foale RA. Myocardial dysfunction in treated adult hypopituitarism: a possible explanation for increased cardiovascular mortality. Br Heart J. 1992;67:92–6.
40. Ito H, Hiroe M, Hirata Y, Tsujino M, Adachi S, Shichiri M, et al. Insulin-like growth factor-i induces hypertrophy with enhanced expression of muscle specific genes in cultured rat cardiomyocytes. Circulation. 1993;87:1715–21.
41. Torella D, Rota M, Nurzynska D, Musso E, Monsen A, Shiraishi I, et al. Cardiac stem cell and myocyte aging, heart failure, and insulin-like growth factor-1 overexpression. Circ Res. 2004;94:514–24.
42. Reiss K, Cheng W, Ferber A, Kajstura J, Li P, Li B, et al. Overexpression of insulin-like growth factor-1 in the heart is coupled with myocyte proliferation in transgenic mice. Proc Natl Acad Sci U S A. 1996;93:8630–5.
43. Delaughter MC, Taffet GE, Fiorotto ML, Entman ML, Schwartz RJ. Local insulin-like growth factor i expression induces physiologic, then pathologic, cardiac hypertrophy in transgenic mice. FASEB J. 1999;13:1923–9.
44. McMullen JR, Shioi T, Huang WY, Zhang L, Tarnavski O, Bisping E, et al. The insulin-like growth factor 1 receptor induces physiological heart growth via the phosphoinositide 3-kinase(p110alpha) pathway. J Biol Chem. 2004;279:4782–93.
45. McMullen JR, Amirahmadi F, Woodcock EA, Schinke-Braun M, Bouwman RD, Hewitt KA, et al. Protective effects of exercise and phosphoinositide 3-kinase(p110alpha) signaling in dilated and hypertrophic cardiomyopathy. Proc Natl Acad Sci U S A. 2007;104:612–7.
46. Redaelli G, Malhotra A, Li B, Li P, Sonnenblick EH, Hofmann PA, et al. Effects of constitutive overexpression of insulin-like growth factor-1 on the mechanical characteristics and molecular properties of ventricular myocytes. Circ Res. 1998;82:594–603.
47. Thorburn J, McMahon M, Thorburn A. Raf-1 kinase activity is necessary and sufficient for gene expression changes but not sufficient for cellular morphology changes associated with cardiac myocyte hypertrophy. J Biol Chem. 1994;269:30580–6.
48. Glennon PE, Kaddoura S, Sale EM, Sale GJ, Fuller SJ, Sugden PH. Depletion of mitogen-activated protein kinase using an antisense oligodeoxynucleotide approach downregulates the phenylephrine-induced hypertrophic response in rat cardiac myocytes. Circ Res. 1996;78:954–61.
49. Clerk A, Michael A, Sugden PH. Stimulation of the p38 mitogen-activated protein kinase pathway in neonatal rat ventricular myocytes by the g protein-coupled receptor agonists, endothelin-1 and phenylephrine: a role in cardiac myocyte hypertrophy? J Cell Biol. 1998;142:523–35.
50. Yamazaki T, Tobe K, Hoh E, Maemura K, Kaida T, Komuro I, et al. Mechanical loading activates mitogen-activated protein kinase and s6 peptide kinase in cultured rat cardiac myocytes. J Biol Chem. 1993;268:12069–76.
51. Choukroun G, Hajjar R, Kyriakis JM, Bonventre JV, Rosenzweig A, Force T. Role of the stress-activated protein kinases in endothelin-induced cardiomyocyte hypertrophy. J Clin Invest. 1998;102:1311–20.
52. Laser M, Kasi VS, Hamawaki M, Cooper G, Kerr CM, Kuppuswamy D. Differential activation of p70 and p85 s6 kinase isoforms during cardiac hypertrophy in the adult mammal. J Biol Chem. 1998;273:24610–9.
53. Ellison GM, Waring CD, Vicinanza C, Torella D. Physiological cardiac remodelling in response to endurance exercise training: cellular and molecular mechanisms. Heart. 2011;98:5–10.
54. Shioi T, Kang PM, Douglas PS, Hampe J, Yballe CM, Lawitts J, et al. The conserved phosphoinositide 3-kinase pathway determines heart size in mice. EMBO J. 2000;19:2537–48.
55. Muslin AJ, DeBosch B. Role of akt in cardiac growth and metabolism. Novartis Found Symp. 2006;274:118–26; discussion 126–31, 152–5, 272–6.
56. Nagoshi T, Matsui T, Aoyama T, Leri A, Anversa P, Li L, et al. Pi3k rescues the detrimental effects of chronic akt activation in the heart during ischemia/reperfusion injury. J Clin Invest. 2005;115:2128–38.
57. Takano H, Komuro I, Zou Y, Kudoh S, Yamazaki T, Yazaki Y. Activation of p70 s6 protein kinase is necessary for angiotensin ii-induced hypertrophy in neonatal rat cardiac myocytes. FEBS Lett. 1996;379:255–9.
58. MacLellan WR, Schneider MD. Death by design. Programmed cell death in cardiovascular biology and disease. Circ Res. 1997;81:137–44.
59. Wang L, Ma W, Markovich R, Chen JW, Wang PH. Regulation of cardiomyocyte apoptotic signaling by insulin-like growth factor i. Circ Res. 1998;83:516–22.
60. Buerke M, Murohara T, Skurk C, Nuss C, Tomaselli K, Lefer AM. Cardioprotective effect of insulin-like growth factor i in myocardial ischemia followed by reperfusion. Proc Natl Acad Sci U S A. 1995;92:8031–5.
61. Palmen M, Daemen MJ, Bronsaer R, Dassen WR, Zandbergen HR, Kockx M, et al. Cardiac remodeling after myocardial infarction is impaired in igf-1 deficient mice. Cardiovasc Res. 2001;50:516–24.
62. Saetrum Opgaard O, Wang PH. Igf-i is a matter of heart. Growth Horm IGF Res. 2005;15:89–94.
63. Parrizas M, Saltiel AR, LeRoith D. Insulin-like growth factor 1 inhibits apoptosis using the phosphatidylinositol 3′-kinase and mitogen-activated protein kinase pathways. J Biol Chem. 1997;272:154–61.
64. Parrizas M, LeRoith D. Insulin-like growth factor-1 inhibition of apoptosis is associated with increased expression of the bcl-xl gene product. Endocrinology. 1997;138:1355–8.

65. Lai HC, Liu TJ, Ting CT, Sharma PM, Wang PH. Insulin-like growth factor-1 prevents loss of electrochemical gradient in cardiac muscle mitochondria via activation of pi 3 kinase/akt pathway. Mol Cell Endocrinol. 2003;205:99–106.
66. Fujio Y, Nguyen T, Wencker D, Kitsis RN, Walsh K. Akt promotes survival of cardiomyocytes in vitro and protects against ischemia-reperfusion injury in mouse heart. Circulation. 2000;101:660–7.
67. Shiraishi I, Melendez J, Ahn Y, Skavdahl M, Murphy E, Welch S, et al. Nuclear targeting of akt enhances kinase activity and survival of cardiomyocytes. Circ Res. 2004;94:884–91.
68. Kajstura J, Leri A, Finato N, Di Loreto C, Beltrami CA, Anversa P. Myocyte proliferation in end-stage cardiac failure in humans. Proc Natl Acad Sci U S A. 1998;95:8801–5.
69. Beltrami AP, Urbanek K, Kajstura J, Yan SM, Finato N, Bussani R, et al. Evidence that human cardiac myocytes divide after myocardial infarction. N Engl J Med. 2001;344:1750–7.
70. Nadal-Ginard B, Kajstura J, Anversa P, Leri A. A matter of life and death: cardiac myocyte apoptosis and regeneration. J Clin Invest. 2003;111:1457–9.
71. Beltrami AP, Barlucchi L, Torella D, Baker M, Limana F, Chimenti S, et al. Adult cardiac stem cells are multipotent and support myocardial regeneration. Cell. 2003;114:763–76.
72. Santini MP, Tsao L, Monassier L, Theodoropoulos C, Carter J, Lara-Pezzi E, et al. Enhancing repair of the mammalian heart. Circ Res. 2007;100:1732–40.
73. Ellison GM, Torella D, Dellegrottaglie S, Perez-Martinez C, Perez de Prado A, Vicinanza C, et al. Endogenous cardiac stem cell activation by insulin-like growth factor-1/hepatocyte growth factor intracoronary injection fosters survival and regeneration of the infarcted pig heart. J Am Coll Cardiol. 2011;58:977–86.
74. Santini MP, Winn N, Rosenthal N. Signalling pathways in cardiac regeneration. Novartis Found Symp. 2006;274:228–38; discussion 239–43, 272–26.
75. Stavropoulou A, Philippou A, Halapas A, Sourla A, Pissimissis N, Koutsilieris M. Upa, upar and tgf-beta(1) expression during early and late post myocardial infarction period in rat myocardium. In Vivo. 2010;24:647–52.
76. Philippou A, Maridaki M, Koutsilieris M. The role of urokinase-type plasminogen activator (upa) and transforming growth factor beta 1 (tgfbeta1) in muscle regeneration. In Vivo. 2008;22:735–50.
77. Khorsandi MJ, Fagin JA, Giannella-Neto D, Forrester JS, Cercek B. Regulation of insulin-like growth factor-i and its receptor in rat aorta after balloon denudation. J Clin Invest. 1992;90:1926–31.
78. Lee WL, Chen JW, Ting CT, Lin SJ, Wang PH. Changes of the insulin-like growth factor i system during acute myocardial infarction: implications on left ventricular remodeling. J Clin Endocrinol Metab. 1999;84:1575–81.
79. Lembo G, Rockman HA, Hunter JJ, Steinmetz H, Koch WJ, Ma L, et al. Elevated blood pressure and enhanced myocardial contractility in mice with severe igf-1 deficiency. J Clin Invest. 1996;98:2648–55.
80. Schulze PC, Spate U. Insulin-like growth factor-1 and muscle wasting in chronic heart failure. Int J Biochem Cell Biol. 2005;37:2023–35.
81. Vasan RS, Sullivan LM, D'Agostino RB, Roubenoff R, Harris T, Sawyer DB, et al. Serum insulin-like growth factor i and risk for heart failure in elderly individuals without a previous myocardial infarction: the Framingham Heart Study. Ann Intern Med. 2003;139:642–8.
82. Laughlin GA, Barrett-Connor E, Criqui MH, Kritz-Silverstein D. The prospective association of serum insulin-like growth factor i (igf-i) and igf-binding protein-1 levels with all cause and cardiovascular disease mortality in older adults: The Rancho Bernardo Study. J Clin Endocrinol Metab. 2004;89:114–20.
83. Sowers JR. Insulin and insulin-like growth factor in normal and pathological cardiovascular physiology. Hypertension. 1997;29:691–9.
84. Copeland KC, Nair KS. Recombinant human insulin-like growth factor-i increases forearm blood flow. J Clin Endocrinol Metab. 1994;79:230–2.
85. Kotlyar AA, Vered Z, Goldberg I, Chouraqui P, Nas D, Fridman E, et al. Insulin-like growth factor i and ii preserve myocardial structure in postinfarct swine. Heart. 2001;86:693–700.
86. Duerr RL, McKirnan MD, Gim RD, Clark RG, Chien KR, Ross J. Cardiovascular effects of insulin-like growth factor-1 and growth hormone in chronic left ventricular failure in the rat. Circulation. 1996;93:2188–96.
87. Kofidis T, de Bruin JL, Yamane T, Balsam LB, Lebl DR, Swijnenburg RJ, et al. Insulin-like growth factor promotes engraftment, differentiation, and functional improvement after transfer of embryonic stem cells for myocardial restoration. Stem Cells. 2004;22:1239–45.
88. Shan YX, Yang TL, Mestril R, Wang PH. Hsp10 and hsp60 suppress ubiquitination of insulin-like growth factor-1 receptor and augment insulin-like growth factor-1 receptor signaling in cardiac muscle: implications on decreased myocardial protection in diabetic cardiomyopathy. J Biol Chem. 2003;278:45492–8.
89. Norby FL, Wold LE, Duan J, Hintz KK, Ren J. Igf-i attenuates diabetes-induced cardiac contractile dysfunction in ventricular myocytes. Am J Physiol Endocrinol Metab. 2002;283:E658–66.
90. Mora A, Davies AM, Bertrand L, Sharif I, Budas GR, Jovanovic S, et al. Deficiency of pdk1 in cardiac muscle results in heart failure and increased sensitivity to hypoxia. EMBO J. 2003;22:4666–76.
91. Cittadini A, Ishiguro Y, Stromer H, Spindler M, Moses AC, Clark R, et al. Insulin-like growth factor-1 but not growth hormone augments mammalian myocardial contractility by sensitizing the myofilament to Ca^{2+} through a wortmannin-sensitive pathway: studies in rat and ferret isolated muscles. Circ Res. 1998;83:50–9.

92. Kovacic S, Soltys CL, Barr AJ, Shiojima I, Walsh K, Dyck JR. Akt activity negatively regulates phosphorylation of amp-activated protein kinase in the heart. J Biol Chem. 2003;278:39422–7.
93. Durzynska J, Philippou A, Brisson BK, Nguyen-McCarty M, Barton ER. The pro-forms of insulin-like growth factor i (igf-i) are predominant in skeletal muscle and alter igf-i receptor activation. Endocrinology. 2013;154:1215–24.
94. Brisson BK, Barton ER. Insulin-like growth factor-i e-peptide activity is dependent on the igf-i receptor. PLoS One. 2012;7:e45588.
95. Vinciguerra M, Santini MP, Martinez C, Pazienza V, Claycomb WC, Giuliani A, et al. Migf-1/jnk1/sirt1 signaling confers protection against oxidative stress in the heart. Aging Cell. 2012;11:139–49.
96. Poudel B, Bilbao D, Sarathchandra P, Germack R, Rosenthal N, Santini MP. Increased cardiogenesis in p19-gfp teratocarcinoma cells expressing the propeptide igf-1ea. Biochem Biophys Res Commun. 2011;416:293–9.
97. Vinciguerra M, Santini MP, Claycomb WC, Ladurner AG, Rosenthal N. Local igf-1 isoform protects cardiomyocytes from hypertrophic and oxidative stresses via sirt1 activity. Aging (Albany NY). 2010;2:43–62.
98. Philippou A, Stavropoulou A, Sourla A, Pissimissis N, Halapas A, Maridaki M, et al. Characterization of a rabbit antihuman mechano growth factor (mgf) polyclonal antibody against the last 24 amino acids of the e domain. In Vivo. 2008;22:27–35.
99. Moschos MM, Armakolas A, Philippou A, Pissimissis N, Panteleakou Z, Nezos A, et al. Expression of the insulin-like growth factor 1 (igf-1) and type i igf receptor mrnas in human hle-b3 lens epithelial cells. In Vivo. 2011;25:179–84.
100. Collins JM, Goldspink PH, Russell B. Migration and proliferation of human mesenchymal stem cells is stimulated by different regions of the mechano-growth factor prohormone. J Mol Cell Cardiol. 2010;49:1042–5.

Calcium Cycling Circuits in Cardiac Physiology and Pathophysiology

12

Kobra Haghighi, Despina Sanoudou, and Evangelia G. Kranias

Abstract

Abnormal calcium cycling is a universal characteristic of human and experimental heart failure. This calcium dys-regulation has been mainly attributed to the impaired function of the cardiac sarcoplasmic reticulum (SR). Abnormal Ca^{2+}-transport by the SR proteins, Ca^{2+}-ATPase (SERCA2a) and phospholamban (PLN), has been shown to have a vital role in cardiac pathophysiology and the progression of heart failure. PLN is an endogenous inhibitor of SERCA2a and as such is a primary player in cardiac relaxation by regulating Ca^{2+}-uptake. Moreover, recent studies identified other regulatory proteins in the SR Ca^{2+}-transport complex, namely inhibitor-1 of protein phosphatase 1 (PP1), the small heat shock protein 20 (Hsp20), the histidine-rich calcium binding protein (HRC), and the HS-1 associated protein X-1 (HAX1). We have shown that these new players could influence the PLN/SERCA activity and consequently, SR Ca^{2+}-transport, cardiomyocyte Ca^{2+}-contractility, cardiac remodeling and cell apoptosis. This article concentrates on the crucial role of the SR Ca^{2+}-handling proteins in the regulation of cardiac function and survival under physiological and pathophysiological conditions. The role of naturally occurring variants in these Ca^{2+}-cycling genes, which may serve as prognostic or diagnostic factors as well as modifiers of heart failure development, is also discussed.

K. Haghighi
Department of Pharmacology and Cell Biophysics, University of Cincinnati, College of Medicine, 231 Albert Sabin Way, Cincinnati, OH 45267-0575, USA

D. Sanoudou
Department of Pharmacology, Medical School, University of Athens and Biomedical Research Foundation of the Academy of Athens, 115-27, Athens, Greece

E.G. Kranias, PhD (✉)
Department of Pharmacology and Cell Biophysics, University of Cincinnati, College of Medicine, 231 Albert Sabin Way, Cincinnati, OH 45267-0575, USA

Academy of Athens Foundation of Biomedical Research, 115-27, Athens, Greece
e-mail: Litsa.Kranias@uc.edu

D.V. Cokkinos (ed.), *Introduction to Translational Cardiovascular Research*,
DOI 10.1007/978-3-319-08798-6_12, © Springer International Publishing Switzerland 2015

Keywords
Calcium • Sarcoplasmic reticulum • Contractility • Heart failure • Human variants

Abbreviations

+dP/dt	Rate of contraction
–dP/dt	Rate of relaxation
AAV9.I-1c	Recombinant adeno-associated viral vector containing I-1c gene
CAMKII	Calmodulin kinase II
CSQ	Calsequestrin
CUPID	Calcium Upregulation by Percutaneous administration of gene therapy In cardiac Disease
DCM	Dilated cardiomyopathy
DHPR	Dihydropyridine receptor
HAX1	HS-1 associated protein X-1
HF	Heart failure
HRC	Histidine-rich calcium binding protein
HSP20	Small heat shock protein 20
HSPs	Heat shock proteins
I-1	Inhibitor-1
I-1c	Constitutively active form of I-1
JCTN	Junctin
KO	Knockout
MI	Myocardial infarction
NCX	Sodium/calcium exchanger
PKA	Protein kinase A
PLN	Phospholamban
PP1	Protein phosphatase 1
RyR	Ryanodine receptor
SERCA2a	Ca^{2+}-ATPase
SR	Sarcoplasmic reticulum
SUMO1	Small ubiquitin-related modifier
TAC	Transverse-aortic constriction
TRDN	Triadin

12.1 Introduction

Cardiovascular disease is the leading cause of morbidity and mortality worldwide, with heart failure representing the fastest growing subcategory over the past decades. Aberrant Ca^{2+} handling is a hallmark of heart failure (HF), which is partially attributed to alterations in the function of the sarcoplasmic reticulum (SR). Coordinated regulation of cytosolic Ca^{2+} by the SR in cardiomyocytes is required during each cycle of cardiac contraction and relaxation. Cytosolic Ca^{2+} is sequestered into the SR lumen by sarcoplasmic reticulum Ca^{2+}-ATPase (SERCA2a), permitting muscle relaxation; subsequently, the stored Ca^{2+} is released through ryanodine receptor channels (RyR) to activate myofilament contraction [1] (Fig. 12.1a). The activity of SERCA2a is reversibly regulated by phospholamban (PLN), a 52 amino acid phosphoprotein [2]. Dephosphorylated PLN interacts with SERCA2a and inhibits Ca^{2+}-pump activity, whereas protein kinase A mediated phosphorylation of PLN through the β-adrenergic pathway relieves its inhibitory effects and augments relaxation [3]. In turn, the restoration of contractility to basal levels is modulated by protein phosphatase 1 (PP1), which dephosphorylates PLN. Interestingly, PP1 is also regulated by an inhibitory phosphoprotein, inhibitor-1 (I-1), which can enhance β-adrenergic mediated phosphorylation of PLN, thereby increasing SERCA2a activity. Recently, the 35-kD anti-apoptotic HS-1 associated protein X-1 (HAX1), a ubiquitously expressed protein that protects cells from programmed cell death, was identified as a binding partner of PLN [4]. Therefore, the HAX1/PLN/SERCA2a interaction has been postulated to regulate contractility and Ca^{2+} cycling in the heart. In addition, of particular interest is a small heat shock protein (~20 kDa) named HSP20. HSP20 overexpression protects the heart from isoproterenol-induced maladaptive remodeling, contractile dysfunction and apoptosis [5, 6] as well as myocardial infarction [7].

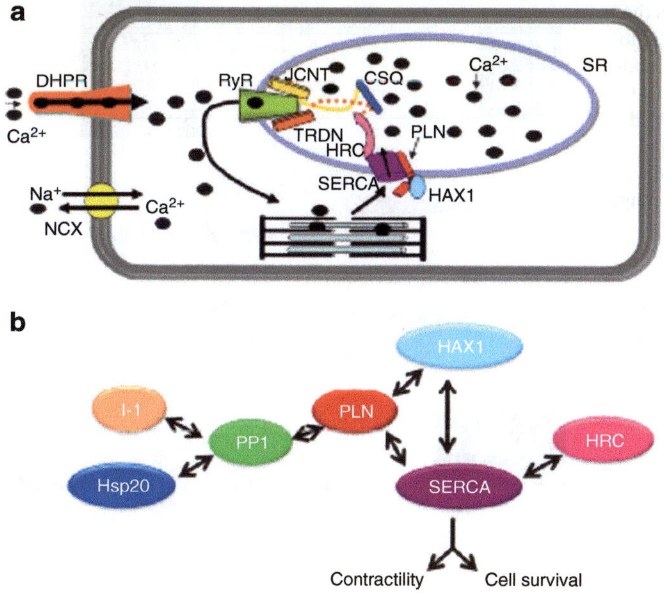

Fig. 12.1 Schematic representation of SR Ca^{2+}-cycling proteins and their global interactions in cardiomyocytes. (**a**) Calcium enters through the dihydropyridine receptor (*DHPR*) and activates the ryanodine receptor (*RyR*) to release calcium from the SR. Intracellular calcium binds to the myofibrils and triggers muscle contraction. Upon relaxation, there is reuptake of calcium by the SR Ca^{2+}-ATPase pump (*SERCA2a*) or removal of the cytosolic Ca^{2+} by the sodium/calcium exchanger (*NCX*). Phospholamban (*PLN*), in its dephosphorylated state, binds to and inhibits SERCA2a activity. HRC interacts with SERCA2a directly and triadin (*TRDN*) and synchronizes SR Ca^{2+} uptake and release. Calsequestrin (*CSQ*) interacts with both TRDN and junctin (*JCTN*) and regulates Ca^{2+} release by RYR. (**b**) Schematic interactions of the SR Ca^{2+}-transport ensemble, including Inhibitor-1 (*I-1*), type 1 protein phophatase (*PP1*), HS-1 associated protein X-1 (*HAX1*), heat shock protein 20 (*Hsp20*), and histidine-rich calcium binding protein (*HRC*). I-1, Hsp20 and PP1 are involved in the regulation of PLN activity; HAX1 interacts with PLN and possibly links SR Ca^{2+} cycling with cell survival

In addition, SR Ca^{2+} cycling is regulated by the histidine-rich calcium binding protein, HRC, which interacts with the ryanodine receptor Ca^{2+} release complex as well as SERCA2a [8]. Importantly, cardiac overexpression of HRC in mice inhibits SR Ca^{2+} uptake and cardiomyocyte relaxation [9], while HRC ablation has opposite effects [10]. Thus, HRC is a key regulator of SR Ca^{2+}-uptake, storage and release.

Collectively, studies on the SR calcium transport regulatory proteins at the intact animal, organ, cellular, and molecular levels (Fig. 12.2) have demonstrated that these proteins are important not only in the physiological cardiac function but also in pathological conditions, and may represent promising therapeutic targets for heart disease.

12.2 Role of SR Calcium Cycling Proteins and Cardiac Function Sarcoplasmic Reticulum Ca^{2+}-ATPase (SERCA)

The 110 kD transmembrane protein, is the major regulator of Ca^{2+} homeostasis and contractility in cardiac and skeletal muscle. SERCA belongs to a family of highly conserved proteins and SERCA2a is primarily expressed in the heart [11]. As mentioned above, the excitation-contraction coupling in the heart is dependent on the Ca^{2+} reuptake function of the SR, which is mainly regulated by the SERCA2a pump. Decreases in SERCA2a gene expression levels and activity have been correlated with defects in

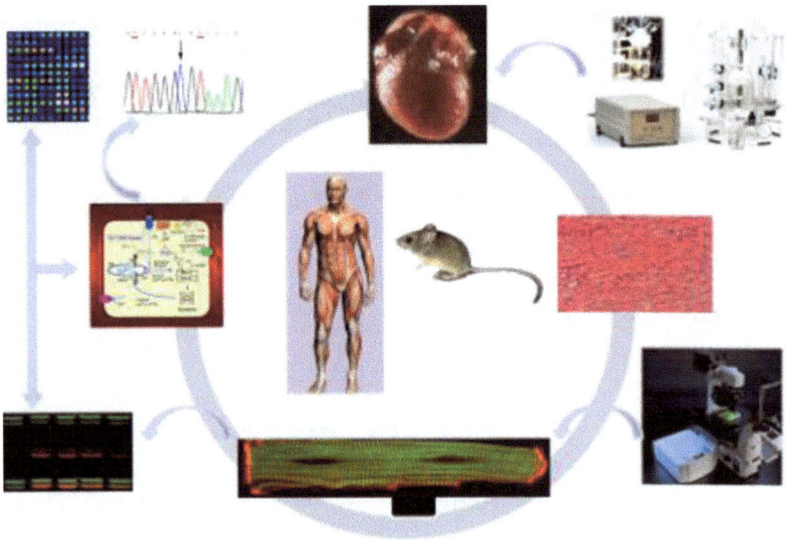

Fig. 12.2 Studies from the clinical side are extended to the bench side. Mouse models are studied at the intact animal, organ, cellular and sub-cellular levels, including genetic and molecular pathways using a wide range of approaches: echocardiography, catheterization, Langendorff perfusion, confocal microscopy, DNA sequencing, whole genome microarrays and a variety of protein assays

SR Ca^{2+}-uptake function in animal and human heart failure [12]. The role of altered SERCA2a levels in the heart has been extensively studied utilizing genetically altered models [13]. Transgenic mice over-expressing SERCA2a demonstrated an enhanced contractile phenotype [14]. Accordingly, disruption of both copies of the SERCA2a gene resulted in early embryonic lethality [15, 16], whereas heterozygous (haplo-insufficient) mice with a single functional allele survived and exhibited impaired cardiac contractility and relaxation without overt heart disease, indicating that heterozygous hearts were able to meet the functional requirements under normal conditions [15, 16]. However, increased hemodynamic stress in these mice resulted in an accelerated pathway to HF, demonstrating that HF occurred more rapidly with reduced SERCA2a levels in conjunction with pressure overload [17]. Generation of the in vivo model systems provided the investigators with the possibilities to explore how changes in SERCA pump levels affected the contraction-relaxation cycle of the heart. Furthermore, these studies suggested that there was a correlation between SERCA2a levels and modulation of cardiac contractility and further supported the notion that SERCA2a function was one of the fundamental determinants of cardiac contractility and an important candidate for gene therapy approaches in failing hearts.

Importantly, a major characteristic of failing human myocardium is abnormal calcium cycling as a consequence of reduced SERCA2a expression and increased inhibition of the pump by dephosphorylated PLN [18, 13]. Although pharmacologic therapies have provided gains in reducing the mortality rates in HF, the rising incidence of the disease indicates that new and novel treatment strategies are urgently needed. Early studies had shown that increasing the activity of SERCA2a via gene transfer resulted in enhanced contractility in isolated failing human cardiac myocytes, and led to improvement in cardiac function in animal models of HF [19–21]. With the advancement of gene vectors, SERCA2a emerged as an attractive clinical target for gene delivery purposes, which is now undergoing clinical testing in HF patients. Using adeno-associated virus constructs, SERCA2a upregulation has been found to improve myocardial function in small and large animal models with HF [21, 22] and these studies paved the way for clinical trials in patients with HF [23–25]. The first-in-human gene therapy trial, Calcium Upregulation by Percutaneous administration of gene therapy In cardiac Disease (CUPID), used an adeno-associated virus carrying SERCA2a in 39 patients with New York Heart Association class III/IV HF. Treatment with the SERCA2a adenovirus resulted in improvement or stabilization in the New York Heart Association class, walking stress test, N-terminal prohormone brain natriuretic peptide levels, peak maximum oxygen consumption and left ventricular end-systolic volume, as well as decreased frequency of cardiovascular events and duration of hospitalizations [24]. More importantly, it was shown that expression of SERCA2a was still observed after 3 years on initial delivery. The long term SERCA2a transgene expression continued to exert beneficial effects in these patients with advanced HF [25]. Thus, adeno-associated virus -mediated delivery of SERCA2a appears safe and effective for treating HF in phase 1 and 2 clinical trials [23, 24]. As a result, this approach has now moved on to the phase 3 trial with a large cohort of patients [25].

Interestingly, additional targets are emerging, which may be considered as candidates for genetic manipulation in diseased hearts. Recently, it was demonstrated that SERCA2a activity could be modulated by post-translational modifications [26]. The small ubiquitin-related modifier (SUMO1) was shown to regulate SERCA2a and act as a SERCA2a-enhancing factor. This regulation seems to be essential for preserving SERCA2a ATPase activity and stability in mouse and human cell modifications [26]. Furthermore, over-expression of SUMO1 in a rodent model of heart failure had favorable effects on myocardial function. Thus, SUMOylation is a critical post-translational modification, which regulates SERCA2a function, and may provide another platform for the design of novel therapeutic strategies for HF.

In summary, increased expression of SERCA2a leads to increases in calcium handling by the SR, which appears to be a benefit that accompanies the improved contractile phenotype of the heart under pathological conditions.

12.2.1 Phospholamban Regulation of SERCA and Cardiac Function

It is well established that SERCA2a activity is directly modulated by a 52-amino acid endogenous inhibitor, PLN. The inhibitory effect of PLN on SERCA2a activity was first revealed using genetically-altered animal models. Cardiac-specific overexpression of PLN inhibited SR Ca^{2+} uptake and reduced systolic Ca^{2+} levels, contractile parameters, and basal systolic function in mice [27]. In contrast, PLN knockout (KO) mice exhibited enhanced Ca^{2+} cycling and myocardial contractility with no gross developmental abnormalities. The elevated contractile parameters were associated with increased affinity of SERCA2a for Ca^{2+} [28]. Furthermore, it was found that the hyperdynamic cardiac function in PLN-KO mice persisted through the aging process. The persistence of hyperdynamic cardiac function over the long term did not induce any pathological or adverse functional consequences, suggesting that PLN may constitute an important target for treatment in heart disease [29].

In addition, comparative analyses with wild type, heterozygous and homozygous PLN-KO mice revealed that the relative PLN levels correlated well with the affinity of SERCA2a for Ca^{2+} and with the rates of relaxation and contraction in cardiomyocytes, intact hearts and in vivo [27, 28, 30, 31]. These findings suggested that the PLN level may impact SR function and cardiac contractility. Indeed, gene transfer approaches to increase the levels of PLN relative to SERCA2a in isolated cardiomyocytes have been reported to significantly alter intracellular calcium handling by prolonging the relaxation phase of the calcium transient, decreasing calcium release, and increasing end-diastolic calcium concentration [32]. Accordingly, antisense strategies to inhibit PLN indicate improved sarcoplasmic reticulum function, calcium mobilization, as well as significantly improved cell shortening in cardiomyocytes isolated from failing human hearts [32, 33]. Furthermore, overexpression of a dominant negative mutant of PLN has been reported to enhance SERCA2a activity [34]. Taken together, these studies suggest that PLN may have a key role in the maintenance of SERCA2a activity and that the PLN/SERCA2a ratio is a critical determinant of basal contractility in cardiomyocytes [35].

The prominent role of PLN in regulation of Ca^{2+}-cycling and excitation-contraction coupling was further supported by the identification of naturally occurring genetic variations in the human PLN gene, which appear to associate with heart failure. There have been four identified naturally occurring mutations in the coding region of the human PLN gene [36–39]. The human V49G point mutation was associated with super-inhibition of SERCA2a and heart failure induction in mouse models [37], while the human R9C-PLN mutation resulted in early death from dilated cardiomyopathy (DCM) in human carriers [36]. The underlying mechanisms included decreases in PLN phosphorylation and chronic inhibition of SERCA2a [36]. The T116G point mutation resulted in a stop codon (L39stop) and homozygosity was associated with DCM at a young age, while the heterozygous individuals exhibited hypertrophy without diminished contractile performance [38]. Another human mutation deleted the arginine 14 amino acid in PLN and heterozygous carriers developed heart failure by mid-age [39]. The R14del-PLN acted as a super-inhibitor of SERCA and cardiac pathology along with early death was observed in mouse models expressing this mutation in the heart [39]. Thus, there are human PLN mutations that are associated with predisposition to dilated cardiomyopathy.

12.2.2 The Anti-apoptotic Protein HAX-1 as a Regulator of Cardiac Function

The HS-1 associated protein X-1 (HAX1) was identified as a new PLN binding protein, using a human cDNA library and the yeast-two-hybrid screening approach [40]. Extensive protein studies led to the identification of the minimal binding domains of HAX1 (residues 203–245) and PLN (residues 16–22), indicating a direct physical interaction (Fig. 12.1b). Phosphorylation of PLN or elevation of the concentration of Ca^{2+} leads to dissociation of HAX1 from PLN, similar to findings on the PLN/SERCA2a interaction, thus indicating a physiological/pathophysiological significance of this association in cardiac muscle. Although HAX1 localizes to mitochondria, in the presence of PLN it becomes redistributed and co-localizes with PLN at the endoplasmic reticulum [40]. Analysis of the anti-apoptotic function of HAX1 revealed that the presence of PLN enhanced the HAX1 protective effects from hypoxia/reoxygenation induced cell death [40]. These findings suggest a potential link between the SR Ca^{2+} handling and cell survival, mediated by the PLN/HAX1 interaction.

12.2.3 The Role of Inhibitor-1 in Cardiac Function

The type-1 phosphatase (PP1) activity is significantly elevated in human and experimental HF. These increases have been suggested to be a contributing factor in the depressed cardiac function and remodeling. Indeed, cardiac overexpression of the catalytic subunit or PP1c in mouse models at similar levels as those observed in human failing hearts resulted in depressed function, remodeling, HF and early death [41]. Thus, it was suggested that inhibition of this enzyme by its endogenous inhibitor 2 and inhibitor 1 may hold promise for targeting the increased PP1 activity in HF. Gene delivery of inhibitor 2 in a rat model prevented HF progression and prolonged survival [42]. In addition, increased activity of inhibitor 1 (I- 1) exhibited therapeutic promise in HF. Inhibitor-1 is activated by protein kinase A (PKA) phosphorylation and this results in potent inhibition of PP1 and increased PLN phosphorylation, leading to enhanced Ca^{2+}-cycling (Fig. 12.3). The role of I-1 in the heart was elucidated by genetically altered mouse models. The I-1 knock-out mouse model (KO) presented with increased PP1 activity, had a depressed cardiac function under basal conditions and attenuated β- adrenergic response [41]. These effects were associated with decreased levels of phosphorylation on Serine 16 and Threonine 17 of PLN [41]. Accordingly, overexpression of a truncated (AA: 1–65) and constitutively active (T35D) form of I-1 (I-1c) demonstrated that I-1c could inhibit PP1 activity, increase Ser16 and Thr17 phosphorylation of PLN and attenuate the hypertrophic response, delaying the onset of HF [43]. In addition, cardiac-specific and inducible expression of I-1c in the adult heart revealed that I-1c enhances basal cardiac function, which is associated with increases in PLN phosphorylation levels [44]. Furthermore, under stress conditions (transverse

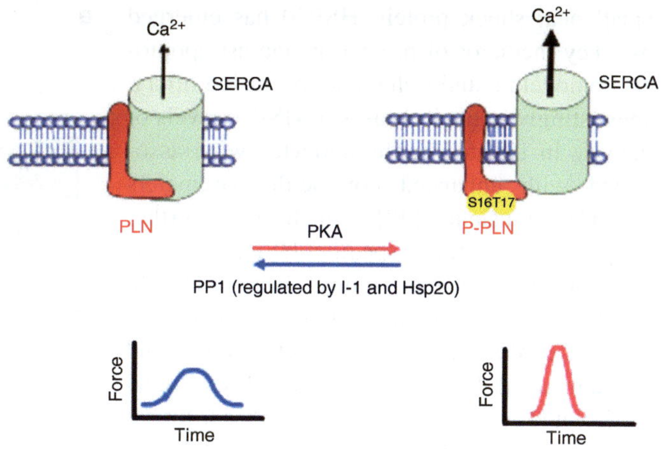

Fig. 12.3 Proposed role of Inhibitor-1 (I-1), PP1 and HSP20 in SR calcium cycling. PLN regulates the activity of the Ca^{2+}-ATPase pump in the SR. Dephosphorylated PLN exhibits an inhibitory effect on SERCA2a. PKA- and CaMKII-dependent phosphorylation of PLN at Ser16 and Thr17, respectively, relieve the inhibition and allow for increased Ca^{2+} pumping into the SR. PP1 is the main phosphatase responsible for dephosphorylating PLN. Inhibitor-1 and Hsp20 suppress PP1 activity, resulting in enhanced contractility

aortic constriction or *in vivo* ischemia/reperfusion), either conventional or inducible expression of I-1c was associated with increased PLN phosphorylation and increased SR Ca^{2+}-transport. This enhanced SR calcium cycling improved the heart's ability to accommodate the hypertrophic stimulus, delay the progression from hypertrophy to failure and impact cell survival under stress conditions. Thus, targeting I-1 may be beneficial in alleviating the detrimental effects of HF, through specific modulation of the PLN-coupled PP1 activity.

Importantly, long-term inducible expression of constitutively active inhibitor-1, I-1c, in the heart (up to 20 months) preserved increased PLN phosphorylation and did not affect survival rates or cardiac remodeling due to chronic increases in Ca^{2+}-cycling and function [45]. Furthermore, long-term expression of I-1c using recombinant adeno-associated virus type 9 gene transfer in rats with HF enhanced contractility and restored remodeling, associated with increased phosphorylation of PLN at Ser16 and Thr17 [45]. Thus, studies in rodent models suggest that chronic inhibition of protein phosphatase 1, through increases in I-1c, does not accelerate age-related cardiomyopathy and gene transfer of this molecule *in vivo* improves function and halts remodeling. These studies were subsequently extended to a large model of HF using gene transfer of I-1c. Heart failure was induced by myocardial infarction (MI) and 1 month post MI, the animals presented with severe failure, as indicated by decreases in ejection fraction, rates of contraction (+dP/dt) and relaxation (−dP/dt). Intracoronary injection of recombinant adeno-associated viral vector containing I-1c (AAV9.I-1c) prevented further deterioration of cardiac function and led to a decrease of scar size [46]. These preclinical studies indicate that cardiac overexpression of I-1c by gene transfer may improve hemodynamic function and improve cardiac remodelling. Interestingly, a naturally occurring genetic variant in I-1 (G147D), which diminishes the cardiomyocyte response to ß- adrenergic stimulation, has been also identified [47] and this indicates that human I-1 genetic variants may contribute to depressed Ca^{2+}-cycling and functional deterioration in HF.

Overall, the studies in small and large animal models indicate that inhibition of the elevated SR PP1 activity in heart disease by active inhibitor-1, I-1c, may constitute a therapeutic strategy to rectify the disturbed Ca^{2+}-homeostasis and function in failing hearts. Finally, the relatively small size of I-1c and its role as an inhibitor of PP1 opens the possibility of pharmacologic manipulation in addition to, or in replacement of, gene therapy.

12.2.4 Role of Hsp20 in SR Ca^{2+}-Cycling

Heat shock proteins (HSPs) are known to enhance cell survival under various stress conditions. In the context of cardiac function, the small heat shock protein HSP20 has emerged as a key mediator of protection against apoptosis, remodeling and ischemia/reperfusion injury. Interestingly, acute increases of HSP20 levels or activity in isolated cardiomyocytes were associated with enhanced contractile parameters and Ca^{2+}-transients [48], which were further supported by cardiac specific HSP20 overexpression in transgenic mouse hearts. HSP20 overexpression resulted in significant enhancement of cardiac function in intact animals, and in augmented Ca^{2+}-cycling and SR Ca^{2+}-load in isolated cardiomyocytes [5]. Accordingly, knockdown of HSP20 by antisense RNA or microRNA-320 resulted in depressed contractility [49]. The enhanced contractility by HSP20 overexpression was associated with specific increases in the phosphorylation of PLN, relieving its inhibitory effect on the apparent Ca^{2+}-affinity of SERCA2a. Interestingly, the activity of PP1, a regulator of PLN signaling, was significantly reduced by HSP20-overexpression, suggesting that the HSP20 stimulatory effects are partially mediated through the PP1/PLN interaction. Further studies revealed an association between HSP20, PP1 and PLN (Fig. 12.1b). Specifically, there is a physical interaction between HSP20 and PP1 [50], which could be indicative of the HSP20 role in the regulation of SR Ca^{2+}-cycling by targeting the PP1/PLN complex (Fig. 12.3). In addition, Hsp20 protects against ischemia/reperfusion-induced cardiac injury, β-agonist-mediated remodeling, and apoptosis [6, 7], introducing an additional role of HSP20 function in the heart. Thus, the enhanced contractility together with the cardioprotective role of HSP20 implies a potential dual benefit of targeting HSP20 in treating heart disease.

A genetic variant in human Hsp20 has also been identified, which results in C59T substitution in exon-1 of Hsp20 and changes a proline residue to leucine, at position 20 (P20L) [51]. This substitution was associated with structural alterations, diminished phosphorylation of Hsp20 and complete reversal of Hsp20's anti-apoptotic effects, suggesting that human carriers of the P20L- HSP20 genetic variant may present with an impaired ability to cope with cellular stress in the heart.

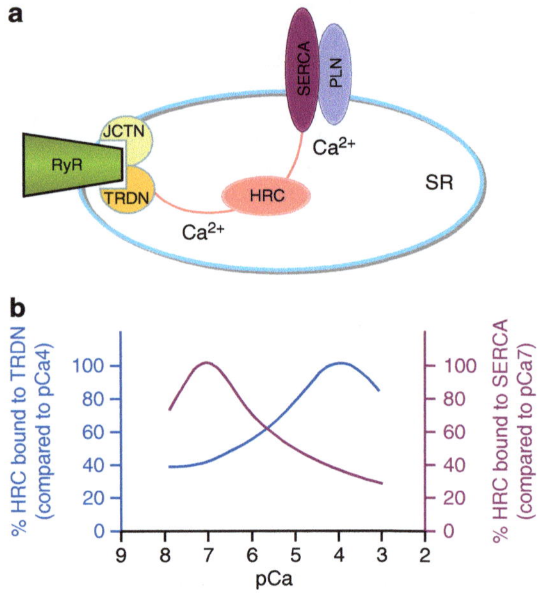

Fig. 12.4 Role of HRC in SR calcium cycling. (**a**) HRC interacts with SERCA2a and triadin (TRDN). (**b**) Increases in Ca^{2+} concentration reduce HRC binding to SERCA2a, while increasing HRC binding to TRDN. Thus, HRC may play a key role in the regulation of SR Ca^{2+} cycling by mediating a fine cross talk between SR Ca^{2+} uptake and release through the RyR in the heart

12.3 The Role of the Histidine-Rich Calcium Protein in the Heart

The histidine-rich calcium binding protein resides (HRC) in the lumen of the SR and has low affinity but high capacity for Ca^{2+}-binding [8]. HRC binds to triadin and associates with the ryanodine receptor Ca^{2+}-complex (Fig. 12.4a). HRC also interacts with SERCA and this binding domain is different than that interacting with triadin (Fig. 12.4a) [8]. Interestingly, binding of HRC to SERCA2a is sensitive to Ca^{2+} alterations [8]. While increases in Ca^{2+} concentration were associated with significant reduction of the HRC binding to SERCA2a, they had opposite effects on the interaction between HRC and triadin (Fig. 12.4b). These findings suggest that HRC may play a key role in the regulation of SR Ca^{2+}-cycling through its direct interactions with SERCA2a and triadin, mediating a fine cross-talk between SR Ca^{2+} uptake and release in the heart.

Indeed, acute overexpression of HRC in rat cardiomyocytes decreased Ca^{2+}-induced Ca^{2+}-release and impaired contractility [9]. In accordance, transgenic mice with cardiac overexpression of HRC presented with impaired SR Ca^{2+} uptake rates (35 %) and attenuated cardiomyocyte Ca^{2+} transient decay (38 %), without alterations in peak Ca^{2+} transients or SR Ca^{2+} load [9]. The underlying mechanism involved inhibition of SERCA2a maximal rates of Ca^{2+}-uptake [9]. The impaired SR Ca^{2+}-uptake led to the development of cardiac hypertrophy and remodeling and ultimately the presentation of congestive HF [9].

Although overexpression of HRC compromised cardiac function, it was protective upon ischemia/reperfusion injury and resulted in reduced infarct size [52]. This cardioprotection was due to reduced apoptosis and necrosis due to reduced SR and mitochondrial Ca^{2+} load [52].

Interestingly, ablation of HRC (HRC-knockout: KO) in mice did not result in any morphological or histological abnormalities [10]. However, cardiomyocytes exhibited significant increases in Ca^{2+}-cycling, contractility, and the maximal rates of SR Ca^{2+}-uptake. The enhanced Ca^{2+}-cycling resulted in increases in Ca^{2+}-spark frequency, the occurrence of Ca^{2+} spontaneous SR Ca^{2+} release and delayed after-depolarizations with ISO in HRC-KO, compared to WT cells [10].

In vivo, after-contractions developed under stress conditions of high-frequency stimulation (5 Hz) in the presence of isoproterenol. Upon transverse-aortic constriction (TAC), the HRC-KO cardiomyocytes showed significantly deteriorated cell contractility and Ca^{2+}-cycling, severe hypertrophy and fibrosis. The KOs developed pulmonary edema and exhibited decreased survival after TAC [10]. Thus, HRC appears to play an essential role in maintaining the integrity of cardiac function.

In humans, an HRC variant (Ser96Ala) was identified upon DNA analysis of 123 Greek patients with DCM and this variant was associated with life-threatening ventricular arrhythmias and sudden death [53]. The Ala/Ala homozygous patients showed an increased number of malignant arrhythmias than the Ser/Ala heterozygotes followed by the Ser/Ser homozygotes. This finding represents the first genetic variant of an SR Ca^{2+}-cycling gene associated with malignant arrhythmias in DCM and could serve as an independent predictor of susceptibility to arrhythmogenesis in the setting of DCM [53]. The underlying mechanisms include: (a) aberrant Ca^{2+}-cycling and depressed SR Ca^{2+}-load; (b) altered interactions of HRC with SERCA2a and triadin associated with impaired function and increased Ca^{2+}-leak by the RyR; and (c) increased Ser2814 phosphorylation of RyR by the calmodulin kinase II (CAMKII), leading to lethal arrhythmias under stress conditions [54], consistent with the phenotype in human carriers.

Conclusions

In summary, several lines of experimental evidence indicate that proper cardiac function is maintained, in part, through the complex regulation of SR calcium cycling. Indeed, the cross-talk between SR Ca^{2+}-cycling proteins mediates signaling pathways, which coordinately regulate cardiac performance. Recent evidence demonstrates that there is "a regulatory SR Ca^{2+}-transport ensemble" composed of SERCA2a, PLN, Hax-1, PP1, Inhibitor-1, Hsp20 and HRC. Disturbances in the fine regulation of these proteins are implicated as important contributors to depressed cardiac function and remodeling in the failing heart and restoring their function may hold promise as therapeutic strategy in heart failure.

Acknowledgements This work was supported by: NIH grants HL-26057 and HL-64018 to E. G. K.; the European Community's Seventh Framework Programme FP7/2007–2013 under grant agreement #HEALTH-F2-2009-241526, "EUTrigTreat" to E.G.K. and D.S.; the Greek General Secretariat for Research and Technology under "ARISTEIA II", the Hellenic Cardiological Society and the John S. Latsis Public Benefit Foundation to D.S.

References

1. MacLennan DH, Kranias EG. Phospholamban: a crucial regulator of cardiac contractility. Nat Rev Mol Cell Biol. 2003;4:566–77.
2. Kranias EG, Bers DM. Calcium and cardiomyopathies. Subcell Biochem. 2007;45:523–37.

3. Kim HW, Steenaart NA, Ferguson DG, Kranias EG. Functional reconstitution of the cardiac sarcoplasmic reticulum Ca^{2+}ATPase with phospholamban in phospholipid vesicles. J Biol Chem. 1990;265:1702–9.
4. Vafiadaki E, Arvanitis DA, Pagakis SN, Papalouka V, Sanoudou D, Kontrogianni-Konstantopoulos A, et al. The anti-apoptotic protein HAX-1 interacts with SERCA2 and regulates its protein levels to promote cell survival. Mol Biol Cell. 2009;20:306–18.
5. Fan GC, Yuan Q, Song G, Wang Y, Chen G, Qian J, et al. Small heat-shock protein Hsp20 attenuates beta-agonist-mediated cardiac remodeling through apoptosis signal-regulating kinase 1. Circ Res. 2006;99:1233–42.
6. Fan GC, Chu G, Mitton B, Song Q, Yuan Q, Kranias EG. Small heat-shock protein Hsp20 phosphorylation inhibits beta-agonist-induced cardiac apoptosis. Circ Res. 2004;94:1474–82.
7. Fan GC, Ren X, Qian J, Yuan Q, Nicolaou P, Wang Y, et al. Novel cardioprotective role of a small heat-shock protein, Hsp20, against ischemia/reperfusion injury. Circulation. 2005;111:1792–9.
8. Arvanitis DA, Vafiadaki E, Fan GC, Mitton BA, Gregory KN, del Monte F, et al. Histidine-rich Ca^{2+}-binding protein interacts with sarcoplasmic reticulum Ca^{2+}-ATPase. Am J Physiol Heart Circ Physiol. 2007;293:H1581–9.
9. Gregory KN, Ginsburg KS, Bodi I, Hahn H, Marreez YM, Song Q, et al. Histidine-rich Ca^{2+} binding protein: a regulator of sarcoplasmic reticulum calcium sequestration and cardiac function. J Mol Cell Cardiol. 2006;40:653–5.
10. Park CS, Chen S, Lee H, Cha H, Oh JG, Hong S, et al. Targeted ablation of the histidine-rich Ca^{2+}-binding protein (HRC) gene is associated with abnormal SR Ca^{2+}-cycling and severe pathology under pressure-overload stress. Basic Res Cardiol. 2013;108:344.
11. Arai M, Matsui H, Periasamy M. Sarcoplasmic reticulum gene expression in cardiac hypertrophy and heart failure. Circ Res. 1994;74:555–64.
12. Meyer M, Schillinger W, Pieske B, Holubarsch C, Heilmann C, Posival H, et al. Alterations of sarcoplasmic reticulum proteins in failing human dilated cardiomyopathy. Circulation. 1995;92:778–84.
13. Kranias EG, Hajjar RJ. Modulation of cardiac contractility by the phopholamban/SERCA2a regulatome. Circ Res. 2012;110:1646–60.
14. He H, Giordano FJ, Hilal-Dandan R, Choi D, Rockman HA, McDonough PM, et al. Overexpression of the rat sarcoplasmic reticulum Ca^{2+} ATPase gene in the heart of transgenic mice accelerates calcium transients and cardiac relaxation. J Clin Invest. 1997;100:380–9.
15. Ji Y, Lalli MJ, Babu GJ, Xu Y, Kirkpatrick DL, Liu LH, et al. Disruption of a single copy of the SERCA2 gene results in altered Ca^{2+} homeostasis and cardiomyocyte function. J Biol Chem. 2000;275:38073–80.
16. Periasamy M, Reed TD, Liu LH, Ji Y, Loukianov E, Paul RJ, et al. Impaired cardiac performance in heterozygous mice with a null mutation in the sarco(endo) plasmic reticulum Ca^{2+} -ATPase isoform 2 (SERCA2) gene. J Biol Chem. 1999;274:2556–62.
17. Schultz Jel J, Glascock BJ, Witt SA, Nieman ML, Nattamai KJ, Liu LH, et al. Accelerated onset of heart failure in mice during pressure overload with chronically decreased SERCA2 calcium pump activity. Am J Physiol Heart Circ Physiol. 2004;286:H1146–53.
18. Gwathmey JK, Yerevanian A, Hajjar RJ. Targeting sarcoplasmic reticulum calcium ATPase by gene therapy. Hum Gene Ther. 2013;24:937–47.
19. del Monte F, Harding SE, Schmidt U, Matsui T, Kang ZB, Dec GW, et al. Restoration of contractile function in isolated cardiomyocytes from failing human hearts by gene transfer of SERCA2a. Circulation. 1999;100:2308–11.
20. del Monte F, Williams E, Lebeche D, Schmidt U, Rosenzweig A, Gwathmey JK, et al. Improvement of survival and cardiac metabolism after gene transfer of sarcoplasmic reticulum Ca^{2+}- ATPase in a rat model of heart. Circulation. 2001;104:1424–9.
21. Miyamoto MI, del Monte F, Schmidt U, Matsui T, Guerrero JL, Gwathmey JK, et al. Adenoviral gene transfer of SERCA2a improves left ventricular function in aortic-banded rats in transition to heart failure. Proc Natl Acad Sci U S A. 2000;97:793–8.
22. Kawase Y, Ly HQ, Prunier F, Lebeche D, Shi Y, Jin H, et al. Reversal of cardiac dysfunction after long-term expression of SERCA2a by gene transfer in a pre-clinical model of heart failure. J Am Coll Cardiol. 2008;51:1112–9.
23. Jaski BE, Jessup ML, Mancini DM, Cappola TP, Pauly DF, Greenberg B, et al. Calcium upregulation by percutaneous administration of gene therapy in cardiac disease (CUPID Trial), a first-in-human phase ½ clinical trial. J Card Fail. 2009;15:171–81.
24. Jessup M, Greenberg B, Mancini D, Cappola T, Pauly DF, Jaski B, et al. Calcium Upregulation by Percutaneous Administration of Gene Therapy in Cardiac Disease (CUPID): a phase 2 trial of intracoronary gene therapy of sarcoplasmic reticulum Ca2+–ATPase in patients with advanced heart failure. Circulation. 2011;124:304–13.
25. Zsebo KM, Yaroshinsky A, Rudy JJ, Wagner K, Greenberg B, Jessup M, et al. Long-term effects of AAV1/SERCA2a gene transfer in patients with severe heart failure: analysis of recurrent cardiovascular events and mortality. Circ Res. 2014;114:101–8.
26. Kho C, Lee A, Jeong D, Oh JG, Chaanine AH, Kizana E, et al. SUMO1-dependent modulation of SERCA2a in heart failure. Nature. 2011;477(7366):601–5.
27. Kadambi VJ, Ponniah S, Harrer JM, Hoit BD, Dorn 2nd GW, Walsh RA, et al. Cardiac-specific overexpression of phospholamban alters calcium kinetics and resultant cardiomyocyte mechanics in transgenic mice. J Clin Invest. 1996;97:533–9.
28. Luo W, Grupp IL, Harrer J, Ponniah S, Grupp G, Duffy JJ, et al. Targeted ablation of the phospholamban gene is associated with markedly enhanced myocardial contractility and loss of beta-agonist stimulation. Circ Res. 1994;75:401–9.

29. Slack JP, Grupp IL, Dash R, Holder D, Schmidt A, Gerst MJ, et al. The enhanced contractility of the phospholamban-deficient mouse heart persists with aging. J Mol Cell Cardiol. 2001;33:1031–40.
30. Luo W, Wolska BM, Grupp IL, Harrer JM, Haghighi K, Ferguson DG, et al. Phospholamban gene dosage effects in the mammalian heart. Circ Res. 1996;78:839–47.
31. Lorenz JN, Kranias EG. Regulatory effects of phospholamban on cardiac function in intact mice. Am J Physiol. 1997;273:H2826–31.
32. del Monte F, Harding SE, Dec GW, Gwathmey JK, Hajjar RJ. Targeting phospholamban by gene transfer in human heart failure. Circulation. 2002;105:904–7.
33. Suckau L, Fechner H, Chemaly E, Krohn S, Hadri L, Kockskamper J, et al. Long-term cardiac-targeted RNA interference for the treatment of heart failure restores cardiac function and reduces pathological hypertrophy. Circulation. 2009;119:1241–52.
34. Ziolo MT, Martin JL, Bossuyt J, Bers DM, Pogwizs SM. Adenoviral gene transfer of mutant phospholamban rescues contractile dysfunction in failing rabbit myocytes with relatively preserved SERCA function. Circ Res. 2005;96:815–7.
35. Brittssan AG, Kranias EG. Phospholamban and cardiac contractile function. J Mol Cell Cardiol. 2000;32:2131–9.
36. Schmitt JP, Kamisago M, Asahi M, Li GH, Ahmad F, Mende U, et al. Dilated cardiomyopathy and heart failure caused by a mutation in phospholamban. Science. 2003;299(5611):1410–3.
37. Haghighi K, Schmidt AG, Hoit BD, Brittsan AG, Yatani A, Lester JW, et al. Superinhibition of sarcoplasmic reticulum function by phospholamban induces cardiac contractile failure. J Biol Chem. 2001;276:24145–52.
38. Haghighi K, Kolokathis F, Pater L, Lynch RA, Asahi M, Gramolini AO, et al. Human phospholamban null results in lethal dilated cardiomyopathy revealing a critical difference between mouse and human. J Clin Invest. 2003;111:869–76.
39. Haghighi K, Kolokathis F, Gramolini AO, Waggoner JR, Pater L, Lynch RA, et al. A mutation in the human phospholamban gene, deleting arginine 14, results in lethal, hereditary cardiomyopathy. Proc Natl Acad Sci U S A. 2006;103:1388–93.
40. Vafiadaki E, Sanoudou D, Arvanitis DA, Catino DH, Kranias EG, Kontogianni-Konstantopoulos A. Phospholamban interacts with HAX-1, a mitochondrial protein with anti-apoptotic function. J Mol Biol. 2007;367:65–79.
41. Carr AN, Schmidt AG, Suzuki Y, del Monte F, Sato Y, Lanner C, et al. Type 1 phosphatase, a negative regulator of cardiac function. Mol Cell Biol. 2002;22:4124–35.
42. Yamada M, Ikeda Y, Yano M, Yoshimura K, Nishino S, Aoyama H, et al. Inhibition of protein phosphatase 1 by inhibitor-2 gene delivery ameliorates heart failure progression in genetic cardiomyopathy. FASEB J. 2006;20:1197–9.
43. Pathak A, del Monte F, Zhao W, Schultz JE, Lorenz JN, Bodi I, et al. Enhancement of cardiac function and suppression of heart failure progression by inhibition of protein phosphatase 1. Circ Res. 2005;96:756–66.
44. Nicolaou P, Rodriguez P, Ren X, Zhou X, Qian J, Sadayappan S, et al. Inducible expression of active protein phosphatase-1 inhibitor-1 enhances basal cardiac function and protects against ischemia/reperfusion injury. Circ Res. 2009;104:1012–20.
45. Pritchard TJ, Kawase Y, Haghighi K, Anjak A, Cai W, Jiang M, et al. Active Inhibitor-1 maintains protein hyper-phosphorylation in aging hearts and halts remodeling in failing hearts. PLoS One. 2013;8:e80717.
46. Fish KM, Ladage D, Kawase Y, Karakikes I, Jeong D, Ly H, et al. AAV9.I-1c delivered via direct coronary infusion in a porcine model of heart failure improves contractility and mitigates adverse remodeling. Circ Heart Fail. 2013;6:310–7.
47. Chen G, Zhou X, Nicolaou P, Rodriguez P, Song G, Mitton B, et al. A human polymorphism of protein phosphatase-1 inhibitor-1 is associated with attenuated contractile response of cardiomyocytes to beta-adrenergic stimulation. FASEB J. 2008;22:1790–6.
48. Chu G, Egnaczyk GF, Zhao W, Jo SH, Fan GC, Maggio JE, et al. Phosphoproteome analysis of cardiomyocytes subjected to beta-adrenergic stimulation: identification and characterization of a cardiac heat shock protein p20. Circ Res. 2004;94:184–93.
49. Ren XP, Wu J, Wang X, Sartor MA, Qian J, Jones K, et al. MicroRNA-320 is involved in the regulation of cardiac ischemia/reperfusion injury by targeting heat-shock protein 20. Circulation. 2009;119:2357–66.
50. Qian J, Vafiadaki E, Florea SM, Singh VP, Song W, Lam CK, et al. Small heat shock protein 20 interacts with protein phosphatase-1 and enhances sarcoplasmic reticulum calcium cycling. Circ Res. 2011;108:1429–38.
51. Nicolaou P, Knöll R, Haghighi K, Fan GC, Dorn 2nd GW, Hasenfub G, et al. Human mutation in the anti-apoptotic heat shock protein 20 abrogates its cardioprotective effects. J Biol Chem. 2008;283:33465–71.
52. Zhou X, Fan GC, Ren X, Waggoner JR, Gregory KN, Chen G, et al. Overexpression of histidine-rich Ca-binding protein protects against ischemia/reperfusion-induced cardiac injury. Cardiovasc Res. 2007;75:487–97.
53. Arvanitis DA, Sanoudou D, Kolokathis F, Vafiadaki E, Papalouka V, Kontrogianni-Konstantopoulos A, et al. The Ser96Ala variant in histidine-rich calcium-binding protein is associated with life-threatening ventricular arrhythmias in idiopathic dilated cardiomyopathy. Eur Heart J. 2008;29:2514–25.
54. Singh VP, Arvanitis DA, Ren X, Gao X, Haghighi K, Gilbert M, et al. Abnormal calcium cycling and cardiac arrhythmias associated with the human Ser96Ala genetic variant of histidine-rich calcium-binding protein. J Am Heart Assoc. 2013;2:e000460.

Inflammation and Atherosclerosis

13

Eva D. Papadimitraki and Dimitrios T. Boumpas

Abstract

Atherosclerosis is a slowly progressing disorder of large- and medium-sized arteries leading to overt disease when significant narrowing or atherosclerotic plaque rupture occurs. Inflammation plays a key role in atherosclerotic plaque formation, progression and rapture. Both innate and adaptive immune responses are important to disease pathogenesis. Toll-like receptors, NOD-like receptors and the inflammasome are key components of LDL and other atherogenic molecule recognition and internalization and the subsequent interaction with components of the adaptive immune response. The NLPR3 inflammasome acts through the activation of caspase, can be primed by TLR activation and seems to have a crucial role in atherosclerosis and other related disorders such as diabetes, obesity and the metabolic syndrome. However, its experimental inactivation/modification has provided conflicting results in animal models of the disease. Lipid perturbations are also important since they can lead to endothelial cell activation and the augmentation of the inflammatory immune response; even high density lipoproteins may lose their atheroprotective capacities. Chronic inflammatory diseases are characterized by accelerated atherosclerosis: Systemic lupus erythematosus, rheumatoid arthritis, Sjogren syndrome and antiphospholipid syndrome patients display an increased incidence of cardiovascular disease not explained by traditional risk factors.

Studying inflammation is achieved through integration of data from animal models, high-throughput technologies and molecular imaging. Emerging and novel therapies target inflammation to achieve atherosclerosis regression. Modulators of cholesteryl ester transfer protein activity and interleukin-1 inhibitors, have produced promising results.

E.D. Papadimitraki, MD
Department of Cardiology,
Laikon General Hospital, Athens, Greece
e-mail: evapapadimitraki@hotmail.com

D.T. Boumpas, MD, FACP (✉)
1st Department of Medicine, Attiko Hospital,
1 Rimini Street, 12462, Chaidari, Athens, Greece
e-mail: boumpasd@med.uoc.gr

D.V. Cokkinos (ed.), *Introduction to Translational Cardiovascular Research*,
DOI 10.1007/978-3-319-08798-6_13,

Keywords
Atherosclerosis • Endothelial dysfunction • Inflammasome • Toll-like receptors • High-throughput technologies

Abbreviations

ACS	Acute coronary syndrome
AID	Autoimmune disease
AMPK	AMP activated kinase
AP-1	Activator protein 1
ApoB100	Apolipoprotein B100
APS	Antiphospholipid syndrome
ASC	Apoptosis associated speck-like protein containing a CARD
ATH	Atherosclerosis
BIR	Baculoviral inhibition of apoptosis repeat domain
CAD	Coronary artery disease
CCL	Chemokine ligand
CCR	C-C chemokine receptor
CD36	Cluster of differentiation 36
CETP	Cholesteryl ester transfer protein
CSF	Colony stimulation factor
CT	Computed tomography
CVD	Cardiovascular disease
CXCL	CX chemokine ligand
DAMP	Damage associated molecular pattern
DC	Dendritic cell
EC	Endothelial cell
ECM	Extracellular matrix
EDA	Ectodysplasin
eNOS	Endothelial NO synthetase
ERK	Extracellular signal regulated kinase
ET	Endothelin
F2LR3	Coagulation factor II (thrombin) receptor-like 3
FDG	18F fluorodeoxyglucose
FFA	Free fatty acid
FoxP3	Forkhead box P3
FXR	Farsenoid X receptor
GPR120	G-protein couplet receptor 120
GWA	Genome wide assay
HDL	High density lipoprotein
HLA	Human leukocyte antigen
HMGB1	High mobility group box 1
HSP	Heat shock protein
IAPP	Islet amyloid polypeptide
ICAM	Intercellular adhesion molecule
IFN	Interferon
IL	Interleukin
IL	Insulin receptor
INFL	Inflammation
IRF	Interferon regulating factor
IRS	Insulin receptor substrate
IVUS	Intravascular ultrasound
LDB	LIM domain binding factor
LDL	Low density lipoprotein
LOX	Lipoprotein scavenger receptor
LpPL	Likpoprotein associated phospholipase
LTB	Leukotriene beta
LXR	Liver X receptor
MACE	Major adverse cardiovascular events
MAD	Mothers against decapentaplegic
MAPK	Mitogen activated protein kinase
MARCO	Macrophage receptor with collagen structure
MCP	Monocyte chemoattractant protein
MCSF	Macrophage colony stimulating factor
MF	Macrophage
MI	Myocardial infarction
miRNA	microRNA
mmLDL	Minimally modified LDL
MRI	Magnetic resonance imaging
MyD88	Myeloid differentiation factor 88
NALP	NACHT, LLR and pyrin domain containing protein
NAMP	Nutrition associated molecular pattern
NASH	Non-alcoholic steatohepatitis

NF-κB	Nuclear factor kappa beta
NIRS	Near-infrared spectroscopy
NLPR	NOD-like protein receptor
NLRs	NOD-like receptors
NO	Nitric oxide
NOD	Nucleotide binding oligomerization domain
OxLDL	Oxidized LDL
PAMP	Protein associated molecular pattern
PCAM	Platelet cell adhesion molecule
PET	Positron emission tomography
PGI	Prostacyclin
PI	Phosphoinositide
PMS	Neutrophil
PPAR	Peroxisome proliferator activated receptor
PSOX	Scavenger receptor that binds phosphatidylserine
RA	Rheumatoid arthritis
RANTES	Regulated on activation, normal T-cell expressed and secreted
RGD	Arginine glycine aspartic acid
ROS	Reactive oxygen species
sICAM	Soluble ICAM
siRNA	Small interfering RNA
SLE	Systemic lupus erythematosus
SMA	Small body size
SMC	Smooth muscle cell
SNP	Single nucleotide polymorphism
SPECT	Single photon emission computed tomography
SRA	Scavenger receptors class A
SRB	Scavenger receptors class B
SREBP	Sterol regulatory element binding protein
SS	Sjogren syndrome
sVCAM	Soluble VCAM
TG	Triglyceride
TGF	Transforming growth factor
T_H	T-helper
TLR	Toll-like receptor
TMAO	Trimethylamine-N-oxide
TNF	Tumor necrosis factor
T_{REGS}	T regulatory cells
TXNIP	Thioredoxin-interacting protein
VCAM	Vascular cell adhesion molecule
VSMC	Vascular smooth muscle cell
β2GP1	Beta 2 glycoprotein 1

13.1 Introduction

Atherosclerosis (ATH), the underlying pathological process of coronary artery (CAD) and cerebrovascular disease, is a slowly progressing chronic disorder of large- and medium – sized arteries, which becomes clinically apparent when significantly narrowing of the vessel lumen or when thrombosis ensues. The concept that ATH constitutes a passive lipid accumulation in the vessel wall, which dominated over the past decades, has recently been challenged by evidence suggesting that ATH is a predominantly low grade chronic inflammatory disorder, where both, innate and adaptive immune responses play a pivotal role throughout initiation, progression and clinical manifestation of the disease [1, 2].

In this chapter, we discuss novel concepts in the physiology of inflammation (INFL) and its role in the initiation and progression of ATH. In this context, we discuss innate and adaptive immune responses with emphasis on the inflammasome and its role in ATH. Endothelial biology is closely linked to both INFL and ATH; we discuss facets of endothelial biology linked to both. Chronic INFL has an impact on lipid metabolism. In turn, lipid metabolism may affect INFL; we critically review the evidence and their importance. We next focus our attention to the chronic autoimmune inflammatory diseases as unique models to study accelerated atherosclerosis in humans and decipher novel mechanisms. To this end, we discuss animal models and novel experimental approaches including high-throughput methods. We conclude with a brief discussion of the rationale behind the development of new therapeutic targets based on the "inflammation hypothesis" of ATH.

13.2 The Immune System in Atherosclerosis

13.2.1 Overview of the Immune Response in Atherosclerosis

Animal experiments, epidemiological studies and clinical investigations have established that high concentrations of cholesterol promote cardiovascular disease (CVD). Cholesterol is transported in the blood by low density lipoprotein (LDL) particles containing esterified cholesterol and triglycerides surrounded by a shell of phospholipids, free cholesterol and apolipoprotein B100 (Apo-B100). Within the arterial intima, Apo-B100 binds to extracellular matrix (ECM) proteoglycans –that is, heavily glycosylated protein/collagen complexes that regulate permeability and molecule binding within the ECM-. Both innate and adaptive immune responses have been described in atherosclerosis.

13.2.1.1 Innate Immune Responses

Subendothelial LDL particles undergo oxidative modifications mediated by myeloperoxidases, lipoxygenases or reactive oxygen species (ROS). Modified phospholipids such as phosphatidylcholine and oxidized 1-palmitoyl-2-arachidonoyl-sn-glycero-30-phosphocholine activate endothelial cells and resident macrophages to express adhesion molecules and cytokines. The internalization of modified LDL particles is mediated by scavenger receptors that recognize oxygenation specific epitopes on oxidized LDL (ox-LDL), such as SRA-1 and SRA-2, MARCO, CD36, SR-B1, LOX-1 and PSOX, and by Toll-like Receptors (TLRs) mainly TLR-2, TLR-4 (but also likely TLR-1, TLR-5, TLR-7 and TLR-9). TLRs either expressed by macrophages or by resident endothelial cells play a major role in ATH. Knockout studies of hypercholesterolemic mice demonstrated a major proatherosclerotic effect of MyD88, an adaptor molecule of TLR signaling. Targeted deletion of the gene encoding TLR-4 also attenuated ATH [3]. Furthermore, genetic variants of specific TLRs are linked to this process. The TLR-4 single nucleotide polymorphism (SNP) Asp299Gly is associated with an increased risk for myocardial infarction. In addition to surface bound TLRs, other receptors of the innate immunity such as the NOD-like receptors (NLRs) may also be involved in the recognition of intracellular triggering stimuli. Some of these assemble into molecular platforms called "inflammasomes" which can trigger the secretion of cytokines such as interleukin (IL)-18 and IL-1β. The NOD-like protein-3 (NLPR-3) inflammasome is activated by cholesterol crystals in macrophages and seems to play a major role in atherosclerosis (see below).

13.2.1.2 TLRs and NLRs

TLRs are transmembrane receptors belonging to the TLR-IL-1 receptor superfamily –also including the Drosophila melanogaster protein Toll and the IL-18 receptor-. They are expressed throughout the body and are mainly found on "professional" innate immune cells but also on endothelial and smooth muscle cells. They initiate conserved signaling pathways involving mitogen-activated protein kinases (MAPKs), and other immune pathways culminating in the activation of nuclear factor (NF)-kB, activator protein 1 (AP-1) and interferon (IFN)-regulating factor (IRF). These transcription factors drive the expression of proinflammatory genes and signals that initiate adaptive immunity. In addition to pathogen derived components, TLRs are also capable of recognizing endogenous inflammatory ligands such as those released during necrotic cell death or the products of degradation of ECM. These endogenous ligands come under the term "damage associated molecular patterns, (DAMPs)" and include heat shock proteins (HSPs), high mobility group box 1 (HMGB1), fibrinogen, heparin sulfate, ectodysplasin (EDA) and nucleic acids. Most of these potential TLR ligands are detected at high levels in atherosclerotic lesions and are reported to be predictive of an increased risk for acute cardiac events. Importantly, minimally modified LDL also activates TLR-4, triggering the expression of pro-inflammatory cytokines such as IL-1β, IL-6 and regulated on activation, normal T-cell expressed and secreted (RANTES) molecule.

Nucleotide binding oligomerization domain (NOD)-like receptors (NLRs) comprise an additional family of innate receptors that drive the immune mechanisms aiming towards the elimination of invading pathogens. In a similar way to TLRs, NLRs activate NF-kB, a key transcription factor for inflammatory and immune gene expression. The NLRs NACHT, LLR and pyrin domain containing protein (NALP)-1 and NALP-3 also activate caspase-1 which is a proinflammatory caspase that processes the pro-forms of IL-1β an IL-18, two crucial proinflammatory cytokines. The TLRs and NOD-1 and NOD-2 can induce pro- IL-1β and IL-18 through NF-kB stimulation. In this context, TLRs prime the caspase-1 containing complexes (termed "inflammasomes") suggesting a complex interplay between TLRs and NLRs for the induction of IL-1β and IL-18. Importantly, the NLPR-3 inflammasome can also be activated by cholesterol crystals and contribute to atherosclerosis.

13.2.2 Hemodynamic Components of the Innate Immune Response

Turbulent flow at arterial branching points or high shear stress –as in the context of hypertension- may also induce endothelial cell activation leading to the expression of adhesion molecules such as E-selectin or vascular cell adhesion molecule 1 (VCAM-1) on the surface of endothelial cells. These act synergistically with chemokines such as CCL2, CCL2, CXCL10, CX3CL1 to attract monocytes, dendritic cells (DCs) and T-cells into the intima. Endothelial cell derived colony stimulating factor (CSF) leads to the differentiation of monocytes into macrophages, a key process in the development of ATH. Once differentiated and activated, macrophages express scavenger receptors that take-up oxidized LDL. The ensuing cholesterol accumulation within these cells leads to the formation of foam cells.

The removal of excess cholesterol from foam cells which is mediated by high density lipoprotein (HDL) and its principal apolipoprotein, apolipoprotein A1 (apoA1) is considered to be atheroprotective. ATP-binding cassette transporters (ABC) A1 (ABCA1) and G1 (ABCG1) are key molecules to cholesterol efflux and cholesterol homeostasis. It has been demonstrated that passive cholesterol diffusion accounts for 30 % of cholesterol efflux from foam cells. The rest 70 % of cholesterol removal is mediated by ABCA1 and ABCG1 through an energy-dependent process accomplished through yet not fully clarified mechanisms. Importantly, genetic deficiencies in either of these two transporters leads to TLR overexpression and inflammatory response which is potentially attributed to cholesterol accumulation in membranes. Of note, although cholesterol efflux is thought to confer some protection against ATH, experiments with different animal models genetically modified not to express ABCA1 or ABCG1 have generated conflicting results.

13.2.2.1 Adaptive Immune Responses

Two molecules have emerged as important potent autoantigens in atherosclerosis; LDL and heat-shock protein 60 (HSP 60) [4, 5]. Whereas under normal conditions DCs tolerize T-cells to antigens, danger signals elicited during atherogenesis, activate DCs switching them from tolerance to the activation of adaptive immunity. During the late stage of monocyte differentiation, oxidized LDL gives rise to mature IL-12 producing DCs that induce syngeneic and allogeneic T-cell stimulation. T-cells are recruited in parallel with macrophages in a T-cell to macrophage ratio between 1:4 and 1:10 and contribute to lesion growth and disease aggravation. In this context, DC driven polarization of T-cells to the T_H1 phenotype leads to the production of IFN-γ, IL-10 and TNF-α which contribute to plaque neovascularization, extracellular matrix (ECM) degradation and increased thrombogenicity, all markers of plaque destabilization, thus conferring to atheroma a propensity to rupture. Although not yet fully established, inflammatory Il-17 producing T cells (T_H17 cells) may also contribute to atherosclerosis progression through the production of inflammatory cytokines. Regulatory, forkhead box P3 (FoxP3) + T cells (T regulatory cells, T_{REGS}) have been found in animal and human atherosclerotic plaques. T_{REGS} may confer atheroprotection through the release of IL-10 and transforming frowth factor beta (TGF-β), two anti-inflammatory cytokines that downregulate inflammatory T_H1 immune response. Although less abundant, B-cells are also present in the adventitial site of the lesions where together with T-cells, macrophages and DCs they form the tertiary lymphoid tissues mostly seen in advanced severe ATH [6] (Fig. 13.1).

13.2.3 The Inflammasome and the Role of NLPR-3 Inflammasome in Atherosclerosis

Inflammasomes are a group of cytosolic multi-protein complexes that recognize inflammation-inducing stimuli including pathogen associated molecular patterns (PAMPs) and DAMPs and control the production of pro-inflammatory cytokines such as IL-1β and IL-18, through the activation of caspase-1. They are also involved in pyroptosis, a form of cell death associated

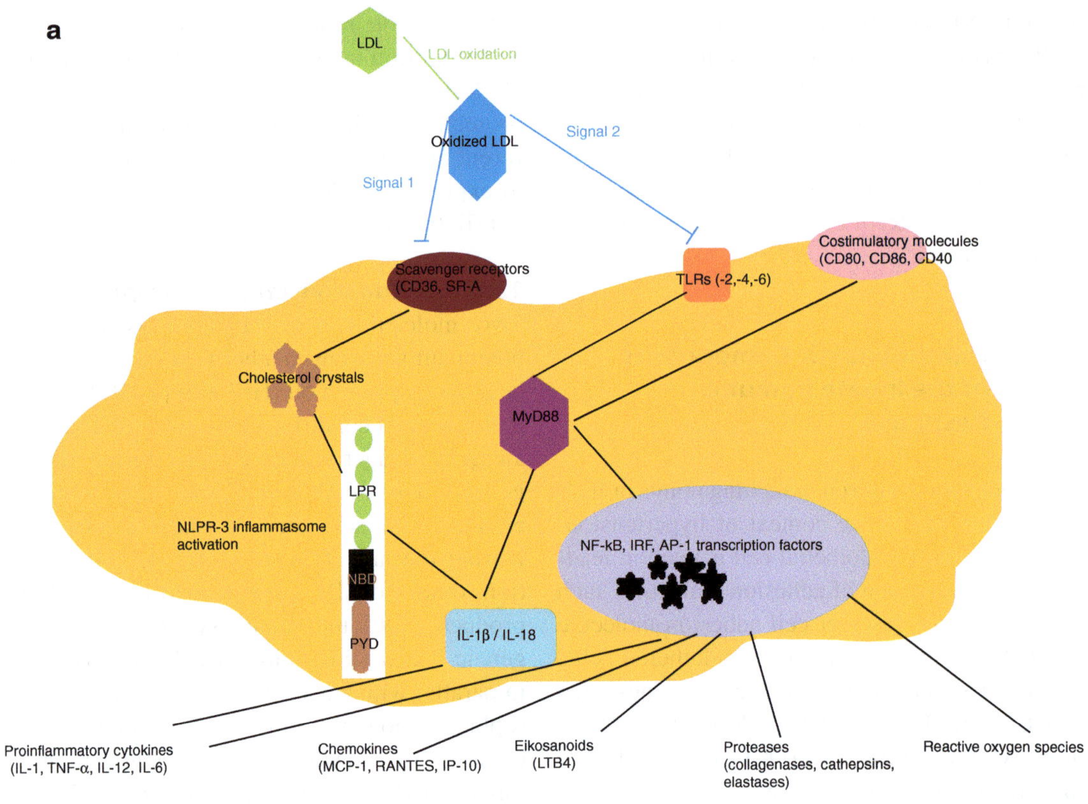

Fig. 13.1 The activation of innate and adaptive immune response in atherosclerosis. (**a**) The innate immune response. Modified LDL particles taken-up by scavenger receptors may activate the inflammasome, leading to IL-1β secretion. Adjunctive signals come from modified LDL activation of TLRs. NF-kB, IRF and AP-1 transcription factors are then activated and a wide variety of proinflammatory molecules is produced. (**b**) The adaptive immune response. Activated DCs present naïve T cells with antigens such as ApoB100. The latter develop into effector T cells that enter the bloodstream. When recruited within atherosclerotic plaques, they are reactivated by antigens presented by local macrophages, DCs or B cells (Adapted by permission from Macmillan Publishers Ltd: Hansson and Henmarsson [6]. Copyright 2012) Abbreviations: *ApoB* apolipoprotein beta, *AP-1* activated protein 1, *DC* dendritic cell, *IL* interleukin, *IRF* insulin related factor, *IP* inositol triphosphate, *LTB4* leukotrien beta, *Mf* macrophage, *MCP* monocyte chemoattractant protein, *MyD88* myeloid differentiation primary response 88, *NLPR3* Nod-like protein 3, *NFkB* nuclear factor kappa beta, *oxLDL* oxidized LDL, *TLR* toll-like receptor, *TNF* tumor necrosis factor

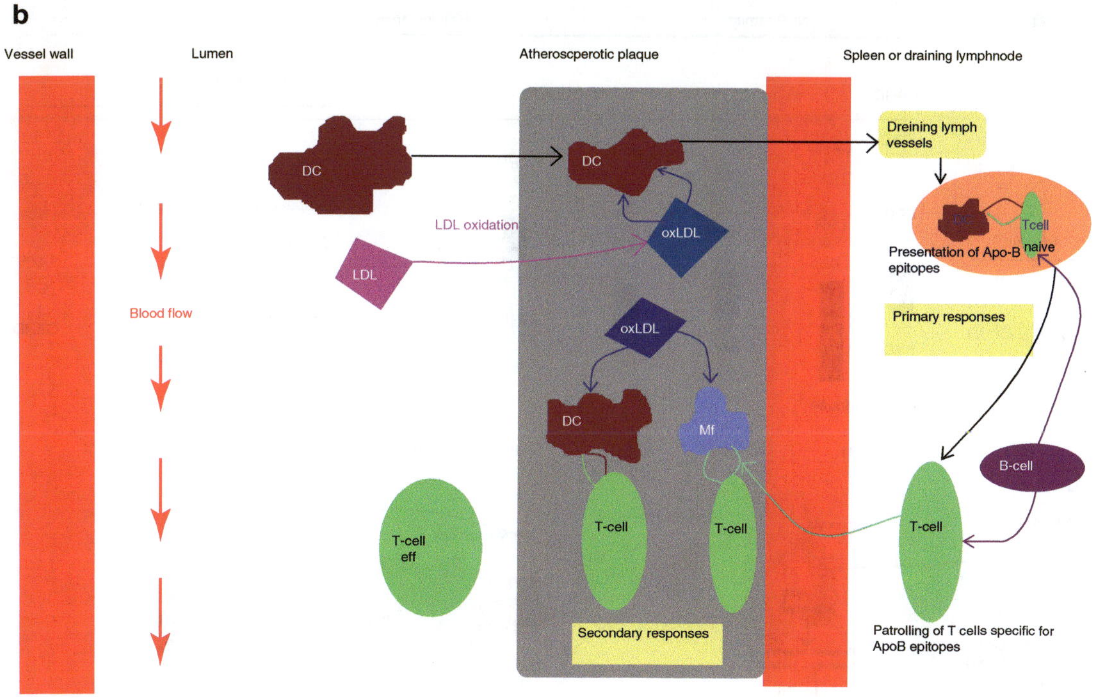

Fig. 13.1 (continued)

with tissue repair. Under normal circumstances, inflammasome activity needs to be tightly regulated to avoid excessive deleterious cytokine production. Indeed, alternative splicing, subcellular location and trafficking of its components, direct sequestration of protein complexes and inducible down-regulation by inflammatory cytokines and CD4+ cells, are some of the mechanisms that protect the cell from the dire consequences of inflammasome overactivation. Inflammasome mediated processes are important for microbial infections as well as metabolic processes and mucosal defense. Inflammasome activation has diverse effects on different cell lineages, namely the production of acute phase proteins by the liver, prostaglandin E2 release by brain, and chemoattraction of neutrophils and platelets within bone tissue (Fig. 13.2a).

The most widely studied is the NLPR-3 inflammasome, normally activated during viral and parasitic infections. The NLPR-3 inflammasome also assembles in response to a diversity of signals. Phagosome- or mitochondria- derived ROS, lysosome aggregates comprising cathepsins B and L and cellular potassium efflux act synergistically to promote NLPR-3 activation. Aberrant activation of NLPR-3 by non-infectious agents is implicated in a wide variety of diseases characterized by sterile INFL such as gout and pseudogout, silica/asbestos related diseases, Alzheimer's disease and in metabolic diseases, but also in ATH.

The contribution of inflammasome to the pathogenesis of ATH may be both direct – through activation by cholesterol crystals- and indirect. In the first case, cholesterol crystals within macrophages activate NLPR-3 through phagolysosome destabilization [7]. In vivo priming of NLPR-3 inflammasome implicates TLR-4/6 and MyD88 dependent pathways and various scavenger receptors; mice deficient in any of these components exhibit less ATH [8]. LDL-receptor deficient mice -which are prone to atherosclerosis- are resistant to disease when genetically modified not to express NLPR-3 or IL-1β. However this finding was not confirmed when APOE-deficient mice –another ATH murine model- were knocked out for NLPR-3 and fed with a very high fat diet

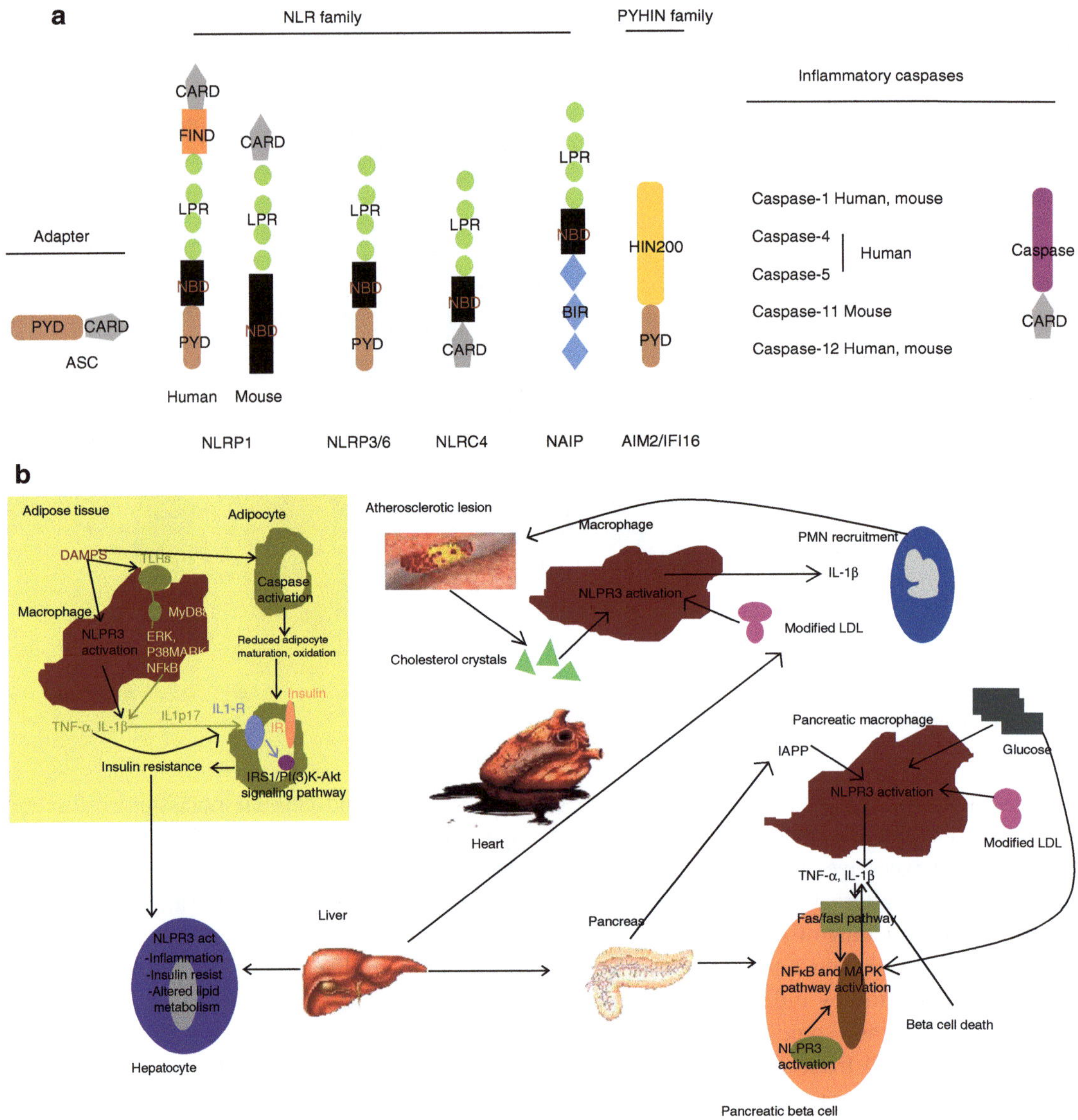

Fig. 13.2 The inflammasome. (**a**) The organization of the inflammasome. Core components of the inflammasome belong to two families, namely NOD-like receptor (NLR) and the PYHIN (pyrin and HIN 200 domain) protein family. The NLR family (NLRP1, NLRP2, NLRP3, NLRP6 and NLRC4 and NLRP12) contain a nucleotide binding domain (*NBD*), carboxy-terminal leucine rich repeat (LRR) and either a PYD or a caspase activation domain (CARD) or both. The PYHIN family members AIM2 and IFI16 have a PYD and a HIN 200 domain commited to ligand binding. (**b**) The role of the inflammasome in metabolic syndrome. DAMPS activate NLPR3 inflammasome in various tissues in obese patients. Palmitate and ceramides activate NLPR3 inflammasome in activated macrophages of adipose tissue. Caspase-1 activation regulates adipocyte differentiation and leads to fatty acid oxygenation. Within the pancreas, both resident macrophages and beta cells secrete IL-1β upon NLPR3 recruitment by IAPP and ROS. Beta cell death and impaired insulin production ensue (Adapted by permission from Macmillan Publishers Ltd: Strowig et al. [2]. Copyright 2012). Abbreviations: *BIR* baculoviral inhibition of apoptosis repeat domain, *DAMP* damage associated molecular pattern, *ERK* extracellular signal related kinase, *FIINF* domain with function to find, *IAPP* islet amyloid polypeptide, *IL* interleukin, *IL-1R* interleukin-1 receptor, *IP(3)-Akt* insulin receptor protein kinase B, *IRS* insulin receptor substrate, *MyD88* myeloid differentiation primary response 88, *NLPR3* nod-like protein 3, *PMN* neutrophil, *p38MAPK* protein 38 mitogen activated protein kinase, *TLR* toll-like receptor, *TNF* tumor necrosis factor

[9]. This discrepancy may imply the existence of potent environmental factors that may alter the course of the disease, the deterministic effect of knocking out genes preferentially at early stages rather than when ATH has been established. This data suggest the presence of yet undefined redundant mechanisms that may account for the activation of the inflammatory cascade independently of the NLPR3 assembly [4].

The indirect effects of inflammasome activation on ATH have emerged from its role in metabolic syndrome, obesity and diabetes (Fig. 13.2b). Insulin resistance, impaired pancreatic beta-cell function, fatty liver disease and ATH are thought to be components of the "metabolic syndrome" and are associated with increased IL-1β and IL-18 production which is the hallmark of NLPR-3 activation. Within adipose tissue, increased levels of palmitate and other saturated free fatty acids reduce the activation of AMP-activated kinase (AMPK), a key regulator of lipid metabolism. This in turn leads to defective mitochondrial autophagy, culminating in the accumulation of dysfunctional mitochondria which release enhanced levels of ROS and DNA into the cytosol. Both these molecules promote the activation of NLPR-3 inflammasome and the release of IL-1β which hampers the function of both, insulin-target cells and pancreatic beta cells. More specifically, IL-1β inhibits the engagement of insulin receptor (IR) by the insulin receptor substrate 1 (IRS1) and the phosphoinositie 3 kinase [PI(3)K-] signaling pathway, which leads to insulin resistance. In the pancreas, islet amyloid polypeptide (IAPP), which is secreted together with insulin, may act synergistically with glucose to induce NLPR-3 mediated macrophage derived IL-1β release, which causes beta cell dysfunction and death through the activation of Fas-FasL pathway and MAPK/NF-κB signaling cascade. Caspase-1 activation is also capable of altering hepatic tissue functions. Enhanced NLPR-3 activation has been demonstrated in patients with non alcoholic steatohepatitis (NASH). A role of the NLPR-3 inflammasome in shaping the adaptive immune response has also been postulated to contribute to the above-mentioned process. In this context, NLPR-3 driven, aberrant accumulation of lymphocytes into adipose tissue, and commitment to the TH_{17} lineage, may further enhance insulin resistance and promote obesity. Along these lines, exercise and calorie restriction were shown to reduce NLPR-3 and IL-1β expression in obese individuals and mice genetically modified not to express NLPR-3 were protected from obesity-induced inflammasome activation in their adipose tissue [10]. Furthermore, inflammasome contributes to the progression of type 2 diabetes, via thioredoxin-interacting protein (TXNIP)-, an ROS sensitive inducer of NLPR3 that senses islet amyloid polypeptide (IAPP)-, which may trigger further inflammasome activation within atherosclerotic lesions and ultimately atherosclerosis progression and plaque destabilization. Of note, glyburide, which is an insulin secretagogue used for the treatment of diabetes, suppresses NLPR-3 mediated IL-1β release which points towards the potential anti-inflammatory actions of the drug as being of major importance for its antidiabetic effects [11].

TLR "priming" of inflammatory cells can provide indispensable adjunct signals for effective inflammasome activation. The significance of TLRs to inflammasome activation is underscored by the fact that under normal circumstances, inflammasome components such as NLPR-3, apoptosis associated speck like protein containing a CARD (ASC) and caspase-1 are expressed at extremely low or even undetectable levels. The necessary induction of the expression of inflammasome components as well as pro-IL-1β and pro-IL-18 seems to be accomplished through TLR activation upon their interaction with DAMPs –such as HSP-60 and HMGB1- or even dietary-derived ligands which come under the term "nutrition associated molecular patterns", (NAMPs). Oxidized LDL ligates to a receptor complex engaging a TLR-4/6 heterodimer and the receptor CD36 to induce IL-1β expression [9]. Minimally modified LDL (mmLDL) also induces TLR-4 dependent Syk- and Nox-2 mediated macrophage derived ROS production, which is another essential signal for inflammasome activation, NLPR-3 up-regulation and IL-1β release.

Another aspect of the combined TLR/NLPR-3 activation in atherosclerosis is related to its unique effect on cellular survival signals. In this context, scavenger receptor class A (SR-A) and TLR-4 combined signaling within endoplasmic reticulum stressed macrophages induces pro-apoptotic signals potentially related to enhanced plaque necrosis and destabilization, which is not the case upon single TLR stimulation. In this case oxLDL, oxidized phospholipids, lipoproteins and saturated fatty acids may act as ligands for the doubly committed pathway. The potentially protective effects of omega-3 poly-unsaturated fatty acids through GPR120 mediated attenuation of inflammasome activation remain to be further established [12].

Genetic variation of inflammasome related loci may also alter the expression profile of several cardiovascular disease related factors such as blood pressure, acute phase proteins and fibrinogen. These data originate from genome wide association and other genetic studies but the precise role of genetic determinants of inflammasome expression on cardiovascular disease burden needs to be better elucidated.

13.3 The Endothelium in Inflammation and Atherosclerosis

The endothelium is the principal regulator of vascular wall homeostasis. Normally, endothelial cells preserve a relaxed vascular tone combined with a low level of oxidative stress. This is accomplished through the release of mediators such as nitric oxide (NO), prostacyclin (PGI2) and endothelin (ET) and the tight control of local angiotensin II activity. In addition, the endothelium actively regulates vascular permeability to plasma constituents, leukocyte and platelet adhesion and aggregation. A wide variety of conditions are capable of altering this balanced endothelial regulation and divert the endothelium from a "homeostatic" to "a non-adaptive" state, which comes under the term "*endothelial dysfunction*". Pro-inflammatory stimuli such as diet rich in saturated fat, obesity, insulin resistance and hypertension activate the endothelium by increasing levels of circulating cytokines such as IL-1 and TNF-α. This up-regulates endothelial expression of adhesion molecules such as intercellular adhesion molecule 1 (ICAM-1), VCAM-1, P-selectin and V-selectin and facilitates the capture, rolling and firm tethering of leukocytes to the endothelial surface. Adhered monocytes then transmigrate into the intima in a monocyte chemoattractant protein 1 (MCP-1) mediated process that also involves macrophage colony stimulating factor (MCSF) and initiates or propagates local INFL. Studies have shown that patients with cardiovascular risk factors, but no overt cardiovascular disease have endothelial dysfunction, which is *per se* an independent predictor of future cardiac events.

13.3.1 LDL and HDL Cholesterol

There is a well documented association between atherogenic lipoproteins (such as some forms of LDL, post-prandial chylomicron remnants and fasting triglyceride-rich particles) and endothelium-dependent responses. Hypercholesterolemia and high levels of LDL are inversely related to endothelium dependent vasodilation whereas anti-atherogenic high density lipoproteins (HDL), apart from mediating reverse cholesterol transport, also seem to modulate endothelial function in a beneficial manner. Oxidized LDL plays a pivotal role in endothelial activation. Accumulated modified LDL molecules retained within the arterial intima activate endothelial cells which up-regulate the expression of adhesion molecules such as VCAM-1 and RANTES, a phenomenon that occurs predominantly at sites undergoing increased hemodynamic stress. This leads to the subsequent recruitment of leukocytes and monocytes, and the propagation of local inflammation. Post-prandial hypertriglyceridemia is also associated with increased levels of TNF-α, IL-6, soluble ICAM-1 (sICAM-1) and sVCAM-1, which imply a pro-inflammatory effect for triglycerides in endothelial dysfunction and atherogenesis.

Plasma levels of HDL are strongly and inversely correlated with ATH. Their atheroprotective effects have been attributed to several mechanisms including reverse cholesterol

Table 13.1 Atheroprotective and antiiflammatory actions of HDL

Reverse cholesterol transport
Inhibition of LDL oxidation
Down-regulation of MCP-1, inhibition of macrophage transmigration to the intima
Alterations in signaling cascades of proiflammatory cytokines (NF-kB, ERK)
Reduction of endothelial SMC proliferation
Enhancement of e-NOS activity and NO production

Abbreviations: *e-NOS* endothelial nitric oxide synthase, *ERK* extracellular signal related kinases, *MCP-1* monocyte chemoattractant protein 1, *NF-kB* nuclear factor kappa beta, *NO* nitric oxide, *SMC* smooth muscle cell

transport, antithrombotic/anti-inflammatory properties and importantly, their effects on endothelial repair.

HDLs have been shown to prevent LDL oxidation and inhibit MCP-1 mediated macrophage transmigration into the intima. They also down-regulate the expression of adhesion molecules and they inhibit the sphingosine kinase, extracellular signal regulated kinase (ERK) and NF-kB signaling cascades of pro-inflammatory cytokine production. Vacular smooth muscle cell proliferation depends on the inflammatory chemokines chemokine ligand 2 (CCL2), CCL5 and CX3CL1. Through NF-kB/Akt and pERK inhibition, HDLs reduce SMC chemokine expression and proliferation contributing to the stabilization of atherosclerotic plaques. It is also postulated that HDL may protect against oxidative damage. Thus, some of its cardioprotective effects may rely on its ability to increase endothelial e-NO synthase (e-NOS) activity and NO production (Table 13.1). HDLs from humans with systemic inflammatory disorders such as systemic lupus erythematosus or rheumatoid arthritis may be incapable of preventing LDL oxidation, suggesting that HDL composition and function may be altered during inflammation and that it can shift from an anti-inflammatory to a pro-inflammatory status under specific conditions (see below). Recent information on the atheroprotective actions of HDLs may justify their use as therapeutic targets for the prevention of atherosclerotic lesion formation and the regression and/or stabilization of the established atherosclerotic plaque [13].

13.4 Interactions Between Inflammation and Lipid Metabolism

Inflammation and dyslipidemia are well established risk factors for the development of ATH. Lipid lowering drugs exert their atheroprotective effects, through the decrease of atherogenic lipids and other "off target", anti-inflammatory actions. On the other hand, anti-inflammatory drugs, may partially restore an abnormal lipid profile in subjects with systemic INFL. High through-put technologies –which are described later- in animal models and in human tissues, have unraveled the existence of an interplay between environmental factors, lipid metabolism and INFL, which is of crucial importance for the pathogenesis of ATH. Free cholesterol and TG, modified LDL and free fatty acids (FFAs) can all alter the "inflammatory status" of an organism through a variety of mechanisms (Fig. 13.3).

Cholesterol feeding elevates markers of INFL such as CRP. Obese patients also exhibit chronic low INFL as evidenced by increased levels of CRP and cytokines such as TNF-α and IL-6. "Metabolic inflammation" is believed to be primarily induced by metabolic endotoxemia, that is, an increased translocation of lipopolysacharide (LPS or endotoxin) through the gut, upon high fat diet. The additive effect of cholesterol and/or TG induced up-regulation of NF-kB mediated cytokine production by several tissues including adipose tissue, liver and vasculature are also important. In addition to high fat diet *per se*, modified lipoproteins may also activate hepatic macrophages and vascular endothelial cells –through the recruitment of the inflammasome- and downregulate the function of T_{REGS}. Importantly, adverse hemodynamic conditions may well activate sterol regulatory element binding protein-2 (SREBP2) –a lipogenic transcriptor factor which is aberrantly regulated in NASH- and induce NLPR-3 inflammasome in endothelial cells within atheroprone vascular areas, thus acting concomitantly with hyperlipidemia to increase ATH [14].

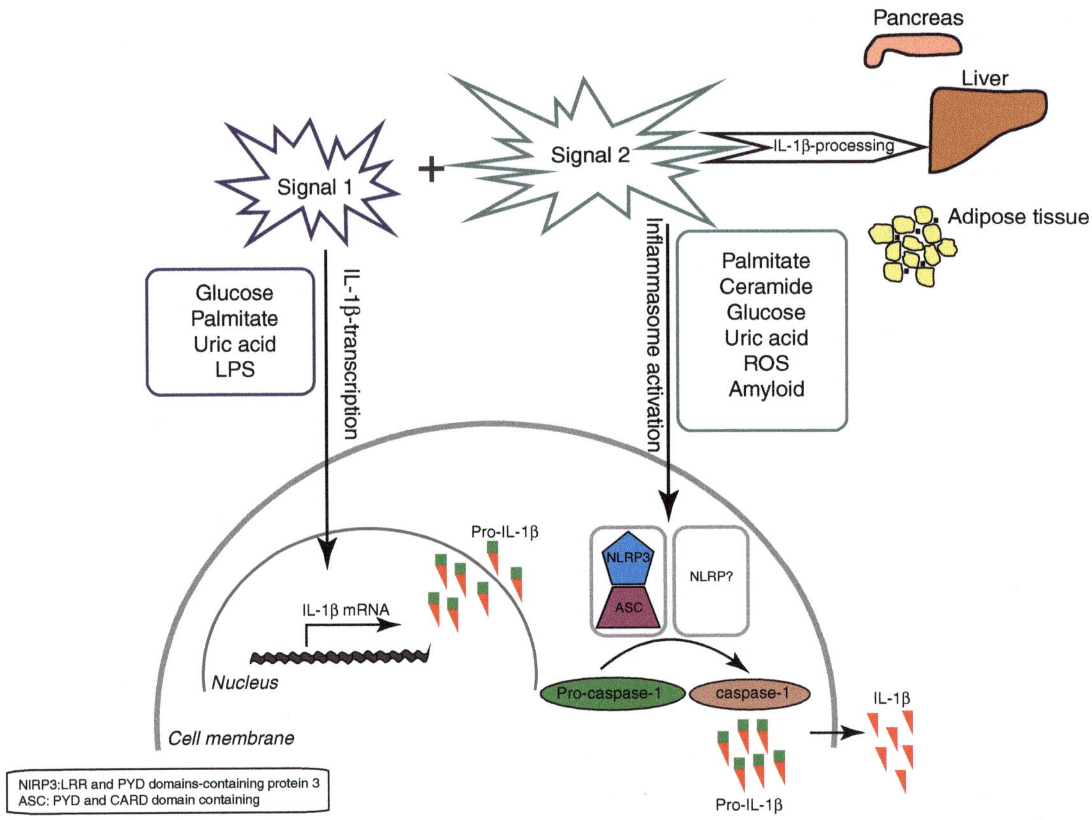

Fig. 13.3 Inflammasome activation in metabolic syndrome*. Overview of the metabolic triggers that may act as primary or secondary signals in inflammasome NLPR3 activation and IL-1β production. This signaling cascade occurs in various tissues such as pancreas, liver, adipose tissue contributing to tissue dysfunction and insulin resistance (Reprinted from Stienstra et al. [1]. Copyright 2012, with permission from Elsevier). Abbreviations: *ASC* apoptosis associated speck like protein containing a CARD, *IL* interleukin, *IL-1R* interleukin-1 receptor, *LPS* lipopolysacharide, *NLPR3* nod-like protein 3, *ROS* reactive oxygen species

Nuclear lipid sensors comprise a specific group of transcription factors that upon recognition of intracellular lipids, regulate the expression of genes implicated in the inflammatory cascade. Peroxisome proliferator activated receptors (PPARs) are fatty acid sensors capable of modifying macrophage response and leukocyte recruitment. Liver X receptors (LXRs) are activated by oxysterols in response to increased intracellular cholesterol levels and exert their anti-inflammatory effects through the activation or reverse cholesterol transport, reduction of inflammatory gene expression and inhibition of T-cell proliferation through control of cholesterol content/membrane synthesis of T-cells. Finally, the farsenoid receptors (FXRs) are activated by endogenous bile acids and expressed at high levels in the liver and the intestine. Their activation regulates bile acid, lipid and glucose metabolism, concurrently leading to FXR binding with inflammatory transcriptional co-repressors or silencing mediators, which ultimately translates into modulation of INFL.

Importantly, lipid metabolism can be modified through epigenetic processes induced by the microbiome, that is the assembly of integrally associated microorganisms colonizing individuals. It has been demonstrated that alterations in the microbial population of the gut can induce metabolic changes favoring the development of metabolic syndrome, obesity and diabetes. Increased plasma levels of trimethylamine-N-oxide (TMAO), an intestinal microbiota-dependent metabolite of choline which is also induced by the farsenoid X receptor, were associated with cardiovascular events in a dose-dependent way in 4,000 individuals studied with elective coronary angiography [15]. The promotion of thiol-dependent oxidant stress, macrophage activation, LDL oxidation and methionine methylation are some of the mechanisms explaining the atherogenic actions of TMAO. Importantly, these complex atherothrombogenic host-microbiota interactions could be potentially modified through dietary changes, the use of probiotics and pharmacological interventions that can suppress the synthesis of TMAO.

Although the effects of lipids on inflammatory pathways have been extensively studied, the role of inflammation on lipid metabolism is addressed only by few studies. Acute inflammation in the context of infection results in increases in TG levels with reduction of both LDL and HDL cholesterol and concomitant increase in oxygenation of LDL particles which facilitate host defense. However, chronic INFL may induce detrimental, atherogenic effects. The most relevant studies come from patients with systemic inflammatory and/or autoimmune conditions, who display an abnormal lipid metabolism and increased incidence of CAD.

13.5 Accelerated Atherosclerosis in Autoimmune Inflammation

Autoimmune diseases (AIDs) are a heterogeneous group of disorders characterized by humoral induced cell-mediated immune responses against self-constituents. The combined effect of complex predisposing genetic factors, immune conditions and environmental triggering events is important to AID manifestations. Among AIDs, systemic lupus erythematosus (SLE), rheumatoid arthritis (RA), antiphospholipid syndrome (APS) and Sjogren syndrome (SS) display augmented ATH linked to an increased cardiovascular morbidity and mortality that cannot be attributed to the classical predisposing risk factors for CAD. There is a growing body of evidence in favor of a causative link between chronic autoimmune inflammation and accelerated atherosclerosis in patients with AIDs.

Cardiovascular disease in SLE patients has been reported with an overall incidence of 6–10 % in various cohorts. Strikingly, women with SLE display a 5- to 9- fold increased risk for CAD compared with their non-diseased counterparts, and premenopausal status does not seem to confer to them adequate cardiovascular protection. Endothelial impairment is one of the key issues in the pathogenesis of ATH in SLE patients. This is induced by the integrated effects of proinflammatory cytokines –such as TNF-α, IFN-γ and IL-10-, the direct toxic actions of cytotoxic T-cells and the autoreactive B-cell mediated complement-dependent attack of the endothelium, all of which synergistically act to destroy its integrity and allow the propagation of inflammation and atherogenesis. Importantly, circulating immune complexes and anti-endothelial autoantibodies are capable of inducing a pro-inflammatory and pro-adhesion endothelial cell phenotype. Defective functions of T_{REGS} – that do not sufficiently suppress autoreactive T-cells- and enhanced T_H17 activity promoting INFL and tissue destruction are also implicated in SLE-related ATH. Interestingly, patients with SLE display increased antibody titers to oxLDLs, and these correlate with disease activity scores and complement activation. Furthermore, antibodies to HDL and apoA1 are also elevated in patients with active SLE. Of note, these correlate inversely with the activity of paraoxonase which normally confers to HDL its anti-oxidant properties [16]. Chronic INFL may cause a decrease in HDL concentration and impair its functions through several alternative mechanisms; these include the enhancement of endothelial lipase and soluble phospholipase A2 activities as well as the replacement of apoA-1 in HDL with serum amyloid A. Modified HDL molecules have been identified as activators of protein kinase Akt, which in turn regulates apoptotic signals on endothelial, smooth muscle cells and pancreatic beta cells, and drives the production of adhesion molecules and NO within the endothelium. Thus, in the context of chronic INFL, HDL may lose its atheroprotective properties and become pro-atherogenic [17]. On the basis of these observations, it can be concluded that, SLE may confer increased cardiovascular risk by instigating both, endothelial damage and alterations in lipid metabolism.

RA is characterized by synovial inflammation and hyperplasia, autoantibody (anti-CCP and RF) production, cartilage tissue and bone destruction and systemic manifestations such as pulmonary or cardiovascular disease. Increased expression of adhesion molecules, pro-inflammatory cytokines and matrix metalloproteases all contribute to joint erosion and atherosclerosis in rheumatoid patients. Tumor necrosis factor alpha (TNF-α) is a key cytokine to RA pathogenesis. This cytokine has a pivotal role in the disruption of microvascular and macrovascular circulation in patients and animal models of the disease. Through NF-kB dependent and independent pathways, it is capable of inducing the expression of various other inflammatory cytokines, chemokines and ROS that contribute to endothelium apoptosis, vascular oxidative stress, impaired NO bioavailability, neovascularization and vascular INFL. It also impairs insulin sensitivity by interfacing with insulin receptor signaling at the level of insulin receptor substrates through activation of kinase enzymes that phosphorylate serine of threonine residues, thus regulating cell proliferation, apoptosis and differentiation, namely serine kinases . Importantly, environmental factors such as diet, smoking and aging have a strong impact on TNF-α production. In addition, some dietary supplements and exercise act favorably on vascular function, since they diminish TNF-α production and inhibit TNF-α mediated signaling [18].

On the basis of the importance of TNF-α for endothelial dysfunction, several clinical trials have investigated the use of the three currently available TNF-α inhibitors (infliximab, etanercept and adalimumab) in vascular disorders that accompany RA and other autoimmune conditions. A growing body of evidence -mainly derived from observational databases and registries- suggests that anti-TNF biologic agents as well as methotrexate, can reduce the risk of future cardiovascular events in patients with RA. Chronic treatment with either of the above-mentioned agents improves endothelial function in RA patients. Anti-TNF-α therapy ameliorates insulin resistance, beta-cell function and insulin signaling in individuals with active RA [19]. In addition to TNF-α inhibitors, various statins (atorvastatin and simvastatin) and the ACE-inhibitor quinapril have been found to decrease circulating levels of TNF-α, which parallels the improvement of endothelial function in patients with type 2 diabetes, congestive heart failure, RA or hyperlipidemia [20, 21]. The role of TNF-α inhibition in CAD and type 2 diabetes remains to be further investigated on the basis of randomized controlled trials.

Antiphospholipid syndrome (APS) is characterized by an excessive production of autoantibodies against phospholipids, mainly cardiolipin and β2-glycoprotein 1 (β2GP1). Circulating immune complexes may lead to the formation of blood clots that are implicated in the pathogenesis of spontaneous abortions and cardiovascular disease. The atherosclerotic plaques of APS patients are infiltrated with β2GP1 in conjunction with CD4+ cells. Immune complexes composed of antibodies against oxLDL/β2GPI are postulated to be taken up by Fcγ receptors, that is specific IgG class recognizing receptors of immune cells that upon binding with their substrate activate an inflammatory immune response. This leads to endothelial activation and promotes the formation of foam cells and ATH [22].

13.6 Studying Inflammation in Atherosclerosis

13.6.1 Animal Models

Murine models are indispensable to study ATH, but some limitations need to be considered when it comes to translate findings from mouse to humans. To cite a few: cholesterol levels in hyperlipidemic atherosclerotic mice greatly exceed the levels found in humans. Mice naturally lack cholesteryl ester transfer protein (CETP) which transfers cholesteryl ester from HDL to apoB-containing lipoproteins in humans. In reference to the immune system, humans lack the clear

T-helper (Th) 1 and Th2 polarization found in mice and markers for M1 and M2 macrophage phenotypes partially differ between both species. Importantly, mouse plaques are not prone to plaque vulnerability and plaque rupture. The latter has been ascribed to differences in vessel size, location of plaques, thrombus formation and size and the fibrinolytic system [23]. Despite their limitations, murine atherosclerosis models represent an important asset to the study of ATH.

13.6.2 High-Throughput Technologies

High-throughput cell biology refers to the use of automation equipment with classical cell biology techniques to address biological questions which would be unattainable using conventional methods. It combines techniques from chemistry, biology, optics and image analysis in order to gain precise insight into cell functions, interactions and disease pathogenesis. High-throughput biology serves as one facet of the so called "omics research", which refers to the interface between large scale biology (genome, proteome, transcriptome), technology and researchers with a view to combine different methods into large scale experiments of good quality and with repetitive results.

Atherosclerosis is a complex biologic process. The widespread application of genomics, transcriptomics, proteomics and epigenomics, aims to model biological processes involved in the pathogenesis of ATH as interconnected networks that would have never been discovered without these new technologies.

In 2007 data from the International HapMap Project and the development of dense genotyping chips enabled genetic epidemiologists to identify gene loci affecting susceptibility to CAD into the region 9p21 of the human genome, a finding that was replicated across multiple international studies [24]. More recently, genome-wide assays (GWAs) have identified INFL related loci associated with CAD risk. These include CXCL12 –relating to the homonymous atheroprotective chemokine-, the ABO locus –which is linked to the expression of cytokine IL-6- and the HLA-C major histocompatibility locus on chromosome 6p21 [25].

Macrodissection and laser-capture microdissection have allowed the isolation and analysis of specific subregions within atherosclerotic lesions (media, adventitia, fibrous cap, etc.) and particular cell types for subsequent genome wide expression profiling, enhancing our understanding of cell type specific functions in atherogenesis. Using expression profiles from human atherosclerotic arterial wall, carotid stenosis and visceral fat, an atherosclerosis-related set of genes linked to transendothelial leukocyte migration pathway and to the transcriptional cofactor LIM domain binding factor 2 (LDB2) were identified as major regulators of the atherogenetic process. Transcriptional analysis of human endothelial cells (ECs), smooth muscle cells (SMCs), and hepatocarcinoma cells treated with atorvastatin or pitavastatin confirmed the statins' impact on coagulation, cell growth and vascular constriction.

MicroRNAs (miRNAs) have recently emerged as a novel class of gene regulators that work via transcriptional degradation and translational inhibition or activation. miRNAs are small noncoding RNA molecules encoded by eukaryotic nuclear DNA that function in transcriptional and post-transcriptional regulation of gene expression. Profiling of miRNAs has also offered insights in atherosclerosis related mechanisms. A variety of functions of endothelial and inflammatory cells involved in angiogenesis, neointimal formation and lipid metabolism have been found to be regulated by miRNAs. Fichtlscherer et al. [26] detected a significant reduction in the plasma concentration of vascular and inflammatory cell-derived miRNAs in patients with CAD whereas cardiac muscle-miRNAs showed an increased trend. miRNA-124 has recently been described as a biomarker for cerebral infarction. Whether microRNAs can be used as diagnostic biomarkers predictive of disease classification and prognosis remains to be further investigated. They are further discussed in Chap. 14.

RNA interference refers to an RNA-dependent gene silencing process resulting in the reduction of mRNA levels. It is initiated by short double stranded RNA molecules, named siRNAs. siRNAs are a valuable tool for the investigation of inflammatory networks and cellular signaling in atherosclerosis. siRNA studies concerning vascular inflammation are mostly based on knocking down on specific genes. Silencing proteins SMA- and MAD- -(intracellular proteins transducing signals from TGF-beta ligands, which are homologues to the *Drosophila* protein *mad*, –mothers against decapentaplegic-, and the *Caenorhabditis elegans* protein *sma*, –small body size-) related signaling in human aortic endothelial cells, down-regulation of TNF-α dependent NF-kB activation or silencing p13-AKT, all had atheroprotective effects. Via transfection of NLPR-3 inflammasome into cultured vascular smooth muscle cells (VSMCs), Wen et al. [27] recently showed that NLPR-3 activation is indispensable for VSMC calcification, which has a significant role in plaque progression and stability. In another interesting study, Nox1 was identified as a pharmacologically accessible target linked to hyperglycemia-induced oxidative stress in diabetic patients [28].

Proteomics involve the study of protein structure, expression, modification and protein-protein interactions. The establishment of LDL-receptor as a key instigator of MAPK and ERK signaling pathway having a major role in ATH has been achieved through proteomics analysis in humans and animal models of the disease.

Metabolomics investigate the whole set of metabolites and their interactions with each other or with diverse regulators.

Lipidomics refers to the study of the lipidome, i.e., the assembly of lipids of an organism, which is of outstanding interest in atherosclerosis research.

Epigenomics involves the study of phenotypic or gene expression changes caused by inheritable mechanisms independent of DNA sequence, *e.g.* DNA methylation and histone posttranscriptional modifications, as well as the study of non-coding RNA alterations which are also considered as epigenetic mechanisms. Importantly, epigenetic alterations depend on a wide variety of intrinsic and extrinsic factors, such as environmental effects or developmental cellular changes. Initial epigenetic studies have addressed vascular-inflammation related epigenetic changes mostly on a global DNA level, and have focused less on specific genes.

DNA methylation is the most thoroughly investigated of all epigenetic mechanisms. It is associated with gene silencing, genome integrity and tissue homeostasis, is mitotically stable and transmitted through cell division with 97–99 % fidelity per mitosis. *De novo* methylation occurs in 3–5 % of mitoses in adult somatic cells. There is substantial evidence indicating that deficient methylation is linked to increased inflammation and atherosclerosis and that cardiovascular risk factors may alter epigenomic patterns related to subclinical or overt cardiovascular disease. For example, genomic DNA within human atherosclerotic lesions has been shown to be hypomethylated. Also, methylation changes have been reported for genes involved in atherogenesis, such as estrogen receptor a, nitric oxide synthase, and 15- lipoxygenase. Interestingly, high through-put, genome wide array based methylation profiling of peripheral DNA from heavy smokers, revealed that these displayed a significantly reduced methylation of F2RL3, a gene with strong impact on cardiovascular mortality in patients with stable CAD [29].

Overall, high-throughput technologies offer a tremendous asset in the field of vascular inflammation and cardiovascular disease research, which is expected to point towards novel ways to prevent or treat CAD in the years to come [30].

13.7 Imaging of Inflammation

Inflammation has a key role in atherosclerotic plaque formation, progression and rupture. Endothelial dysfunction, vascular INFL, atherosclerotic plaque composition and vulnerability can all be studied using multiple invasive or noninvasive imaging modalities. The combination of cardiovascular and molecular imaging is rapidly evolving and current developments in cardiovascular biology and imaging allow the noninvasive molecular evaluation of atherosclerotic plaque characteristics and prediction of future events. Positron emission tomography (PET) and single photon emission computed tomography (SPECT) are readily used in clinical practice. Magnetic resonance (MRI), computed tomography (CT) and ultrasound (U/S) have primarily been used for the visualization of anatomical structures. The development of targeted contrast agents enables molecular imaging using these techniques.

Molecular contrast agents consist of a ligand and a contrast element. The ligand is usually an antibody, –antibody-fragment, peptide, oligosaccharide- with a specific binding capacity to a molecular target. It retains the contrast element at the site of interest. The attached contrast element is specific to the imaging modality used, for example, a radionuclide tracer for PET and SPECT, iodine for CT, gadolinium for MRI, or microbubbles for ultrasound. The contrast element can either be attached directly to the carrier, or via a carrier vehicle, such as micelle, nanoparticle, or microbubble [31].

13.7.1 PET/CT Scan

Positron emission tomography (PET) using [18F]-fluorodeoxy-glucose (FDG) has been recently advocated as a means of measuring vascular INFL. FDG is a glucose analogue, and the method relies on the ability of FDG-PET to highlight areas of increased glucose metabolism, a feature of macrophages in ATH, particularly in high risk, "activated' plaques. The uptake of FDG is directly proportional to macrophage density and activation which are hallmarks of plaque activation. PET/FDG uptake correlates with markers of systemic INFL and risk factors for atherosclerosis and can accurately quantify INFL in aorta, iliac and peripheral arteries. The small lumen of coronary arteries, combined with cardiac and respiratory motion during data acquisition and myocardial cell FDG uptake, compromise the efficiency of the method in defining coronary artery plaque characteristics. Furthermore, the use of radionuclide tracers is associated with ionizing radiation, which limits the method's clinical utility. The method is still under development and further ameliorations/manipulations with ongoing efforts to reduce the dose radiation or dose equivalent are expected to provide adequate and accurate coronary image data with a safe total radiation dose in the near future [32].

The combined assessment of FDG and 18F-sodium fluoride (18F NaF) –an agent that effectively recognizes regions of active calcification- has recently emerged as a very promising method for the identification of active INFL and concomitant active calcification, both markers of a "vulnerable atheroclerotic plaque" [33]. In addition to FDG and 18 NaF, several other probes detecting a wide variety of markers of vulnerable atherosclerotic plaques are under experimental and even clinical evaluation. These include markers of apoptosis (Annexin 5), lectin-like oxidized LDL receptor (LOX-1), matrix metalloproteases (MMPs), thrombus formation (tissue factors, TFs), intraplaque vascularization (^{18}F Galacto RGD, a ligand of $\alpha\nu\beta3$ integrin), and vascular INFL (VCAM-1, MCP-1, labeled LDL, etc.).

13.7.2 IVUS and Contrast Enhanced Ultrasound

The morphologic features of a stenosis and reference segment can be assessed by intravascular ultrasound (IVUS). Besides precise dimensional measurements, IVUS can locate determinants of plaque vulnerability such as a thin fibrous cap, the presence of a necrotic core in contact with the lumen, a high eccentricity index, the presence of echolucent zones within the plaque representing large necrotic pools, and the existence of a prominent enlargement of the vessel referred to as "positive remodeling", all indirect evidence of an ongoing inflammatory process.

Targeted contrast ultrasound relies on the selective retention of the contrast agent after clearance of the freely circulating non-attached population. Microbubbles designed for molecular imaging targeted to antigens expressed on endothelial cells, adherent leukocytes or platelets are under development. Contrast enhanced ultrasound is under development and is expected to make a major contribution to understanding, accurate diagnosis and therapeutics of atherosclerosis [34].

13.7.3 OCT and NIRS

Even more detail of structure and plaque composition can be obtained with optical coherence tomography (OCT). Intracoronary OCT is a catheter-based optical imaging modality capable of providing high-resolution cross sectional images of the coronary wall employing near infra-red light. It has a superior resolution for evaluating features of the vulnerable plaque such as plaque rupture, intracoronary thrombus, thin-capped fibroatheroma and the presence of macrophages within the fibrous caps [35]. In a study by Jefferson et al. [36], contrast enhanced OCT using microparticles of iron oxide, successfully detected the presence of VCAM-1 and platelet cell adhesion molecule 1 (PCAM-1) in cultured endothelial cells under conditions of increased shear-stress ex-vivo. Using a catheter system similar to that of IVUS, near infrared wave-length light can be employed to detect cholesterol content in a vessel, based on the molecule's distinct "spectroscopic signature". Near-infrared spectroscopy (NIRS) is at present a clinical research tool providing a well validated "chemographic" map of coronary vessels [37].

13.8 Targeting Inflammation in Atherosclerosis

Current therapies in atherosclerosis are largely restricted to alleviating hypertension and hyperlipidemia or controlling hemostasis to prevent thrombotic complications. Established, emerging and future directions in the treatment of atherosclerosis as an "inflammatory disease" are subsequently discussed.

13.8.1 Established Therapies

Benefits gained from the administration of statins rely on their pluri-potent actions which may well extend beyond their lipid-lowering effects. Along these lines, statins improve endothelial function and reduce plaque lipids and thrombogenicity thereby limiting and stabilizing atherosclerotic plaques. Aggressive lipid-lowering with atorvastatin reduced high sensitivity CRP (hs-CRP) and entailed regression of atherosclerotic lesions assessed by IVUS [38], whereas in acute coronary syndrome (ACS) patients, aggressive statin treatment may independently reduce the incidence of subsequent myocardial infarction, with concurrent LDL and hsCRP reduction. Shifting the lipid balance in favor of HDL cholesterol using nicotinic acid achieves regression of carotid intima-media thickness owing to the anti-inflammatory effects entailed by binding of niacin to its receptor GPR109A [39]. Finally, b-blockers and ACE inhibitors may also have a role in the regression of endothelial dysfunction and inflammation.

13.8.2 Emerging Therapies

Artificial HDL-mimetic complexes promote cholesterol efflux by avidly binding oxidized lipids, exert anti-inflammatory effects and may mediate regression of CAD. The selective Lp-PLA inhibitor daraplatib prevented the expansion of plaque related necrotic core in patients with CAD [40]. Torcetrabib, a cholesteryl ester transfer protein (CETP) inhibitor, effectively increased HDL cholesterol, but was associated with an increased mortality, subsequently thought to be due to compound specific "off-target" effects which included a rise in blood pressure and vascular INFL [41]. A 24-month double-blind-placebo controlled randomized trial employing 130 subjects assessed the safety profile and the efficiency of dalcetrabib, a novel modulator of CETP activity, in modifying vessel enlargement using MRI and PET/CT data. Dalcetrabib exhibited a good safety profile and achieved a reduction in vascular inflammation and in vessel enlargement over 24 months, but long term data are required to establish the clinical efficacy and safety of this agent [42].

13.8.3 Experimental Therapies

Based on data coming from high through-put studies, a variety of therapeutic schemes employing modulators of INFL including cytokine and

Table 13.2 Emerging therapies targeting inflammation in atherosclerosis

Drug	Therapeutic action	Mechanism	Effects	Human studies	Reference
Canakinumab	Inhibition of IL-1	IL-1β neutralizing ab	Reduced stent restenosis	Yes	[43]
Anakinra	Inhibition of IL-1	IL-1r antagonist	Reduced HF after MI	Yes	[44]
Tocilizumab	Inhibition of IL-6	IL-6r antagonist	Improved endothelial function in RA, adverse lipid effects	Not in atherosclerosis	[45]
VIA 2291 (Atreleuton)	Reduces leukotriene production	5-Lipoxygenase inhibitor	Reduced plaque volume and new plaque formation in recent MI	Yes	[46]
DG031	Reduces leukotriene production	Inhibitor of 5 Lipoxygenase activating protein	Reduced inflammatory markers in patients with risk variants for leukotrien genes	Not evaluated for MACE reduction	[47]
Daraplatib	Inhibition of lipoprotein phospholipase	LpPLA2 inhibitor	Reduced IL-6 and CRP in CAD	Yes, ongoing STABILITY and SOLID/TIMI 52 trial	[48]
Dorcetlabib	Cholesteryl ester transfer protein (CETP) inhibitor	HDL mimetic complex	Reduced vascular inflammation and vessel enlargement in CAD	Yes	[42]
MLN1212	CCR2 antagonism	CCR2 monoclonal ab	Reduces hsCRP in CAD	Not evaluated for MACE reduction	[49]
Immunization	Tolerisation against plausible antigens	Immunization with DCs pulsed with diverse molecules such as LDL, apoB100, HSP fragments	Conflicting results	No	[50]

Abbreviations: *apoB100* apolipoprotein B 100, *CAD* coronary artery disease, *DC* dendritic cell, *HSP* heat shock protein, *MACE* major adverse cardiovascular events

chemokine modulation (IL-1 and IL-6; CCR-2 antagonist), selective phospholipase and leukotriene inhibitors and others are currently under experimental evaluation. Most of these are presented in Table 13.2 [44–50].

13.8.3.1 Interleukin-1 Inhibitors

In humans atherosclerotic arteries show elevated levels of IL-1 and the IL-1 receptor antagonist gene was associated with a lower incidence of restenosis after coronary stenting. A large secondary prevention trial [Canakinumab Anti-Inflammatory Thrombosis Outcomes Study (CANTOS)] with canakinumab, a neutralizing antibody of IL-1β is ongoing [43]. In addition, the Medical Research Council- Interleukin-1 receptor antagonist-HEART study will compare short term use of Anakinra, an IL-1 receptor antagonist to placebo in patients with myocardial infarction. Preliminary results from anakinra in MI patients imply a lower incidence of subsequent heart failure in treated subjects versus controls, but this remains to be confirmed by long term more solid data [44].

Conclusions

The concept that ATH constitutes a passive lipid accumulation in the vessel wall, which dominated over the past decades, has been challenged by evidence suggesting that ATH is a predominantly low grade chronic inflammatory disorder, where both, innate and adaptive immune responses play a pivotal role throughout initiation, progression and clinical manifestation of the disease. Endogenous ligands like DAMPs and NAMPs as well as modified cholesterol molecules, partially through TLR activation, lead to NLPR-3 inflammasome upregulation, caspase activation and inflammatory cytokine release. Lipid metabolism has a crucial role in this process. Largely influenced by modifiable extrinsic factors –such as diet intake- as well as intrinsic processes –such as microbiome associated engagement of nuclear lipid receptors- it may determine the magnitude and quality of the ensuing immune response. Adaptive immunity, hemodynamic parameters and endothelial activation act synergistically with lipid metabolism to orchestrate the inflammatory response culminating in atherosclerosis.

Patients with systemic inflammatory and/or autoimmune conditions display abnormal lipid metabolism and increased incidence of CAD. Endothelial damage, autoantibodies against lipid components, loss of atheroprotective HDL properties, increased systemic INFL resulting in impaired insulin resistance, obesity and metabolic syndrome are implicated in increased CAD burden of these patients. Based on data coming from high through-put studies, therapeutic schemes employing modulators of INFL that were originally utilized as immune-suppressors for systemic inflammatory conditions, are currently under experimental evaluation. Among these therapies, schemes based on IL-1R antagonism have produced promising results.

References

1. Stienstra R, Tack CJ, Kanneganti T-D, Joosten LA, Netea MG. The inflammasome puts obesity in the danger zone. Cell Metab. 2012;15:10–8.
2. Strowig T, Henao-Mejia J, Elinav E, Flavell R. Inflammasomes in health and disease. Review. Nature. 2012;481:278–86.
3. Michelsen KS, Wong MH, Shah PK, Zhang W, Yano J, Doherty TM, et al. Lack of Toll like receptor-4 or myeloid differentiation factor 88 reduces atherosclerosis and alters phenotype in mice deficient in apolipoprotein E. Proc Natl Acad Sci U S A. 2004;101:10679–84.
4. Teixeira PC, Cutler P, Vuilleimier N. Autoantibodies to apolipoprotein A-1 in cardiovascular diseases: current perspectives. Clin Devel Immunol. 2012; Article ID 868251:7 pages.
5. Galkina E, Ley K. Immune and inflammatory mechanisms of atherosclerosis. Annu Rev Immunol. 2009;27:165–97.
6. Hansson GK, Hermansson A. The immune system in atherosclerosis. Nat Immunol. 2009;12:204–12.
7. Duewell P, Kono H, Rayner KJ, Sirois CM, Vladimer G, Bauernfeind FG, et al. NLPR3 inflammasomes are required for atherogenesis and activated by cholesterol crystals. Nature. 2010;464:1357–61.
8. Stewart CR, Stewart LM, Wilkinson K, van Gils GM, Deng J, Halle A, et al. CD36 ligands promote sterile inflammation through assembly of a Toll-like receptor 4 and 6 heterodimer. Nat Immunol. 2010;11:155–61.
9. Menu P, Pellegrin M, Aubert JF, Bouzourene K, Tardivel A, et al. Atherosclerosis in ApoE-deficient mice progresses independently of the NLPR3 inflammasome. Cell Death Dis. 2011;2:e137.
10. Vandanmagsar B, Youm YH, Ravussin A, Galgani JE, Stadler K, Mynatt RL, et al. The NLPR3 inflammasome instigates obesity-induced inflammation and insulin resistance. Nat Med. 2011;17:179–88.
11. Lamkanfi M, Mueller JL, Vitari AC, Misaghi S, Fedorova A, Deshayes K, et al. Glyburide inhibits the cryopyrin/Nalp3 inflammasome. J Cell Biol. 2009;187:61–70.
12. Seimon TA, Nadolski MJ, Liao X, Magallon J, Nguyen M, Feric NT, et al. Atherogenic lipids and lipoproteins trigger CD36-TLR2-dependent apoptosis in macrophages undergoing endoplasmic reticulum stress. Cell Metab. 2010;12:467–82.
13. Yasuda T, Ishida T, Rader DJ. Update on the role of endothelial lipase in high density lipoprotein metabolism, reverse cholesterol transport and atherosclerosis. Circ J. 2010;74:2263–70.
14. Xiao H, Lu M, Lin TY, Chen Z, Chen G, Wang WC, et al. Sterol regulatory element binding protein 2 activation of the NLPR3 inflammasome in endothelium mediates hemodynamic-induced atherosclerosis susceptibility. Circulation. 2013;128:632–42.
15. Wilson-Tang WH, Wang Z, Levison BS, Koeth RA, Britt EB, Fu W, et al. Intestinal microbial metabolism of phosphatidylcholine and cardiovascular risk. N Engl J Med. 2013;368:1575–84.
16. Narshi CB, Giles IP, Rahman A. The endothelium: an interface between autoimmunity and atherosclerosis in systemic lupus erythematosus? Lupus. 2011;20:5–13.
17. Rohrer R, Hersberger M, von Eckardstein A. High density lipoproteins in the intersection of diabetes mellitus, inflammation and cardiovascular disease. Curr Opin Lipidol. 2009;15:269–78.
18. Zhang H, Park Y, Wu J, Chen XP, Lee S, Yang J, Dellsperger KC, et al. Role of TNF-α in vascular dysfunction. Clin Sci. 2009;116:219–30.
19. Stagakis I, Bertsias G, Karvounaris S, Kavousanaki M, Virla D, Raptopoulou A, et al. Anti-tumor necrosis factor therapy improves insulin resistance, beta cell function and insulin signaling in active rheumatoid arthritis patients with high insulin resistance. Arthritis Res Ther. 2012;14:R141.

20. Sola S, Mir MQ, Lerakis S, Tandon N, Khan BV. Atorvastatin improves left ventricular systolic function and serum markers of inflammation in nonischemic heart failure. J Am Coll Cardiol. 2006;47:332–7.
21. Kovacs I, Toth J, Tarjan J, Koller A. Correlation of flow mediated dilation with inflammatory markers in patients with impaired cardiac function. Beneficial effects of inhibition of ACE. Eur J Heart Fail. 2006;8: 451–9.
22. George J, Harats D, Gilburd B, Afek A, Levy Y, Schneiderman J, et al. Immunolocalization of beta2-glycoprotein I (apolipoprotein H) to human atherosclerotic plaques: potential implications for lesion progression. Circulation. 1999;99:2227–30.
23. Hewing B, Fisher E. Preclinical mouse models and methods for the discovery of the causes and treatments of atherosclerosis. Expert Opin Drug Discov. 2012;7:207–16.
24. Broadbent HM, Peden JF, Lorkowski S, Goel A, Ongen H, Green H, et al. Susceptibility to coronary artery disease and diabetes is encoded by distinct, tightly linked SNPs in the ANRIL locus on chromosome 9p. Hum Mol Genet. 2008;17:806–14.
25. McPherson R, Davies RW. Inflammation and coronary artery disease. Insights from genetic studies. Can J Cardiol. 2012;28:662–6.
26. Firchtscherer S, De Rosa S, Fox H, Schwietz T, Fischer A, Liebertrau C, et al. Circulating microRNAs in patients with CAD. Circ Res. 2010;107: 677–84.
27. Wen C, Yang X, Yan Z, Zhao M, Yue X, Cheng X, et al. Nalp 3 inflammasome is activated and required for vascular smooth muscle cell calcification. Int J Cardiol. 2013;168:2242–7.
28. Gray SP, Di Marco E, Okabe J, Szyndralewietz C, Heitz F, Montezano AC, et al. Nox1 plays a key role in diabetes associated atherosclerosis. Circulation. 2013;127:1888–902.
29. Breitling LP, Salzmann K, Rothenbacher D, Burwinkel B, Brenner H. Smoking, F2RL3 methylation and prognosis in stable coronary heart disease. Eur Heart J. 2012;33:2841–8.
30. Doring Y, Noels H, Weber C. The use of high-throughput technologies to investigate vascular inflammation and atherosclerosis. Arterioscler Thromb Vasc Biol. 2012;32:182–95.
31. ten Kate GL, Sijbrands EJG, Valkema R, ten Cat FJ, Feinstein SB, van de Steen AF, et al. Molecular imaging of inflammation and intraplaque vasa vasorum: a step forward to identification of vulnerable plaques? J Nucl Cardiol. 2010;17:897–912.
32. Joshi F, Rosenbaum D, Bordes S, Rudd JH. Vascular imaging with positron emission tomography. J Intern Med. 2011;270:99–109.
33. Dweck MR, Chow MWL, Joshi NV, Williams MC, Jones C, Fletcher AM, et al. Coronary arterial 18F-sodium fluoride uptake. A novel marker of plaque biology. J Am Coll Cardiol. 2012;59: 1539–48.
34. Inaba Y, Lindner JR. Molecular imaging of disease with targeted ultrasound contrast imaging. Transl Res. 2012;159:140–8.
35. Kern MJ, Hodgson JM, Seto A. Nonangiographic coronary lesion assessment: FFR, IVUS, OCT, NIRS. In: The interventional cardiac catheterization handbook. 3rd ed. Philadelphia: Elsevier. Saunders. 2013; p. 244–89.
36. Jefferson A, Wijesurendra RS, McAteer MA, Digby JE, Douglas G, Bannister T, et al. Molecular imaging with optical coherence tomography using ligand-conjugated microparticles that detect activated endothelial cells: Rational design through target qualification. Atherosclerosis. 2011;219: 579–87.
37. Waxman S, Sixon SR, L'Allier P, Moses JW, Petersen JL, Cutlip D, et al. In vivo validation of a catheter-based near-infrared spectroscopy system for detection of lipid core coronary plaques: initial results of the SPECTACL study. JACC Cardiovasc Imaging. 2009;2:858–68.
38. Nissen SE. Effect of intensive lipid lowering on progression of coronary atherosclerosis: evidence for an early benefit from the Reversal of Atherosclerosis with Aggressive Lipid Lowering (REVERSAL) trial. Am J Cardiol. 2005;96:61F–8.
39. Digby JE, Ruparelia N, Choudhury RP. Niacin in cardiovascular disease. Recent preclinical and clinical developments. Arterioscler Thromb Vasc Biol. 2012;32:582–8.
40. Serruys P, Garcia-Garcia HM, Buszman P, Erne P, Verheye S, Aschermann M, et al. Effects of the direct lipoprotein-associated phospholipase A2 darapladib on human coronary atherosclerotic plaque. Circulation. 2008;118:1172–82.
41. Barter PJ, Caulfield M, Eriksson M, Grundy SM, Kastelein JJ, Komajda M, et al. Effects of torcetrabib in patients at high risk for coronary events. N Engl J Med. 2007;357:2109–22.
42. Fayad ZA, Mani V, Woodward M, Kallend D, Abt M, Burguess T, et al. Safety and efficacy of dalcetrabib on atherosclerotic disease using novel non-invasive multimodality imaging (dal-PLAQUE): a randomized clinical trial. Lancet. 2011;378:1547–59.
43. Ridker PM, Thuren T, Zalewski A, Libby P. Interleukin-1 beta inhibition and the prevention of recurrent cardiovascular events: rationale and design of the Canakimumab Anti-Inflammatory Thrombosis Outcomes Study (CANTOS). Am Heart J. 2011;162:597–605.
44. Abbate A, Van Tassell BW, Biondi-Zoccai G, Kontos MC, Grizzard JD, Spillman DW, et al. Effects of interleukin-1 blocking with anakinra on adverse cardiac remodeling and heart failure after acute myocardial infarction [from the Virginia Commonwealth University Anakinra Remodeling Trial (2) (VCU-ART2) Pilot Study. Am J Cardiol. 2013;111:1394–400.
45. Protogerou AD, Zampeli E, Fragiadaki K, Stamatelopoulos K, Papamichael C, Sfikakis P. A pilot study of endothelial dysfunction and aortic stiffness

after interleukin-6 receptor inhibition in rheumatoid arthritis. Atherosclerosis. 2011;219:734–6.
46. Tardif JC, Lallier PL, Ibrahim R, Gregoire JC, Nozza A, Cossette M, et al. Treatment with lipoxygenase 5 inhibitor VIA 2291 (Atreleuton) in patients with recent acute coronary syndrome. Circ Cardiovasc Imaging. 2010;3:298–307.
47. Kakonarson H, Thorvaldsson S, Helgadottir A, Gudbjardsson D, Zink F, Andresdottir M, et al. Effects of a 5-lipoxygenase activating protein inhibitor on biomarkers associated with risk of myocardial infarction: a randomized trial. JAMA. 2005;293: 2245–56.
48. van der Valk FM, van Wijk DF, Stroes ESG. Novel anti-inflammatory strategies in atherosclerosis. Curr Opin Lipidol. 2012;23:532–9.
49. Gilbert J, Lekstrom-Himes J, Donaldson D, Lee Y, Hu M, Xu J, et al. Effect of CC chemokine receptor 2 CCR2 blockade on serum C-reactive protein in individuals in atherosclerotic risk with a single nucleotide polymorphism of the monocyte chemoattractant protein 1 promoter region. Am J Cardiol. 2011;107:906–11.
50. Weber C, Noels H. Atherosclerosis: current pathogenesis and therapeutic options. Nat Med. 2011;17: 141–2.

Stress Proteins and the Adaptive Response of the Heart

14

Theodora Tzanavari and Katia P. Karalis

Abstract

Stressors may be major contributors to cardiovascular disease. The systemic adaptive response to stressors, referred as "stress response", is primarily mediated by the activation of the hypothalamic-pituitary-adrenal (HPA) axis and the catecholaminergic system. At the cellular level, cardiomyocytes have developed various mechanisms to counterbalance stressors affecting their contractile, metabolic and other functions. These mechanisms include remodeling and activation of the fetal gene program. Here we describe the fundamentals of the stress response, we review the implications of stressors such as oxidative, endoplasmic and metabolic on heart function and we discuss the effects of specific hormonal mediators of the stress response in heart function. We particularly refer to the cardiovascular effects of Corticotropin Releasing Hormone and its related peptides in supporting the adaptive response, a potentially therapeutic strategy to overcome stressors threatening homeostasis and driving disease development.

Keywords

Stress • Homeostasis • Adaptive response • Hypothalamic-pituitary-adrenal (HPA) axis • Corticotropin-releasing hormone (CRH)

Abbreviations

AMPK	5' AMP-activated protein kinase
ANP	Atrial natriuretic peptide
ATH	Atherosclerosis
BNP	Brain natriuretic peptide
CDCM	Congenital dilated cardiomyopathy
CRH	Cortioctropin-releasing hormone
CT-1	Cardiotrophin-1
CVD	Cardiovascular disorder
ER	Endoplasmic reticulum
ETCs	Electron transport chains
GPCRs	G-protein coupled receptors
GREs	Glucocorticoid responsive elements
Hif1α	Hypoxia-inducible factor 1-alpha
HPA	Hypothalamic-pituitary-adrenal
HSP90	Heat shock protein 90

T. Tzanavari, PhD (✉) • K.P. Karalis, MD, PhD
Developmental Biology Lab, Center of Basic Research I, Biomedical Research Foundation of the Academy of Athens, 4 Soranou Efessiou Street, Athens 11527, Greece
e-mail: ttzanavari@bioacademy.gr; kkarali@bioacademy.gr

D.V. Cokkinos (ed.), *Introduction to Translational Cardiovascular Research*,
DOI 10.1007/978-3-319-08798-6_14,

IGF-1	Insulin-like growth factor 1
$iPLA_2$	Calcium insensitive phospholipase A_2
IκBK	IκB kinase
JNK	jun N-terminal kinase
K_{ATP}	ATP-sensitive potassium channel
MAPK	Mitogen activated protein kinase
MCPIP	Monocyte chemoattractant protein-induced protein
MI	Myocardial infarction
MPTP	Mitochondrial permeability transition pore
mROS	Mitochondrial ROS
NFκB	Nuclear factor κ light-chain enhancer of activated B cells
PGC1α	Peroxisome proliferator-activated receptor gamma coactivator 1-alpha
PI3K	Phosphoinositide-3-kinase
PKCε	Protein kinase C epsilon
REM	Remodeling
ROS	Reactive oxygen species
SNS	Sympathetic nervous system
SOCE	Store-operated Ca^{2+} entry
STIM1	Stromal interaction molecule 1
UCN	Urocortin
UPR	Unfolded protein response

14.1 Introduction: Definition of Stress

Living organisms survive by maintaining a complex dynamic and harmonious equilibrium, or homeostasis, that is constantly challenged by intrinsic or extrinsic disturbing forces or stressors. In this context, stress may be defined as a 'state of disharmony, or threatened homeostasis'. Although minimum at normal levels, stress is an important part of normal daily life, as it enables the organism to cope with changes in the environment. However, excess stress, either physical or psychological, is a cause of harm [1].

As already described in Chap. 6, Hans Selye, who was the first to define stress, conceived the General Adaptation Syndrome, as "the non-specific response by the body to any demand", physical or psychological [2]. The General Adaptation Syndrome represents a "chronological development of the stress response to stressors when their action is prolonged". It consists of an initial "alarm reaction" or "shock" phase, a second "resistance" phase and a final "exhaustion" phase. According to Selye, during the second phase the body is allowed to compensate and restore homeostasis. In addition, Selye distinguished eustress (healthy stress) from distress (pathogenic stress). Distress resulting from an excessive or inappropriate response to a stressor can lead to stress-induced maladies [3]. The adaptive responses can be either specific to the stressor or nonspecific. Along these lines, Chrousos and Gold described the activity of the stress system as a sigmoidal dose-response curve with stressor potency and stress response related in a nonlinear manner. This concept can be modified to show stressor potency as an independent variable and the stress response as the dependent variable. The activity of the stress response will need a threshold to be activated, beyond which a quasilinear relationship commences. As expected, beyond a given point, the activity of the stress response does not increase despite further increase in stressor potency. This dose-response sigmoid curve is individual-specific [4]. The latter is the core of the theory of "allostasis", which is defined as the "stability obtained through changes". This concept which was developed by Sterling and Eyer refers to the active processes via which the body responds to daily events to maintain homeostasis [5]. The concept of allostasis suggests that when an organism is threatened, effector systems are activated to promote adaptation to a new equilibrium, rather than a return to the previous, no-longer-existing condition. Various allostatic mechanisms may be triggered by any given condition. Depending on the actual mechanisms triggered some sort of adaptation will be affected; this is the allostatic load to which the organism is submitted. Under normal conditions, allostasis is the mechanism that protects the body, promotes improved health and guarantees survival. When the allostatic load is excessively strong or lasts for a long period, it becomes allostatic overload, with the continued activation of the effector systems, which is extremely harmful, resulting in maladaptation and the appearance of stress related diseases [4]. Stress increases the susceptibility of the body to infection, autoimmune diseases, chronic fatigue syndrome, psychiatric illnesses, cancer, and chronic diseases. Depending on the individual situation and predisposition, stress can be a major contributor to the development of cardiovascular disorders (CVD), such as ischemic heart disease, arrhythmia and sudden death [6].

14.2 Hormonal Regulation of the Adaptive Response

The stress system is organized into central, peripheral, and cellular systems within a network of anatomical regions that work together to keep the body both informed and ready to react to encountered changes in either external or internal cellular environments [1]. The hypothalamic-pituitary-adrenal (HPA) axis and the sympathetic nervous system (SNS) constitute the main effector pathways of the stress system [7, 8].

The HPA axis is the principal endocrine axis regulating the stress response [4]. Stressors of different origins activate the hypothalamic corticotropin-releasing hormone (CRH), which stimulates pituitary ACTH secretion and finally release of glucocorticoid from the adrenal gland [9]. In parallel, the catecholaminergic system is activated both at the locus coeruleus and the adrenal medulla, leading in the release of norepinephrine and epinephrine. The HPA axis operates via forward positive feedback system, so that following its activation, glucocorticoid, the end-product of its activation, exerts negative feedback on CRH and ACTH. CRH has anxiogenic properties and coordinates the adaptive, behavioral, and physical changes that occur during stress. Glucocorticoid, the final mediator of the HPA axis, plays a crucial role in mounting the adaptive response to stress and are crucial for the appropriate termination of every stress response. Glucocorticoid, via their receptors, act on positive or negative glucocorticoid responsive elements (GREs) to activate or suppress the expression of various genes, which are either directly or indirectly implicated in vital metabolic pathways [10, 11]. Cortisol, the primary glucocorticoid in humans, is continuously secreted by the adrenal cortex and its release increases significantly during environmental stressors [12].

The SNS, the other principal effector component of the stress system, provides a mechanism which allows rapid regulation of vital functions, such as cardiovascular, respiratory, gastrointestinal, renal, and endocrine functions [13, 14]. Cytokines, in particular IL-6, are potent activators of the central stress response, forming a feedback loop through which the immune/inflammatory system communicates with the brain [15].

When stress, which moderates the proteome of the cytosol, endoplasmic reticulum (ER) and mitochondria, is sensed in one tissue, it can activate responses in different tissues in a non-autonomous way. This way, mechanisms that protect against and mechanisms that promote disease progression rely on coordination and communication between cells and tissues. The control of intercellular communication and cell-autonomous regulation is subject to neuroendocrine regulation through HPA activation. Chronic activation of the stress system, together with its associated catabolic, anti-reproductive, antigrowth and immunosuppressive effects, may prove detrimental for the organism. A cellular stress response may thus develop into a systemic stress response through activation of the hypothalamic-pituitary-adrenal (HPA) axis and release of glucocorticoid. Results of chronic stress include behavioral changes affecting physical activity and dietary habits leading to weight gain and the metabolic syndrome, and thus to abnormalities of glucose and lipid metabolism [16], induction of chronic hypercortisolemia that can in the long run cause visceral fat accumulation, decreased lean body mass, and insulin resistance [17, 18], and increased sympathoadrenal system activity. The latter contributes to impaired glucose tolerance and to increased risk for acute cardiovascular events [19].

14.3 Stress and Cardiovascular Disease

The concept of stress being involved as risk factor for CVD dates back more than 100 years ago and has been thoroughly investigated using a combination of epidemiological, mechanistic, psychophysiological experiments and clinical studies. Adaptation to stressors is an integral part of cardiovascular physiology, whereas stress can be a major contributor in the development of cardiovascular disorders, such as ischemic heart disease, arrhythmia and sudden death [6]. Chronic stress, either at early life or adulthood, has been associated with a 40–60 % excess risk of cardiovascular disorder [20].

Cardiomyocytes have developed various mechanisms to deal with stressors affecting their contractile performance and/or energy supply. The success of these mechanisms depends to a large extent on the nature and duration of the stress. At the cellular level, stress results in adverse rearrangement of cytoskeletal structures, a process known as remodeling (REM), together with the accumulation of dysfunctional mitochondria and ER. Success or failure of these cellular adaptive mechanisms, which will be discussed in detail in the following paragraphs, may lead to repair of the injury or propagation of the damage often progressing to heart failure (HF).

14.3.1 Cardiomyocyte Remodeling in Response to Stress

At the cellular level, REM causes stress to the cardiomyocyte as a whole, by altering energy metabolism, the structure of the contractile apparatus and the cytoskeleton. Thus, cardiomyocytes lose the characteristics of mature (differentiated) cardiomyocytes and re-express genes from embryonic or fetal developmental stages REM is intimately connected to cellular dedifferentiation. It has been proposed that by dedifferentiation or sarcomeric disassembly, cardiomyocytes gain resistance to altered metabolic and/or hypoxic stress [21–24]. Dedifferentiation provides cardiomyocytes with a plasticity which allows the myocardium to cope much better with hypoxia-induced or overload-induced cell death, preventing the progression from compensated hypertrophy to HF [25]. Parallel activation of the fetal gene program is characterized by the up-regulation of early cardiac-specific transcription factors, including MEF2c, NFAT, GATA and Nkx2.5 [26], as well as the stem cell markers c-kit, Runx1 and Dab2. Numerous other genes, including destrin, a-SM-actin, the natriuretic peptides ANP and BNP, smooth-muscle actin (ACTN1), moiesin, and oncostatin M (OSM) are also re-expressed. The fetal gene program also shows induced expression of ER chaperones such as BiP/GRP78, GRP94 and calreticulin during early development, and also triggers significant changes in metabolic programs [27]. These changes are also described in Chap. 17.

In diseased states, compensatory REM is accompanied by certain maladaptive processes including inflammatory infiltration, increased interstitial connective tissue (increasing the oxygen diffusion distance and wall stiffness), reduction of cardiomyocyte cell contacts, and apoptotic cell death, eventually reducing the ventricular ejection capacity [28–30]. The degree of cardiomyocyte degeneration and loss of differentiation markers can be correlated with the extent of inflammatory infiltration [23, 31].

Myocyte dedifferentiation, including loss of myoglobin, reduces oxygen-dependent generation of ATP, but maintains the ability of heart cells to generate energy by glycolysis. Cardiac REM and metabolic adaptation are closely interconnected, as reflected by the characteristic switch from fatty acid oxidation to glucose utilization in stressed cardiomyocytes. Interestingly, although changes in mitochondrial metabolism seem initially beneficial to sustain contractility and survival, increasing evidence suggests that metabolic reprogramming might eventually result in mitochondrial dysfunction and cardiac failure [32].

A good method to study and understand compensatory REM in animal models is cardiac ischemia, as it comprises response mechanisms caused by the lack of oxygen and includes secondary inflammatory infiltration. Importantly, REM affects both ischemic and non-ischemic regions of the ventricle leading to changes in chamber size, shape and function. Smaller damages may only lead to hypertrophy of remaining cardiomyocytes in order to normalize wall stress, while large infarcts cause significant changes in heart architecture [33–35].

14.3.2 Cardiomyocytes and Oxidative Stress

The accumulation of dysfunctional mitochondria is characteristic of a wide spectrum of cardiac diseases. Mitochondria are important cellular energy components. In addition to producing energy through respiration, mitochondria regulate cellular metabolism and produce reactive oxygen species (ROS) through electron transport chains (ETCs). Although the adrenergic system plays a central role in stress signaling and stress is often associated with increased production of ROS, ROS overproduction generates oxidative stress, a key part of various common pathological conditions, including the metabolic syndrome and numerous cardiovascular diseases, such as coronary artery disease, heart failure, left ventricular hypertrophy, diabetic cardiomyopathy and hyperkinetic arrhythmias.

ROS are reactive chemical units involving two main categories: (a) free radicals such as superoxide (O_2^-), hydroxyl (OH) and nitric oxide (NO); and (b) non-radical derivatives of O_2 such as hydrogen peroxide (H_2O_2) and peroxynitrate ($ONOO^-$) [36]. Under normal conditions, ROS control several physiological processes, including host defense, hormone biosynthesis, fertilization and cell signaling. Oxidative stress causes protein, lipid and DNA damage leading to cellular dysfunction. Excessive O_2^- may decrease nitric oxide (NO) availability, leading to endothelial dysfunction and endothelium-dependent vasodilation decrease [37]; while oxidative protein modification may result in the formation of nitrotyrosine that represents a powerful and autonomous marker of cardiovascular diseases. O_2^- is also implicated in the generation of oxidized LDL, a key initiator of atherosclerosis (ATH) [38].

ROS can cause posttranslational protein modifications to regulate signaling pathways. Redox modifications may affect mitochondrial function either directly or indirectly by acting on mediators involved in most mitochondrial activities. For example, STAT3 seems to preserve ETC activity by preventing ROS leakage at complex I. In mice, cardiac-specific deletion of STAT3 results in the development of cardiac inflammatory fibrosis, dilated cardiomyopathy and heart failure with advancing age; while lack of STAT3 eliminates the cardioprotective effects of ischemic preconditioning, contrary to its overexpression in cardiomyocytes, which protects mice against doxorubicin toxicity that involves mitochondrial dysfunction [39]. Expression of a recombinant form of STAT3 that targets mitochondria and lacks the DNA-binding domain protected the heart from ischemic damage by decreasing mitochondrial ROS (mROS) production and attenuating cytochrome c release in a model of ischemia. mROS is of a dual nature. Very high quantities of mROS directly damage proteins, lipids and nucleic acids. Lower levels, however, function as signaling molecules to adapt to stress, and even lower amounts of mROS are required for normal cell function. For example, mROS are involved in cardioprotective preconditioning pathways, and antioxidants render ischemic preconditioning ineffective [40].

Emerging evidence points to the role of NAPDH oxidase (NOX) family of enzymes, a major source of ROS in both metabolic and cardiovascular dysfunction [41]. As very well established, β-adrenergic signaling is markedly attenuated in conditions such as heart failure, with downregulation and desensitization of the receptors and their uncoupling from adenylyl cyclase. Transgenic activation of β_2-adrenoreceptor leads to elevation of NADPH oxidase activity, with greater ROS production and p38 MAPK phosphorylation. Inhibition of NADPH oxidase or ROS significantly reduces the p38 MAPK signaling cascade. βAR stimulation antagonizes the protective effect of the Akt pathway through inhibition of hypoxia-inducible factor 1-alpha (Hif1a) and Sirt1 induction, key elements in cell survival [42]. Sirtuins, a family of seven highly conserved class III histone deacetylases that regulate a wide range of cellular processes, such as transcription, inflammation, apoptosis, and aging [43], are involved in modulating the cellular stress response directly by deacetylation of some factors. Lately, the role of Sirt1 (also called NAD^+ – dependent protein deacetylase) as the most important factor in the pathway of mitochondrial biogenesis and a key regulator of cellular defense and survival has been recognized [44]. Sirt1 increases cellular stress resistance, by induction of insulin sensitivity, decrease in circulating free fatty acids and insulin-like growth factor 1 (IGF-1), induction of 5' AMP-activated protein kinase (AMPK) and peroxisome proliferator-activated receptor gamma coactivator 1-alpha (PGC1a) activity, and mitochondrial genesis. Resveratrol, a therapeutic agent and an activator of SIRT1, suppresses ROS production and induces the expression of the mitochondrial protein NDUFA13 [45, 46].

14.3.3 Endoplasmic Reticulum Stress

The endoplasmic reticulum (ER) is an intracellular organelle with major contribution to protein synthesis and metabolism of nutrients and toxic metabolic products. ER stress developing in states of overwhelming load of the ER is associated with a variety of states such as oxidative stress, ROS production, viral infection, environmental toxins, heat, drugs, inflammatory cytokines, lipotoxicity, Ca^{2+} depletion, metabolic starvation and aging. ER stress has been also identified as a key contributor in the pathogenesis of cardiac and vascular diseases [27, 47–50]. Tight control of metabolic homeostasis that is necessary for normal function of all tissues is particularly important for the cardiac tissue and involves Ca^{2+}, K^+, Na^+, Cl^-, oxygen, glucose, amino acids, and fatty acids. Disruption of metabolic homeostasis can lead to ER stress. For example, disruption of Ca^{2+} homeostasis is directly responsible for ER stress and activation of cardiac REM, leading to cardiac hypertrophy. Cardiomyocytes monitor Ca^{2+} homeostasis in regard to excitation-contraction versus ER stress by, at least in part, the regulation of store-operated Ca^{2+} entry (SOCE) and an ER membrane-associated Ca^{2+} sensor, stromal interaction molecule 1 (STIM1) [51]. In rats, SOCE is abundant in neonatal cardiomyocytes, while it is absent in adult cardiomyocytes [52], correlating with STIM1 mRNA and protein expression. Stress-triggered STIM1 re-expression and consequent SOCE activation are critical elements in the upstream, Ca^{2+} -dependent control of pathological cardiac hypertrophy [52]. In states of thoracic aortic constriction (TAC) and in neonatal cardiomyocytes under induced hypetrophy, STIM1 protein and mRNA levels are significantly increased. The above is an example of the molecular pathways mediating mobilization of Ca^{2+} -signaling molecules and pathways and their interconnection to the preservation of ER function, all contributing to support normal cardiac function in normal and adverse conditions.

There is a constant, interactive relation between active inflammation and ER stress, underlying a spectrum of diseases with insulin resistance the most widely studied [53]. Increase of the unfolded protein response (UPR), ROS production, Ca^{2+} release from the ER, and the activation of the nuclear factor κ light-chain enhancer of activated B cells (NF-κB) and of Jun N-terminal kinase (JNK) can trigger the inflammatory response associated with ATH and CVD [54–56]. Briefly, upon tissue damage, inflammatory cells such as neutrophils and macrophages are recruited to the site of damage, initiating inflammatory cytokine production and ROS generation, protein folding disruption and ER stress triggering. When ER stress is prolonged, NF-κB initiates apoptosis, thereby shifting the outcome of the compensatory mechanism from an adaptive to a maladaptive one. NF-κB activation is initiated via the action of IκB kinase (IκBK), which phosphorylates and inactivates IκB-α. Its inactivation in turn results in NF-κB nuclear translocation and in the expression of inflammation-related genes, such as those encoding the potent inflammatory cytokines TNFα and IL-6 [54, 56]. Specific to cardiomyocytes, NFκB deletion promotes an adaptive response to ER stress, whereas once NFκB is activated, cardiomyocytes undergo inflammation, fibrosis and apoptosis. The angiogenic factor MCP-1 is linked to inflammation and the activation of autophagy in the heart. During chronic inflammation, increased MCP-1 expression induces oxidative stress by upregulating monocyte chemoattractant protein-induced protein (MCPIP), a novel zinc finger protein, which causes oxidative stress via iNOS activation and ROS production, followed by the induction of ER stress-responsive genes and autophagy [57]. Gene-silencing experiments have demonstrated that MCPIP reduction decreases MCP-1 induced cell death in cardiac myoblasts. MCP-1 recruits monocytes and differentiates monocytic lineage cells into endothelium-like cells, thus promoting vascular growth and angiogenesis [58].

ER stress is highly associated with various CVD. Myocardial infarction (MI) provides a classic example; it results in severe complications associated with hypoxia and fuel starvation in the muscle tissue, generation of a buildup of misfolded protein, and thus disruption of ER homeostasis and generation of ER stress. Furthermore, during ischemia, ER stress results in the degeneration of cardiac myocytes and over time in cell death. However, if preconditioning, such as mild heat stress, is applied, damage may be prevented, most possibly due to the activation of an adaptive coping response, consequently limiting the amount of damage generated during the subsequent insult. Similarly, hypertension or aortic construction or stenosis, also resulting in pressure overload, induce ER stress. The list of CVD implicating ER stress is growing rapidly. Congenital dilated cardiomyopathy (CDCM) is linked to a mutation in the KDEL receptor, which leads to a buildup of misfolded proteins and results in ER stress [59]. Reports show that disruptions in the excitation-contraction coupling, with abnormal Ca^{2+} homeostasis, result in ER stress and congestive HF. Atherosclerosis results from the accumulation of misfolded proteins due to the oxidation of lipids, the upregulation of homocysteine in vascular cells, and inclusion of large amounts of cholesterol esters in macrophages. ER stress may also play a role in cardiac amyloidosis. It is thus obvious that ER stress and CVD are intimately intertwined and therefore therapeutic interventions to cope with ER stress provide a promising venue in the fight against detrimental chronic diseases [60].

14.3.4 Effects of the Hormonal Mediators of the Stress Response in the Cardiovascular System

HPA axis is the principal endocrine axis regulating the stress response. Stressors of different origins activate the hypothalamic CRH, which stimulates pituitary ACTH secretion and finally release of glucocorticoid from the adrenal gland. In parallel, the catecholaminergic system is activated both at the locus coeruleus and peripheral sites leading to the release of norepinephrine and epinephrine. The HPA axis operates via forward positive feedback system, while the end-product, glucocorticoid exerts negative feedback regulation of CRH and ACTH. All different components of the HPA axis affect, directly or indirectly, heart function and may precipitate disease development. A summary of HPA axis and CRH regulation is shown in Fig. 14.1. Below, we give a brief summary of the effects of glucocorticoid and the CRH family of peptides in the regulation of cardiovascular function.

14.3.4.1 Glucocorticoid

Cardiomyocytes participate actively in the adaptive stress response via initiating a cascade of pathways to secure homeostasis. Failure to do so, results in extensive tissue damage, disease development and eventually HF. Glucocorticoid act by synchronizing the metabolic, autonomic, psychological, hemostatic and cardiovascular components of the stress response via its multiple tissue-specific genomic and non-genomic effects. These actions facilitate the vascular and metabolic effects of other stress hormones, such as catecholamines, glucagon and angiotensin-II, through stimulation of $\alpha 1$ adrenergic and angiotensin II receptor expression, and increase in the affinity and binding capacity of β-adrenergic receptors. In parallel, glucocorticoid suppresses associated processes such as inflammation, cellular proliferation and tissue repair processes. Finally, glucocorticoid prepare the organism for prolonged nutritional deprivation by facilitating proteolysis and support development of insulin resistance at the muscle level, while inducing

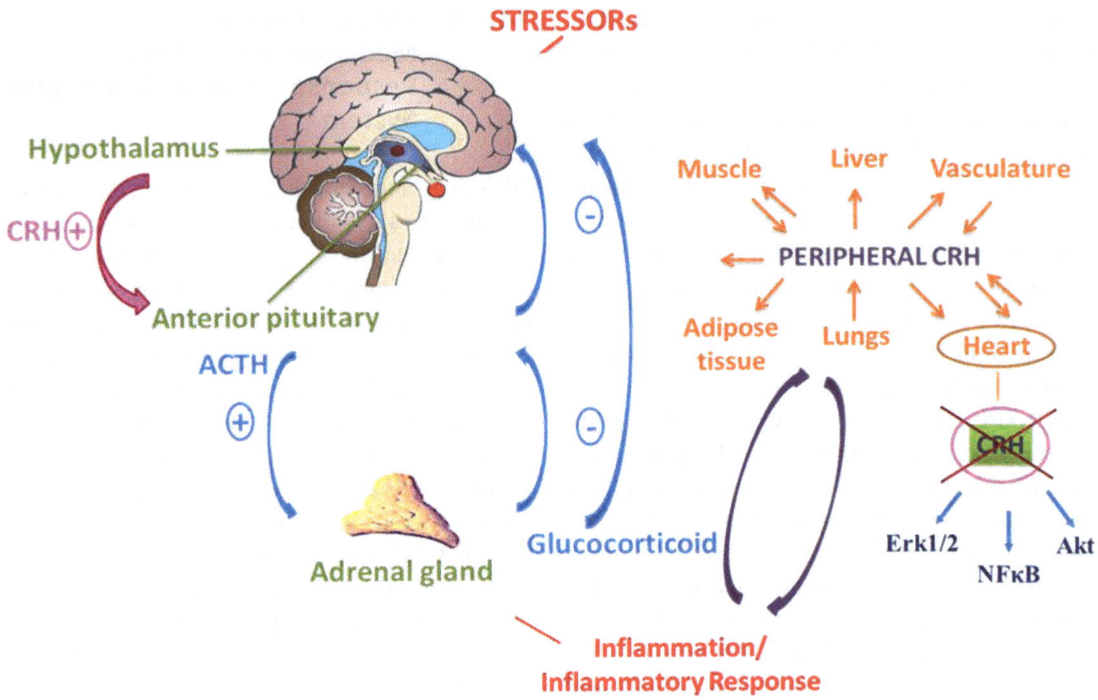

Fig. 14.1 HPA axis is the principal endocrine axis regulating the stress response. Stressors of different origins activate the hypothalamic CRH, which stimulates pituitary ACTH secretion and finally release of glucocorticoid from the adrenal gland. The HPA axis operates via forward positive feedback system, while the end-product, glucocorticoid exerts negative feedback regulation of CRH and ACTH. In addition to its expression in the central nervous system, several functions in peripheral sites have been identified. Genetic ablation of CRH (*Crh* knockout, *Crh−/−* mouse) in the heart negatively affects cardiac function, through the *Erk1/2*, *Akt* and *NFκB* signaling pathways

gluconeogenesis and lipolysis. This pleiotropic action of glucocorticoid may be harmful for the cardiovascular system because of increased blood pressure and insulin resistance. Corticosteroid excess is associated with adverse cardiovascular outcomes. Patients with Cushings's syndrome and primary aldosteronism, two conditions characterized by glucocorticoid excess and inappropriately high aldosterone production respectively, have increased risk for CVD. Prior to treatment of Cushing's syndrome, it has not been uncommon for patients to experience early death from MI or stroke. In animal models, excess glucocorticoid can induce ATH. In humans, it has been suggested that corticosteroid-treated patients with rheumatoid arthritis and lupus erythematosus develop significantly more ATH than those not treated with steroids and the risk of ATH is related to the cumulative dose of corticosteroid. There have also been cases of adverse outcomes of steroid-dependent rheumatoid arthritis patients treated with thrombolytic agents for acute MI, possibly due to increased risk of myocardial rupture. However, there has been no consensus on the proposed adverse effects of glucocorticoid given acutely in MI [61].

On the other hand, glucocorticoid deficiency may result in hypotension, weight loss, hypoglycemia and death, particularly during stress; while glucocorticoid excess can lead to hypertension, insulin resistance, hyperglycemia and weight gain [62–64]. The vascular effects of glucocorticoid seem to be achieved by enhancing adrenergic stimulation, angiotensin II and possibly endothelin-1. Glucocorticoid upregulate angiotensin II type I receptor expression and α1 adrenergic receptors in rat vascular smooth muscle cells and potentiate the vasoconstrictive actions of angiotensin-II and norepinephrine in animals [65]

14.3.4.2 Crh and CRH-Related

In addition to its expression in the central nervous system, CRH has been identified in peripheral sites with functions not completely elucidated yet. So far, a dual, both anti- and pro- proinflammatory role for peripheral CRH has been identified. Its significant expression in inflamed human and rodent tissues due to the corresponding neutrophil and polymorphonuclear cell accumulation has been shown [66], and its effects have been confirmed in transgenic animal models [67–70]. Angiogenic effects of CRH, both *in vivo* and *in vitro,* have been shown [71, 72].

CRH belongs to an extended family of CRH-related peptides, which includes urocortins (UCN) (I, II and III). These peptides share significant homology with CRH, while they all bind the same family of receptors (CRHR1 and CRHR2), with CRH and UCN I binding both receptors, although with different affinities, and UCN II and III binding CRHR2 exclusively. UCNs and CRHRs are also widely expressed in a variety of tissues. CRH receptors belong to the G-protein coupled receptors (GPCRs) family and upon activation stimulate various intracellular pathways, in a time- and tissue-dependent manner. Expression of both CRHRs and UCN have been identified in the endothelium and the heart with CRHR2 robustly [73] and CRHR1 minimally if at all expressed [74]. Activation of phosphoinositide-3-kinase (PI3K)/Akt (protein kinase B/Akt) and mitogen-activated protein kinases (MAPK) in endothelial cells by CRHR2 links its expression with specific biological effects, while protective effects in cardiomyocytes during experimental ischemia have been shown [75, 76]. Furthermore we have recently found stimulation of VEGF by CRH via CRHR2 in endothelial cells [72, 77].

Cardioprotective effects of UCNs have been well documented in several experimental systems. In general, urocortins exhibit potent vasodilatory effects in arteries of different species through regulation of intracellular Ca^{2+} levels, increase heart contractility and evoke positive inotropic and lusitropic effects. More specifically, UCNs protect the heart from ischemia and reperfusion injury via improvement of post-ischemic cardiac performance, such as cardiac contractility, prevention from Ca^{2+} overload and reduction of cardiac cell death. These effects involve the activation of several signaling pathways targeting both cytoplasmic and mitochondrial processes. In particular UCN1, by initially binding to GPCRs, initiates the activation of PI3K, protein kinase A (PKA), Akt, protein kinase C (PKC) and MAPKs. Activation of these kinase pathways alters the activity of various channels including the mitochondrial permeability transition pore (MPTP), which is involved in the induction of cell death [78, 79], as described in Sects. 15.2.1 and 15.2.2. Apart from their acute effects, UCNs exert more prolonged, modulatory actions, such as transcriptional and translational effects on mitochondrial ATP-sensitive potassium channel (K_{ATP}), calcium insensitive phospholipase A_2 (iPLA_2) and protein kinase C epsilon (PKCε), all three involved in cardioprotection [80–84]. UCN1 acts via a p42/p44 MAPK (Erk1/2)-dependent signaling pathway in protecting both *in vitro* primary cell models and *ex vivo* and *in vivo* rodent heart from reperfusion injury. Erk1/2 phosphorylation and activation is mediated by the MAP kinase MEK1/2 following UCN1 treatment; while its inhibition disrupts UCN1-mediated cardioprotection [85, 86]. PI3K and its downstream effector Akt are crucial for UCN-stimulated increase in survival of cardiomyocytes [87]. Both MEK1/2 and PI3K are responsible for preventing pro-caspases -9 and -3 from being cleaved into their active forms [88, 89]. UCN2 and UCN3 also act through the PI3K pathway [75]. In addition to the protective effects, UCN treatment of both neonatal and adult rat cardiomyocytes stimulates the secretion of atrial natriuretic peptide (ANP) and brain natriuretic peptide (BNP), both of which are markers of hypertrophy [90, 91]. Another significant contribution of UCN1-mediated cardioprotection involves *de novo* protein synthesis. For example, expression of the cardioprotective heat shock protein 90 (HSP90) has been reported to be induced by UCN1, a specific effect blocked by the MK1/2 inhibitor PD98059 [92]. The expression of cardiotrophin-1 (CT-1), an additional cardioprotective peptide, is also increased upon exposure of cells to UCN 1 [93].

Based on the above experimental evidence for the cardioprotective role of urocortins and on the reported role of CRH on various peripheral sites, a possible role for CRH in the cardiac adaptive response to stressors has recently been explored by our group. The absence of CRH in mice leads to low levels of ACTH and corticosterone and a blunted HPA response. Thus, CRH regulates adrenal function as well as responses to stress mediated via the HPA axis. Genetic ablation of CRH (*Crh*-knockout, *Crh−/−*, mice) leads to inability of the cardiovascular system to cope with a mild stressor, resulting in death. Similar to those described for UCNs, signaling pathways involved in this process, include Erk1/2, Akt, and AMPK. *Crh* deletion also results in increased infiltration of the heart tissue with inflammatory cells and apoptosis. Metabolic dysregulation evident by significantly compromised ability for fatty acid oxidation may underlie, at least, the latter, and possibly drive the compromised function of the *Crh−/−* heart [94].

Conclusion

Heart is a tissue where different pathways activated by various stressors convey and alter its functions, often resulting in remodeling, chronic inflammation, metabolic dysfunction and ultimately, heart failure. Given the active participation of the heart in the adaptive response to stressors, and the effects of specific mediators of the adaptive response on these processes, the possibility they represent promising targets for novel therapeutic schemes is raised. New models taking into account the contribution of these factors at both the cell and systemic responses and proposing novel therapeutic strategies need to be validated.

References

1. Cuesta JM, Singer M. The stress response and critical illness: a review. Crit Care Med. 2012;40:3283–9.
2. Selye H. What is stress? Metabolism. 1956;5: 525–30.
3. Selye H. The stress concept. Can Med Assoc J. 1976;115:718.
4. Chrousos PG, Gold PW. The concepts of stress and stress system disorders. JAMA. 1992;267:1244–52.
5. Sterling P, Eyer J. Biological basis of stress-related mortality. Soc Sci Med E. 1981;15:3–42.
6. Davis AM, Natelson BH. Brain-heart interactions. The neurocardiology of arrhythmia and sudden cardiac death. Tex Heart Inst J. 1993;20:158–69.
7. Gold PW, Goodwin F, Chrousos GP. Clinical and biochemical manifestations of depression: relationship to the neurobiology of stress, part 1. N Engl J Med. 1988;319:348–53.
8. Gold PW, Goodwin F, Chrousos GP. Clinical and biochemical manifestations of depression: relationship to the neurobiology of stress, part 2. N Engl J Med. 1988;319:413–20.
9. Dallman MF, Yates FE. Dynamic asymmetries in the corticosteroid feedback path and distribution-metabolism-binding elements of the adrenocortical system. Ann N Y Acad Sci. 1969;156:696–721.
10. De Kloet ER, Vreugdenhil E, Oitzl MS, Joels M. Brain corticosteroid receptor balance in health and disease. Endocr Rev. 1998;19:269–301.
11. Boumpas DT, Chrousos GP, Wilder RL, Cupps TE, Balow JE. Glucocorticoid therapy for immune-mediated diseases: basic and clinical correlates. Ann Intern Med. 1993;119:1198–208.
12. Mastorakas G, Chrousos GP, Weber JS. Recombinant interleukin-6 activates the hypothalamic-pituitary-adrenal axis in human. J Clin Endocrinol Metab. 1993;77:1690–4.
13. Kvetnansky R, Sabban EL, Palkovits M. Catecholaminergic system in stress: structural and molecular genetic approaches. Physiol Rev. 2009;89:535–606.
14. Gilbey MP, Spyer KM. Essential organization of the sympathetic nervous system. Baillieres Clin Endocrinol Metab. 1993;7:259–78.
15. Turnbull AV, Rivier CL. Sprague-Dawley rats obtained from different vendors exhibit distinct adrenocorticotropin responses to inflammatory stimuli. Neuroendocrinology. 1999;70:186–95.
16. Adam TC, Epel ES. Stress, eating and the reward system. Physiol Behav. 2007;91:449–58.
17. Björntorp P. Do stress reactions cause abdominal obesity and comorbidities? Obes Rev. 2001;2:73–86.
18. Rosmond R, Dallman MF, Björntorp P. Stress-related cortisol secretion in men: relationships with abdominal obesity and endocrine metabolic and hemodynamic abnormalities. J Clin Endocrinol Metab. 1998;83:1853–9.
19. Grippo AJ, Johnson AK. Stress, depression and cardiovascular dysregulation: a review of neurobiological mechanisms and the integration of research from preclinical disease models. Stress. 2009;12:1–21.
20. Steptoe A, Kivimäki M. Stress and cardiovascular disease. Nat Rev Cardiol. 2012;9:360–70.
21. Bersell K, Arab S, Haring B, Kühn B. Neuregulin1/ErbB4 signaling induces cardiomyocyte proliferation and repair of heart injury. Cell. 2009;138:257–70.
22. Engel FB, Schebesta M, Duong MT, Lu G, Ren S, Madwed JB, et al. p38 MAP kinase inhibition enables

proliferation of adult mammalian Cardiomyocytes. Genes Dev. 2005;19:1175–87.
23. Kubin T, Pöling J, Kostin S, Gajawada P, Hein S, Rees W, et al. Oncostatin M is a major mediator of cardiomyocyte dedifferentiation and remodeling. Cell Stem Cell. 2011;9:420–32.
24. Taegtmeyer H, Sen S, Vela D. Return to the fetal gene program: a suggested metabolic link to gene expression in the heart. Ann N Y Acad Sci. 2010;1188: 191–8.
25. Hein S, Arnon E, Kostin S, Schönburg M, Elsässer A, Polyakova V, et al. Progression from compensated hypertrophy to failure in the pressure-overloaded human heart: structural deterioration and compensatory mechanisms. Circulation. 2003;107:984–91.
26. Zhang Y, Li TS, Lee ST, Wawrowsky KA, Cheng K, Galang G, et al. Dedifferentiation and proliferation of mammalian cardiomyocytes. PLoS One. 2010;5:e12559.
27. Groenendyk J, Sreenivasaiah PK, Kim DH, Agellon LB, Michalak M. Biology of endoplasmic reticulum stress in the heart. Circ Res. 2010;107:1185–97.
28. Mann N, Rosenzweig A. Can exercise teach us how to treat heart disease? Circulation. 2012;126:2625–35.
29. Hou J, Kang YJ. Regression of pathological cardiac hypertrophy: signaling pathways and therapeutic targets. Pharmacol Ther. 2012;135:337–54.
30. Kostin S, Hein S, Arnon E, Scholtz D, Schaper J. The cytoskeleton and related proteins in the human failing heart. Heart Fail Rev. 2000;5:271–80.
31. Pöling J, Gajawada P, Lörchner H, Polyakova V, Szibor M, Böttger T, et al. Tha Janus face of OSM-mediated cardiomyocyte dedifferentiation during cardiac repair and disease. Cell Cycle. 2012;11:439–45.
32. Verdejo HE, del Campo A, Troncoso R, Gutierrez T, Toro B, Quiroga C, et al. Mitochondria, myocardial remodeling, and cardiovascular disease. Curr Hypertens Rep. 2012;14:532–9.
33. Seino Y, Ikeda U, Takahashi M, Hojo Y, Irokawa M, Kasahara T, et al. Expression of monocyte chemoattractant protein-1 in vascular tissue. Cytokine. 1995;7:575–9.
34. Apostolakis S, Lip GY, Shantsila E. Monocytes in heart failure: relationship to a deteriorating immune overreaction or a desperate attempt for tissue repair? Cardiovasc Res. 2010;85:649–60.
35. van Amerongen MJ, Harmsen MC, van Rooijen N, Petersen AH, van Luyn MJ. Macrophage depletion impairs wound healing and increases left ventricular remodeling after myocardial injury in mice. Am J Pathol. 2007;170:818–29.
36. Paravicini TM, Touyz RM. NADPH oxidases, reactive oxygen species, and hypertension: clinical implications and therapeutic possibilities. Diabetes Care. 2008;31 Suppl 2:S170–80.
37. Huang PL. Unraveling the links between diabetes, obesity, and cardiovascular disease. Circ Res. 2005;96:1129–31.
38. Beckman JS, Koppenol WH. Nitric oxide, superoxide, and peroxynitrite: the good, the bad, and ugly. Am J Physiol. 1996;271:C1424–37.
39. Jacoby JJ, Kalinowski A, Liu MG, Zhang SS, Gao Q, Chai GX, et al. Cardiomyocyte-restricted knockout of STAT3 results in higher sensitivity to inflammation, cardiac fibrosis, and heart failure with advanced age. Proc Natl Acad Sci U S A. 2003;100:12929–34.
40. Wojtovich AP, Nadtochiy SM, Brookes PS, Nehrke K. Ischemic preconditioning: the role of mitochondria and aging. Exp Gerontol. 2012;47:1–7.
41. Fortuno A, San José G, Moreno MU, Beloqui O, Díez J, Zalba G. Phagocytic NADPH oxidase overactivity underlies oxidative stress in metabolic syndrome. Diabetes. 2006;55:209–15.
42. Khan M, Mohsin S, Avitabile D, Siddiqi S, Nguyen J, Wallach K, et al. β-Adrenergic regulation of cardiac progenitor cell death versus survival and proliferation. Circ Res. 2013;112:476–86.
43. Pantazi E, Zaouali MA, Bejaoui M, Folch-Puy E, Ben Abdennebi H, Roselló-Catafau J. Role of sirtuins in ischemia-reperfusion injury. World J Gastroenterol. 2013;19:7594–602.
44. Motta MC, Divacha N, Lemieux M, Kamel C, Chen D, Gu W, et al. Mammalian SIRT1 represses forkhead transcription factors. Cell. 2004;116:551–63.
45. Hosoda R, Kuno A, Hori YS, Ohtani K, Wakamiya N, Oohiro A, et al. Differential cell-protective function of two resveratrol (trans-3, 5, 4'- trihydroxystilbene) glucosides against oxidative stress. J Pharmacol Exp Ther. 2013;344:124–32.
46. Li YG, Zhu W, Tao JP, Xin P, Liu MY, Li JB, et al. Resveratrol protects cardiomyocytes from oxidative stress through SIRT1 and mitochondrial biogenesis signaling pathways. Biochem Biophys Res Commun. 2013;438:270–6.
47. Glembotski CC. Endoplasmic reticulum stress in the heart. Circ Res. 2007;101:975–84.
48. Kimata Y, Kohno K. Endoplasmic reticulum stress-sensing mechanisms in yeast and mammalian cells. Curr Opin Cell Biol. 2011;23:135–42.
49. Hetz C. The unfolded protein response: controlling cell fate decisions under ER stress and beyond. Nat Rev Mol Cell Biol. 2012;13:89–102.
50. Tabas I, Ron D. Integrating the mechanisms of apoptosis induced by endoplasmic reticulum stress. Nat Cell Biol. 2011;13:184–90.
51. Hogan PG, Lewis RS, Rao A. Molecular basis of calcium signaling in lymphocytes: STIM and ORAI. Annu Rev Immunol. 2010;28:491–533.
52. Luo X, Hojayev B, Jiang N, Wang ZV, Tandan S, et al. STIM1-dependent store-operated Ca^{2+} entry is required for pathological cardiac hypertrophy. J Mol Cell Cardiol. 2012;52:136–47.
53. Hasnain SZ, Lourie R, Das I, Chen AC, McGuckin MA. The interplay between endoplasmic reticulum stress and inflammation. Immunol Cell Biol. 2012;90:260–70.
54. Li Y, Schwabe RF, DeVries-Seimon T, Yao PM, Gerbod-Giannone MC, et al. Free cholesterol-loaded macrophages are an abundant source of tumor necrosis factor-α and interleukin-6: model of NF-κB- and MAP kinase-dependent inflammation in advanced atherosclerosis. J Biol Chem. 2005;280:21763–72.

55. Hansson GK, Libby P. The immune response in atherosclerosis: a double-edged sword. Nat Rev Immunol. 2006;6:508–19.
56. Zhang K, Kaufman RJ. From endoplasmic-reticulum stress to the inflammatory response. Nature. 2008;454:455–62.
57. Kolattukudy PR, Niu J. Inflammation, endoplasmic reticulum stress, autophagy, and the monocyte chemoattractant protein-1/CCR2 pathway. Circ Res. 2012;110:174–89.
58. Niyama H, Kai H, Yamamoto T, Shimada T, Sasaki K, et al. Roles of endogenous monocyte chemoattractant protein-1 in ischemia-induced neovascularization. JAm Coll Cardiol. 2004;44:661–6.
59. Hamada H, Suzuki M, Yuasa S, Mimura N, Shinozuka N, Takada Y, et al. Dilated cardiomyopathy caused by aberrant endoplasmic reticulum quality control in mutant KDEL receptor transgenic mice. Mol Cell Biol. 2004;24:8007–17.
60. Minamino T, Komuro I, Kitakaze M. Endoplasmic reticulum stress as a therapeutic target in cardiovascular disease. Circ Res. 2010;107:1071–82.
61. Walker BR. Glucocorticoids and cardiovascular disease. Eur J Endocrinol. 2007;157:545–59.
62. Bamberger CM, Schulte HM, Chrousos GP. Molecular determinants of glucocorticoid receptor function and tissue sensitivity to glucocorticoids. Endocr Rev. 1996;17:245–61.
63. Dostert A, Heinzel T. Negative glucocorticoid receptor response elements and their role in glucocorticoid action. Curr Pharm Des. 2004;10:2807–16.
64. Degawa-Yamauchi M, Moss KA, Bovenkerk JE, Shankar SS, Morrison CL, Lelliott CJ, et al. Regulation of adiponectin expression in human adipocytes: effects of adiposity, glucocorticoids, and tumour necrosis factor alpha. Obes Res. 2005;13:662–9.
65. Ht L, Long CS, Gray MO, Rokosh DG, Honbo NY, Karliner JS. Cross talk between angiotensin AT1 and alpha 1-adrenergic receptors: angiotensin II downregulates alpha 1a-adrenergic receptor subtype mRNA and density in neonatal rat cardiac myocytes. Circ Res. 1997;81:396–403.
66. Karalis K, Sano H, Redwine J, Listwak S, Wilder RL, Chrousos GP. Autocrine or paracrine inflammatory actions of corticotropin-releasing hormone in vivo. Science. 1991;254:421–3.
67. Chrousos GP. The hypothalamic-pituitary-adrenal axis and immune-mediated inflammation. N Engl J Med. 1995;332:1351–62.
68. Karalis KP, Kontopoulos E, Muglia LJ, Majzoub JA. Corticotropin-releasing hormone deficiency unmasks the proinflammatory effect of epinephrine. Proc Natl Acad Sci U S A. 1999;96:7093–7.
69. Venihaki M, Dikkes P, Carrigan A, Karalis KP. Corticotropin-releasing hormone regulates IL-6 expression during inflammation. J Clin Invest. 2001;108:1159–66.
70. Benou C, Wang Y, Imitola J, VanVlerken L, Chandras C, Karalis KP, et al. Corticotropin-releasing hormone contributes to the peripheral inflammatory response in experimental autoimmune encephalomyelitis. J Immunol. 2005;174:5407–13.
71. Arbiser JL, Karalis K, Viswanathan A, Koike C, Anand-Apte B, Flynn E, et al. Corticotropin-releasing hormone stimulates angiogenesis and epithelial tumor growth in the skin. J Invest Dermatol. 1999;113:838–42.
72. Im E, Rhee SH, Park YS, Fiocchi C, Taché Y, Pothoulakis C. Corticotropin-releasing hormone family of peptides regulates intestinal angiogenesis. Gastroenterology. 2010;138:2457–67.
73. Kimura Y, Takahashi K, Totsune K, Muramatsu Y, Kaneko C, Darnel AD, et al. Expression of urocortin and corticotropin-releasing factor receptor subtypes in the human heart. J Clin Endocrinol Metab. 2002;87:340–6.
74. Baigent SM, Lowry PJ. mRNA expression profiles for corticotrophin-releasing factor (CRF), urocortin, CRF receptors and CRF-binding protein in peripheral rat tissues. J Mol Endocrinol. 2000;25:43–52.
75. Brar BK, Jonassen AK, Egorina EM, Chen A, Negro A, Perrin MH, et al. Urocortin-II and urocortin-III are cardioprotective against ischemia reperfusion injury: an essential endogenous cardioprotective role for corticotropin releasing factor receptor type 2 in the murine heart. Endocrinology. 2004;145:24–35.
76. Huang M, Kempuraj D, Papadopoulou N, Kourelis T, Donelan J, Manola A, et al. Urocortin induces interleukin-6 release from rat Cardiomyocytes through p38 MAP kinase, ERK and NF-kappaB activation. J Mol Endocrinol. 2009;42:397–405.
77. Chaniotou Z, Giannogonas P, Theocharis S, Teli T, Gay J, Savidge T, et al. Corticotropin-releasing factor regulates TLR4 expression in the colon and protects mice from colitis. Gastroenterology. 2010;139:2083–92.
78. Townsend PA, Davidson SM, Clarke SJ, Khaliulin I, Carroll SJ, Scarabelli TM, et al. Urocortin prevents mitochondrial permeability transition in response to reperfusion injury indirectly by reducing oxidative stress. Am J Physiol Heart Circ Physiol. 2007;293:H928–38.
79. Baines CP. The mitochondrial permeability transition pore as a target of cardioprotective signaling. Am J Physiol Heart Circ Physiol. 2007;293:H903–4.
80. Lawrence KM, Chanalaris A, Scarabelli T, Hubank M, Pasini E, Townsend PA, et al. K(ATP) channel gene expression is induced by urocortin and mediates its cardioprotective effect. Circulation. 2002;106:1556–62.
81. Lawrence KM, Scarabelli TM, Turtle L, Chanalaris A, Townsend PA, Carroll CJ, et al. Urocortin protects cardiac myocytes from ischemia/reperfusion injury by attenuating calcium-insensitive phospholipase A2 gene expression. FASEB J. 2003;17:2313–5.
82. Lawrence KM, Townsend PA, Davidson SM, Carroll CJ, Eaton S, Hubank M, et al. The cardioprotective effect of urocortin during ischaemia/reperfusion involves the prevention of mitochondrial damage. Biochem Biophys Res Commun. 2004;321:479–86.

83. Lawrence KM, Kabir AM, Bellahcene M, Davidson S, Cao XB, McCormick J, et al. Cardioprotection mediated by urocortin is dependent on PKCepsilon activation. FASEB J. 2005;19:831–3.
84. Downey JM, Davis AM, Cohen MV. Signaling pathways in ischemic preconditioning. Heart Fail Rev. 2007;12:181–8.
85. Schulman D, Latchman DS, Yellon DM. Urocortin protects the heart from reperfusion injury via upregulation of p42/p44 MAPK signaling pathway. Am J Physiol Heart Circ Physiol. 2002;283:H1481–8.
86. Latchman DS. Urocortin protects against ischemic injury via a MPK-dependent pathway. Trends Cardiovasc Med. 2001;11:167–9.
87. Brar BK, Stephanou A, Knight R, Latchman DS. Activation of protein kinase B/ Akt by urocortin is essential for its ability to protect cardiac cells against hypoxia/ reoxygenation-induced cell death. J Mol Cell Cardiol. 2002;34:483–92.
88. Cardone MH, Roy N, Stennicke HR, Salvesen GS, Franke TF, Stanbridge E, et al. Regulation of cell death protease caspase-9 by phosphorylation. Science. 1998;282:1318–21.
89. Terada K, Kaziro Y, Satoh T. Analysis of Ras-dependent signals that prevent caspase-3 activation and apoptosis induced by cytokine deprivation in hematopoietic cells. Biochem Biophys Res Commun. 2000;267:449–55.
90. Chanalaris A, Lawrence KM, Townsend PA, Davidson S, Jamshidi Y, Stephanou A, et al. Hypertrophic effects of urocortin homologous peptides are mediated via activation of the Akt pathway. Biochem Biophys Res Commun. 2005;328:442–8.
91. Railson JE, Liao Z, Brar BK, Buddle JC, Pennica D, Stephanou A, et al. Cardiotrophin-1 and urocortin cause protection by the same pathway and hypertrophy via distinct pathways in cardiac myocytes. Cytokine. 2002;17:243–53.
92. Brar BK, Railson J, Stephanou A, Knight RA, Latchman DS. Urocotin increases the expression of heat shock protein 90 in rat cardiac myocytes in a MEK1/2-dependent manner. J Endocrinol. 2002;172:283–93.
93. Janjua S, Lawrence KM, Ng LL, Latchman DS. The cardioprotective agent urocortin induces expression of CT-1. Cardiovasc Toxicol. 2003;3:255–62.
94. Tzanavari T, Varela A, Theocharis S, Pantos C, Cokkinos D, Karalis K. CRH regulates cardiac function in normal and inflammatory states. In: Abstract of XXII Journées Européennes de la Societé Française de Cardiologie, Paris, 12–14 Jan 2012.

The Mechanisms and Modalities of Cell Death

15

Dennis V. Cokkinos

Abstract

Cell death is involved in many aspects of cardiovascular disease. Its main representatives are Apoptosis, which is characterized by nucleus condensation, Necrosis, characterized by cytosolic membrane rupture, which induces inflammation and innate immunity activation, and Autophagy which is an energy and membrane-sparing and mitochondrial preservation process. These three modalities are interconnected with significant cross-talk among them, especially between Necrosis and Apoptosis, acting on the Mitochondrial Permeability Transition Pore. They are involved in acute myocardial infarction with the resultant ischemia/reperfusion injury, chronic heart failure, especially post-infarct, pressure and volume cardiac overload and antineoplastic therapy. The diagnostic elements of Cardiac death modalities are briefly described and the continuous advance in therapeutic approaches is underlined.

Abbreviations

AMI	Acute myocardial infarction
APO	Apoptosis
AUTO	Autophagy
CD	Cell death
CHF	Heart Failure
DR	Death Receptor
ER	Endoplasmic reticulum
HF	Heart Failure
HMG	High Mobility Group
HSP	Heat Shock Protein
I/R	Ischemia/Reperfusion
LMP	Lysosome membrane permeabilization
MCU	Mitochondrial calcium uniporter
MI	Myocardial Infarction
MITO	Mitochondria
MPTP	Myocardial Permeability Transition P…
N	Necrosis
PARP	Poly-ADP ribose polymerase
REM	Myocardial Remodeling
TLRs	Toll like receptors
UPS	Ubiquitin Proteasome System

15.1 Introduction

Cell death (CD) is a main player in cardiovascular disease. In the myocardium its various forms lead to cardiomyocyte loss, which, especially when

D.V. Cokkinos MD, FESC
Heart and Vessel Department, Biomedical Research Foundation Academy of Athens, Athens, Greece
e-mail: dcokkinos@bioacademy.gr

D.V. Cokkinos (ed.), *Introduction to Translational Cardiovascular Research*,
DOI 10.1007/978-3-319-08798-6_15,

replaced by fibrotic tissue leads to cardiac remodeling (REM), chronic heart failure (CHF), and death. It is beyond the scope of this article to stress the increasing incidence of CHF. However, it must also be realized that during organ and specifically cardiac development many cells and cellular formations disappear or are transformed through various processes. This review cannot in any way be all-inclusive. The outline of the main operative mechanisms will be given, always with a view towards their clinical and translational aspects.

Galluzzi et al. [1] very elegantly describe that in human health and disease conditions, CD plays a very prominent role; thus myocardial infarction, (MI) stroke, inflammation, atherosclerosis, immunologic factors, AIDS, are involved in the cardiovascular field. In the chapter of oncology, interplay is vastly more complex.

Before trying to describe the various modalities, the difficulty in their definition should be underlined. The Nomenclature Committee on Cell Death in 2005 and more detailed report in 2009 [2], in order to circumvent these difficulties, which any reader who is not an expert in this field will duly appreciate, actually decided to use purely morphological criteria (Table 15.1), although as Galluzzi et al. [1] point out CD can also be classified apart from morphologic appearance according to: enzymological criteria, functional aspects, as programmed or accidental, physiological, pathological or immunological characteristics. The Nomenclature Committee itself [2] expresses the wish that morphological aspects should be replaced by biochemical and functional criteria.

The term CD includes three modalities leading to this result. Some atypical forms will be described at the end of this chapter.

15.2 Apoptosis

Here it must be reminded, as Whelan et al. [3] and other authors point out, that apoptotic programmed CD in the nematode Caenorhabditis elegans has been conserved over 600 million years during the development of this organism.

Moreover, since it involves the Mitochondria (MITO) it gives a significant insight into the function of these important organelles, as will be further described.

Its name derives from the Greek, meaning falling (ptosis)-off (apo). While necrosis (N) is characterized by cell swelling due to plasma membrane rupture, this membrane in Apoptosis (APO) remains intact (not to be confused with the rupture of the outer mitochondrial membrane) while the cell shrinks, together with the nucleus. Morphologic characteristics of the nucleus in APO are chromatin condensation, and nuclear fragmentation. In a further stage, the nucleus break-up is also called karyorrhexis (rhexis = rupture).

The cells emit processes or pseudopodia (budding) which contain pyknotic nuclear fragments, as described 20 years ago by Majno and Joris [4] who mention that the first microscopic picture of APO probably appeared in 1886. These "buds" are phagocytosed by local resident cells, usually without causing an inflammatory response.

Kroemer et al. [2] as well as Kostin [5] describe plasma membrane "blebs" as typical of APO

Apoptotic bodies contain fragments of both cytoplasm and nucleus.

Whelan et al. [3] and Crow et al. [6] from the group of Richard Kitsis describe the two pathways which mediate cell death in APO and which are intimately entwined:

(a) Extrinsic pathway or death receptor (DR) pathway [7]. This is effected by the binding of death ligands, Fas and TNF-α being prime examples. Fas binds to the cell surface receptors, binding to the adaptor protein FADD (Fas- associated via death domain). FADD recruits procaspases-8 and-10 through the DISC (multiprotein death inducing complex) which activates procaspase-3 and Bid, (BH3 – interacting domain death agonist) which activates pro-to caspase-3.

    Kostin [5] has also given a concise description of the two pathways. The death receptor activation is effected-apart from Fas, and TNFα by AT II and β1 adrenergic receptors, which are further discussed in Chap. 5.

(b) The intrinsic pathway or canonical or mitochondrial pathway. It also involves the endoplasmic reticulum (ER). This combines extra-cellular and intra-cellular stresses of

Table 15.1 Cell death methodology

Definition	Notes	Methods of detection [3–5]
Molecular or morphological criteria lo define dead cells		
Loss of plasma membrane integrity	Plasma membrane has broken down, resulting in the loss of cell's identity	(IF) Microscopy and/or FACS to assess the exclusion of vital dyes, *in vitro*
Cell fragmentation	The cell (including its nucleus) has undergone complete fragmentation into discrete bodies (usually referred to as apoptotic bodies)	(IF) microscopy FACS quantification of hypodiploid events (sub-G_1 peak)
Engulfment by adjacent cells	The corpse or its fragments have been phagocytosed by neighboring cells	(IF) microscopy FACS colocalization studies
Proposed points-of-no return to define dying cells		
Massive activation of caspases	Caspases execute the classic apoptotic program, yet in several instances, caspase- independent death occurs. Moreover, caspases are involved in non-lethal processes including differentiation and activation of cells	Immunoblotting FACS quantification by means of fluorogenic substrates or specific antibodies
$\Delta\Psi_m$ dissipation	Protracted $\Delta\Psi_m$ loss usually precedes MMP and cell death; however, transient dissipation is not always a lethal event	FACS quantification with $\Delta\Psi_m$, -sensitive probes Calcein-cobalt technique
MMP	Complete MMP results in the liberation of lethal catabolic enzymes or activators of such enzymes. Nonetheless, partial permeabilization may not necessarily lead to cell death	IF colocalization studies Immunoblotting after subcellular fractionation
PS exposure	PS exposure on the outer leaflet of the plasma membrane often is an early event of apoptosis, but may be reversible. PS exposure occurs also in T-cell activation, without cell death	FACS quantification of Annexin V binding
Operative definition of cell death, in particular in cancer research		
Loss of clonogenic survival	This method does not distinguish cell death from long-lasting or irreversible cell cycle arrest	Clonogenic assays

From Kroemer et al. [2] by permission from Nature Publishing Group
Abbreviations: *$\Delta\Psi_m$* mitochondrial transmembrane permeabilization, *FACS* fluorescence-activated cell sorter, *IF* immunofluorescence, *MMP* mitochondrial membrane permeabilization, *PS* phosphatidylserine

any type; however in the former, deficiency of nutrients, radiation, drugs and physical stress predominate, while in the latter the main factors are oxidative stress, DNA damage and protein misfolding. Both types of signals are transmitted to the MITO by the BH3 only proteins which will be further described. These stimulate the release of cytochrome-c and other apoptogens as described by Baines [7].

Apoptotic stimuli are ultimately mediated through the proapoptotic Bcl-2 protein family. This family is differentiated as follows:

1. The antiapoptotic members, of which Bcl-2 (B cell Leukemia/lymphoma 2) and Bcl-XL (long isoform) are the representatives.
2. The proapoptotic members, which include many proteins:Main players are (Bax (Bcl-2 associated X protein), Bak (Bcl-2- homologous antagonist killer and BH3-only (Bcl-2 homology domain 3-only) proapoptotic proteins: Bid (BH3 interacting domain death agonist), Bad (Bcl-2-antagonist of cell death). Bim (Bcl-2-interacting mediator of cell death). Bmf (Bcl-2 modifying factor), Noxa, Smac/DIABLO which will be discussed further on, Puma (p 53 upregulated modulator of APO), which is essential for DNA damage-induced APO, BNIP3 (Bcl-2 and 19 kDa interacting protein-3). Either Bax or Bak are necessary for this process; they are translated to the outer mitochondrial membrane (MOM). They stim-

ulate the release of cytochrome c and other apoptogenic mitochondrial proteins into the cytosol. Bax activation may be mediated through calpain; as this protein will also be mentioned as an effector of N, its participation in both processes may represent another link in the crosstalk of the two processes. Bax and Bak, which are located at the ER as well as the MITO increase ER Ca^{+2} stores, while Bcl-2 decreases them. The increased ER Ca^{2+} increases the release of Ca^{2+} in the cytoplasm, causing APO [6].

Cytochrome c and other apoptogens (importantly procaspase-9) are gathered in the apoptosome, activating pro-caspase 9, which activates caspase-3, the main mediator of apoptotic CD. Many other effectors are involved in this process, as described by Whelan et al. [3] and Crow et al. [6].

According to Whelan et al. [3] the main inhibitor of APO in the intrinsic pathway are the Bcl-2 proteins. However, the IAP proteins (inhibitor of APO family) are also important, since they inhibit activated caspase-3 and −7.

Other APO inhibitors are: FLIP (FLICE-like Fas associated death domain protein-like-interleukin-1-converting enzyme like inhibitory protein), and ARC (apoptosis repressor with a CARD).

Apart from their role in APO, several BH3 only members also regulate cell-cycle, DNA repair and metabolism, but are also involved in the crosstalk of APO with the third cell death process to be discussed next, autophagy (AUTO) by liberating Beclin 1 from its binding within the Bcl-2/Bcl-XL complexes.

Crompton [8] underlines the multifaceted actions of the Bcl-2 family proteins, with the Bcl-2/Bax ratio determining resistance to APO. This ratio is very widely used in REM myocardium studies.

The JNKs (superfamily of MAP-kinases) are instrumental in both cell proliferation and APO; the balance can be tilted by many factors.

Dhanasekaran and Reddy [9] point out that JNK signals APO by various mechanisms: It increases expression of TNF-α, Fas and Bak. It also phosphorylates the p53 family of proteins. It is also critical for the release of cytochrome c, and induces cleavage of Bid; it promotes the release of Smac/DIABLO, which antagonizes cytosolic IAPs, from the inter-membrane space to the cytosol, stimulating caspase activation.

The mitochondria production of APO is to a large extent mediated by the MITO. A description of their structure and function is considered helpful.

They are located into the intermyofibrillar spaces, underneath the sarcolemma. Their location permits more efficient ATP supply to the myofibrils.

The MITO drive two different CD mechanisms (APO and N) through the mitochondrial permeability transition pore (MPTP). They are surrounded by two membranes [7, 8, 10], with a narrow intermembrane space between them.

15.2.1 The Outer Membrane (MOM or OMM)

It has many pores based on protein, which allow passage of ions and molecules. It drives APO.

This is the action site of the already mentioned pro-death members of the Bcl-2 family. Under the response to noxious stimuli, Bax which normally resides in the cytosol, is translocated to MOM and the endoplasmic reticulum (ER).

Thus it causes MOM permeabilization and the release of pro-apoptotic proteins from the inter-membrane space into the cytosol, such as cytochromes, Smac/DIABLO and endonuclease-G (endo G). Cytochrome c binds to the cytosolic protein apaf 1 and thus causes the formation of the "apoptosome" which activates the caspase-9 and −3 system [7].

15.2.2 The Inner Membrane (MIM or IMM)

This has more restricted permeability, much like the cell plasma membrane. It is involved in electron transport and ATP synthesis, and is spanned by the Mitochondrial Permeability Transition Pore (MPTP) which drives N.

This pore is inhibited by low pH <7:0 thus it is closed during ischemia, which corresponds clinically to persistent artery occlusion. When reperfusion occurs, there is restitution of pH and acceleration of cytosolic Ca^{2+} increase (which is slow during ischemia). The cell deals with this explosive Ca^{2+} increase by taking it up into the mitochondria via the MITO Ca^{2+} uniporter a protein that uses the negative $\Delta\Psi m$ to drive Ca^{2+} into the matrix [12].

There exist many MPTP activators, such as Ca^{2+}, ROS, Pi inorganic phosphate which uses after adenine nucleotides are depleted after the onset of ischemia and a reduction of the ATP/ADP ratio. From the pharmacological agents cyclosporine-A is a typical inhibitor; its beneficial effects on I/R injury [8] will be discussed later.

The MPTP is very well described by Baines [7], Crompton [8], Lemasters et al. [10], and Weiss et al. [11]: They state that the MITO use electron transport to develop an electrochemical gradient across the MIM (membrane space and matrix). This is formed by the MIM membrane potential ($\Delta\Psi m$ or ΔCm according to Weiss et al. [11] ≈ -200 mV), and a proton gradient (ΔpH). The electrochemical gradient is employed by ATP synthase to phosphorylate ADP to ATP. When MPTP opens, $\Delta\Psi m$ depolarizes, and the synthase actually starts consuming ATP in a (futile) attempt the restore the proton gradient; solutes up to 15 kDa pass the MIM, and cause MITO swelling. As MITO swell, the MIM stretches, but actually it is the MOM which ruptures: The surface of MIM is enhanced by the cristae, parallel invaginating membrane structures. The MOM rupture effects the release of pro-apoptotic proteins from the inter-membrane space, notably cytochrome c, Smac/DIABLO and endonuclease – G (endoG). Cytochrome c binds to the cytosolic protein apaf1, creating the "apoptosome" which activates the Caspase-9 and 3 protease system, while EndoG translates to the nucleus, mediating DNA fragmentation, as described by Baines [7], who also points out that the Bcl-2 proteins permeabilize the MOM while ROS and Ca^{2+} the MIM. The role of ROS production is complex. MITO ROS can trigger MPTP opening, with further ROS release creating a cascading process known as ROS-induced ROS release mechanism.

Some further molecular characteristics of the MPTP should be given:

(a) The voltage-dependent anion channel (VDAC) resides in the MOM. This protein facilitates efficient transport of ATP/ADP across MOM; According to Baines [7], this protein, although very abundant, is not an essential component of the MPTP.
(b) The Adenine nucleotide translocase (ANT) family resides in the MIM and facilitates the exchange of ATP and ADP across it. It is considered an essential factor, although recently some doubts have emerged about its central role. Crompton [9] points out that VDAC and ANT can interact strongly in junctional sites between the two membranes. They form a complex which can recruit additional proteins. One of these is Cyclophilin-D (CYPD).

15.2.3 Cyclophilin-D

This protein resides in the MITO matrix. Its activation opens the MPTP, while its inhibition (by cyclosporine-A or sangliferin A) is cardioprotective [12]. Interestingly according to Lemasters et al. [10] CsA prevents both N and APO.

The MITO phosphate carrier (PiC) is a CypD-interacting protein which regulates ATP synthesis. Its overexpression induces APO.

Apart from the MPTP, another death channel has been described, the mitochondrial apoptosis channel, which is regulated by the Bcl-2 protein family [12]: The Mitochondrial calcium uniporter (MCU), through which. normally, Ca^{2+} enter the MITO. As Pan et al. [13] describe, under normal conditions entry of Ca^{2+} in the MITO augments their ATP production to match its demand up to 10–20 fold. However, larger increases can induce CD. Normally, most unstimulated cells maintain Ca^{2+} in the range of 100–200 nM in the cytosol and the MITO through the function of pumps in the plasma membrane and the ER.

The MCU blockade can prevent abnormal increase Ca^{2+} (and Fe^{2+} entry).

Thus it is suggested that MCU is required to cope with increased Ca^{2+} cycling.

During ischemia, the closed state of the MPTP, effected by a decrease in pH, activation of Pi, and a mild increase of Ca^{2+} and ROS results into limited damage. At reperfusion, the opening of the MPTP is characterized by an increase of the pH, the Pi, the Ca^{2+} and an explosive increase of ROS resulting into irreversible damages.

Lemasters et al. [10] recapitulate that the MPTP is involved in both APO and N.

Another question which has been advanced is whether APO can be induced without the all-important caspase-3 activation [3, 12].

Studies in mice and C. elegans provide evidence for caspase independent CD. The apoptosis-inducing factor (AIF) is such a candidate.

Susin et al. [14] have shown that AIF can cause a picture of mitochondrial- effected APO which cannot be prevented by a wide ranging caspase inhibitor. It does not need Apaf 1 or pro-caspase-9 for its action. However, AIF is required for cell death mediated by poly-ADP ribose polymerase (PARP), which is a main component of N, as will be further described. It also interacts with cyclophilin A, and triggers the release of cytochrome c. They suggest that it has a direct effort on isolated nuclei, effecting chromatin condensation and fragmentation which can be caspase-independent. They also postulate that BH3-domain only protein may act independently of Apaf-1 and caspases.

15.2.4 Other Pathways Involved in APO

15.2.4.1 The Tumor Suppressor p53

It exerts its pro-apoptotic action through activation of multiple pro-apoptotic genes, i.e. Bax, Bid, Puma, apaf-1, caspase 6 and Fas.

The endoplasmic (or sarcoplasmic in muscle cells) reticulum pathway ER.

It causes an increase in intracellular Ca^{2+}; its stores are increased by Bax and Bak which-apart from the outer mitochondrial membrane –are also located in the ER, together with the anti-apoptotic Bcl-2 which has an opposing effect.

The HSP-70 which a well known cardioprotective chaperone reduces ER stress. It also reduces the apoptosome formation and AIF activation.

15.3 Necrosis

Necrosis (N) to the non-researcher has been considered the prevalent form of CD. It derives from the Greek νεκρός = corpse, dead person) It is usually considered to be non-programmed, in contrast to the two forms of Programmed Cell Death (PCD), Apoptosis and Autophagy.

However it will be subsequently shown that this distinction is not absolute.

Thus, some authors are bringing back the originally employed term oncosis, which is a predominantly morphologic term [6, 15]. The morphologic differences of the two modalities are well presented by Feuerstein et al. [15] (Fig. 15.1).

The main causes of N are: The impact of a stress or insult beyond the protective capacity of the cell, which causes rupture of the plasma membrane and swelling of the MITO and endoplasmic reticulum (this is why the term oncosis has also been used. It is accompanied by nuclear pyknosis. However, the nuclear chromatin condensation is not as intense as seen in APO (Fig. 15.1).

The increased membrane permeability and rupture has two results: cellular and extracellular.

1. Cellular
   The cell and its organelles swell, as already described.
2. Extracellular
   Necrotic cells release their intracellular content, thus they induce inflammatory reactions, both of adjacent cells but also systemically. This causes activation of innate immunity, as will be further described.

N occurs because ATP cellular supply is exhausted. In what sequence this is associated with membrane rupture is difficult to ascertain, as will be further discussed. The decline in function of the ATP-dependent ion pumps in the membrane lead to the opening of the “death channel”

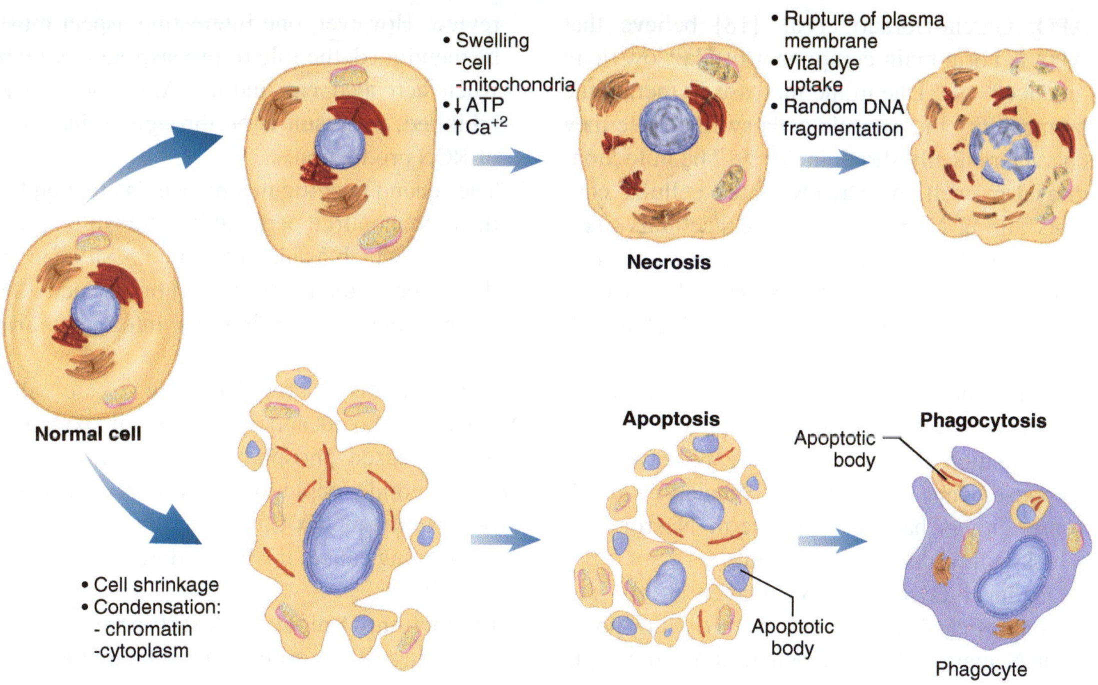

Fig. 15.1 Morphological differentiation of necrosis from apoptosis. This figure illustrates cardinal features of the histological appearances of cell death by either necrosis or apoptosis. The integrity of the plasma membrane and cell swelling are marked in necrosis, whereas cell shrinkage and fragmentation are most common in apoptosis. Most notable is the discrete process of phagocytosis of the "apoptotic bodies" by resident cells eliminating apoptosis, whereas cell eruption and content leakage (events triggering inflammation) are the final outcome of necrosis (Reproduced from Feuerstein et al. [15], copyright 1997 with permission from Elsevier)

which results in colloid osmotic forces and entry of cations inside the membrane,

The "death channel" is selectively permeable to cations and inhibitable by glycine [16].

Hotchkiss et al. [12] very pertinently point out that acute and profound decreases in ATP induce N, while modest yet chronic decreases of ATP induce APO.

Various types of insults have been described: Loss of blood flow is what mostly concerns the cardiologist, but physical trauma, heat, and radiation are also significant factors.

In what instances is N seen in the heart?

In the cardiovascular context, it is mainly caused by the abrupt interruption of blood flow, especially during coronary occlusion in the course of an acute myocardial infarction (AMI). The emergence of APO was widely identified when reperfusion was introduced in the therapy of MI.

Baines [7] reviews work showing that the MPTP is inhibited by low pH, and that it is quiescent during ischemia (occlusion).

However N is also seen as a result of combination of ischemic and reperfusion injury.

Early on it must be stressed that the limits between N and APO are becoming less distinct. Thus, very experienced workers refer to cell death as occurring through "necrosis or apoptosis" in I/R [17].

A main component of cell N is calcium overload during reperfusion [5, 6].

Also, Baines [7] points out that if a stress is severe and/or prolonged ATP (which is required for APO) will be significantly depleted and N will occur.

It is proposed that the hypercontraction caused by I/R in early experiments is a characteristic component of contraction band necrosis [3].

It is postulated that Ca^{2+} overload at higher magnitudes can cause N and at lower

APO. Garcia-Dorado et al. [18] believe that APO is not a main component of Ca^{2+} overload –induced. CD. Due to the increase of membrane permeability the necrotic cells swell (while they characteristically shrink in APO). The mitochondria also swell. As already stated cellular contents during N spill into the extracellular space (and can be detected the periphery-plasma) inducing an inflammatory response [13]. This is mostly ascribed to molecules such as high mobility group protein B1 (HMGB 1).

Zong and Thompson [19] point out that N may enter the fate cycle of a cell and that the inflammation that it elicits may be a warning response. Thus, according to Whelan et al. [3] some authors have used the term Necroptosis, which will be discussed later on.

Galluzzi et al. [1], Whelan et al. [3] and Hotchkiss et al. [12] stress an intriguing point: That N may be less accidental and more regulated than originally thought.

Thus Galluzzi et al. [1] postulate that there exists a stereotyped cascade of events in the various models of N. Another aspect which they refer to is that N can occur during mammalian development, i.e. the death of chondrocytes during bone growth, or in the adult the loss of intestinal epithelial cells.

Luke et al. [20] have described that the intracellular serpin-6 which "regulates" N, exibits a prosurvival function by blocking N, protecting against hypotonic shock, heat shock, oxidative stress, and cation channel hypertrophy, thus casting doubt on its completely accidental nature.

15.3.1 Necrotic Pathways

According to Whelan et al. [3] N can be signaled by two pathways:

1. The first involves death receptors, such as Tumor Necrosis Factor-α receptor 1 (TMFR1). This receptor can promote survival, APO or N. Laster et al. [21] stress the complex nature of the cytotoxic response that it can induce: In the rat fibroblast F17 cell line it induced typical APO while in the L-M line it caused N. Further details are beyond the scope of this review. However, one interesting aspect must be mentioned, the role of procaspase-8, which when activated can induce APO, but when inhibited, the result is N, through an increase of ROS production.
2. The second necrotic mechanism is effected by the mitochondrial permeability transition pore (MPTP) which as already stated is situated in the inner mitochondrial membrane, actually on its inner leaf facing the intermembrane space.

This process is regulated by Cyclophilin D. MPTP can be opened by increases in oxidative stress, increased phosphate concentration, adenine nucleotide depletion, and importantly an increase of the matrix Ca^{2+}.

Its opening causes the break-down of intracellular ATP.

Cyclophilin-D regulates MPTP pore opening and swelling of the mitochondria hallmark of N and cell death.

Cytoplasmic Ca^{2+} through MPTP opening can lead to N, in the worm and in the mammal through the proteases calpains, which are activated by Ca^{2+}, and cathepsins which are released from the lysosomes during stress.

According to Zong and Thompson [19] calpain activation leads to N through cleavage of the Na^+/Ca^{2+} exchanger in the plasma membrane and a sustained secondary intracellular Ca^{2+} overload.

However, according to Whelan et al. [3] calpain can also induce APO through Bax and Bid, and autophagy, through cleavage of Atg 5 (autophagy related 5 homolog) which will be described later. According to the same authors, the lysosomal cathepsins leak out explosively of the lysosomes, digest molecules and lead to N; under less abrupt conditions; partial lysosomal rupture leads to APO. They point out that N, APO and AUTO can be initiated by the lysosomes, whose integrity is preserved by HSP70.

Syntichaki et al. [22] point out that they are the result of perturbation of intercellular Ca^{2+}.

Hotchkiss et al. [12] delineate the following mediators of N: ROS, Ca^{2+}-activated non-lysosomal proteases calpains and cathepsins. These proteases are activated by oxidative stress and Ca^{2+} overload. Prolonged elevation of catecholamines Ang II and other vasoactives hormones may well be involved.

Whelan et al. [3] describe how ischemia-induced hypoxia increases intracellular acidosis, which extrudes H^+ from the cell by Na^+/H^+ exchange leading to an increase of intracellular Na^+, which through the Na^+/Ca^{2+} exchanger leads to an intercellular Ca^{2+} increase, with the cell swelling effects which have already been described.

At reperfusion, Ca^{2+} induced Ca^{2+} release is effected through the ER(SR), or sarcoplasmic reticulum and MPTP opening is induced in some forms of N, such as DNA damage from alkylating agents mainly through ATP depletion. They also describe that HMGβ1, which as already stated is released as an inflammatory elicitor during N, can provide a switch from APO to N.

Opening of the MPTP pore is a major component of necrotic cell death. At R, APO cell death occurs at a lower incidence than N, but for a more extended time: APO occurs as early as 30 min and as late as 3 days after R initiation [23].

According to Whelan et al. [3], Poly-ADP-ribose-polymerase (PARP) is a main player in N occurring through DNA damage from alkylating agents.

15.4 Autophagy

This term derived from the Greek (auto = self and phagy = eat), delineates a process of death triggered by a sub-lethal stress involving nutrient deprivation. This causes the cell to recycle its own non-essential redundant or damaged organelles. Kroemer et al. [2] point out that probably one should define CD not occurring <u>through</u>, but <u>with</u> AUTO. The same authors point out that cells with the characteristics of autophagic CD can still recover when the noxious stimulus is withdrawn.

According to Clarke et al. [24], AUTO occurs regularly during the development of an organism, as in the amphibian tail during metamorphosis.

Three forms have been described: <u>Macroautophagy</u> will be further discussed. <u>Chaperone mediated AUTO</u> refers to a process mediated through chaperone proteins, such as HSC70 and Heart Shock Protein (HSP)70; these bind selectively to the substrate and deliver it to the lysosomes for degradation. <u>In micro-autophagy</u>, the material to be phagocytized is surrounded by invagination of the lysosomal membrane. From this point on, <u>macro-autophagy</u> will be described, in which the material to be phagocytized is sequestered within the characteristic body, the "autophagosome" contained by a double membrane vesicle.

This body can be well seen with electron microscopy. Its formation is governed by autophagy-regulating (atg) proteins, one of which interestingly a hallmark of AUTO-is Beclin-1(atg 6) [25]. Characteristically Beclin-1 is a BH3-only protein already described to be active in APO. Moreover, the anti-apoptotic proteins Bcl-2 and Bcl-XL can also inhibit starvation-induced AUTO.

Thus Bcl-2 plays a dual role: it can be pre-survival in the MITO, by blocking APO, and detrimental in the ER, by inhibiting AUTO.

Additional factors are the phosphatidylinosital-3-kinase (PI-3 K) and the mammalian target of rapamycin (mTOR) which inhibits autophagosome formation.

Whelan et al. [3] point out that under energy availability (fed condition) mTOR inhibits AUTO by phosphorylating and activating Atg proteins.

However, under starvation, reduced PI3K-Akt signaling decreases mTOR activity and activates AUTO.

After inclusion in the autophagosome, its components are lysed by the action of the lysosomes, providing the cell with amino acids, free fatty acids and energy.

Nucleus pyknosis can be seen, but is not so prominent as in APO. Thus, nucleus pyknosis is a characteristic of all three death modalities. Autophagosomes fuse with the lysosomes, the enclosed cytoplasmic material is degraded by acid hydrolysis, and the nutrients are released to the cytosol for recycling

Wang et al. [26] describe the multiple ways in which AUTO participates in metabolic remodeling: It provides amino acids, nucleotides, sugars and lipids. The former enter the tricarboxylic (TCA) acid cycle. Nucleotides can be recycled into new nucleic acids or enter the pentose phosphate pathway (PPP). Sugars can participate into new glucose synthesis and glycolysis, while lipids undergo β-oxidation. Together with energy production, the above processes contribute to new membrane generation biosynthesis. Starvation nutrient deprivation, hypoxia, ROS, damaged organelles and protein aggregates can induce AUTO, in an mTOR dependent process.

According to Dhesi et al. [27], the process of AUTO involves five steps:

1. Formation of the isolation membrane or phagophore.
2. Expansion of the phagophore.
3. Formation of the double membrane.
4. Fusion of the autophagosome with a lysosome to form the autolysosome.
5. Digestion of the content together with the inner membrane layer by the lysosome hydrolases.

However, there is some discussion if these processes can actually cause CD, converting AUTO from a survival to a death process, if it is overexpressed. The increased number of autophagosomes in dying cells might signify that they are associated with CD, but it can well be a sign of failure of the cell to survive despite sacrificing its vital components, according to Hotchkiss et al. [12].

Thus, Dhesi et al. [27] believe that it is a beneficial process under most conditions. They also describe ER-phagy, or reticulo-phagy which selectively targets the ER, which actually forms the dual membranes described.

Gottlieb and Mentzer [28] also point out that it is a beneficial process under most conditions. Notably they enumerate many cardioprotective agents which induce AUTO (diazoxide, ranolazine, rapamycin, statins). They describe an additional term, mitophagy which is a specialized form which causes elimination of the MITO, which have been reported to be contained within the autophagosomes. Thus, they could be protected from "a mitochondrial stampede" causing widespread cell death by the "ROS begetting ROS production" process already described. They further stress that this may be the more important mechanism, since the amount of energy production may not be critical. They further enlarge upon the adaptive versus maladaptive instances, some of which will be further described. They conclude that the bulk of available evidence supports the protective role of AUTO.

Another question has arisen whether AUTO can be an adaptive response in desmin-related cardiomyopathy which is characterized by overexpression of mutated ab crystalin (cry ABR120G). It is being discussed by two investigative groups.

Tannous et al. [29] believe that AUTO increases by twofold in order to cope with the increase of misfolded protein aggregates seen in this disorder. Blunting AUTO dramatically hastened progression to heart failure.

Maloyan et al. [30] remark that mice with this cardiomyopathy show progressive MITO abnormalities and activation of CD through APO. By preventing APO through crossing this mice with transgenic stains with cardiac-specific Bcl-2 overexpression, they found decreased MITO abnormalities, attenuation of APO, reduction of protein aggregation, restitution of cardiac function, prevention of cardiac hypertrophy and a prolongation of survival by 20 %. However, the animals still died prematurely, thus inhibition of APO resulted in AUTO upregulation and increased N according to the authors, as detected by an increase of Evan Blue Dye cells, a technique which detects necrotic CD-related abnormalities. It is not clear from their work if CD is overall reduced or not.

Zhu et al. [31] have a different opinion as regards hemodynamic stress and AUTO: They consider that AUTO increases after transverse aortic constriction representing a maladaptive process. These questions will be further addressed when the three forms of death are assessed in the principal cardiological conditions.

Ferdous et al. [32] provide a very comprehensive review. They differentiate among three forms of AUTO activity: Basal, which is adaptive. This includes homeostatic protein control, ROS detoxification and removal of defective MITO. Maladaptive, which consists of excessive catabolism, MITO elimination, adverse REM, and reduced cell survival, or complete AUTO absence.

These authors point out the role of FoxO (Forehand box-containing protein, O subfamily) in governing AUTO.

Cao et al. [33] describe the role of this protein, which is activated by mechanical unloading and acts through the AUTO-lysosomal and ubiquination-proteasomal pathways to produce cardiac atrophy. Interestingly, it triggers BNIP-3 (Bcl-2 and 19-kDa interacting protein 3) which is also involved in APO.

15.4.1 The Role of the Ubiquitin Proteasome System (UPS)

It is often mentioned, but its actual role has not been adequately defined. Calise and Powell [34] provide a recent inclusive review.

This system, in parallel with the various mechanisms involved in CD has definite roles in cell-cycle control, protein turnover and quality control, cell signaling and APO.

According to the authors, the system is closely involved in myocardial ischemia. Its four components include the proteasome, ubiquitin (UB), the ubiquitination machinery and the deubiquitinases. It is an energy-requiring (ATP) process.

The proteasome can be involved in the removal and clearing of oxidized and damaged proteins. It can also form a hybrid, the "immunoproteasome", since the ubiquitin system is also involved in immune response and antigen presentation.

Ubiquitin (Ub) is involved in protein degradation.

The UPS and specifically the proteasome, becomes dysfunctional in ischemia, both myocardial and cerebral. Its ATP-dependent activity is mainly affected, decreasing proteasome activity. It is also affected by oxidative damage. As in so many aspects of CD, the authors describe that whether a proteasome inhibitor has beneficial or detrimental effects is dose and time dependent. Thus, the inhibitor bortezomib, indicated for multiple myeloma treatment, may demonstrate cardiovascular toxicity.

The UPS becomes dysfunctional during ischemia, while its function is preserved by ischemic preconditioning.

The UPS exerts a parallel function to AUTO, which also prevents proteotoxic stress, but targets mostly macromolecular structures and organelles. Moreover, AUTO is upregulated while the UPS becomes dysfunctional at ischemia. Actually, it is suggested that there is an inverse relationship between UPS and autophagic flux.

15.4.2 Efforts at CD Modality Clarification

It must be pointed out that the efforts to further clarify the various modalities of CD continue.

Thus the nomenclature Committee on Cell Death has issued Recommendations in 2005 and 2009 [2]. They state that it is important to discriminate between dying as a process and death as an end point (Table 15.1).

They also suggest that exact description of various characteristics should replace the mention of the modality itself i.e. TUNEL positive cells % instead of APO %. Similarly they recommend that "double membraned microvesicles" should be described instead of AUTO.

Galluzzi et al. [1] as many other authors have, describe that N is a negative definition i.e. cell death with no signs of APO or AUTO. Moreover they suggest limiting the use of the term oncosis. However, Kostin [5] extensively uses this term.

The Committee authors [2] also describe the term: Mitotic catastrophe which occurs after a dysregulated of failed mitosis and is morphologically accompanied by micro- and multinucleosis.

Also in their Table 15.2 they describe "cornification".

They also comment on the validity of the term "programmed cell death".

Table 15.2 Distinct modalities of cell death

Cell death mode	Morphological features
Apoptosis	Rounding-up of the cell
	Retraction of pseudopodes
	Reduction of cellular and nuclear volume (pyknosis)
	Nuclear fragmentation (karyorrhexis)
	Minor modification of cytoplasmic organelles
	Plasma membrane blebbing
	Engulfment by resident phagocytes, *in vivo*
Autophagy	Lack of chromatin condensation
	Massive vacuolization of the cytoplasm
	Accumulation of (double-membraned) autophagic vacuoles
	Little or no uptake by phagocytic cells, *in vivo*
Cornification	Elimination of cytosolic organelles
	Modifications of plasma membrane
	Accumulation of lipids in F and L granules
	Extrusion of lipids in the extracellular space
	Desquamation (loss of corneocytes) by protease activation
Necrosis	Cytoplasmic swelling (oncosis)
	Rupture of plasma membrane
	Swelling of cytoplasmic organelles
	Moderate chromatin condensation

Adapted from Kroemer et al. [2] by permission by Nature Publishing Group

They point out that "genetic programming" characterizes APO during development and aging. They recommend that the terms developmental, etoposide, osmotic shock-induced cell death etc. should be used.

Moreover, they give a useful suggestion as to when a cell can be considered dead (Table 15.1).

1. When it has lost the integrity of its plasma membrane.
2. When including the nucleolus. it has undergone complete fragmentation into discrete bodies.
3. Its corpse or its fragments has been engulfed by an adjacent cell in vivo.

In their Table 15.2 they give morphologic characteristics of APO, AUTO, and N.

15.4.3 Cross Talk Among Processes

Before finishing this description of the various forms of CD, the common pathways of the cross-talk among the three processes, which has already been referred to, and addressed by most expert groups [1–3, 12] must be further discussed.

Kung et al. [35] described experiments both in C. elegans and mammalian cells.

They stress that the process of N is as old as APO, and that Virchow first described the "unregulated" or 'accidental" form of N. They describe that in APO the main mechanism is permeabilization of the MOM, while in N the opening of the MPTP, which spans the MIM. They also point out that the same death ligands that can activate APO (TNFα, Fas ligand TRAIL-TNF-related APO-inducing ligand) can also stimulate N, and that TNFα can induce survival, APO or N. They also remind how, when caspase-8 is deleted or inhibited, APO cannot be initiated and programmed N emerges through TNFR1 ligation. They also remind that apart from Ca^{2+} overload, Fe^{2+} cystolic increase can lead to TNFα-induced N. They also remind that APO and N are connected at the death receptor and MITO pathways, and that the MOM and MIM are separated by only microns, promoting these cross-talks.

A number of expert researchers has been discussing to what extent N death can be considered to be programmed.

Konstandinidis et al. [36] from the Richard N. Kitsis group also stress that MITO and the ER are central to both APO and N signaling; the Bcl-2 family proteins can be implicated both in APO and N. Also, they stress that the ER can mediate both APO and N, and that the proapoptotic proteins Bax and Bak have been shown to also regulate N.

Proskuryakov et al. [37] underline that various stimuli (cytokines, ischemia, heat irradiation, pathogens) can cause both APO and N. Also, protective mechanisms (Bcl-2/Bcl – XL, HSPs) are equally effective against both forms of CD. Finally, they stress that a main difference between the two forms of CD are the inflammatory response caused by N. This will be discussed further.

The question whether and how much. N can be programmed-thus merging towards APO-is being posed with increasing frequency.

Kung et al. [35] and Konstandinidis et al. [36] point out a significant difference: In APO the central mitochondrial event is permeabilization of the MOM while in N the opening of the MIM and the MPTP which is regulated by Cyclophilin D.

The same authors describe that programmed N can be activated by the same ligands as APO (TNFa, FasL, TRAIL), and that the intrinsic mitochondrial death pathway is the more ancient, conserved in C. elegans.

The same authors stress that regulated-or programmed-N is an important factor of CD in MI or CHF, as will be further discussed.

Linkerman and Green [38] use another term for programmed cell death-Necroptosis-which is dependent on the activity of the Receptor-interacting protein interacting protein 3 (RIP3) which through various processes death binds to the TNF and (FADD). This kinase is necessary for programmed N. In contrast, Necrostatin (Nec)-1 is a small molecule inhibitor of programmed N, which inhibits the kinase activity of the RIP. Kinase 3 (RIPK3).

Necroptosis was initially recognized as a defensive mechanism against viral infection. However, according to the authors it is operative also in I/R injury, myocardial infarction, atherosclerosis among others. It is characterized by the necrosome. It is caspase-independent and can actually be triggered by TNF in the presence of caspase-8 inhibition. It is inhibited by necrostatin 1 which is an inhibitor of RIPK1(receptor increasing protein kinase 1) which after a series of interactions) promotes CD. The authors point out that necroptosis and APO may occur in the same organ.

Finally, it should be realized that N death is predominant in the ubiquitous cardiovascular involvement of atherosclerosis, but APO also contributes.

The great majority of dying cells in human atherosclerotic plaques undergo N. Oxidative stress, depletion of ATP and increased Ca^{2+} together with decreased clearance of APO cells promotes this process, which in turn, through the release of various substances, further promotes inflammation.

15.4.4 The Induction of Inflammation by Various Modalities of Cell Death

Traditionally, as already described, N has been considered as causing inflammation through the rupture of the cell membrane and the spilling of intracellular contents in the intercellular space. APO was traditionally considered as not causing inflammation actually causing "anergy" [12]. Konstantinidis et al. [36] characteristically describe that in APO, when phagocytosis by macrophages or occasionally neighboring cells is efficient, inflammation is avoided.

The inflammatory response after I/R is well known. Again, this process is not solely noxious, because it contributes to healing, as pointed by Timmers et al. [39].

These authors refer to the endogenous alarm signals produced by I/R as Danger-associated Molecular Patterns. These include HSPs, high-mobility group box-1, hyaluronic acid and fibronectin fragments.

Here it must be pointed out that the activation of Toll-like receptors (TLRs) can also have a beneficial effect, if not prolonged. Otherwise, it exerts a deleterious action.

However, APO has another effect: it contributes to the production and secretion of microparticles which modulate the innate and acquired immune system.

Kostin [5] remarks that an essential part of APO is timely removal of the dying cell before it causes a secondary inflammation.

Here it must be stressed again that the role of CD is not the same for all pathologic conditions. What is bad for the heart may be good for cancer.

As regards AUTO, it was also long regarded a "clean" process. However, Oka et al. [40] showed that mitochondrial DNA escaping from AUTO leading to TLR-9 mediated inflammatory cardiomyocyte responses.

On the other hand, inflammation itself can trigger APO [41].

Kung et al. [35] further describe "silent" vs "noisy" removal. In the former, phagocytosis is predominant. In "noisy" removal, N factors released (protein and nucleic acid) modify the inflammation response. The high-mobility group protein β1(HMG β1) is such a protein which acts through the well known TLRs and RAGEs (Receptor for advanced Glucation End-products).

Linkermann and Green [38] point out that N triggers inflammation, and innate and adaptive immune responses. They further describe that: Necroptosis, as already described, is a main element of ischemia-reperfusion-injury, and alloimmune injury in organ transplantation. They also note that RIPK3 confers resistance against a viral load. However, absence of these mechanisms prevented various types of inflammatory lesions (intestinal epithelial cells, atherosclerotic lesions through high-fat diets). The authors consider Necroptosis as a second-line defense mechanism against viruses which however can result in maladaptive inflammatory response.

15.4.5 The Role of HSPs

These protective chaperones delay lysosome membrane permeabilization (LMP) and N induced by TNF and oxidative stress. LPM leads to a release of ROS, free cytosolic iron –which is important for TNFα induced N and release of cathepsins which leads to N.

Kroemer et al. [2] give some more additional definitions of atypical CD.

Pyroptosis is an APO type of death seen in macrophages infected with Salmonella typhimurium, Yersinia, P. aeruginosa, and other pathogens, mainly through caspase-1 activation. The macrophages involved exhibit morphological features of APO, but also some traits of N. It is induced by the inflammasome [42], which is described by Boumpas and Papademetraki in Chap. 13 of this book.

Excitotoxicity is a death of neurons through glutamate or related excitatory amino acids. It overlaps with APO and N.

15.5 Cell Death in Various Conditions

Up to now a general description of CD modalities has been given. However, it is obvious that there are many situations which can affect cell survival in different ways. Many authors [3, 36] give a list of these conditions.

15.5.1 Acute Myocardial Infarction (AMI)

In the human this dramatic event has been the subject of intense research regarding its pathophysiology and treatment. Many older observations are no longer pertinent, since currently in the vast majority of cases reperfusion (R) is employed, either by thrombolysis or by primary angioplasty. It is thus very interesting that most descriptions are based on the work of Kajstura et al. [23] which is 18 years old but still widely referred to. They studied AMI post left coronary artery ligation in rats. At that time they studied only APO and N, not AUTO. They found that at 2 h the former was responsible for the death of 2.8 million (M) cells while the latter for the death of only 90.000. APO was still the major component of cardiomyocyte death at 4.5 h, killing 6.6 M myocytes. Myocytes showing both APO and N were prominent only after 6 h. N peaked at 1 day, involving 1.1 M myocytes, remained elevated up to 2 days and decreased sharply at 7 days. However, it must be noted that the researchers did not study the border zone, which is important area between necrotic and remote myocardium.

The most important point concerning this work is that the authors used permanent coronary artery ligation without re-opening it, i.e. without employing reperfusion. Few direct comparisons exist, performed by the same team, between permanent occlusion and occlusion/reperfusion. Gottlieb et al. [17] performed such a study in the rabbit: They compared animals undergoing 30 min of ischemia (I) and 4 h of reperfusion (R) compared to those undergoing 4.5 h of continuous ischemia only. They also studied other groups of animals which will be discussed further on.

Their main findings can be summarized as follows: Seven rabbits underwent I/R. They all showed a typical nucleosome ladder on DNA electrophoresis, in the ischemic LV area but not outside it. In this group 50 % of cells developed CD in the ischemic area at risk, by TTC (triphenyl tetrazolium chloride) staining which mainly signifies N. In the five rabbits undergoing continuous occlusion, no nucleosome cleavage suggestive of APO was detected. This is in agreement with the suggestions of Baines [7] that APO cannot occur with persistent ischemia, during which he suggests that the MPTP is quiescent.

Gotlieb et al. [17] also studied two more subgroups: At 5 min of ischemia only, no CD was detected, nor was APO detected at only 5 min of ischemia and 4 h R. Additionally, the authors subjected three animals to 30 min I only without R. No DNA nucleosomal fragmentation was found. They did not specifically study N in this subgroup.

The authors also postulate that APO may be converted to N by polymorphonuclear attachment to the ischemic area activation. This brings into focus an aspect of the I/R injury discussed by Whelan et al. [3]: They note that both the extrinsic and intrinsic pathways are involved, with the latter playing a more central role, as evidenced by the effects of various manipulations of Bcl-2 and Bax and their inhibitors. In describing N, the authors point at that cyclophilin D, a factor affecting APO is also involved in N through explosive MPTP opening.

One aspect that has not been adequately discussed is the contribution of inflammation in the I/R injury. Yellon and Hausenloy [43] gave a very detailed review. They describe the following potential mediators of reperfusion injury:

The O_2 paradox, part of which is oxidative stress.

Oxidative stress reduces the bioavailability of NO. Here the authors remind the inconclusive results of antioxidant treatment in R injury.

The calcium paradox

At R, the abrupt increase in intracellular Ca^{2+} occurs. It is the result of sarcolemmal membrane damage and ER dysfunction. The explosive Ca^{2+} overload opens MPTP and causes CD.

The pH paradox

Reperfusion normalizes the pH mainly by washing out lactic acid, activating the Na^+-H^+ exchanger and the Na^+-bicarbonate symporter.

Baines [7] has very well described the effects of pH normalization.

The authors also point that a fourth, important component of R injury exists:

15.5.2 Inflammation

The release of chemoattractant attracts neutrophils into the infarct zone. These cells have very important effects: They induce vascular plugging and also release degrading enzymes and ROS.

It has already been described that during N, due to the rupture of the cytoplasmic membrane, cell contents leaking into the intercellular space elicit a systemic reaction Timmers et al. [39] have termed it an innate immunity activation.

Dutta et al. [44] showed that an index MI accelerates atherosclerosis. They ascribe this finding to activation of sympathetic nervous system, signaling expression of Interleukin-6, MMP-9, myeloperoxidase and LY-6c in atherosclerosis plaques after an acute infarct.

Another protective mechanism which sheds light on I/R injury is the active protein Phosphatase-1 Inhibitor-1 which attenuates the ER stress response, which, when induced in the ischemic heart contributes to APO through altered Ca^{2+} homeostasis [45]. Murphy and Steenbergen [46] discuss the relative roles of the CD modalities in I/R. They also stress that this injury can be a mixture of all three, and that the MPTP is a major regulator of both APO and N.

Further evidence suggesting that at I/R both APO and N are induced are given by other authors.

Ong and Gustafsson et al. [47] stress that N, APO, and AUTO all contribute to call death in the reperfused heart. They re-iterate that during ischemia N is the main component, due to long-lasting oxygen deprivation and ATP depletion. At reperfusion (R) both APO and N are rapidly activated.

Park and Lucchesi [48] point out, in accordance with the findings of Gotlieb et al. [17], that N occurs only if R is initiated after 20 min of occlusion. They also stress the activation of the complement cascade, which triggers the already mentioned innate immunity, and the neutrophil/endothelium interaction as a major component of the inflammatory response.

Eltzsching and Eckle [49] gave a translational review.

They also stress the role of the innate immune responses, representing a "sterile inflammation".

They further underline that I/R dues not operate only during the course of an acute MI. The kidney, intestine, and brain undergo similar processes, while cardiac and vascular surgery create similar conditions.

Additionally, multi-organ I/R injury may be seen in trauma, resuscitation after cardiac arrest, sickle cell disease and sleep apnea.

In accordance with this Whelan et al. [3] state that cyclophilin D, a major factor in APO, according to Crompton [9] is also involved in N. They also describe the role of necrostatin-1, which reduces infarct size after I/R through RPI-RIP3 signalling.

Whelan et al. [3] also suggest that during occlusion AMPK is activated inhibiting the AUTO inhibitor mTOR thus AUTO is induced. However at reperfusion Beclin-1 induced AUTO as already suggested by Matsui et al. [50] may be detrimental.

Again, the interplay between AUTO and APO in hypoxia has been described by Azad et al. [51] in cancer cells which underwent cell death hypoxia. This was reduced by AUTO but not with caspase inhibitors. This autophagic death was effected through a mechanism involving BNIP3.

Konstantinidis et al. [36] point out that many paradigms of pharmacologic or genetic manipulations of CD exist in the setting of MI. Thus, lack of Fas and Bax and Bak in mice results into smaller infarcts; the same is seen with Bcl-2 overexpression. The lack of cyclophilin-D has the same effect. The protective role of cyclophilin-D inhibition by cyclosporine A or sanglifehrin A has already been discussed.

15.5.3 Myocardial Remodeling

The development of post-MI CHF is linked to the emergence of myocardial remodeling (REM).

Mani and Kitsis [52] give an excellent editorial comment. They cite 13 animal and human studies which point out the main role played by APO in this aspect.

Sam et al. [53] studying the mouse heart, have very pertinently shown that at 6 months post-MI REM APO can co-exist with increased wall thickness in areas remote from the infarct.

We [54] and others have shown that APO is mainly expressed in the border zone surrounding the infarct, in the experimental animal [55] and in the human [56]. The subject has been studied very extensively.

Slezak et al. [57] postulate that AUTO is a prosurvival mechanism in the hibernating myocardium.

Gotlieb and Mentzer [17] cite numerous studies suggesting that AUTO is protective against post-MI REM

Interestingly, Fallavolita et al. [58] have shown that APO and reduced SERCA-2 underlie the transition from chronically stunned to hibernating myocardium.

Kung et al. [35] and Konstandinidis et al. [36] point out that N probably participates in post-MI heart failure but that further data are needed. The MITO are strongly involved in CHF.

However, although the post-MI is the prime paradigm of REM and CHF in which APO is strongly involved, other causes have been noted. Thus: Pacing induced HF involves APO, i.e. caspase-3, AIF, and the nuclear-localized marker p53 and p21, according to Marin-Garcia et al. [59] who stress that:

In rapid atrial fibrillation induced for 3 weeks in the dog, an increase of APO TUNEL and molecular markers caspases-3 and 8, reduced Bcl-2 is seen at the atria.

APO can be seen in volume overload produced by an A-V shunt in rats, especially the males [60].

Pressure overload can also produce APO, in the spontaneous hypertensive rat and after aortic banding [61].

The antineoplastic drug doxorubicin significantly induces APO, characterized by Caspase-3 activation and Bcl-XL decrease [62].

15.5.4 The Aging Heart

In Fischer 344 hearts, Kajstura et al. [63] in the left ventricular free wall at 24 months found 13,600 myocytes undergoing N but only 874 cells undergoing APO. A combination of both processes involved 14,500 cells. Olivetti et al. [64] in 106 human hearts found that in aging men 64 M cells had been lost in both right (19 M) and left side (45 M). They did not differentiate between N and APO.

In a specific form of CHF, acromegalic cardiomyopathy Frustaci at al [65] found a massive increase in APO (495 fold in the myocytes and 305 fold in the non myocytes). They also found collagen accumulation indicative of previous N. Only the magnitude of cardiomyocyte APO correlated with the degree of myocardial dysfunction.

Myocarditis is an uncommon but significant cause of acute heart failure. Its main manifestation is the presence of necrotic myocytes. In the subacute phase the myocardium is infiltrated by natural killer cells. TNFa and IL-1 B and IL-2 are produced. Cytotoxic T lymphocytes can lyse virus-infected cardiocytes [66].

Brunner et al. [67] have shown APO in virus-induced dilated cardiomyopathy in mice.

It is interesting that a vicious feed-back cycle has been postulated in acute myocarditis, since cardiac myosin, liberated through an initial insult can promote chronic immunity and chronic inflammation through TLRs [68].

As Whelan et al. [3] point out, autophagosomes are increased in this condition; however it cannot be determined whether this is compensatory or deleterious, This has already been discussed in the context of hemodynamic overload states.

Knaapen et al. [69] have found in cardiac tissue of pts with terminal CHF due to both ischemic and dilated cardiomyopathy autophagic cell death by granular cytoplasmic ubiquitin inclusions but no APO or N indications.

Park et al. [70] addressed the question whether cardiomyocytes are the only heart cells involved in cardiac injury.

They point out that, by cell number 75 % of cells in the heart are non-myocytes. In a primate model of chronic heart failure produced first by experimental MI and subsequently rapid pacing for 2–6 months, they found, as expected an increase in APO with the emergence of HF. However, the TUNEL-positive nonmyocytes were eightfold higher than cardiomyocytes in the borderzone and ninefold higher in the remote area.

15.5.5 Therapeutic Implications

This is the translational investigator's dream.

Whelan et al. [3] and Hotchkis et al. [12] dedicate parts in their extensive reviews.

The first group of authors [3] concentrates mostly on acute MI, which according to their postulation requires treatment for a limited period of time. They focus on the promise of small molecule polycaspase inhibitors which reduce infarct size by 21–52 % following I/R.

In the already cited reviews by Whelan et al. [3] the following findings can be underlined: Bcl-2 overexpression, Bax ablation and caspase inhibition reduce I/R injury, through APO reduction.

They also mention that Akt reduces infarct size. However, its adenoviral transduction seems difficult to apply.

On this subject of acute MI excellent reviews have been written: The Working Group of Cellular Biology of the Heart of the European Society of Cardiology states that "there is currently no effective therapy for protecting the heart against the detrimental effects of acute I/R injury [71].

Possibly the drug giving the greatest promise is cyclosporine A, which inhibits N by inhibiting MPTP [72]. This clinical beneficial result is supported by experimental data with cyclosporine A but also by sanglifehrin –A another powerful inhibitor by the MPTP.

Hydrogen sulfide is a drug which in small doses may protect against I/R injury [73].

Necrostatin –1 which decreases N by inhibiting the activity of RIP1 may prove a promising agent [74].

It is interesting that a modality widely employed in the past therapeutic, glucose-insulin-potassium, reduces APO in AMI by soluble Fas and sFas measurements [75].

Further data are given in this book by Wang and Fragogiannis in Chap. 16.

15.5.6 Mechanisms of Conditioning

This very important cytoprotective mechanism, a universal phenomenon, decreases CD through all its three forms (N, APO and AUTO).

A pertinent review is given in this volume by Iliodromitis et al. in Chap. 28 and very recently by Ovize et al. [76].

In the first review, the major signaling pathways underlying cardioprotection are noted. The authors point out that “conditioning” (pre-, peri- and post-) is effected by two endogenous cardioprotective pathways:

RISK: Reperfusion Injury Salvage Kinase

SAFE: Survival Activating Factor Enhancement

The former is exerted through MEK1/2-E881/2 and PI3K-Akt while the latter by the TNFα receptor and STAT3.

Both pathways relay these signals from cell membrane reception to the MITO and MPTP inhibition.

It has been shown by many authors that it decreases N, evidenced by decrease of LDH and CK production and tetrazolium staining [77, 78].

Ischemic preconditioning (IPC) also induces AUTO which exerts a protective role, at I/R [79].

It both increased Beclin-1 AUTO and decreased APO in a rat I/R model [80].

Heat damage of H9c2 cells by temperatures of 40–44 °C at 90–180 min caused N, APO and AUTO, which was diminished by HSP70 induction through mild heat preconditioning [81].

15.5.7 Other Cardioprotective Interventions

Hypothermia has been tried against both myocardial and cerebral ischemia. It was found to ameliorate APO in rat hearts undergoing experimental transplantation [82].

Exercise training can upregulate AUTO [83].

15.5.8 Pharmaceutic Interventions

Minocyclin protects against hypoxia-ischemia-against APO: it inhibits MITO Ca^{2+} uptake [84].

Cardiac damage is produced by antineoplastic treatment. In doxorubicin-induced cardiotoxicity both APO and N are seen [60]. Here it must be repeated that the intrinsic apoptotic pathway activity is downregulated as the heart matures with age.

In a tumor-bearing mouse model, augmentation of AUTO by rapamycin attenuates doxorubicin induced cardiotoxicity [85].

It has already been stated that while N triggers inflammation [4]; inflammation also contributes to death in heart failure. Christia and Frangogiannis [41] have given an excellent account, with therapeutic implications.

Chen et al. [86] have shown that T3 treatment for 3 days in experimental MI in rats decreased border area APO through phosphorylation of Akt.

We have shown the same results but at 2 weeks after AMI in the rat [87].

Ferreyra et al. have shown the same in acute tubular necrosis induced by I/R in the rat [88].

This drug is now being used in a multicenter European trial in post-infarct patients. However, the results are not uniform in all organs. Hyperthyroidism has been found to induce hepatic injury. Kumar et al. have found that it also induces APO in the rat liver [89], while Sinha et al. [90] also showed that thyroid hormone stimulates hepatic lipid catabolism via activation of autophagy.

Another promising drug is Bendavia which is an overall MITO protective agent: It has shown beneficial effect early post-MI in the dog [91].

15.5.9 Chronic Treatment-Prevention of Remodeling

Although most efforts are directed at acute MI, the very important problem of REM characterized by cardiac enlargement and leading to CHF and death should not be underestimated. It is postulated that 30 % of anterior infarcts, despite primary angioplasty and the administration of the four main drugs, ACE inhibitors or Angiotensin Receptor blockers, aldosterone inhibitors and b-blockers. Thus, a large number of drugs has been and is still being tried to prevent or reverse this process. The concept of REM is being described by Swyngedaw in Chap. 17, and Wang and Frangogiannis et al. in Chap. 16 in this book.

Gajarsa and Kloner gave recently a very pertinent review [92].

The authors describe extensively the benefits of β-blocker therapy, clarifying that β1 receptors induce hypertrophy and APO, while β2 receptor stimulation may be antiapoptotic, up to a year in the rat, but only with concominant β1 blockade. They also describe the beneficial anti-angiotensin-II and antialdosterone therapy. Both these substances induce APO and fibrosis.

The authors also describe attempts at MMP inhibition; the PREMIERE study in which a broad MMP inhibitor PG-116800 showed no effect. Before further describing therapeutic attempts against post-MI REM and CHF one must be reminded that in real-life most of these patients already receive anti-adrenergic, anti-angiotensin and anti-aldosterone treatment in their great majority.

Statins, although they possess anti-necrotic anti-flammatory and anti-apoptotic qualities, have proven disappointing in HF trials.

Tousoulis et al. [93] describe the efforts at nitric oxide manipulation, with emphasis on sildenafil, an NO synthase transcription enhancers.

TNFα neutralization would be an obvious target. However, it was not successful in the RENEWAL and ATTACH trials [94, 95].

Another long-used drug, Pentoxifilline, which modulates TNFα mRNA expression, has proven successful in a small trial [96].

Also, Interleukin-1 blockade by Anakinra prevented REM after MI, without evidence of impaired healing [97].

The n-3 polyunsaturated fatty acids (PUFA) have been to anti-apoptotic in many studies;. α-linolenic acid prevents APO in cardiomyopathic hamsters [98].

Kanamori et al. [99] found that Resveratrol reverses REM in rat hearts with large, old myocardial infarctions through enhanced AUTO.

A drug which has been tried in patients with heart failure with preserved ejection fraction is relaxin. This agent decreases APO in the swine acute MI model while also decreasing N, and inflammation, and improving the cardiac index [100].

Valproic acid, a drug widely used in psychiatric treatment, has been shown to ameliorate post-MI REM in the rat, by HDAC inhibition [101].

MAO inhibitors have a strong MITO protective action and have been shown to exert anti-REM activity in pressure overload [102].

We have shown favorable results with Rasagiline at 4 weeks post-MI in the rat.

Very recently Unsöld et al. [103] have shown that melusin, a chaperone protein improves post-MI remodeling.

Some other drugs to be considered are Ranolazine which is emerging as an anti-ischemic drug. Erythropoetin has been very successful in the animal but has disappointed in the human.

This brings into focus the great variety of therapies available for therapy of post-MI REM. The review by Dorn [104] emphasizes that in ventricular REM all three modalities of CD are involved.

Here it must be reminded that in the post-MI heart three distinct zones have been delineated: The infarct, the border, and the remote zone. Each has distinct characteristics.

Thus the difficulty of managing post-MI REM can be readily appreciated.

15.6 Imaging of Cell Death

After enumerating these 3 CD modalities and the complexity of their interactions and their cross-talk and the interventions pertaining to their prevention or reversal it should be stressed that their detection is equally complex. As Kroemer et al. in their review [2] point out, their detection is based on many methods as shown in their Table 15.3, reproduced here (Table 15.3).

Table 15.3 Biochemical aspects of distinct modalities of cellular catabolism

Cell death mode	Biochemical features	Methods for detection [3–5]
Apoptosis	Activation of proapoptotic Bcl-2 family proteins (e.g. Bax, Bak, Bid)	IF microscopy localization studies
		Immunoblotting with conformation-specific antibodies
	Activation of caspases	Colorimetric/fluorogenic substrate-based assays in live cells
		Colorimetric/fluorogenic substrate-based assays of lysates in microtiter plates
		FACS/IF microscopy quantification with antibodies specifically recognizing the active form of caspases
		FACS/IF microscopy quantification with antibodies specific for cleaved caspase substrates
		FACS/IF microscopy quantification with fluorogenic substrates
		Immunoblotting assessment of caspase-activation state
		Immunoblotting assessment of the cleavage of caspase products
	$\Delta\Psi_m$ dissipation	Calcein-cobalt technique (FACS/IF microscopy)
		FACS/IF microscopy quantification with $\Delta\Psi_m$-sensitive probes
		Oxygen-consumption studies (polarography)
	MMP	Colorimetric techniques to assess the accessibility of exogenous substrates to IM-embedded enzymatic activities
		FACS-assisted detection of IMS proteins upon plasma membrane permeabilization
		FACS-assisted detection of physical parameters of purified mitochondria
		HPLC-assisted quantification of mitochondrial alterations in purified mitochondria
		IF microscopy colocalization studies of IMS proteins (e.g. Cyt *c*) with sessile mitochondrial proteins (e.g., VDACI)
		IF (video) microscopy with Cyt *c*-GFP fusion protein
		Immunoblotting detection of IMS proteins (e.g. Cyt *c*) upon cellular fractionation
	Oligonucleosomal DNA fragmentation	DNA ladders
		FACS quantification of hypodiploid cells (sub-G_1, peak)
		TUNEL assays
	Plasma membrane rupture	Colorimetric/fluorogenic substrate-based assays of culture supernatants in microtiter plates to determine the release of cytosolic enzymatic activities (e.g. LDM)
		FACS quantification with vital dyes
	PS exposure	FACS quantification of Annexin V binding
	ROS overgeneration	FACS/IF microscopy quantification with ROS-sensitive probes
	ssDNA accumulation	FACS quantification with ssDNA-specific antibodies
Autophagy	Beclin-1 dissociation from Bcl-2/X_L	Co-immunoprecipitation studies
	Dependency on *atg* gene products	Genetic studies (e g., knockout models, RNA interference, plasmid-driven overexpression systems)
	LC3-I to LC3-II conversion	IF microscopy with GFP-LC3 fusion protein
		Immunoblotting with LC3-specific antibodies
	$p62^{Lck}$ degradation	Immunoblotting with p62-specific antibodies
Cornification	Expression of TGs	Immunoblotting with antibodies specific for TG type 1, 3 and 5 qRT-PCR
	Expression of TG substrates	Immunoblotting with antibodies specific for TG substrates (e.g. loricrin, SPR, involucrin, keratins) qRT-PCR
	Crosslinking activity	HPLC detection of K-L isodipeptide bonds
		Monodansyl-cadaverine incorporation to detect TG activity in tissues
		Radiolabeled putrescine incorporation to detect TG activity in cell extracts

Table 15.3 (continued)

Cell death mode	Biochemical features	Methods for detection [3–5]
Necrosis	Activation of calpains	Colorimetric/fluorogenic substrate-based assays of cell lysates in microtiter plates
	Activation of cathepsins	Colorimetric/fluorogenic substrate-based assays in live cells
		Colorimetric/fluorogenic substrate-based assays of cell lysates in microtiter plates
	Drop of ATP levels	Luminometric assessments of ATP/ADP ratio
	HMGB-1 release	Immunoblotting of culture medium with HMGB-1-specific antibodies
	LMP	FACS quantification with lysomorphotropic probes
	Plasma membrane rupture	Colorimetric/fluorogenic substrate-based assays of culture supernatants in microtiter plates to determine the release of cytosolic enzymatic activities (e.g., LDH)
		FACS quantification with vital dyes
	RIP1 phosphorylation	Immunoblotting with phosphoneoepitope-specific antibodies
	RIP1 ubiquitination	Immunoprecipitation with anti-RIP1 antibodies followed by immunoblotting with anti-ubiquitin antibodies
	ROS overgeneration	FACS quantification with ROS-sensitive probes
	Specific PARP1 cleavage pattern	Immunoblotting with PARP1-specific antibodies

From Kroemer et al. [2] by permission from Nature Publishing Group

Abbreviations: $\Delta\Psi_m$ mitochondrial transmembrane permeabilization, *Cyt c* cytochrome c, *FACS* fluorescence-activated cell sorter, *GFP* green fluorescent protein, *HPLC* high-pressure liquid chromatography, *IF* immunofluorescence, *IM* mitochondrial inner membrane, *IMS* mitochondrial intermembrane space, *LDH* lactate dehydrogenase, *LMP* lysosomal membrane permeabilization, *MMP* mitochondrial membrane permeabilization, *PS* phosphatidylserine, *qRT-PCR* real-time quantitative reverse transcription PCR, *ROS* reactive oxygen species, *RNAi* RNA interference, *TG* transglutaminase, *TUNEL* terminal deoxynucleotidyl transferase-mediated dUTP nick-end labeling, *VDACI* voltage-dependent anion channel I

The author being primarily a clinical cardiologist wishes to stress the importance of imaging for detecting many of the aspects involved in CD, such as APO and inflammation.

Cell death imaging can include many modalities which are extensively described in Chaps. 22 and 23 of this book.

Finally, the huge and continuously expanding aspect of peripheral biomarkers is beyond the scope of this chapter.

Conclusion

It is obvious that supplemental technologies incrementally used in CD prevention and reversal are expected to be incrementally important for the human. However, the continued importance of basic research findings is obvious.

Acknowledgments The author wishes to thank Dr. Klitos Konstandinidis for carefully reviewing this chapter and Professor Richard N. Kitsis for his suggestions.

References

1. Galluzzi L, Maiuri MC, Vitale I, Zischka H, Castedo M, Zitvogel L, et al. Cell death modalities: classification and pathophysiological implications. Cell Death Differ. 2007;14:1237–43.
2. Kroemer G, Galluzzi L, Vandenabeele P, Abrams J, Alnemri ES, Baehrecke EH, et al. Classification of cell death: recommendations of the Nomenclature Committee on Cell Death 2009. Cell Death Differ. 2009;16:3–11.
3. Whelan RS, Kaplinskiy V, Kitsis RN. Cell death in the pathogenesis of heart disease: mechanisms and significance. Annu Rev Physiol. 2010;72:19–44.
4. Majno G, Joris I. Apoptosis, oncosis, and necrosis. An overview of cell death. Am J Pathol. 1995;146:3–15.
5. Kostin S. Pathways of myocyte death: implications for development of clinical laboratory biomarkers. Adv Clin Chem. 2005;40:37–98.
6. Crow MT, Mani K, Nam YJ, Kitsis RN. The mitochondrial death pathway and cardiac myocyte apoptosis. Circ Res. 2004;95:957–70.
7. Baines CP. The mitochondrial permeability transition pore and ischemia-reperfusion injury. Basic Res Cardiol. 2009;104:181–8.

8. Crompton M. Mitochondrial intermembrane junctional complexes and their role in cell death. J Physiol. 2000;529:11–21.
9. Dhanasekaran DN, Reddy EP. JNK signaling in apoptosis. Oncogene. 2008;27:6245–51.
10. Lemasters JJ, Theruvath TP, Zhong Z, Nieminen AL. Mitochondrial calcium and the permeability transition in cell death. Biochim Biophys Acta. 2009;1787:1395–401.
11. Weiss JN, Korge P, Honda HM, Ping P. Role of the mitochondrial permeability transition in myocardial disease. Circ Res. 2003;93:292–301.
12. Hotchkiss RS, Strasser A, McDunn JE, Swanson PE. Cell death in disease. Mechanisms and emerging therapeutic concepts. N Engl J Med. 2009;361:1570–83.
13. Pan X, Liu J, Nguyen T, Liu C, Sun J, Teng Y, et al. The physiological role of mitochondrial calcium revealed by mice lacking the mitochondrial calcium uniporter. Nat Cell Biol. 2013;15:1464–72. doi:10.1038/incb2868.
14. Susin SA, Lorenzo HK, Zamzami N, Marzo I, Snow BE, Brothers GM, et al. Molecular characterization of mitochondrial apoptosis-inducing factor. Nature. 1999;397:441–6.
15. Feuerstein G, Ruffolo Jr RR, Yue TL. Apoptosis and congestive heart failure. Trends Cardiovasc Med. 1997;7:249–55.
16. Nishimura Y, Lemasters JJ. Glycine blocks opening of a death channel in cultured hepatic sinusoidal endothelial cells during chemical hypoxia. Cell Death Differ. 2001;8:850–8.
17. Gottlieb RA, Burleson KO, Kloner RA, Babior BM, Engler RL. Reperfusion injury induces apoptosis in rabbit cardiomyocytes. J Clin Invest. 1994;94:1621–8.
18. Garcia-Dorado D, Ruiz-Meana M, Inserte J, Rodriguez-Sinovas A, Piper HM. Calcium-mediated cell death during myocardial reperfusion. Cardiovasc Res. 2012;94:168–80.
19. Zong WX, Thompson CB. Necrotic death as a cell fate. Genes Dev. 2006;20:1–15.
20. Luke CJ, Pak SC, Askew YS, Naviglia TL, Askew DJ, Nobar SM, et al. An intracellular serpin regulates necrosis by inhibiting the induction and sequelae of lysosomal injury. Cell. 2007;130:1108–19.
21. Laster SM, Wood JG, Gooding LR. Tumor necrosis factor can induce both apoptic and necrotic forms of cell lysis. J Immunol. 1988;141:2629–34.
22. Syntichaki P, Xu K, Driscoll M, Tavernarakis N. Specific aspartyl and calpain proteases are required for neurodegeneration in C. elegans. Nature. 2002;419:939–44.
23. Kajstura J, Cheng W, Reiss K, Clark WA, Sonnenblick EH, Krajewski S, et al. Apoptotic and necrotic myocyte cell deaths are independent contributing variables of infarct size in rats. Lab Invest. 1996;74:86–107.
24. Clarke PG. Developmental cell death: morphological diversity and multiple mechanisms. Anat Embryol (Berl). 1990;181:195–213.
25. Glick D, Barth S, Macleod KF. Autophagy: cellular and molecular mechanisms. J Pathol. 2010;221:3–12.
26. Wang ZV, Ferdous A, Hill JA. Cardiomyocyte autophagy: metabolic profit and loss. Heart Fail Rev. 2013;18:585–94.
27. Dhesi P, Tehrani F, Fuess T, Schwarz ER. How does the heart (not) die? The role of autophagy in cardiomyocyte homeostasis and cell death. Heart Fail Rev. 2015;15:15–21.
28. Gottlieb RA, Mentzer Jr RM. Autophagy: an affair of the heart. Heart Fail Rev. 2013;18:575–84.
29. Tannous P, Zhu H, Johnstone JL, Shelton JM, Rajasekaran NS, Benjamin IJ, et al. Autophagy is an adaptive response in desmin-related cardiomyopathy. Proc Natl Acad Sci U S A. 2008;105:9745–50.
30. Maloyan A, Sayegh J, Osinska H, Chua BH, Robbins J. Manipulation of death pathways in desmin-related cardiomyopathy. Circ Res. 2010;106:1524–32.
31. Zhu WZ, Wang SQ, Chakir K, Yang D, Zhang T, Brown JH, et al. Linkage of beta1-adrenergic stimulation to apoptotic heart cell death through protein kinase A-independent activation of Ca^{2+}/calmodulin kinase II. J Clin Invest. 2003;111:617–25.
32. Ferdous A, Battiprolu PK, Ni YG, Rothermel BA, Hill JA. FoxO, autophagy, and cardiac remodeling. J Cardiovasc Transl Res. 2010;3:355–64.
33. Cao DJ, Jiang N, Blagg A, Johnstone JL, Gondalia R, Oh M, et al. Mechanical unloading activates FoxO3 to trigger Bnip3-dependent cardiomyocyte atrophy. J Am Heart Assoc. 2013;2(2):e000016. doi:10.1161/JAHA.113.000016.
34. Calise J, Powell SR. The ubiquitin proteasome system and myocardial ischemia. Am J Physiol Heart Circ Physiol. 2013;304:H337–49.
35. Kung G, Konstantinidis K, Kitsis RN. Programmed necrosis, not apoptosis, in the heart. Circ Res. 2011;108:1017–36.
36. Konstantinidis K, Whelan RS, Kitsis RN. Mechanisms of cell death in heart disease. Arterioscler Thromb Vasc Biol. 2012;32:1552–62.
37. Proskuryakov SY, Konoplyannikov AG, Gabai VL. Necrosis: a specific form of programmed cell death? Exp Cell Res. 2003;283:1–16.
38. Linkermann A, Green DR. Necroptosis. N Engl J Med. 2014;370:455–65.
39. Timmers L, Paster Kamp G, de Hoog VC, Arslan F, Appleman Y, de Kleijn DPV. The innate immune response in reperfused myocardium. Cardiovasc Res. 2012;94:276–83.
40. Oka T, Hikoso S, Yamaguchi O, Taneike M, Takeda T, Tamai T, et al. Mitochondrial DNA that escapes from autophagy causes inflammation and heart failure. Nature. 2012;485:251–5. doi:10.1038/nature10992.
41. Christia P, Frangogiannis NG. Targeting inflammatory pathways in myocardial infarction. Eur J Clin Invest. 2013;43:986–95.
42. Cunha LD, Zamboni DS. Subversion of inflammasome activation and pyroptosis by pathogenic bacteria. Front Cell Infect Microbiol. 2013;3:76.

43. Yellon DM, Hausenloy DJ. Myocardial reperfusion injury. N Engl J Med. 2007;357:1121–35.
44. Dutta P, Courties G, Wei Y, Leuschner F, Gorgatov R, Robbins C, et al. Myocardial infarction accelerates atherosclerosis. Nature. 2012;487:325–9.
45. Nicolaou P, Rodriguez P, Ren X, Zhou X, Qian J, Sadayappan S, et al. Inducible expression of active protein phosphatase-1 inhibitor-1 enhances basal cardiac function and protects against ischemia/reperfusion injury. Circ Res. 2009;104:1012–20.
46. Murphy E, Steenbergen C. Mechanisms underlying acute protection from cardiac ischemia-reperfusion injury. Physiol Rev. 2008;88:581–609.
47. Ong SB, Gustafsson AB. New roles for mitochondria in cell death in the reperfused myocardium. Cardiovasc Res. 2012;94:190–6.
48. Park JL, Lucchesi BR. Mechanisms of myocardial reperfusion injury. Ann Thorac Surg. 1999;68:1905–2012.
49. Eltzsching HK, Eckle T. Ischemia and reperfusion from mechanism to translation. Nat Med. 2011;17:1393–401.
50. Matsui Y, Takagi H, Qu X, Abdellatif M, Sakoda H, Asano T, et al. Distinct roles of autophagy in the heart during ischemia and reperfusion: roles of AMP-activated protein kinase and Beclin 1 in mediating autophagy. Circ Res. 2007;100:914–22.
51. Azad MB, Chen Y, Henson ES, Cizeau J, McMillan-Ward E, Israels SJ, et al. Hypoxia induces autophagic cell death in apoptosis-competent cells through a mechanism involving BNIP3. Autophagy. 2008;4:195–204.
52. Mani K, Kitsis RN. Myocyte apoptosis: programming ventricular remodelling. J Am Coll Cardiol. 2003;41:761–4.
53. Sam F, Sawyer DB, Chang DL, Eberli FR, Ngoy S, Jain M, et al. Progressive left ventricular remodeling and apoptosis late after myocardial infarction in mouse heart. Am J Physiol Heart Circ Physiol. 2000;279:H422–8.
54. Pantos C, Mourouzis I, Galanopoulos G, Gavra M, Perimenis P, Spanou D, et al. Thyroid hormone receptor alpha1 downregulation in postischemic heart failure progression: the potential role of tissue hypothyroidism. Horm Metab Res. 2010;42:718–24.
55. Palojoki E, Saraste A, Eriksson A, Pulkki K, Kallajoki M, Voipio-Pulkki LM, et al. Cardiomyocyte apoptosis and ventricular remodeling after myocardial infarction in rats. Am J Physiol. 2001;280:H2726–31.
56. Abbate A, Biondi-Zoccai GG, Baldi A. Pathophysiologic role of myocardial apoptosis in post-infarction left ventricular remodeling. J Cell Physiol. 2002;193:145–53.
57. Slezak J, Tribulova N, Okruhlicova L, Dhingra R, Bajaj A, Freed D, Singal P. Hibernating myocardium: pathophysiology, diagnosis, and treatment. Can J Physiol Pharmacol. 2009;87:252–65.
58. Fallavollita JA, Lim H, Canty Jr JM. Myocyte apoptosis and reduced SR gene expression precede the transition from chronically stunned to hibernating myocardium. J Mol Cell Cardiol. 2001;33:1937–44.
59. Marín-García J, Goldenthal MJ, Damle S, Pi Y, Moe GW. Regional distribution of mitochondrial dysfunction and apoptotic remodeling in pacing-induced heart failure. J Card Fail. 2009;15:700–8.
60. Dent MR, Tappia PS, Dhalla NS. Gender differences in apoptotic signaling in heart failure due to volume overload. Apoptosis. 2010;15:499–510.
61. Sun M, Chen M, Dawood F, Zurawska U, Li JY, Parker T, et al. Tumor necrosis factor-alpha mediates cardiac remodeling and ventricular dysfunction after pressure overload state. Circulation. 2007;115:1398–407.
62. Negoro S, Oh H, Tone E, Kunisada K, Fujio Y, Walsh K, et al. Glycoprotein 130 regulates cardiac myocyte survival in doxorubicin-induced apoptosis through phosphatidylinositol 3-kinase/Akt phosphorylation and Bcl-xL/caspase-3 interaction. Circulation. 2001;103:555–61.
63. Kajstura J, Cheng W, Sarangarajan R, Li P, Li B, Nitahara JA, et al. Necrotic and apoptotic myocyte cell death in the aging heart of Fischer 344 rats. Am J Physiol. 1996;271:H1215–28.
64. Olivetti G, Giordano G, Corradi D, Melissari M, Lagrasta C, Gambert SR, et al. Gender differences and aging: effects on the human heart. J Am Coll Cardiol. 1995;26:1068–79.
65. Frustaci A, Chimenti C, Setoguchi M, Guerra S, Corsello S, Crea F, et al. Cell death in acromegalic cardiomyopathy. Circulation. 1999;99:1426–34.
66. Kawai C, Matsumori A. Dilated cardiomyopathy update: infectious-immune theory revisited. Heart Fail Rev. 2013;18:703–14.
67. Brunner S, Theiss HD, Leiss M, Grabmaier U, Grabmeier J, Huber B, et al. Enhanced stem cell migration mediated by VCAM-1/VLA-4 interaction improves cardiac function in virus-induced dilated cardiomyopathy. Basic Res Cardiol. 2013;108:388.
68. Zhang P, Cox CJ, Alvarez KM, Cunningham MW. Cutting edge: cardiac myosin activates innate immune responses through TLRs. J Immunol. 2009;183:27–31.
69. Knaapen MW, Davies MJ, De Bie M, Haven AJ, Martinet W, Kockx MM. Apoptotic versus autophagic cell death in heart failure. Cardiovasc Res. 2001;51:304–12.
70. Park M, Shen YT, Gaussin V, Heyndrickx GR, Bartunek J, Resuello RR, et al. Apoptosis predominates in nonmyocytes in heart failure. Am J Physiol. 2009;297:H785–91.
71. Hausenloy DJ, Bøtker HE, Condorelli G, Ferdimandly P, Grurcia-Dorado D, Heusch G, et al. Translating cardioprotection for patient benefit: position paper from the Working Group of Cellular Biology of the Heart of the European Society of Cardiology. Cardiovasc Res. 2013;98:7–22.
72. Piot C, Croisille P, Staat P, Thibault H, Rioufol G, Mewton N, et al. Effect of cyclosporine on reperfusion injury in acute myocardial infarction. N Engl J Med. 2008;359:473–81.
73. Soha NR, Clement RT, Feng J, Liu Y, Bianchi C, Horvath EM, et al. The effects of therapeutic sulfide on myocardial apoptosis in response to

ischemia-reperfusion injury. Eur J Cardiothorac Surg. 2008;33:906–13.
74. Smith CC, Davidson SM, Lim SY, Simkin JC, Hothersall JS, Yellon DM. Necrostatin: a potential novel cardioprotective agent? Cardiovasc Drugs Ther. 2007;21:227–33.
75. Zhang L, Zhang L, Li YH, Zhang HY, Chen ML, Gao MM, et al. High-dose glucose-insulin-potassium treatment reduces myocardial apoptosis in patients with acute myocardial infarction. Eur J Clin Invest. 2005;35:164–70.
76. Ovize M, Thibault H, Przyklenk K. Myocardial conditioning: opportunities for clinical translation. Circ Res. 2013;113:439–50.
77. Yellon DM, Downey JM. Preconditioning the myocardium: from cellular physiology to clinical cardiology. Physiol Rev. 2003;83:1113–51.
78. Pantos CI, Davos CH, Carageorgiou HC, Varonos DV, Cokkinos DV. Ischaemic preconditioning protects against myocardial dysfunction caused by ischaemia in isolated hypertrophied rat hearts. Basic Res Cardiol. 1996;91:444–9.
79. Yan WJ, Dong HL, Xiong LZ. The protective roles of autophagy in ischemic preconditioning. Acta Pharmacol Sin. 2013;34:636–43.
80. Peng W, Liu Y, Xu WJ, Xia QH. Role of Beclin 1-dependent autophagy in cardioprotection of ischemic preconditioning. J Huazhong Univ Sci Technolog Med Sci. 2013;33:51–6.
81. Hsu SF, Chao CM, Huang WT, Lin MT, Cheng BC. Attenuating heat-induced cellular autophagy, apoptosis and damage in H9c2 cardiomyocytes by pre-inducing HSP70 with heat shock preconditioning. Int J Hyperthermia. 2013;29:239–47.
82. Al-Amran FG. Apoptosis amelioration through hypothermic reperfusion in heart transplant. J Pharmacol Pharmacother. 2013;4:275–80.
83. Fiuza-Luces C, Delmiro A, Soares-Miranda L, González-Murillo A, Martínez-Palacios J, Ramírez M. Exercise training can induce cardiac autophagy at end-stage chronic conditions: Insights from a graft-versus-host-disease mouse model. Brain Behav Immun. 2013. doi:10.1016/j.bbi.2013.11.007. pii: S0889-1591(13)00538-2.
84. Tao R, Kim SH, Honbo N, Karliner JS, Alano CC. Minocycline protects cardiac myocytes against simulated ischemia–reperfusion injury by inhibiting poly (ADP-ribose) polymerase-1. J Cardiovasc Pharmacol. 2010;56:659–68.
85. Sishi BJ, Loos B, van Rooyen J, Engelbrecht AM. Autophagy upregulation promotes survival and attenuates doxorubicin-induced cardiotoxicity. Biochem Pharmacol. 2013;85:124–34.
86. Chen YF, Kobayashi S, Chen J, Redetzke RA, Said S, Liang Q, et al. Short term triiodo-L-thyronine treatment inhibits cardiac myocyte apoptosis in border area after myocardial infarction in rats. J Mol Cell Cardiol. 2008;44:180–7.
87. Pantos C, Mourouzis I, Saranteas T, Clavé G, Ligeret H, Noack-Fraissignes P, et al. Thyroid hormone improves postischaemic recovery of function while limiting apoptosis: a new therapeutic approach to support hemodynamics in the setting of ischaemia-reperfusion? Basic Res Cardiol. 2009;104:69–77.
88. Ferreyra C, Vargas F, Rodríguez-Gómez I, Pérez-Abud R, O'Valle F, Osuna A. Preconditioning with triiodothyronine improves the clinical signs and acute tubular necrosis induced by ischemia/reperfusion in rats. PLoS One. 2013;8:e74960. doi:10.1371/journal.pone.0074960.
89. Kumar A, Sinha RA, Tiwari M, Singh R, Koji T, Manhas N, et al. Hyperthyroidism induces apoptosis in rat liver through activation of death receptor-mediated pathways. J Hepatol. 2007;46:888–98.
90. Sinha RA, You SH, Zhou J, Siddique MM, Bay BH, Zhu X, et al. Thyroid hormone stimulates hepatic lipid catabolism via activation of autophagy. J Clin Invest. 2012;122:2428–38.
91. Sabbah HN, Wang M, Zhang K, Gupta RC, Rastogi S. Long-term therapy with Bendana (MTP-131), a novel mitochondria-targeting peptide, improves left ventricular systolic function in dogs with chronic heart failure in dogs with chronic heart failure. European Society of Cardiology Congress Amsterdam, 31 Aug–4 Sept 2013.
92. Gajarsa JJ, Kloner RA. Left ventricular remodeling in the post-infarction heart: a review of cellular, molecular mechanisms, and therapeutic modalities. Heart Fail Rev. 2011;16:13–21.
93. Tousoulis D, Papageorgiou N, Briasoulis A, Androulakis E, Charakida M, Tsiamis E, et al. Conflicting effects of nitric oxide and oxidative stress in chronic heart failure: potential therapeutic strategies. Heart Fail Rev. 2012;17:65–79.
94. Mann DL, McMurray JJ, Packer M, Swedberg K, Borer JS, Colucci WS, et al. Targeted anticytokine therapy in patients with chronic heart failure: results of the Randomized Etanercept Worldwide Evaluation (RENEWAL). Circulation. 2004;109:1594–602.
95. Chung ES, Packer M, Lo KH, Fasanmade AA, Willerson JT, Anti-TNF Therapy Against Congestive Heart Failure Investigators. Randomized, double-blind, placebo-controlled, pilot trial of infliximab, a chimeric monoclonal antibody to tumor necrosis factor-alpha, in patients with moderate-to-severe heart failure: results of the anti-TNF Therapy Against Congestive Heart Failure (ATTACH) trial. Circulation. 2003;107:3133–40.
96. Sliwa K, Woodiwiss A, Candy G, Badenhorst D, Libhaber C, Norton G, et al. Effects of pentoxifylline on cytokine profiles and left ventricular performance in patients with decompensated congestive heart failure secondary to idiopathic dilated cardiomyopathy. Am J Cardiol. 2002;90:1118–22.
97. Abbate A, Van Tassell BW, Biondi-Zoccai G, Kontos MC, Grizzard JD, Spillman DW, et al. Effects of interleukin-1 blockade with Anakinra on adverse cardiac remodeling and heart failure after acute myocardial infarction [from the Virginia Commonwealth University-Anakinra Remodeling Trial (2) (VCU-ART2) pilot study]. Am J Cardiol. 2013;111:1394–400.

98. Carotenuto F, Minieri M, Monego G, Fiaccavento R, Bertoni A, Sinigaglia F, et al. A diet supplemented with ALA-rich flaxseed prevents cardiomyocyte apoptosis by regulating caveolin-3 expression. Cardiovasc Res. 2013;100:422–31.
99. Kanamori H, Takemura G, Goto K, Tsujimoto A, Ogino A, Takeyama T, et al. Resveratrol reverses remodeling in hearts with large, old myocardial infarctions through enhanced autophagy-activating AMP kinase pathway. Am J Pathol. 2013;182: 701–13.
100. Di Lascio G, Harmelin G, Targetti M, Nanni C, Bianchi G, Gasbarri T, et al. Cellular retrograde cardiomyoplasty and relaxin therapy for postischemic myocardial repair in a rat model. Tex Heart Inst J. 2012;39:488–99.
101. Lee TM, Lin MS, Chang NC. Inhibition of histone deacetylase on ventricular remodeling in infarcted rats. Am J Physiol. 2007;293:H968–77.
102. Kaludercic N, Carpi A, Menabò R, Di Lisa F, Paolocci N. Monoamine oxidases (MAO) in the pathogenesis of heart failure and ischemia/reperfusion injury. Biochim Biophys Acta. 1813;2011:1323–32.
103. Unsöld B, Kaul A, Sbroggiò M, Schubert C, Regitz-Zagrosek V, Brancaccio M, et al. Melusin protects from cardiac rupture and improves functional remodelling after myocardial infarction. Cardiovasc Res. 2014;101:97–107.
104. Dorn 2nd GW. Apoptotic and non-apoptotic programmed cardiomyocyte death in ventricular remodelling. Cardiovasc Res. 2009;81:465–73.

Repair of the Infarcted Myocardium

16

Junhong Wang and Nikolaos G. Frangogiannis

Abstract

The adult mammalian heart has negligible regenerative capacity; thus, sudden death of a large number of cardiomyocytes in the infarcted myocardium leads to replacement of dead cells with collagen-based scar. Repair of the infarcted heart can be divided into three distinct, but overlapping phases: the inflammatory phase, the proliferative phase and the maturation phase. Cardiomyocyte necrosis and matrix fragmentation in the infarcted myocardium release damage-associated molecular patterns (DAMPs) that activate innate immune cascades and trigger the inflammatory reaction. Induction of chemokines and cytokines is a hallmark of the post-infarction inflammatory response mediating recruitment of neutrophils and mononuclear cells in the myocardium. As infiltrating leukocytes clear the wound from dead cells and matrix debris, pro-inflammatory signaling is repressed and fibroblasts undergo myofibroblast conversion. Induction of specialized matricellular proteins that modulate growth factor and cytokine responses plays a critical role in activation of reparative cells and in formation of the scar. Cross-linking of the collagen-based matrix marks the end of the proliferative phase, as the scar matures and most fibroblasts and vascular cells in the wound undergo apoptosis. This chapter provides an overview of the phases of repair in the infarcted heart. Moreover, we discuss challenges and opportunities in targeting the inflammatory and reparative response following infarction in order to attenuate adverse remodeling and to prevent progression of post-infarction heart failure.

J. Wang • N.G. Frangogiannis, MD (✉)
Department of Medicine (Cardiology),
The Wilf Family Cardiovascular Research Institute,
Albert Einstein College of Medicine,
1300 Morris Park Avenue Forchheimer G46B,
Bronx, NY 10461, USA
e-mail: nikolaos.frangogiannis@einstein.yu.edu

D.V. Cokkinos (ed.), *Introduction to Translational Cardiovascular Research*,
DOI 10.1007/978-3-319-08798-6_16, © Springer International Publishing Switzerland 2015

Keywords
Cardiac remodeling • Chemokine • Cytokine • Extracellular matrix Inflammation • Leucokyte • Matricellular proteins • Myocardial infarction Myofibroblast

Abbreviations

AMI	Acute myocardial infarction
DAMPs	Damage-associated molecular patterns
GM-CSF	Granulocyte Macrophage-Colony Stimulating Factor
HF	Heart failure
HIF-1α	Hypoxia-Inducible Factor
HSPs	Heat shock proteins
ICAM-1	Intercellular Adhesion Molecule 1
IL	Interleukin
INFL	Inflammation
IRAK-M	Interleukin-1 receptor associated kinase
MCP	Monocyte Chemoattractant Protein
M-CSF	Macrophage-Colony Stimulating Factor
MI	Myocardial infarction
MMP	Matrix metalloproteinase
PAI-1	Plasminogen Activator Inhibitor
REM	Cardiac remodeling
ROS	Reactivate Oxygen Species
SCF	Stem Cell Factor
SDF	Stromal Derived Factor
SOD	Superoxide dismutase
TGF-β	Transforming growth factor-β
TIMP-1	Tissue Inhibitor of Metalloproteinases
TLRs	Toll-like receptors
TNF-α	Tumor Necrosis Factor-α
TSP-1	Thrombospondin-1
VEGF	Vascular Endothelial Growth Factor

16.1 Introduction

Acute myocardial infarction (AMI) is a major cause of morbidity and mortality in both industrial nations and in the developing world. Despite advances in coronary care and the introduction of new treatment modalities, approximately 16 % of patients who experience an AMI will die within 1 year of hospitalization [1]. In patients suffering an AMI, prolonged sudden occlusion of a coronary artery triggers a series of events that culminates in death of ischemic cardiomyocytes. Adult mammalian hearts have negligible regenerative capacity; thus, extensive necrosis of ischemic cardiomyocytes in the infarcted myocardium activates an inflammatory cascade that not only serves to clear the dead cells and matrix debris, but also results in healing and replacement of the damaged tissue with scar. Therefore, inflammation (INFL) after AMI is an important component of the reparative response [2]. However, in addition to its role in repair of the infarcted myocardium and in scar formation, the inflammatory cascade is also involved in post-infarction cardiac remodeling (REM), a constellation of geometric and functional alterations that involves both cardiomyocytes and interstitial cells and is associated with progression of heart failure (HF), development of ventricular arrhythmias and death. The extent of adverse remodeling is dependent not only on the size of the infarct, but also on the qualitative characteristics of the wound. It is clear that the molecular and morphologic changes associated with infarct healing directly influence REM and affect prognosis in patients with AMI.

Although recent advances have resulted in the development of novel strategies that salvage myocardium and improve early mortality in patients with myocardial infarction (MI), approaches directly targeting the healing process are lacking. Therefore, understanding of the specific events involved in infarct healing is crucial in order to design novel therapeutic strategies aiming at optimizing cardiac repair and attenuating post-infarction remodeling. The current chapter summarizes the cellular and molecular events associated with infarct healing and describes the pathways implicated in REM of the infarcted heart.

16.1.1 The Phases of Cardiac Repair

For descriptive purposes, the reparative response following myocardial infarction can be divided into three distinct, but overlapping phases: the inflammatory phase, the proliferative phase and the maturation phase [3]. Necrosis of a large number of cardiomyocytes in the infarcted myocardium releases danger signals activating an innate immune response that results in infiltration of the infarct with abundant neutrophils, monocytes and lymphocytes. As professional phagocytes clear the infarct from dead cells and matrix debris, the inflammatory reaction is repressed and mesenchymal cells are recruited into the infarct, leading to the proliferative phase. Fibroblasts differentiate into myofibroblasts and deposit extracellular matrix proteins in the infarcted area. Maturation of the scar follows, as matrix proteins are cross-linked and fibroblasts become apoptotic leading to formation of a stable scar with a low cellular content.

16.2 The Inflammatory Phase

16.2.1 Initiation of the Post-infarction Inflammatory Response

Ischemic myocardial injury results in decreased oxygen tension and subsequent loss of oxidative phosphorylation leading to decreased generation of ATP. Cessation of aerobic metabolism, ATP depletion and accumulation of products of anoxic metabolism occur within only 10 s of occlusion. Striking myocardial dysfunction occurs almost simultaneously and is evident within 60 s. Five to ten minutes after the onset of ischemia reversible ultrastructural cardiomyocyte changes appear, including depletion of cytoplasmic glycogen stores and mitochondrial swelling. After 20–40 min of sustained ischemia, irreversible cardiomyocyte injury occurs (involving first the more susceptible subendocardial cardiomyocytes), evidenced by sarcolemmal disruption and by the presence of small amorphous mitochondrial densities [4]. Acute sudden necrosis of cardiomyocytes in the infarcted heart activates the innate immune system and initiates an intense inflammatory response (Fig. 16.1). Necrotic cardiomyocytes release endogenous "danger" signals, known as damage-associated molecular patterns (DAMPs) [5]. High-mobility group box-1 (HMGB1), heat shock proteins (HSPs), ATP and matrix fragments (including low molecular hyaluronic acid, and fibronectin fragments) serve as DAMPs following infarction activating the immune response [6]. DAMPs signal through activation of Toll-like receptors (TLRs), a family of transmembrane receptors that trigger downstream pro-inflammatory pathways. Moreover, activation of the complement cascade and generation of reactive oxygen species (ROS) also contribute to activation of the inflammatory reaction in the infarcted myocardium.

16.2.2 Role of Complement Activation in Post-infarction Inflammation

The complement system is a first line of defense with a central role to the innate immune response. Involvement of the complement system in MI was first demonstrated in a rat MI model by Hill and Ward [7]. Since then, numerous studies documented that activation of complement is an early event in postinfarction inflammation and healing [8]. In the infarcted myocardium, subcellular substances released by dying cardiomyocytes (such as cardiolipin) can activate complement. On the basis of extensive experimental evidence, inhibition of the complement system seems to be a promising therapeutic target to reduce myocardial injury and limit the infarct size. Consumptive depletion of complement [9], antibody-induced inhibition of individual complement components (e.g. C5), or infusion of modified native complement components that block complement activation exhibited protective actions in experimental animal models of AMI [10, 11]. The effectiveness of such approaches in animal models generated considerable interest leading to clinical trials testing the effectiveness of C5 inhibition in patients with MI. Most clinical studies have

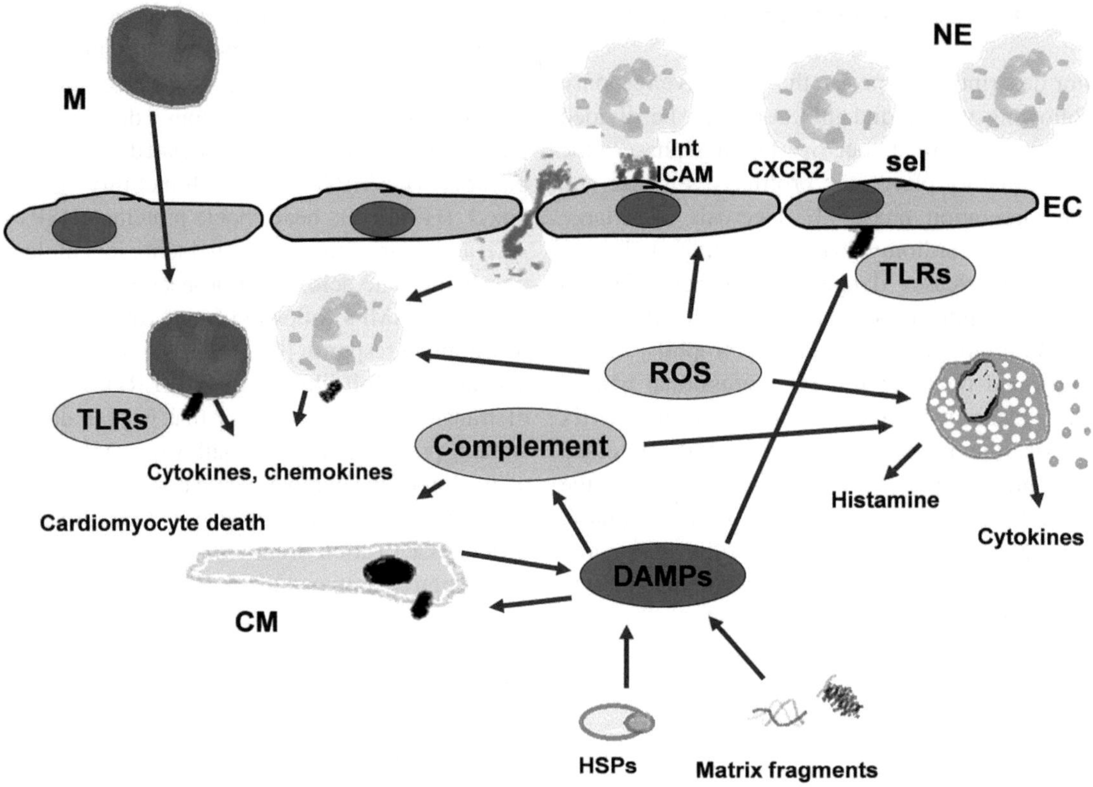

Fig. 16.1 The inflammatory phase of cardiac repair. Release of damage-associated molecular patterns (DAMPs) by dying cardiomyocytes and matrix fragments activates innate immune pathways leading to recruitment of leukocytes in the healing infarct. Mast cells, neutrophils and mononuclear cells, but also endothelial cells, fibroblasts and cardiomyocytes contribute to the pro-inflammatory environment

focused on pexelizumab, a humanized single chain variable fragment (scFv) to complement C5. Although some favorable results of pexelizumab were reported as adjunctive therapy to reduce reperfusion injury in coronary artery bypass surgery [12], most of the clinical data, showed no benefit in patients with AMI [13].

16.2.3 The Role of ROS Generation

Reactivate Oxigen species (ROS) are atoms or molecules with unpaired electrons in their outer orbit; they are highly reactive entities and can participate in a variety of biochemical reactions [14]. ROS react directly with cellular lipids, proteins and DNA causing cell injury and death, and are critically involved in the oxidative burst reaction, which is essential for phagocyte function. The normal heart possesses substantial ability to counterbalance the generation of ROS through inhibitory enzymatic pathways and through activation of intracellular antioxidants. The antioxidant defenses, however, are overwhelmed following infarction, resulting in net generation of free radicals that may cause myocardial contractile dysfunction and structural damage [15]. Generation of ROS can activate the immune cells in the infarcted heart and trigger cytokine and chemokine release partially through activation of NF-κB system [16]. Overactive ROS-mediated signaling has the potential for detrimental actions in the infarcted heart mediated through matrix degradation and by inducing cardiomyocyte apoptosis.

Free radical scavengers have been widely used to study the role of ROS in the pathophysiology of MI; their effects generated interest in possible clinical applications. Jolly et al. [17] demonstrated protective effects of combining the antioxidant enzymes superoxide dismutase (SOD) and catalase in reduction of infarct size in dogs undergoing coronary occlusion and reperfusion. Recently, transgenic mice with specific overexpression of extracellular SOD (ecSOD) in cardiomyocytes exhibited significant protection from post-ischemic/reperfusion injury [18]. In addition, mice overexpressing manganese SOD (MnSOD) demonstrated a significant decrease in infarct size in Langendorff-perfused hearts undergoing coronary artery ligation [19]. However, not all experimental evidence suggests a deleterious effect of ROS in the infarcted heart [20]. The timing of administration, the dosage of the antioxidant, and the pleiotropic effects of ROS may be responsible for contradictory findings in experimental studies. Thus, it is not surprising that studies using antioxidant therapy in myocardial infarction have produced discouraging results in the clinical arena. A small clinical study using recombinant human SOD in patients with AMI undergoing balloon angioplasty [21] demonstrated no significant improvement in left ventricular function.

16.2.4 TLR Signaling in the Post-infarction Inflammatory Reaction

DAMPs exert their pro-inflammatory actions by activating members of the TLR family; binding of danger signals to the respective TLRs induces activation of several kinases and of the NF-κB cascade. Of the 13 known mammalian TLRs, TLR-2, -3 and -4 has been identified to play an important role in mediating the inflammatory response in the infarcted heart [22–24]. Deletion of TLR-4 [25] or disruption of TLR-2 signaling [23] by specific antibodies have decreased infarct size and suppressed inflammation following MI, identifying TLR-2 and -4 as key components of the innate immune response in the heart. Thus, TLR-dependent activation of inflammatory cells plays an important role in the innate immune response following MI.

16.2.5 NF-κB Activation in Myocardial Infarction

TLR-mediated, complement-activated and ROS-induced pathways converge on the activation of the transcription factor NF-κB, an important signaling component for early inflammatory activation that triggers cytokine, chemokine and adhesion molecule expression in the ischemic myocardium. Activation of the NF-κB system has been demonstrated in models of experimental myocardial ischemia and reperfusion. Although some studies have suggested injurious pro-inflammatory actions of NF-κB in the infarcted myocardium, other investigations indicated that the NF-κB pathway may also mediate cytoprotective responses in the ischemic heart [26]. Activation of the NF-κB signaling cascade in multiple parallel processes involving various cell types, critical for infarct healing, complicates understanding of its role in myocardial infarction. In vivo studies examining the role of cell-specific NF-κB activation at different stages of the reparative response would greatly contribute to our understanding of cardiac injury and repair.

16.2.6 Inflammatory Signals and Cellular Events During the Inflammatory Phase of Infarct Healing: Chemokine Signaling in the Infarcted Heart

Induction of chemokines is a prominent feature of the post-infarction inflammatory response [27–29]. The chemokines are small polypeptides with molecular weights in the range of 8–14 kDa that play an important role in leukocyte trafficking. From a structural perspective, chemokines are divided into subfamilies on the basis of the number and sequential relationship of their conserved cysteine residues (CXC, CC, XC and CX_3C chemokines) [3]. CXC chemokines that contain the ELR (elastin-like recombinamer) motif, such as IL-8/CXCL8, mediate neutrophil migration, whereas CC chemokines, such as Monocyte Chemoattractant Protein (MCP)-1/CCL2 recruit mononuclear cells. The effects of chemokines extend beyond actions on cells of hematopoietic origin. For example, the CXC chemokine Stromal Derived Factor (SDF)-1 is implicated in angiogenesis and fibrous tissue deposition [30]. On the other hand, another ELR-negative CXC chemokine, Interferon-inducible Protein (IP)-10/CXCL10 exerts direct inhibitory actions on fibroblast migration, serving as an antifibrotic agent [31], and may also act as an angiostatic mediator [32]. Using a mouse model of reperfused infarction, our laboratory demonstrated that endogenous IP-10/CXCL10 is an essential inhibitory signal that regulates the cellular composition of the healing infarct, preventing uncontrolled fibrosis and attenuating adverse REM through direct actions on fibroblast migration and function [33].

Monocyte Chemoattractant Protein (MCP)-1/CCL2 is the best-studied CC chemokine. In addition to its critical role in mononuclear cell recruitment, MCP-1 has been suggested to exert important actions on non-hematopoietic cells, inducing angiogenic and arteriogenic effects [34] and modulating fibroblast phenotype and activity by increasing collagen expression and by regulating matrix metalloproteinase synthesis [35]. Using both antibody neutralization studies and genetic disruption models, we have documented a crucial role of MCP-1 on macrophage recruitment and activation, cytokine synthesis and myofibroblast accumulation in healing infarcts [36]. MCP-1 −/− mice demonstrated decreased and delayed macrophage infiltration accompanied by impaired phagocytosis and delayed replacement of injured cardiomyocytes by granulation tissue in the healing infarct.

16.2.7 Expression and Role of the Cytokines in Myocardial Infarction

Activation of cytokine cascades is a prominent characteristic of the post-infarction inflammatory reaction. Complement activation, TLR signaling, free radical generation and NF-κB activation are capable of stimulating cytokine expression in both resident and blood-derived cells, resulting in marked cytokine upregulation in the infarcted area. Cytokines are highly pleiotropic and are capable of modulating phenotype and function of all cell types involved in cardiac repair. Their multifunctional and context-dependent properties have hampered understanding of their role in the infarcted myocardium.

As the prototypical pro-inflammatory cytokine, interleukin (IL)-1 mediates synthesis of other cytokines, chemokines, growth factors, and adhesion molecules in the infarct and stimulates leukocyte recruitment [37]. Marked IL-1β upregulation has been reported in experimental models of MI and in patients suffering an AMI [38]. Activation of the inflammasome, the molecular platform involved in IL-1 activation, is noted in both cardiomyocytes and non-cardiomyocytes in the infarcted heart [39, 40]. IL-1 is a central mediator in the post-infarction inflammatory response; disruption of IL-1 signaling markedly reduces infiltration of the infarcted myocardium with leukocytes and attenuates MMP expression decreasing dilative REM [37]. IL-1 also critically regulates fibroblast phenotype in the infarct, delaying conversion of fibroblasts into myofibroblasts and promoting a matrix-degrading phenotype [41]. Because of its central role in mediating post-infarction INFL, matrix degradation and dilative REM, the IL-1 system may be a promising therapeutic target in patients with AMI [42].

The pro-inflammatory cytokine Tumor Necrosis Factor-α (TNF-α) is released early in the infarcted myocardium [43], and (much like IL-1) may stimulate expression of other inflammatory mediators by leukocytes and endothelial cells. TNF-α deficient mice undergoing MI protocols had reduced expression of chemokines and adhesion molecules suggesting an important role for TNF-α in mediating the post-infarction inflammatory response [44]. However, as a highly pleiotropic mediator, TNF-α does not simply serve as a trigger of a cytokine cascade, but may also modulate cell survival pathways. Experimental studies exploring effects of TNF signaling on cardiomyocyte survival have produced contradictory results. Kurrelmeyer et al. [45] demonstrated that TNFR1/TNFR2 double receptor knockout mice undergoing left coronary artery ligation had significantly increased infarct size exhibiting accentuated cardiomyocyte apoptosis when compared with wild-type controls. In contrast,

Sugano et al. [46] reported that reduction of bioactive TNF-α through local delivery of sTNFR1 inhibited cardiomyocyte apoptosis in a rat model of ischemia/reperfusion. Attempts to implement anti-TNF approaches in patients with AMI have been disappointing, possibly reflecting the pleiotropic actions of the cytokine that may exert both injurious effects (through accentuation of inflammation) and protective pro-survival actions on cardiomyocytes.

16.2.8 The Cellular Immune Response in the Infarcted Myocardium

16.2.8.1 The Neutrophils

Early recruitment of abundant neutrophils is a hallmark of the post-infarction inflammatory reaction. Neutrophils release oxidants and proteases, secrete mediators that may amplify inflammatory cell recruitment, and phagocytose dead cells and debris. Early experimental studies suggested that neutrophil depletion in ischemia-reperfusion models markedly reduced infarct size [47] suggesting a role for neutrophils in extension of ischemic injury. However, more recent studies using genetic models associated with marked reduction in neutrophil infiltration in the infarct did not confirm these observations suggesting that neutrophil-mediated injury may not increase the size of the infarct [48].

Neutrophil transmigration in the infarcted myocardium requires specific interactions between the leukocytes and the endothelium, mediated through activation of a multistep adhesive cascade (Fig. 16.1). Each step of the cascade requires either upregulation, or activation, of distinct sets of adhesion molecules. First, leukocytes are captured by endothelial cells or roll on the endothelial surface via interactions that involve members of the selectin family. The selectin family includes L-, P- and E-selectin. L-selectin (CD62L) is expressed in neutrophils, whereas P-selectin (GMP-140, CD62P) and E-selectin (CD62E) are expressed in the endothelial surface. Although extensive evidence suggests the role of the selectins in supporting leukocyte margination under shear stress, the effects of selectin-related interventions in experimental models of myocardial ischemia have been inconsistent [48].

As leukocytes roll on the endothelium through selectin-mediated actions, they "sense" chemokines immobilized on the endothelial surface and engage into a firm adhesive interaction with endothelial cells through activation of the integrins [49]. The integrins are a family of heterodimeric membrane glycoproteins that consist of an α and a β subunit. Activated neutrophil β2 (CD18) integrins interact with endothelial Intercellular Adhesion Molecular (ICAM)-1 resulting in firm adhesion of leukocytes into the vascular endothelial layer. After firm adhesion, transmigration of activated neutrophils follows. The transmigration step is dependent on adhesion molecules, such as ICAM-1, Vascular endothelial (VE)-cadherin and members of the Junctional Adhesive Molecular (JAM) family. Because of the critical role of the integrins in neutrophil adhesion and transmigration, integrin-targeting strategies have been utilized to mitigate post-reperfusion inflammation in various experimental models. In animal models of experimental MI, inhibition of CD11/CD18 integrin resulted in significant reduction of infarct size [50]. However, despite the promising findings of the experimental studies, in small clinical trials leukocyte integrin inhibition was not effective in reducing infarct size and acute injury [51].

16.2.8.2 Monocytes and Macrophages

Monocytes and macrophages are key cellular effectors in the post-infarction inflammatory and reparative response [52]. Distinct monocyte subpopulations are sequentially recruited in the infarcted myocardium [53]. The CC chemokine CCL2/MCP-1 plays an important role in chemotactic attraction of pro-inflammatory monocytes that express the chemokine receptor CCR2 and have prominent phagocytic properties [36]. Other mediators including complement, Transforming growth factor (TGF)-β, free radicals and other CC chemokines may also play a role in regulating monocyte infiltration; their role in recruitment of specific monocyte subsets remains unknown. The recruited monocytes are predominantly bone

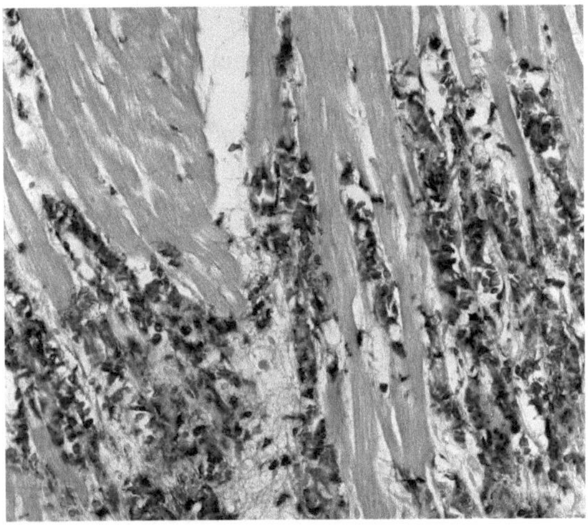

Fig. 16.2 Immunohistochemical staining with the macrophage-specific antibody PM-2K identifies an abundant macrophage population in canine infarcts after 1 h of coronary occlusion and 72 h of reperfusion

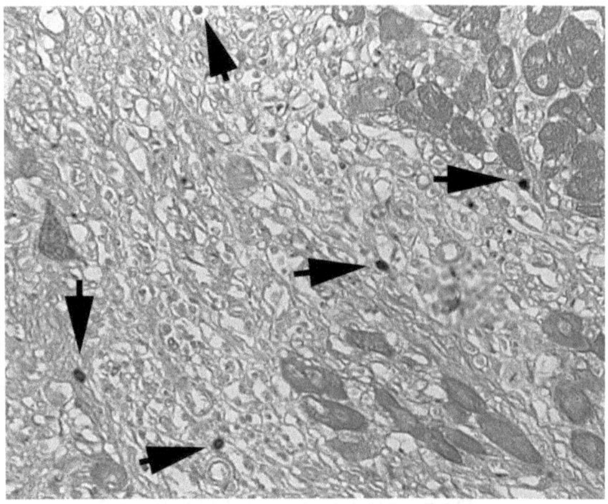

Fig. 16.3 Toludine blue staining identifies mast cells accumulating in the infarcted canine heart (*arrows*)

marrow-derived; however, in mouse models extramedullary sources (such as the spleenic monocyte reservoir) may also mobilize monocyte subpopulations [54, 55]. Recruited monocytes undergo phenotypic changes and may differentiate into macrophages (Fig. 16.2) in response to microenvironmental factors, such as cytokines and growth factors. The maturation of monocytes into mature macrophages is a complex and poorly understood process, that involves growth factors such as Macrophage-Colony Stimulating Factor (M-CSF) and Granulocyte Macrophage-Colony Stimulating Factor (GM-CSF) [56]. In addition to the clearance of the infarct from dead cells and matrix debris, macrophages have several additional functions including: (a) the production of a wide range of growth factors and cytokines that stimulate fibroblast and endothelial cell proliferation and may regulate the healing response and angiogenesis and (b) remodeling of the extracellular matrix network through the production of matrix metalloproteinases and their inhibitors.

16.2.8.3 The Mast Cells: Versatile Cells with a Potential Role in Infarct Healing

Mast cells are multifunctional cells that contain a wide range of mediators, including cytokines, growth factors, tryptase, chymase and histamine. Due to their strategic location, mast cells are likely to play an important role in initiating the inflammatory response through the release of pro-inflammatory mediators, capable of triggering the cytokine cascade. Mast cells release histamine and TNF-α in the early stages of the ischemic response and may play an important role in initiating the cytokine cascade [43]. As the infarct heals, induction of Stem Cell Factor (SCF) attracts mast cell progenitors, leading to a marked increase in mast cell numbers in the infarcted area (Fig. 16.3) [57]. Mast cell-derived mediators, have potent pro-inflammatory, angiogenic and fibrogenic actions. Although other cell types can produce growth factors and cytokines, histamine and the proteases tryptase and chymase are uniquely secreted by mast cells and may play an important role in cardiac repair [58].

16.3 The Proliferative Phase of Healing

16.3.1 Resolution of the Post-infarction Inflammatory Response

During the inflammatory phase of infarct healing, infiltration with activated neutrophils and mononuclear cells plays a crucial role in phagocytotic removal of dead cells and debris. However, effective repair is dependent on timely repression and resolution of the inflammatory reaction and on spatial containment of post-infarction inflammation in the infarcted area. Unrestrained, prolonged or expanded inflammatory activity could have catastrophic consequences in the injured heart, leading to adverse dilative REM and to the development of systolic and/or diastolic dysfunction. Repression of inflammation is an active process that requires timely activation of endogenous "STOP" signals that suppress the inflammatory reaction and trigger reparative cascades. From a cell biological perspective, timely resolution of inflammation following MI requires the coordinated actions of several different cell types including neutrophils, mononuclear cells, endothelial cells and pericytes. Alterations in the extracellular matrix network also participate to the resolution of inflammation after myocardial infarction.

16.3.2 Activation of Inhibitory "STOP" Signals in the Infarcted Heart: Expression of Decoy Receptors to Terminate Inflammation in Myocardial Healing

Cytokines and chemokines play important roles in post-infarction inflammation by interacting with their receptors, thus activating downstream intracellular pathways. However, for several members of the cytokine and chemokine family, receptors have been identified that bind to the corresponding inflammatory mediators with high affinity, but do not transduce a signal, thus serving as a molecular trap to remove the cytokine or chemokine from the local microenvironment. Although induction of decoy receptors to limit INFL is an intriguing mechanism for negative regulation of the inflammatory reaction, the role of such receptors in MI remains largely unknown. D6 is a chemokine decoy receptor that specifically binds and scavenges inflammatory CC-chemokines. Recently, Cochain et al. [59] found that D6 is upregulated in the infarcted myocardium, and that D6 –/– mice have increased chemokine levels in the infarct heart associated with enhanced infiltration with neutrophils and monocytes. As a result of the accentuated inflammatory reaction, D6 null mice were more susceptible to cardiac rupture prone after myocardial infarction. These findings suggest that induction of decoy receptors may protect the infarcted heart from uncontrolled inflammation following infarction.

16.3.3 Activation of Intracellular Pathways That Inhibit the Innate Immune Response

As uncontrolled TLR activation may stimulate a broad spectrum of inflammatory signals, several distinct pathways have evolved to negatively regulate TLR-mediated responses. Interleukin-1 receptor associated kinase (IRAK)-M, is a member of the IRAK family, predominantly expressed in macrophages, that lacks kinase activity but functions as a decoy to limit TLR- and IL-1 mediated inflammatory responses [60]. Our recent experiments demonstrated that IRAK-M is upregulated in macrophages and fibroblasts in the infarcted myocardium. IRAK-M null mice showed accentuated dilative REM with increased infiltration of pro-inflammatory monocytes and overactived MMP activity, suggesting that endogenous IRAK-M may attenuate adverse postinfarction remodeling by suppressing inflammatory activity and by inhibiting fibroblast-mediated matrix degradation in the infarcted heart [61].

16.3.4 The Role of Soluble Inhibitory Mediators in Suppression of the Post-infarction: Inflammatory Response the Role of TGF-Β

TGF-β is a multifunctional cytokine that exerts a wide range of biological effects in regulation of cell proliferation, differentiation, and apoptosis and has profound modulatory actions in the immune response. Because of its effects on both inflammatory and reparative cells, TGF-β is ideally suited as a "master switch" mediator in the transition from inflammation to fibrous tissue deposition in healing infarcts. TGF-β suppresses cytokine and chemokine synthesis by stimulated macrophages and endothelial cells, while promoting myofibroblast transdifferentiation and activation [62], In addition, TGF-β exerts matrix-preserving actions, decreasing expression of proteinases and increasing synthesis of proteinase inhibitors, such as Plasminogen Activator Inhibitor (PAI)-1 and TIMP-1. Unfortunately, the complex biology of TGF-β activation and its multiple cellular actions have hampered our efforts to understand its role in infarct healing.

TGF-β is markedly upregulated in MI and is predominantly localized in the infarct border zone [63]. Early TGF-β inhibition has deleterious consequences on the infarcted heart, presumed due to enhanced pro-inflammatory cytokine synthesis [64]. Thus, timely activation of TGF-β signaling may be important for suppression of inflammatory mediator synthesis following infarction. GDF-15 belongs to the TGF-β superfamily, is induced in the infarcted heart and has been reported to suppress chemokine-triggered integrin activation, thus limiting the inflammatory leukocyte adhesion to the endothelium. GDF-15 null mice undergoing coronary artery ligation protocols exhibited enhanced recruitment of neutrophils into the infarcted myocardium and an increased incidence of cardiac rupture [65], suggesting an important role of this growth factor in negative regulation of the post-infarction inflammatory reaction.

16.3.5 The Potential Role of IL-10

IL-10, a cytokine with potent anti-inflammatory properties, is predominantly expressed by activated Th2 lymphocytes and a subset of macrophages infiltrating the infarct [66]. Its expression shows a late and prolonged time course in the infarcted canine and mouse heart [66]. Monocytes and macrophages are particularly responsive to the anti-inflammatory actions of IL-10. In addition, IL-10 may play a significant role in extracellular matrix remodeling by promoting Tissue Inhibitor of Metalloproteinases (TIMP)-1 synthesis, leading to stabilization of the matrix [67]. Yang et al. demonstrated that IL-10 −/− mice had an enhanced inflammatory response and increased mortality following myocardial infarction [68]. In contrast, our laboratory found comparable survival and post-infarction remodeling in WT and IL-10 null mice undergoing reperfused infarction protocols. When compared with WT animals IL-10 null mice had elevated myocardial MCP-1 and TNF-α expression [69]; suggesting a relatively subtle effect of IL-10 in repression of the post-infarction inflammatory reaction that is not critical for the reparative response.

16.3.6 The Extracellular Matrix as a Regulator of the Post-infarction Inflammatory Reaction

16.3.6.1 Removal of Matrix Fragments Modulates the Inflammatory Response in Healing Myocardium

Extracellular matrix proteins not only provide structural and mechanical support to the tissue, but also modulate cell signaling through interactions with specific surface receptors. During infarct healing, the cardiac extracellular matrix undergoes dynamic changes that drive the inflammatory and reparative response [70]. During the first few hours after MI, matrix fragments are generated in the infarcted area and stimulate the inflammatory mediator synthesis. Evidence from our lab suggested that hyaluronan, a key component of the cardiac extracellular matrix, may undergo degradation in the infarcted area, leading to accumulation of pro-inflammatory low molecular weight hyaluronan fragments in infarcted area. The hyaluronan fragments may activate endothelial cells and macrophages inducing synthesis of cytokines and chemokines. Removal of the low molecular weight hyaluronan fragments from the infarcted area attenuates inflammation in the infarcted heart triggering inhibitory signals through interactions involving CD44 [71].

16.3.6.2 The Role of the Matricellular Proteins

Matricellular proteins are a family of structurally unrelated macromolecules that do not play a structural role, but bind to the matrix and

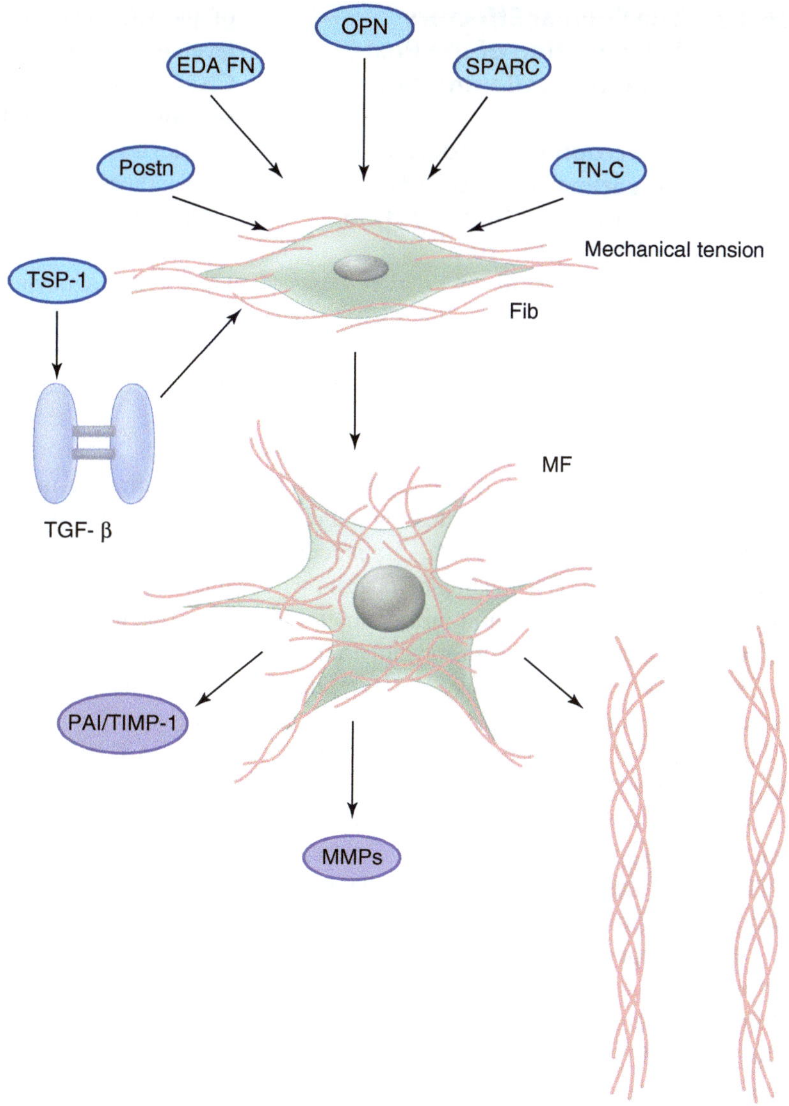

Fig. 16.4 The matricellular proteins osteopontin, SPARC, tenascin-C, periostin and thrombospondin-1 regulate fibroblast phenotype and activity in the healing infarct. Other specialized matrix proteins (such as ED-A fibronectin) also play a critical role in myofibroblast conversion

modulate cell-cell and cell-matrix interactions [72]. Temporally and spatially restricted induction and deposition of matricellular proteins is observed in the proliferative phase of infarct healing. Our laboratory has demonstrated that the matricellular protein thrombospondin (TSP)-1, a crucial TGF-β activator with potent angiostatic and anti-inflammatory properties, is strikingly upregulated in the border zone of the infarct [73]. TSP-1 null mice exhibited enhanced and prolonged expression of chemokines in the infarcted heart and showed expansion of the inflammatory infiltrate into the noninfarcted area. These findings suggest an important role for TSP-1 in suppression and containment of the inflammatory reaction following infarction. Therefore, localized induction of TSP-1 in the infarct border zone may form a "barrier" preventing expansion of the inflammatory infiltrate into the noninfarcted area. Other matricellular proteins, such as TSP-2, SPARC/osteonectin, osteopontin (OPN), tenascin-C and periostin are also upregulated in the infarcted heart and modulate the reparative response (Fig. 16.4) [72].

16.3.7 The Cellular Effectors in Resolution of the Post-infarction Inflammation

16.3.7.1 Macrophage-Mediated Clearance of Apoptotic Neutrophils in Resolution of Post-infarction Inflammation

Clearance of apoptotic cells in the injured tissue may be a crucial cellular mechanism for resolution of inflammation. Neutrophils infiltrating the infarct are programmed to undergo apoptosis, and clearance of apoptotic neutrophils by phagocytes ingesting is associated with active suppression of inflammation and release of large amounts of inhibitory mediators. Apoptotic granulocytes attenuate inflammation in healing myocardium by releasing mediators that inhibit further neutrophil recruitment, or by activating an anti-inflammatory program in macrophages. Macrophages phagocytosing neutrophils release large amounts of IL-10, TGF-β and proresolving lipid mediators [2]. Although the fundamental biology of the inflammatory response suggests that macrophage-mediated clearance of apoptotic infiltrating neutrophils may be crucial in triggering anti-inflammatory and proresolving signals, direct evidence supporting this concept in vivo is lacking. Recently, Wan and co-workers demonstrated that clearance of apoptotic (efferocytosis) in the ischemic myocardium through activation of myeloid-epithelial-reproductive tyrosine kinase (Mertk) in myeloid cells promotes resolution of inflammation protecting from adverse remodeling [74].

16.3.8 Mononuclear Cell Subsets as Negative Regulators of Inflammation Following Myocardial Infarction

16.3.8.1 Inhibitory Monocytes/Macrophages in Resolution of Inflammation

Two main subsets of monocytes have been identified in mice: (1) a subpopulation of Ly6C^{hi} pro-inflammatory monocytes that exhibit high levels of the CC chemokine receptor CCR2 and low level of expression of the fractalkine receptor, CX3CR1 (Ly6C^{hi} CCR2^{hi} CX3CR1^{low}); (2) a subset of Ly6C^{low}CCR2$^{low/neg}$CX3CR1^{hi} resident monocytes. Following myocardial infarction, early induction of CCR2 ligands (such as MCP-1) recruits the proinflammatory Ly6C^{hi} cells into the injured site; these cells secrete inflammatory cytokines and phagocytose dead cells and debris [53]. Inhibiting Ly6C^{hi} monocytes infiltration into the infarcted has been suggested as a promising therapeutic strategy to suppress the inflammatory response in healing myocardium [75, 76]. However, attenuation of pro-inflammatory monocyte infiltration may delay phagocytotic removal of dead cardiomyocytes. CX3CR1 (+) monocytes also infiltrate the myocardium and may play a reparative role; however, the mechanisms of their recruitment are poorly understood [77]. In human patients, CD16- monocytes have the same proinflammatory character as murine Ly6C^{hi} cells. Recently, the presence and localization of CD14+CD16– and CD14+CD16+ monocyte subsets was studied in human AMI [78]. In the inflammatory phase after AMI, CD14+ cells were identified in the infarct border zone, adjacent to cardiomyocytes, and consisted predominantly of CD14+CD16– cells. In contrast, during the proliferative phase, the infiltrate of CD14+ cells was localized mainly in the infarct core, and contained about 60 % CD14+CD16– cells and 40 % CD14+CD16+ monocytes. Further clinical data have demonstrated that circulating proinflammatory CD14+/CD16- cells exhibit an early peak in patients with ST elevation myocardial infarction and are negatively correlated with recovery of function 6 months after the acute event [79].

In response to the dynamic alteration in cytokine and growth factor expression in the infarct, the infiltrated monocytes undergo phenotypic changes. Upregulation of macrophage-colony stimulating factor induced monocyte to macrophage differentiation [56]. Macrophages can secrete inhibitory mediators to suppress inflammation during resolution of post-infarction healing. On the other hand, as they phagocytose apoptotic cells, macrophages acquire pro-resolving properties secreting anti-inflammatory mediators. In a somewhat simplified classification, macrophages are classified into proinflammatory M1 and inhibitory/reparative M2 subsets. In the healing infarct, M1 macrophages are abundant during the first 3 days after AMI, whereas M2 macrophages represented the predominant macrophage subset after 5 days [80].

16.3.9 Regulatory T Cells in Resolution of Inflammation

Subpopulations of T cells with suppressive properties (such as regulatory T cells/Tregs) may also be involved in negative regulation of postinfarction inflammation. Recent evidence suggested that Tregs infiltrate the infarcted heart and may play an important role in suppression of postinfarction inflammation, ameliorating pathologic cardiac remodeling [81, 82]. Chemokine receptor CCR5 null mice exhibited reduced myocardial infiltration with Tregs, associated with increased inflammation after myocardial infarction, indicating that Tregs may play a role in suppression of postinfarction inflammation [81]. Recently, Tang and his coworker [82] demonstrated that in rats undergoing infarction protocols, cell therapy with Tregs improved cardiac function. In addition, infiltration of neutrophils, macrophages and lymphocytes and expression of TNF-α and IL-1β were also significantly decreased in the rats that received Tregs. Take together, those data demonstrate that Treg cells may serve to protect against adverse ventricular remodeling and may contribute to improve cardiac function after myocardial infarction via inhibition of inflammation, or direct protection of cardiomyocytes.

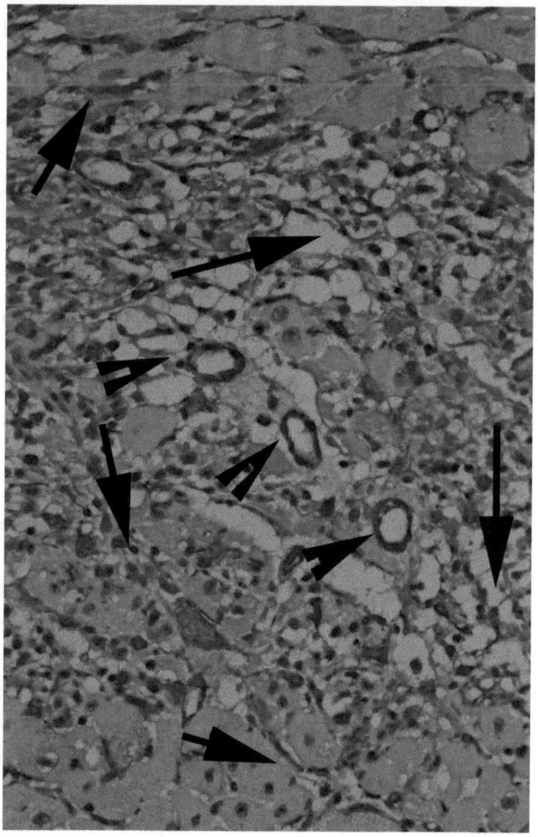

Fig. 16.5 Myofibroblasts infiltrating the infarcted mouse heart (1 h ischemia/72 h reperfusion) are identified as α-smooth muscle actin (α-SMA)-positive spindle shaped cells located outside the media of vessels (*arrows*). Vascular smooth muscle cells are also labeled through α-SMA staining (*arrowheads*)

16.3.10 Formation of Granulation Tissue in the Healing Infarct

16.3.10.1 Myofibroblast Activation in Infarct Healing

In adult mammalian hearts, fibroblasts are the most abundant non-cardiomyocytes located in the interstitial and perivascular space. In normal hearts, the resident fibroblasts play a role in maintenance the homeostatic of extracellular matrix network. During the proliferative phase of myocardium healing, fibroblasts undergo dramatic phenotypic changes, exhibiting high proliferative activity, increased migration through the provisional matrix network of the infarct, conversion into myofibroblasts (Fig. 16.5) through expression and incorporation of contractile proteins in the cytoskeleton, and increased synthesis of both structural and matricellular extracellular matrix proteins [83]. Mechanical tension, TGF-β and altered extracellular matrix composition are responsible for myofibroblast conversion. Activated myofibroblasts in the healing infarcts produce large amounts of extracellular matrix proteins (such as collagens and fibronectin) [84]. Myofibroblasts also deposit matricellular proteins, thus modulating cytokine and growth factor signaling, and regulate matrix metabolism by expressing MMPs and their inhibitors.

Animal model studies have suggested promising new approaches that may prevent adverse remodeling following myocardial infarction by targeting fibroblast functions [85]. Limiting fibroblast-mediated inflammatory and matrix-degrading activity by using IL-1 inhibition, or blocking fibrogenic growth factor-mediated cascades, such as TGF-β1/Smad3 signaling or FGF-2 may attenuate remodeling and dysfunction of the infarcted heart [86, 87]. Targeting fibroblasts may also provide an effective tool to inhibit arrhythmogenesis. Evidence suggests that conversion of fibroblasts into myofibroblasts during the proliferative phase is associated with generation of arrhythmias [88]. However, it should be noted that pharmacological disruption of fibroblast function may have adverse consequences because of the potential interference with scar formation. While excessive matrix deposition in the infarcted heart causes diastolic dysfunction, exaggerated matrix degradation may induce chamber dilation and systolic dysfunction. Thus, caution is needed when targeting fibroblast-mediated matrix deposition to selectively target excessive fibrosis, while avoiding matrix loss that may have catastrophic consequences on cardiac geometry and function.

16.3.11 Infarct Angiogenesis for Myocardial Healing

Wound healing is associated with intense angiogenesis that serves to provide oxygen and nutrients to the metabolically active cells of the healing wound. Angiogenic growth factors are expressed in the ischemic heart where they may stimulate vascular formation promoting cardiac repair. bFGF and Vascular Endothelial Growth Factor (VEGF) are induced and released during the first few hours following myocardial ischemia and may mediate neovessel growth [32]. Hypoxia-Inducible Factor (HIF)-1α, an upstream initiator of ischemia-induced angiogenesis, is also expressed by cardiomyocytes, endothelial and inflammatory cells early after myocardial infarction [89]. HIF-1α activation induces VEGF expression and release, playing an important role in mediating endothelial sprouting in the healing infarct [90]. Several other mediators, such as the angiopoietins and members of the chemokine family are also capable of modulating angiogenesis, and may participate in the complex process of neovessel formation following myocardial infarction [33, 91].

16.4 The Maturation Phase

As a matrix network comprised of mature cross-linked collagen is formed, signals inhibiting fibrosis are activated and mark the transition to the maturation phase of infarct healing. The pathways involved in suppression of the fibrotic response are poorly understood and may involve a wide of range of signals implicated in suppression of growth factor signaling. Fibroblasts in the mature scar become quiescent and may undergo apoptosis as they become deprived of key pro-survival signals transduced through matricellular proteins and fibrogenic growth factors. Moreover, the infarct vasculature matures, as infarct neovessels acquire a coat comprised of pericytes [92]. During the proliferative phase of healing, a rich network of capillaries is formed along with enlarged pericyte-poor "mother vessels" [93]. As the vasculature matures, some infarct neovessels are coated with pericytes, whereas uncoated vessels regress [94].

16.4.1 Targeting the Inflammatory and Reparative Response in Myocardial Infarction

Despite growing understanding of the role of inflammatory mediators in cardiac repair, implementation of strategies targeting inflammation in patients with AMI has not been successful. Early application of broad anti-inflammatory strategies (such as corticosteroids) in AMI patients had deleterious effects [95], suggesting the need for selective anti-inflammatory approaches to achieve effective suppression of harmful effects without interfering with the reparative response. In the 1980s and 1990s a large amount of experimental evidence suggested that inflammation may extend acute ischemic injury and that targeting specific inflammatory pathways may markedly reduce the size of the infarct. Antibody neutralization approaches in large animal models identified integrin inhibition as a highly promising and effective strategy in reducing infarct size following ischemia and reperfusion [50]. These studies generated great enthusiasm about the potential use of anti-inflammatory strategies in patients with AMI. Unfortunately, translation of this highly promising concept in human patients has been unsuccessful, as three small clinical trials targeting β2 integrins in human patients did not show beneficial effects [51]. Approaches targeting other key inflammatory mediators were equally disappointing. A large clinical trial targeting the complement system, a pathway critical in activation of the post-infarction inflammatory reaction failed to protect patients undergoing percutaneous interventions for AMI [13]. In recent years the development and availability of genetically manipulated mice showed that, in most cases, attenuation of inflammation does not significantly affect the size of the acute infarct [36, 37, 48], challenging the early pharmacologic studies. However, the apparent disconnect between animal experimentations and clinical investigations had a lasting effect on the field and dampened enthusiasm about the potential usefulness of approaches targeting the inflammatory reaction in patients with AMI. This is unfortunate because the critical role of key inflammatory cascades in post-infarction remodeling has not been exploited therapeutically.

How should we proceed to translate our knowledge on the reparative response following myocardial infarction into therapy for patients with AMI? Successful translation requires understanding the fundamental biology of the reparative response and insights into the complexities and pathophysiologic heterogeneity of the clinical context. Unlike animal models, AMI in human patients is characterized by a wide range of pathophysiologic responses, dependent on characteristics of the patient (age, gender, genetic profile, etc.) and the disease (pattern of the disease, presence or absence of comorbidities). There is a need for development of biomarker-based strategies to identify patient subpopulations with distinct pathophysiologies. Overactive inflammation induces matrix degradation in the myocardium, causing chamber dilation and systolic dysfunction. On the other hand, accentuated pro-fibrotic signaling is associated with excessive matrix deposition and diastolic dysfunction. The association between persistent elevations of pro-inflammatory chemokines in the serum of patients with acute coronary syndromes and increased mortality may reflect the adverse consequences of prolonged inflammation on cardiac remodeling [96]. These patients may benefit from treatment with anti-MCP-1 or anti-IL-1 agents (such as anakinra) [86]. On the other end of the spectrum, certain patient subpopulations (such as diabetics) develop post-infarction heart failure in the absence of significant dilation [97], predominantly associated with diastolic dysfunction [98]. The pathologic changes observed in these individuals may reflect activation of the pro-fibrotic TGF-β/Smad axis. These patients may benefit from cautious inhibition of Smad signaling.

Conclusion

The recent focus of the cardiovascular community on cardiac regeneration following infarction has raised hopes for the development of effective therapies that stimulate new cardiomyocyte growth. Much like the past experience with anti-inflammatory strategies, cell therapy approaches demonstrated impressive effectiveness in animal models; however, clinical investigations have been much less encouraging. The field has moved from the early notion that cell therapy can induce myocardial regeneration to the concept that cells can be used as tools for modulation of the inflammatory or reparative response. Eventually, growth in our understanding of the biology of progenitor cells will lead to effective and practical approaches to regenerate the heart. This effort will likely require decades of work and may be a long journey through failed attempts and occasional successful experiences. There is no doubt however, that understanding of the endogenous reparative response will remain critical for successful implementation of regenerative strategies.

Acknowledgments Dr Frangogiannis' laboratory is funded by NIH grants R01 HL76246 and R01 HL85440 and by the Wilf Family Cardiovascular Research Institute.

References

1. Lloyd-Jones D, Adams R, Carnethon M, De Simone G, Ferguson TB, Flegal K, et al. Heart disease and stroke statistics–2009 update: a report from the American Heart Association Statistics Committee and Stroke Statistics Subcommittee. Circulation. 2009;119:480–6.
2. Frangogiannis NG. Regulation of the inflammatory response in cardiac repair. Circ Res. 2012;110:159–73.
3. Frangogiannis NG. The mechanistic basis of infarct healing. Antioxid Redox Signal. 2006;8:1907–39.
4. Jennings RB, Murry CE, Steenbergen Jr C, Reimer KA. Development of cell injury in sustained acute ischemia. Circulation. 1990;82:II2–12.
5. Arslan F, de Kleijn DP, Pasterkamp G. Innate immune signaling in cardiac ischemia. Nat Rev Cardiol. 2011;8:292–300.
6. Frangogiannis NG. The immune system and the remodeling infarcted heart: cell biological insights and therapeutic opportunities. J Cardiovasc Pharmacol. 2014;63:185–95.
7. Hill JH, Ward PA. The phlogistic role of C3 leukotactic fragments in myocardial infarcts of rats. J Exp Med. 1971;133:885–900.
8. Banz Y, Rieben R. Role of complement and perspectives for intervention in ischemia-reperfusion damage. Ann Med. 2010;44:205–17.
9. Maroko PR, Carpenter CB, Chiariello M, Fishbein MC, Radvany P, Knostman JD, et al. Reduction by cobra venom factor of myocardial necrosis after coronary artery occlusion. J Clin Invest. 1978;61:661–70.
10. Tanhehco EJ, Lee H, Lucchesi BR. Sublytic complement attack reduces infarct size in rabbit isolated hearts: evidence for C5a-mediated cardioprotection. Immunopharmacology. 2000;49:391–9.
11. Zacharowski K, Otto M, Hafner G, Marsh Jr HC, Thiemermann C. Reduction of myocardial infarct size with sCR1sLe(x), an alternatively glycosylated form of human soluble complement receptor type 1 (sCR1), possessing sialyl Lewis x. Br J Pharmacol. 1999;128:945–52.
12. Smith PK, Shernan SK, Chen JC, Carrier M, Verrier ED, Adams PX, et al. Effects of C5 complement inhibitor pexelizumab on outcome in high-risk coronary artery bypass grafting: combined results from the PRIMO-CABG I and II trials. J Thorac Cardiovasc Surg. 2011;142:89–98.
13. Armstrong PW, Granger CB, Adams PX, Hamm C, Holmes Jr D, O'Neill WW, et al. Pexelizumab for acute ST-elevation myocardial infarction in patients undergoing primary percutaneous coronary intervention: a randomized controlled trial. JAMA. 2007;297:43–51.
14. Giordano FJ. Oxygen, oxidative stress, hypoxia, and heart failure. J Clin Invest. 2005;115:500–8.
15. Kleikers PW, Wingler K, Hermans JJ, Diebold I, Altenhofer S, Radermacher KA, et al. NADPH oxidases as a source of oxidative stress and molecular target in ischemia/reperfusion injury. J Mol Med (Berl). 2012;90:1391–406.
16. Xuan YT, Tang XL, Banerjee S, Takano H, Li RC, Han H, et al. Nuclear factor-kappaB plays an essential role in the late phase of ischemic preconditioning in conscious rabbits. Circ Res. 1999;84:1095–109.
17. Jolly SR, Kane WJ, Bailie MB, Abrams GD, Lucchesi BR. Canine myocardial reperfusion injury. Its reduction by the combined administration of superoxide dismutase and catalase. Circ Res. 1984;54:277–85.
18. Obal D, Dai S, Keith R, Dimova N, Kingery J, Zheng YT, et al. Cardiomyocyte-restricted overexpression of extracellular superoxide dismutase increases nitric oxide bioavailability and reduces infarct size after ischemia/reperfusion. Basic Res Cardiol. 2012;107:305.
19. Chen Z, Siu B, Ho YS, Vincent R, Chua CC, Hamdy RC, et al. Overexpression of MnSOD protects against myocardial ischemia/reperfusion injury in transgenic mice. J Mol Cell Cardiol. 1998;30:2281–9.
20. Betge S, Lutz K, Roskos M, Figulla HR. Oral treatment with probucol in a pharmacological dose has no beneficial effects on mortality in chronic ischemic heart failure after large myocardial infarction in rats. Eur J Pharmacol. 2007;558:119–27.
21. Flaherty JT, Pitt B, Gruber JW, Heuser RR, Rothbaum DA, Burwell LR, et al. Recombinant human superoxide dismutase (h-SOD) fails to improve recovery of ventricular function in patients undergoing coronary angioplasty for acute myocardial infarction. Circulation. 1994;89:1982–91.
22. Timmers L, Sluijter JP, van Keulen JK, Hoefer IE, Nederhoff MG, Goumans MJ, et al. Toll-like receptor 4 mediates maladaptive left ventricular remodeling and impairs cardiac function after myocardial infarction. Circ Res. 2008;102:257–64.
23. Arslan F, Smeets MB, O'Neill LA, Keogh B, McGuirk P, Timmers L, et al. Myocardial ischemia/reperfusion injury is mediated by leukocytic toll-like receptor-2 and reduced by systemic administration of a novel anti-toll-like receptor-2 antibody. Circulation. 2010;121:80–90.
24. Lu C, Ren D, Wang X, Ha T, Liu L, Lee EJ, et al. Toll-like receptor 3 plays a role in myocardial infarction and ischemia/reperfusion injury. Biochim Biophys Acta. 1842;2014:22–31.

25. Oyama J, Blais Jr C, Liu X, Pu M, Kobzik L, Kelly RA, et al. Reduced myocardial ischemia-reperfusion injury in toll-like receptor 4-deficient mice. Circulation. 2004;109:784–9.
26. Gordon JW, Shaw JA, Kirshenbaum LA. Multiple facets of NF-kappaB in the heart: to be or not to NF-kappaB. Circ Res. 2011;108:1122–32.
27. Frangogiannis NG, Smith CW, Entman ML. The inflammatory response in myocardial infarction. Cardiovasc Res. 2002;53:31–47.
28. Frangogiannis NG. The role of the chemokines in myocardial ischemia and reperfusion. Curr Vasc Pharmacol. 2004;2:163–74.
29. Frangogiannis NG. Chemokines in the ischemic myocardium: from inflammation to fibrosis. Inflamm Res. 2004;53:585–95.
30. Liehn EA, Tuchscheerer N, Kanzler I, Drechsler M, Fraemohs L, Schuh A, et al. Double-edged role of the CXCL12/CXCR4 axis in experimental myocardial infarction. J Am Coll Cardiol. 2011;58:2415–23.
31. Shiraha H, Glading A, Gupta K, Wells A. IP-10 inhibits epidermal growth factor-induced motility by decreasing epidermal growth factor receptor-mediated calpain activity. J Cell Biol. 1999;146:243–54.
32. Frangogiannis NG, Mendoza LH, Lewallen M, Michael LH, Smith CW, Entman ML. Induction and suppression of interferon-inducible protein 10 in reperfused myocardial infarcts may regulate angiogenesis. FASEB J. 2001;15:1428–30.
33. Bujak M, Dobaczewski M, Gonzalez-Quesada C, Xia Y, Leucker T, Zymek P, et al. Induction of the CXC chemokine interferon-gamma-inducible protein 10 regulates the reparative response following myocardial infarction. Circ Res. 2009;105:973–83.
34. Salcedo R, Ponce ML, Young HA, Wasserman K, Ward JM, Kleinman HK, et al. Human endothelial cells express CCR2 and respond to MCP-1: direct role of MCP-1 in angiogenesis and tumor progression. Blood. 2000;96:34–40.
35. Gharaee-Kermani M, Denholm EM, Phan SH. Costimulation of fibroblast collagen and transforming growth factor beta 1 gene expression by monocyte chemoattractant protein-1 via specific receptors. J Biol Chem. 1996;271:17779–84.
36. Dewald O, Zymek P, Winkelmann K, Koerting A, Ren G, Abou-Khamis T, et al. CCL2/Monocyte Chemoattractant Protein-1 regulates inflammatory responses critical to healing myocardial infarcts. Circ Res. 2005;96:881–9.
37. Bujak M, Dobaczewski M, Chatila K, Mendoza LH, Li N, Reddy A, et al. Interleukin-1 receptor type I signaling critically regulates infarct healing and cardiac remodeling. Am J Pathol. 2008;173:57–67.
38. Herskowitz A, Choi S, Ansari AA, Wesselingh S. Cytokine mRNA expression in postischemic/reperfused myocardium. Am J Pathol. 1995;146:419–28.
39. Kawaguchi M, Takahashi M, Hata T, Kashima Y, Usui F, Morimoto H, et al. Inflammasome activation of cardiac fibroblasts is essential for myocardial ischemia/reperfusion injury. Circulation. 2011;123:594–604.
40. Mezzaroma E, Toldo S, Farkas D, Seropian IM, Van Tassell BW, Salloum FN, et al. The inflammasome promotes adverse cardiac remodeling following acute myocardial infarction in the mouse. Proc Natl Acad Sci U S A. 2011;108:19725–30.
41. Saxena A, Chen W, Su Y, Rai V, Uche OU, Li N, et al. IL-1 Induces Proinflammatory Leukocyte Infiltration and Regulates Fibroblast Phenotype in the Infarcted Myocardium. J Immunol. 2013;191:4838–48.
42. Bujak M, Frangogiannis NG. The role of IL-1 in the pathogenesis of heart disease. Arch Immunol Ther Exp (Warsz). 2009;57:165–76.
43. Frangogiannis NG, Lindsey ML, Michael LH, Youker KA, Bressler RB, Mendoza LH, et al. Resident cardiac mast cells degranulate and release preformed TNF-alpha, initiating the cytokine cascade in experimental canine myocardial ischemia/reperfusion. Circulation. 1998;98:699–710.
44. Maekawa N, Wada H, Kanda T, Niwa T, Yamada Y, Saito K, et al. Improved myocardial ischemia/reperfusion injury in mice lacking tumor necrosis factor-alpha. J Am Coll Cardiol. 2002;39:1229–35.
45. Kurrelmeyer KM, Michael LH, Baumgarten G, Taffet GE, Peschon JJ, Sivasubramanian N, et al. Endogenous tumor necrosis factor protects the adult cardiac myocyte against ischemic-induced apoptosis in a murine model of acute myocardial infarction. Proc Natl Acad Sci U S A. 2000;97:5456–61.
46. Sugano M, Tsuchida K, Hata T, Makino N. In vivo transfer of soluble TNF-alpha receptor 1 gene improves cardiac function and reduces infarct size after myocardial infarction in rats. FASEB J. 2004;18:911–3.
47. Romson JL, Hook BG, Kunkel SL, Abrams GD, Schork MA, Lucchesi BR. Reduction of the extent of ischemic myocardial injury by neutrophil depletion in the dog. Circulation. 1983;67:1016–23.
48. Briaud SA, Ding ZM, Michael LH, Entman ML, Daniel S, Ballantyne CM. Leukocyte trafficking and myocardial reperfusion injury in ICAM-1/P-selectin-knockout mice. Am J Physiol Heart Circ Physiol. 2001;280: H60–7.
49. Middleton J, Patterson AM, Gardner L, Schmutz C, Ashton BA. Leukocyte extravasation: chemokine transport and presentation by the endothelium. Blood. 2002;100:3853–60.
50. Lefer DJ, Shandelya SM, Serrano Jr CV, Becker LC, Kuppusamy P, Zweier JL. Cardioprotective actions of a monoclonal antibody against CD-18 in myocardial ischemia-reperfusion injury. Circulation. 1993;88:1779–87.
51. Faxon DP, Gibbons RJ, Chronos NA, Gurbel PA, Sheehan F. The effect of blockade of the CD11/CD18 integrin receptor on infarct size in patients with acute myocardial infarction treated with direct angioplasty: the results of the HALT-MI study. J Am Coll Cardiol. 2002;40:1199–204.
52. Nahrendorf M, Swirski FK. Monocyte and macrophage heterogeneity in the heart. Circ Res. 2013;112:1624–33.
53. Nahrendorf M, Swirski FK, Aikawa E, Stangenberg L, Wurdinger T, Figueiredo JL, et al. The healing myocardium sequentially mobilizes two monocyte

subsets with divergent and complementary functions. J Exp Med. 2007;204:3037–47.
54. Swirski FK, Nahrendorf M, Etzrodt M, Wildgruber M, Cortez-Retamozo V, Panizzi P, et al. Identification of splenic reservoir monocytes and their deployment to inflammatory sites. Science. 2009;325:612–6.
55. Ismahil MA, Hamid T, Bansal SS, Patel B, Kingery JR, Prabhu SD. Remodeling of the mononuclear phagocyte network underlies chronic inflammation and disease progression in heart failure: critical importance of the cardiosplenic axis. Circ Res. 2014; 114:266–82.
56. Frangogiannis NG, Mendoza LH, Ren G, Akrivakis S, Jackson PL, Michael LH, et al. MCSF expression is induced in healing myocardial infarcts and may regulate monocyte and endothelial cell phenotype. Am J Physiol Heart Circ Physiol. 2003;285:H483–92.
57. Frangogiannis NG, Perrard JL, Mendoza LH, Burns AR, Lindsey ML, Ballantyne CM, et al. Stem cell factor induction is associated with mast cell accumulation after canine myocardial ischemia and reperfusion. Circulation. 1998;98:687–98.
58. Somasundaram P, Ren G, Nagar H, Kraemer D, Mendoza L, Michael LH, et al. Mast cell tryptase may modulate endothelial cell phenotype in healing myocardial infarcts. J Pathol. 2005;205:102–11.
59. Cochain C, Auvynet C, Poupel L, Vilar J, Dumeau E, Richart A, et al. The chemokine decoy receptor D6 prevents excessive inflammation and adverse ventricular remodeling after myocardial infarction. Arterioscler Thromb Vasc Biol. 2012;32:2206–13.
60. Kobayashi K, Hernandez LD, Galan JE, Janeway Jr CA, Medzhitov R, Flavell RA. IRAK-M is a negative regulator of Toll-like receptor signaling. Cell. 2002; 110:191–202.
61. Chen W, Saxena A, Li N, Sun J, Gupta A, Lee DW, et al. Endogenous IRAK-M attenuates postinfarction remodeling through effects on macrophages and fibroblasts. Arterioscler Thromb Vasc Biol. 2012;32: 2598–608.
62. Dobaczewski M, Chen W, Frangogiannis NG. Transforming growth factor (TGF)-beta signaling in cardiac remodeling. J Mol Cell Cardiol. 2011;51: 600–6.
63. Dean RG, Balding LC, Candido R, Burns WC, Cao Z, Twigg SM, et al. Connective tissue growth factor and cardiac fibrosis after myocardial infarction. J Histochem Cytochem. 2005;53:1245–56.
64. Ikeuchi M, Tsutsui H, Shiomi T, Matsusaka H, Matsushima S, Wen J, et al. Inhibition of TGF-beta signaling exacerbates early cardiac dysfunction but prevents late remodeling after infarction. Cardiovasc Res. 2004;64:526–35.
65. Kempf T, Zarbock A, Widera C, Butz S, Stadtmann A, Rossaint J, et al. GDF-15 is an inhibitor of leukocyte integrin activation required for survival after myocardial infarction in mice. Nat Med. 2011;17:581–8.
66. Frangogiannis NG, Mendoza LH, Lindsey ML, Ballantyne CM, Michael LH, Smith CW, et al. IL-10 is induced in the reperfused myocardium and may modulate the reaction to injury. J Immunol. 2000; 165:2798–808.
67. Lacraz S, Nicod LP, Chicheportiche R, Welgus HG, Dayer JM. IL-10 inhibits metalloproteinase and stimulates TIMP-1 production in human mononuclear phagocytes. J Clin Invest. 1995;96:2304–10.
68. Yang Z, Zingarelli B, Szabo C. Crucial role of endogenous interleukin-10 production in myocardial ischemia/reperfusion injury. Circulation. 2000;101:1019–26.
69. Zymek P, Nah DY, Bujak M, Ren G, Koerting A, Leucker T, et al. Interleukin-10 is not a critical regulator of infarct healing and left ventricular remodeling. Cardiovasc Res. 2007;74:313–22.
70. Dobaczewski M, de Haan JJ, Frangogiannis NG. The extracellular matrix modulates fibroblast phenotype and function in the infarcted myocardium. J Cardiovasc Transl Res. 2012;5:837–47.
71. Huebener P, Abou-Khamis T, Zymek P, Bujak M, Ying X, Chatila K, et al. CD44 is critically involved in infarct healing by regulating the inflammatory and fibrotic response. J Immunol. 2008;180:2625–33.
72. Frangogiannis NG. Matricellular proteins in cardiac adaptation and disease. Physiol Rev. 2012;92:635–88.
73. Frangogiannis NG, Ren G, Dewald O, Zymek P, Haudek S, Koerting A, et al. Critical role of endogenous thrombospondin-1 in preventing expansion of healing myocardial infarcts. Circulation. 2005;111: 2935–42.
74. Wan E, Yeap XY, Dehn S, Terry R, Novak M, Zhang S, et al. Enhanced efferocytosis of apoptotic cardiomyocytes through myeloid-epithelial-reproductive tyrosine kinase links acute inflammation resolution to cardiac repair after infarction. Circ Res. 2013;113:1004–12.
75. Zouggari Y, Ait-Oufella H, Bonnin P, Simon T, Sage AP, Guerin C, et al. B lymphocytes trigger monocyte mobilization and impair heart function after acute myocardial infarction. Nat Med. 2013;19:1273–80.
76. Anzai A, Anzai T, Nagai S, Maekawa Y, Naito K, Kaneko H, et al. Regulatory role of dendritic cells in postinfarction healing and left ventricular remodeling. Circulation. 2012;125:1234–45.
77. Jung K, Kim P, Leuschner F, Gorbatov R, Kim JK, Ueno T, et al. Endoscopic time-lapse imaging of immune cells in infarcted mouse hearts. Circ Res. 2013;112:891–9.
78. van der Laan AM, Ter Horst EN, Delewi R, Begieneman MP, Krijnen PA, Hirsch A, et al. Monocyte subset accumulation in the human heart following acute myocardial infarction and the role of the spleen as monocyte reservoir. Eur Heart J. 2014; 35:376–85.
79. Tsujioka H, Imanishi T, Ikejima H, Kuroi A, Takarada S, Tanimoto T, et al. Impact of heterogeneity of human peripheral blood monocyte subsets on myocardial salvage in patients with primary acute myocardial infarction. J Am Coll Cardiol. 2009;54:130–8.
80. Yan X, Anzai A, Katsumata Y, Matsuhashi T, Ito K, Endo J, et al. Temporal dynamics of cardiac immune cell accumulation following acute myocardial infarction. J Mol Cell Cardiol. 2013;62:24–35.

81. Dobaczewski M, Xia Y, Bujak M, Gonzalez-Quesada C, Frangogiannis NG. CCR5 signaling suppresses inflammation and reduces adverse remodeling of the infarcted heart, mediating recruitment of regulatory T cells. Am J Pathol. 2010;176:2177–87.
82. Tang TT, Yuan J, Zhu ZF, Zhang WC, Xiao H, Xia N, et al. Regulatory T cells ameliorate cardiac remodeling after myocardial infarction. Basic Res Cardiol. 2012;107:232.
83. Shinde AV, Frangogiannis NG. Fibroblasts in myocardial infarction: a role in inflammation and repair. J Mol Cell Cardiol. 2014;70:74–82.
84. Squires CE, Escobar GP, Payne JF, Leonardi RA, Goshorn DK, Sheats NJ, et al. Altered fibroblast function following myocardial infarction. J Mol Cell Cardiol. 2005;39:699–707.
85. Shinde AV, Frangogiannis NG. Fibroblasts in myocardial infarction: A role in inflammation and repair. J Mol Cell Cardiol. 2014;70C:74–82.
86. Abbate A, Kontos MC, Grizzard JD, Biondi-Zoccai GG, Van Tassell BW, Robati R, et al. Interleukin-1 blockade with anakinra to prevent adverse cardiac remodeling after acute myocardial infarction (Virginia Commonwealth University Anakinra Remodeling Trial [VCU-ART] Pilot study). Am J Cardiol. 2010;105: 1371–1377.e1.
87. Bujak M, Frangogiannis NG. The role of TGF-beta signaling in myocardial infarction and cardiac remodeling. Cardiovasc Res. 2007;74:184–95.
88. Rohr S. Arrhythmogenic implications of fibroblast-myocyte interactions. Circ Arrhythm Electrophysiol. 2012;5:442–52.
89. Cochain C, Channon KM, Silvestre JS. Angiogenesis in the infarcted myocardium. Antioxid Redox Signal. 2013;18:1100–13.
90. Fukuda S, Kaga S, Sasaki H, Zhan L, Zhu L, Otani H, et al. Angiogenic signal triggered by ischemic stress induces myocardial repair in rat during chronic infarction. J Mol Cell Cardiol. 2004;36:547–59.
91. Dobaczewski M, Frangogiannis NG. Chemokines and cardiac fibrosis. Front Biosci (Schol Ed). 2009;1: 391–405.
92. Katare R, Riu F, Mitchell K, Gubernator M, Campagnolo P, Cui Y, et al. Transplantation of human pericyte progenitor cells improves the repair of infarcted heart through activation of an angiogenic program involving micro-RNA-132. Circ Res. 2011;109: 894–906.
93. Ren G, Michael LH, Entman ML, Frangogiannis NG. Morphological characteristics of the microvasculature in healing myocardial infarcts. J Histochem Cytochem. 2002;50:71–9.
94. Dobaczewski M, Akrivakis S, Nasser K, Michael LH, Entman ML, Frangogiannis NG. Vascular mural cells in healing canine myocardial infarcts. J Histochem Cytochem. 2004;52:1019–29.
95. Roberts R, DeMello V, Sobel BE. Deleterious effects of methylprednisolone in patients with myocardial infarction. Circulation. 1976;53:I204–6.
96. de Lemos JA, Morrow DA, Blazing MA, Jarolim P, Wiviott SD, Sabatine MS, et al. Serial measurement of monocyte chemoattractant protein-1 after acute coronary syndromes: results from the A to Z trial. J Am Coll Cardiol. 2007;50:2117–24.
97. Carrabba N, Valenti R, Parodi G, Santoro GM, Antoniucci D. Left ventricular remodeling and heart failure in diabetic patients treated with primary angioplasty for acute myocardial infarction. Circulation. 2004;110:1974–9.
98. Aronson D, Musallam A, Lessick J, Dabbah S, Carasso S, Hammerman H, et al. Impact of diastolic dysfunction on the development of heart failure in diabetic patients after acute myocardial infarction. Circ Heart Fail. 2010;3:125–31.

Pathways to Cardiac Remodeling

17

Bernard Swynghedauw

Abstract

"Re-modelling" implies changes which result in the re-arrangement of normally existing structures. The present review focuses only on permanent modifications in relation to clinical dysfunction in cardiac remodelling (CR) secondary to myocardial infarction and/or arterial hypertension, and includes a special chapter on the senescent heart, since it is mainly a disease of the elderly.

From a biological point of view CR is determined by (i) the general process of adaptation which allows both the myocyte and the collagen network to adapt to new working conditions; (ii) ventricular fibrosis, i.e. increased collagen concentration, which is multifactorial and caused by ischemia, senescence, diabetes, various hormones and inflammatory processes; (iii) cell death, a parameter linked to fibrosis, is usually due to necrosis and apoptosis, and occurs in nearly all models of CR.

The process of adaptation is associated with various changes in genetic expression, including a general activation which causes hypertrophy, isogenic shifts which result in the appearance of a slow isomyosin and a new Na^+, K^+ ATPase with a low affinity for sodium, reactivation of genes encoding for ANF and the renin-angiotensin system, and a diminished concentration of SERCA, -adrenergic receptors and the K^+ channel responsible for I_{to}.

The senescent heart is a remodelled heart sharing many similarities with cardiac hypertrophy in the compensated state. Nevertheless, the phenotype of these two remodelled hearts differs in some crucial points. The senescent heart is indeed much more fibrotic and arrhythmogenic, and has several specificities.

B. Swynghedauw, PhD, MD
INSERM, U 942-INSERM Hôpital Lariboisière,
Paris 75475, France
e-mail: Bernard.Swynghedauw@inserm.fr

D.V. Cokkinos (ed.), *Introduction to Translational Cardiovascular Research*,
DOI 10.1007/978-3-319-08798-6_17, © Springer International Publishing Switzerland 2015

From a clinical point of view, fibrosis is for the moment a major marker for HF, and a crucial determinant of myocardial heterogeneity, increasing diastolic stiffness, and the propensity for reentry arrhythmias. In addition, systolic dysfunction is facilitated by slowing of the calcium transient and the down-regulation of the entire adrenergic system. Modifications of intracellular calcium movements are the main determinants of the triggered activity and automaticity which cause arrhythmias and alterations in relaxation.

Keywords
Cardiac remodeling • Cardiac torsion – Cardiocytes Cardiac hypertrophy • Laplace law • Initial shortening velocity • Muscle economy • Adaptation Senescent heart • Myocardial fibrosis

Abbreviations

ANF	Atrial natriuretic factor
AP	Action potential
	ATPase of the Sarcoplasmic Reticulum
BNP	Brain-natriuretic factor
CR	Cardiac remodeling
EC	Endothelial cells
ECG	Electrocardiogram
HF	Heart Failure
HYP	Hypertrophy
LV	Left ventricular
MI	Myocardial infarction
MMPs	Matrix Metalloproteinases
NYHA	New York Heart Association
PP	Phenotypic plasticity
QT	QT interval duration
SERCA	Sarcoplasmic reticulum calcium ATPase
TIMP	Tissue Inhibitors of MMP

17.1 Definitions

Re-modelling qualifies changes which result in the re-arrangement of normally existing structures. The above-definition includes gestational and developmental aspects, and also the so-called physiological cardiac hypertrophy which follows intensive exercise. Cardiac remodelling, (CR), concerns the two components of the cardiovascular system, namely the coronary vessels and the myocardium itself. In current practice myocardium remodelling is mainly utilised to describe the changes in cardiac structures that followed myocardial infarction, (MI.) The word was subsequently extended and used to qualify a variety of conditions including pure mechanical overload, as well as hypertensive, valvular cardiopathy, familial hypertrophic and dilated cardiomyopathy. Transgenic manipulations [1], experimental or clinical hormonal influence (i.e. due to thyroxin, angiotensin II, or aldosterone) [2] are also able to remodel the myocardium. CR is, at least in part, a reversible process. This has considerable links to clinical and basic pharmacology and has been extensively reviewed [2–11].

CR is triggered by mechanical stretch; nevertheless after myocardial ischemia there are also several different factors including the changes directly induced by ischemia, diabetes, obesity, senescence, hormones and vasoactive peptides, which can modify the consequences of the mechanical factor. Currently, the most common clinical situation during which remodelling is known to occur is a rather complex biological mixture of stretch due to mechanical overload, aging, myocardial ischemia, stress due myocardial scar and increased plasma levels of hormones or vasoactive peptides. An additional factor has to be listed, namely the unknown signal which provides to the heart the information concerning the amount of substance which has been lost after a MI.

17.2 Cellular Remodeling

The first demonstration that, in adults, cardiac myocytes (Fig. 17.1) hypertrophy (HYP) and cardiac non-muscular cells both hypertrophy and divide by mitosis in response to cardiac overload was made using thymidine-labelling in the laboratory of Murray Rabinowitz and Radovan Zak [3]. This finding provided the basis for the general belief that postnatal growth of cardiocytes occurs through myocyte hypertrophy, and that cardiac myocytes are terminally differentiated cells which are unable to re-enter the cell cycle. In contrast, in the non muscle cells, which include both fibroblasts and endothelial cells (EC), a hyperplastic component persists. Then during mechanical overloading the heart hypertrophies and this process is due to cardiocyte HYP. This was the credo in cell cardiology during 30 years despite the repeated observations of rare mitotic figures and several polyploid cardiocytes, mainly in very bulky human hearts (references quoted in Ref. [6]). These mitotic images do not necessarily mean that cardiocytes multiply; there are many other explanations, nevertheless the above-credo remains alive for many years.

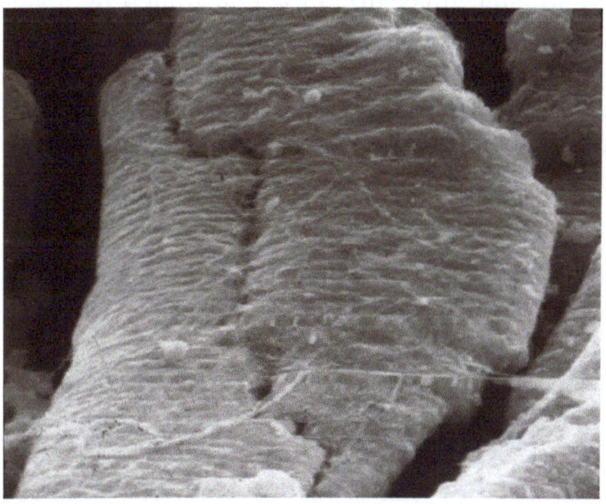

Fig. 17.1 Electron micrograph of an isolated adult cardiocyte

A second thesis was supported since a long time by the group of Piero Anversa [12] (Fig. 17.2). According to Anversa cardiocytes remain able to multiply during all their life and are still capable to regenerate, even in old persons. In addition, there are a substantial amount of stem cells within the heart and these stem cells remain active in adult and even in aged hearts, which may have practical consequences for regenerative surgery. A technological revolution has recently bring strong support to this view, the retrospective C^{14} cellular birth dating. Surprisingly such a revolution was due to the Cold War and the nuclear

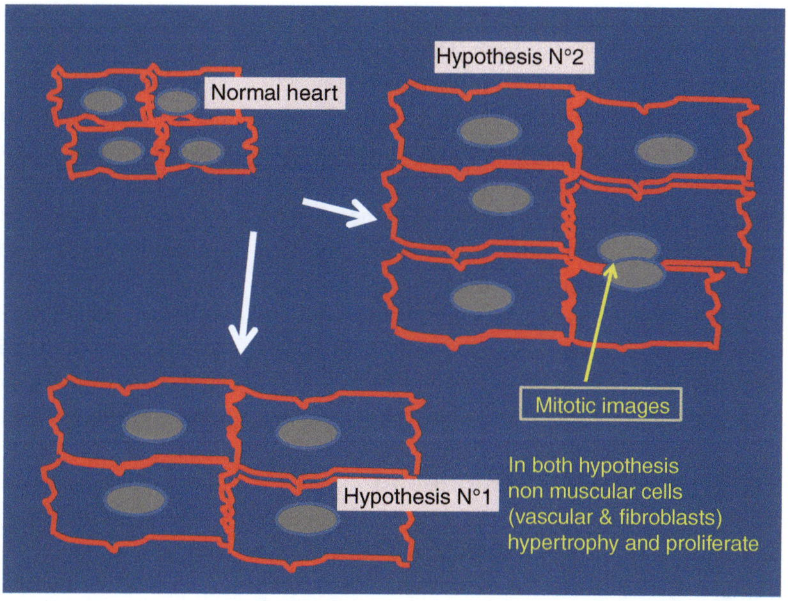

Fig. 17.2 The two hypothesis concerning the role of cardiocyte hypertrophy. Hypothesis N°1 is from Zak and Rabinowitz's Group [3] hypothesis N° 2 is that of Anversa et al. [12]

bomb [13, 14]. Before the Cold War the atmospheric radioactive C^{14} concentration was very low and stable. In 1963, the occurrence of nuclear assays acutely enhanced this concentration. In 1970, nuclear assays stopped which results in an exponential decay in atmospheric concentration in the isotope. C^{14} is found in every tissue of individuals born after this date [13] and it is therefore possible to quantitate the turn-over of a given category of cells providing the method to quantitate the radioactive compound is sensitive enough. The group of Anversa was able to measure the turn-over of cardiocytes on human hearts and found that, approximately, the age of these cardiocytes was 8 months in children, 8 years in adults and 2 years and a half in aged persons. The conclusion was that the turn-over rate of aged cardiocytes is accelerated (probably by the increased aortic impedance that causes an impedance mechanical overload in aged hearts, see below [15]). In addition, they found that, between the age of 20 and 80 years cardiocytes, EC and fibroblasts of the myocardium were respectively replaced 8, 6 and 8 times. Mechanical overload enhances this turn-over rate.

Cardiocyte HYP is the result of a sarcomeric reorganisation. Dilation of the heart is associated with myocyte lengthening mediated by the generation of new sarcomeres in series. The result is a pronounced enhancement of the length/width ratio of the myocytes. The same phenomenon is observed in the rat 2 or 6 days after birth. This would suggest that during CR a foetal gene program involving activation of the cytoskeletal proteins is initiated which regulates the overall shape of the myocyte by preferentially directing lengthening of the cell. In contrast, HYP of cardiocytes is the result of the addition of new sarcomeres in parallel. Such a hypothesis is favoured by the observation made by J.-L. Samuel et al. showing a reversible rearrangement of the microtubular network during the early stage of cardiac overload [16].

17.2.1 Anatomical Remodeling

The current belief that the heart is a sphere or a rugby balloon, is against evidence. The human heart and the bird heart, are more like a mop and hypertrophy or dilatation are not simply an exaggeration of the balloon structure but have also modified the structure of the mop. Ventricles do not contract homogeneously; during contraction the apex does not move despite the fact that it is free, while the basis, that is attached, is moving periodically up and down. The diastolic filling cannot be explained using the balloon image and requires a model in which filling is an active process and this is the case in such a model: In Spain, an anatomist named F. Torrent-Guasp provided the response by showing that in fact the ventricular myocardium is constituted by a single contractile band that is submitted during embryogenesis to several modifications. The final result is a double helix structure of the ventricles [17, 18]. It is possible to quantify the torsion of the heart [19], but such a measure is not routinely performed despite the fact that this likely to provide a better estimation of myocardial performance than the classical ejection fraction.

The contractile band is unique and begins below the pulmonary artery and then takes a rightward direction to form the right ventricle, the posterior wall of the left ventricle, followed by the descending and the ascending fibers of the left ventricle to end as an apical loop; the subepicardium becomes subendocardium during the formation of the loop [17, 20]. CR strongly modifies the "mop" structure of the heart, especially during dilatation. Fibers progressively lose their helicoidal shape by becoming parallel which per se will seriously impair the contractile performance. The mop effect is also strongly attenuated by fibrotic bands and the loss of homogeneity [17].

The increase in left ventricular (LV) mass and volume is accompanied by a change in the shape of the ventricle. If the process is triggered by a MI, the remodelling is asymmetric and is associated with infarct expansion. Early ventricular remodelling following coronary occlusion is dominated by infarct expansion which is an acute dilation caused by death and slippage of the myocytes; it dramatically alters ventricular volume and geometry.

Ventricular remodelling after MI is the result of infarct expansion and volume-overload hypertrophy

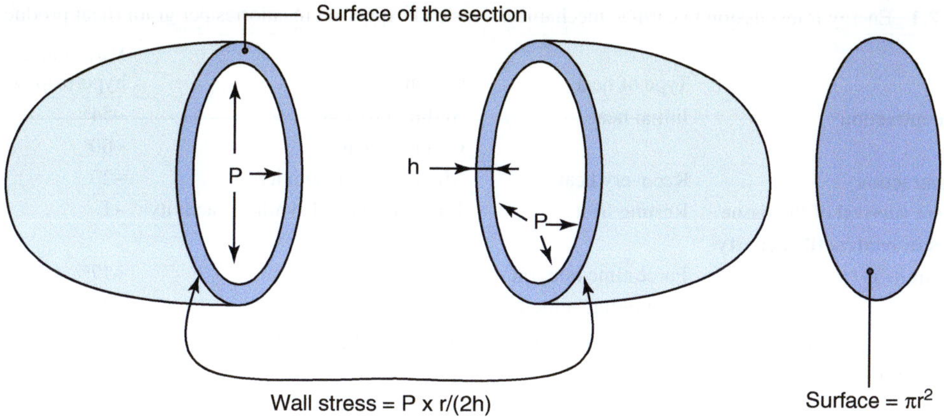

Fig. 17.3 The Laplace law: dilatation of the heart requires hypertrophy to maintain a normal wall stress

of non-infarcted myocardium. Later on CR is associated to additional enlargement and sphericity of the ventricle, a decrease in stroke volume and impaired diastolic filling [this aspect of remodeling has been developed in 7]. Systolic impairment secondary to the loss of contractile material results in an increased end-systolic volume, an increased cardiac size and a secondary augmentation of the diastolic filling pressure and distensibility. As the fibrosis increases, the distensibility decreases resulting in an increase in diastolic pressure and volume. Peripheral mechanisms including vasoconstriction subsequently increase both preload and afterload; this produces an increased wall stress and a progressive thinning of the area. Simultaneously in non-infarcted segments, elevation of the end-diastolic stress causes volume-overload HYP which tends to normalise the wall stress according to Laplace's law. The extent and location of the infarction, therapy or associated diseases, may considerably modify remodelling [21]. Ventricular HYP remains symmetric and concentric when the cause of CR is pressure overload due to arterial hypertension or aortic stenosis, by contrast volume overload creates dilatation and renders the fibers more parallel and attenuates the loop structure [7].

17.2.1.1 Physiological Mechanisms of Adaptation

In every organ or organism, the so-called "phenotypic plasticity" is a general mechanism widely utilized in nature to adapt organs to new environmental conditions [8, 22]. In muscle physiology, biological adaptation is an evolutionary process by which an organ structure, i.e. the structure of a muscle is modified to obtain a thermodynamic status adapted to the new mechanical conditions. Skeletal or cardiac muscles are equally "plastic" and equally capable to adapt to changes in chronic loading conditions by both increasing the contractile mass and modifying their maximum shortening velocity. In terms of economy, the myocardium is slightly continuously different from the skeletal muscle: (i) it has indeed to contract day and night and then requires a highly efficient oxygen-dependent source of energy as mitochondria; (ii) it has a more or less "spheric shape" as already described, and as such respond to the Laplace law (Fig. 17.3).

In the heart, changing loading conditions, for example during pressure overload after aortic stenosis, is just like increasing the load on a skeletal muscle fiber (or the load on a car). To maintain contraction (or, for the car, to pursue the trip), the cardiac contraction velocity becomes slower (the driver has to slow his car), and, in the same time, the muscle economy (the amount of work per mol of Adenosine Tri-Phosphate, ATP) drops [5].

This adaptation process begins very rapidly and is dominated by several changes in genetic expression which allow the heart to recover a normal economy and to maintain a normal contraction for a long period of time. Quantitative modifications lead to cardiac hypertrophy, and, according to Laplace's law, will normalise the wall stress (Fig. 17.3). Simultaneously, molecular

Table 17.1 Energy transmission in cardiac mechanical overload expressed in calories per gram (heat produced)

	Type of heat	Origin	Variation in hypertrophy (%)
During contraction	Initial heat	Sliding process	−54[a]
		Ca movements	−60[a]
After contraction	Recovery heat	Mitochondrial activity	−20
Permanent survival of the tissue	Resting heat	Ionic milieu and synthesis activity	−1
Changes in contractile activity			
Force (N/mm^2)	Force-time integral		+17[a]
	Shortening velocity		−48[a]

This schematic view has been rearranged from the different data published by N. Alpert
[a]Highly significant

changes will allow the myocardial fibre to contract more slowly and to recover a normal economy by having a lower maximum shortening velocity, Vmax (see further) [5]. The permanent changes in genetic expression simultaneously have, even at the beginning, both beneficial effects in terms of muscular economy and detrimental, or even useless, consequences. Heart Failure, (HF), when it occurs, indicates the limits of the process of biological adaptation.

Such a change in the phenotype is the same in a variety of conditions, including foetal development, volume and pressure-overload, senescence or hypothyroidism. The same programme is always used simply because this is the only developmental program available in the heart; (in contrast, in the skeletal muscle, two programs are available, a foetal and an embryonic program, they both are re-expressed during mechanical overload [23]).

17.2.2 Cardiac Hypertrophy

Cardiac HYP enables the heart to adapt the new working conditions by both multiplying the contractile units and reducing the wall stress according to Laplace's law. The activation of protein synthesis is a rapid and rather homogeneous phenomenon, it belongs the foetal reprogramming as well, and, for example, the first signs of an activated synthesis can be observed within half an hour after banding the aorta of a rabbit [4] (Tables 17.1 and 17.2). Others have shown that total protein, myosin, myoglobin, and collagen synthesis, were activated after 3 h of increased aortic pressure. The accumulation of total proteins or myosin is due to an increased rate of synthesis, nevertheless the rate of degradation is also augmented in parallel; such a paradoxical wasting effect is a general feature in protein metabolism [references in 6].

Table 17.2 The fetal reprogramming in cardiac overload

Changes in gene expression	Consequences
Global increase in gene expression	Hypertrophy and normalization of wall stress
Activation of microRNAs (non coding)	Fine tuning of the foetal program
Genes induced or re-expressed	
Increased expression of beta myosin heavy chain, ANF and BNP, neuronal NO synthase and caveoline; anaerobic switch (LDH-M, CK-B)	Decreased myosin ATPase and Vmax; decreased exercise performances, better recovery period Increased Economy
Increased alpha-3 subunit of Na-K-ATPase	Decreased Na affinity
Increased genes coding the apoptotic pathway	"Eat-me" signal occurs at the early beginning after an overload
Genes expression blunted (the concentration of the corresponding protein diminishes)	
Ca-ATPase of SR (SERCA2), early transient K current It0, alpha myosin heavy chain;	Increased action potential duration and relaxation time
Beta-1 adrenergic and muscarinic receptor	Decreased contractility during exercise
Myoglobin	Participates in the anaerobic switch

17.2.2.1 Thermodynamic Adaptation

In order to quantitate the economy of a system, it is necessary to measure the mechanical performance indices such as force, or force/time integrals, or work (economy is then termed efficiency) and the corresponding energy flux. The energy flux can be quantitated by measuring ATP, or oxygen consumption, or heat production (the heat production is an index of economy according to the second Carnot principle in thermodynamic, see [5] for further explanations). A major technical progress was made following the invention of a microthermopile which allowed N. Alpert's group to measure heat production on a rabbit papillary muscle as well as in strips of human cardiac muscle on a beat-to-beat basis.

The heart, as any other muscle, utilizes energy: (i) for the simple survival of the tissue, such as protein synthesis and ion movements ("resting heat"); (ii) resynthesis of the high-energy phosphate stores which mainly occurs in mitochondria, but can depend on the anaerobic glycolytic pathway during ischemia ("recovery heat"); (iii) contraction ("initial heat"), including ATP hydrolysis for cross-bridge cycling ("tension-dependent initial heat"), and excitation-contraction coupling ("tension-independent initial heat") (Table 17.1).

The fundamental process of adaptation which occurs during mechanical overload, both in human and in experimental models, includes a slowing of Vmax with a diminution of the heat produced per g of active tension during contraction. Both the resting and recovery heats remain unchanged. Special experimental protocols allow one to partition heat produced by the sliding process, from that produced by the movement of calcium and the activity of the different calcium pumps. Both systems are used during contraction and both function more economically during cardiac HYP in animal models and in end-stage HF in humans [5].

To conclude: (i) the reduction in Vmax is the main basic process responsible for myocardial adaptation to mechanical overload. Thermodynamic data has suggest that this reduction is due to a decreased recruitment of myosin cross-bridges. Such modifications already exist in the compensated stage. (ii) In sharp contrast with the current bedside opinion, the diminution of Vmax (the initial shortening velocity, which is also the maximum shortening velocity and is obtained by extrapolation of the shortening velocity/load curve) has a beneficial event at least at the myofiber level, since it allows the cardiac fiber to contract at a normal energy cost. Nevertheless at the organ level the diminution of Vmax is also the first step which will finally lead to a decrease in cardiac output and finally to failure. (iii) Perturbed mitochondrial oxidative phosphorylation or anaerobic energy metabolism are both unlikely candidates to cause HF since the "recovery heat" remains unchanged (despite a non statistically significant 20 % decrease) even during end-stage HF in dilated cardiomyopathy. Hence, investigations concerning the adaptational process have to focus on energy utilisation rather than energy production (Table 17.1).

17.3 Molecular Remodeling

The necessary foetal reprogramming is directly triggered by the mechanical effect; mechanotransduction is a general evolutionary process which exists also in plants and finally results in foetal reprogramming. There are several clinical tools that allow the clinician to fully appreciate this mechanism.

17.3.1 The Foetal Reprogramming

The foetal program is the only alternative available for the myocardium, and, by chance (!), it allows the muscle to have a slower maximum shortening velocity (Vmax, the shortening velocity for an unloaded muscle) which will improve economy and, from a thermodynamic point of view, allows the adaptation process to occur. The foetal program includes the reprogramming of genes that have been expressed during the foetal life and were blunted during adulthood, as the isomyosin shift. The shift results in the expression of the slow form of isomyosin, the beta isomyosin with a low ATPase that corresponds to the slow maximum contractile velocity, Vmax

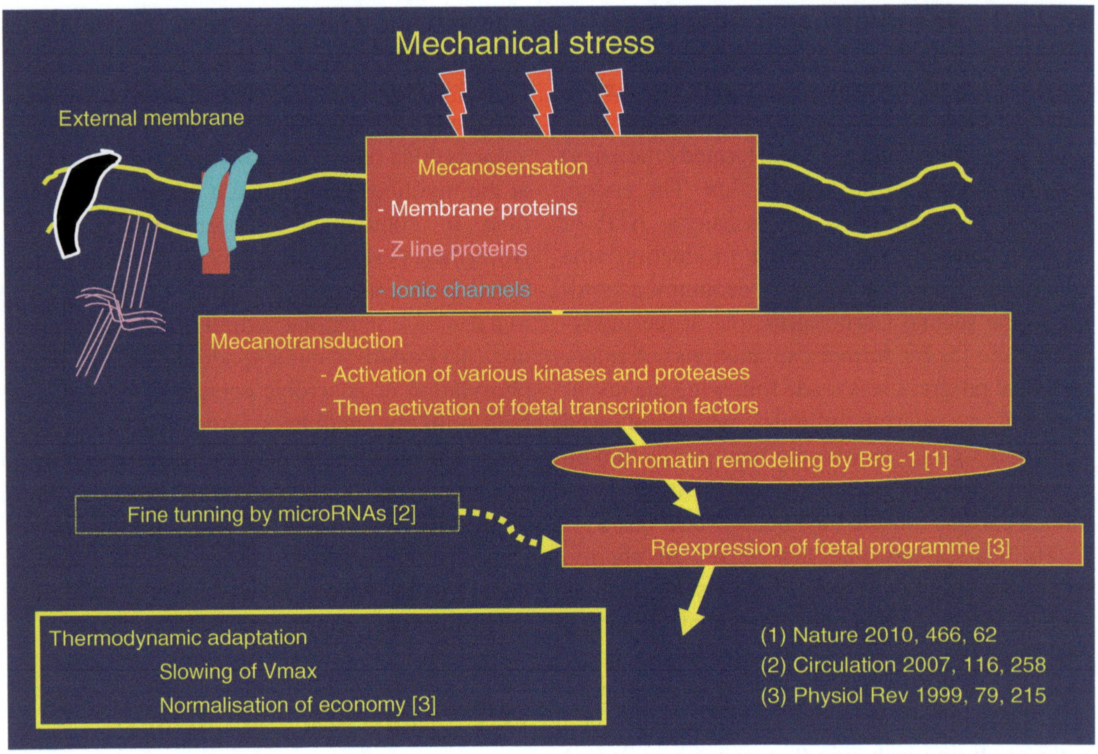

Fig. 17.4 Mechanosensation and mechanotransduction

[24]. It also includes both the reactivation of a program still expressed during normal adulthood as synthesis of the collagen and contractile proteins (that finally causes cardiac hypertrophy), and the non activation of genes that are not activated in the foetus, which will result in a diminution of the concentration (per g of tissue) of the corresponding protein, a receptor for example. They include genes encoding the beta adrenergic receptors, some potassium channels (see following paragraph) and the calcium activated ATPase of the Sarcoplasmic Reticulum, SERCA [25]. The changes in SERCA were not the only modifications in membrane proteins that were responsible for the adaptation of the intracellular calcium movements, others exist (see Table 17.2).

17.3.2 Mechanosensation and Mechanotransduction

The myocardial cells are able to sense mechanical stimuli and, by so-doing, to reactivate the foetal program. The so-called mechanosensation allows mechanical stimuli to stimulate nuclear sensors (Fig. 17.4). Some of these transcription factors were already identified as factors used during normal development or after hormonal induction. Others have been recently discovered including various kinases but also various microRNAs which may, potentially, have a clinical interest, in other disease states they can currently be measured in the blood.

Several groups have evidenced that numerous microRNAS are able to promote HYP and that it is possible to inhibit the hypertrophic process either by using transgenic knock-out of microRNA genes or by using specific “antagomirs”. In addition one group has shown an increased expression of dozen of microRNA after cardiac overloading. Interestingly the microRNAs that were overexpressed were the same described during cardiac development which represents a new argument in favor of the foetal reprogramming. It is generally accepted that microRNAs do not control the general process of adaptation but constitute a sort of fine tuning of the gene expression in this condition [26–28].

17.3.3 Clinical Markers of Reprogramming

Two markers are easily available: the plasma levels of the atrial natriuretic factor, ANF, or the brain-natriuretic factor, BNP, and the QT internal duration (QT).

ANF has been discovered by Hatt in 1976 [29]. It forms small grains in normal atria and is physiologically regulated by water availability. Mechanical overload induces the ventricular expression of genes coding for ANF and is responsible for the enhanced plasma levels of ANF. BNP is normally expressed in both atria and ventricles and mechanical overload also enhances its plasma level of BNP is a more sensitive biomarker for mechanical overload and has now been widely adopted by clinicians. An enhanced level of BNP indicates cardiac overload and, *stricto* sensu, is not a marker of HF as generally believed. *Stricto* sensu, the definition of HF is indeed purely functional and does not include an elevated plasma level of BNP (or ANF).

Another, frequently forgotten, direct marker of the adaptational process is the lengthening of the QT interval in the electrocardiogram (ECG), and its equivalent on action potential (AP), the lengthening of the action potential duration. The increased QT (or QTc, if corrected for heart rate) interval duration in the ECG and the enhanced action potential duration in isolated cardiomyocytes are well-documented characteristics of the hypertrophied heart and cardiocyte. The AP potential shape and duration depends on the activity of several ion channels and can increase either when an outward current is depressed or when an inward current is enhanced. The modifications of these current activities result from changes in the expression of genes encoding ion channels. These genes were not expressed in the foetus. Acquired modifications of the repolarisation time reflect the adaptational response compensating for the mechanical overload such as the isomyosin shift. An important contribution concerning CR was the discovery that the electrophysiological modifications of the two components of the transient outwork K^+ current Ito, Ito-s (regulating slow recovery from inactivation) and Ito-f (regulating fast recovery from inactivation), reflect changes in the genetic expression of the corresponding K^+ channels at the level of both the protein and the mRNA. The expression of Kv1.4 and Kv2.1, which are genes encoding Ito-s, and that of Kv4.2, which is the gene encoding Ito-f, are decreased by 60 and 54 % respectively suggesting that the diminution of Ito, and the corresponding lengthening of both action potential and QT are in fact transcriptionally regulated and participate in the adaptational process. During HF in humans convincing reports have shown that the prolongation of the duration of the AP is, at least in part, caused by I_{to} since 3 mM 4-aminopyridine, a specific inhibitor of I_{to}, does not entirely restore a normal duration. Moreover, there is a co-ordinated decrease in I_{to} and I_{K1}. The delayed rectifier is hardly detectable and plays only a minor role in the human cardiocyte [see detailed references in 30].

17.3.4 Deleterious Aspects of Cardiac Remodeling

The less controversial definition of HF is "ventricular dysfunction with symptoms" [31] which means that HF is a disease state with both abnormalities in the myocardial structure (i.e. CR) and clinical symptoms due to fluid retention. The severity of the disease is commonly appreciated using the New York Heart Association (NYHA) classification which is entirely based on functional symptoms. HF indicates the limits of the adaptational process and also the development of myocardial fibrosis which is an additional deleterious process linked to the new determinants of CR, including senescence, diabetes, and ischemia. Therefore CR is both beneficial and deleterious, the so-called Yin and Yang paradox.

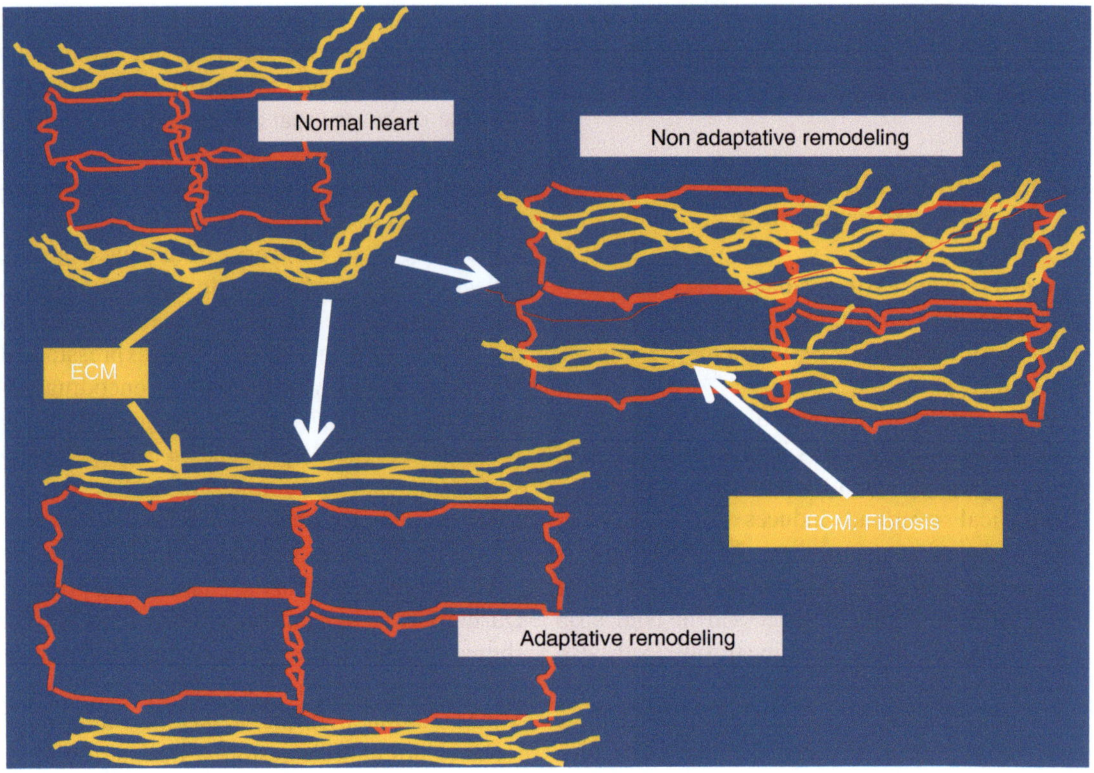

Fig. 17.5 Role of fibrosis in cardiac remodeling

17.3.4.1 The Deleterious Consequences of Foetal Reprogramming

Heart failure may indicate the limits of the above-defined adaptational process. Every phenotypic modification has a limit, e.g. the beneficial effects, in terms of myocardial economy. For example, the isomyosin shift is maximal when the fast myosin has been completely replaced by the slow isoform (Table 17.2).

17.3.4.2 Cell Death and Fibrosis

Fibrosis is multifactorial and is caused by myocardial ischemia or hypoxia, senescence (see below), inflammatory processes, diabetes, hormones, vasoactive peptides. Failure is also caused by a loss of muscle due to necrosis or apoptosis and above all by replacement fibrosis [11]. A main myocardial marker of HF is the concentration of collagen, the main component of the myocardial extra-cellular matrix whose concentration indicates fibrosis. The wound healing response of the myocardium after myocardial infarction involves both reparative fibrosis, which is organised as a scar, and, in the surrounded area, reactive fibrosis and compensatory myocyte HYP.

Tissue injury is initially associated with inflammatory cells, mainly macrophages, which transform interstitial fibroblasts into myofibroblasts detectable 4 days after injury. Myofibroblasts have a high density of angiotensin II receptors, and contain various forms of collagenases (or Matrix MetalloProteinases, MMPs) and collagen-linked proteases and proteases regulatory proteins as TIMP (Tissue Inhibitors of MMP). These various components regulate the rather complex collagen metabolism (Fig. 17.5) [11].

Vasoactive peptides and aldosterone which are secreted during CR are all able to activate fibrogenesis and represent models currently utilised in experimental models [2, 11]. Non-insulin dependent diabetes is associated with interstitial ventricular fibrosis, resulting from an increased type III collagen [32].

17.4 Cardiovascular Senescence

As compared to adult heart, the senescent heart is different and is both an organ submitted to the consequences of the senescent arterial system and a senescent organ. The senescence process generates arterial stiffness and increases aortic impedance and, by so-doing, creates an impedance overloading of the left ventricle. Nevertheless, senescence is also a general process that affects directly the myocardium and causes cardiocyte loss and replacement fibrosis.

The normal load of the LV is a rather complex parameter, called aortic impedance which includes aortic stiffness, blood pressure and viscosity and the effects of aortic elasticity on aortic distensibility. The senescent heart is very much alike a left ventricular pressure overload model such as that due to aortic stenosis. Nevertheless, in senescence, the load is aortic impedance, not only arterial hypertension as frequently thought. In 26-month old rats, it was shown that the LV is modified and, from a thermodynamic point of view, there is a compensatory cardiac CR. This is caused by the same phenotypic modifications of contractile and membrane proteins as in the pressure-overloaded heart [33]. The LV of aged persons is normally hypertrophied and also submitted to the general process of adaptation. The force-time integral of the individual myosin cross-bridge cycle is correlated with the age of the patient with non-failing myocardium, suggesting that, even in man, ageing is associated with an improved economy. Finally, recent data also suggest that the turn-over rate of myocytes is augmented in aged senescent human hearts [15].

Phenotypic modifications of the myocardium predominate in the LV. Nevertheless, the senescent heart is not exactly the same as an overloaded young myocardium in at least three points: the high incidence of arrhythmias, cell death, and an important fibrosis. Clinical and experimental studies have demonstrated a prevalence of supraventricular and ventricular ectopic beats and an attenuation of heart rate variability. Arrhythmias result from both fibrosis and changes in the membrane phenotype responsible for the increased duration of the AP and calcium transient [34, 35].

The aged heart contains fewer myocytes than younger hearts. Based on autopsy findings, it has been suggested that the process is gender-specific and does not occur in women [36]. The cause of death includes both ischemic necrosis due, in part, to the aged-related reduction in coronary reserve. Necrosis is the predominant cause of cell death; quantification has indeed shown that there are about 1,000 times more necrotic cells than apoptotic cells. Apoptosis during ageing is localised into the LV suggesting that it is initiated by mechanical factors. Myocardial fibrosis is a constant finding in healthy senescent hearts both in rats and humans. Cardiac fibrosis in this condition is certainly, at least in part, a reparative process related to myocyte death and predominates in the subendocardium. Nevertheless, the regulation of myocardial concentration of collagen during ageing is a complex phenomenon. Different studies have provided converging results and have shown a paradoxically inverse relationship between the protein and mRNA content of collagen in aged hearts; the lower the mRNA concentration, the higher the protein levels [37], which is in contrast with the situation observed with another component of the extra-cellular matrix, fibronectin. In addition a 40–45 % diminution of both collagenase (MMP) 2 and MMP 1 has recently been evidenced in 22–24 month old rat hearts, suggesting that collagen accumulation is, at least in part, regulated at the level of the degradative pathway. A recent paper [38] had explored the collagen turn-over in a sheep model of tachycardia-induced HF in young and aged animals. As compared to young controls, the collagen content of the myocardium is augmented in senescent controls and in failing young animals. Nevertheless and surprisingly, the increase in myocardial collagen was less pronounced in the old failing animals and this is due to a reduction of collagenase inhibitor activity.

The senescent heart, even in the absence of arterial hypertension or coronary insufficiency, is potentially a diseased heart. Myocardial function in the elderly is still normal because of the various adaptational mechanisms. Nevertheless the laboratory of Sophie Besse able to demonstrate that very old rats (28 month old) were potentially failing with a very high diastolic pressure while rats do not suffer from coronary atherosclerosis [39]. As such it resembles compensatory cardiac hypertrophy occurring before NYHA stage I during the course of an arterial hypertension.

Conclusions

CR results from interactions between mechanical factors which cause adaptational modifications of the cardiocyte, and numerous etiologic, epidemiological or neurohormonal factors which all are capable to modify the cardiocyte phenotype, can cause cell death and trigger the fibrotic process. The slowing of the shortening velocity is a consequence of the general process of adaptation, and is a major factor to improve the thermodynamic status of an overloaded heart An important clinical consequence is that, in chronic HF, the target of therapy should be economy, not inotropy. Chronic HF rarely occurs in the absence of several additional factors, namely fibrosis or cell death. In clinical practice, CR and HF are diseases of aged people with myocardial infarction and/or arterial hypertension. From a biological point of view, cardiocyte modifications, cell death and fibrosis are combined in the failing human heart. Fibrosis renders the myocardium stiffer and mechanically and electrically heterogeneous and this plays a crucial role in the genesis of arrhythmias and deterioration of both systolic and diastolic function. For the moment, therefore fibrosis is the best marker of heart failure.

Dedication This chapter is dedicated to the memory of three great friends, Pierre-Yves Hatt (Paris, F), Radek Zak (Chicago, USA) and Norman Alpert (Burlington, USA) who, all, were pioneers in this field of medical research. Without them such a chapter could not be written and they all were determinant in the genesis of the concept of remodelling and adaptation. All three had in common modesty, a very rare quality.

References

1. Swynghedauw B. Transgenic models of myocardial dysfunction. Heart Fail Rev. 1996;1:277–90.
2. Delcayre C, Swynghedauw B. Molecular mechanisms of myocardial remodeling. The role of aldosterone. J Mol Cell Cardiol. 2002;34:1577–84.
3. Grove D, Zak R, Nair KG, Aschenbrenner V. Biochemical correlates of cardiac Hypertrophy IV. Observations on the cellular organization of growth during myocardial hypertrophy in the rat. Circ Res. 1969;25:473–85.
4. Hatt PY, Berjal G, Moravec J, Swynghedauw B. Heart failure: an electron microscopic study of the left ventricular papillary muscle in aortic insufficiency in the rabbit. J Mol Cell Cardiol. 1970;1:235–40.
5. Alpert NR, Mulieri LA, Hasenfuss G. Myocardial Chemo-Mechanical energy transduction. In: Fozzard HA, Haber E, Katz AM, Jennings R, Morgan E, editors. The heart and cardiovascular system. New York: Raven press pub; 1992. p. 111–28.
6. Swynghedauw B. Molecular mechanisms of myocardial remodeling. Physiol Rev. 1999;79:215–62.
7. Opie LH, Commerford PJ, Gersh BJ, Pfeffer MA. Controversies in ventricular remodeling. Lancet. 2006;367:356–67.
8. Swynghedauw B. Phenotypic plasticity of adult myocardium: molecular mechanisms. J Exp Biol. 2006; 209:2320–7.
9. Swynghedauw B, Delcayre B, Samuel JL, Mebazaa A, Cohen-Solal A. Molecular mechanisms In evolutionary cardiology. Heart failure. Ann N Y Acad Sci. 2010;1188:58–67.
10. Cokkinos D, Pantos C. Myocardial remodeling, and overview. Heart Fail Rev. 2011;16:1–4.
11. Weber KT, Sun Y, Bhattachyara SK, Ahokas RA, Gerling IC. Myofibroblast-mediated mechanisms of pathological remodeling of the heart. Nat Rev Cardiol. 2013;10:15–26.
12. Anversa P, Palackal T, Sonnenblick EH, Olivetti G, Meggs LG, Capasso JM. Myocyte cell loss and myocyte cellular hyperplasia in the hypertrophied aging rat heart. Circ Res. 1990;67:871–85.
13. Spalding KL, Buchholz BA, Bergman L-E, Druid H, Frisén J. Forensics: age-written in teeth by nuclear tests. Nature. 2005;437:333–4.
14. Bergmann O, Bhardwaj RD, Bernard S, Zdunek S, Barnabé-Heider F, Walsh S, et al. Evidence for cardiomyocyte renewal in humans. Science. 2009;324:98–102.
15. Kajstura J, Rota M, Cappetta D, Ogórek B, Arranto C, Bai Y, et al. Cardiomyogenesis in the aging and failing heart. Circulation. 2012;126:1869–81.
16. Samuel JL, Marotte F, Delcayre C, Rappaport L. Microtubule reorganization is related to the rate of heart myocyte hypertrophy. Am J Physiol. 1986;251: H1118–25.
17. Torrent-Guasp F, Buckberg GD, Clemente C, Cox JL, Coghlan HC, Gharib M. The structure and function of the helical heart and its buttress wrapping. I The normal macroscopic structure of the heart. Semin Thorac Cardiovasc Surg. 2001;13:301–19.
18. Torrent-Guasp F, Kocica MJ, Corno A, Komeda M, Cox J, Flotats A, et al. Review. Systolic ventricular filling. Eur J Cardiothorac Surg. 2004;25:376–82.

19. Helle-Valle T, Crosby J, Edvardsen T, Lyseggen E, Amundsen BH, Smith HJ, et al. New noninvasive method for assessment of left ventricular rotation. Speckle tracking echocardiography. Circulation. 2005;112:3149–56.
20. Buckberg GD, Weisfeld ML, Ballester M, Beyar R, Burkhoff D, Coghlan HC, et al. Left ventricular form and function. Scientific priorities and strategic planning for development of new views of the disease. Circulation. 2004;110:e333–6.
21. McKay RG, Pfeffer MA, Pasternak RC, Markis JE, Come PC, Nakao S, et al. Left ventricular remodeling after myocardial infarction: a corollary to infarct expansion. Circulation. 1986;74:693–702.
22. DeWitt TJ, Scheiner SM. Phenotypic variation from single genotypes. In: DeWitt TJ, Scheiner SM, editors. Phenotypic plasticity. New York: Oxford University Press; 2004. p. 1–9.
23. Swynghedauw B. Developmental and functional adaptation of contractile proteins in cardiac and skeletal muscle. Physiol Rev. 1986;66:710–71.
24. Lompré AM, Schwartz K, d'Albi J, Lacombe G, Van Thiem N, Swynghedauw B. Myosin isozymes redistribution in chronic heart overloading. Nature. 1979;282:105–7.
25. Lompré AM, de la Bastie D, Boheler KR, Schwartz K. Characterisation and expression of the rat heart sarcoplasmic reticulum Ca^{2+} ATPase mRNA. FEBS Lett. 1989;249:35–41.
26. van Rooij E, Sutherland LB, Qi X, Richardson JA, Hill J, Olson EN. Control of stress-dependent cardiac growth and gene expression by a microRNA. Science. 2007;316:575–9.
27. Thum T, Galuppo P, Wolf C, Fiedler J, Kneitz S, van Laake LW, et al. MicroRNAs in the human heart: a clue to fetal gene reprogramming in heart failure. Circulation. 2007;116:258–67.
28. Engelhardt S. Small RNA, biomarkers come of age. J Am Coll Cardiol. 2012;60:300–3.
29. Marie JP, Guillemot H, Hatt PY. Le degré de granulation des cardiocytes auriculaires. Etude planimétrique au cours des différents apports d'eau et de sodium chez le rat. Pathol Biol (Paris). 1976;24:549–55.
30. Swynghedauw B, Coraboeuf E. Cardiac JN hypertrophy and failure: basic aspects. In: Willerson JT, Cohn JN, editors. Cardiovascular Medicine. New York: Churchill Livingstone; 2000. p. 955–78.
31. Poole-Wilson PA, Colucci WS, Massie BM, et al., editors. Heart failure. Scientific principles and clinical practice. New York: Churchill Livingstone; 1997. p. 13–31.
32. Shimizu M, Umeda K, Sugihara N, Yoshio H, Ino H, Takeda R, et al. Collagen remodeling in myocardia of patients with diabetes. J Clin Pathol. 1993;46:32–6.
33. Besse S, Assayag P, Delcayre C, Carre F, Cheav SL, Lecarpentier Y, et al. Normal and hypertrophied senescent rat heart. Mechanical and molecular characteristics. Am J Physiol. 1993;265:H183–90.
34. Carré F, Rannou F, Sainte-Beuve C, Chevalier B, Moalic JM, Swynghedauw B, et al. Arrhythmogenicity of the hypertrophied and senescent heart and relationship to membrane proteins involved in the altered calcium handling. Cardiovasc Res. 1993;27:1784–9.
35. Levy D, Anderson KM, Savage DD, Balkus SA, Kannel WB, Castelli WP, et al. Risk of ventricular arrhythmias in left ventricular hypertrophy: the Framingham heart study. Am J Cardiol. 1987;6:560–5.
36. Olivetti G, Giordano G, Corradi D, Melissari M, Lagrasta C, Gambert SR, et al. Gender differences and aging: effects on the human heart. J Am Coll Cardiol. 1995;26:1068–79.
37. Besse S, Rober V, Assayag P, Delcayre C, Swynghedauw B. Non-synchronous changes in myocardial collagen mRNA and protein during aging. Effect of DOCA-salt hypertension. Am J Physiol. 1994;267:H2237–44.
38. Horn MA, Graham HK, Richard MA, Clarke JD, Greensmith DJ, Briston SJ, et al. Age-related divergent remodeling of the cardiac ECM in heart failure: collagen accumulation in the young and loss in the aged. J Mol Cell Cardiol. 2012;53:82–90.
39. Rozenberg S, Tavernier B, Riou B, Swynghedauw B, Page CL, Boucher F, et al. Severe impairment of ventricular compliance accounts for advanced age-associated hemodynamic dysfunction in rats. Exp Gerontol. 2006;41:289–95.

A Translational Approach to Probe the Arrhythmic Potential of the Heart: Therapeutic Considerations

18

Faisal M. Merchant, Omid Sayadi, Dheeraj Puppala, Jagmeet P. Singh, E. Kevin Heist, Theofanie Mela, and Antonis A. Armoundas

Abstract

Electrocardiographic alternans, a phenomenon of beat-to-beat alternation in cardiac electrical waveforms, has been implicated in the pathogenesis of ventricular arrhythmias and sudden cardiac (SCD). However, rather than merely being associated with an increased risk for SCD, several lines of pre-clinical and clinical evidence suggest that cardiac alternans may play a causative role in generating the electrophysiologic substrate necessary for the onset of ventricular arrhythmias. In the clinical setting, a positive microvolt T-wave alternans (MTWA) test has been associated with a heightened risk of arrhythmic mortality and SCD during *medium*- and *long*-term follow-up. Although deficiencies in Ca^{2+} transport processes have been implicated in the genesis of alternans at the sub-cellular and cellular level, the specific underlying mechanisms have not been fully elucidated. In this chapter we propose a framework of conditions necessary to give rise to alternans from the myocyte to the whole heart level. It supports the idea that alternans results from a synergistic interaction between a vulnerable substrate and an inciting trigger event. Lastly, the potential clinical utility of modulating repolarization alternans via electrical or pharmacologic therapies to prevent life threatening arrhythmias is explored.

F.M. Merchant, MD
Cardiology Division, Emory University School of Medicine, Atlanta, GA, USA

O. Sayadi, PhD • D. Puppala, MD
A.A. Armoundas, PhD (✉)
Cardiology Division, Cardiovascular Research Center, Massachusetts General Hospital, 149 13th Street, Charlestown, Boston, MA 02129, USA
e-mail: aarmoundas@partners.org

J.P. Singh, MD, PhD • E.K. Heist, MD, PhD
T. Mela, MD
Cardiology Division, Massachusetts General Hospital, Boston, MA, USA

D.V. Cokkinos (ed.), *Introduction to Translational Cardiovascular Research*, DOI 10.1007/978-3-319-08798-6_18, © Springer International Publishing Switzerland 2015

Keywords
Sarcoplasmic reticulum • Ryanodine receptor • Cardiac myocyte • Cellular alternans • Mechanisms of alternans • Alternans suppression

Abbreviations

($[Ca^{2+}]_i$)	Intracellular calcium concentration
AP	Action potential
APD	Action potential duration
CICR	Calcium-induced-calcium-release
DAD	Delayed after depolarization
ECG	Electrocardiogram
EGM	Electrogram
ICD	Implantable cardioverter-defibrillator
LVEF	Left ventricle ejection fraction
MI	Myocardial infarction
MTWA	Microvolt T-wave alternans
NCX	Na^+/Ca^{2+} exchanger
RA	Repolarization alternans
RyRs	Ryanodine receptors
SCD	Sudden cardiac death
sEADs	Spontaneous early after-depolarizations
SERCA2a	Sarcoplasmic reticulum Ca^{2+} ATPase
SR	Sarcoplasmic reticulum
VT/VF	Ventricular tachycardia/ventricular fibrillation
VTE	Ventricular tachyarrhythmic events

18.1 Introduction

Electrocardiographic alternans, a phenomenon of beat-to-beat oscillation in the morphology and/or duration of electrocardiographic waveforms, was first described by Hering in 1908 [1]. Much of the interest in the alternans phenomenon has focused on alternans during the repolarization phase of the ventricles, also known as repolarization alternans (RA). More specifically, RA has been associated with an increased risk for malignant ventricular arrhythmias and sudden cardiac death (SCD) across a wide range of pathophysiological conditions including both ischemic and non-ischemic congestive heart failure with impaired left ventricle ejection fraction (LVEF) and recent myocardial infarction (MI) [2, 3]. Cardiac alternans can also be produced in structurally normal hearts under conditions of chronotropic stimulation [4, 5] or significant metabolic stress [6].

This chapter aims to present a contemporary understanding of the sub-cellular and cellular processes underlying the genesis of cardiac alternans and potential therapeutic applications based on this mechanistic understanding.

18.2 Mechanisms of Alternans in Isolated Myocytes

Two major hypotheses have been developed to explain the alternans phenomenon at the cellular level. The first hypothesis suggests that alternation in sarcolemmal currents, membrane voltage and action potential (AP) morphology leads to beat-to-beat fluctuations in intracellular calcium concentration. In support of this hypothesis, it has recently been shown that the modulation of sarcolemmal Ca^{2+} [7] and K^+ [8, 9] currents based on changes in AP morphology [10] has a significant effect on the stability of Ca^{2+} handling processes and the transition to stable [11] alternans. In contrast, the second major hypothesis suggests that alternation of intracellular calcium concentration ($[Ca^{2+}]_i$) is the primary event which then secondarily leads to alternans of membrane voltage and AP morphology [6, 10, 12–16]. According to the second hypothesis, $[Ca^{2+}]_i$ alternans can result from stress-induced [5, 12] perturbations in any number of Ca^{2+} transport processes including Ca^{2+} entry into the cytoplasm [9], recovery of ryanodine receptors (RyRs) from inactivation, triggering of sarcoplasmic reticulum (SR) Ca^{2+} release [6, 13], SR Ca^{2+} uptake [17], intra-SR Ca^{2+} redistribution [18] and linking of intracellular

Ca^{2+} handling to surface membrane voltage [10] (Fig. 18.1). The mechanisms that give rise to cardiac alternans may reside anywhere along this multi-step process of intracellular calcium cycling. A preponderance of recent data has emerged in support of the second hypothesis, suggesting the primacy of perturbations in Ca^{2+} handling processes as the fundamental event in the genesis of cellular alternans.

Among the many steps involved in calcium cycling, alternation of calcium entry into the cell via incomplete recovery from inactivation of the L-type calcium channel ($I_{Ca,L}$) could theoretically lead to $[Ca^{2+}]_i$ alternans [9, 19]. However, a number of studies have demonstrated that peak $I_{Ca,L}$ is unchanged during alternans [6, 13, 20, 21], and equally importantly, $I_{Ca,L}$ has been shown to be unaltered in myocytes from diseased hearts [22], making this a less likely mechanism for the lower alternans threshold observed in the failing heart. Furthermore, alternans of $[Ca^{2+}]_i$ can be elicited in a high-frequency stimulated myocyte during AP-clamp with similar AP morphology [23], also suggesting that the Ca^{2+} influx trigger of calcium-induced-calcium-release (CICR) is not the primary event in inducing alternans. The use of small depolarizing pulses [20] to induce alternans may account for alternans encountered at very high stimulation frequencies when most of the L-type Ca^{2+} channels are unavailable, and thus provide a plausible explanation for the presence of alternans in the normal heart at unusually high stimulation frequencies [4, 5].

Beat-to-beat fluctuations in SR Ca^{2+} content have also been implicated as a potential mechanism for alternans. SR Ca^{2+} measurements made during alternans using the indirect approach of measurement of the caffeine-evoked Na^+/Ca^{2+} exchanger (NCX) current have suggested that SR Ca^{2+} alternates [20, 24, 25]. However, others have shown that while $[Ca^{2+}]_{SR}$ exerts a major influence on SR Ca^{2+} release, beat-to-beat alternation in $[Ca^{2+}]_{SR}$ is not required for $[Ca^{2+}]_i$ alternans to occur [6, 21].

The rate of recovery of the RyR from a refractory (adapted or inactivated) state is another step in the calcium cycling machinery that may give rise to alternans. Given that calcium-induced calcium release is a slower process than either sarcoplasmic reticulum Ca^{2+}-ATPase (SERCA2a) mediated Ca^{2+} uptake or $I_{Ca,L}$ recovery [26] incomplete RyR recovery on alternate beats at high stimulation frequencies may produce chronotropically induced alternans. With increased steepness of the released Ca^{2+}-SR Ca^{2+} content relationship, as may occur in diseased hearts [22], small changes in $[Ca^{2+}]_{SR}$ should result in large changes in the beat-to-beat $[Ca^{2+}]_i$, even for a constant $I_{Ca,L}$ trigger [26, 27]. As such, a large $[Ca^{2+}]_i$ would be produced when the $[Ca^{2+}]_{SR}$ is relatively high and a disproportionately small $[Ca^{2+}]_i$ when the $[Ca^{2+}]_{SR}$ content is relatively low. A large $[Ca^{2+}]_i$ would then cause enhanced Ca^{2+} mediated L-type current inactivation, thus suppressing Ca^{2+} entry, as well as enhanced Ca^{2+} extrusion from the myocyte via the NCX [25], all of which results in a lower SR Ca^{2+} content and hence lower $[Ca^{2+}]_i$ on the next beat. The lower $[Ca^{2+}]_i$ then results in decreased Ca^{2+} mediated L-type current inactivation and reduced Ca^{2+} extrusion through the NCX, leading to increased SR Ca^{2+} content and a return to the higher $[Ca^{2+}]_i$ on the following beat. This sequence sets the stage for *concordant cellular* alternans between $[Ca^{2+}]_i$ and membrane voltage/action potential duration (APD) such that both oscillate *in-phase* (i.e. large $[Ca^{2+}]_i$ corresponds to a long APD and vice versa).

While the use of small depolarizing pulses to induce alternans [20] may differ significantly from the often encountered chronotropic induction of alternans, the biphasic rise in $[Ca^{2+}]_i$ [25] has been attributed to an initial steep rise in activation of the RyRs, while the second slower phase has been attributed to wave like propagation. We [25] and others [28] have ascribed this secondary slower phase to secondary RyR openings [25, 29]. We have shown that elevated SR Ca^{2+} content results in both aberrant SR Ca^{2+} release and $[Ca^{2+}]_i$ alternans, and also gives rise to an inward depolarizing current that results in spontaneous early after-depolarizations (sEADs) and APD prolongation which correlates directly with the magnitude and timing of the aberrant Ca^{2+} release. We have also shown the presence of *discordant cellular* alternans between $[Ca^{2+}]_i$ and

APD at the myocyte level and the importance of $[Ca^{2+}]_i$ in defining the in- or out-of-phase relationship between $[Ca^{2+}]_i$ and AP (Fig. 18.1b).

In aggregate, these findings support the primacy of alternation in $[Ca^{2+}]_i$ in driving APD alternans and also in determining the presence of concordance or discordance between $[Ca^{2+}]_i$ and AP morphology within the individual myocyte. Furthermore, experimental evidence suggests that the same Ca^{2+} cycling perturbations that give rise to cellular alternans can be viewed as inherently coupled processes of an intracellular pathophysiological substrate and trigger events (i.e. transient β-stimulation bursts), which in concert create the necessary conditions for the establishment of cellular alternans.

Many studies have suggested that RyRs are more likely to be triggered by cytosolic Ca^{2+} when SR luminal Ca^{2+} is elevated [30, 31] and that increasing SR Ca^{2+} content increases spontaneous SR Ca^{2+} release [32] and delayed afterdepolarizations (DAD) amplitude towards the threshold to trigger an AP [33, 34]. Furthermore, triggered activity arising from DADs in response to high stimulation rates [35] or to catecholamines has been demonstrated in normal ventricular myocytes [36], experimental heart failure preparations [37] and cardiomyopathic human hearts [38]. These studies provide a plausible justification for the hypothesis that SR Ca^{2+} "stabilization" at a sub-maximal value is the primary reason for abolishing alternans in studies in which thapsigargin and ryanodine treatment of myocytes markedly suppressed $[Ca^{2+}]_i$ and prevented APD alternans [12], and ryanodine treatment alone abolished both tension and AP alternans in papillary muscles [18].

In that context, in the normal heart, CICR is manifest by an operational baseline $[Ca^{2+}]_{SR}$ that is lower than the threshold to trigger spontaneous Ca^{2+} release. However, high stimulation frequency or β-adrenergic stimulation trigger SR Ca^{2+} overload that raises the SR Ca^{2+} baseline level close to or above the threshold at which spontaneous sub-threshold Ca^{2+} release may occur. In the diseased heart, although the baseline SR Ca^{2+} level is decreased, the $[Ca^{2+}]_{SR\text{-threshold}}$ for RyR opening is also decreased. Although β-adrenergic responsiveness is impaired in the diseased heart [39], even a moderate residual or transient β-adrenergic responsiveness [37] may result in spontaneous sub-threshold Ca^{2+} release at a lower $[Ca^{2+}]_{SR.}$ The lower than normal $[Ca^{2+}]_{SR\text{-threshold}}$ for RyR opening in diseased hearts may explain the presence of electrocardiographic alternans at lower heart rates than in normal hearts (Fig. 18.2).

Further justification for the role of SR Ca^{2+} content in the genesis of alternans comes from the recent study by Xie and Weiss [28] demonstrating that under control conditions, myocytes become susceptible to Ca^{2+} overload during rapid pacing and that interactions between spontaneous Ca^{2+} waves and AP-triggered $[Ca^{2+}]_i$ produce *sub-cellular spatially discordant* alternans (SDA) and even more complex sub-cellular $[Ca^{2+}]_i$ patterns. Therefore, the genesis [35, 40] and propagation [41] of Ca^{2+} waves, which are in general associated with increased SR Ca^{2+} content through increased luminal Ca^{2+} sensitization of the RyR to cytosolic Ca^{2+} and perhaps through increased ability of cytosolic Ca^{2+} to activate adjacent RyR sites, may essentially reset local $[Ca^{2+}]_{SR}$ [28], and give rise to sub-cellular alternans. According to this mechanism, a partially propagated Ca^{2+} wave triggers a gradient in SR refractoriness when the next AP occurs. In the region of the myocyte through which the Ca^{2+} wave has already passed, the affected SR is empty and partially refractory, thus minimizing Ca^{2+} release. In contrast, the region into which the Ca^{2+} wave has not entered causes the release of a normal amount of SR Ca^{2+}, resulting in a spatially non-uniform $[Ca^{2+}]_i$. In the next beat, both $[Ca^{2+}]_{SR}$ content and excitability of the refractory region will have recovered, producing a large release, therefore perpetuating the presence of sub-cellular spatially discordant alternans.

The presence of sub-cellular spatially discordant $[Ca^{2+}]_i$ leads to increased dispersion of sub-cellular electrophysiologic properties and, in the setting of an appropriate trigger, may lead to an arrhythmia at the cellular level. Although sub-cellular spatially discordant alternans is usually preceded by sub-cellular spatially concordant alternans, under certain circumstances

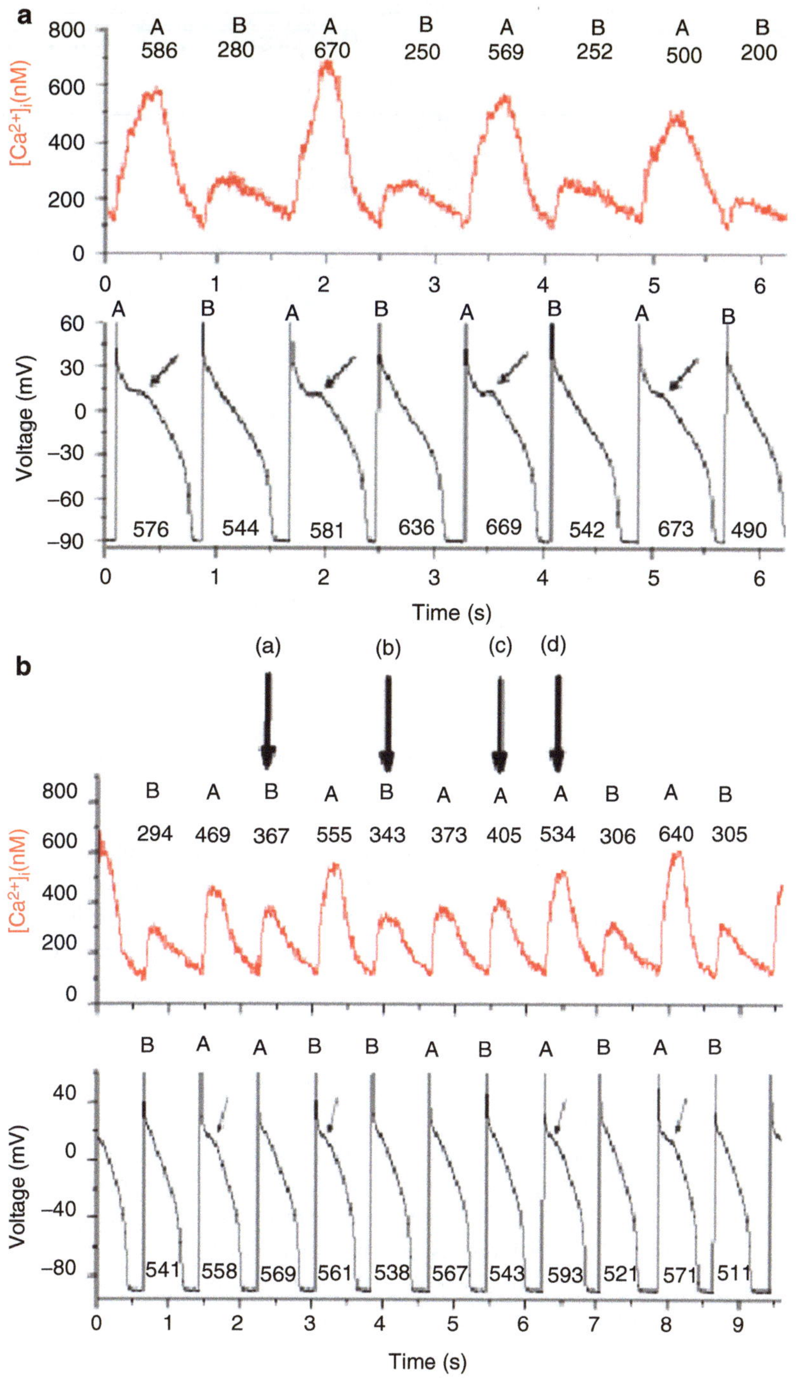

Fig. 18.1 Representative examples of $[Ca^{2+}]_i$ and AP alternans. (**a**) Representative example of concordant $[Ca^{2+}]_i$ and AP alternans in a left ventricular canine myocyte stimulated every 0.8 s. The arrows indicate a subthreshold early after-depolarization; (**b**) representative example of phase transitions (*a*)–(*d*) between $[Ca^{2+}]_i$ and AP alternans obtained during the same data record as (**a**). In-phase (concordant) $[Ca^{2+}]_i$ and AP alternans leads to out-of-phase (discordant) alternans (*a*) and (*c*) and back again to in-phase alternans (*b*) and (*d*). "A" and "B" denote large and small $[Ca^{2+}]_i$ or long and short APD respectively; the peak $[Ca^{2+}]_i$ and APD for these beats are also shown [25, 29]

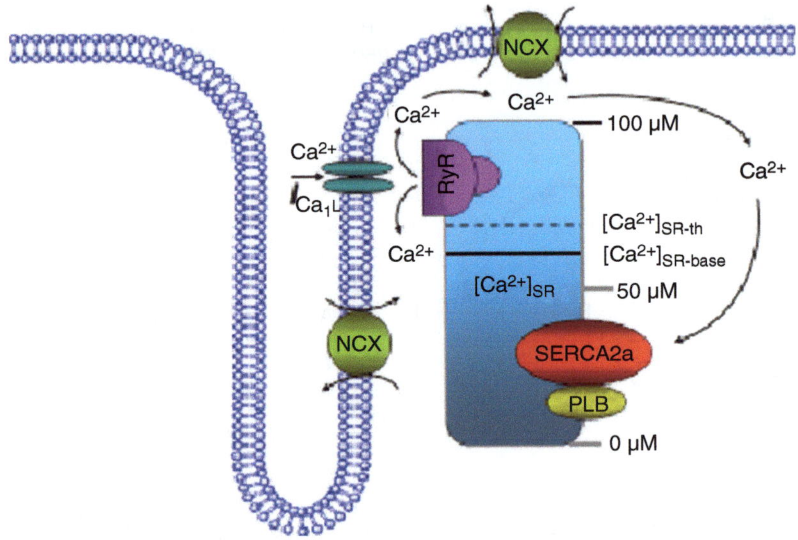

Fig. 18.2 Relationship between cellular calcium content and alternans threshold. Schematic diagram of the effect of the SR Ca^{2+} content on a proposed model for cellular alternans. Ca^{2+} cycling though calcium-induced-calcium-release (CICR) includes the L-type Ca^{2+} channel, the SR Ca^{2+} ATPase pump (*SERCA2a*), phospholamban (*PLB*), the ryanodine receptor (*RyR*) channel and the Na^+/Ca^{2+} exchanger (*NCX*). The solid line shows the SR Ca^{2+} baseline ($[Ca^{2+}]_{SR\text{-base}}$) and the dashed line shows the threshold SR Ca^{2+} ($[Ca^{2+}]_{SR\text{-th}}$) content at which Ca^{2+} release occurs. In the normal heart, CICR is manifested by an operational baseline of $[Ca^{2+}]_{SR}$ that is lower than the threshold to trigger spontaneous Ca^{2+} release. However, high stimulation frequency or β-adrenergic stimulation results in SR Ca^{2+} overload that raises the SR Ca^{2+} baseline level above the threshold such that spontaneous sub-threshold Ca^{2+} release may occur

sub-cellular spatially discordant alternans may arise spontaneously [28].

In support of the concept of sub-cellular spatially discordant alternans, it is also possible that as SERCA2a, NCX and RyR function is dynamically regulated on a beat-to-beat basis by many metabolic and ionic factors in the microdomain of the SR [42, 43], SR Ca^{2+} uptake and release is also dynamically changing, especially in the diseased heart [28, 37, 44], thus creating differential spatial heterogeneity of thresholds for the onset of alternans in different regions of the myocyte [28, 42]. In such cases, small differences of SR Ca^{2+} content in different parts of the myocyte may exist under basal conditions and these differences may be amplified once the steepness of the relationship between Ca^{2+} release and SR Ca^{2+} content begins to rise.

In summary, these data suggest that in the diseased heart, cellular alternans requires a trigger event (such as increased β-stimulation or a Ca^{2+} wave) and an appropriate sub-cellular substrate to develop. Increasing the probability of RyR opening alone does not produce arrhythmogenic Ca^{2+} release due to an accompanying decrease in SR Ca^{2+} content. β-adrenergic stimulation increases SR Ca^{2+} content and thereby allows the increased RyR open probability to produce Ca^{2+} release [44]. A trigger event alone may be sufficient to induce alternans in the normal heart; however, it requires supra-physiologic heart rates in order to create a heterogeneous (fragmented) sub-cellular Ca^{2+} release profile. In the diseased heart, however, perturbations in the intracellular calcium cycling machinery create a sufficiently heterogeneous sub-cellular substrate leading to development of alternans at lower heart rates and predisposing to arrhythmogenesis.

18.2.1 Mechanisms of Alternans in the Intact Heart

As discussed above, the current paradigm suggests that perturbations in cellular calcium cycling processes lead to alternation in cytosolic Ca^{2+} levels, which then secondarily lead to oscillations in membrane voltage and AP duration. In a manner analogous to *sub-cellular* spatially concordant and discordant alternans of $[Ca^{2+}]_i$, APD alternans at the tissue or whole heart level can also be spatially concordant or discordant.

Studies in normal hearts using optical mapping techniques have shown that discordant AP alternans (reflecting two adjacent areas of the myocardium that oscillate with opposite phase) is associated with a state of marked cardiac electrical instability, as evidenced by the fact that when ventricular fibrillation occurs following alternans, it only occurs after discordant APD alternans, but never concordant APD alternans [5]. This unstable electrical substrate is consistently induced at a critical heart rate threshold and is largely independent of the pacing site [5], suggesting that it is caused by heterogeneities of cellular repolarization properties and not heterogeneous propagation delay. Interestingly, in this study, alternans most commonly involved the slope of the AP plateau and the onset of final repolarization, timing during CICR that coincides with the timing of aberrant RyR release during alternans observed by our group [25] and others [13].

Recently a two-photon confocal imaging study in the intact rat ventricle [45] has shown that the spatial distribution of $[Ca^{2+}]_i$ alternans within the myocyte is time-dependent. Specifically, areas that mark the boundaries between regions of the myocyte that are out of phase during alternans can drift within the myocyte. These phase-mismatched myocyte regions are essentially driven by the myocyte membrane potential, defined by a spatial average potential of all myocytes within the electrotonic space constant, and thus providing a spatial constraint to the region of discordant alternans. Furthermore, the same study [45] has shown that rapid pacing synchronized Ca^{2+} waves in a sufficient mass of neighboring myocytes to cause DADs at the tissue level. In contrast, sporadic Ca^{2+} waves in individual myocytes at slow rates had no effect on membrane potential due to source-sink mismatch, wherein the magnitude of the Ca^{2+} wave (source) is insufficient to overcome diffusion into adjacent myocytes (sink), such that the wave fails to propagate. Thus, if myocytes in a region of tissue synchronously develop Ca^{2+} waves [45], resulting in sub-cellular alternans, it is possible that the amplitude and the phase of APD alternans in that region may change relative to the surrounding tissue, thus increasing dispersion of APD and generating a potentially arrhythmogenic substrate.

Based on this evidence, it is conceivable that following cardiac "injury", during the remodeling phase of the heart, the compensatory increase in β-adrenergic stimulation results in progressively increased SR Ca^{2+} content and a higher probability of inducing alternans. Although in end-stage heart failure the loss of β-adrenergic responsiveness is almost complete [39], in moderate cardiac dysfunction, it is likely that residual β-adrenergic responsiveness results in higher $[Ca^{2+}]_{SR}$ content and spontaneous SR Ca^{2+} release [37]. As the heart transitions from the compensatory phase to clinical heart failure, cardiac remodeling progresses to the point that the slope of the released SR Ca^{2+}-SR Ca^{2+} content relationship is steep enough that despite the loss of β-adrenergic responsiveness [39], transient/residual β-adrenergic responsiveness [37] may result in higher $[Ca^{2+}]_{SR}$ content, increased incidence of fractionated, aberrant SR Ca^{2+} release and Ca^{2+} waves, and higher probability of alternans occurrence.

In summary, it appears that AP alternans begins in a localized area in the heart and gives rise to micro-volt level alternans [46]. When this region of AP alternans extends to a significant portion of the myocardium (such that it is large enough to overcome the three-dimensional current sink problem) and becomes sufficiently synchronous, it can then be seen on the surface electrocardiogram as repolarization alternans [47]. Localized alternation in APD in turn is associated with delayed recovery on an every other beat basis, resulting in spatial dispersion of recovery, fractionation of depolarization wavefronts and setting the stage for the development of re-entry and arrhythmia onset (Fig. 18.3) [2, 15, 48].

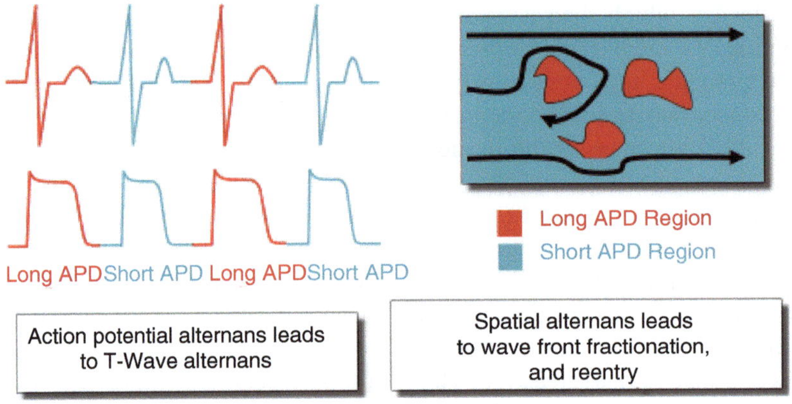

Fig. 18.3 Functional relationship of alternans and reentry. Localized action potential alternans is manifested as repolarization alternans on the electrocardiogram. Localized regions of tissue exhibiting action potential alternans are associated with delayed recovery on an every other beat basis. These tissue areas of delayed recovery may lead to wavebreak and the development of reentry

18.3 Repolarization Alternans and Clinical Arrhythmia Susceptibility

Microvolt T-wave alternans (MTWA) testing has traditionally been used as a marker of medium- and long-term risk of ventricular tachyarrhythmic events (VTEs) and SCD. T-wave alternans represents an alternating fluctuation in the morphology of cardiac repolarization (ST-segment and T-wave) on the body-surface electrocardiogram (ECG).

The alternans analysis algorithm for the estimation of RA has been previously described in detail [49–53]. Briefly, following R-wave detection and alignment, ST-segment and T-wave annotations are obtained using the wavelet transform and RA is estimated using a rolling 128-beat window that is shifted one beat at a time (Fig. 18.4). Spectral alternans analysis is performed on a beat-by-beat basis for each 128-beat data sequence using a 512-point power spectrum to improve the frequency-domain resolution. To account for the spatial variability of RA, spectral analysis is independently performed for each lead.

Repolarization alternans indices are estimated as follows:

$$\text{alternans voltage}(\mu\text{V}) = \sqrt{\text{alternans peak} - \mu_{\text{noise}}}$$

$$K_{\text{score}} = \frac{\text{alternans peak} - \mu_{\text{noise}}}{\sigma_{\text{noise}}}$$

where, the alternans peak is the peak in the aggregate power spectrum corresponding to 0.5 cycles/beat and the mean (μ_{noise}) and the standard deviation (σ_{noise}) of spectral noise are estimated from a predefined aggregate power spectrum noise window (0.40–0.46 cycles/beat), as shown in Fig. 18.4. The alternans voltage is a direct measure of the presence of alternans while the alternans K_{score} is a measure of the statistical significance of the alternans voltage.

18.3.1 Repolarization Alternans and Medium-/Long-Term Arrhythmia Susceptibility

Clinical MTWA testing identifies microvolt-level alternation during low-level exercise or chronotropic stimulation. A robust body of literature has identified a close association between heightened levels of MTWA and risk of VTE/SCD [2, 3, 54, 55]. TWA is believed to represent an electrocardiographic manifestation of spatiotemporal APD heterogeneity and the cellular and sub-cellular mechanisms which give rise to APD alternans (discussed above) likely provide the physiologic substrate for TWA identified on ECG

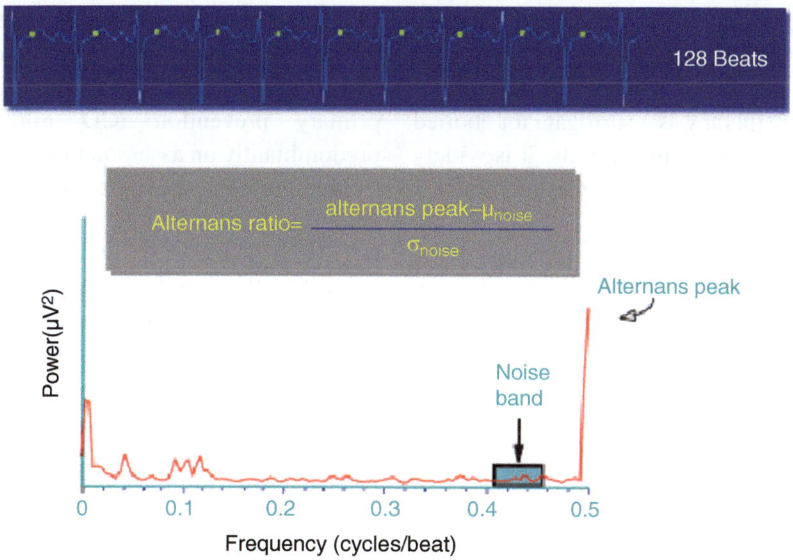

Fig. 18.4 Representative example of the algorithm used to estimate repolarization alternans

(for a more detailed discussion of clinical MTWA testing, please see Verrier et al. [55] and Rosenbaum et al. [54]).

18.3.1.1 Clinical Value of Microvolt T Wave Alternans

A robust body of clinical literature has demonstrated that MTWA can be used to stratify patients for risk of VTE/SCD with positive and negative predictive values that are comparable to invasive electrophysiologic testing [54]. In general, these studies have demonstrated that patients with a positive MTWA test have a significantly increased risk of VTE/SCD compared to those with a negative MTWA test result. Furthermore, the negative predictive value of MTWA testing has been excellent and consistent with the observation that even among patients with impaired left ventricular ejection fraction (LVEF) (i.e. ≤35 %), those with a negative MTWA have a very low risk of VTE/SCD, on the order of about 1 % per year [56]. In light of this data, there was significant optimism that MTWA testing could serve as a useful tool for identifying patients who were most or least likely to benefit from primary prevention implantable cardioverter-defibrillators (ICDs) [3]. However, more recent studies, including larger percentages of patients implanted with primary prevention ICDs, have raised some doubt about the utility of MTWA testing for this purpose. In particular the MASTER study enrolled 575 patients meeting Multicenter Automatic Defibrillator Implantation Trial II (MADIT-II) criteria for ICDs [57]. All patients underwent MTWA testing followed by ICD implantation. Over 3 years of follow-up, MTWA was not a significant predictor of the primary endpoint of documented VTE, SCD or "appropriate" ICD shocks. In a similar study design, the Sudden Cardiac Death in Heart Failure Trial (SCD-HeFT) investigators performed MTWA testing in a subset of 490 patients enrolled in the overall trial [58]. Again, MTWA testing was not a significant predictor of the same primary endpoint (documented VTE, SCD or appropriate ICD therapy).

Several possible explanations have been proposed to explain the discrepancy between earlier trials in which MTWA testing appeared to be a useful tool for VTE/SCD risk stratification and the more recent studies (MASTER, SCD-HeFT substudy) in which MTWA has not been a significant predictor. Although differences in the management of β-blockers at the time of MTWA testing

[59] may have contributed to differences in study results, it seems likely that the primary cause for the apparent discrepancy involves the use of appropriate ICD therapy as a surrogate for aborted SCD as an endpoint in clinical trials. It is widely acknowledged that appropriate ICD therapy is a relatively poor surrogate for SCD and in the Defibrillators in Non-Ischemic Cardiomyopathy Treatment Evaluation (DEFINITE) trial, the frequency of appropriate ICD therapies among patients randomized to ICDs was more than two-fold greater than the rate of SCD in the control arm [60]. This observation has been attributed to the fact that many appropriate ICD therapies treat arrhythmias that would have self-terminated or that ICDs may induce arrhythmias that they subsequently treat [60, 61]. Therefore, in studies that include a high percentage of patients implanted ICDs, the use of appropriate ICD therapy as an endpoint may confound the capacity of MTWA testing to predict risk of VTE/SCD.

In support of this hypothesis, a recent systematic analysis demonstrated that MTWA testing was a significant predictor of VTE/SCD in studies where a relatively small percentage (i.e. ≤15 %) of patients are implanted with ICDs but was a much less robust predictor in studies with higher percentages of ICDs [61]. Furthermore, in a pooled analysis of over 2,800 patients without ICDs, the 2 year risk of SCD among patients with a non-negative MTWA test was over four-fold higher than patients with a negative test result [56]. Both the MASTER trial and the SCD-HeFT sub-study included a large percentage of patients with ICDs and this observation may provide a plausible explanation for the discrepancy between these and earlier studies. Despite the potentially confounding effect of ICDs in recent MTWA studies, the aggregate of clinical data strongly supports the notion that an increased magnitude of RA, as detected by MTWA testing, is closely associated with the substrate that gives rise to VTE/SCD over medium and long-term follow-up. In light of these findings, it is plausible that MTWA testing is best utilized for patients who do not already have ICDs in order to determine whether they are at risk and should be considered for ICD therapy.

There has also been recent interest in the use of MTWA as part of a multi-marker strategy for SCD risk stratification. Current guidelines for primary prevention ICD implantation rely predominantly on assessment of LVEF. However, as highlighted in the recent National Heart, Lung and Blood Institute and Heart Rhythm Society (HLBI/HRS) report on SCD prediction and prevention [62], there is widespread recognition that LVEF reflects only one aspect of the complex electro-anatomic substrate that gives rise to ventricular arrhythmias and in isolation, LVEF is a sub-optimal risk stratification tool. Specifically, among patients who are currently candidates for primary prevention ICD therapy (i.e. LVEF ≤35 %), only a small percentage of patients (~2–5 %/year) will suffer a ventricular arrhythmia resulting in SCD [62], demonstrating that the positive predictive value and specificity of low LVEF for predicting SCD is quite limited. Conversely, the majority of SCD events occur in patients with only mildly impaired or even preserved LV systolic function [63], thus highlighting the limited negative predictive value and low sensitivity of impaired LVEF for determining SCD risk.

In light of this, we have hypothesized that multi-marker SCD risk profiling may provide better risk stratification than individual risk markers used in isolation. In a cohort of over 3,000 patients, we developed a multi-marker profile to predict risk of SCD at 24 months based on three variables: LVEF, MTWA status and presence of coronary artery disease [64]. We sought to characterize the limitations of LVEF for SCD risk prediction by comparing it to the multi-marker model. In Fig. 18.5 we compared the *predicted* and *observed* SCD free survival at 24 months for patients with LVEF ≤ or >35 %. Using the multivariate model, patients were divided into four groups based on *predicted* risk of 24 month SCD: <1, 1–5, 5–10 and >10 %. For patients in each of the four predicted risk groups, the *observed* rate of SCD was then plotted using Kaplan-Meier estimates. From Fig. 18.5, it is evident that the risk of SCD is not homogeneous for patients stratified by LVEF and important overlap exists between patients above and below

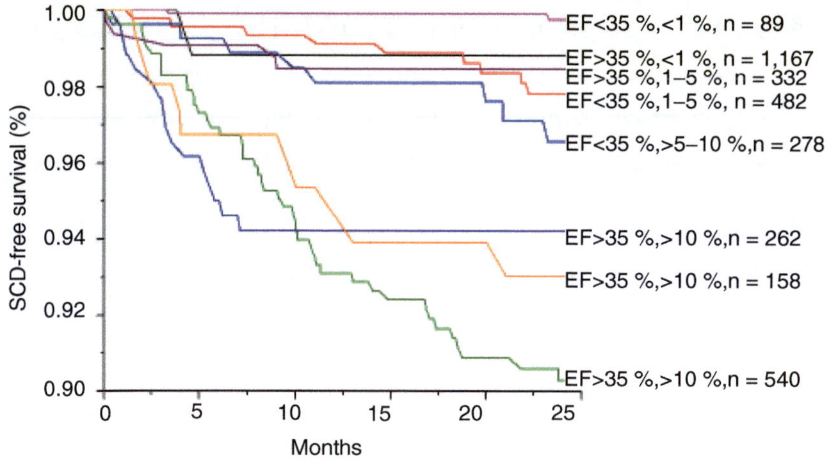

Fig. 18.5 Kaplan-Meier event-free survival curves for the primary endpoint of sudden cardiac death, stratified by *predicted* SCD risk based on the multivariate model. Using the multivariate model, patients with left ventricle ejection fraction (LVEF) ≤ or >35 % were further stratified into one of four groups based on predicted SCD risk at 24 months: <1, 1–5, 5–10 and >10 %. The survival curves demonstrate that even among patients stratified by LVEF, there is still significant heterogeneity in SCD risk, which can be accurately predicted by the multivariate model. The p value by log-rank test is <0.001, suggesting a significant difference in survival across subgroups

the LVEF 35 % threshold. Specifically, among patients with LVEF ≤35 %, approximately 39 % (540 out of 1,389) were predicted to be in the highest quartile of SCD risk based on the multivariate model and the observed event rate in this subgroup approaches 10 % at 24 months, confirming the heightened level of risk. However, a significant minority of patients with LVEF ≤35 % was predicted to be at relatively low risk of SCD at 24 months. Out of 1,389 patients with LVEF ≤35 %, 89 (6 %) had a predicted risk of <1 % and 482 (35 %) had a predicted risk of 1–5 %. The very low observed event rates in these subgroups highlight the significant heterogeneity of risk even among patients with impaired LV systolic function and support the notion of multivariate risk prediction. Figure 18.5 also demonstrates a similarly heterogeneous risk profile among patients with LVEF >35 %. Although the majority of patients with LVEF >35 % (1,167 out of 1,919, 61 %) are predicted to, and observed to, have a very low risk of SCD (<1 % at 24 months), it is evident from the survival curves that a subset of patients with LVEF >35 % can be identified who demonstrate significantly increased SCD risk. Nearly 22 % of patients with LVEF >35 % (420 out of 1,919) are predicted to have a 24 month SCD risk of either 5–10 or >10 % and the observed events rates in these patients clearly seen to exceed the risk among many of the patients with LVEF ≤35 %. With the use of the multi-marker model, this subgroup of patients can be identified as being at heightened risk of SCD but would be missed with the use of LVEF alone.

18.3.2 Repolarization Alternans and Acute Arrhythmia Susceptibility

In addition to a role in risk stratifying patients for ICD therapy, recent clinical observations have also suggested that heightened RA may be an important predictor of short-term arrhythmia susceptibility. Analysis of ambulatory body-surface electrograms (Holter monitors) from patients with coronary artery disease has demonstrated a sharp upsurge in RA magnitude (measured by time-domain techniques) within minutes prior to spontaneous VTE [65]. TWA amplitude reached a peak about 10 min prior to the onset of ventricular arrhythmia with a peak magnitude about 25 % higher than during a mean baseline obtained 60–120 min prior

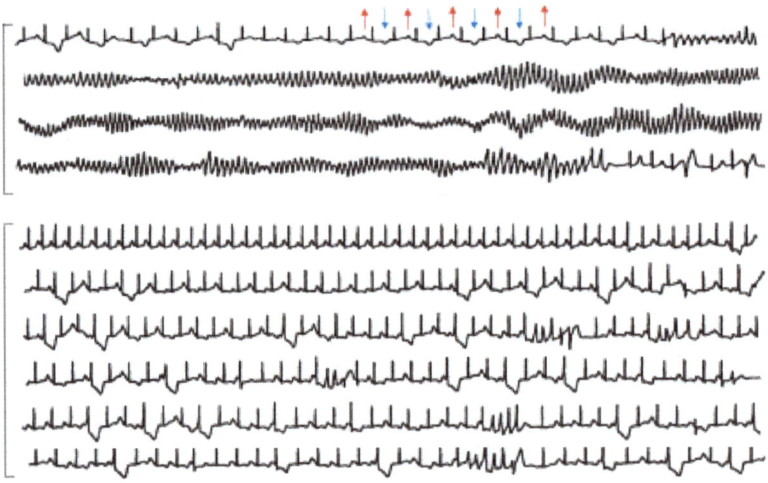

Fig. 18.6 Visible T-wave polarity alternans preceding and following self-terminating torsade de pointes ventricular tachycardia (**a**) captured on holter monitor of a 72 year old female patient with a history of resuscitated cardiac arrest [80]. In panel (**b**), three minutes of continuous ECG monitoring after the termination of ventricular tachycardia shows persistent T-wave alternans and several runs of non-sustained ventricular tachycardia

the VTE. Sharp upsurges in T-wave alternans immediately preceding spontaneous ventricular arrhythmias have also been documented from body-surface ECGs (leads V1, V5 and aVF) in patients hospitalized for acute heart failure [66]. In this study, TWA increased from a baseline of 18.6±2.1 μV to 27.9±4.6 μV ($p<0.05$) during the 15–30 min prior to arrhythmia onset and remained elevated until the occurrence of VTE; results were similar across all three body surface leads.

Although the magnitude of surges in TWA measured from body-surface leads is less than that measured from intra-cardiac electrograms (EGMs), the aforementioned data support the idea that significant increases in T-wave alternans prior to the onset of spontaneous VTE can be measured from body-surface electrodes and may be used to predict acute arrhythmia susceptibility (Fig. 18.6). However, given the significantly larger magnitude of RA measured from intra-cardiac EGMs, it seems likely that the use of intra-cardiac data will provide a much more robust assessment of the link between surges in RA and acute arrhythmogenesis. Importantly, simultaneous measurement of RA from body-surface and intra-cardiac electrograms by our group [53] and others [67] has shown a high degree of correlation suggesting that these measurements are detecting the same electrical phenomenon.

Analysis of intra-cardiac EGMs from ICDs has demonstrated a sharp increase in RA magnitude immediately prior to spontaneous ventricular arrhythmias [49, 68]. However, a similar upsurge in RA has not been observed prior to induced ventricular arrhythmias or preceding inappropriate ICD shocks [68]. A recent prospective, multicenter study has extended these observations by analyzing intra-cardiac EGMs from patients with ICDs [69]. In this study, due to the limited number of beats stored by the ICD prior to the onset of the VTE, repolarization dynamics were estimated using a simple averaging method which measures both alternans and non-alternans T-wave variability (TWA/V). Although this method is less specific for determining alternans periodicity than the better validated spectral-analytic method, given the significantly larger amplitude of T-wave alternans measured from ICD shock electrograms compared to body-surface ECGs, the simple averaging method can provide a measure of T-wave dynamics without extensive signal processing and with a limited number of beats to analyze prior to arrhythmia onset. The magnitude of TWA/V immediately prior to VTE was compared to four control data segments: baseline rhythm, rapid pacing (at 105 bpm), time-matched ambulatory EGMs from the same time of day at which spontaneous VTE occurred and EGMs

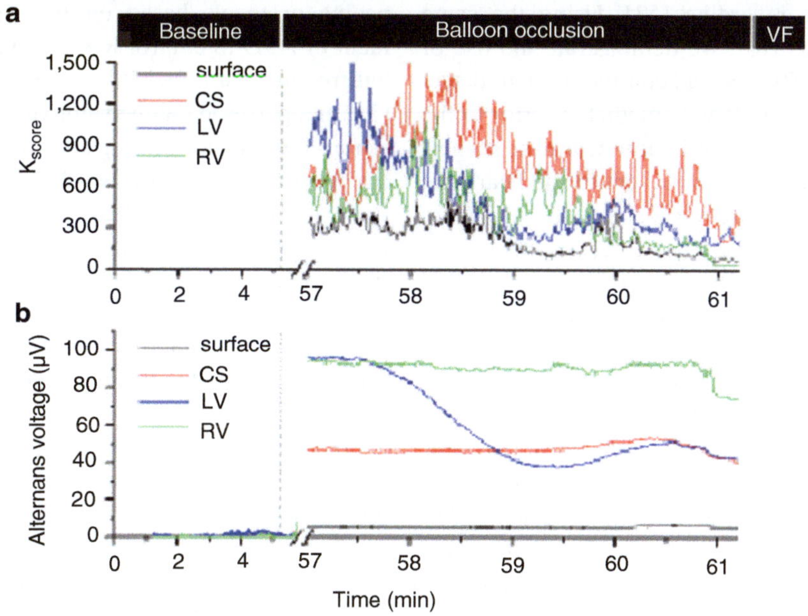

Fig. 18.7 Significant repolarization alternans (RA) induced by angioplasty-balloon occlusion of the circumflex coronary artery preceding ventricular fibrillation. Alternans voltage (**a**) and K_{score} (**b**) estimated from an intra-cardiac system of far-field bipolar leads (CS3CS8, RV2CS3 and RV2CS8) of catheters in the right ventricle and the coronary sinus. The vertical line corresponds to the start of the occlusion. A marked elevation in alternans voltage and K_{score} is observed during several minutes prior to VF, demonstrating that these markers can be accurately measured immediately prior to the onset of arrhythmia and may be used as a trigger to initiate "upstream" anti-arrhythmic therapy

prior to supraventricular tachycardia (SVT) onset. The magnitude of TWA/V prior to spontaneous VTE was significantly greater than during any of the four control data segments. Furthermore, in logistic regression models, each 10 μV increase in TWA/V was associated with an increase in odds of VTE of 2.2. These data show a close temporal association between surges in T-wave alternans/variability and onset of spontaneous ventricular arrhythmias.

In aggregate, several lines of evidence support the idea that surges in RA, measured either from body-surface or intra-cardiac electrodes, are closely associated with an increase in acute ventricular, and potentially atrial arrhythmia susceptibility. These data suggest that the heart either passes through a state of heightened RA on the way to ventricular tachycardia/ventricular fibrillation (VT/VF) or heightened RA occurs in close conjunction with developing VT/VF [15, 16]. In either scenario, these findings suggest that detecting significantly elevated levels of RA may serve as an important *short*-term predictor of impending arrhythmias and also raise the possibility of using upstream therapies to abort VT/VF prior to arrhythmia onset.

18.3.3 Utility of Repolarization Alternans to Guide Therapy

Repolarization alternans in vivo is known to be a spatially and temporally heterogeneous phenomenon and therefore, any attempt to deliver upstream suppressive therapy is predicated on the ability to accurately detect alternans regardless of where in the heart it originates. Our group has identified a novel lead configuration for the optimal spatio-temporal detection of intra-cardiac RA (based on two leads positioned in the RV and the CS), using the spectral technique (more details on this method can be found in [53]). Although there are dynamic fluctuations in RA magnitude during acute ischemia, we have shown that there is a surge of RA that remains significantly elevated compared to baseline within the first

5 min of the recording [53]. Using the same model, in Fig. 18.7, we demonstrate the use of the triangular RV-CS lead configuration to detect temporal surges in RA, immediately prior to the onset of ventricular fibrillation. Our data suggest that if significant RA is present in the heart, the RV-CS lead configuration is able to detect it more than 85 % of the time. Therefore, despite the significant spatiotemporal heterogeneity of RA, using this novel lead configuration, RA can be detected with a high degree of sensitivity when it is present in the heart. The use of the RV-CS lead configuration also has important clinical applicability since many currently utilized implantable devices (i.e. cardiac resynchronization therapy platforms) already employ RV and CS leads. The ability to detect heightened levels of RA from implantable intra-cardiac devices opens the door to the possibility of delivering upstream therapy to suppress RA and prevent a favorable substrate for arrhythmogenesis from developing. Upstream therapy also has the important potential benefit of preventing the need for ICD shocks, which have an adverse impact on quality of life and may also have a detrimental effect on heart failure disease progression [70].

Various forms of upstream therapy [71] have been proposed including adaptive pacing protocols [51, 72, 73] that might be incorporated into existing implantable device platforms such that if the device detects an unstable myocardial substrate (as evidenced by heightened RA magnitude), the adaptive pacing protocol would be activated to deliver electrical therapy to re-stabilize the electrical substrate so that even if a trigger event occurred (i.e. a premature beat), that trigger would no longer encounter a vulnerable electrical substrate and the onset of arrhythmia would be prevented. The adaptive pacing protocol could be terminated when the RA magnitude falls below a predetermined threshold.

Prior studies have investigated the use of dynamic pacing protocols based on real-time measurement of APD to control alternans. Simulation studies in one-dimensional cable geometry have suggested that RA control is limited to a maximum cable length due to the formation of standing wave patterns of alternans [74]. In vitro studies have utilized dynamic pacing protocols based on real-time measurement of APD to control RA in small sections of bullfrog myocardium [75], canine Purkinje fibers [73] and perfused canine right ventricular preparations [76], demonstrating alternans control over a region of tissue as large as ~2–2.5 cm. However, these studies were limited in controlling alternans in spatially constrained models. The only in vivo demonstration of dynamic pacing therapy to control alternans, demonstrated control of AV nodal conduction alternans in five patients undergoing clinically-indicated electrophysiology studies [72]. However, AV nodal conduction alternans remains a spatially limited phenomenon and does not recapitulate the complex spatial-temporal nature of alternans during ventricular repolarization. Therefore, the ability to control ventricular alternans, in-vivo, in the diseased heart has been elusive until recently.

Data from our group on the use of adaptive pacing to suppress RA are presented in Fig. 18.8. Using the acute coronary artery occlusion model in swine, we plot the alternans voltage (Fig. 18.8a) and K_{score} (Fig. 18.8b) of the triangular intra-cardiac bipolar lead configuration CS2CS8, LV4CS2 and LV10CS2. In intervention "a", one observes significant spontaneously occurring RA. Upon detection of significant RA, we estimated the phase of RA [52] and applied in-phase R-wave triggered pacing with positive polarity from a catheter lead in the right ventricle apex with the following parameters: amplitude: +4 mA; pulse width: 10 ms; pulse coupling: 10 ms, on every even beat (intervention "b"). We observe that R-wave triggered pacing results in a significant reduction of spontaneous RA during acute ischemia (77.59 % average reduction across the three leads of the alternans voltage compared to baseline, $p<0.0001$; 92.55 % average reduction across the three leads of the K_{score} compared to baseline, $p<0.0001$). In intervention "c", R-wave triggered pacing is discontinued, leading to an increase of the alternans voltage and K_{score} (68.62 % average increase across the three leads of the alternans voltage compared to RA suppression, $p<0.0001$; 87.06 % average increase across the three leads of the K_{score}, compared to RA suppression, $p<0.0001$).

These findings are further supported by our recent observation [51] that pacing during the absolute refractory period on an every beat basis induces a consistent, lead-dependent modulation on ventricular repolarization. These data provide an important proof of concept that the phase of RA is a critical parameter that can be estimated in real-time and used to suppress spontaneously occurring RA. Pacing on every beat does not suppress RA because it fails to account for the importance of phase (i.e. long or short action potential) in the pathogenesis of alternans. Importantly, pacing on every beat in this model does not decrease the level of alternans (data not shown).

In Fig. 18.8c, we present the change of ECG morphology from baseline during sinus rhythm

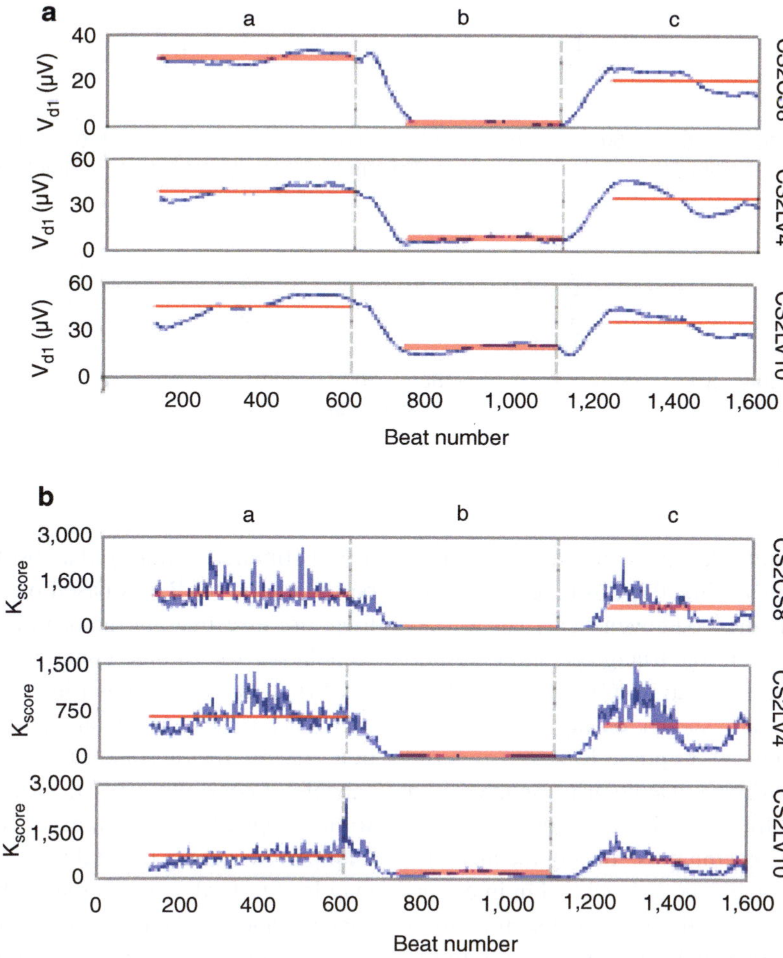

Fig. 18.8 Example of spontaneously occurring alternans suppression in sinus rhythm during acute myocardial ischemia. Alternans voltage (**a**) and K_{score} (**b**) are plotted for the intra-cardiac lead configuration CS2CS8, CS2LV4 and CS2LV10. Alternans suppression pacing is delivered from the right ventricle apex (RV12; amplitude: +4 mA, width: 10 ms, coupling to R-wave: 10 ms). *a*: spontaneously occurring alternans is visible at baseline, *b*: R-wave triggered pacing is delivered from RV12 on every even beat with a positive polarity pulse, which results to significant reduction of RA (77.59 % reduction of the alternans voltage compared to baseline, $p<0.0001$; 92.55 % reduction of the K_{score} compared to baseline, $p<0.0001$), *c*: R-wave triggered pacing is discontinued and both alternans voltage and K_{score} increase to the baseline level during sinus rhythm. Transitions *a* to *c* occur correspondingly at times marked by solid vertical black lines, while the colored horizontal lines during each intervention indicate the mean value of the alternans voltage and K_{score} during that intervention. In (**c**) ECG morphology changes during the corresponding recordings *a–c*, above; *panels* show the median odd (*red*)/ even(*blue*) beats in a 128-beat sequence of the triangular intra-cardiac bipolar lead configuration CS2CS8, CS2LV4 and CS2LV10 during each intervention

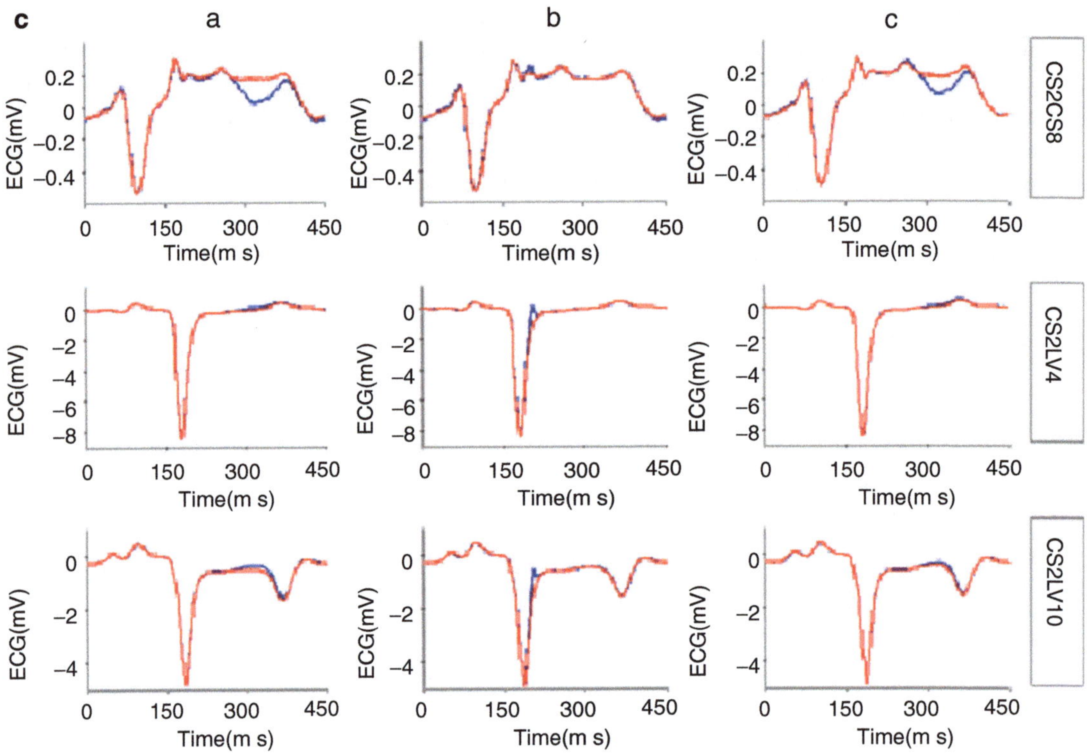

Fig. 18.8 (continued)

(when significant RA is present), to RA suppression by pacing during the absolute refractory period. The median odd/even beats (in a 128-beat sequence) of the triangular intra-cardiac bipolar lead configuration CS2CS8, CS2LV4 and CS2LV10 are shown during spontaneous RA (intervention A), in-phase R-wave triggered pacing with positive pulse polarity (intervention "b") and baseline RA (intervention "c"). The presence of the pacing pulse during the absolute refractory period can be appreciated in intervention "b", along with the loss of discrimination between odd and even beats, consistent with the suppression of RA. While visible RA is present during both baselines (interventions "a" and "c"), intervention "b" demonstrates a significant reduction in the alternans level, to the extent that RA is no longer visible.

These data provide an important proof of concept that adaptive pacing protocols can be used in real-time to suppress RA and potentially prevent the formation of a pro-arrhythmic substrate. The use of stimulation during the absolute refractory period to control RA is based on a vast body of literature investigating the use of non-excitatory stimulation for cardiac contractility modulation (CCM). It has been shown in computer simulations [77] and experimental studies that stimulation during the absolute refractory period is capable of controlling APD. Specifically, pacing stimuli applied during the early absolute refractory period appear to modulate I_{to} [78], which may lead to further activation of the L-type Ca^{2+} channel and modulation of calcium transients [78]. Therefore, the use of sub-threshold stimulation to control APD and RA may share common mechanisms with the pathogenesis of RA at the cellular level.

Beyond adaptive pacing protocols, detection of RA by implantable devices may also be coupled to other forms of therapy. For instance, there is significant interest in coupling micro-electromechanical systems (MEMS) to implantable devices to facilitate localized delivery of pharmacologic agents for treating various aspects of chronic heart failure i.e. neurohormonal antagonists, diuretics, anti-arrhythmic agents [79]. It is conceivable that timely and potentially localized delivery of anti-arrhythmic agents may also be capable of suppressing RA and re-stabilizing the electrical substrate.

Conclusions

The prevailing hypothesis of repolarization alternans is that dynamic sub-cellular perturbations in intracellular Ca^{2+} homeostatic mechanisms occurring on a beat-to-beat basis give rise to $[Ca^{2+}]_i$ alternans, which in turn gives rise to APD alternans and electrocardiographic alternans. At the whole heart level, the presence of discordant APD alternans is associated with increased spatial dispersion of refractoriness, wavefront fractionation and under certain circumstances, the onset of reentrant arrhythmias. This paradigm suggests that rather than being merely associated with *medium-* and *long*-term risk of VTE/SCD, surges in RA may play a more proximate role in creating the conditions necessary for *acute* arrhythmogenesis. The temporal association between RA and acute arrhythmia susceptibility may also have important clinical implications for early detection of impending arrhythmias and for guiding upstream anti-arrhythmic therapies.

Acknowledgments This work was supported by National Institutes of Aging (NIA) grant 1R21AG035128 and a Founders Affiliate Post-doctoral Fellowship (#12POST9310001) from the American Heart Association. This work was also supported by a Fellowship and a Science Award from the Center for Integration of Medicine and Innovative Technology (CIMIT), the Deane Institute for Integrative Research in Atrial Fibrillation and Stroke and the Cardiovascular Research Society.

References

1. Hering HE. Das Wesen des Herzalternans. Munch Med Wchenschr. 1908;4:1417–21.
2. Armoundas AA, Tomaselli GF, Esperer HD. Pathophysiological basis and clinical application of T Wave alternans. J Am Coll Cardiol. 2002;40: 207–17.
3. Armoundas AA, Hohnloser SH, Ikeda T, Cohen RJ. Can microvolt T-wave alternans testing reduce unnecessary defibrillator implantation? Nat Clin Pract Cardiovasc Med. 2005;2:522–78.
4. Turitto G, Caref EB, El-Attar G, Hellal M, Mohamed A, Pedalino RP, et al. Optimal target heart rate for exercise-induced T-wave alternans. Ann Noninvasive Electrocardiol. 2001;6:123–8.
5. Laurita KR, Pastore JM, Rosenbaum DS. How restitution, repolarization, and alternans form arrhythmogenic substrates: insights from high-resolution optical mapping. In: Zipes DP, Jalife J, editors. Cardiac electrophysiology: from cell to bedside. 2nd ed. Philadelphia: W.B.Saunders; 1999. p. 239–48.
6. Hüser J, Wang YG, Sheehan KA, Cifuentes F, Lipsius SL, Blatter LA. Functional coupling between glycolysis and excitation-contraction coupling underlies alternans in cat heart cells. J Physiol. 2000;524(Pt 3):795–806.
7. Mahajan A, Sato D, Shiferaw Y, Baher A, Xie LH, Peralta R, et al. Modifying L-type calcium current kinetics: consequences for cardiac excitation and arrhythmia dynamics. Biophys J. 2008;94:411–23.
8. Hua F, Johns DC, Gilmour Jr RF. Suppression of electrical alternans by overexpression of HERG in canine ventricular myocytes. Am J Physiol Heart Circ Physiol. 2004;286:H2342–51.
9. Fox JJ, McHarg JL, Gilmour Jr RF. Ionic mechanism of electrical alternans. Am J Physiol. 2002; 282:H516–30.
10. Jordan PN, Christini DJ. Action potential morphology influences intracellular calcium handling stability and the occurrence of alternans. Biophys J. 2006; 90:672–80.
11. Allen DG, Orchard CH. Myocardial contractile function during ischemia and hypoxia. Circ Res. 1987; 60:153–68.
12. Goldhaber JI, Xie LH, Duong T, Motter C, Khuu K, Weiss JN. Action potential duration restitution and alternans in rabbit ventricular myocytes: the key role of intracellular calcium cycling. Circ Res. 2005;96:459–66.
13. Diaz ME, Eisner DA, O'Neill SC. Depressed ryanodine receptor activity increases variability and duration of the systolic Ca2+ transient in rat ventricular myocytes. Circ Res. 2002;91:585–93.
14. Kockskamper J, Zima AV, Blatter LA. Modulation of sarcoplasmic reticulum Ca2+ release by glycolysis in cat atrial myocytes. J Physiol. 2005;564:697–714.
15. Pastore JM, Girouard SD, Laurita KR, Akar FG, Rosenbaum DS. Mechanism linking T-wave alternans to the genesis of cardiac fibrillation. Circulation. 1999;99:1385–94.
16. Pastore JM, Rosenbaum DS. Role of structural barriers in the mechanism of alternans-induced reentry. Circ Res. 2000;87:1157–63.
17. Kameyama M, Hirayama Y, Saitoh H, Maruyama M, Atarashi H, Takano T. Possible contribution of the sarcoplasmic reticulum Ca(2+) pump function to electrical and mechanical alternans. J Electrocardiol. 2003;36:125–35.

18. Lab MJ, Lee JA. Changes in intracellular calcium during mechanical alternans in isolated ferret ventricular muscle. Circ Res. 1990;66:585–95.
19. Shiferaw Y, Watanabe MA, Garfinkel A, Weiss JN, Karma A. Model of intracellular calcium cycling in ventricular myocytes. Biophys J. 2003;85:3666–86.
20. Diaz ME, O'Neill SC, Eisner DA. Sarcoplasmic reticulum calcium content fluctuation is the key to cardiac alternans. Circ Res. 2004;94:650–6.
21. Picht E, DeSantiago J, Blatter LA, Bers DM. Cardiac alternans do not rely on diastolic sarcoplasmic reticulum calcium content fluctuations. Circ Res. 2006;99:740–8.
22. Belevych AE, Terentyev D, Viatchenko-Karpinski S, Terentyeva R, Sridhar A, Nishijima Y, et al. Redox modification of ryanodine receptors underlies calcium alternans in a canine model of sudden cardiac death. Cardiovasc Res. 2009;84:387–95.
23. Chudin E, Goldhaber J, Garfinkel A, Weiss J, Kogan B. Intracellular Ca^{2+} dynamics and the stability of ventricular tachycardia. Biophys J. 1999;77:2930–41.
24. Eisner DA, Choi HS, Diaz ME, O'Neill SC, Trafford AW. Integrative analysis of calcium cycling in cardiac muscle. Circ Res. 2000;87:1087–94.
25. Armoundas AA. Discordant calcium transient and action potential alternans in a canine left ventricular myocyte. IEEE Trans Biomed Eng. 2009;56:2340–4.
26. Trafford AW, Diaz ME, Sibbring GC, Eisner DA. Modulation of CICR has no maintained effect on systolic Ca2+: simultaneous measurements of sarcoplasmic reticulum and sarcolemmal Ca2+ fluxes in rat ventricular myocytes. J Physiol. 2000;522(Pt 2):259–70.
27. Bassani JW, Yuan W, Bers DM. Fractional SR Ca release is regulated by trigger Ca and SR Ca content in cardiac myocytes. Am J Physiol. 1995;268(5 Pt 1):C1313–9.
28. Xie LH, Weiss JN. Arrhythmogenic consequences of intracellular calcium waves. J Physiol. 2009;297: H997–1002.
29. Armoundas AA. Mechanism of abnormal sarcoplasmic reticulum calcium release in canine left ventricular myocytes results in cellular alternans. IEEE Trans Biomed Eng. 2009;56:220–8.
30. Li Y, Kranias EG, Mignery GA, Bers DM. Protein kinase A phosphorylation of the ryanodine receptor does not affect calcium sparks in mouse ventricular myocytes. Circ Res. 2002;90:309–16.
31. Gyorke I, Gyorke S. Regulation of the cardiac ryanodine receptor channel by luminal Ca2+ involves luminal Ca2+ sensing sites. Biophys J. 1998;75:2801–10.
32. Satoh H, Blatter LA, Bers DM. Effects of [Ca2+]i, SR Ca2+ load, and rest on Ca2+ spark frequency in ventricular myocytes. Am J Physiol. 1997;272(2 Pt 2):H657–68.
33. Kass RS, Tsien RW. Fluctuations in membrane current driven by intracellular calcium in cardiac Purkinje fibers. Biophys J. 1982;38:259–69.
34. Orchard CH, Eisner DA, Allen DG. Oscillations of intracellular Ca2+ in mammalian cardiac muscle. Nature. 1983;304(5928):735–73.
35. Pogwizd SM, Bers DM. Cellular basis of triggered arrhythmias in heart failure. Trends Cardiovasc Med. 2004;14:61–6.
36. Priori SG, Corr PB. Mechanisms underlying early and delayed afterdepolarizations induced by catecholamines. Am J Physiol. 1990;258(6 Pt 2):H1796–805.
37. Pogwizd SM, Schlotthauer K, Li L, Yuan W, Bers DM. Arrhythmogenesis and contractile dysfunction in heart failure: roles of sodium-calcium exchange, inward rectifier potassium current, and residual beta-adrenergic responsiveness. Circ Res. 2001;88:1159–67.
38. Gilmour Jr RF, Heger JJ, Prystowsky EN, Zipes DP. Cellular electrophysiologic abnormalities of diseased human ventricular myocardium. Am J Cardiol. 1983;51:137–44.
39. Bristow MR, Ginsburg R, Minobe W, Cubicciotti RS, Sageman WS, Lurie K, et al. Decreased catecholamine sensitivity and beta-adrenergic-receptor density in failing human hearts. N Engl J Med. 1982;307:205–11.
40. Venetucci LA, Trafford AW, O'Neill SC, Eisner DA. The sarcoplasmic reticulum and arrhythmogenic calcium release. Cardiovasc Res. 2008;77:285–92.
41. Lukyanenko V, Subramanian S, Gyorke I, Wiesner TF, Gyorke S. The role of luminal Ca2+ in the generation of Ca2+ waves in rat ventricular myocytes. J Physiol. 1999;518(Pt 1):173–86.
42. Aistrup GL, Shiferaw Y, Kapur S, Kadish AH, Wasserstrom JA. Mechanisms underlying the formation and dynamics of subcellular calcium alternans in the intact rat heart. Circ Res. 2009;104:639–49.
43. Zima AV, Kockskamper J, Mejia-Alvarez R, Blatter LA. Pyruvate modulates cardiac sarcoplasmic reticulum Ca2+ release in rats via mitochondria-dependent and -independent mechanisms. J Physiol. 2003;550(Pt 3):765–83.
44. Venetucci LA, Trafford AW, Eisner DA. Increasing ryanodine receptor open probability alone does not produce arrhythmogenic calcium waves: threshold sarcoplasmic reticulum calcium content is required. Circ Res. 2007;100:105–11.
45. Fujiwara K, Tanaka H, Mani H, Nakagami T, Takamatsu T. Burst emergence of intracellular Ca2+ waves evokes arrhythmogenic oscillatory depolarization via the Na+–Ca2+ exchanger: simultaneous confocal recording of membrane potential and intracellular Ca2+ in the heart. Circ Res. 2008;103:509–18.
46. Smith JM, Clancy EA, Valeri CR, Ruskin JN, Cohen RJ. Electrical alternans and cardiac electrical instability. Circulation. 1988;77:110–21.
47. Lewis T. Notes upon alternation of the heart. Q J Med. 1910;4:141–4.
48. Restivo M, Caref EB, Kozhevnikov DO, El-Sherif N. Spatial dispersion of repolarization is a key factor in the arrhythmogenicity of long QT syndrome. J Cardiovasc Electrophysiol. 2004;15:323–31.
49. Armoundas AA, Albert CM, Cohen RJ, Mela T. Utility of implantable cardioverter defibrillator electrograms to estimate repolarization alternans

preceding a tachyarrhythmic event. J Cardiovasc Electrophysiol. 2004;15:594–7.
50. Armoundas AA, Mela T, Merchant FM. On the estimation of T-wave alternans using the spectral fast fourier transform method. Heart Rhythm. 2012;9:449–56.
51. Armoundas AA, Weiss EH, Sayadi O, Laferriere S, Sajja N, Mela T, et al. A novel pacing method to suppress repolarization alternans in vivo: implications for arrhythmia prevention. Heart Rhythm. 2013;10:564–72.
52. Sayadi O, Merchant FM, Puppala D, Mela T, Singh JP, Heist EK, et al. A novel method for determining the phase of T-wave alternans: diagnostic and therapeutic implications. Circ Arrhythm Electrophysiol. 2013;6:818–26.
53. Weiss EH, Merchant FM, d'Avila A, Foley L, Reddy VY, Singh JP, et al. A novel lead configuration for optimal spatio-temporal detection of intracardiac repolarization alternans. Circ Arrhythm Electrophysiol. 2011;4(407):407–17.
54. Rosenbaum DS, Jackson LE, Smith JM, Garan H, Ruskin JN, Cohen RJ. Electrical alternans and vulnerability to ventricular arrhythmias. N Engl J Med. 1994;330:235–41.
55. Verrier RL, Klingenheben T, Malik M, El-Sherif N, Exner DV, Hohnloser SH, et al. Microvolt T-wave alternans physiological basis, methods of measurement, and clinical utility–consensus guideline by International Society for Holter and Noninvasive Electrocardiology. J Am Coll Cardiol. 2011;58: 1309–24.
56. Merchant FM, Ikeda T, Pedretti RF, Salerno-Uriarte JA, Chow T, Chan PS, et al. Clinical utility of microvolt T-wave alternans testing in identifying patients at high or low risk of sudden cardiac death. Heart Rhythm. 2012;9:1256–64.
57. Chow T, Kereiakes DJ, Onufer J, Woelfel A, Gursoy S, Peterson BJ, et al. Does microvolt T-wave alternans testing predict ventricular tachyarrhythmias in patients with ischemic cardiomyopathy and prophylactic defibrillators? The MASTER (Microvolt T Wave Alternans Testing for Risk Stratification of Post-Myocardial Infarction Patients) trial. J Am Coll Cardiol. 2008;52:1607–15.
58. Gold MR, Ip JH, Costantini O, Poole JE, McNulty S, Mark DB, et al. Role of microvolt T-wave alternans in assessment of arrhythmia vulnerability among patients with heart failure and systolic dysfunction: primary results from the T-wave alternans sudden cardiac death in heart failure trial substudy. Circulation. 2008;118:2022–8.
59. Chan PS, Gold MR, Nallamothu BK. Do Beta-blockers impact microvolt T-wave alternans testing in patients at risk for ventricular arrhythmias? A meta-analysis. J Cardiovasc Electrophysiol. 2010;21:1009–14.
60. Ellenbogen KA, Levine JH, Berger RD, Daubert JP, Winters SL, Greenstein E, et al. Are implantable cardioverter defibrillator shocks a surrogate for sudden cardiac death in patients with nonischemic cardiomyopathy? Circulation. 2006;113:776–82.
61. Hohnloser SH, Ikeda T, Cohen RJ. Evidence regarding clinical use of microvolt T-wave alternans. Heart Rhythm. 2009;6(3 Suppl):S36–44.
62. Fishman GI, Chugh SS, Dimarco JP, Albert CM, Anderson ME, Bonow RO, et al. Sudden cardiac death prediction and prevention: report from a National Heart, Lung, and Blood Institute and Heart Rhythm Society Workshop. Circulation. 2010;122:2335–48.
63. Stecker EC, Vickers C, Waltz J, Socoteanu C, John BT, Mariani R, et al. Population-based analysis of sudden cardiac death with and without left ventricular systolic dysfunction: two-year findings from the Oregon Sudden Unexpected Death Study. J Am Coll Cardiol. 2006;47:1161–6.
64. Merchant FM, Zheng H, Bigger T, Steinman R, Ikeda T, Pedretti RF, et al. A combined anatomic and electrophysiologic substrate based approach for sudden cardiac death risk stratification. Am Heart J. 2013;166:744–52.
65. Shusterman V, Goldberg A, London B. Upsurge in T-wave alternans and nonalternating repolarization instability precedes spontaneous initiation of ventricular tachyarrhythmias in humans. Circulation. 2006; 113:2880–7.
66. Nearing BD, Wellenius GA, Mittleman MA, Josephson ME, Burger AJ, Verrier RL. Crescendo in depolarization and repolarization heterogeneity heralds development of ventricular tachycardia in hospitalized patients with decompensated heart failure. Circ Arrhythm Electrophysiol. 2012;5:84–90.
67. Paz O, Zhou X, Gillberg J, Tseng HJ, Gang E, Swerdlow C. Detection of T-wave alternans using an implantable cardioverter-defibrillator. Heart Rhythm. 2006;3:791–7.
68. Kim JW, Pak HN, Park JH, Nam GB, Kim SK, Lee HS, et al. Defibrillator electrogram T wave alternans as a predictor of spontaneous ventricular tachyarrhythmias in defibrillator recipients. Circ J. 2009;73:55–62.
69. Swerdlow C, Chow T, Das M, Gillis AM, Zhou X, Abeyratne A, et al. Intracardiac electrogram T-wave alternans/variability increases before spontaneous ventricular tachyarrhythmias in implantable cardioverter-defibrillator patients: a prospective, multi-center study. Circulation. 2011;123: 1052–60.
70. Moss AJ, Schuger C, Beck CA, Brown MW, Cannom DS, Daubert JP, et al. Reduction in inappropriate therapy and mortality through ICD programming. N Engl J Med. 2012;367:2275–83.
71. Garfinkel A, Spano ML, Ditto WL, Weiss JN. Controlling cardiac chaos. Science. 1992; 257(5074):1230–5.
72. Christini DJ, Stein KM, Markowitz SM, Mittal S, Slotwiner DJ, Scheiner MA, et al. Nonlinear-dynamical arrhythmia control in humans. Proc Natl Acad Sci U S A. 2001;98:5827–32.
73. Christini DJ, Riccio ML, Culianu CA, Fox JJ, Karma A, Gilmour Jr RF. Control of electrical alternans in canine cardiac purkinje fibers. Phys Rev Lett. 2006;96:104101.

74. Echebarria B, Karma A. Instability and spatiotemporal dynamics of alternans in paced cardiac tissue. Phys Rev Lett. 2002;88:208101.
75. Hall GM, Gauthier DJ. Experimental control of cardiac muscle alternans. Phys Rev Lett. 2002;88:198102.
76. Kanu UB, Iravanian S, Gilmour Jr RF, Christini DJ. Control of action potential duration alternans in canine cardiac ventricular tissue. IEEE Trans Biomed Eng. 2011;58:894–904.
77. Li M, Otani NF. Controlling alternans in cardiac cells. Ann Biomed Eng. 2004;32:784–92.
78. Greenstein JL, Wu R, Po S, Tomaselli GF, Winslow RL. Role of the calcium-independent transient outward current I(to1) in shaping action potential morphology and duration. Circ Res. 2000;87:1026–33.
79. Merchant FM, Dec GW, Singh JP. Implantable sensors for heart failure. Circ Arrhythm Electrophysiol. 2010;3:657–67.
80. Armoundas AA, Nanke T, Cohen RJ. Images in cardiovascular medicine. T-wave alternans preceding torsade de pointes ventricular tachycardia. Circulation. 2000;101:2550.

Part IV

Man and Animals

Animal Models of Cardiovascular Disease

19

Inês Falcão-Pires and Adelino F. Leite-Moreira

Abstract

Cardiovascular diseases (CVD) often lead to heart failure (HF). HF prevalence is continuously rising and represents one of the leading causes of death and an economic burden in the western societies. The study of potential novel therapeutic options and interventions requires reliable animal models to evaluate myocardial progressive structural and functional changes. Indeed, during the past 40 years, basic and translational scientists have used small animal models to understand the pathophysiology of HF and improve prevention and treatment of patients suffering from congestive HF (CHF). Each species and animal model has advantages and disadvantages and the choice of one model over another should take them into account for a good experimental design.

The aim of this chapter is to describe and highlight the features of some commonly used animal models of cardiovascular diseases with a particular emphasis on the ones leading to HF, including nongenetically and genetically engineered models. Larger animal models will be briefly mentioned and compared to rodents but this chapter will mostly focus on rat and mouse models.

Keywords

Animal models • Rodents • Heart failure • Metabolic syndrome • Cardiovascular disease

Abbreviations

ATH	Atherosclerosis
CHF	Congestive heart failure
CVD	Cardiovascular diseases
DCM	Dilated cardiomyopathy
DM	Diabetes mellitus
DOCA	Deoxycortcosterone acetate
DOX	Doxorubicin

I. Falcão-Pires, MSc, PhD (✉)
A.F. Leite-Moreira, MD, PhD
Department of Physiology and Cardiothoracic Surgery, Faculty of Medicine, Universidade do Porto, Alameda Prof Hernâni Monteiro, Porto 4200-319, Portugal
e-mail: ipires@med.up.pt; amoreira@med.up.pt

D.V. Cokkinos (ed.), *Introduction to Translational Cardiovascular Research*,
DOI 10.1007/978-3-319-08798-6_19,

EF	Ejection fraction
EMCV	Encephalomyocarditid virus
HF	Heart failure
HFpEF	Heart failure with preserved ejection fraction
HFrEF	Heart failure with reduced ejection fraction
HT	Hypertension
HYP	Hypertrophy
LAD	Left anterior descending
LV	Left ventricle
MCT	Monocrotaline
MI	Myocardial infarction
MS	Metabolic syndrome
RAAS	Renin-angiotensin-aldosterone system
REM	Remodeling

19.1 Introduction

Cardiovascular diseases (CVD) represent the leading cause of deaths worldwide, though since the 1970s, cardiovascular mortality rates have declined in western society countries. CVD includes all the diseases of the heart and circulation including coronary heart disease, congenital heart disease and stroke among other. The increasing prevalence of risk factors such as hypertension, obesity and diabetes has led to a striking rise in CVD, often progressing towards HF. In turn, this syndrome can be defined as an abnormality of cardiac structure or function leading to failure of the heart to deliver oxygen at a rate commensurate with the requirements of the metabolizing tissues, despite normal filling pressures (or only at the expense of increased filling pressures) [1]. It is the common symptomatic end stage of a number of distinct CVD and thus is considered a multifactorial and polygenetic syndrome.

Heart failure is often divided in two distinct entities, namely HF with reduced ejection fraction (EF, HFrEF) and HF with preserved EF (HFpEF). Despite the controversy on the definition of each entity, HFrEF is related to systolic dysfunction and characterized by an inability of the myocardium to contract and eject blood. In turn, HFpEF is associated to diastolic dysfunction and so refers to a disturbance in accommodating blood volume during diastole at low filling pressures, due to impaired ventricular relaxation (primarily affecting early diastole) or increased myocardial stiffness (primarily affecting late diastole) [2]. Besides being rather difficult to replicate pure HFpEF in animal models, these are also more demanding and time consuming than HFrEF. Therefore, the great majority of animal models have been developed for HFrEF. Simillarly, cardiac failure can affect the right, the left or both ventricles. Nevertheless most animal models were developed to exhibit left ventricular failure.

19.2 Animal Models of Cardiovascular Disease

19.2.1 Vascular Dysfunction and Atheroscrosis

The hypothesis that macrovascular disease is due to hypercholesterolemic dyslipidemia has been a powerful concept that has fostered the development of cholesterol-lowering therapeutics, most notably statins. However, despite recent thepeutical progresses that effectively control plasma cholesterol concentrations, a major reduction in the incidence of CV Diseases was not observed. Animal models of vascular dysfunction and atherosclerosis are hard to achieve without highly abnormal diets or genetically modified mice. Such is the case of the JCR:La-Cp derived from Koletsky corpulent rats inbred over many generations to produce a rat presenting significant ATH, hyperlipidemia, insulin-resistance-induced micro/macrovascular lesions, ischemic myocardial lesions and spontaneous myocardial infarction (Fig. 19.1) (MI). Also, knockout mice such as *ApoE*$^{-/-}$ and *LDLR*$^{-/-}$ are widely used as models of ATH. *ApoE*$^{-/-}$ mouse presents hypercholesterolemia and exhibits advanced intima lesions confined to aortic root area, which may spread upon a high-cholesterol diet. Similarly, the C57BL/6 mouse develops some ATH in the aortic root when fed with a high-fat or high-cholesterol diet. In turn *LDLR*$^{-/-}$ mouse is a model of the familial hypercholesterolemia due to a muta-

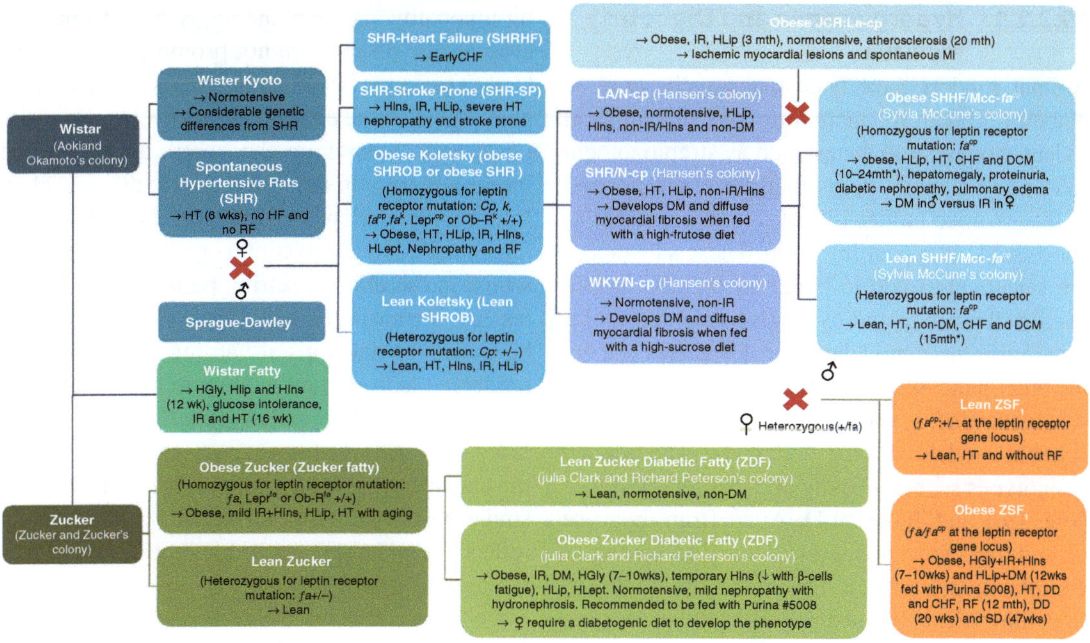

Fig. 19.1 Relationship between different strains of rats whose selective crossing over several generations gave rise to different animal models of diabetes, hypertension, obesity and metabolic syndrome. Currently male obese ZDF, obese ZSF_1, Koletsky and obese SHHF/Mcc-*fa*^{cp} rats are accepted as good animal models of metabolic syndrome. *: the timing depends on the gender and genotype. *CHF* congestive heart failure, *DCM*, dilated cardiomyopathy, *DD* diastolic dysfunction, *DM* diabetes mellitus, *HF* heart failure, *HGly* hyperglycemia, *HLep* hyperleptinemia, *HLip* hyperlipidemia, *HIns* Hyperinsulinemia, *HT* hypertension, *IR* insulin resistance, *MI* myocardial infarction, *mth* months, *RF* renal failure, *SD* systolic dysfunction, *wks* weeks

tion affecting the LDL receptor, developing extremely high plasma cholesterol levels. Similar to untreated humans, these mice exhibit xanthomas and extensive atherosclerotic lesions in several vessels [3].

Of note is the fact that most of diet-induced ATH models do not present occlusive coronary artery disease, myocardial infarction, cardiac dysfunction and premature death, which are a rather common feature of human atherosclerotic disease that may lead to congestive HF.

19.2.2 Metabolic Syndrome

The metabolic syndrome (MS) is diagnosed whenever three of the following disorders: obesity, hypertension, insulin resistance, hyperglycemia or dyslipidemia are found in the same individual. This triad represents a threatening and complex disorder, which is the leading cause of CV morbidity and mortality in modern societies. Over the last four decades, two significant mutations (i.e. *fa* and *cp*) that elicit obesity have been identified in rats. The *fa* mutation, originally described by Zucker in 1961 [4] has been backcrossed into several strains (Fig. 19.1). The *cp* mutation described originally by Koletsky has been also backcrossed into several strains, including SHHF/Mcc-*fa*^{cp} rats [5]. Several strains have been selectively inbred and backcrossed for many generations to select particular features, such as hypertension, obesity or hyperglycemia, giving rise to a huge variety of models whose relationship can be difficult to establish and comprising a part or the whole metabolic syndrome phenotype as illustrated in Fig. 19.1.

This chapter will address separately animal models of hyperglycemia and diabetes mellitus, hypertension and obesity, highlighting those that might represent good animal models of the metabolic syndrome.

19.2.2.1 Hyperglycemia and Diabetes Mellitus

Animal models have been extensively used in diabetes research, including pharmacological rodent models of diabetes such as streptozotocin (STZ) and alloxan, drugs that when administred to rats or mice induce diabetes mellitus (DM) as soon as 24–48 h post-injection. These substances are selectively toxic to pancreas β-cells, induce insulin deficiency and hyperglycemia and therefore represents a model of type-1 diabetes [6]. On the other hand, selective inbreeding has produced several strains of animal that are considered reasonable models of type 2 diabetes and related phenotypes such as obesity and insulin resistance (Fig. 19.1 and Table 19.1). Apart from their use in studying the pathogenesis of the disease and its complications, all new treatments for diabetes, including islet cell transplantation and preventive strategies, are initially investigated in animal models. In recent years, a large number of new genetic animal models for the study of diabetes, including knockin or generalized and tissue-specific knockout mice have been described. Rodent models of type-2 diabetes include the Zucker fatty rat, as well as db/db and ob/ob mice, all of which display dysfunctional or absent leptin homeostasis and therefore develop insulin resistance at different timepoints (Table 19.1).

These rodent models share many features of human diabetic cardiomyopathy. For example, rodent models of obesity, insulin resistance and type 2 diabetes present left ventricle (LV) hypertrophy, diastolic dysfunction, increased cardiac fatty acid uptake and utilization, decreased cardiac efficiency, impaired mitochondrial energetics, increased myocardial lipid storage and impaired Ca^{2+} handling [7]. Moreover, depending on the model, in vivo studies have revealed susceptibility to systolic and diastolic dysfunction assessed by echocardiography and hemodynamics [8] as well as propensity to ischemia/reperfusion injury following ligation/unligation of the left anterior descending coronary artery (LAD), which occurs in conjunction with structural and functional changes to the LV [9].

However, there are several limitations when comparing these models to human diabetic cardiomyopathy, as spontaneous ischemia and atherosclerotic disease are not prominent in rodents [10]. The latter becomes simultaneously a valuable aspect as the effects of obesity, insulin resistance and diabetes on the heart can be studied independently of coronary artery disease [11]. Importantly, rodent models present sudden and uncontrolled hyperglycemia or insulin resistance, whilst in the clinical setting patients with diabetes are increasingly well controlled. Moreover, because DM develops at varying stages in these models, it is important to keep in mind that studies performed in animals before the onset of diabetes may reflect changes that are secondary to the underlying obesity and insulin resistance, and studies performed after the onset of diabetes may reflect the added effects of hyperglycemia of different durations.

19.2.2.2 Systemic Hypertension

Spontaneously Hypertensive Rats SHR

Systemic hypertension is another relevant risk factor for human congestive HF. Spontaneous hypertension is a natural model of pressure overload, in which systemic hypertension leads to HF with ageing. Hypertensive vascular lesions appear within 6–7 weeks, being more severe in males than in females. For the first 12 months, hypertrophy is compensated and contractility is preserved, but after 18–24 months there is overt congestive HF characterized by fibrosis, LV dilation and reduced systolic function [12]. These structural and functional changes occur together with a marked rise in cytokine levels such as TNF-α and interleukin-6 [13]. Transition to failure has been suggested to depend on significant alterations in the expression of genes encoding extracellular matrix proteins, oxidative stress and increased apoptosis of myocytes [12]. The gradual onset of hypertension with ageing makes this model suitable for studying the transition from hypertrophy to CHF and for reproducing hypertension-induced CHF in humans [14]. It has the advantage of avoiding the complications associated with surgical or pharmacological interventions, while mimicking the changes found in human essential hypertension [12]. Indeed, the SHR is a very useful model of genetic hyperten-

Table 19.1 Summary of the characteristics of the most usual diabetes mellitus animal models

Model	Type	DM type	Specie	Pathophysiologic changes	Advantages	Disadvantages
Alloxan	P	1	Mouse	Significant hyperglycemia	Fast, economic and consistent	High mortality rate
			Rat	Ketosis and/or ketoacidosis		Alloxan has a very short half-life (<1 min)
				Glycosuria, hyperlipidemia, polyphagia, polydipsia		Hyperglycemia frequently reverts by pancreatic regeneration
				Neuropathy and cardiomyopathy		
Streptozotocin	P	1	Mouse	Significant hyperglycemia	Fast, economic and consistent	High mortality rate
			Rat	Polyuria, polydipsia		Very severe model
				Muscular atrophy		
				Neuropathy		
OLETF – Otsuka Long-Evans Tokushima Fatty	G	2	Rat	Hyperglycemia	Progressive DM:	Late DM development
				Polyuria, polydipsia	Initial phase (0–9 wk): Pancreatic islet hyperplasia and lymphocytes' infiltration	Only males develop DM
				Mild obesity	Intermediate phase (10–40 wk): Pancreatic islet fibrosis	
				Diastolic dysfunction	Advanced phase (>40 wk): pancreatic islet atrophy. Type 1 DM	
				Diabetic nephropathy with nodular glomerulosclerosis (30 wk)		
ZDF – Zucker Diabetic Fatty	G	2	Rat	Dysfunctional leptin receptor	Very common model	Mild nephropathy with hydronephrosis
				Hyperphagia, hyperlipidemia, hyperglycemia	ZDF were selectively bred from Zucker rat which are similar but without hyperglycemia and DM	Due to different genetic backgrounds, no comparisons can be made between ZDF and Zucker rats
				Glucose intolerance and hyperinsulinemia (10–12 wk).that progresses to impaired insulin secretion with β-cells fatigue		
				Mild hypertension and obesity	Females develop DM upon a high-fat diet	Useful for studies on the efficacy of drugs directed at macrovascular function, nephropathy, myocardial injury and lipidemia
				Loss of both GLUT-2 glucose transporters in pancreatic β-cells and GLUT-4 in the muscle (25–55 %)		
				Impaired cardiac contractility and diastolic function (~20 wk)		
				Increased LV mass and fatty acid oxidation		
				Microvascular damage leading to glomerular sclerosis and retinopathy		
				Evidence of vascular dysfunction in the aorta, coronary arteries, and mesenteric arteries in middle-aged obese ZDF rats probably related to frank diabetes		

(continued)

Table 19.1 (continued)

Model	Type	DM type	Specie	Pathophysiologic changes	Advantages	Disadvantages
GK – Goto-Kakizaki	G	1	Rat	Mild fast hyperglycemia	Stable degree of glucose intolerance	Non obese
				Hyperinsulinemia and insulin resistance	Useful for studying advanced diabetic nephropathy	
				Decreased insulin production	Wistar rats are the control group	
				Retinopathy, microangiopathy, neuropathy and nephropathy		
Wistar Fatty	G	1/2	Rat	Hyperglycemia, hyperlipidemia e hyperinsulinemia (12 wk)	Wistar rats are the control group	Only males develop type-2 DM
				Glucose intolerance and insulin resistance		
				Hypertension (16 wk)		
				Wistar × Zucker selective breeding		Not commercially available
Db/db	G	2	Mouse	Leptin receptor deficiency	Advantages associated with mice reduced size (see text)	Glucose levels progressively increase until the 16th week
				Hyperlipidemia and obesity (8 wk)		
				Polyphagia, polyuria and polydipsia		
				Insulin resistance, hyperinsulinemia (2 wk) and hyperglycemia (8 wk)		
				Peripheral neuropathy		
				Diabetic cardiomyopathy		
				Impaired diastolic function, mitochondrial energetic, Ca2+ homeostasis and cardiac efficiency		
				Impaired endothelial and vascular function		
				Increased LV mass, fatty acid oxidation and RAAS activation		
Ob/ob	G	2	Mouse	Leptin deficiency	Advantages associated with mice reduced size (see text)	Certain degree of infertility
				Hyperphagia and obesity (4 wk)	Allows the evaluation of the early effects of obesity and insulin resistance on cardiac function and the effects of additional hyperglycemia at older ages	Reduced metabolism and hypothermia
				Hyperglycemia and hyperinsulinemia (15 wk, following obesity)		
				Insulin resistance and glucose intolerance		
				Impaired diastolic function, mitochondrial energetic, Ca2+ homeostasis and cardiac efficiency		
				Increased LV mass, fatty acid oxidation and lipid content		

Pancreatectomy	S	1	All	Mild hyperglycemia	Useful for pancreatic regeneration studies	Risk of infection.
				No weight or insulin levels reduction	Can be used in all animal model species	Post-operative precautions
					Avoids pharmacologic toxicity of DM-induction drugs	Digestive complications
					Similar to type-2 DM due to pancreatic degeneration	
High fat diet C57BL/6 J	HFD	2	Mouse	Leptin and insulin resistance	Advantages associated with mice reduced size (see text)	Reduced metabolism and hypothermia
				Hyperphagy and obesity	Present many genetic and environmental features of the human disease	Long high fat diet period
				Hyperglycemia and hyperinsulinemia (following obesity)		Mild hyperglycemia
				Glucose intolerance	High fat diet C57BL/6 J mice change myocardial substrate utilization prior to obesity and severe insulin resistance	
				Cardiac dysfunction (20 wk)	Useful for pharmacologic tests	
CIRKO, Akita and OVE 26	T	2,1,1	Mouse	Please check Table 19.2		

Adapted from Gomes et al. [15] with permission

DM diabetes mellitus, *G* genetic model (selective breeding), *HFD* high-fat-diet model, *P* pharmacologic model, *S* surgical model, *T* transgenic, *wk* week sion because drugs that lower blood pressure in SHR also decrease blood pressure in essential hypertension, being this one of the main reasons why researchers have used it extensively. Nonetheless, the long period required for developing CHF poses a great limitation, making it a time-consuming and consequently an expensive model. Moreover, Wistar Kyoto (WKY) is currently accepted as the "normotensive" control of SHR but it shows considerable genetic differences displayed and thus no ideal control exists for SHR.

The SHR stroke prone (SHR-SP) was selectively bred from a substrain of the SHR that showed even higher levels of blood pressure and a strong tendency to die from stroke [16]. SHR-SP rats also display nephropathy, insulin resistance, hyperinsulinemia, hypertriglyceridemia and hypercholesterolemia. Moreover, despite comparable degrees of hypertension among males and females, stroke-related mortality is greater in males than females. Renal vascular disease including thrombotic microangiopathy affecting glomeruli and microvessels as well as cardiac damage are more prominent in male SHR-SP [17].

Spontaneously Hypertensive HF Prone Rats (SHHF)

These animals were developed by backcrossing the obese SHR (SHROB) rat to the SHR/N rat and afterwards selectively bred to decrease the age at which animals developed CHF. The obese offspring carries the *facp* corpulent gene, which encodes a defective leptin receptor gene, and therefore they develop obesity and HF. The time for the development of HF depends on *facp* genotype and gender (male animals are more prone to HF than females [18]) but, in general, SHHF rats present HF earlier than the SHR strain, with loss of cardiac function starting at the age of 15 months [19]. The obese SHHF display hypertension, nephropathy, obesity, insulin resistance, hyperinsulinemia, type 2 DM, hypertriglyceridemia and hypercholesterolemia. Controls are SHHF lean that also exhibits HF characteristics but at a different age from the SHHF obese. All SHHF, regardless of genotype or gender, eventually develop spontaneous dilated cardiomyopathy (DCM). These animals present alterations in the renin-angiotensin-aldosterone system (RAAS) and also in calcium metabolism [20]. The greatest advantage of this strain, which is considered a good model of metabolic syndrome, is the possibility of studying drug interventions in an extended range of cardiovascular risk factors like obesity, diabetes and renal dysfunction [21].

Dahl Salt-Sensitive Rats

This is a mutant strain of Sprague–Dawley rats that is characterized by hypersensitivity to sodium intake [22]. When placed on a high salt diet since the 6th week of age they develop concentric LV hypertrophy (HYR) without chamber dilation around the 11th week and decompensate HF with marked ventricular dilation between the 15th and the 20th week [23]. Failure is associated with reduced myocardial performance as evidenced by the lower performance of muscle strip preparations and the short lifetime of failing rats [24].

Interestingly, it has been shown that introducing high-salt diet at 7 or 8 weeks of age can result in distinct HF phenotypes. Indeed, the 7-week starting rats showed a steeper elevation in blood pressure and progressive LV hypertrophy, falling into overt HFpEF at approximately 19 weeks. On the other hand, the 8-week starting rats showed a gradual rise in blood pressure and less progressive LV hypertrophy, developing HFrEF at approximately 26 weeks. Therefore, these two different models of overt HF may be useful as models of isolated HFpEF and HFrEF based on the same hypertensive heart disease, which could be relevant to the pathophysiologic and molecular characterization of each HF subtype [25]. Another report found that the development of HF was dissociated from changes in passive diastolic and active systolic properties, suggesting that volume overload plays an important pathophysiological role in development of congestion despite preserved overall ventricular pump function in this model of chronic hypertension [23].

This model is suitable to study the transition from compensated HYR to failure. Moreover, it is often used to identify the role of several pathways and molecular mechanisms like oxidative stress, extracellular matrix degradation, calcium handling impairment, redox regulated transcription factors and apoptotic factors activation [15].

Deoxycorticosterone Acetate (DOCA) Hypertensive Rats

The deoxycorticosterone acetate (DOCA) salt-induced model of hypertension is a typical representative of pharmacologically-induced hypertension. A very high subcutaneous dose of DOCA is required to induce hypertension in rats. Isotonic saline is the sole drinking fluid, which hastens and aggravates the progression to hypertension [26]. Despite being salt-dependent in its initiation, this model frequently needs surgical renal mass reduction or unilateral nephrectomy. DOCA-salt hypertension is a low renin and volume overload form of hypertension. The combination of DOCA-salt and unilateral nephrectomy results in hypertension, renal HYP, nephrosclerosis, cardiac hypertrophy and perivascular fibrosis within 4–5 weeks of chronic treatment [27]. Several studies report diastolic dysfunction in these rats [28].

The pathophysiologic mechanisms underlying the development and maintenance of DOCA-salt hypertension include increased levels of arginine, vasopressin [29], angiotensin II/aldosterone [30], endothelin [31] and oxidative stress [32], excessive activation of the sympathetic nervous system [33] and nitric oxide synthase (NOS) uncoupling due to oxidative depletion of its cofactor tetrahydrobiopterin (BH4) [28]. Nonetheless, the cardiac consequences are minimal during the development of DOCA-salt hypertension-induced HYP [34]. This is in contrast with the decreased cardiac performance reported in other rat models of cardiac HYP and in the failing human heart. Therefore, hypertrophy in hearts of DOCA-salt hypertensive rats does not reproduce the changes observed in the failing human heart [34]. Besides this disadvantage, other DOCA-salt model limitations are (1) the need to employ a large amount of drug, (2) the requirement for surgical reduction of renal mass and (3) the dependence on a strictly controlled ingestion of a high NaCl dose. On the other hand, its advantage is the potential to investigate the role of sodium in the developmental stages of hypertension. In an attempt to overcome some of these limitations, more recently, a group published a mouse model that combines transverse aortic constriction (TAC) with DOCA administration under a normal-salt diet. Compared with TAC mice, TAC plus DOCA mice had similarly normal LV systolic pressure and fractional shortening but more hypertrophy, fibrosis, oxidative stress and diastolic dysfunction with increased lung weights, consistent with HFpEF. Therefore, these authors suggest that pressure-overload HYP sensitizes the heart to mineralocorticoid excess, promoting the transition to HFpEF without activation of the classic mineralocorticoid receptor-dependent gene transcription [35].

Two-Kidneys, One-Clip (2K1C) or One-Kidney, One-Clip (1K1C) Rats

Since 1934, when Goldblatt and his co-workers induced an elevation of blood pressure by partial constriction of the renal artery of the dog [36], many successful models of renal-induced experimental hypertension have been developed in rats. In general, the procedure includes two-kidney Goldblatt hypertension (constriction of one renal artery while the contralateral kidney is left intact) and one-kidney Goldblatt hypertension (one renal artery is constricted and the contralateral kidney is removed) [26]. Clipping one renal artery, while leaving the contralateral kidney untouched, induces systemic hypertension and LV concentric remodeling within 8 weeks [37]. Histologic studies revealed extensive LV fibrosis while echocardiography and hemodynamic data consistently showed diastolic dysfunction [37]. Indeed, inhibition of matrix metalloproteinase activity in these hypertrophic hearts has been shown to provide beneficial effects in terms of structure and function [38]. At cellular level, several changes in the energy metabolism, actin-myosin cross-bridge cycle and protein expression were identified in renovascular hypertensive rats [37]. In addition, the central role of activation of the RAAS [39] and the sympathetic nervous system [40] has been thoroughly studied. In the one-kidney model, no compensatory increase in sodium and water excretion can occur, and hence, fluid volume is retained, which means this model is thus a sodium-fluid volume-dependent model. Therefore, it would be valuable for studying the role of volume expansion in the development of hypertension [41]. During the early developmental stage, if the clip is removed arterial blood pressure returns to normal in both models, suggesting that renovascular hypertension is both reversible and reproducible [42].

ZSF1 Obese Rats

The obese ZSF1 is commonly used to study renal failure with additional disease complications. However, these rats also represent a robust animal model of metabolic syndrome since they comprise hypertension, obesity, type 2 DM, insulin resistance, hyperinsulinemia, hypertriglyceridemia, hypercholesterolemia and even HF. Considering such features, this cardiometabolic risk animal model has recently been shown to develop diastolic dysfunction and HF, having therefore been considered a robust animal model of HFpEF by their 20th week of age. At this age no renal failure was yet observed in obese ZSF1 despite the diastolic dysfunction as confirmed by increased myocardial stiffness mostly due to myofilamentary changes, since myocardial fibrosis was absent. Lean ZSF1 also display hypertension but no diastolic dysfunction, obesity, DM nor the associated metabolic disturbances [43]. Other reports have suggested that obese ZSF1 present decreased LV contractility indices by the 45th week of age.

19.2.2.3 Obesity

Obesity is associated with premature death by increasing the risk of many chronic diseases, including type 2 DM, CV disease and certain cancers. Thus, not surprisingly, many obesity animal models are also diabetic and held major CV abnormalities (Fig. 19.2). As previously mentioned, many available models of obesity derive from selective crossings between rats comprising one out of the two most significant mutations in leptin receptor (i.e. *fa* and *cp*). Such is the case of Zucker fatty rats, the *fa* (fatty) gene "family", whose obesity is not as marked as in SHROB or JCR:La-cp, the *cp* (corpulent) gene "family". Figure 19.1 display several rat models of obesity derived from selective crossings among and between these two "families". Many obese animal models, such as Zucker fatty rat, SHROB or even SHHF, are also models of hypertension or MS and thus were mentioned in previous sections. Another example is the Otsuka Long-Evans Tokushima Fatty (OLETF) rat obtained by selecting spontaneously diabetic rats

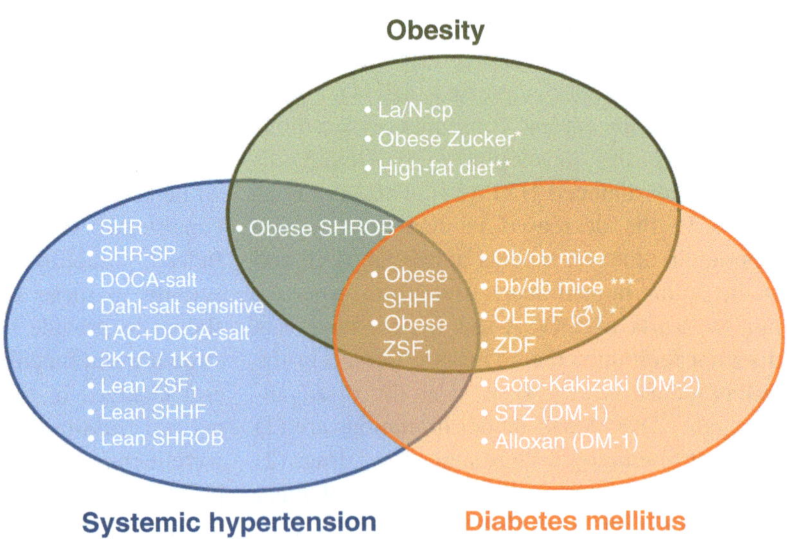

Fig. 19.2 Overview of some of the most important animal models of cardiovascular or cardiovascular-related diseases and their features. *DM-1* type 1 diabetes mellitus, *DM-2* type 2 diabetes mellitus

exhibiting polyuria, polydipsia and obesity from an out-bred colony of Long-Evans rats. These rats exhibit obesity, hyperglycemia (at the adult age, 18 weeks), hyperinsulinemia, chronic DM, which is first non-insulin dependent but that over time progresses to insulin dependent. The control strain, LETO appears to share some of diabetogenic genes with OLETF rats [44].

In the human setting, the development of obesity and metabolic syndrome is mostly linked with increased caloric intake and lack of physical activity, in addition to genetic predisposition. Thus it would be relevant to study the pathogenesis of CV disease resulting from abnormal food intake. Many models of obesity are induced by the consumption of modified diets, such as high-fat or high-carbohydrate diets, therefore representing potentially more relevant pathophysiological models of the human disease. Such is the case of C57BL/6 mouse fed with a high-fat diet described previously as an animal model or vascular dysfunction and atherosclerosis. Still regarding mice, *ob/ob* mice [45], with leptin deficiency, and *db/db* mice [46], presenting a mutation in leptin receptor, constitute the most used models of obesity, which also display hyperglycemia and hyperlipidemia without hypertension and thus represent a good animal model of metabolic syndrome.

Apart from these models, other genetic modifications gave rise to a whole range of transgenic including knockout and knockin mice, which are briefly described throughout Table 19.1, wherein the most usual DM animal models are also described.

19.2.3 Cardiac Hypertrophy

Cardiac hypertrophy may subside as a response of the heart to hemodynamic overload, during which terminally differentiated cardiomyocytes increase in size without undergoing cell division. This subchapter will only describe animal models of LV hypertrophy, while the subchapter regarding "pulmonary hypertension, emphysema and right ventricular failure" will address animal models of right ventricular HYP.

19.2.3.1 Pressure-Overload Induced Hypertrophy

Aortic constriction (banding) is a well-established surgical technique to induce LV chronic pressure overload and hypertrophy. Initially, aortic banding imposes almost no restriction to aortic flow but as the animal grows, the severity of the constriction gradually increases, resulting in cardiac hypertrophy. Banding in several aortic segments (ascending (AAC), transverse (TAC) or supra/infra-renal abdominal aorta) has been used to mechanically reproduce the cardiac consequences of aortic stenosis, coarctation of the aorta and systemic hypertension [47]. The timeline of the disease progression depends on the selected specie, age, gender, anatomic locations or degree of the constriction (Fig. 19.3).

Changes in nitric oxide (NO) pathway are believed to play an important role in the pressure-overloaded heart and pathological cardiac remodelling (REM). In fact, reports showed that the phosphodiesterase-5 inhibitor sildenafil reduces LV HYP and dilatation in a mouse TAC model [48]. Additionally, the exogenous administration of the NOS cofactor BH4, has been shown to reduce LV HYP, fibrosis, and cardiac dysfunction in mice with pre-established pressure-overload hypertrophy. In this setting, BH4 re-coupled endothelial NOS, with subsequent reduction of NOS-dependent oxidative stress and reversal of maladaptive remodelling [49].

Among the major advantages that these banding models share compared to other hypertensive or HF models, is the ability to manipulate the degree of pressure overload by changing the constriction severity [50]. Concerning the thoracic aorta constrictions the main advantage is the similarities to human HF progression, especially to aortic stenosis patients. Accordingly, it is characterized by initial compensatory phase, with concentric LV hypertrophy followed by an enlargement of cardiac chambers associated with a further deterioration of LV function [51]. Another advantage is the extensive information regarding TAC model: it was first described in 1994 by Rockman [52] and it has been extensively used since then, especially in mice either by traditional thoracotomy approach or by mini-

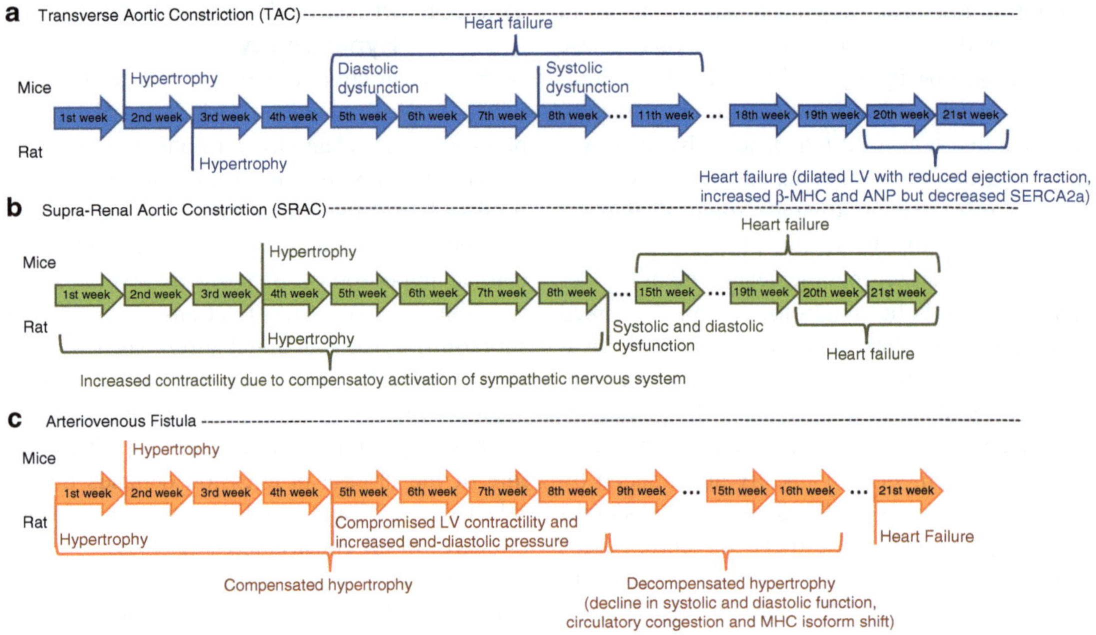

Fig. 19.3 Timeline progression of three animal models of left ventricular hypertrophy in mice and rat: Transverse aortic constriction (*TAC*), Supra-renal aortic constriction (*SRAC*) and arteriovenous fistula

mally invasive aortic banding through a small incision in the proximal sternum [15]. Finally, this method permits the quantification of the pressure gradient across the aortic constriction and the stratification of LV hypertrophy [13]. However, the TAC model has several drawbacks such as the prolonged duration of the protocols (Fig. 19.3), inter-individual variability in the response to pressure overload, high proportion of debanding due to internalization of the constriction knot [15]. These two last disadvantages require the use of large experimental groups and the use of accessory methods for visualization of the constriction integrity and progression of disease, such as echocardiography. Both AAC and TAC models have a common disadvantage resultant from the complex surgical method and equipment necessary for open-chest microsurgery. The lack of such an extended learning curve is the major advantage of abdominal constriction model, alongside with the lower mortality rate associated with banding (10 %). Activation of RAAS might however limit the use of abdominal aorta constriction in some studies [53]. Moreover, decrease of LV relaxation rates makes such models valuable for the evaluation of diastolic dysfunction, which is an important factor in the progression of LV failure [54]. In addition, the stimulus for HF is gradual in onset as is the progression from compensated HYP to HF in humans, thus making it clinically more relevant.

19.2.3.2 Volume-Overload Induced Hypertrophy

Arteriovenous shunts or fistulas have been used to induce volume overload, HYP and later DCM and HF in rodents. Femoral artery to femoral vein or aorta to cava fistulas lead to HF, but present a mortality rate above 25 % in all studies [55]. The more recent aortocaval shunt is a relatively simpler and a faster alternative to induce HF with good survival rates and no need to perform thoracotomy [56]. Compared to the rat, reports on the cardiac consequences of arteriovenous shunts in mice are still scarce. The progression of myocardial changes is represented in Fig. 19.3. Notably conflicting observations have been reported probably due to differences in the techniques utilized to induce volume overload, duration and size of the shunt or even the stage of cardiac hypertrophy. This procedure has the advantage of being fast and usually well tolerated, despite the limitation of requiring a laparotomy. Nonetheless, shunt closure has been reported in 7 % of the cases, which means that it is necessary to confirm the patency of the shunt at the end of investigation.

Another procedure used to induce volume overload in rats is aortic valve regurgitation, in which an aortic valve cusp is punctured [57].

19.2.4 Dilated Cardiomyopathy

Engineered mice with mutations or lacking certain cytoskeleton genes are known to cause dilated cardiomyopathy (DCM). Such is the case of dystrophin and utrophin knockout mice that develop severe muscular dystrophies and cardiomyopathy similar to humans. Also knockout mice for muscle LIM protein, melusin, tumor necrosis factor-α (TNF-α), protein kinase C-β2 (PKC-β2) and calmodulin kinase II display phenotypic features of the human DCM (Table 19.2) [58]. Besides genetically modified mice only a few animal models are able to satisfactorily mimic DCM, such as SHHF/Mcp-*fa*^{cp} which, regardless of the gender or genotype, eventually develop spontaneous DCM accompanied by subcutaneous edema, dyspnea, cyanosis, lethargy, enlarged hearts, thickened ventricles, dilated heart chamber, ascites, pulmonary edema and pleural effusion. Moreover, several animal models used for other CV diseases developed DCM, that is, myocarditis or myocardial ischemia. Apart from rodents, DCM can be induced by chronic rapid pacing at a frequency three- to fourfold higher than the spontaneous heart rate and is mostly applied to dogs, but also to pigs, sheep and monkeys [58].

19.2.4.1 Doxorubicin

Doxorubicin (DOX) is an anthracycline widely used in cytostatic treatments. One of the major long-term consequences of DOX therapy is the development of dose-dependent cardiomyopathy and ultimately congestive HF either in humans as in various animal species. Therefore, understanding the pathogenesis of cardiotoxic cardiomyopathy is essential to the development of new measures to prevent cardiotoxicity associated with antineoplastic therapies [15].

DOX administration once a week for 6 weeks or on alternate days for 2 weeks has been shown to induce cardiomyopathy and HF in rodent, while in rabbits the first abnormalities are observed after 3 months' injections twice weekly. Interestingly, a single intravenous administration of DOX has been shown to induce significant LV dysfunction in mice after 5 days, while its intracoronary injection allows a smaller dose of DOX to induce HF without systemic toxicity [15].

DOX-induced cardiomyopathy is characterized by ventricular wall thinning and dilatation (reduced mass-to-volume ratio), and depressed systolic and diastolic function accompanied by fluid retention and by neurohumoral activation. At the cardiac muscle level, DOX promotes intrinsic contractile dysfunction and reduced contractile reserve. Furthermore, DOX impairs vascular, as well as cardiac endothelial function and induces inflammatory reactions in the heart, leading to thrombosis in the atria and myocarditis [15].

Multiple pathways of antracycline-induced cardiac cellular injury have been proposed, such as the release of cardiotoxic substances which subsequently accumulate in cardiomyocytes, the generation of free radical, lipid peroxidation and suppression of DNA, RNA and protein synthesis. Other studies suggest that cardiotoxicity pathways include abnormalities in Ca^{2+} handling; induction of mitochondrial DNA lesions; degradation of myofilamental and cytoskeletal proteins, including titin and dystrophin; interference with various pro-survival kinases [59] and changes in adrenergic and adenylate cyclase function. All these mechanisms may contribute to cardiac cell damage, ultimately leading to myocyte death, either by necrosis or by apoptosis [15].

DOX model has a short time course of induction of HF and also the advantages of being technically simple, reproducible, non-invasive, and economical. Additionally, it can be used in several animal species to promote either chronic or acute HF [60]. The main limitations of this model

Table 19.2 Brief description of the most important genetically engineered mouse models used for heart failure research

	Gene		Mechanism	Structural changes	Functional changes	Comments
Cytoskeletal and sarcomeric proteins	Melusin [62]		Knockout	Cardiac chamber dilation and relative wall thinning	Depressed systolic function and myocardial contractility, pulmonary congestion and impaired adrenal responsiveness	Melusin is a muscle specific integrin β1-interacting protein. Probably required for LVH induced by biochemical stress but not by humoral stimulation No effect on cardiac structure or basal function in physiologic conditions or in response to ATII or phenylephrine Leads to LVH and favours the transition toward dilated cardiomyopathy and contractile dysfunction in response to chronic pressure overload
	Muscle LIM protein (MLP) [63]		Knockout	Myofiber disarray, severe LV hypertrophy and dilation and fibrosis	Systolic dysfunction and CHF Blunted response to β-agonist stimulation	Suitable model for long-term observation of drug effects on cardiac function and remodelling (near normal life span). Mutations in MLP were identified in patients with DCM or hypertrophic cardiomyopathy [64]
	Proteins linked to FHC (β-MHC, troponin T, MyBP-C) [65]		Knockout	These models are important to study the mechanisms linking the primary mutation and the secondary development of CHF. Moreover, environmental or genetic factors play a role in the development of each phenotype		
	Proteins linked to heritable dilated cardiomyopathy (actin, β-MHC, troponin T) [66]	Desmin	Knockout	Severe disorganization of muscle architecture associated with degeneration [67]		Mutation in β-cristallin (a molecular chaperone heat shock protein essential for cytoskeletal integrity) causes a desmin-related myopathy [68]
		Cardiac actin		Reduced number of actin filaments and myofiber disarray	Early postnatal death [69]	
		Dystrophin			DCM only in the presence of concomitant urotrophin deficiency [70]	

Neurohumoral receptors	Sympathetic nervous system	α1B-AR [71, 72]	Mutation	Ventricular hypertrophy increased ANF expression (sufficient for hypertrophy development)		Clinical studies with α1-AR selective blockers or activators of central α2-ARs have so far provided disappoint results [73] The activation of subtype-specific α2-AR at peripheral nerves has not been tried yet [74]
		α2A or α2C-AR [75]	Knockout		Faster progression to CHF and death when challenged with pressure overload (TAC) than wild-type or α2B knockout mice	Feedback pre-synaptic inhibition seems to be important to attenuate the detrimental effect of catecholamines
		β1-AR	Overexpression [76, 77]	Significant hypertrophy of the myocytes, altered nuclear morphology and concomitant fibrosis, with increased expression of apoptotic proteins in fibrosis areas	Elevated basal heart frequency and increased contractility in young animals; at 35 weeks of age the contractility decreases and many animals present clinical signs of HF and die before the age of 14 months. Contractile dysfunction is preceded by impaired calcium handing [78]	Chronic activation clearly implicated in CHF development in both animal and clinical studies In a model with concomitant deletion of PLB gene, mice did not die prematurely anymore, the cardiac hypertrophy and fibrosis were inhibited, LV function was preserved and also the disturbed Ca^{2+} handling was restored. These findings show that the β1-adrenoceptor–PLB-signalling cascade is a crucial regulator of cardiac contractility [79, 80]

(continued)

Table 19.2 (continued)

Gene		Mechanism	Structural changes	Functional changes	Comments
	β2-AR	Overexpression [81]	Myocardial hypertrophy that could not be prevented [82–84]	Increased basal contractility; LV dP/dtmax, relaxation and heart rate were increased [85–88]. The improved contractility could be attributed to better Ca^{2+} cycling of the SR, which showed decreased PLB expression [89, 90]	In CHF there is selective down-regulation of β1-AR and desensitization of both β1-AR and β2-AR (mediated by β-ARK1)
				Other studies showed that mice die earlier from severe HF indicated by cardiac dilation, pulmonary congestion and pleural effusion [91, 92]	Mice subjected to pressure overload through aortic constriction showed higher mortality and incidence of heart failure
	β-ARK1 [93]	Knockout	Mice do not survive		
	β-ARK peptide inhibitor [93]	Overexpression		Increased cardiac contractility	Cross-breeding with cardiomyopathic MLP-knockout mice restores the responsiveness to β-agonist stimulation and enhances cardiac contractility [94]
					Cross-breeding with mice overexpressing calsequestrin enhances cardiac function and reduces mortality. Combination with the β-blocker metoprolol has an additive effect [95]. β-ARK1 seems to be a putative therapeutic target

Neurohumoral receptors	Renin-angiotensin system	AT-1 [96]	Overexpression	Significant cardiac hypertrophy and remodelling with increased expression of ANF and interstitial collagen deposition	CHF in the absence of blood pressure changes	This model attests the direct role of AII in cardiac hypertrophy
	Cytokines	TNF-α [18, 97]	Overexpression	Biventricular dilation, fibrosis, interstitial infiltrates and hypertrophy	Marked decline in cardiac function and blunted responsiveness to β-agonist stimulation	Clinical trials with TNF-α inhibitors failed to achieve beneficial results [98, 99]
		IL-6 and gp130 (receptor) [100, 101]	Overexpression	Ventricular hypertrophy	No progression to CHF	Gp130 signalling cascade could be a potential therapeutic target because of its cardioprotective effect
			Disruption	Myocardial apoptosis	Accelerated transition to CHF when subjected to pressure overload	
Cellular signalling proteins	Heterotrimeric G proteins	Gαq	Overexpression [102]	Cardiac hypertrophy with increased expression of ANF and β-MHC	Blunted response to β-agonist stimulation	Gαq signalling is necessary and sufficient to the development of cardiac hypertrophy
			Modest			Mice with attenuated hypertrophic response to pressure overload (expression of Gαq peptide inhibitor or lack of norepinephrine) have increased wall stress but no decline in cardiac function [103]
			High		Overt CHF	
			Transient expression of constitutively active Gαq [104]	Cardiac hypertrophy	Dilated cardiomyopathy	Gq signalling pathway could be an interesting therapeutic target to prevent cardiac hypertrophy and CHF
			Inhibition (overexpression of a dominant-negative Gαq) [105, 106]	Resistance to hypertrophy induced by pressure overload		

(continued)

Table 19.2 (continued)

Gene			Mechanism	Structural changes	Functional changes	Comments
		Gαs	Modest overexpression [107]	Cardiomyopathy similar to that induced by chronic catecholamine administration in elderly mice (cellular degeneration, necrosis, replacement fibrosis)		
		Gi	Conditional expression of Gi-coupled receptor ($R_0$1) [108]		High-level of expression causes hyperactive Gi signalling with systolic dysfunction. Suppression of $R_0$1 expression after 8 weeks prevents further myocardial degeneration and partially improves systolic function and CHF	It is still matter of controversy if up-regulation of Gi pathway is a compensatory response to hyperactive Gs signalling
Cellular signalling proteins	Small GTPases	Ras [109]	Ventricular expression of a constitutively active form	Hypertrophy	Diastolic dysfunction	
		RhoA [110]	Overexpression		Sinus and atrioventricular nodal dysfunction and contractile failure without ventricular hypertrophy	
		Rac1 [111]	Myocardial expression of constitutively active form	Transient hypertrophy resolving with age	Lethal dilated cardiomyopathy	

	Protein kinases	PKC-β2 [112]	Overexpression	Cardiac dilation and fibrosis	Reduced cardiac function	
		PKC-α [113]	Knockout		Less systolic dysfunction and LV dilation in response to LAD	Cardiomyocyte-specific expression of a PKC-α inhibitor leads to the same results of knockout [114]
		PKC-ε [115]	Overexpression	Mild concentric hypertrophy without fibrosis	Normal cardiac function	
		PKA [116]	Expression of catalytic subunit in heart		Dilated cardiomyopathy with arrhythmias and reduced cardiac function	Enhanced Ca release from SR in response to β-AR signalling
		Calmodulin kinase II [117]	Overexpression	Progressive LV hypertrophy and dilation	Overt CHF	CaMKII contributes to heart failure progression. Expression of a cardiomyocyte-specific CaMKII inhibitory peptide reduces LV hypertrophy and dilation and systolic dysfunction. [118] A pharmacological inhibitor of CaMKII (KN93) attenuated LV dilation and improved systolic function post-MI in wild-type rats suggesting that this kinase could be a potential interesting therapeutic target [119]
		Calmodulin [120]	Overexpression	Myocardial hypertrophy	No CHF	Other downstream pathways of calmodulin signalling could prevent the progression to CHF
		Calcineurin [113]	Overexpression	Myocardial hypertrophy	CHF development within 2 months	
Calcium-regulating proteins	L-type Ca channels [121]		Overexpression	Ventricular hypertrophy, apoptosis and fibrosis	Overt CHF within 8 months and death of CHF within 12 months in the majority of mice	
	Calsequestrin [122, 123]		Overexpression	Hypertrophy	Progressive CHF – increased SR Ca storage and decreased systolic Ca transients	Restoration of β-AR signalling improves cardiac function and reduces mortality in these mice [95]

(continued)

Table 19.2 (continued)

Gene		Mechanism	Structural changes	Functional changes	Comments
SERCA2A		Knockout [124]	Lethal in embryonic period		SERCA2a overexpression improves systolic function and contractile reserve in mice with aortic constriction [125]
		Heterozygous (null mutation) [124]		Impaired cardiac function	
		Overexpression [127, 128]		Enhanced cardiac relation and contractility	Restoring adequate levels of SERCA2A expression in failing hearts improves LV systolic function, remodelling and survival [126]
Phospholamban (PLN)		Overexpression		Increased adrenergic drive and mildly reduced ventricular contractility at the age of 3 months; overt CHF and death with ageing [131]	Mutation PLNR9C identified in inherited human cardiomyopathy and the phenotype can be reproduced in mice. [129]
		Knockout	Reverses cardiac remodelling and enhances cardiac function in mice overexpressing calsequestrin [130]	Increased contractility [132]	PLN inhibition could be a potential therapeutic target but it is not certain if the beneficial effect would be the same in all types of congestive HF
				Preserves cardiac contractility and left ventricular chamber size close to normal in MLP-deficient mice [133]	Ablation of PLN in Gαq overexpressing and mutant MyBP-C expressing mice does not correct global cardiac dysfunction Studies in animal models similar to most common forms of CHF in humans are needed
S100A1 [134]		Overexpression		Restoring expression of S100A1 to normal levels in post-MI rats improved LV function and reduced LV dilation	S100A1 is a calcium-regulatory protein that facilitates calcium transport across sarcoplasmic reticulum by optimizing activity of ryanodine receptor and SERCA2A
RyR [135]	FKBP12.6	Knockout	Cardiac hypertrophy	Disregulation of Ca release in the myocytes	A benzothiazepine derivative JTV519 prevents the decrease of RyR2-bound FKBP12.6, improves cardiac function and avoids cardiac remodelling in a canine model of CHF raising the question of it could be a novel therapeutic target [136]

ECM proteins	B1-integrin [137]		Knockout (cardiac selective)	Myocardial fibrosis	Congestive HF	Inhibition of MMP could be a potential therapeutic target in CHF but it is necessary to identify the specific MMP members related to each CHF etiology
	MMP-2 [138]		Knockout	Decreased LV dilation and rupture	Better cardiac function and survival rate in mice subjected to coronary artery ligation	
	MMP-9 [139]		Knockout	Reduced LV dilation and collagen accumulation following LAD occlusion		
	TIMP-1 [140]		Knockout	Increased LV remodelling after myocardial infarction		
Oxidative-stress	Mn-SOD [141, 142]		Tissue-specific conditional knockout	Dilated cardiomyopathy with fibrosis at 4 months of age	Reduced contractility	Molecular defects in mitochondrial respiration and suggested that administration of anti-oxidants could restore cardiac contractility
Insulin signalling pathways	Cardiomyocyte selective insulin receptor	CIRKO	Knockout	Reduction in myocyte size	Reduced rates of glucose utilization	Gene deleted shortly after birth
				Decreased capillary density in the myocardium [144]	Metabolic features including glycolysis and decreased fatty acid oxidation [143]	Persistence of the fetal program
				Dilated ventricles, reduced relative wall thickness	LV systolic dysfunction upon hemodynamic stress or in aged mice	Animal model of insulin resistance [145]
					Higher relative LV wall stress [47]	
		Akita	Spontaneous mutation	Preserved systolic function in the absence of interstitial fibrosis and hypertrophy [146]	Type 1 diabetes Severe hyperglycemia, hypoinsulinemia, and polydipsia [147]	Animal model of insulin resistance. Type 1 diabetic cardiomyopathy which is characterized by diastolic dysfunction associated with lipotoxic cardiomyopathy [145]
	Calmodulin minigene regulated by the rat insulin II promoter	OVE 26	Overexpression	Islet cell destruction and an insulin-deficient state [148]	Type 1 DM Severe hyperglycemia	Animal model of insulin resistance. These mice have been reported to develop diabetic cardiomyopathy [149]

Adapted from Gomes et al. [15] with permission

are related to the variable degree of ventricular dysfunction and the high incidence of arrhythmias that contributes to the high mortality rate. Importantly, it is known that doxorubicin cardiotoxicity is dose-dependent and may appear either during and within 2–3 days of its administration or later within 30 days of administration of its last dose. In humans, it may occur even after 6–10 years after its administration [61]. Anthracycline administration also has undesirable bone marrow, gastrointestinal and renal toxicity that can however be avoided by the intracoronary injection of the drug [60].

19.2.4.2 Isoproterenol

Excessive doses of catecholamines, such as isoproterenol, produce diffuse myocardial destruction with cardiomyocyte necrosis and extensive fibrosis in both animals and humans [150]. The mechanism underlying myocardial damage is likely related to an imbalance between oxygen supply versus demand due to myocardial hyperactivity [151]. In mice, infusion of isoproterenol for 7 days has been shown to induce cardiac dysfunction [152]. In rats, subcutaneous administration of isoproterenol for 3 days leads to a dose-dependent impairment of cardiac function and neurohumoral activation [153], with cardiomyocyte necrosis and extensive LV hypertrophy and dilation and after 2 and 12 weeks, respectively [154]. However, isoproterenol administration before ischemia exerts a cardioprotective effect in rats [154]. The advantages of this model are its technical simplicity and excellent reproducibility in association with a satisfactory low mortality. Nonetheless, it seems not suitable for inducing an overt state of CHF because higher doses of catecholamines can increase the mortality rate up to 80 % [153].

19.2.5 Myocardial Infarction-Induced Heart Failure

Since ischemic heart disease is the most important cause of human HF, coronary artery occlusion is the most common method of inducing acute myocardial damage in animal models. LAD coronary Ligation artery or one of its branches remains the most preferred and acceptable method of inducing regional injury and subsequent HF in rodents as well as to gain further insight into pathophysiology of post-myocardial infarction (MI) cardiac remodelling (REM) [13]. The mechanisms responsible for cardiac REM are mostly related to changes in extracellular matrix and cardiomyocytes of the remaining overloaded myocardium and neurohumoral activation [155].

Surviving mice gradually develop HF within the 4 weeks following the surgical procedure [156]. In rats, a significant decrease up to 25 % in cardiac output is observed 8 weeks after LAD ligation [157]. The infarct size varies significantly (between 10 and 45 %) and is directly related to the degree of LV function impairment [158], influencing the time course of CHF development [155]. Generally, the infarct extension needs to affect at least 30 % of the LV mass in order to present the typical characteristics of CHF and to induce considerable increases in the molecular markers of hypertrophy [155]. Age also exerts a noteworthy effect on the time course of CHF development, with young animals tolerating well LAD ligation without CHF signs, in spite of the larger infarct size [159]. Some recent studies showed that female mice undergo less extensive ventricular REM, suggesting the influence of sex hormones as a putative explanation for gender differences [160].

In both mice and rats, mortality ranges between 35 and 50 % and occurs within the first hour after MI due to ventricular fibrillation and severe acute HF. Furthermore, in rats, it seems to be strain dependent with Lewis inbred rats producing a uniform infarct size and surviving more than Sprague-Dawley rats. Moreover, LAD occlusion performed in adult Sprague-Dawley rats as been described to induce cardiac cachexia [15].

Contrary to the clinical situation, in which the patient has progressive non-occlusive coronary artery obstruction, MI in this model is due to the sudden occlusion of a normal coronary artery. Therefore, efforts have been made to create a model of chronic myocardial ischemia, more similar to the clinical reality. To overcome this limitation, coronary microembolization using intracoronary infusion of microspheres have been attempted in larger animals [161].

Protocols of temporary LAD occlusion have been developed to reproduce human ischemia-reperfusion injury. This model has confirmed the benefits of reperfusion since infarct size was found to be significantly smaller than after permanent occlusion of the coronary artery. However, they also revealed the diversity of results as a consequence of the high variability of mouse left coronary anatomy [162]. The procedure was further modified to analyze ischemic preconditioning of the heart. In this method, LAD is repeatedly occluded to subject the heart to several rounds of brief ischemia and reperfusion before permanent occlusion. Molecular analyses identified various ischemia-induced genes that confer tolerance to subsequent more severe ischemic event [163].

The cost and simplicity confer important advantages to LAD ligation. On the other hand, rats differ from humans in terms of electrophysiology, coronary circulation, cardiac protein isoforms and time course of MI evolution. In fact, available data suggests a faster onset of healing and termination processes in rats [164], which mean results must be interpreted with caution. Even so, most therapeutic approaches to MI have emerged from this experimental model.

An alternative model of MI was cryoinfarction, which induces a series of cryo-injuries in the epicardium of mice and rats [165]. However, it has not caught the interest of the scientific community and thus it is no longer used.

19.2.5.1 Myocarditis-Induced Hear Failure

Viral myocarditis may cause of DCM and HF. The Coxsackie-B3 virus (CB3) and the encephalomyocarditis virus (EMCV) have been used to induce myocarditis in rodents [166]. EMCV infection can lead to myocyte necrosis and significant biventricular dilation during the phase of viremia, while typical signs of CHF appear after 7 to 14 days of virus inoculation [167]. This model is limited to Balb/c and DBA/2 mice because other mouse strains are resistant to virus infection [74]. Virus inoculation in genetic engineered mice has been shedding light on the molecules involved in the pathogenesis of viral myocarditis. Indeed, the administration of an exogenous anti-TNF-α antibody reduced myocardial lesion and improved survival, mitigating the effect of the observed increase in TNF-α expression [168]. A retrovirus model of encephalitis and myocarditis in mice showed that nuclear factor-kB activation confers protection against viral-mediated apoptosis and its expression is preserved in the presence of interferon-B. The absence of any of these molecules in the myocardium leads to striking viral infection and cell death [15]. Transgenic knockout models of components of the immune system have provided interesting insights in the pathogenesis of viral myocarditis [169].

Another pathogenic agent capable of causing myocarditis and DCM is the protozoan parasite *Trypanosoma cruzi*, which causes Chagas disease, a major form of HF in Latin America [170]. The infection causes generalized vascular inflammation, which stimulates the production of endothelin-1 and thromboxane-A2, further enhancing coronary vasospasm and myocardial ischemia [171].

Autoimmune myocarditis has been induced by an immunization process with different intracellular antigens. In rats, hemodynamic deterioration and myocarditis have been reported after 3 weeks of immunization with cardiac α-myosin or α-myosin peptides [172]. This was associated with increased expression and activity of inducible nitric oxide synthase (iNOS) and an inhibitor of that enzyme effectively attenuated the histopathological changes, thus pointing out to a relevant pathophysiologic role of NO [173]. In mice, immunization with a monoclonal anti-dog SERCA-2a antibody caused myocarditis [174].

Immunization of mice with recombinant murine cardiac troponin I (mcTnI) resulted in myocardial deposition and elevated serum levels of anti-mcTnI autoantibodies, accompanied by myocardial inflammation (both humoral and cellular immune response), cardiac dilatation, contractile failure and increased mortality rates [175].

19.2.5.2 Pulmonary Arterial Hypertension, Emphysema and Right Ventricular Failure

Monocrotaline-Induced Pulmonary Hypertension

Monocrotaline (MCT) is a plant toxin derived from *Crotalaria spectabilis* that can be administered by intraperitoneal, subcutaneous, or intravenous injection to induce right ventricular dysfunction and HF within 4–6 weeks [176]. Current hypotheses of the pathogenesis of MCT-induced pneumotoxicity suggest that MCT is transformed in a bioactive pyrrole metabolite in the liver and is then transported by red blood cells to the lung, where it initiates endothelial injury. The metabolite has a half-life of ~3 s in aqueous media and primarily affects the pulmonary vascular bed as lungs are the first major vascular bed after the liver [177]. Nonetheless, MCT can injury other structures such as liver [178] or kidney [179]. In the pulmonary vasculature MCT induces perivascular inflammation, platelet activation, and endothelial dysfunction, generally leading to increased pulmonary arterial pressure. These changes are accompanied by an increase in RV systolic and diastolic pressures, hypertrophy and ultimately HF [180]. Besides inducing HF, MCT is a simple model, which, at an earlier phase, presents relevant similarities with human pulmonary hypertension. Also, it is considered as an animal model of cachexia-secondary to HF.

19.2.5.3 Heart Failure with Preserved Ejection Fraction

In spite of the rising prevalence of HFpEF, currently there exist no evidence-based treatment strategies capable of changing its natural history, reflecting our poor understanding of this HF subtype [181]. Therefore, animal models of diastolic dysfunction and HFpEF care urgently headed for the development and preclinical evaluation of new effective therapies for this disease. However, animal models of HFpEF are rather scarce, thus leading to the utilization of diastolic dysfunction models, which are more widely published and very similar regarding the basic pathophysiological mechanisms [182]. Furthermore, these models have been most commonly created in large animals, such as canine, sheep and swine. Nonetheless, there have been some successful rodent models that deserve to be highlighted in this chapter.

Thus, researchers have tried to reproduce the paramount factors typically documented to cause diastolic dysfunction and HFpEF, namely ageing, diabetes mellitus and hypertension [183]. In fact, the alterations in myocardial relaxation and stiffness associated with chronic hypertension and diabetes have been already mentioned above in the appropriate models, namely Dahl-salt sensitive rats, DOCA-salt rats, obese ZSF1 and diabetic cardiomyopathy.

Despite the great difficulty in developing an animal model of age-induced HFpEF, a recent study has characterized a model demonstrating isolated diastolic dysfunction associated with accelerated aging [184]. This mouse model is a spontaneous senescence model that displays many common geriatric disorders in the human population and recapitulates diastolic dysfunction as it naturally occurs in the elderly. Diastolic dysfunction, accompanied by fibrosis and an increase in pro-fibrotic cytokines, develops between 3 and 6 months of age, which is an early time point in the life span of these animals. This suggests that the abnormality manifests over a relatively short period of time and, from an experimental standpoint, adds an advantage as it allows for a more rapid study of pathophysiologic mechanisms. The senescence-accelerated mouse model will probably turn to be a useful model for future studies of age-related diastolic dysfunction, since the better insight into its underlying mechanisms could pave the way for designing specific pharmacological strategies to prevent or treat this pathology [184].

The association between aging and diastolic dysfunction had already been addressed in a previous study which compared adult (6-month-old) and old (24-month-old) Fischer 344/BNF1 rats after either 12 weeks of treadmill training or normal sedentary cage life [185]. Echocardiographic indices of LV relaxation were significantly impaired in the old rats, but with training, they returned back to the levels seen in the adults. LV stiffness measured in isolated perfused hearts, was not affected by age or training, but increased more rapidly during low-flow ischemia in the old hearts than in the younger adults. Again, training eliminated this age-associated difference in the response to ischemia, although it was not ascertained if the improvement was due to reversal of ageing consequences or superimposition of some other effects. These findings indicate that in rats some age-associated changes in diastolic function are reversible and thus may not be intrinsic to ageing but instead secondary to other processes, such as deconditioning [185].

With regard to diastolic dysfunction, it should be emphasized that rodent models generally progress to HFpEF within a variable amount of time, which means in those animals HFpEF is only a temporary step in the progression towards HFrEF. Therefore, small animal models could be misleading because they suggest that HFpEF invariably progress to HFrEF, which in fact seldom happens in humans. Additionally, in humans, HFpEF is a condition typically associated with ageing and the diastolic dysfunction/DHF animal models herein mentioned are relatively young.

19.3 Genetically Engineered Mouse Models

The development of molecular biology offers the opportunity to study the impact of overexpression or deletion of specific genes involved in the pathophisyology of congestive HF. Indeed, transgenic mice models will help understanding the molecular basis of congestive HF which might open the door for the development of novel molecular targets for its treatment. A wide number of genetic modifications have been successfully introduced in mice, both in terms of gain of function and loss of function. Besides the genetically engineered mouse models summarized in Table 19.2, other selective inbreed and other genetic animal models were presented in previous sections whenever appropriate.

Transgenic mice could be useful to study the molecular basis of HF due to the availability of many genetically engineered strains made possible by their well characterized genome and the easy introduction and stable transmission of gene mutations. Moreover, since 99 % of the human genes have direct murine orthologs it is possible to generate transgenic mice models to mimic human disorders [186]. Care should be taken when dealing with genetically engineered mice. Besides taking into account strain and gender issues, high levels of overexpression must be carefully interpreted [15]. In fact, transgenic mice that express a biologically inert green fluorescent protein in a cardiomyocyte-specific fashion develop LV hypertrophy, dilatation and systolic dysfunction in a manner directly related to the level of protein expression. Therefore, non-specific effects on LV structure and function may result from vast overexpression of even biologically inactive proteins [187]. Furthermore, certain phenotypes depend on the expression level of the gene concerned, which means it is necessary to develop multiple transgenic lines to establish a gene-dosage effect. Development of compensatory mechanisms could be triggered in response to gene overexpression or deletion at a very early stage after manipulation, masking the direct effects of the targeted gene. The use of inducible and conditional gene activation or deactivation could be a good way of overcoming this problem [74]. In conclusion, despite the inherent pitfalls in transgenesis, many of them can be circumvented by creating additional transgenic lines that can be used as controls to check dosage or epigenetic sequelae, as has been recently reviewed [188].

19.4 Discussion and General Considerations

Not many diseases exhibit a line of causality in which a given antecedent elicits a particular disorder. Indeed, the pathophysiology of nearly all CVD is mostly represented by a web of causality in which a complex network of interactions and progressive disorders underlie the course of the disease progression. Most scientists though have uncritically adopted the "line-of-causality" approach to study a particular disease discarding the complex pathophysiology underlying it. In this regard, transgenic mice represent "dangerous" models to mimic human disease.

Besides ethical and philosophical questions, the use of animal models of CVD needs careful consideration not only because the studied disease may be associated with discomfort and pain to the animal but also results from animal studies are not readily transferable to human patients. Apart from species differences as well as their advantages and disadvantages (Table 19.3), some general considerations should be taken into account when using animal models: (1) most animal models are developed to study chronic and LV failure, (2) experiments conducted in rodents have limited genetic/cultural variability, (3) surgical interventions introduce variability, (4) surgical aggression triggers changes in behaviour, physiology and neuroendocrine activation and

Table 19.3 Advantages and disadvantages of different species for animal experimentation in comparison with human CV changes

Specie	Advantages	Disadvantages
Primates	Phylogenetically close to humans	Long life-cycle (require long protocols for the establishment of the disease)
	Similar omnivorous diet	Expensive to maintain
	Have similar metabolism	Carry viral zoonoses
	Develop metabolic syndrome and CV diseases with ageing	Significant ethical issues
		Expensive therapeutic protocols – large amounts of experimental agents are required
Swine	Susceptibility to atherosclerosis	Size and handling difficulties of adults
	Similar dietary preferences	Spontaneous development of metabolic syndrome and insulin resistance rarely occurs. Expensive therapeutic protocols – large amounts of experimental agents are required
	Similar gastrointestinal system and metabolism	Coronary circulation similar to a young-human heart
	Widely used as an animal model of dilated cardiomyopathy	
Dog	Similar aging CV alterations	Significant cultural and ethical issues
	Good animal model for revascularization studies	Resistant to high-lipid diets ad atherosclerosis due to its carnivorous diets
	Widely used as an animal model of dilated cardiomyopathy	Resistance to myocardial infarction due to extensive myocardial collateral circulatory system
	Similar excitation-contraction coupling	Expensive therapeutic protocols – large amounts of experimental agents are required
		Coronary circulation similar to an old-human heart
Rabbit	Small and relatively inexpensive	The common respiratory disease of rabbits "snuffles" (*Pasteurella multocida*) has atherogenic consequences
	Good animal model of atherosclerosis upon high-cholesterol diet	Less resistant to infections
	Watanabe strain comprises a defective LDL receptor and develops extreme hypercholesterolemia and advanced atherosclerosis	
	Prevalence of β-MHC isoform	
	Similar excitation-contraction coupling	
	Similar hemodynamic behaviour	

(continued)

Table 19.3 (continued)

Specie	Advantages	Disadvantages
Rat	Small and low housing and maintenance costs (allowing increasing the number of animals included in a given study and improving its statistical power)	Resistance to atherosclerosis
	Genome sequenced	Substantial differences in myocardial Ca^{2+} homeostasis and ATP usage
	Very robust animal	Very short action potential without a plateau phase
	Bigger amount of post-mortem myocardial tissue for several studies when compared to other rodents	
Mouse	Small and low housing and maintenance costs	Resistant to CV disease
	Easy to manipulate genetically – great number of transgenic mice models of CV disease	Small size is challenging for CV function assessment
	Cheapest pharmacologic protocols – small amounts of experimental agents are required	Small amount of myocardial tissue available
	Rapid gestation period (21 days), large litter size and a short life cycle allowing to follow the disease at an accelerated pace	Substantial differences in myocardial Ca^{2+} homeostasis and ATP usage
	Faster metabolism and faster disease progression	Heart rate is five times higher than that of humans with an inverse relationship between force and frequency
		α-MHC predominates in the myocardium
Hamster	Small and low housing and maintenance costs	Animal models of CV disease require highly abnormal diets or cytotoxic chemical agents
	Similar lipid metabolism	Substantial differences in myocardial Ca^{2+} homeostasis and ATP usage
	Good animal model of mild atherosclerosis	
	Fed with a very-high (60 %) fructose diet become insulin-resistant	
	β-cells destruction with streptozotocin creates type 1 DM with significant atherosclerosis and glomerular sclerosis in cholesterol-fed animals that can evolve to aortic lesions	
Sand Rat	Small and low housing and maintenance costs	Does not develop advance atherosclerotic lesions
	Placed on an energy-rich diet (laboratory chow) becomes obese, insulin-resistant and exhibits VLDL hyperlipidemis and type 2 DM	Substantial differences in myocardial Ca^{2+} homeostasis and ATP usage
	Good animal model of insulin-resistance metabolic disturbances	

CV cardiovascular, *DM* diabetes mellitus

(5) procedures among different operators should be standardized as much as possible.

Another drawback of rodent models of CVD is that many protocols produce a sudden onset of HF due to a surgical or drug intervention, whereas human HF generally develops over a period of several years. Most models also use young adult animals, while human patients are usually old. In addition, human HF is often associated with atherosclerosis, hypertension, diabetes or obesity, but the development of atherosclerosis is rather rare in most rodent strains [154].

Even though rodent models have been extremely useful in developing concepts concerning the pathogenesis of HF, they have not predicted outcomes in phase III clinical trials. Although translation of findings to clinical trials requires pre-clinical studies where the appropriate animal model is used for either acute or chronic HF, therapeutic results obtained in small animal models are not necessarily predictive of outcomes in human patients but can provide a potential future approach in the human context. Finally, the majority of the numerous genetic studies performed in mice has not resulted in any clinically approved treatment in humans so far [188]. However, it is not uncommon for a drug to take over 20 years from inception to clinical application. Given that genetically modified mouse models have only recently become a mainstay approach, it may take many more years before approaches based on this technology are introduced into clinical practice.

In summary, animal studies are vital to the understanding of disease mechanisms and for testing safety and efficacy interventions. Nevertheless, these studies are heterogeneous, and more so than a typical clinical trial. A successfully translation of experimental findings to humans diseases depends largely upon an understanding and awareness of these sources of heterogeneity and their impact on effect size. Meta-analysis is a useful tool for this purpose when the data are systematically identified and surely will help to overcome some of the above-mentioned limitations of animal studies. Thus performing meta-analysis and review of experimental and preclinical data would definitely provide valuable information that could help to plan clinical trial design, or try to explain discrepancies between preclinical and clinical trial results. Indeed, systematic reviews of data from preclinical literature are important for a number of reasons. First their purpose is to reduce bias by outlining transparent aims and methodology. This approach enables to identify all of the published literature to answer a particular research question. In turn this may highlight gaps in knowledge which can be fulfilled by further preclinical experimentation, or it can help to avoid unnecessary replication which is unethical and of limited benefit. Secondly, clinical trials of novel interventions should not proceed without a rigorous evaluation of the preclinical data and systematic reviews which deliver important information about the efficacy of any given intervention as well as its limitations. All of these should be taken into account in clinical trial design.

Conclusion

The use of animal models has proven to be an extremely valuable tool in understanding the pathophysiology of complex CVD mimicking congestive HF. The ideal animal model of cardiovascular disease will mimic the human subject metabolically and pathophysiologically, will be large enough to permit physiological and metabolic studies, and will develop end-stage disease comparable to those in humans. Given the complex multifactorial nature of CVD, no species or animal model will be similar to the human disease and thus the models should be chosen according to the study aim. However, due to the constant development of invasive and noninvasive techniques to evaluate hemodynamics in human patients, animal models of HF are becoming less important to study hemodynamics, neurohumoral activation and myocardial function. Furthermore, with cardiac transplantation and left ventricular assist device placement, surgery, end-stage human myocardium became available for molecular and biochemical studies. Nevertheless, animal models remain critically important to study myocardial changes during compensated, initial stages of congestive HF, during transition from HYP to failure and during the process of REM, all of which are currently difficult or even impossible to follow serially in human patients. Animal models may also be relevant to study the effects of new pharmacological interventions on hemodynamics, neurohumoral activation and survival under preclinical conditions.

At present, transgenic models of congestive HF are essential for understanding the molecular alterations underlying the development of the disease, as they allow the identification of genes that are causative for HF and to characterize molecular mechanisms responsible for the development and progression of the disease.

Finally, animal models which mimic distinct features of human HF will play an important role in unravelling the consequences of gene transfer and molecular techniques to correct disturbed subcellular processes in the failing heart. These experiments are indispensable and these rodent models will continue to held an important role, not only in expanding our knowledge about the mechanisms underlying HF, but also in developing novel therapeutic strategies for this syndrome.

References

1. McMurray JJ, Adamopoulos S, Anker SD, Auricchio A, Bohm M, Dickstein K, et al. ESC guidelines for the diagnosis and treatment of acute and chronic heart failure 2012: The Task Force for the Diagnosis and Treatment of Acute and Chronic Heart Failure 2012 of the European Society of Cardiology. Developed in collaboration with the Heart Failure Association (HFA) of the ESC. Eur J Heart Fail. 2012;14:803–69.
2. Leite-Moreira AF. Current perspectives in diastolic dysfunction and diastolic heart failure. Heart. 2006;92:712–8.
3. Russell JC, Proctor SD. Small animal models of cardiovascular disease: tools for the study of the roles of metabolic syndrome, dyslipidemia, and atherosclerosis. Cardiovasc Pathol. 2006;15:318–30.
4. Zucker LM, Zucker TF. Fatty, a new mutation in the rat. J Hered. 1961;52:275–8.
5. McCune S, Baker P, Stills H. SHHF/Mcc-cp rat: model of obesity, non-insulin-dependent diabetes, and congestive heart failure. ILAR J. 1990;32(3): 23–7.
6. Rerup C, Tarding F. Streptozotocin- and alloxan-diabetes in mice. Eur J Pharmacol. 1969;7:89–96.
7. Bugger H, Abel ED. Molecular mechanisms for myocardial mitochondrial dysfunction in the metabolic syndrome. Clin Sci (Lond). 2008;114: 195–210.
8. Van den Bergh A, Flameng W, Herijgers P. Type II diabetic mice exhibit contractile dysfunction but maintain cardiac output by favourable loading conditions. Eur J Heart Fail. 2006;8:777–83.
9. Greer JJ, Ware DP, Lefer DJ. Myocardial infarction and heart failure in the db/db diabetic mouse. Am J Physiol Heart Circ Physiol. 2006;290:H146–H153.
10. Boudina S, Abel ED. Diabetic cardiomyopathy revisited. Circulation. 2007;115:3213–23.
11. Ishibashi S, Goldstein JL, Brown MS, Herz J, Burns DK. Massive xanthomatosis and atherosclerosis in cholesterol-fed low density lipoprotein receptor-negative mice. J Clin Invest. 1994;93:1885–93.
12. Bing OH, Brooks WW, Robinson KG, Slawsky MT, Hayes JA, Litwin SE, et al. The spontaneously hypertensive rat as a model of the transition from compensated left ventricular hypertrophy to failure. J Mol Cell Cardiol. 1995;27:383–96.
13. Patten RD, Hall-Porter MR. Small animal models of heart failure: development of novel therapies, past and present. Circ Heart Fail. 2009;2:138–44.
14. Mitchell GF, Pfeffer JM, Pfeffer MA. The transition to failure in the spontaneously hypertensive rat. Am J Hypertens. 1997;10:120S–6.
15. Gomes AC, Falcao-Pires I, Pires AL, Bras-Silva C, Leite-Moreira AF. Rodent models of heart failure: an updated review. Heart Fail Rev. 2013;18:219–49.
16. Okamoto K, Yamamoto K, Morita N, Ohta Y, Chikugo T, Higashizawa T, et al. Establishment and use of the M strain of stroke-prone spontaneously hypertensive rat. J Hypertens Suppl. 1986;4: S21–4.
17. Masineni S, Chander P, Singh G, Powers C, Stier CJ. Male gender and not the severity of hypertension is associated with end-organ. Am J Hypertens. 2005;18:878–84.
18. London B, et al. Calcium-dependent arrhythmias in transgenic mice with heart failure. Am J Physiol Heart Circ Physiol. 2003;284(2):H431–41.
19. Heyen JR, Blasi ER, Nikula K, Rocha R, Daust HA, Frierdich G, et al. Structural, functional, and molecular characterization of the SHHF model of heart failure. Am J Physiol Heart Circ Physiol. 2002;283:H1775–84.
20. Gomez AM, Valdivia HH, Cheng H, Lederer MR, Santana LF, Cannell MB, et al. Defective excitation-contraction coupling in experimental cardiac hypertrophy and heart failure. Science. 1997;276:800–6.
21. Schlenker EH, Kost Jr CK, Likness MM. Effects of long-term captopril and L-arginine treatment on ventilation and blood pressure in obese male SHHF rats. J Appl Physiol. 2004;97:1032–9.
22. Dahl LK, Heine M, Tassinari L. Role of genetic factors in susceptibility to experimental hypertension due to chronic excess salt ingestion. Nature. 1962;194:480–2.
23. Klotz S, Hay I, Zhang G, Maurer M, Wang J, Burkhoff D. Development of heart failure in chronic hypertensive Dahl rats: focus on heart failure with preserved ejection fraction. Hypertension. 2006;47:901–11.
24. Inoko M, Kihara Y, Morii I, Fujiwara H, Sasayama S. Transition from compensatory hypertrophy to dilated, failing left ventricles in Dahl salt-sensitive rats. Am J Physiol. 1994;267:H2471–82.
25. Doi R, Masuyama T, Yamamoto K, Doi Y, Mano T, Sakata Y, et al. Development of different phenotypes of hypertensive heart failure: systolic versus diastolic failure in Dahl salt-sensitive rats. J Hypertens. 2000;18:111–20.
26. Sun ZJ, Zhang ZE. Historic perspectives and recent advances in major animal models of hypertension. Acta Pharmacol Sin. 2005;26:295–301.
27. Grobe JL, Mecca AP, Mao H, Katovich MJ. Chronic angiotensin-(1–7) prevents cardiac fibrosis in DOCA-salt model of hypertension. Am J Physiol Heart Circ Physiol. 2006;290:H2417–23.
28. Silberman GA, Fan TH, Liu H, Jiao Z, Xiao HD, Lovelock JD, et al. Uncoupled cardiac nitric oxide synthase mediates diastolic dysfunction. Circulation. 2010;121:519–28.
29. Intengan HD, Park JB, Schiffrin EL. Blood pressure and small arteries in DOCA-salt-treated genetically AVP-deficient rats: role of endothelin. Hypertension. 1999;34:907–13.

30. Van den Berg DT, de Kloet ER, de Jong W. Central effects of mineralocorticoid antagonist RU-28318 on blood pressure of DOCA-salt hypertensive rats. Am J Physiol. 1994;267:E927–33.
31. Schiffrin EL. Role of endothelin-1 in hypertension and vascular disease. Am J Hypertens. 2001;14:83S–9.
32. Li L, Chu Y, Fink GD, Engelhardt JF, Heistad DD, Chen AF. Endothelin-1 stimulates arterial VCAM-1 expression via NADPH oxidase-derived superoxide in mineralocorticoid hypertension. Hypertension. 2003;42:997–1003.
33. Katholi RE, Naftilan AJ, Oparil S. Importance of renal sympathetic tone in the development of DOCA-salt hypertension in the rat. Hypertension. 1980;2:266–73.
34. Brown L, Ooi SY, Lau K, Sernia C. Cardiac and vascular responses in deoxycorticosterone acetate-salt hypertensive rats. Clin Exp Pharmacol Physiol. 2000;27:263–9.
35. Mohammed SF, Ohtani T, Korinek J, Lam CS, Larsen K, Simari RD, et al. Mineralocorticoid accelerates transition to heart failure with preserved ejection fraction via "nongenomic effects". Circulation. 2010;122:370–8.
36. Goldblatt H, Lynch J, Hanzal RF, Summerville WW. Studies on experimental hypertension: I. The production of persistent elevation of systolic blood pressure by means of renal ischemia. J Exp Med. 1934;59:347–79.
37. Junhong W, Jing Y, Jizheng M, Shushu Z, Xiangjian C, Hengfang W, et al. Proteomic analysis of left ventricular diastolic dysfunction hearts in renovascular hypertensive rats. Int J Cardiol. 2008;127:198–207.
38. Rizzi E, Castro MM, Prado CM, Silva CA, Fazan Jr R, Rossi MA, et al. Matrix metalloproteinase inhibition improves cardiac dysfunction and remodeling in 2-kidney, 1-clip hypertension. J Card Fail. 2010;16:599–608.
39. Freeman RH, Davis JO, Watkins BE, Stephens GA, DeForrest JM. Effects of continuous converting enzyme blockade on renovascular hypertension in the rat. Am J Physiol. 1979;236:F21–4.
40. Burke SL, Evans RG, Head GA. Effects of chronic sympatho-inhibition on renal excretory function in renovascular hypertension. J Hypertens. 2011;29: 945–52.
41. Berg RG, Leenen FH, de Jong W. Plasma renin activity and sodium, potassium and water excretion during reversal of hypertension in the one-clip two-kidney hypertensive rat. Clin Sci (Lond). 1979;57: 47–52.
42. Kuwajima I, Kardon MB, Pegram BL, Sesoko S, Frohlich ED. Regression of left ventricular hypertrophy in two-kidney, one clip Goldblatt hypertension. Hypertension. 1982;4:113–8.
43. Hamdani N, Franssen C, Lourenco A, Falcao-Pires I, Fontoura D, Leite S, et al. Myocardial titin hypophosphorylation importantly contributes to heart failure with preserved ejection fraction in a rat metabolic risk model. Circ Heart Fail. 2013;6:1239–49.
44. Fellmann L, Nascimento AR, Tibirica E, Bousquet P. Murine models for pharmacological studies of the metabolic syndrome. Pharmacol Ther. 2013;137: 331–40.
45. Ingalls AM, Dickie MM, Snell GD. Obese, a new mutation in the house mouse. J Hered. 1950;41:317–8.
46. Hummel KP, Dickie MM, Coleman DL. Diabetes, a new mutation in the mouse. Science. 1966;153:1127–8.
47. Hu P, Zhang D, Swenson L, Chakrabarti G, Abel ED, Litwin SE. Minimally invasive aortic banding in mice: effects of altered cardiomyocyte insulin signaling during pressure overload. Am J Physiol Heart Circ Physiol. 2003;285:H1261–9.
48. Takimoto E, Champion HC, Li M, Belardi D, Ren S, Rodriguez ER, et al. Chronic inhibition of cyclic GMP phosphodiesterase 5A prevents and reverses cardiac hypertrophy. Nat Med. 2005;11:214–22.
49. Moens AL, Ketner EA, Takimoto E, Schmidt TS, O'Neill CA, Wolin MS, et al. Bi-modal dose-dependent cardiac response to tetrahydrobiopterin in pressure-overload induced hypertrophy and heart failure. J Mol Cell Cardiol. 2011;51:564–9.
50. Moens AL, Leyton-Mange JS, Niu X, Yang R, Cingolani O, Arkenbout EK, et al. Adverse ventricular remodeling and exacerbated NOS uncoupling from pressure-overload in mice lacking the beta3-adrenoreceptor. J Mol Cell Cardiol. 2009;47:576–85.
51. Boluyt MO, Robinson KG, Meredith AL, Sen S, Lakatta EG, Crow MT, et al. Heart failure after long-term supravalvular aortic constriction in rats. Am J Hypertens. 2005;18:202–12.
52. Rockman HA, Wachhorst SP, Mao L, Ross Jr J. ANG II receptor blockade prevents ventricular hypertrophy and ANF gene expression with pressure overload in mice. Am J Physiol. 1994;266:H2468–75.
53. Rodriguez-Iturbe B, Quiroz Y, Kim CH, Vaziri ND. Hypertension induced by aortic coarctation above the renal arteries is associated with immune cell infiltration of the kidneys. Am J Hypertens. 2005;18:1449–56.
54. Falcao-Pires I, Palladini G, Goncalves N, van der Velden J, Moreira-Goncalves D, Miranda-Silva D, et al. Distinct mechanisms for diastolic dysfunction in diabetes mellitus and chronic pressure-overload. Basic Res Cardiol. 2011;106:801–14.
55. Ozek C, Zhang F, Lineaweaver WC, Chin BT, Eiman T, Newlin L, et al. A new heart failure model in rat by an end-to-side femoral vessel anastomosis. Cardiovasc Res. 1998;37:236–8.
56. Garcia R, Diebold S. Simple, rapid, and effective method of producing aortocaval shunts in the rat. Cardiovasc Res. 1990;24:430–2.
57. Drolet MC, Lachance D, Plante E, Roussel E, Couet J, Arsenault M. Gender-related differences in left ventricular remodeling in chronic severe aortic valve regurgitation in rats. J Heart Valve Dis. 2006;15: 345–51.
58. Recchia FA, Lionetti V. Animal models of dilated cardiomyopathy for translational research. Vet Res Commun. 2007;31 Suppl 1:35–41.

59. Peng X, Chen B, Lim CC, Sawyer DB. The cardiotoxicology of anthracycline chemotherapeutics: translating molecular mechanism into preventative medicine. Mol Interv. 2005;5:163–71.
60. Monnet E, Chachques JC. Animal models of heart failure: what is new? Ann Thorac Surg. 2005;79: 1445–53.
61. Volkova M, Russell 3rd R. Anthracycline cardiotoxicity: prevalence, pathogenesis and treatment. Curr Cardiol Rev. 2011;7:214–20.
62. Brancaccio M, et al. Melusin, a muscle-specific integrin beta1-interacting protein, is required to prevent cardiac failure in response to chronic pressure overload. Nat Med. 2003;9(1):68–75.
63. Arber S, et al. MLP-deficient mice exhibit a disruption of cardiac cytoarchitectural organization, dilated cardiomyopathy, and heart failure. Cell. 1997;88(3): 393–403.
64. Mohapatra B, et al. Mutations in the muscle LIM protein and alpha-actinin-2 genes in dilated cardiomyopathy and endocardial fibroelastosis. Mol Genet Metab. 2003;80(1–2):207–15.
65. Marian AJ, Roberts R. The molecular genetic basis for hypertrophic cardiomyopathy. J Mol Cell Cardiol. 2001;33(4):655–70.
66. Seidman JG, Seidman C. The genetic basis for cardiomyopathy: from mutation identification to mechanistic paradigms. Cell. 2001;104(4):557–67.
67. Milner DJ, et al. Disruption of muscle architecture and myocardial degeneration in mice lacking desmin. J Cell Biol. 1996;134(5):1255–70.
68. Vicart P, et al. A missense mutation in the alphaB-crystallin chaperone gene causes a desmin-related myopathy. Nat Genet. 1998;20(1):92–5.
69. Kumar A, et al. Rescue of cardiac alpha-actin-deficient mice by enteric smooth muscle gamma-actin. Proc Natl Acad Sci U S A. 1997;94(9):4406–11.
70. Grady RM, et al. Skeletal and cardiac myopathies in mice lacking utrophin and dystrophin: a model for Duchenne muscular dystrophy. Cell. 1997;90(4):729–38.
71. Milano CA, et al. Myocardial expression of a constitutively active alpha 1B-adrenergic receptor in transgenic mice induces cardiac hypertrophy. Proc Natl Acad Sci U S A. 1994;91(21):10109–13.
72. Akhter SA, et al. Transgenic mice with cardiac overexpression of alpha1B-adrenergic receptors. In vivo alpha1-adrenergic receptor-mediated regulation of beta-adrenergic signaling. J Biol Chem. 1997;272(34): 21253–9.
73. Cohn JN. Sympathetic nervous system in heart failure. Circulation. 2002;106(19):2417–8.
74. Wang QD, Bohlooly YM, Sjoquist PO. Murine models for the study of congestive heart failure: implications for understanding molecular mechanisms and for drug discovery. J Pharmacol Toxicol Methods. 2004;50(3):163–74.
75. Brede M, et al. Feedback inhibition of catecholamine release by two different alpha2-adrenoceptor subtypes prevents progression of heart failure. Circulation. 2002;106(19):2491–6.
76. Engelhardt S, et al. Progressive hypertrophy and heart failure in beta1-adrenergic receptor transgenic mice. Proc Natl Acad Sci U S A. 1999;96(12): 7059–64.
77. Engelhardt S, et al. Early impairment of calcium handling and altered expression of junctin in hearts of mice overexpressing the beta1-adrenergic receptor. FASEB J. 2001;15(14):2718–20.
78. Muller FU, et al. Junctional sarcoplasmic reticulum transmembrane proteins in the heart. Basic Res Cardiol. 2002;97 Suppl 1:I52–5.
79. Engelhardt S, et al. Altered calcium handling is critically involved in the cardiotoxic effects of chronic beta-adrenergic stimulation. Circulation. 2004;109(9): 1154–60.
80. MacLennan DH, Kranias EG. Phospholamban: a crucial regulator of cardiac contractility. Nat Rev Mol Cell Biol. 2003;4(7):566–77.
81. Schwarz B, et al. Altered calcium transient and development of hypertrophy in beta2-adrenoceptor overexpressing mice with and without pressure overload. Eur J Heart Fail. 2003;5(2):131–6.
82. Schwinger RH, Bohm M, Erdmann E. Evidence against spare or uncoupled beta-adrenoceptors in the human heart. Am Heart J. 1990;119(4):899–904.
83. Du XJ, et al. beta(2)-adrenergic receptor overexpression exacerbates development of heart failure after aortic stenosis. Circulation. 2000;101(1):71–7.
84. Schwinger RH, et al. Unchanged protein levels of SERCA II and phospholamban but reduced Ca2+ uptake and Ca(2+)-ATPase activity of cardiac sarcoplasmic reticulum from dilated cardiomyopathy patients compared with patients with nonfailing hearts. Circulation. 1995;92(11):3220–8.
85. Du XJ, et al. Response to cardiac sympathetic activation in transgenic mice overexpressing beta 2-adrenergic receptor. Am J Physiol. 1996;271(2 Pt 2):H630–6.
86. Milano CA, et al. Marked enhancement in myocardial function resulting from overexpression of a human beta-adrenergic receptor gene. J Thorac Cardiovasc Surg. 1995;109(2):236–41.
87. Bittner HB, et al. Functional analysis of myocardial performance in murine hearts overexpressing the human beta 2-adrenergic receptor. J Mol Cell Cardiol. 1997;29(3):961–7.
88. Bond RA, et al. Physiological effects of inverse agonists in transgenic mice with myocardial overexpression of the beta 2-adrenoceptor. Nature. 1995;374(6519):272–6.
89. Zhou YY, et al. Constitutive beta2-adrenergic signalling enhances sarcoplasmic reticulum Ca2+ cycling to augment contraction in mouse heart. J Physiol. 1999;521(Pt 2):351–61.
90. Rohrer DK, et al. Cardiovascular and metabolic alterations in mice lacking both beta1- and beta2-adrenergic receptors. J Biol Chem. 1999;274(24): 16701–8.
91. Du XJ, et al. Age-dependent cardiomyopathy and heart failure phenotype in mice overexpressing

beta(2)-adrenergic receptors in the heart. Cardiovasc Res. 2000;48(3):448–54.
92. Liggett SB, et al. Early and delayed consequences of beta(2)-adrenergic receptor overexpression in mouse hearts: critical role for expression level. Circulation. 2000;101(14):1707–14.
93. Koch WJ, et al. Cardiac function in mice overexpressing the beta-adrenergic receptor kinase or a beta ARK inhibitor. Science. 1995;268(5215):1350–3.
94. Rockman HA, et al. Expression of a beta-adrenergic receptor kinase 1 inhibitor prevents the development of myocardial failure in gene-targeted mice. Proc Natl Acad Sci U S A. 1998;95(12):7000–5.
95. Harding VB, et al. Cardiac beta ARK1 inhibition prolongs survival and augments beta blocker therapy in a mouse model of severe heart failure. Proc Natl Acad Sci U S A. 2001;98(10):5809–14.
96. Paradis P, et al. Overexpression of angiotensin II type I receptor in cardiomyocytes induces cardiac hypertrophy and remodeling. Proc Natl Acad Sci U S A. 2000;97(2):931–6.
97. Kubota T, et al. Dilated cardiomyopathy in transgenic mice with cardiac-specific overexpression of tumor necrosis factor-alpha. Circ Res. 1997;81(4):627–35.
98. McMurray J, Pfeffer MA. New therapeutic options in congestive heart failure: Part I. Circulation. 2002;105(17):2099–106.
99. McMurray J, Pfeffer MA. New therapeutic options in congestive heart failure: Part II. Circulation. 2002;105(18):2223–8.
100. Hirota H, et al. Loss of a gp130 cardiac muscle cell survival pathway is a critical event in the onset of heart failure during biomechanical stress. Cell. 1999;97(2):189–98.
101. Hirota H, et al. Continuous activation of gp130, a signal-transducing receptor component for interleukin 6-related cytokines, causes myocardial hypertrophy in mice. Proc Natl Acad Sci U S A. 1995;92(11):4862–6.
102. D'Angelo DD, et al. Transgenic Galphaq overexpression induces cardiac contractile failure in mice. Proc Natl Acad Sci U S A. 1997;94(15):8121–6.
103. Esposito G, et al. Genetic alterations that inhibit in vivo pressure-overload hypertrophy prevent cardiac dysfunction despite increased wall stress. Circulation. 2002;105(1):85–92.
104. Mende U, et al. Transient cardiac expression of constitutively active Galphaq leads to hypertrophy and dilated cardiomyopathy by calcineurin-dependent and independent pathways. Proc Natl Acad Sci U S A. 1998;95(23):13893–8.
105. Akhter SA, et al. Targeting the receptor-Gq interface to inhibit in vivo pressure overload myocardial hypertrophy. Science. 1998;280(5363):574–7.
106. Wettschureck N, et al. Absence of pressure overload induced myocardial hypertrophy after conditional inactivation of Galphaq/Galpha11 in cardiomyocytes. Nat Med. 2001;7(11):1236–40.
107. Iwase M, et al. Adverse effects of chronic endogenous sympathetic drive induced by cardiac GS alpha overexpression. Circ Res. 1996;78(4):517–24.
108. Redfern CH, et al. Conditional expression of a Gi-coupled receptor causes ventricular conduction delay and a lethal cardiomyopathy. Proc Natl Acad Sci U S A. 2000;97(9):4826–31.
109. Hunter JJ, et al. Ventricular expression of a MLC-2v-ras fusion gene induces cardiac hypertrophy and selective diastolic dysfunction in transgenic mice. J Biol Chem. 1995;270(39):23173–8.
110. Sah VP, et al. Cardiac-specific overexpression of RhoA results in sinus and atrioventricular nodal dysfunction and contractile failure. J Clin Invest. 1999;103(12):1627–34.
111. Sussman MA, et al. Altered focal adhesion regulation correlates with cardiomyopathy in mice expressing constitutively active rac1. J Clin Invest. 2000;105(7): 875–86.
112. Wakasaki H, et al. Targeted overexpression of protein kinase C beta2 isoform in myocardium causes cardiomyopathy. Proc Natl Acad Sci U S A. 1997;94(17): 9320–5.
113. Molkentin JD, et al. A calcineurin-dependent transcriptional pathway for cardiac hypertrophy. Cell. 1998;93(2):215–28.
114. Jeong D, et al. PICOT inhibits cardiac hypertrophy and enhances ventricular function and cardiomyocyte contractility. Circ Res. 2006;99(3):307–14.
115. Takeishi Y, et al. Transgenic overexpression of constitutively active protein kinase C epsilon causes concentric cardiac hypertrophy. Circ Res. 2000;86(12): 1218–23.
116. Antos CL, et al. Dilated cardiomyopathy and sudden death resulting from constitutive activation of protein kinase a. Circ Res. 2001;89(11):997–1004.
117. Ling H, et al. Requirement for Ca2+/calmodulin-dependent kinase II in the transition from pressure overload-induced cardiac hypertrophy to heart failure in mice. J Clin Invest. 2009;119(5):1230–40.
118. Anderson ME. Calmodulin kinase signaling in heart: an intriguing candidate target for therapy of myocardial dysfunction and arrhythmias. Pharmacol Ther. 2005;106(1):39–55.
119. Yoo B, et al. Beta1-adrenergic receptors stimulate cardiac contractility and CaMKII activation in vivo and enhance cardiac dysfunction following myocardial infarction. Am J Physiol Heart Circ Physiol. 2009;297(4):H1377–86.
120. Gruver CL, et al. Targeted developmental overexpression of calmodulin induces proliferative and hypertrophic growth of cardiomyocytes in transgenic mice. Endocrinology. 1993;133(1):376–88.
121. Muth JN, et al. A Ca(2+)-dependent transgenic model of cardiac hypertrophy: a role for protein kinase Calpha. Circulation. 2001;103(1):140–7.
122. Jones LR, et al. Regulation of Ca2+ signaling in transgenic mouse cardiac myocytes overexpressing calsequestrin. J Clin Invest. 1998;101(7): 1385–93.
123. Sato Y, et al. Cardiac-specific overexpression of mouse cardiac calsequestrin is associated with depressed cardiovascular function and hypertrophy in transgenic mice. J Biol Chem. 1998;273(43):28470–7.

124. Periasamy M, et al. Impaired cardiac performance in heterozygous mice with a null mutation in the sarco(endo)plasmic reticulum Ca2+-ATPase isoform 2 (SERCA2) gene. J Biol Chem. 1999;274(4): 2556–62.
125. Ito K, et al. Transgenic expression of sarcoplasmic reticulum Ca(2+) atpase modifies the transition from hypertrophy to early heart failure. Circ Res. 2001;89(5):422–9.
126. Tsuji T, et al. Rescue of Ca2+ overload-induced left ventricular dysfunction by targeted ablation of phospholamban. Am J Physiol Heart Circ Physiol. 2009;296(2):H310–7.
127. He H, et al. Overexpression of the rat sarcoplasmic reticulum Ca2+ ATPase gene in the heart of transgenic mice accelerates calcium transients and cardiac relaxation. J Clin Invest. 1997;100(2):380–9.
128. Baker DL, et al. Targeted overexpression of the sarcoplasmic reticulum Ca2+-ATPase increases cardiac contractility in transgenic mouse hearts. Circ Res. 1998;83(12):1205–14.
129. Schmitt JP, et al. Dilated cardiomyopathy and heart failure caused by a mutation in phospholamban. Science. 2003;299(5611):1410–3.
130. Sato Y, et al. Rescue of contractile parameters and myocyte hypertrophy in calsequestrin overexpressing myocardium by phospholamban ablation. J Biol Chem. 2001;276(12):9392–9.
131. Dash R, et al. Interactions between phospholamban and beta-adrenergic drive may lead to cardiomyopathy and early mortality. Circulation. 2001;103(6): 889–96.
132. Luo W, et al. Targeted ablation of the phospholamban gene is associated with markedly enhanced myocardial contractility and loss of beta-agonist stimulation. Circ Res. 1994;75(3):401–9.
133. Minamisawa S, et al. Chronic phospholamban-sarcoplasmic reticulum calcium ATPase interaction is the critical calcium cycling defect in dilated cardiomyopathy. Cell. 1999;99(3):313–22.
134. Pleger ST, et al. S100A1 gene therapy preserves in vivo cardiac function after myocardial infarction. Mol Ther. 2005;12(6):1120–9.
135. Xin HB, et al. Oestrogen protects FKBP12.6 null mice from cardiac hypertrophy. Nature. 2002;416(6878):334–8.
136. Yano M, et al. FKBP12.6-mediated stabilization of calcium-release channel (ryanodine receptor) as a novel therapeutic strategy against heart failure. Circulation. 2003;107(3):477–84.
137. Shai SY, et al. Cardiac myocyte-specific excision of the beta1 integrin gene results in myocardial fibrosis and cardiac failure. Circ Res. 2002;90(4): 458–64.
138. Hayashidani S, et al. Targeted deletion of MMP-2 attenuates early LV rupture and late remodeling after experimental myocardial infarction. Am J Physiol Heart Circ Physiol. 2003;285(3):H1229–35.
139. Ducharme A, et al. Targeted deletion of matrix metalloproteinase-9 attenuates left ventricular enlargement and collagen accumulation after experimental myocardial infarction. J Clin Invest. 2000;106(1):55–62.
140. Creemers EE, et al. Deficiency of TIMP-1 exacerbates LV remodeling after myocardial infarction in mice. Am J Physiol Heart Circ Physiol. 2003;284(1):H364–71.
141. Shimizu T, et al. Model mice for tissue-specific deletion of the manganese superoxide dismutase gene. Geriatr Gerontol Int. 2010;10 Suppl 1:S70–9.
142. Ikegami T, et al. Model mice for tissue-specific deletion of the manganese superoxide dismutase (MnSOD) gene. Biochem Biophys Res Commun. 2002;296(3):729–36.
143. Belke DD, et al. Insulin signaling coordinately regulates cardiac size, metabolism, and contractile protein isoform expression. J Clin Invest. 2002;109(5): 629–39.
144. McQueen AP, et al. Contractile dysfunction in hypertrophied hearts with deficient insulin receptor signaling: possible role of reduced capillary density. J Mol Cell Cardiol. 2005;39(6):882–92.
145. Velez M, Kohli S, Sabbah HN. Animal models of insulin resistance and heart failure. Heart Fail Rev. 2014;19(1):1–13.
146. Basu R, et al. Type 1 diabetic cardiomyopathy in the Akita (Ins2WT/C96Y) mouse model is characterized by lipotoxicity and diastolic dysfunction with preserved systolic function. Am J Physiol Heart Circ Physiol. 2009;297(6):H2096–108.
147. Yoshioka M, et al. A novel locus, Mody4, distal to D7Mit189 on chromosome 7 determines early-onset NIDDM in nonobese C57BL/6 (Akita) mutant mice. Diabetes. 1997;46(5):887–94.
148. Epstein PN, Overbeek PA, Means AR. Calmodulin-induced early-onset diabetes in transgenic mice. Cell. 1989;58(6):1067–73.
149. Shen X, et al. Cardiac mitochondrial damage and biogenesis in a chronic model of type 1 diabetes. Am J Physiol Endocrinol Metab. 2004;287(5): E896–905.
150. Teerlink JR, Pfeffer JM, Pfeffer MA. Progressive ventricular remodeling in response to diffuse isoproterenol-induced myocardial necrosis in rats. Circ Res. 1994;75:105–13.
151. El-Demerdash E, Awad AS, Taha RM, El-Hady AM, Sayed-Ahmed MM. Probucol attenuates oxidative stress and energy decline in isoproterenol-induced heart failure in rat. Pharmacol Res. 2005;51: 311–8.
152. Oudit GY, Crackower MA, Eriksson U, Sarao R, Kozieradzki I, Sasaki T, et al. Phosphoinositide 3-kinase gamma-deficient mice are protected from isoproterenol-induced heart failure. Circulation. 2003;108:2147–52.
153. Grimm D, Elsner D, Schunkert H, Pfeifer M, Griese D, Bruckschlegel G, et al. Development of heart failure following isoproterenol administration in the rat: role of the renin-angiotensin system. Cardiovasc Res. 1998;37:91–100.
154. Halapas A, Papalois A, Stauropoulou A, Philippou A, Pissimissis N, Chatzigeorgiou A, et al. In vivo

models for heart failure research. In Vivo. 2008;22:767–80.
155. Bayat H, Swaney JS, Ander AN, Dalton N, Kennedy BP, Hammond HK, et al. Progressive heart failure after myocardial infarction in mice. Basic Res Cardiol. 2002;97:206–13.
156. Gao XM, Dart AM, Dewar E, Jennings G, Du XJ. Serial echocardiographic assessment of left ventricular dimensions and function after myocardial infarction in mice. Cardiovasc Res. 2000;45:330–8.
157. Hwang GS, Oh KS, Koo HN, Seo HW, You KH, Lee BH. Effects of KR-31378, a novel ATP-sensitive potassium channel activator, on hypertrophy of H9c2 cells and on cardiac dysfunction in rats with congestive heart failure. Eur J Pharmacol. 2006;540:131–8.
158. Pfeffer MA, Pfeffer JM, Fishbein MC, Fletcher PJ, Spadaro J, Kloner RA, et al. Myocardial infarct size and ventricular function in rats. Circ Res. 1979;44:503–12.
159. Gould KE, Taffet GE, Michael LH, Christie RM, Konkol DL, Pocius JS, et al. Heart failure and greater infarct expansion in middle-aged mice: a relevant model for postinfarction failure. Am J Physiol Heart Circ Physiol. 2002;282:H615–21.
160. Wu JC, Nasseri BA, Bloch KD, Picard MH, Scherrer-Crosbie M. Influence of sex on ventricular remodeling after myocardial infarction in mice. J Am Soc Echocardiogr. 2003;16:1158–62.
161. Skyschally A, Leineweber K, Gres P, Haude M, Erbel R, Heusch G. Coronary microembolization. Basic Res Cardiol. 2006;101:373–82.
162. Michael LH, Entman ML, Hartley CJ, Youker KA, Zhu J, Hall SR, et al. Myocardial ischemia and reperfusion: a murine model. Am J Physiol. 1995;269:H2147–54.
163. West MB, Rokosh G, Obal D, Velayutham M, Xuan YT, Hill BG, et al. Cardiac myocyte-specific expression of inducible nitric oxide synthase protects against ischemia/reperfusion injury by preventing mitochondrial permeability transition. Circulation. 2008;118:1970–8.
164. Krzeminski TF, Nozynski JK, Grzyb J, Porc M. Wide-spread myocardial remodeling after acute myocardial infarction in rat. Features for heart failure progression. Vascul Pharmacol. 2008;48:100–8.
165. Ryu JH, Kim IK, Cho SW, Cho MC, Hwang KK, Piao H, et al. Implantation of bone marrow mononuclear cells using injectable fibrin matrix enhances neovascularization in infarcted myocardium. Biomaterials. 2005;26:319–26.
166. Heymans S, Pauschinger M, De Palma A, Kallwellis-Opara A, Rutschow S, Swinnen M, et al. Inhibition of urokinase-type plasminogen activator or matrix metalloproteinases prevents cardiac injury and dysfunction during viral myocarditis. Circulation. 2006;114:565–73.
167. Nishio R, Sasayama S, Matsumori A. Left ventricular pressure-volume relationship in a murine model of congestive heart failure due to acute viral myocarditis. J Am Coll Cardiol. 2002;40:1506–14.
168. Matsumori A, Sasayama S. Immunomodulating agents for the management of heart failure with myocarditis and cardiomyopathy–lessons from animal experiments. Eur Heart J. 1995;16:140–3.
169. Liu P, Penninger J, Aitken K, Sole M, Mak T. The role of transgenic knockout models in defining the pathogenesis of viral heart disease. Eur Heart J. 1995;16:25–7.
170. Cunha-Neto E, Dzau VJ, Allen PD, Stamatiou D, Benvenutti L, Higuchi ML, et al. Cardiac gene expression profiling provides evidence for cytokinopathy as a molecular mechanism in Chagas' disease cardiomyopathy. Am J Pathol. 2005;167:305–13.
171. Carvalho KA, Guarita-Souza LC, Hansen P, Rebelatto CL, Senegaglia AC, Miyague N, et al. Cell transplantation after the coculture of skeletal myoblasts and mesenchymal stem cells in the regeneration of the myocardium scar: an experimental study in rats. Transplant Proc. 2006;38:1596–602.
172. Wakisaka Y, Niwano S, Niwano H, Saito J, Yoshida T, Hirasawa S, et al. Structural and electrical ventricular remodeling in rat acute myocarditis and subsequent heart failure. Cardiovasc Res. 2004;63: 689–99.
173. Hirono S, Islam MO, Nakazawa M, Yoshida Y, Kodama M, Shibata A, et al. Expression of inducible nitric oxide synthase in rat experimental autoimmune myocarditis with special reference to changes in cardiac hemodynamics. Circ Res. 1997;80:11–20.
174. Halapas A, Pissimissis N, Lembessis P, Rizos I, Rigopoulos AG, Kremastinos DT, et al. Molecular diagnosis of the viral component in cardiomyopathies: pathophysiological, clinical and therapeutic implications. Expert Opin Ther Targets. 2008;12:821–36.
175. Goser S, Andrassy M, Buss SJ, Leuschner F, Volz CH, Ottl R, et al. Cardiac troponin I but not cardiac troponin T induces severe autoimmune inflammation in the myocardium. Circulation. 2006;114: 1693–702.
176. Usui S, Yao A, Hatano M, Kohmoto O, Takahashi T, Nagai R, et al. Upregulated neurohumoral factors are associated with left ventricular remodeling and poor prognosis in rats with monocrotaline-induced pulmonary arterial hypertension. Circ J. 2006;70:1208–15.
177. Plestina R, Stoner HB. Pulmonary oedema in rats given monocrotaline pyrrole. J Pathol. 1972;106:235–49.
178. Kay JM, Smith P, Heath D. Electron microscopy of Crotalaria pulmonary hypertension. Thorax. 1969;24:511–26.
179. Schoental R, Head MA. Pathological changes in rats as a result of treatment with monocrotaline. Br J Cancer. 1955;9:229–37.
180. Hessel MH, Steendijk P, den Adel B, Schutte CI, van der Laarse A. Characterization of right ventricular function after monocrotaline-induced pulmonary hypertension in the intact rat. Am J Physiol Heart Circ Physiol. 2006;291:H2424–30.
181. Wood P, Piran S, Liu PP. Diastolic heart failure: progress, treatment challenges, and prevention. Can J Cardiol. 2011;27:302–10.

182. Dubi S, Arbel Y. Large animal models for diastolic dysfunction and diastolic heart failure-a review of the literature. Cardiovasc Pathol. 2010;19:147–52.
183. Zile MR, Brutsaert DL. New concepts in diastolic dysfunction and diastolic heart failure: part I: diagnosis, prognosis, and measurements of diastolic function. Circulation. 2002;105:1387–93.
184. Reed AL, Tanaka A, Sorescu D, Liu H, Jeong EM, Sturdy M, et al. Diastolic dysfunction is associated with cardiac fibrosis in the senescence-accelerated mouse. Am J Physiol Heart Circ Physiol. 2011;301:H824–31.
185. Brenner DA, Apstein CS, Saupe KW. Exercise training attenuates age-associated diastolic dysfunction in rats. Circulation. 2001;104:221–6.
186. Finck BN, Lehman JJ, Leone TC, Welch MJ, Bennett MJ, Kovacs A, et al. The cardiac phenotype induced by PPARalpha overexpression mimics that caused by diabetes mellitus. J Clin Invest. 2002;109:121–30.
187. Huang WY, Aramburu J, Douglas PS, Izumo S. Transgenic expression of green fluorescence protein can cause dilated cardiomyopathy. Nat Med. 2000;6:482–3.
188. Molkentin JD, Robbins J. With great power comes great responsibility: using mouse genetics to study cardiac hypertrophy and failure. J Mol Cell Cardiol. 2009;46:130–6.

In vitro Experimental Assessment of Cardiac Function

20

Inês Falcão-Pires and Adelino F. Leite-Moreira

Abstract

The increasing number of animal models available has undoubtedly contributed to the great advances in cardiovascular research. Not with standing the development of these valuable tools, it is important to properly assess myocardial function both in physiological and in pathological conditions as well as in response to certain drugs. It is clear from recent literature that significant technological progresses to evaluate cardiac function has been made over the last 10 years. This progress has substantially overcome many of the difficulties associated with cardiovascular function assessment in disease models. Moreover by means of a reductionist approach it has been possible to dissect the complexities of in vivo heart function using more detailed and sensitive in vitro techniques that are able to exclude confounding factors of the in vivo setting. Thus many new questions are constantly arising and additional experiments and methodologies urge.

Keywords

Cardiac function • Rodents • Single cardiomyocytes • Multicellular preparations • Langendorff/Working heart

Abbreviations

AT	Active tension
dT/dt_{max}	Maximum velocity of tension rise
dT/dt_{min}	Maximum velocity of tension decline
F_{active}	Maximal Ca^{2+}-activated (active) force stiffness
$F_{passive}$	Passive force
FT	Force transducer
HF	Heart Failure
LV	Left ventricle
LVP	Left ventricle pressure
LV-PV	Left Ventricular Pressure-Volume
pCa_{50}	Myofilaments Ca^{2+} sensitivity of isometric force

I. Falcão-Pires, MSc, PhD (✉)
A.F. Leite-Moreira, MD, PhD
Department of Physiology and Cardiothoracic Surgery, Faculty of Medicine, University of Porto, Alameda Prof Hernâni Monteiro, Porto 4200-319, Portugal
e-mail: ipires@med.up.pt; amoreira@med.up.pt

D.V. Cokkinos (ed.), *Introduction to Translational Cardiovascular Research*,
DOI 10.1007/978-3-319-08798-6_20,

20.1 Introduction

In the last 20 years alternative strategies have been developed to overcome interspecies differences as well as various issues related to animal experimentation, especially ethical concerns. These approaches include studying the changes at the cellular and tissue level in human biopsies (whenever possible) or in smaller animal samples to reduce, refine and replace animal experimentation. This approach has encouraged a progressive refinement of methodologies to accurately assess cardiac function in vitro on a smaller level of complexity and to properly integrate and translate the results to the whole body.

For researchers, especially those in the fields of physiology, pharmacology and toxicology, the choice of the correct in vitro technique/methodology to experimentally evaluate cardiac function is crucial. With the rising field of translational research, even primarily molecular biology laboratories aim to correlate their molecular findings with functional data. Thus a correct functional evaluation provides a valuable tool to evaluate the physiological and pathophysiological consequences derived from molecular, cellular, and tissue biology advances and for predicting the effectiveness and safety of new interventions in humans. This chapter aims to provide an overview of the most commonly used techniques to assess cardiac function in vitro in the context of cardiovascular disease and heart failure (HF). For each technique we will provide a brief description, its applications, advantages, disadvantages, derived parameters as well as some innovative studies. For the sake of simplicity, the detailed methodological protocols will be omitted, but the appropriate references will be suggested.

20.2 In Vitro and Ex Vivo Assessment of Cardiac Function

20.2.1 Single Cardiomyocytes

A great deal of effort has been spent in developing methodologies to evaluate cardiac performance in intact isolated single cardiomyocytes as well as investigating the mechanical and contractile properties of these cells [1].

Classically, passive and active properties of cardiac muscle have been measured mostly in multicellular preparations such as papillary muscles and trabeculae. Intact, multicellular strips of cardiac muscle comprise a population of contractile cells having an unknown distribution of orientation and force generation, intimately surrounded by a connective tissue matrix (see Sect. 20.2.2 in this Chapter). Moreover, because contractile function is strongly dependent on sarcomere length and cross-bridge cycling, the absence of direct visualization of the sarcomeres and the inhomogeneity present in multicellular preparations substantially limits the interpretations of sarcomere performance and cross-bridge function as well as its contractile properties. Thus, it would desirable to investigate muscle mechanics directly in single isolated cardiac cells. A preparation devoid of collagen and containing relatively few myofibrils in a single cohesive structure would allow almost direct access to the measurement of sarcomere length and cross-bridge contractile responses. Indeed the current ability to isolate cardiomyocytes for mechanical studies simplified this problem opening new avenues for in vitro assessment of cardiac function. The use of isolated cardiomyocytes has a number of additional advantages such as the ability to select cells from different areas of the heart including the atria, left and right ventricles, the conductive system or a specific region of the infarcted heart. Also, while imaging techniques are often limited in multicellular preparations, isolated cells are well-suited for experiments aimed at visualizing cellular structure and the precise localization of intracellular molecules. Isolated cardiomyocytes are also routinely used for studies examining intracellular Ca^{2+} homeostasis, cellular mechanics, and protein biochemistry, can easily be infected or transfected for gene transfer studies. Nevertheless, the inherent challenges of isolating and/or attaching the cell non-injuriously, recording force measurement at microgram levels, and obtaining appropriate optical sarcomere resolution are still a matter of concern in some commercial systems currently available [1]. These challenges have delayed the progression of isolated cardiac myocyte functional research; however, alternative mechanical measurements, such as shortening of unattached cells, auxotonic responses of cells attached to relatively compliant force transducers, stiffness measurements (see Sects. 20.2.1.1 and 20.2.1.2), cardiomyocytes cell culture, and labelled antibody staining of cytoskeletal and intermediate filaments, are leading to more detailed knowledge in myocardial contractile process [1].

Despite these concerns, almost four decades ago some investigators, advanced the state of the art by introducing the single isolated cell preparation, which allowed measurements to be made on a finer scale [2, 3]. The isolated cardiac myocyte preparation enabled to unravel fundamental mechanisms of contraction and excitation-contraction coupling in a preparation that excludes the confounding effects of the extracellular matrix or the endocardial endothelium. It has also made it possible to carefully assess several cell-specific phenomena, such as cellular biochemical processes, gap junction communication using neighbor cells, gene and protein expression/function which may be difficult or even impossible to understand in multicellular systems [4]. Further refinements include myocyte culture, the use of embryonic stem cell systems, the assessment of cell-cell interactions with endothelial or neuronal cells [4]. Nevertheless these methodologies are beyond the scope of this chapter.

The use of isolated cardiac myocytes holds several advantages over larger preparations due to uniformity in myofibril alignment and stress-strain distribution. Moreover, because the myofibrils are approximately 1 μm and range from 20 to 40 μm in diameter, diffusion coefficients allow a fast and nearly uniform ion distribution and even more in permeabilized cells; thus, activation should be essentially uniform [5]. Altogether, interpretation of data from single myofibril experiments appears to be particularly straight forward even considering the disadvantages of this technique. The first is related to the fact that most preparations are devoid of significant external mechanical load, thus load-dependent effects on contractile properties cannot be properly addressed [4]. To overcome this, a new technique was recently developed that uses intact cardiomyocytes glued between a force transducer and a motor in combination with an optical sarcomere spacing detector to provide a precise regulation of the sarcomere length in loaded intact cardiomyocytes [6]. This quite physiological system allows for assessment of tetanus, cardiac work loops, length dependent activation, force-velocity relationship, afterload and constant load contraction studies combined with calcium imaging, sarcomere spacing or even NAD/NADH and FAD/FADH studies. A second limitation concerns the fact that in some single skinned preparations or unloaded preparations, sarcomere length might not always be precisely controlled depending on how visible the sarcomeres are after the mechanical cell isolation procedure. Thus, length-dependent effects on contractile function are sometimes not possible to address. Thirdly, in unloaded preparations, the contribution of passive tension (stiffness) and restoring forces to the shortening responses of myocytes requires careful attention. Since the externally unloaded myocyte will usually shorten below slack length, the contribution of this passive tension may be most relevant in terms of resistance to shortening and in generating restoring forces, whereas in isometric preparations (whether single or multi-cellular), resistance to stretch is of greater relevance [1, 6]. In any case the myofibrillar macromolecule titin plays a major role in the myocardium, acting as a bidirectional spring [7].

It should be noted that, passive tension is relevant in all intact myocardial preparations (single or multi-cellular), but the precise influence on systolic and diastolic function varies between these preparations. While this cellular component of passive tension may not necessarily make a very large contribution to overall elasticity in most physiological circumstances, it becomes significant in pathological conditions such as pressure-overload-induced hypertrophy and HF with preserved ejection fraction [8–10]. In multicellular preparations, in addition to myofilaments passive stiffness, extracellular components play a role in myocardial stiffness, becoming particularly important for higher sarcomere lengths [11].

In summary, contractile and mechanical non-uniformities of multicellular cardiac preparations anticipate the need to evaluate cardiac sarcomere performance directly in simpler cardiac preparations. The single cardiac cell represents the simplest intact cardiac preparation and it can provide the opportunity for direct studies of cardiac sarcomere performance, since sarcomere length can easily be measured and the force for each sarcomere level is fairly well defined compared to the situation in more complex preparations. Often the measurement of contractile function in isolated cardiomyocytes rely on the optical assessment of unloaded cells shortening or in procedures technically more demanding, such as the measurement of force production, external loading and control of sarcomere length [5, 3, 12]. These procedures will be next described.

20.2.1.1 Intact Cardiomyocytes

It has been previously demonstrated that isolated single cardiac myocytes retain the Ca^{2+}-dependent systolic and diastolic properties of intact muscle regarding their resting membrane potential and excitability, spontaneous Ca^{2+} release from the sarcoplasmic reticulum and the effects of changes in stimulation frequency or extracellular Ca^{2+} concentration [4]. It was also shown that measurements of isolated single cell properties correlated properly with many properties of intact muscle, such as passive tension as well as maximum inotropy achieved with a variety of Ca^{2+}-elevating interventions [10, 13]. There is a large body of evidence showing that myocyte shortening responses to a wide variety of interventions parallel those observed in more complex preparation, such as the responses to α- and β-adrenergic stimulation, endothelin, Ca^{2+} sensitisers and desensitisers, modulation of sarcoplasmic reticular function, acidosis, alkalosis, hypoxia-reoxygenation, electrical tetanisation and stimulation of the nitric oxide/cGMP pathway [4]. This similar pattern of response between myocytes and intact multicellular muscle is consistent with the findings that, over a wide range of cell and sarcomere lengths, changes in cell length are linearly related to changes in force [14].

The utility of the single myocyte preparation has been enormously enhanced by advances that have enabled measurement with high spatial and temporal resolution of variables such as membrane currents (with voltage clamp techniques) and intracellular ion (Ca^{2+}, H^{+}, Na^{+}) concentrations, (with fluorescence spectrometry, FRET, imaging and confocal microscopy [15, 16]. Indeed, much of the current understanding of the mechanisms of excitation-contraction coupling is based largely on studies in single cells. Likewise, major advances in understanding Ca^{2+} transients and cellular mechanisms of arrhythmias derive from studies in single cells. Simultaneous measurements of cytosolic Ca^{2+} and cell shortening have also provided significant information regarding the inter-relationship between these variables, especially with respect to a variety of inotropic interventions [17]. These valuable methodologies enable measurement of the "steady-state" relationship between these variables during tetanisation of intact cells, as an approach to the assessment of myofilament response to Ca^{2+} in intact cells with intact signaling pathways [4]. This is in fact a major advantage of this technique, while detailed analyses of Ca^{2+}-myofilament interaction and crossbridge cycling are only possible in skinned tissue. However, the latter lacks membranes, membrane receptors or even sarcoplasm and thus most signaling pathways cannot be studied (See Sect. 20.2.1.2).

Assessment of shortening in unattached cells as a measure of contractility has been the subject of a wide variety of successful studies, gathering relevant information on cardiac cellular physiology. Nevertheless, these cells, largely devoid of collagen, are extremely sensitive to external mechanical stress, which make difficult its attachment to any equipment [1]. Recently a biocompatible, cellular adhesive was developed to overcome this limitation providing a method for securely attaching single cardiomyocyte to any research tool without damaging the cell [6].

Studying the mechanical properties of the isolated cardiac myocyte is also a way to understand the kinetics of crossbridge cycling. However, this preparation only provides an indirect assessment of crossbridges properties [1]. For instance, to measure myocyte force or stiffness it is necessary to attach the cardiomyocyte and this process is known to produce distorting strains or stresses that influence the contractile response [1]. Also, it is necessary to circumvent the small forces developed by the isolated myocyte with high-sensitive systems. On the other hand, measuring shortening in unattached myocytes only provides the assessment of the maximum turnover rate of the crossbridges without sizing neither internal viscous loading and loading by longitudinal and radial elastic elements, nor external cell orienting or stabilizing forces against which the cycling cross bridges are working [1].

20.2.1.2 Skinned Cardiomyocytes

An alternative approach to assess cardiac function is, as previously described, to measure force under isometric conditions by fixing one end of the cell and attaching the other end to a sensing probe by using isolated skinned cardiomyocytes systems. This system consists of an electromagnetic motor and a force transducer. The motor's movement is used to adjust cardiomyocyte length, while the force transducer measures isometric cardiomyocyte contraction. A single permeabilized (skinned) cardiomyocyte is mounted between these two elements and a specially developed optical system is used to determine cardiomyocyte sarcomere length and morphology from both the horizontal and the vertical directions (Fig. 20.1a).

The experimental protocol usually consists of a series of force measurements upon Ca^{2+} stimuli (using Ca^{2+} buffer solutions with a pCa ($-\log[Ca^{2+}]$) ranging from 9.0 to 4.5), the determination of actin-myosin crossbridge kinetics and the measurement of the passive tension of the mounted cardiomyocytes for certain sarcomere lengths. For example, isolated rat cardiac cells have a length of ~70–170 μm and diameters between 20 and 40 μm, often with irregular cross sections (Fig. 20.1b). They develop maximal isometric forces of ~12 μN. The rate constant of force redevelopment following rapid release-restretch maneuvers is ~5 s^{-1} after a length change of 20 % of the total cell length in 2.5 ms (Fig. 20.1c). Basic experiments, such as isometric force measurements, require a force sensor system that resolves forces below 0.1 μN, yet is sufficiently stiff so isometric conditions are maintained and sarcomere length is changed by less than ~0.1 %. Over time, several force transducers have been developed for mechanical measurements on single cardiomyocytes such as capacitive force transducers, optical fibers, suction pipettes, glass needles, and microfabricated polysilicon beams as cantilevers [1, 2, 18, 19]. Force can be estimated either with an open loop system using a relatively non-compliant probe whose displacement is a measure of force [1, 2, 19] or a closed loop system in which a feedback control loop is used to stabilize the position of the probe, with the resulting control signal being a measure of force [12]. Cells are attached directly to the force transduces and the motor either by impalement, mechanical knots, wax or silicone glue, suction or polylysine [12].

A good force transducer is designed to comprise the following features: (1) high sensitivity with sufficient frequency response (resonant frequency around 250 Hz), (2) freedom to select any 3-D orientation of the transducer, (3) a simple and fast calibration procedure, (4) continuous analog signal, (5) little temperature drift and (6) good linearity and dynamic range [12]. Indeed, the transducer is the key element in the isolated skinned cardiomyocytes technique, enabling to measure several force and force related parameters produced by cardiac myofilaments. This system is well suited to evaluate contractility, stiffness and Ca^{2+} sensitivity baseline or upon stimulation with drugs acting directly on myofilaments. Many skinned cardiomyocytes apparatus allow attaching cells to a small amount of glue which is placed on the tip of micropipettes attached to a force transducer and to a length controller (Fig. 20.1b).

Most isolated skinned cardiomyocytes systems control and measure force and length, maximal Ca^{2+}-activated force (F_{active}), stiffness ($F_{passive}$), myofilaments Ca^{2+} sensitivity of isometric force (pCa_{50}, using different Ca^{2+} containing solutions to construct pCa versus force curves, Fig. 20.1d), actin-myosin turnover rate assessed by isometric tension redevelopment

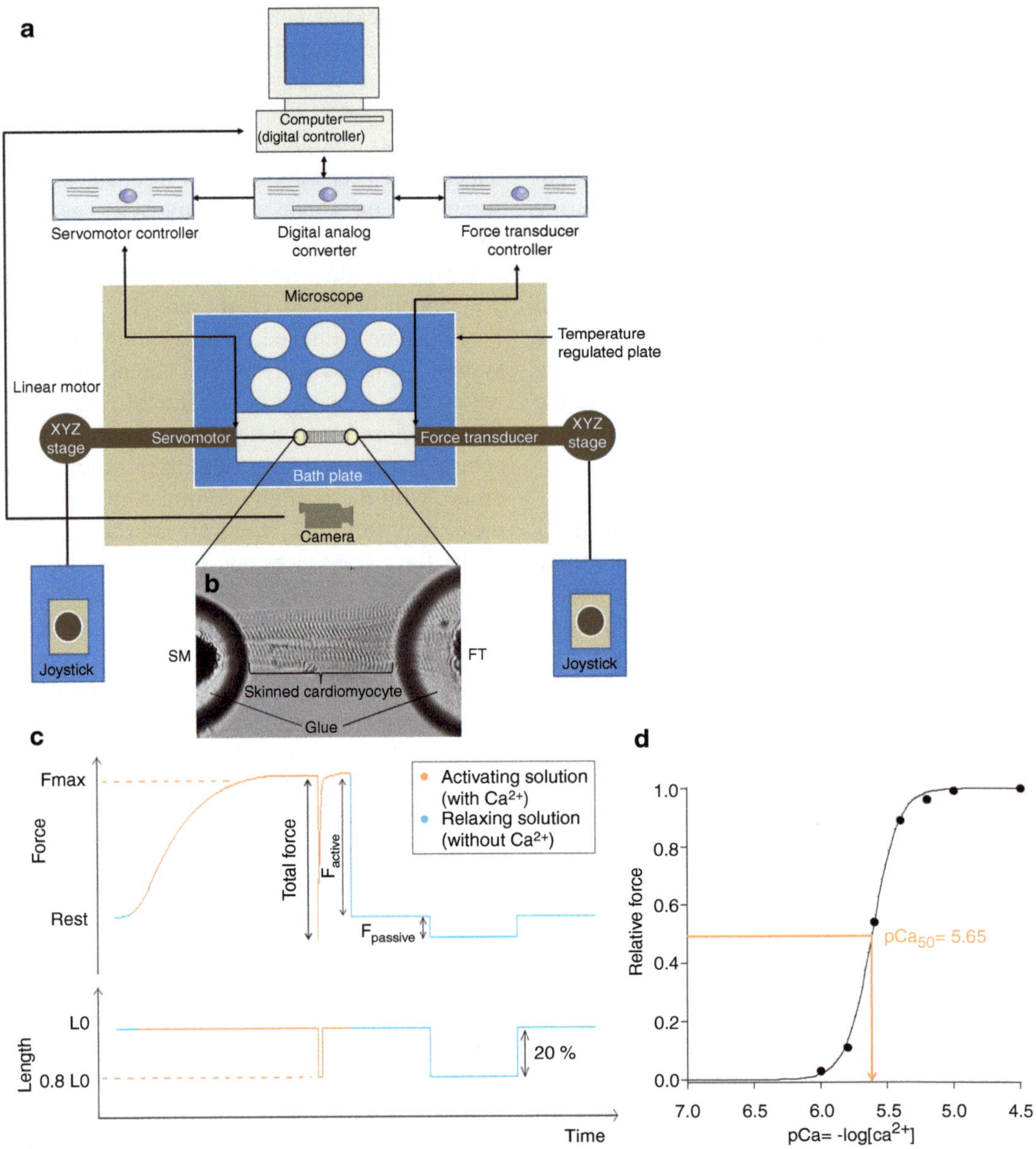

Fig. 20.1 Representation of several components of a single skinned cardiomyocyte setup (**a**) where a permeabilized (skinned) cardiomyocyte (**b**) is glued between a force transducer (*FT*) and a servomotor (*SM*) allowing assessment force and force-derived parameters under isometric conditions. A typical contraction-relaxation sequence is shown in (**c**). After transferring the myocyte from relaxing to activating solution (*red line*), isometric force starts to develop. Once a steady-state force level has been reached, the cell is shortened within 1 ms to 80 % of its original length (slack test) to determine the baseline of the force transducer. The distance between the baseline and the steady force level is the total force ($F_{total} = F_{active} + F_{passive}$). After 20 ms, the cell is restretched and returns to the relaxing solution (*blue line*), in which a second slack test of 10-s duration is performed to determine resting or passive force ($F_{passive}$). Using several Ca^{2+}-containing solutions it is possible to extract and normalize the value of F_{active} to maximal Factive and construct a pCa versus force curve (**d**). From this graph is calculated the value of pCa_{50} (-log[Ca^{2+}] for half-maximum force) and this parameter represents an index of myofilaments Ca^{2+} sensitivity

rate (kTR), myofilaments cooperativity (nHill) and sarcomere length dependence of F_{active}, $F_{passive}$, pCa_{50}, nHill, kTR.

The advantages of this system include the possibility to: (1) use diminute amounts of frozen tissue (transported and stored at ≤−80°C) as a source of cardiomyocytes; (2) test a wide range of species, including mice, rats, rabbits, guineas pigs, pigs and humans; (3) reproduce physiological (e.g. stretch) and pathophysiological (e.g. oxidative stress) conditions in vitro; (4) conduct inexpensive experiments as pharmacological studies use very small amount of drugs or enzymes and (5) assume and rely on an uniform alignment of the myofibrils.

Other similar setups were developed prior to this one. Le Guennec et al. [20] presented a technique that allowed controlling preload of a cardiomyocyte fixed to carbon fibers. Thus it was possible to increase the length of the sarcomere homogeneously and calculate the passive and active forces by optically monitoring changes of the carbon fibers curvature under an auxotonic contraction. More recently, Nishimura et al. [21] modified Le Guennec technique presenting a system that controlled force and length. This method can be used in isolated cardiomyocytes during isometric, isotonic and auxotonic contractions. Two carbon fibers anchor the cell – one fiber is stiff, serving as a mechanical anchor, whereas the bending motion of the compliant fiber is monitored for force length measurement. Furthermore, by controlling the position of the compliant fiber using a piezoelectric translator, it is possible to change load dynamically during contractions. This apparatus allowed performing for the first time physiological force-length loops in isolated myocytes. A disadvantage of this technique is the absence of control of the position of cardiomyocytes thus biasing sarcomere length accurate assessment.

Basic physiology of cardiac muscle can also be studied at the level of the sarcomere. Cardiac myofilament activity, the ultimate determinant of cellular dynamics and force, is a central player in the integration and regulation of pathways crucial to cardiac function and can be assessed by atomic force microscopy. Most atomic force microscopy sensors utilize small silicon cantilever beams with dimensions in the range of several micrometers. They have high resonance frequencies (often >10 kHz) and high stiffness (~10–1,000 N/m). With the appropriate detection system (i.e., laser beam deflection, tunneling current, interferometer), these sensors can reach the required nN resolution necessary for experiments on cardiac myocytes [18]. Despite these excellent properties, atomic force microscopy sensors are not well suited for measurements on cardiac myocytes. First, the diameters of single cardiac cells approach the dimensions of the cantilever of typical atomic force microscopy sensors [18]. It is therefore difficult to attach single myocytes exactly to the end of the beam and to accurately define the loading and the effective length of the cantilever. Second, the glue necessary to attach the cell must be distributed over a relatively large area of the beam such that its mechanical properties are changed. Third, atomic force microscopy sensors are fragile. Removal of glue residue and cell debris from the beam is not possible, and a new sensor is required for each cell [18].

20.2.2 Multicellular Preparations

In vitro studies have traditionally used multicellular preparations, such as papillary muscle or trabeculae, for the evaluation of cardiac mechanical properties including inotropic, lusitropic as well as basic electrophysiological and pharmacological properties. Actually, these preparations represent one of the oldest techniques used for the assessment of myocardial contractility and many fundamental concepts of muscle mechanics have been based on studies in this preparation, dating back more than 60 years [4]. Multicellular preparation data closely correlate with qualitatively results obtained from intact ventricle studies and thus become an invaluable tool to assess myocardial performance in conditions such as cardiomyopathy or heart failure. In these circumstances, parameters such as pressure and volume, which apply to the whole heart, are replaced by force or tension and length. By definition, force means the absolute amount of contractile strength, measured

a Isotonic contraction

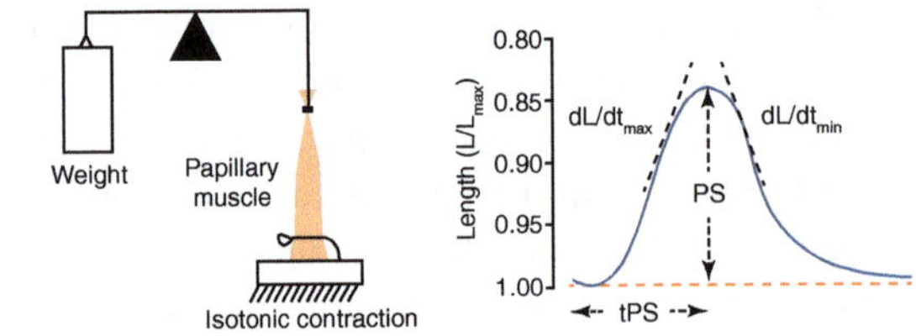

Isotonic parameters	Description
PS	Peak shortening (L/L_{max})
tPS	Time to peak shortening (ms)
VC (dL/dt_{max})	Maximal velocity of shortening (L_{max}/s)
tVC	Time to maximal velocity of shortening (ms)
VR (dL/dt_{min})	Maximal velocity of lengthening (L_{max}/s)
tVR	Time to maximal velocity of lengthening (ms)

b Isometric contraction

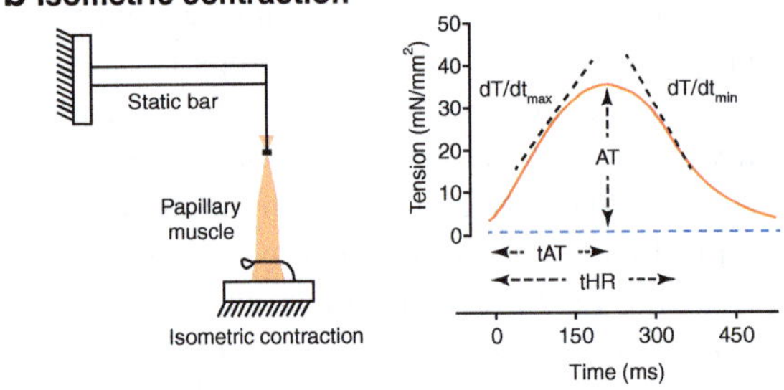

Isometric parameters	Description
AT	Active tension (mN/mm^2)
tAT	Time to active tension (ms)
tHR	Time to half relaxation (ms)
Pdf (dT/dt_{max})	Maximal velocity of tension rise (mN/mm^2.s)
tPdF	Time to maximal velocity of tension rise (ms)
NdF (dT/dt_{min})	Maximal velocity of tension decline (mN/mm^2.s)
tNdF	Time to maximal velocity of tension decline (ms)

Fig. 20.2 Isotonic (**a**) and isometric (**b**) contraction in multicellular preparations. *Left*: different setups to assess mechanical properties of papillary muscles using isotonic or isometric contraction. In the isotonic contraction the preloaded muscle lifts the load/weight by shortening the contractile element without distension of the elastic component. In the isometric contraction the muscle develops tension by shortening the contractile element and thereby stretching the elastic component, with the overall length of the muscle remaining constant. *Middle*: the upper panel represents length of the muscle twitch over time while the lower panel represents tension of the muscle twitch over time. During an isotonic contraction (*blue lines*) the tension remains constant (*blue dotted line* in the *lower panel*) but the muscle length changes (*blue full line* in the *upper panel*). During an isometric contraction (*orange lines*) the length remains constant (*orange dotted line* in the *upper panel*) but the muscle tension changes (*orange full line* in the *lower panel*). Some parameters represented in these panels are: *AT* active tension, dL/dt_{max} maximal velocity of shortening, dL/dt_{min} maximal velocity of lengthening, dT/dt_{max} maximal velocity of tension rise, dT/dt_{min} maximal velocity of tension decline, *PS* peak shortening, *tAT* time to active tension, *tHR* time to half relaxation, *tPS* time to peak shortening. All velocity parameters are obtained by the first derivative of tension or length over time. *Right*: Isotonic and isometric contractions derived parameters and the respective units. All parameters are normalized to muscle cross sectional area

in newtons (N), whereas tension is force related to cross sectional area, measured in newtons per squared millimetre (N/mm^2).

Protocols aimed to assess cardiac function in multicellular preparations typically involve muscle twitches (contraction–relaxation sequences) of either isotonic or afterloaded isometric contractions, but the frequency of contraction is very low compared to the physiological frequencies [22]. An isolated papillary muscle preparation responds to an electrical stimulus of suprathreshold intensity with an isotonic, an isometric or an auxotonic contraction (Fig. 20.2).

During contraction of a muscle in an isotonic setup, the muscle is fixed to the base, while the other end is attached to a loose transducer. Thus, when the muscle is electrically stimulated to contract under isotonic conditions there will be a displacement of the transducer and this movement is registered [23] (Fig. 20.2a).

During an isometric force measurement, force develops while shortening is prevented because the muscle is attached to two fixed ends one of which is a transducer. Upon electrical stimulation, the developed force is recorded under isometric conditions by the transducer. An important parameter to assess in such in vitro preparations is the L_{max} – the length for which the muscle develops maximal force (Fig. 20.2b).

In these multicellular setups mechanical load, such as preload and afterload are controlled and influence the pattern of contraction of the muscles. Also quick changes in load and length have been used to give information about cardiac muscle mechanics. The preload is responsible for the initial muscle stretch and thus its length. After stimulation, the contractile elements of the muscle begin to shorten, but the length does not change: the muscle fibers shorten at the expense of the interaction of the myofilaments. The stretching of the elastic members results in a progressive increase of the force developed, but no muscle shortening. When the contractile force equals the load (afterload), the muscle shortens without increasing the developed force. The speed and force of contraction are dependent on the concentration of intracellular free Ca^{2+}. Muscle force and speed are inversely related, so without load the speed is maximal but the force is residual. In contrast, in isometric contractions muscle does not shorten, its velocity of shortening is zero but develops maximal force [24].

These experiments are usually performed in organ bath heated to physiological temperatures containing oxygenated carbonate buffers (see Sect. 20.2.3.1). At the bottom of the bath there is a small device to oxygenate the solution or instead oxygen can be dissolved in the carbonate buffer that is perfusing the tissue. The pH of this solution should be strictly monitored and kept between 7.37 and 7.42 by altering the 95 % O_2/5 % CO_2 bubbling intensity. The base of the papillary muscle/trabeculae is fixed by a clamp, while the opposite end is attached to a transducer. In the organ bath there is a sensor that, together with a heater, controls the bath temperature [25]. The papillary muscles need to be stimulated electrically. Since the solution contains salts, it is possible that electrolytic processes occurring at the electrodes could lead to polarization and release of metals from the electrodes. This is usually prevented by using non polarizable electrodes such as platinum [25]. The buffer solution(s) chosen for the dissection and maintenance of the tissue is important as it will affect the viability of the preparation and hence the experimental protocol.

The basic procedure to obtain a stable preparation before starting any protocol typically includes the intravenous administration of anesthesia and heparin to the animal, to avoid the deposition of blood clots that potentially damage the endocardial endothelium. A thoracotomy is performed followed by the excision and fast immersion of the heart in the carbonate buffer. The heart is allowed to contract for a few beats to eject all the blood kept inside the ventricles coronary circulation and then is transferred to a similar solution but containing a cardioplegic agent to arrest the heart. Cardioplegia allows a safe dissection of the trabeculae or papillary muscles, which are subsequently transferred to the heated organ bath. The electric stimulation is turned on and the cardioplegic solution is replaced by normal carbonate buffer. During all this procedure the temperature should be kept as close as possible to the physiologic temperature of the animal.

Usually the derived parameters include active tension, maximum velocity of tension rise (dT/dt_{max}), maximum velocity of tension decline (dT/dt_{min}), peak shortening, time to peak shortening, maximum velocity of shortening (dL/dt_{max}), maximum velocity of lengthening (dL/dt_{min}) and time to half relaxation (Fig. 20.2). However other parameters can be derived from these, such as coefficients R1 and R2. Because changes in the contraction phase induce coordinated changes in the relaxation phase, variations in contraction and relaxation must be considered simultaneously to quantify drug induced changes in lusitropy [26]. Coefficient $R1 = dL/dt_{max}/dL/dt_{min}$ evaluates the lusitropy under isotonic conditions where the amplitude of sarcomere shortening is greater than that observed under isometric conditions [27]. Because of the lower sensitivity of myofilament for calcium when cardiac muscle is markedly shortened under low load, relaxation proceeds more rapidly than contraction, apparently due to the rapid uptake of calcium by the sarcoplasmatic reticulum. Thus, R1 tests sarcoplasmic reticulum uptake function [28]. Coefficient $R2 = dT/dt_{max}/dT/dt_{min}$ evaluates the lusitropy under a high load. When the muscle contracts isometrically, the sarcomeres shorten very little [27]. Because of the higher sensitivity of myofilament for calcium [29], the time course of relaxation is determined by calcium release from troponin C rather than by calcium sequestration by the sarcoplasmatic reticulum. Thus, R2 indirectly reflects myofilament calcium sensitivity [28].

Some of the advantages of the multicellular preparations include their great usefulness in elucidating the myocardial effects and mechanisms of action of certain drugs and neurohumoral agents while excluding the influence of systemic and other neurohumoral processes that occur in intact animals. Thus, they represent a classical pharmacological tool to assess dose response relationships in contractile tissue which is widely used in preclinical safety studies. Secondly, these preparations allow to measure and control force and length in preparations with relatively uniform fiber orientation, more than in the whole heart but less than in single cardiomyocytes, and to measure isotonic or isometric muscle performance independently of geometric constraints and interaction with blood flow and vascular tone. The results obtained from these organ bath systems are generally more consistent, reproducible and useful for measurement of concentration response curves. Finally, papillary muscles or trabeculae can be excised with minimal mechanical injury and remain stable for hours.

Some limitations of this preparation include the fact that: (1) the papillary muscle preparation has a higher elasticity than the one assumed due to end compliance, related to injured muscle extremities and the compliance of attached recording devices. This often results in significant mid-segmental shortening (up to 12 % L_{max}) during supposedly isometric contractions [4]; (2) the resultant spatial inhomogeneity of sarcomere length and intracellular Ca^{2+} may invalidate many of the assumptions required for cardiac function assessment; (3) there is no simple relationship between active and passive elements in this preparation; (4) it is not possible to undertake voltage clamp studies, thus greatly diminishing its usefulness in studying excitation-contraction coupling processes [4]; (5) there is a potential inadequacy of oxygenation and substrate supply by the carbonate buffer to the inner parts of the muscles (hypoxic core) and (6) the accumulation of metabolites, such as inorganic phosphate, and concentration gradients in the organ bath [4]. In this regard, an appropriate selection of muscles with relatively low cross-sectional areas (<0.5 mm thick) is critical and may surpass these limitations.

Regarding the influence of endothelial cells on myocardial function, it is important to account for the important functional differences between endocardial and coronary vascular endothelial cells [30]. Moreover, the coronary vascular endothelial cells, unless perfused, are probably non-functional in this preparation [31] in contrast to the endocardial endothelial cells whose interaction with the myocardium has been quite well studied in the papillary muscle [30]. In addition, important and relevant aspects of endothelial function, such as cyclical mechanotransduction mediated by shear stress are largely inoperative.

Despite these limitations, a number of recent technical breakthroughs provide the potential to overcome some of these problems. Among the most important of these is the ability to accurately assess sarcomere length, as well as, to obtain true isosarcometric contractions using laser diffraction to monitor sarcomere length and adaptive control systems to regulate it [32]. Interestingly, this approach demonstrated that many “isometric” conditions assumed in previous studies may not be totally reliable. Laser diffraction analysis coupled with force measurements provides important information about muscle contractile properties. Moreover, the incorporation of objective measurement of variables such as intracellular Ca^{2+} transients, ATPase activity, heat production and O_2 consumption [32, 33] are a major advance over much less precise and speculative interpretative assessments based solely on mechanical correlates. Other progresses include the use of skinned fibres with careful, uniform control of Ca^{2+} levels for studying Ca^{2+}-myofilament interaction, and the use of caged compounds [34]. In addition, information about the availability of stored calcium to activate muscle contraction is studied using rapid cooling contracture techniques. Rapid cooling contractures are also useful for assessing sarcoplasmic reticulum Ca^{2+}, especially in multicellular preparations where slow caffeine diffusion to all the cells limits the utility of the caffeine approach. Cooling to 0 °C inhibits Ca^{2+} pumping and also causes rapid sarcoplasmic reticulum Ca^{2+} release (presumably due to very long ryanodine receptor openings). Then, one can measure either $\Delta[Ca^{2+}]i$ or contractile force (which develops slowly at 0 °C). This technique is less quantitative concerning absolute amounts of Ca^{2+} but is useful for measuring changes in sarcoplasmatic reticulum Ca^{2+} content under different conditions.

20.2.3 The Isolated Perfused Heart

The ex vivo isolated perfused heart includes two different preparations: the Langendorff preparation, first described by Oskar Langendorff in 1895 [35] who demonstrated that the heart receives its nutrients and oxygen from blood via the coronary arteries and that cardiac mechanical function is reflected by changes in the coronary circulation and the ejecting heart or "working heart" system developed by Howard Morgan and James Neeley in 1967 to investigate the metabolism of the heart and coronary regulation [36].

20.2.3.1 Langendorff Preparation

In the Langendorff preparation, blood or more commonly crystalloid perfusates (nutrient solution), are delivered into the heart through a cannula inserted in the ascending aorta, either at constant pressure or constant flow. Retrograde (reverse) flow in the aorta closes the aortic valve and, as a result, the entire perfusate enters the coronary arteries via the ostia, located just outside the valve at the aortic root, thus maintaining the viability of the heart muscle. After passing through the coronary circulation the perfusate drains into the right atrium via the coronary sinus and tends to drip from the apex of the heart making it easily available for collection (Fig. 20.3a). This preparation is useful for cardiomyocyte isolation as well as for physiological monitoring of cardiac function using a system where stable preparations perfusion of several hours is usual.

All media has to be oxygenated and if a system other than whole blood is used, the media must be buffered, either with the traditional carbonate buffers such as Krebs-Henseleit, Locke's or Tyrode's or with variations of these formulas using HEPES or MES buffers. A substrate such as glucose is necessary and, depending on experimental design, other energy substrates can be utilized, such as pyruvate, lactate, fatty acids, and amino acids. The ionic components of the media will vary with the species; potassium and calcium are the most variable and critical of the ions. Dextran, polyvinyl pyrrolidone or albumin may be added to the perfusate to maintain oncotic pressure (8–25 mmHg). Temperature is also an important factor, can be manipulated depending on the experimental model being used: e.g., 4.5 °C for cryogenic studies; 37.5 °C for physiological studies and >37.5 °C for heat shock studies.

In the Langendorff system, because the cardiovascular system is no longer a closed loop, the ventricles do not fill with the perfusate and therefore do not perform pressure-volume work. Left ventricular pressure can however still be measured inside the balloon with the use of a catheter connected to a pressure transducer. Once inserted, the ventricle can contract isovolumetrically against the balloon, which can be made easily using items such as ultrathin food wrap that is the most recommended material. The balloon is placed into the left ventricle (LV) and inflated until a resting pressure of 3–10 mmHg is achieved (Fig. 20.3a) and should have the following characteristics: (*1*) appropriate size of the rodent heart, the balloon should be inflated to greater than the size of the stretched mouse/rat ventricular lumen to guarantee that the balloon itself is not contributing to the LV pressure; (*2*) highly flexible to follow the contours of the ventricular lumen; (*3*) highly compliant and thin to efficiently and accurately transmit LV pressures to the fluid in the balloon; and (*4*) highly linear frequency response of the pressure measurement system (balloon and transducer including tubing and attachments) to ensure faithful recording of LV pressures. Commercial latex balloons or the use of condom tips should be avoided as they do not meet all these criteria [37].

Once the heart is cannulated and successfully beating, there are several physiological, morphological, biochemical and pharmacological parameters that can be measured and recorded from the Langendorff preparation including: (1) mechanical parameters (LV pressure and volume and derived indices); (2) coronary vascular function; (3) cardiac metabolism; (4) bioelectrical parameters (ECG, monophasic injury potentials) and

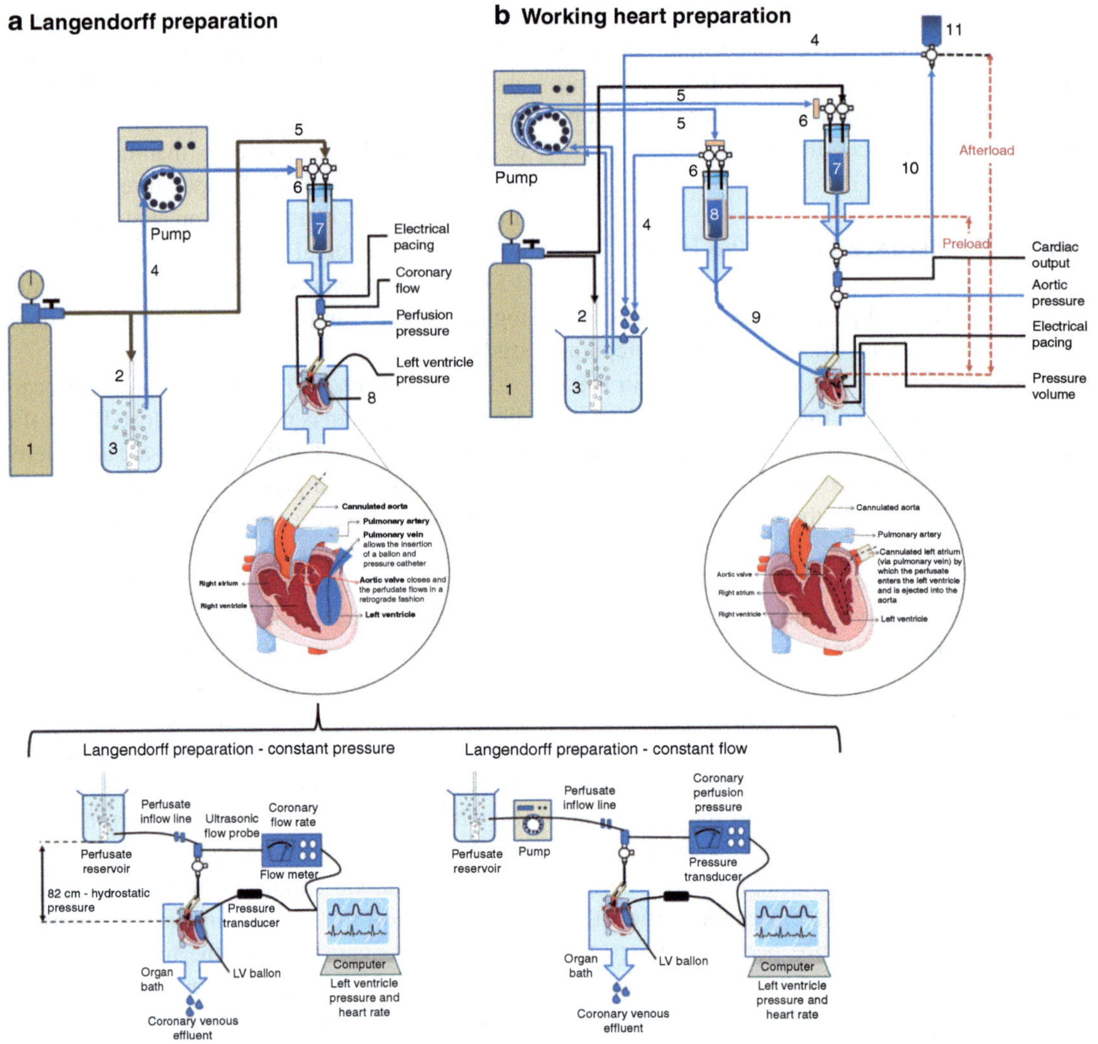

Fig. 20.3 The isolated perfused heart includes two different preparations: the Langendorff (**a**) working at constant perfusion pressure or constant flow and the ejecting heart or "working heart" preparation (**b**). In the **Langendorff apparatus**: (*1*) 95 % O_2–5 % CO_2 tank, (*2*) gas dispersion tube, (*3*) carbonate buffer reservoir, (*4*) perfusate line, (*5*) pressure line, (*6*) filter disc, (*7*) compliance chamber, (*8*) balloon. The carbonate buffer reservoir is warmed to 37 °C, and the compliance chamber and heart chamber are maintained at 37 °C by circulating warm water through the water-jacketed chambers. The heart is electrically paced via platinum electrodes placed on the epicardial surface of the right ventricle. Coronary flow is measured by placing an in-line flow probe in the aortic perfusion line. Coronary perfusion pressure is measured via a sidearm connected to a pressure transducer. Left ventricular (LV) pressure is measured via a balloon inserted in the LV chamber and connected via polyethylene tubing to a pressure transducer. An additional sidearm can be added to the aortic perfusion line for infusion of pharmacological drugs. In the **working heart apparatus**: (*1*) 95 % O_2–5 % CO_2 tank, (*2*) gas dispersion tube, (*3*) Carbonate buffer reservoir, (*4*) recirculation line, (*5*) perfusate line, (*6*) filter disc, (*7*) windkessel, (*8*) atrial reservoir, (*9*) preload line, (*10*) afterload line, and (*11*) overflow reservoir. The atrial reservoir, Windkessel, and heart chamber are maintained at 37 °C by circulating warm water through the water-jacketed chambers. The heart is electrically paced via platinum electrodes placed on the epicardial surface of the right ventricle. Cardiac output is measured by placing an in-line flow probe in the afterload line. Aortic pressure is measured via a sidearm connected to a pressure transducer. An additional in-line flow probe and pressure transducer sidearm can be placed in the preload line to measure atrial flow rate and atrial pressure. LV pressures and volumes can be simultaneously measured via a 1.4-Fr high-fidelity transducer inserted into the apex of the LV and sutured. Cardiac preload and afterload can be adjusted by varying the heights of the atrial reservoir and overflow reservoir

(5) cardiac cycle rhythm. Langendorff system applications include studies on global or regional ischemia, stunning, preconditioning, arrhythmias and proarrhythmic potential of drugs as well as studies on ischemia-reperfusion and storage conditions for preparing hearts for transplantation [38]. Indeed, the isolated perfused heart model represents an invaluable tool to test new interventions leading to improved heart preservation and to attenuation of ischemia-reperfusion injuries. However, the model is also widely used for physiologic, pathophysiologic and pharmacologic studies requiring assessment of cardiac function and/or coronary circulation (Table 20.1).

With constant perfusion pressure (Fig. 20.3a) the heart maintains the ability to autoregulate coronary vascular tone, which is important during ischemia-reperfusion injury experiments when perfusion to part of the vascular bed is restricted (or eliminated in the case of permanent coronary ligation). In this scenario, constant flow during reperfusion maintained at the same rate before

Table 20.1 Isolated perfused heart breakthroughs

Significant studies
The mechanisms underlying the involvement of reactive oxygen and nitrogen species in ischemia–reperfusion injury have been studied in the isolated rat hearts showing that oxidative stress via formation of peroxynitrite is a critical determinant to the early injury of the heart during reperfusion following ischemia [44].
Several interesting investigations in the field of cell-based therapy have been made within the last few years with the use of the isolated perfused heart as a tool to evaluate its impact on cardiac mechanical function. The underlying principle of the method is based on delivering cells, which have a potential to proliferate and differentiate into cardiomyocytes in the injured heart. Suzuki et al. developed a method for cell transplantation through the coronary artery instead of their direct intramuscular injection. In their experimental model, hearts were isolated from the donor animal, perfused with cells, and then transplanted into recipient animals. This method was further elaborated and improved to in vivo intracoronary infusion of cells, making the method more applicable from the clinical point of view [45]. Ohno et al. investigated the transplantation of skeletal myoblasts and vascular smooth muscle into the hearts of cardiomyopathic hamsters. On the basis of this experiment, Ohno et al. also elaborated a method of cell cryostorage [46].
Langendorff-mode isolated heart perfusion, in conjunction with ^{31}P NMR spectroscopy, combines the fields of biochemistry and physiology into one experiment. The protocol allows for the dynamic measurement of high-energy phosphate content and turnover in the heart while concurrently monitoring physiologic function. When performed correctly, this is a valuable technique in the assessment of cardiac energetics [47]. http://www.jove.com/video/2069/assessment-cardiac-function-energetics-isolated-mouse-hearts-using
Recently, two optical mapping systems, the panoramic imaging system, and the dual (voltage and calcium) imaging modality were described in Langendorff-perfused rabbit heart. The panoramic mapping system is used to map the entire epicardium of the rabbit heart, providing a global view of the evolution of reentrant circuits during arrhythmogenesis and defibrillation, and has been used to study the mechanisms of arrhythmias and antiarrhythmia therapy. The dual mapping system is used to map the action potential and calcium transient simultaneously from the same field of view. This approach fosters the understanding of the role of calcium in the electrical alternans and the induction of arrhythmia [48]. http://www.jove.com/video/3160/multiparametric-optical-mapping-langendorff-perfused-rabbit
When studying the metabolic effects of myocardial injury, such as ischemia, it is often necessary to identify the location of the affected tissue. This can be done by imaging the fluorescence of NADH (the reduced form of nicotinamide adenine dinucleotide), a coenzyme found in large quantities in the mitochondria. NADH fluorescence (fNADH) displays a near linearly inverse relationship with local oxygen concentration and provides a measure of mitochondrial redox state. fNADH imaging during hypoxic and ischemic conditions has been used as a dye-free method to identify hypoxic regions and to monitor the progression of hypoxic conditions over time. The objective of the method is to monitor the mitochondrial redox state of biventricular working hearts during protocols that alter the rate of myocyte metabolism or induce hypoxia or create a combination of the two. The combination of the heart model and fNADH imaging provides a new and valuable experimental tool for studying acute cardiac pathologies within the context of realistic physiological conditions [49]. http://www.jove.com/video/4115/nadh-fluorescence-imaging-isolated-biventricular-working-rabbit
A biventricular working heart system allows for ex vivo studies of diseases characterized by pulmonary vascular dysfunction and right heart pathophysiology. In addition to the ejecting left heart, which is now supplying perfusate to the coronaries and thus maintaining heart muscle viability, the right heart is also performing the low pressure ejection, whereby the perfusate enters the right atrium, flows into the right ventricle and exits through the pulmonary artery. Additional measurements of right ventricular pressure or right ventricular pressure-volume can now be taken independently or simultaneously with LVP/LV-PV [50].

ischemia would force a greater volume of perfusate through the compromised vascular bed, thus shearing and potentially damaging the coronary arteries. Conversely, autoregulatory mechanisms that attempt to increase coronary flow under increased workload conditions are overcome by constant flow, which carries a risk of developing low-grade ischemia. The advantage of constant flow perfusion using a high-fidelity peristaltic pump is that precise and reproducible degrees of low flow can be induced to study the effect of low-flow ischemia in the heart [39]. Constant flow is also particularly well suited for studying the effect of vasoactive substances on coronary vasomotor tone; coronary pressure is a sensitive parameter that is easily monitored, and the coronary vascular resistance is derived from this measurement using Ohm's law [39, 40] (Fig. 20.3a). Switching between constant flow and constant pressure modes of perfusion is not straightforward and, with simple apparatus, may not be feasible within a single experimental protocol.

One may choose to have a non-recirculating (single pass) system or a recirculating system. A single pass system is useful when an experimenter wishes to apply several agents in sequence and then allow their effects to dissipate as the agent is washed out of the heart. This approach is also useful when measuring the uptake or release of various drugs, neurotransmitters or metabolites. A recirculating system is useful when it is necessary to reduce the total volume of perfusate when utilizing expensive drugs or substrates.

Moreover, one must decide on whether the heart will be paced or allowed to beat spontaneously. Pacing is used to maintain a standard contractile response and metabolic demand, while spontaneous beating may permit the experimenter to measure changes in heart rate and rhythm that will occur with various drugs or manipulations. To pace a heart, the stimulus rate must exceed the natural cardiac pacemaker rate. Often the sinoatrial node is crushed or the right atrium excised to eliminate the contribution of the primary intrinsic pacemaker. Pacing voltage is determined as a set percentage (normally 110–150 %) above the voltage required to capture (pace) the heart and should not have to exceed 3–5 V, with duration of 0.1–1 ms.

The advantages of this methodology include its high reproducibility, the fact that the preparations are neither time-consuming nor technically demanding and the costs of experiments are relatively low. Despite the fact that hearts are isolated from the body, the method remains reasonably physiological and the heart spontaneously beats based on the myogenic nature of impulse initiation [41]. Another feature that can be considered an advantage is the fact that the preparation is free of the influence of other organs, the systemic circulation and signals from both circulating neurohormones and the central and the autonomic nervous systems, revealing potential direct actions of the drugs of interest on various cardiac parameters [41]. As drugs concentration can be precisely controlled, this method allows for very accurate determination of concentration-response relationships. It is also valuable for assessing the cardiotoxicity of test drugs and it is especially useful in distinguishing direct versus indirect cardiac injury [42]. Additionally, the preparation readily allows for the induction of ischemia, anoxia and hypoxia at various degrees and arrhythmia, making it a very important tool in studies of pathological conditions, which would normally pose a threat to the survival of the animal in an in vivo experiment [43].

The limitations of the method include the absence of normal humoral influences and neuronal regulation, as well as high coronary flow and edema when using cell free perfusate. The dramatically different rheology of crystalloid buffer and the higher flow rates alter sheer stress along the endothelium of coronary arteries. Some have modified the method by supplementing the Krebs–Henseleit buffer with red blood cells, resulting in the normalization of coronary flow rates. Lack of colloidal osmotic pressure of such perfusates may lead to tissue edema of the heart [41]. The lack of several blood derived antioxidants and glucocorticosteroids causes the preparation to be vulnerable to ambient immune stimuli, in particular bacterial endotoxin which is difficult to eliminate and will result in the stimulation of inducible nitric oxide synthase as well as endogenous peroxynitrite generation, resulting in the accelerated deterioration of heart function [43]. Additionally, the preparation requires a certain degree of skill and gentleness as the heart is highly vulnerable to injuries. There is a significant possibility of inadvertently preconditioning the heart during its isolation and instrumentation. The retrograde flow of perfusate in the aorta may lead to incompetence of the aortic valve (at very high perfusion pressures) and thus the entire perfusate may not pass through the coronary circulation [41]. A detailed description of the technique is provided in Bell et al. and Skrzypiec-Spring et al. [38, 41].

20.2.3.2 Ejecting Heart or Working Heart Preparation

Even though the Langendorff-perfused isolated heart is beating, the LV chamber is contracting isovolumetrically and the preparation is considered nonworking since no work is performed, as no perfusate is ejected from the heart (there is force generation, but no shortening). Neely and Morgan made a major modification in the isolated heart model and described an isolated rat heart preparation that performed physiologically relevant mechanical work. In this model, the aorta of a rat heart is attached via a cannula to an aortic outflow line and initially perfused in the Langendorff mode via a sidearm to the aortic line. A second cannula is inserted into the left atrium, and heart work is initiated by clamping the retrograde perfusion line while simultaneously unclamping the atrial inflow and aortic outflow lines. The atrial inflow line delivers perfusate at a constant preload hydrostatic pressure via the left atrium to the LV, and as the LV fills and contracts, perfusate is ejected out the aortic outflow line against a constant afterload hydrostatic pressure (Fig. 20.3b). Myocardial perfusion is achieved in a more physiological manner; during the course of ventricular relaxation, the aortic hydrostatic pressure leads to orthograde perfusion of the coronary vasculature of the heart. This method presents the advantage to provide accurate control of ventricular preload and afterload [36]. In the working heart model, contractile function can be assessed by the initial ejection pressure at the aorta and the concomitant ability to pump against an afterload as adjusted via the compliance chamber and/or reach a set ejection pressure with a preload set by adjusting the height of the atrial reservoir. This way a more physiological assay of ventricular contractility is possible as the left ventricle is now fully-ejecting and performing pressure-volume and acceleration work. Multiple parameters can be obtained from the working heart system including aortic pressure and flow, cardiac output, LV pressure, dP/dt_{max} and dP/dt_{min}, LV end-diastolic and end-systolic pressures and end-diastolic pressure-volume derived parameters, ECG, heart rate, amongst others. In order to fully exploit this advantage, recent equipment include a specialized pathway, which easily allows introduction of a pressure (LVP) or pressure-volume (LV-PV) catheter directly into the left ventricle via the aorta or via an apical puncture. Pressure-volume work is determined by the product of developed pressure with the total volume of fluid ejected by the ventricle in a cardiac cycle. In any of these cases, the experimenter should determine the appropriate amount of resting force or pressure required to maintain the heart on the ascending limb of the Starling curve and avoid overstretching the heart muscle.

Table 20.2 Useful parameters for isolated perfused heart in rat

Perfusion pressure	(60, 70) mmHg
Flow rate	(7–9) ml/min
Balloon diameter	3–4 mm
Pressure inside the balloon (diastolic pressure)	(5, 10) mmHg
Oxygen tension	(550, 600) mmHg
Initial preload	Height of 10 cmH_2O (6.5 mmHg)
Afterload height	60–80 mmHg
Coronary flow	8–12 ml/min/g wet weight of tissue
Spontaneous heart rate	250–300 bpm

Some important parameters for the correct assembling of isolated perfused heart system in rats are depicted in Table 20.2.

20.3 Discussion and General Considerations

Adequate evaluation and understanding of cardiac performance is not limited simply to studying cardiac muscle, or contractile function, or even just the mechanical properties of myocardial tissue.

Frequently, researchers become acquainted with a methodology establish in their own laboratory and consequently succumb to the temptation of searching for questions that might be addressed using their favorite preparation. This is certainly not the best option for scientific advance; instead real progress in research is achieved by first defining the question/hypothesis and then identifying the most appropriate experimental preparation to answer that question.

Moreover, no single experimental approach is exclusively suited to the physiologic, pharmacological or pathophysiological evaluation of myocardial performance. Indeed, each experimental approach present advantages and disadvantages and thus, appropriate integration of data derived from multiple complementary methodologies is the best approach.

Conclusion

Given the complexity of cardiac physiology and pathophysiology, it is unlikely that any single methodology could provide enough information to complete a study. Thus, appropriate integration of data, acquired using multiple complementary approaches and techniques, will certainly help to clarify the complexity of the cardiovascular system. Each successive reduction in the methodology scale inevitably results in the loss of some variables that normally influence function in the intact organ, while allowing a more refine assessment of the remaining variables. Knowledge integration demands considering the advantages and drawbacks of individual methodologies, the limits of extrapolation to other model systems as well as the necessity to confirm and validate data or hypotheses in other systems and ultimately in humans.

References

1. Brady AJ. Mechanical properties of isolated cardiac myocytes. Physiol Rev. 1991;71(2):413–28.
2. Fabiato A, Fabiato F. Techniques of skinned cardiac cells and of isolated cardiac fibers with disrupted sarcolemmas with reference to the effects of catecholamines and of caffeine. Recent Adv Stud Cardiac Struct Metab. 1976;9:1–94.
3. Tarr M. Mechanical and contractile properties of isolated single intact cardiac cells. Adv Exp Med Biol. 1983;161:199–216.
4. Shah AM, Sollott SJ, Lakatta EG. Physiopharmacological evaluation of myocardial performance: an integrative approach. Cardiovasc Res. 1998;39(1):148–54.
5. Linke WA, Popov VI, Pollack GH. Passive and active tension in single cardiac myofibrils. Biophys J. 1994;67(2):782–92.
6. Prosser BL, Ward CW, Lederer WJ. X-ROS signaling: rapid mechano-chemo transduction in heart. Science. 2011;333(6048):1440–5.
7. Labeit S, Kolmerer B, Linke WA. The giant protein titin. Emerging roles in physiology and pathophysiology. Circ Res. 1997;80(2):290–4.
8. Falcao-Pires I, Goncalves N, Moura C, Lamego I, Eloy C, Lopes JM, et al. Effects of diabetes mellitus, pressure-overload and their association on myocardial structure and function. Am J Hypertens. 2009;22(11):1190–8.
9. Borbely A, Falcao-Pires I, van Heerebeek L, Hamdani N, Edes I, Gavina C, et al. Hypophosphorylation of the Stiff N2B titin isoform raises cardiomyocyte resting tension in failing human myocardium. Circ Res. 2009;104(6):780–6.
10. Borbely A, van der Velden J, Papp Z, Bronzwaer JG, Edes I, Stienen GJ, et al. Cardiomyocyte stiffness in diastolic heart failure. Circulation. 2005;111(6):774–81.
11. Linke WA, Fernandez JM. Cardiac titin: molecular basis of elasticity and cellular contribution to elastic and viscous stiffness components in myocardium. J Muscle Res Cell Motil. 2002;23(5–6):483–97.
12. Tung L. An ultrasensitive transducer for measurement of isometric contractile force from single heart cells. Pflugers Arch. 1986;407(1):109–15.
13. Capogrossi MC, Stern MD, Spurgeon HA, Lakatta EG. Spontaneous Ca2+ release from the sarcoplasmic reticulum limits Ca^{2+}-dependent twitch potentiation in individual cardiac myocytes. A mechanism for maximum inotropy in the myocardium. J Gen Physiol. 1988;91(1):133–55.
14. Holubarsch C, Ludemann J, Wiessner S, Ruf T, Schulte-Baukloh H, Schmidt-Schweda S, et al. Shortening versus isometric contractions in isolated human failing and non-failing left ventricular myocardium: dependency of external work and force on muscle length, heart rate and inotropic stimulation. Cardiovasc Res. 1998;37(1):46–57.
15. Stern MD. Theory of excitation-contraction coupling in cardiac muscle. Biophys J. 1992;63(2):497–517.
16. Bers DM. Cardiac excitation-contraction coupling. Nature. 2002;415(6868):198–205.
17. Krueger JW, Forletti D, Wittenberg BA. Uniform sarcomere shortening behavior in isolated cardiac muscle cells. J Gen Physiol. 1980;76(5):587–607.
18. Tasche C, Meyhofer E, Brenner B. A force transducer for measuring mechanical properties of single cardiac myocytes. Am J Physiol. 1999;277(6 Pt 2):H2400–8.

19. Tarr M, Trank JW, Leiffer P, Shepherd N. Sarcomere length-resting tension relation in single frog atrial cardiac cells. Circ Res. 1979;45(4):554–9.
20. Le Guennec JY, Peineau N, Argibay JA, Mongo KG, Garnier D. A new method of attachment of isolated mammalian ventricular myocytes for tension recording: length dependence of passive and active tension. J Mol Cell Cardiol. 1990;22(10):1083–93.
21. Nishimura S, Yasuda S, Katoh M, Yamada KP, Yamashita H, Saeki Y et al. Single cell mechanics of rat cardiomyocytes under isometric, unloaded, and physiologically loaded conditions. Am J Physiol Heart Circ Physiol. 2004;287(1):H196–202.
22. Mellors LJ, Barclay CJ. The energetics of rat papillary muscles undergoing realistic strain patterns. J Exp Biol. 2001;204(Pt 21):3765–77.
23. Jewell BR, Rovell JM. Influence of previous mechanical events on the contractility of isolated cat papillary muscle. J Physiol. 1973;235(3):715–40.
24. Levy MN, Berne RM, Koeppen BM, Stanton BA. Berne & Levy principles of physiology. 4th ed. St. Louis: Elsevier Mosby; 2006. p. 1–836.
25. Dhein S, Mohr FW, Delmar M. Practical methods in cardiovascular research. Berlin/New York: Springer; 2005. p. 1–500.
26. Chemla D, Lecarpentier Y, Martin JL, Clergue M, Antonetti A, Hatt PY. Relationship between inotropy and relaxation in rat myocardium. Am J Physiol. 1986;250(6 Pt 2):H1008–16.
27. Lecarpentier Y, Martin JL, Claes V, Chambaret JP, Migus A, Antonetti A, et al. Real-time kinetics of sarcomere relaxation by laser diffraction. Circ Res. 1985;56(3):331–9.
28. Coudray N, Beregi JP, Lecarpentier Y, Chemla D. Effects of isoproterenol on myocardial relaxation rate: influence of the level of load. Am J Physiol. 1993;265(5 Pt 2):H1645–53.
29. Housmans PR, Lee NK, Blinks JR. Active shortening retards the decline of the intracellular calcium transient in mammalian heart muscle. Science. 1983;221(4606):159–61.
30. Brutsaert DL, Andries LJ. The endocardial endothelium. Am J Physiol. 1992;263(4 Pt 2):H985–1002.
31. Lamberts RR, van Rijen MH, Sipkema P, Fransen P, Sys SU, Westerhof N. Increased coronary perfusion augments cardiac contractility in the rat through stretch-activated ion channels. Am J Physiol Heart Circ Physiol. 2002;282(4):H1334–40.
32. Janssen PM, de Tombe PP. Uncontrolled sarcomere shortening increases intracellular Ca2+ transient in rat cardiac trabeculae. Am J Physiol. 1997;272(4 Pt 2): H1892–7.
33. Hasenfuss G, Mulieri LA, Allen PD, Just H, Alpert NR. Influence of isoproterenol and ouabain on excitation-contraction coupling, cross-bridge function, and energetics in failing human myocardium. Circulation. 1996;94(12):3155–60.
34. Homsher E, Millar NC. Caged compounds and striated muscle contraction. Annu Rev Physiol. 1990;52:875–96.
35. Langendorff O. Untersuchungen am uberlebenden Saugethierherzen. Pflugers Arch. 1895;61:291–332.
36. Neely JR, Liebermeister H, Battersby EJ, Morgan HE. Effect of pressure development on oxygen consumption by isolated rat heart. Am J Physiol. 1967;212(4):804–14.
37. Liao R, Podesser BK, Lim CC. The continuing evolution of the Langendorff and ejecting murine heart: new advances in cardiac phenotyping. Am J Physiol Heart Circ Physiol. 2012;303(2):H156–67.
39. Bell RM, Mocanu MM, Yellon DM. Retrograde heart perfusion: the Langendorff technique of isolated heart perfusion. J Mol Cell Cardiol. 2011;50(6):940–50.
39. Assayag P, Charlemagne D, Marty I, de Leiris J, Lompre AM, Boucher F, et al. Effects of sustained low-flow ischemia on myocardial function and calcium-regulating proteins in adult and senescent rat hearts. Cardiovasc Res. 1998;38(1):169–80.
40. Dijkman MA, Heslinga JW, Sipkema P, Westerhof N. Perfusion-induced changes in cardiac contractility and oxygen consumption are not endothelium-dependent. Cardiovasc Res. 1997;33(3):593–600.
41. Skrzypiec-Spring M, Grotthus B, Szelag A, Schulz R. Isolated heart perfusion according to Langendorff – still viable in the new millennium. J Pharmacol Toxicol Methods. 2007;55(2):113–26.
42. Anderson PG, Digerness SB, Sklar JL, Boor PJ. Use of the isolated perfused heart for evaluation of cardiac toxicity. Toxicol Pathol. 1990;18(4 Pt 1):497–510.
43. Ferdinandy P, Panas D, Schulz R. Peroxynitrite contributes to spontaneous loss of cardiac efficiency in isolated working rat hearts. Am J Physiol. 1999;276(6 Pt 2):H1861–7.
44. Ferdinandy P, Schulz R. Nitric oxide, superoxide, and peroxynitrite in myocardial ischaemia-reperfusion injury and preconditioning. Br J Pharmacol. 2003;138:532–43.
45. Suzuki K, Murtuza B, Fukushima S, Smolenski RT, Varela-Carver A, Coppen SR, et al. Targeted cell delivery into infarcted rat hearts by retrograde intracoronary infusion: distribution, dynamics, and influence on cardiac function. Circulation. 2004;110:225–30.
46. Ohno N, Fedak PW, Weisel RD, Mickle DA, Fujii T, Li RK. Transplantation of cryopreserved muscle cells in dilated cardiomyopathy: effects on left ventricular geometry and function. J Thorac Cardiovasc Surg. 2003;126:1537–48.
47. Kolwicz SC, Jr., Tian R. Assessment of cardiac function and energetics in isolated mouse hearts using 31P NMR spectroscopy. J Vis Exp. 2010;(42).
48. Lou Q, Li W, Efimov IR. Multiparametric optical mapping of the Langendorff-perfused rabbit heart. J Vis Exp. 2011;(55).
49. Asfour H, Wengrowski AM, Jaimes R, 3rd, Swift LM, Kay MW. NADH fluorescence imaging of isolated biventricular working rabbit hearts. J Vis Exp. 2012;(65).
50. Demmy TL, Magovern GJ, Kao RL. Isolated biventricular working rat heart preparation. Ann Thorac Surg. 1992;54:915–20.

In Vivo Experimental Assessment of Cardiac Function

21

André P. Lourenço, Inês Falcão-Pires, and Adelino F. Leite-Moreira

Abstract

The increasing number of cardiovascular disease animal models has enabled great advances in heart failure and cardiovascular research. This was possible due to a parallel development of highly sophisticated methodologies for functional assessment and phenotyping of these same animal models. Since almost all research is currently carried out in rodents who have very high heart rates and small size, extremely precise and sophisticated equipment along with developed technical skills are needed for an accurate assessment of cardiac function. Main techniques described are telemetry, echocardiography, and hemodynamic evaluation, including pressure-volume curves.

Keywords

Cardiac function • Rodents • Telemetry • Echocardiography • Hemodynamics

Abbreviations

E	Early wave of transmitral flow
Ea	Effective arterial elastance
ECG	Electrocardiography
ECHO	Echocardiography
Ees	End-systolic elastance
Emax	Maximum elastance
F	Frequency
G	Conductance
IVCT	Isovolumetric contraction time
IVRT	Isovolumetric relaxation time
L	Length
LV	Left ventricular
Pmax	Maximum pressure
TEL	Telemetry

A.P. Lourenço, MD, PhD (✉)
I. Falcão-Pires, MSc, PhD
A.F. Leite-Moreira, MD, PhD
Department of Physiology and Cardiothoracic Surgery, Faculty of Medicine of University of Porto, 4200-319 Porto, Portugal
e-mail: aplourenco@yahoo.com; ipires@med.up.pt; amoreira@med.up.pt

21.1 Introduction

Cardiovascular research has since its origin strongly relied on animal models of disease. These have evolved from the early large animal

D.V. Cokkinos (ed.), *Introduction to Translational Cardiovascular Research*, DOI 10.1007/978-3-319-08798-6_21, models to the recent rodent models and also from surgically produced or pathogen-related models to genetically modified models. The methods for functional assessment in vivo have evolved as well. Three of the main, most widespread and well-established advances in functional assessment in cardiovascular research have been the application of telemetric technology, modern echocardiographic techniques and of conductance-based pressure-volume hemodynamic evaluation assessment in rats and mice. In this chapter our goal is to summarize key concepts, possibilities, potential biases, "tricks" and new developments in rodent telemetry, echocardiography and hemodynamic assessment for cardiovascular research.

21.2 Experimental In Vivo Assessment of Cardiac Function

21.2.1 Telemetry

Radiotelemetry has been in use since the 1950s with recent improvements in implantable device manufacturing as a result of technology progress (Table 21.1). It represents the state of the art for monitoring physiological functions in conscious and freely moving laboratory animals while minimizing stress artefacts, such as restraining, anaesthesia or animals proximity to the investigator. Moreover, this technology has been sufficiently validated as a useful tool for an accurate and reliable measurement of

Table 21.1 Telemetry breakthroughs

Significant studies
Combination of cardiovascular telemetry data collection with calorimetry studies allowed to determine metabolic rates in rodents [46]
Combination of telemetric blood pressure measurement with flowprobes to simultaneously monitor pressure and cardiac output, or pressure and renal flow simultaneously, though the flow measurement still requires external leads and tether connections [47]
Miniaturization of transmitters capable of being use in cases in which space in the abdominal cavity is particularly limited such as during pregnancy and small mice [48]
Studies that involve collecting respiratory data have generally required restraining the animals and placing a pneumotach on their face to collect respiratory data. This method can be stressful for the animal and thus limits data collection to short periods of time. Alternatively, with external telemetry and respiratory inductive plethysmography (RIP), the animal is unrestrained and is therefore presumably less stressed, allowing data to be collected continuously [49]
A new transmitter enables simultaneous collection up to four parameters, such as body temperature, activity, blood pressure, ECG, and other biopotentials in small animal models, besides information about battery life, animal identification, and calibration information. This contrasts with previous transmitters that could measure either blood pressure or ECG parameters. This new device eliminates the need for separate animal groups for assorted measurements and allows for a more complete cardiovascular assessment [50, 51]. http://www.jove.com/video/3260/implantation-radiotelemetry-transmitters-yielding-data-on-ecg-heart
Simultaneously measurement of pulmonary and systemic blood pressure and the electrocardiogram in rats using dual blood-pressure telemetry transmitter. The transmitter was implanted in normotensive and monocrotaline-induced pulmonary hypertensive Wistar rats, with sensing catheters placed in the pulmonary artery and descending aorta. Biopotential electrodes were positioned to record an apex-based lead II electrocardiogram [52]
Merging cardiovascular telemetry data collection with metabolic treadmill studies in rodents to determine VO_2/CO_2 consumption combined with telemetry-derived parameters
Implantable blood pressure telemetry combined with cutting-edge echocardiography to combine arterial pressure measurements with cardiac output, assessing pressure-diameter curves, amongst other parameters
Synchronizing data collected from a respiratory chamber and an implantable telemetry (intra-pleural pressure telemetry signal) obtaining more complex respiratory data

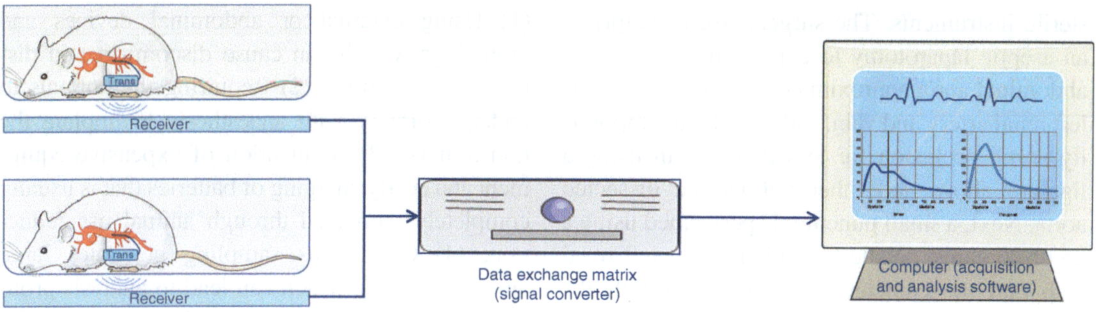

Fig. 21.1 Diagram of a radiotelemetry system. A rat implanted with a transmitter on its abdominal cavity, capable of monitoring blood pressure via the abdominal aorta. The transmitter emits a radio signal that is detected by a receiver beneath the cage. This signal is sent to a data exchange matrix (signal converter) and afterwards to the computer where the acquisition and analysis software displays the results (These images were created using Servier Medical Art and licensed under a Creative Commons Attribution 3.0 Unported License)

a growing number of physiological parameters such as locomotor activity, electrocardiography (ECG), electroencephalography (EEG), electromyography (EMG) and electrooculography (EOG), heart rate, respiratory inductive plethysmography, temperature (core body, brain, tail, brown fat, etc.) and pressure by using a sensor tipped catheter to assess left ventricular pressure, systolic arterial pressure, central venous pressure, pulmonary artery pressure, pleural pressure, intra-ocular pressure, bladder pressure, pulse wave velocity, etc.

Telemetry (TEL) minimizes interanimal variability and the number of animals per protocol as the same animal can be its own internal control and several tests can be repeated in the same animals. Thus this technology represents the most humane method of assessing physiological parameters in laboratory animals, contributing to animal welfare (reduction and refinement alternatives) and reducing overall animal research costs [1].

Telemetry transmitters are surgically implanted or externally mounted devices that sense, process and transmit physiological information via electromagnetic radio waves (3 Hz–300 GHz), from a freely moving animal to a located receiver. Traditional implantable TEL devices range in size from approximately 1–35 cm^3, are biocompatible, typically have permanently affixed leads, and can transmit signals up to 5 m. External devices are approximately 150–200 cm^3; the larger size accommodates a bigger battery and the electronics required to transmit many signals from a single animal in a room that may contain up to 36 animals. Transmitters for blood pressure measurements utilize fluid filled catheter technology for arterial placement, containing a biocompatible gel that transduces blood pressure fluctuations back to the transmitter. Once the signal is received, it is transferred to a data acquisition computer for processing. Data collection is initiated by touching the animal with a magnet, switching on the transmitter. The acquisition program collects data signals sent to the computer from the converters and receivers. This program can either collect data for a specific period of time at regular intervals or sample continuously and save the data on the computer's hard drive. As the range and the quality of the emitted signal depends strongly on the material composition of the cage and surrounding equipment, it is suggested that the receiver plate is placed as close to the animal as possible. After the data have been gathered and stored, they can be plotted, listed and analysed for a variety of different parameters using the analysis program (Fig. 21.1).

The animal surgical protocol for a blood pressure transmitter implantation in the abdominal aorta includes fasting the animal 12 h before surgery and preparing it for aseptic surgery using sterile instruments. The surgery itself comprises an aseptic laparotomy to expose and dissect the abdominal aorta approximately 15 mm below the left renal artery and vein, followed by a temporarily aortic occlusion for less than 1 min using a ligature above and other bellow the dissected aorta. Next, a small puncture is performed using a 25 or 26 gauge needle 5 mm below the left renal vein and the catheter tip inserted through the puncture into the aorta. After hemostatic closure of the aortic puncture with medical glue, the occluding ligatures are released. Finally, the telemetric transmitter is placed within the abdominal cavity or subcutaneously. For ECG and EEG measurements the positive and negative electrodes are placed subcutaneously. For blood pressure measurements one or more fluid-filled catheters are placed into the appropriate blood vessel (usually the carotid artery, thoracic aorta, femoral artery, pulmonary artery, or abdominal aorta). For measurements of respiratory pressure changes, a fluid-filled catheter is introduced into the pleural cavity. Once the equipment is placed and checked for proper function, all incisions are closed and the animals are permitted 1–2 weeks recovery from surgery with appropriate analgesics before studies are conducted. Potential adverse effects resulting from this procedure may include anaesthetic related respiratory distress, infection of the subcutaneous pocket, abdominal cavity or catheter insertion site, dehiscence of the surgical site, seroma formation around the transmitter, hind limb paresis or paralysis related to ischemia or nerve damage and hemorrhage due to leaking of the vessel around the catheter insertion site.

Advantages of TEL include: (1) Enabling long-term recordings; (2) Monitoring conscious rats in natural environments; (3) Reducing handling-induced stress artefacts; (4) Allowing to use animals sequentially as their own controls or in multiple studies (number reduction); (5) Decreasing animal maintenance costs; (6) Allowing to understand the complex physiological interactions between cardiovascular, respiratory and central nervous system; (7) Providing objective biological data on animal wellbeing to help implement humane endpoints (refinement). However, this methodology presents some disadvantages such as: (1) Using external or abdominal devices and mountings, which can cause discomfort and distress to the animal; (2) Requiring the animals to undergo surgery with anaesthesia to implant the transmitters; (3) Acquisition of expensive equipment and costly charging of batteries that is usually completely recovered through animal use reduction; (4) Continuous sampling generates large amounts of data, which can lead to analysis problems and (5) Requiring appropriate surgical training to implant a TELE device in an animal. Measures that can be taken to refine surgical implantation procedures include ensuring that the animals have adequate recovery time, using appropriate anaesthetics (inhalatory anaesthetics such as sevoflurane or isoflurane are recommended for telemetry procedures), using appropriate analgesia, and proper aseptic technique [2].

In conclusion, TELE systems are versatile and enable valuable physiological information to be collected from animals for a variety of different research needs. Combining telemetry with other methodologies has boosted and significantly improved in vivo assessment of cardiovascular function, providing important tools to maximise the information gained and thus understand the pathophysiology of cardiac disease in animal models.

21.2.2 Echocardiography

Echocardiographic evaluation is a powerful tool for non-invasive evaluation of both cardiovascular structure and function. It is a relatively quick and versatile method that allows serial assessment. Considerable developments in technology and equipment in the last decade have made possible a thorough evaluation of cardiac structure and function even in mice. New transducer with small footprints, capable of both high frame-rates and improved near-field imaging are now available which enable fabulous views with outstanding temporal resolution even in small rodents [3]. This equipment however is extremely expensive and many cardiovascular function parameters can still be evaluated with more affordable echocardiography machines. Moreover, we must point out that ECHO is not an automated procedure. It is highly operator dependent and relies on the proper acquisition and interpretation of results by an examiner who is familiar with the principles, capabilities, and limitations of ultrasound imaging rather than on the equipment itself [4]. Because of the important operator dependency in experimental settings whenever possible the examiner should be blinded.

21.2.2.1 Principles of Echocardiography

It is beyond the scope of this chapter to exhaustively revise the principles of ultrasound imaging. Briefly, image is formed by tissue reflection of sound waves above the range of human hearing generated by piezoelectric crystals. Echocardiography probes or transducers interconvert electrical energy in ultrasound upon emission and reception. The piezoelectric crystals deform when exposed to a strong electrical field and emit ultrasound. Then again they also deform mechanically when they receive the echoes of emitted ultrasound and generate a voltage. The oscillation upon electrical stimulation has a specific frequency that varies inversely with crystal thickness. Crystals in transducers are covered by damping materials and acoustic lenses. The ultrasound waves are sent out in a cylindrical pattern up to a certain distance, the near-field, and then diverge conically in the far-field. The lateral edges of the ultrasound beam are not abrupt. Beam width defines lateral space resolution which is the minimum distance at which two separate reflectors will be perceived as such by generating separate echoes. Beam width decreases with increasing frequencies. The more recent ECHO machines use a method called harmonic imaging to further reduce beam width and artefactual images from multiple reverberations by filtering the received signals. Strong reflectors such as metal are usually perceived further to the edge of the beam and thus appear larger, an artefact called blooming. Despite all adjustments diffraction phenomenon still generate oblique weaker secondary beams known as side lobes that are responsible for side-lobe artefacts. To increase the width and tissue depth of the image crystals are usually grouped and closely spaced in the probe. Additionally, they can be rotated in a fan-like fashion by mechanical sector scanners. Moreover pulses of ultrasound waves can lag between each of the crystals (phased array) so that during sector scanning the wave fronts from the crystals form an arc which constitutes a slice or wedge of the scanned object. Phased arrays increase the ability to scan wide fields of tissue in deeper planes. If the crystals emit simultaneously a (linear phase) beam is formed perpendicular to the probe and a rectangular tissue section is imaged. Linear arrays are informative on a wide region of tissue close to the transducer and are usually used for superficial imaging.

Ultrasound waves change pressure within the medium which they traverse periodically over time and space with both a set frequency which is the reciprocal of their period, or time between successive pressure peaks and a set wavelength which is the distance between pressure peaks of an ultrasound wave. The wavelength (λ) relates to the frequency (f) depending on the speed of propagation within the medium (c):

$$c = f(\lambda)$$

The speed of propagation varies proportionally to materials or tissues stiffness and therefore it is higher in solids and lower in gases. Wavelength is the determinant of space resolution. Higher frequencies therefore provide better resolution. Additionally waves also have an amplitude that relates both to the changes in pressure within the tissue they traverse and to the power and voltage of emission and reading, respectively, in the ECHO machine. For most purposes, including 2D ECHO ultrasound, waves are released in pulses interspersed by long periods of silence for returning echo analysis. Therefore ultrasound waves also have pulse duration, pulse repetition frequency and a duty cycle or the percentage of time that the pulse of ultrasound is on. Duty cycle and wave amplitude are the determinants of power output.

The image is formed upon reception of the echoes. In 2D or brightness mode (B-mode) echocardiography a selected group of crystals emit ultrasound as defined by the sector scan, with a certain pulse repetition frequency. When waves are emitted they perform a round-trip travel from probe to tissue and back. For an accurate analysis there must only be one pulse of ultrasound in the tissue in every period of analysis. This means that higher pulse repetition frequencies do not allow time for tissue penetration. To increase temporal resolution (frame rate) in order to assess fast-moving objects, both sector scan and sector depth should be reduced to enable high pulse repetition frequencies. The highest frame rate is achieved by reducing sector scan to a single line as in motion-mode (M-mode). In this case visual representation is a plotting of brightness along that line as a function of time. This view allows the best temporal resolution when measuring distances between rapidly moving objects. Nonetheless, storage in video format has a lower rate; for higher rate storage digital storage media must be used. Echo signals are converted digitally to pixels in a grey scale. The dynamic range is the ratio between the strongest and weakest echo signals that can be distinguished in this scale. The higher resolution component in ECHO machines is range resolution, or axial resolution along the beam, which depends mostly on frequency. For better range or axial resolution the surfaces of interest should be as perpendicular as possible to the beam. When measuring the axial distances between objects in M-mode or 2D-echocardiography the aspect of resolution should also be taken in account, contrasting interfaces between surfaces will appear as a trail with a leading and a trailing edge, measurements should be made between the leading edges to minimize errors in estimation and by convention (leading edge-to-leading-edge) [5].

Ultrasound images are formed mostly by wave reflections from tissues which define the major anatomic features, and by tissue scattering which defines the texture of tissues. Reflections occur mainly due to sudden differences in acoustic impedance which is mainly dependent on density. When these differences are too pronounced they prevent imaging in deeper planes, this is the case of the tissue-air and tissue-bone interfaces in the lung and rib-cage. Reflections are maximal when the interface is perpendicular to the direction of ultrasound and is almost absent when it is parallel. This is why endocardial and epicardial borders and poorly viewed in the 3 and 9 o'clock positions in a cross-sectional short-axis left ventricular view. Scattering is more important in non-homogeneous tissues such as the myocardium and less in blood, which appears echo-lucent. During deeper tissue penetration ultrasound waves suffer attenuation this is to say they progressively lose amplitude (power) because the ultrasound energy is converted in heat within tissues and part of it is reflected or scattered. To compensate for this loss most ECHO machines allow automatic or manual time-gain compensation that increases the intensity of images in deeper tissues.

Besides blooming and side-lobe artefacts, other typical sham images are ladder–like or comet tail appearances which result from unusually strong reflections or reverberation between two highly reflecting structures. Particular cases are the mirror image which is typical of vessel structures and consists of a duplication of a strongly reflecting interface at an equal distance but further away from the probe and the near-field clutter when highly reflecting structures are near the probe. Another common artefact is shadowing beyond an unusually reflective structure which is due to reduction in ultrasound energy.

Although we previously stated scattering was less important in blood it is the weak backscattering from blood cells that is used to perform Doppler ECHO. Blood cells are much smaller than the wavelengths of the ultrasound waves and actually have no reflection at all but only very weak scattering signals. The Doppler effect first described for light by Christian Doppler, is the wave frequency change that takes place when the emitter and reflector are in motion relative to each other. In a simplistic view, frequency increases when they approach because wave fronts are squeezed foreshortening the wavelength and increasing the frequency. When the emitted signal is combined with the received signal in the ECHO machine a difference, or Doppler shift, is computed. According to the original Doppler equation the frequency of emission (f_0) is changed to a Doppler frequency (f_D) as a function of the velocity of motion between the emitter and the receptor (v), which must be accounted for twice, and the speed of propagation in the medium (c):

$$f_D = f_0 * 2 * v / (c - v)$$

As an approximation since v is of a very lower magnitude compared to c, the equation is usually simplified to:

$$f_D = f_0 * 2 * v / c \text{ and therefore } v = c / 2 * f_D / f_0$$

Doppler's equation however only applies to objects that move in a straight line towards each other. For oblique movements only the vector component of velocity that falls in the line directly connecting the objects should be taken in account and the angle of movement must be corrected for (θ):

$$v = c / (2 * \cos\theta) * f_D / f_0$$

Corrections to θ <20° are usually minimal otherwise the software of the machine usually allows manual insertion of an angle for correction. Nevertheless since the flow is actually tridimensional the researcher should try to get several readings and stick with the highest value. For Doppler ECHO recordings the ultrasounds are of lower frequency and higher amplitude to increase the strength of the scattered signal and the main output is to ascertain velocity from the frequency change or shift. The Doppler shift is in the human hearing range and can be converted to sound. Alternatively using a Fourier transformation the echocardiography machine analyses the full spectrum of returned frequencies (or velocities) and their corresponding strengths and plots them as a function of time. Spectral analysis is required because scattering occurs in a pool of sampled blood and tissue and therefore frequencies/velocities vary. In every vertical line all velocities are represented and their strength is reported by a grey scale. To prevent strong low-velocity reflections from tissue a low-velocity wall-filter is usually applied. Spectral analysis and display can be done either with continuous-wave or pulsed-wave Doppler. In continuous-wave Doppler some crystals continuously emit ultrasound whereas others receive them. The spectrum received results from superimposition of all the echoes returning from all depths along the ultrasonic beam continuously and therefore higher-speed signals can be recorded unambiguously but not their precise location. In contrast to continuous-wave Doppler pulsed wave Doppler uses the same crystals as emitters and receivers in a pulse and repetition manner and can be viewed along with a 2D-ECHO image at a low rate. The researcher can select the targeted sample blood volume area along the Doppler line and then toggle to spectral Doppler view with higher temporal resolution. The spectral reading is usually more linear because velocities are more homogeneous unless an area of turbulent flow is selected. Pulsed-wave Doppler in contrast to continuous-wave Doppler, however, does not measure maximum velocities as accurately and if these are fast such as those across a stenotic or banded vessel or across the tricuspid valve in regurgitation it is unable to measure them at all. When the Doppler shift exceeds half the pulse repetition frequency, the velocity of objects falls outside the limits of display and gives rise to a false record usually indicating reversal of flow. This phenomenon is called aliasing and the limit of velocity for its occurrence is the Nyquist limit. The Nyquist limit can be increased to avoid aliasing by lowering frequency and diminishing depth. In the device the scale and baseline should also be adjusted. In rodents, some speeds can only be recorder with continuous-wave Doppler, for instance when a banding is applied to high pressure vessels such as the aorta or pulmonary artery or when assessing tricuspid regurgitation velocity. This poses a problem to the application to rodents of high-frequency linear probes commonly used for superficial structure and soft-part imaging in the clinics, because these do not have the possibility for continuous-wave Doppler. To gauge flow dynamics coding can also be done with colour superimposed on the 2D-image, with a lower temporal resolution. The scale goes from red to blue signalling velocity of approximation or departure from the probe, respectively. As for aliasing the same principles of pulsed-wave Doppler apply to colour-Doppler. Since the frequencies applied with Doppler are lower and the signal is weak it is exquisitely sensitive to electrical interference.

The same Doppler principle can be applied to tissue motion but in this case the velocities are quite lower and the signal is stronger. By adjusting scales and filters tissue Doppler images can be viewed either spectrally in pulsed-wave or in colour-mode. The velocity scale must be reduced to values near the 1–2 cm s^{-1}, wall-filters should be removed and gain minimized. Tissue motion analysis by Doppler has many limitations; the structures in the heart are constantly moving, the myocardium contracts both longitudinally and circumferentially, and passive movements are not separable from active motion. Usually analysis is performed at the myocardium near the mitral or tricuspid annuli to assess the areas with greater excursion with pulsed-wave Doppler that is able to record maximum velocities with a better temporal resolution.

Analysis of myocardial deformation or strain and its velocity or strain rate in ECHO initially arose with tissue Doppler by comparing velocities at two distinct myocardial regions. The main advantages are the ability to better distinguish active contraction from passive motion and segmental analysis. With new software developments these can also be computed from 2D-echocardiography by tracking of speckles in the image. These are naturally occurring acoustic marks due to particular patterns of ultrasound scattering in the myocardium [6].

21.2.2.2 Tips for a Good Echocardiography Exam

Attention to details can have an important role in image optimization. Ultrasound route to the target tissue should be as clear as possible. The fur must be completely shaved and if possible a depilatory cream should be applied to minimize artefacts. The animal should be positioned in order to approximate the heart from the chest wall and increase the area not covered by the lungs which usually requires left lateral decubitus and thoracic extension. A generous ECHO gel layer or even a gel containing rubber covering the tip of the probe can minimize signal loss, increase the contact surface area between animal and probe, and serve as acoustic standoffs that gain millimetres in depth for proper tissue focus. Settings should be adjusted to obtain the optimal image or velocity recording following the previously outlined principles. Artefacts are very common in small animals several strategies can minimize them. Reducing power output and repositioning the probe usually reduces artefactual images. When doubts arise several planes and depth settings should be analysed to ascertain which images are indeed real. On screen image is usually improved simply by reducing ambient light and avoiding reflection. A simultaneous ECG acquisition is invaluable while assessing timing of phenomena along the cardiac cycle, particularly in what concerns flow and tissue motion. When analysing 2D-images with low resolution moving the stored cine images back and forth usually helps defining the endocardial and epicardial contours. When acquiring functional parameters changes with breathing should be taken in account in the selection for analysis.

21.2.2.3 Anaesthesia

Echocardiography recordings should be as physiological as possible. It is crucial to maintain animal temperature to preserve heart rate and cardiovascular function. With anaesthesia, shaving and application of ECHO gel animals rapidly become hypothermic. If possible the ECHO gel should be heated as well as local environment. In an attempt to reach readings closest to physiology many researchers perform ECHO in restrained unanaesthetised animals usually after previous animal training sessions. The main drawbacks are animal stress, variations in stress response between groups, and poor technical conditions to perform the exam. Other researchers minimally sedate animals and perform the exam under spontaneous ventilation. In these conditions care must be taken to avoid compressing the thorax because the animal's respiration is already depressed, and the irregular breathing patterns make image acquisition difficult. Another alternative is to perform assisted breathing in order to prevent hypoxia or hypoventilation in a lightly anaesthetised animal without remarkably disturbing cardiovascular physiology.

Again the probe should be applied gently to the chest to avoid animal reactions and to minimize cardiovascular reflexes elicited by chest compression such as bradycardia and hypotension. Deep anaesthesia and controlled ventilation are not advisable. As for the anaesthetic to choose, most researchers now prefer halogenated gases due to their easy titration, rapid reversibility and minimal cardiovascular depression.

21.2.2.4 Echocardiographic Views in Rodents

Each researcher will adopt and become familiarized with his/her own protocol but we briefly describe the most standard views. A parasternal long-axis view can easily be obtained (Fig. 21.2A1). In this view it is possible to measure aortic root dimensions and left ventricular (LV) long axis, from the mitral annulus to LV endocardial surface at the apex (Fig. 21.2A1a). Care must be taken not to foreshorten the distance to the apex by ensuring that the longer axis is visualized (Fig. 21.2B1b). The left atrium and mitral valve function can also be gauged in this view and closer to the probe and adjacent to the aorta the right ventricular outflow tract is also visualized. Slightly tilting the probe can reveal the right heart and the pulmonary artery. While both ascending aortic banding and pulmonary artery banding can be easily visualized in this view the alignment for Doppler measurements is only adequate for the pulmonary artery (Fig. 21.2A1b). By rotating the probe 90° a parasternal short axis view is obtained (Fig. 21.2A2), the probe can then be moved gently either cephalad to view first the left and right ventricular outflow tracts (Fig. 21.2A2b), the origin of the great vessels and the aortic and pulmonary valves, then the main pulmonary artery branching (Fig. 21.2A2a) and finally the aortic arch or caudally to view the papillary muscles (Fig. 21.2A2d) and myocardial apex. Fractional shortening, ejection fraction and wall-thickness estimation are usually performed by most researchers with M-mode (Fig. 21.2B2b) with the cursor placed at the longest LV crossing near the tip of the papillary muscles (Fig. 21.2A2c). Slightly tilting the probe usually allows the identification of the roundest LV contour but minimal deviations can result in errors of estimation (Fig. 21.2B1a). Fractional area change can also be computed from 2D-echocardiography at this view with a lower temporal-resolution (Fig. 21.2A2c). Left ventricular mass can be estimated from M-mode tracings or 2D-echocardiography tracings based on distinct geometric assumptions such as the cubed method, the area-length method or the truncated ellipsoid, for a review see Collins et al. [7]. The four chamber view can be obtained by placing the probe where the apex is expected to be and directing the ultrasound beam medially, cephalad and posteriorly to traverse both the LV and right ventricular walls, both atria, and the interatrial and interventricular septa (Fig. 21.23a). This view enables reasonably good orientation of a Doppler mitral and tricuspid flow signal and also the acquisition of tissue Doppler signals near the mitral and tricuspid valve annuli. Is also permits good alignment of the mitral and tricuspid annuli to assess their motion in M-mode (Fig. 21.2B2a). With training the researcher will also realize that a slight deviation or tilting of the probe can usually reveal the left ventricular outflow tract and aorta (Fig. 21.2A3b) in an angle that is convenient for Doppler assessment of velocity of flow (Fig. 21.2B3b). When two orthogonal long-axis views or even combined short and long axis views of the LV are available measurement of areas in systole and diastole allows determination of ejection fraction by a method similar to the biplane, stacked discs or modified Simpson method [8]. Another view that is useful for assessing a successful transverse aortic constriction is the suprasternal view of the aortic arch and its main branches (Fig. 21.2A4a).

21.2.2.5 Functional Indexes

It is beyond the scope of this chapter to describe all research work on functional evaluation by ECHO. We will summarize briefly some of the most commonly employed functional indices. Fractional shortening, fractional area shortening and ejection fraction have already been mentioned. These are highly load dependent indexes

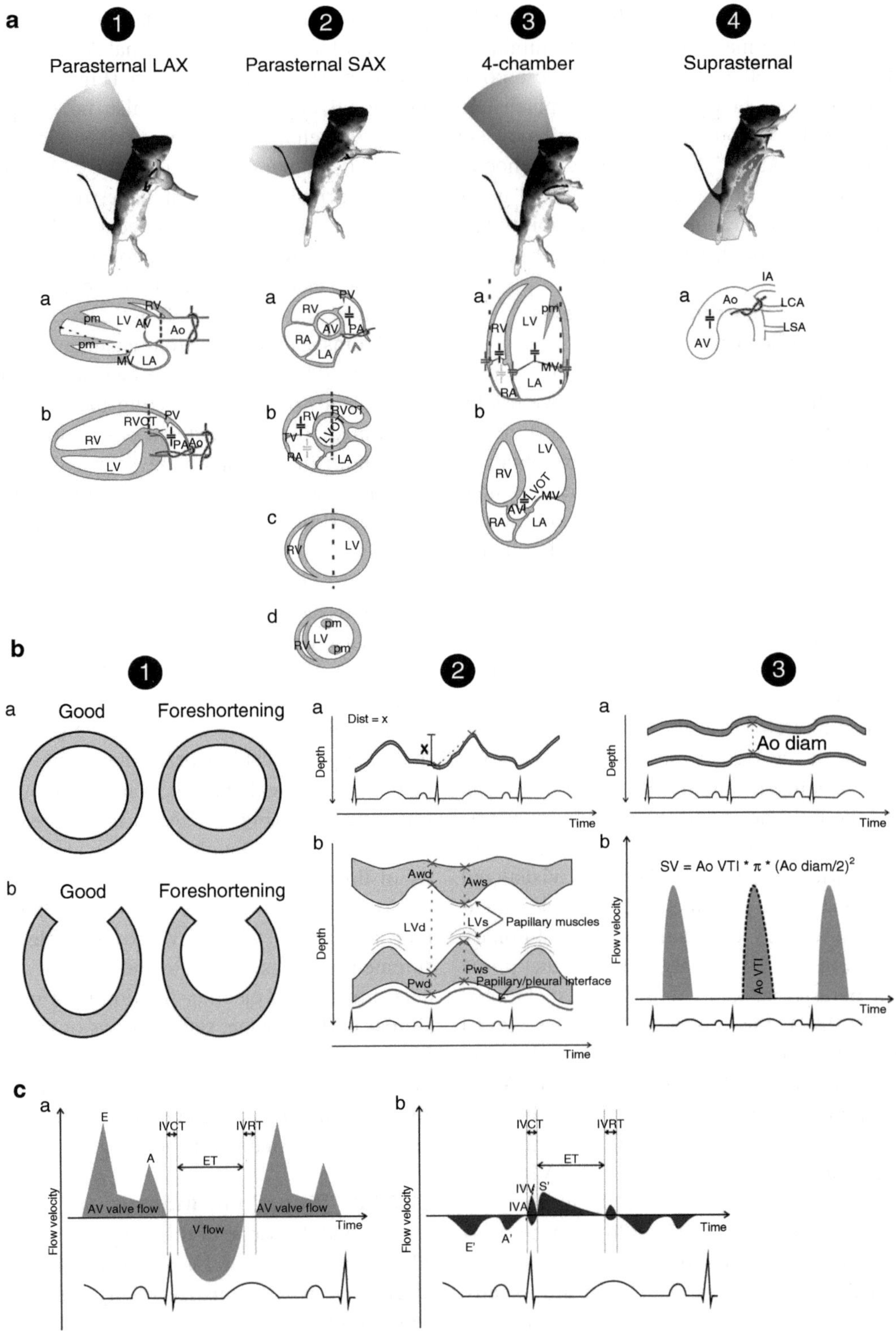
a
1 Parasternal LAX
2 Parasternal SAX
3 4-chamber
4 Suprasternal
Ao diam
SV = Ao VTI * π * (Ao diam/2)^2
Papillary muscles
Papillary/pleural interface
Good
Foreshortening
Dist = x
Depth
Time
Flow velocity
AV valve flow
V flow
IVCT
IVRT
ET

and prone to errors in estimation due to their inability to fully scope segmental changes and their reliance on geometrical assumptions of ventricular volumes. Cardiac output can be assessed by multiplying heart rate by stroke volume. Stroke volume can be measured by integrating the velocity of flow over time in an aortic (Fig. 21.2B3b) or LV outflow tract pulsed-wave Doppler acquisition and multiplying it by the cross-sectional area of the aorta (Fig. 21.2B3a) or left ventricular outflow tract, respectively [7]. When there are large differences in animal weight cardiac output should be normalized for body surface area, which is then named cardiac index [9]. The myocardial performance index originally described by Tei et al. evaluates overall LV or right ventricular myocardial function simply based on Doppler-derived intervals without any assumption of volume. It can be calculated from both blood flow Doppler (Fig. 21.2Ca) or tissue Doppler derived readings (Fig. 21.2Cb). Briefly it is derived by dividing the difference of the time from cessation to onset of mitral inflow with duration of ejection by the duration of ejection, or alternatively by dividing the sum of the isovolumetric contraction and relaxation periods (IVCT and IVRT, respectively) by ejection time (ET) [10]:

$$\text{Myocardial performance}\left(\text{Tei}\right)\text{index} = \left(\text{IVCT} + \text{IVRT}\right) / \text{ET}$$

The underlying rationale is that both isovolumetric periods are energy dependent but do not produce work. Myocardial dysfunction usually prolongs the isovolumetric periods yielding higher values for this index compared to the healthy heart. Another approach that does not rely on volume estimation is the measurement of mitral or tricuspid annuli plane systolic excursion [11]. Nevertheless, annular excursion only assesses longitudinal motion at the base of the ventricles. Although it can also be evaluated in 2D-ECHO it is usually measured in M-mode because of the better temporal resolution (Fig. 21.2B2a). A better assessment of systolic function relies on assessing tissue-Doppler motion in the myocardium near the annuli of atrioventricular valves, peak systolic motion (S′)

Fig. 21.2 *Experimental echocardiography in rodents. Standard echocardiographic views* (**A**): (*1*) parasternal long-axis (LAX), (*2*) parasternal short-axis (SAX), (*3*) 4-chamber view, and (*4*) suprasternal view Variations in standard views are signalled by *a*, *b*, *c*, and *d*, see text for details. Typical locations for banding visualization are signalled with a knot; left ventricular long axis dimension measurement is marker in *panel 1a*; M-mode readings of dimensions or annuli displacement are marked with dashed lines; usual sites for Doppler recordings are indicated by the cursor (+): *black*, *dark grey*, and *light grey cursors* indicate pulsed-wave flow Doppler, pulsed-wave tissue-Doppler Doppler, and continuous-wave Doppler, respectively, *dark grey cursor. Ao* aorta, *AV* aortic valve, *IA* innominate artery, *LA* left atrium, *LCA* left common carotid artery, *LV* left ventricle, *LVOT* LV outflow tract, *LSA* left subclavian artery, *MV* mitral valve, *PA* pulmonary artery, *pm* papillary muscle, *PV* pulmonary valve, *RA* right atrium, *RV* right ventricle, *RVOT* RV outflow tract, *TV* tricuspid valve. *Particular 2D, M-mode and pulsed-wave Doppler recordings* (**B**): (*1*) illustration on the importance of not foreshortening left ventricular dimensions in short-axis (*a*) or long-axis (*b*), (2) M-mode image of atrioventricular valve annulus excursion (dist=x) (*a*) and left ventricular short axis for fractional-shortening measurement (*b*), (*3*) M-mode measurement of aortic dimensions (*a*) and pulsed-wave Doppler of aortic flow (*b*). Stroke volume (*SV*) can be retrieved from the aortic velocity of flow-time integral (*Ao VTI*) and aortic diameter (*Ao diam*). AWd and AWs, anterior wall dimension at end-diastole and end-systole, respectively; LVd and LVs, left ventricular cavity dimensions in end-diastole and end-systole, respectively; PWd and PWs, posterior wall dimensions at end-diastole and end-systole, respectively. *Atrioventricular (AV) valve flow Doppler (a) and corresponding tissue-Doppler (b) at the myocardium adjoining the annulus* (**C**): ventricular (*V*) flow usually contaminates the recording enabling the determination of ejection time (*ET*) in the AV valve flow Doppler. Isovolumetric acceleration (*IVA*) is estimated as the slope of velocity rise in myocardial motion during isovolumetric contraction. *A* peak-velocity of late or atrial transAV flow, *A′* late velocity of diastolic myocardial motion, *E* early velocity of transAV flow, *E′* early velocity of diastolic myocardial motion, *IVCT* isovolumetric contraction time, *IVRT* isovolumetric relaxation time, *IVV* maximum isovolumetric velocity, *S′* maximum velocity of myocardial motion during ejection during ejection can be used as an index of contractility, but isovolumetric acceleration is a more load-independent index since it is recorded during the isovolumetric contraction period [12] (Fig. 21.2Cb). Diastolic function has traditionally been assessed by the transmitral flow pattern and the isovolumetric relaxation period duration (Fig. 21.2Ca). With the ready availability of tissue Doppler imaging the paradigm has shifted towards a more straightforward approach. Myocardial motion in early diastole as assessed by E′ is a good measure of diastolic function (Fig. 21.2Cb). It depends mostly on left ventricular relaxation kinetics whereas the early wave of transmitral flow (E) depends not only on relaxation but also on the driving force, the pressure gradient between left atrium and left ventricle. E to E′ ratio is therefore a good estimator of left ventricular filling pressures that has been adopted as one of the criteria for clinical diagnosis of heart failure with preserved ejection fraction [13] and applied successfully to small animal studies [9]. Better estimates of function both systolic and diastolic may be derived from strain analysis but there is still a long way to go to make this approach more easily available, straightforward and less laborious to researchers and physicians [6].

Right ventricular function evaluation is challenging due to the right ventricle's complex geometry and its retrosternal location but new methods of high-resolution echocardiography have made it possible to substitute for invasive hemodynamic recordings in many scenarios [14]. Estimation of systolic pulmonary artery pressure from the velocity of tricuspid regurgitation based on Bernoulli's equation that is customary in the clinics is rarely feasible in rodent models because measurable regurgitation appears late in the course of disease and because high-frequency probes do not allow for continuous-wave Doppler which would be mandatory to record such high velocities (Fig. 21.2A3a). Although it requires good time resolution, balanced gain-scale settings, and correction for cycle or ejection length pulmonary artery acceleration time is a reliable alternative for mean pulmonary artery pressure estimation in animal models [14]. An estimation of right ventricular hypertrophy and ejection fraction can usually be obtained at the right ventricular outflow tract (Fig. 21.2A2b).

Myocardial Volumes and Structure

High-frequency probes have allowed a better estimation of myocardial volume and structure measurements. Additionally, echo-contrast and 3D-ECHO which relies on the ability of 3D-reconstruction after automated steering and acquisition of electrocardiography-gated serial 2D-slices without altering transducer position in several beats can define volumes with higher accuracy without the need for geometrical assumptions even in mice [15].

21.2.3 Hemodynamics

Hemodynamic evaluation aims at in situ cardiovascular function assessment by means of pressure and flow or volume measurements. The high heart rate and small dimension of rodents mandates solid state or catheter-tip transducers, which offer superior frequency response and more precise pressure recording compared with fluid-filled catheter transducers. These catheters are however fragile, expensive, temperature-sensitive, and require calibration against an external standard. Load independent assessment of cardiac function, work and ventriculo-vascular coupling requires simultaneous and complex recording of pressure and volume during load manipulation that is also farther complex in rodents.

If an accurate comparison between experimental groups and minimal interference with biological function is envisaged a painstaking experimental preparation with conservation of normovolemia, normothermia, normoventilation, and anaesthesia tailored to achieve both minimum cardiovascular depression and animal comfort is required. This, of course, is only possible in a laboratory equipped with modern equipment suitable for rodents: (1) a ventilator, (2) inhaled anaesthetic vaporizers, (3) temperature monitoring, (4) animal and fluid warming-devices, (5) syringe-pumps, (6) respiratory monitoring such as oximetry and capnography or blood gas exam, and (7) ECHO. Room temperature is cornerstone to preserve animal temperature. Fluid therapy should aim at optimal cardiac output and take in account maintenance requirements due to fasting and insensitive water losses, additional deficits whenever bodily cavities and organ surfaces are exposed, and replacement of estimated blood losses. For such small animals with high surface area to volume ratio maintenance fluid therapy can be as high as 8 mL Kg^{-1} h^{-1}, and fluid replacement for thoracotomy can surmount to 32–64 mL Kg^{-1} h^{-1}. Blood should be replaced in a 4 to 1 ratio. Electrolyte balanced crystalloid solutions are favoured and prevent acidosis. Since skin incision and tissue dissection are necessary, a surgical anaesthesia plane should be ensured. As minimum requirements rodents should be non-reactive to toe pinch. Deepness of anaesthesia can be higher during surgical aggression and then down-titrated until a stable preparation with minimum cardiovascular depression is attained.

If recovery is expected additional care should be taken to ensure regaining of normoventilation, balanced nutritional status, proper organ function, and alleviation of pain. This usually requires orotracheal intubation as an alternative to tracheostomy, maintenance of positive-end expiratory pressure to prevent post-operative atelectasis, draining all the air from the chest-cavity, early refeeding or administration of glucose and sodium containing fluids, ocular care by either moistening or eyelid closure to prevent corneal injury, minimally invasive interventions that reduce tissue injury and blood loss, and timely administration of analgesics. Strong opioid class analgesics are needed for thoracotomy or laparotomy approaches.

According to the researchers' needs, hemodynamic recordings can be done through a central vessel, with a closed-chest cavity, or under direct vision through the apex, with an open-chest approach. Major advantages and disadvantages of these approaches are summarized in Table 21.2.

The right carotid artery approach to access the LV is relatively straightforward and compatible with recovery. Right ventricular access through the right jugular vein is technically more challenging with straight rigid catheters but can be eased by custom made catheters, a flexible introducer sheath, and careful animal positioning. A closed-chest preparation can also be achieved through the tendinous part of the diaphragm. If acute load manipulations are needed, the closed-chest preparation still requires surgical access to the inferior vena cava. The carotid approach precludes isovolumetric afterload manipulations because the catheter passes through the aorta. The open-chest approach is preferable when access to both ventricles, extensive load manipulations, and minimum ventricular interaction are needed. It is customary to advance or withdraw the catheter in order to get a systemic arterial pressure tracing, in open and closed-chest preparations, respectively, but the most informative preparation would be to insert a second pressure catheter through another artery and to advance it into the aorta in order to get continuous and simultaneous recording of systemic arterial pressure. As a useful rule of thumb, end-systolic pressure is highly correlated with mean arterial systemic pressure and can be used as its surrogate in pressure-volume recordings.

Baseline recordings should be done once the preparation is stable and all acquisitions

Table 21.2 Comparison of the closed and open-chest approaches to haemodynamic assessment

Open-chest	Closed-chest
Minimizes	Preserves
Ventricular interaction	Ventricular interaction
Ventilation interference	Ventilation interference
Better access to	Worse access to
RV, load manipulation, CO measurement	RV, load manipulation, CO measurement
Demands controlled ventilation	Can be done under spontaneous or assisted ventilation
Less physiological	More physiological
Deeper anaesthesia	Lighter anaesthesia or no anaesthesia at all
Higher fluid losses	Lower fluid losses
Venous return/CO is reduced	Preserves venous return/CO
Harder to perform recovery and redo assessment	Compatible with recovery and redo assessment

RV right ventricle, *CO* cardiac output

should be done with ventilation suspended at -end-expiration to minimize ventilation interference. Respiratory drive and cumbersome respiratory movements can be problematic, particularly in mice. These can be dealt with by hyperventilation, increasing anaesthetic doses, or mechanical attempts to minimize diaphragmatic movements. The use of muscle blockers is not advised unless strictly necessary, and all care must be taken to ensure an adequate deepness of anaesthesia.

21.2.3.1 Hemodynamic Parameters Derived from Pressure Recordings

Several functional indices can be derived from simple analysis of pressure recordings. The maximum rates of pressure rise and fall, dP/dt_{max} and dP/dt_{min}, respectively, can be used as rough indices of contractility and relaxation. Excluding extreme cases of severe ventricular dysfunction or marked vasodilation dP/dt_{max} happens during isovolumetric contraction and is therefore afterload independent. Otherwise, a related index, the ratio of dP/dt_{max} to maximum pressure (P_{max}) can be used. DP/dt_{max} is highly sensitive to changes in inotropic state but also to preload thus it is more useful for serial evaluation of ventricular contractility when preload changes are excluded. As for dP/dt_{min}, it is both preload and afterload dependent and frequently falls out of the isovolumetric relaxation period thus its value is very limited. Another index can be derived from isovolumetric ventricular pressure fall tracings, the time constant τ of isovolumetric relaxation. Although it is not load independent as initially held it is still the gold standard measure of LV relaxation. Weiss first derived it by fitting pressure fall beyond dP/dt_{min} to a monoexponential function of time with two parameters and a null asymptote. The constant was calculated by logarithmic transformation or by deriving the negative reciprocal of the slope of a semilogarithmic plot of pressure fall with time. Glantz introduced a third parameter, a non-zero asymptote or an addictive baseline shift to account for external pericardial and pleural pressure and intrinsic LV pressure after complete relaxation. Time constant was also derived in a geometrically more convenient way by plotting pressure phase plane plots (derivative of pressure as a function of pressure) and deriving a linear fit to the isovolumetric relaxation phase, whose negative slope reciprocal represents τ. Since in many circumstances this fit was not ideal Matsubara et al. [16] later proposed an empirical logistic fit. In this case calculation of τ is mathematically cumbersome and only feasible with software applications. Changes of pressure tracing with load manipulations, particularly single-beat afterload elevations, can be more informative on intrinsic myocardial performance [17]. The healthy heart responds to suddenly increased afterload with faster relaxation over a wide pressure range, whereas the diseased heart with systolic dysfunction has a limited ability to generate high systolic pressures, and responds to afterload elevations with impaired relaxation and elevated end-diastolic pressures (afterload-induced diastolic dysfunction) [18].

21.2.3.2 Joint Measurements of Pressure and Volume

Volume can be assessed in various ways. In rodents, imaging methods can be used, but not in real-time or simultaneously with pressure recordings in order to allow a direct acquisition of load-independent indexes by load-manipulation. Sonomicrometry is an invasive alternative that is unable to account for complex geometry and changes in wall thickness. The most straightforward approach for simultaneous pressure and volume measurement in rodents relies on the conductance methodology for volume determination and pressure-volume catheters [19]. Although changes in impedance with each heartbeat had been reported since the beginning of the twentieth century, the conductance methodology is grounded on the pioneering works of Baan et al. [20] who measured pressure-volume relationships in situ in dogs and humans replicating previous works of Suga and Sagawa [21] in the excised dog LV. It was hard to obtain a ventriculogram simultaneously with ventricular pressure, and the conversion from the angiography to time-varying ventricular volume was complex, time consuming and not suitable for continuous pump function monitoring during interventions thus

Baan et al. developed a catheter with several electrodes spaced along the left ventricular long axis and successfully applied it to dogs and patients. The two outermost electrodes emitted current thus creating an electrical field that was sensed by pairs of inner electrodes as voltage.

All materials (or tissues) have an intrinsic resistivity to electrical current (ρ), a quantifiable property (Ω.m) that opposes electrical current flow as well as its reciprocal conductivity or specific conductance (σ) whose units are S.m.

$$\sigma = 1/\rho$$

Cylindrical electrical conductors, such as electrical cables, resist electric conductance not only depending on the material itself but also on their length (L) and cross-sectional area (A), this property is resistance (R):

$$R = \rho * L / A$$

As a natural consequence, their conductance (G), whose units are S, is:

$$G = A/(L * \rho) \text{ or } G = \sigma * A / L$$

If the ventricular chamber is viewed as an electric conductor, and the emitting electrodes are assumed to be end-plates, the voltage sensed between each inner electrode pair relates to tissue conductivity, to the cross sectional area of surrounding conductive tissue (A), and to the inter-electrode distance (L). With a subtle mathematical transformation, which consists of multiplying both numerator and denominator by L, we then derive the volume (V) of the cylinder contained between each electrode pair:

$$G = \sigma * A / L = \sigma * V / L^2 \Leftrightarrow V = G * L^2 / \sigma \; or \; V = G * L^2 * \rho$$

The summation of the conductances from stacked cylinders (G_i) is proportional to the whole chamber volume (V_t) if the outermost electrodes span the range from apex to base:

$$V_t = \sum_i \left[\left(G_i * L^2 / \sigma \right) \right]$$

Pressure-volume catheter systems have been miniaturized for application in rodents but such small animals do not require several pairs of sensing electrodes (segments) [22]. Rodent catheters have only two pairs of electrodes, an outer emitting pair and an inner sensing pair.

The change in sensed voltage during each heartbeat is caused by changes in conductance between electrodes as a result of the variation of cross-sectional area of conducting tissue. Voltage increases during diastole because there is more blood in the cavity and blood conducts electrical current approximately three times faster than the myocardium.

Nonetheless, part of the electrical conductance is due to the myocardium or far-field, so-called parallel conductance. Baan et al. directly recorded this conductance by suctioning canine left ventricles to zero volume and later estimated it by injecting small volumes of hypotonic glucose solutions or hypertonic salt solutions to transiently and progressively reduce or increase blood conductivity during a few heartbeats, respectively. Such small volumes could not change loading conditions or ejection fraction but definitely altered conductance by changing blood conductivity. Moreover, the change was more pronounced in end-diastolic conductance because in diastole there is more blood in the heart. By plotting a regression between end-diastolic and end-systolic conductances during these transient changes and intercepting it with the identity line (end-systolic and end-diastolic conductances are equal), they mathematically derived conductance at zero ventricular volume (Fig. 21.3A1).

To quantify actual ventricular cavity volume this parallel conductance (G_p) must be subtracted from overall conductance (G_t).

$$V = \left(G_t - G_p \right) * L^2 / \sigma$$

Many studies have shown that parallel conductance remains reasonably constant throughout any experimental determination since it only depends on myocardial wall thickness and also that injection of hypertonic solution can be done not only from the pulmonary artery but also from any central or peripheral vein as long as there is no change to hemodynamic performance. Parallel conductance is increasingly more relevant in larger animals due to the influence of the contralateral ventricle and surrounding structures (far field); in large animals and man it can surmount to almost 70 % of total conductance signal, but has a relatively minor influence in mice [23]. Parallel conductance estimation in mice demands fast but careful injection of very small volumes (<20 μL) of hypertonic saline (10–30 %) which is technically demanding, can lead to volume loading, depress myocardial function and alter blood resistivity. More recently alternative methods to estimate parallel conductance have used dual frequency catheter excitation. Blood has a constant conductivity

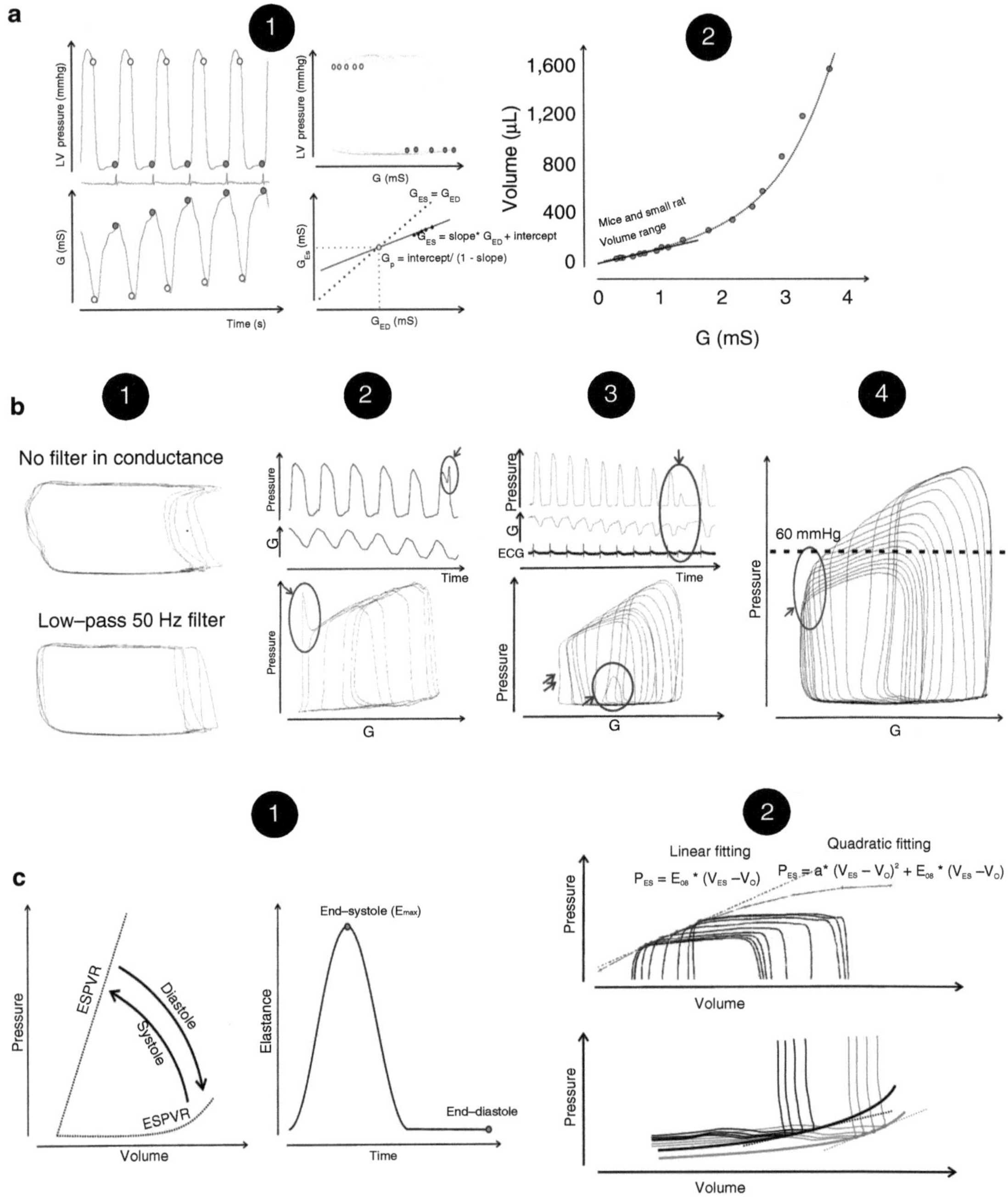

over the range of frequencies from 2 to 100 kHz, whereas muscle is more conductive at frequencies of 12 kHz and becomes very resistive at lower frequencies, so dissipation of current beyond the blood pool decreases. Geougakopoulos and Kass [23] used alternate 2 and 20 kHz excitation frequency in mice, the conductance signal was higher at 20 kHz and the difference was highly correlated with G_p without any bias. This method allows repeated estimations during any procedure or even continuous real-time acquisition without the need for hypertonic saline injection. It also clearly demonstrated slight variations in parallel conductance throughout the cardiac cycle. Other authors questioned the validity of the dual-frequency excitation methodology in large animals showing that parallel conductance measured at lower frequencies is not negligible [24]. Another alternative is the admittance technique. Admittance like conductance is also a measure of how easily a circuit or device will allow current flow but further takes into account dynamic effects, or reactance, whereas conductance applies to steady current. Since the myocardium is closer to the electrodes at end-systole it receives more current than in end-diastole. Also, the percentage of blood in the myocardium during systole is lower than in diastole. Moreover, admittance takes into account the dynamic effects of the material's susceptance to polarization, which is of course higher in the myocardium which as intrinsic capacitance when exposed to electrical current. The underlying assumption behind this technology is that the myocardium has capacitive properties while the blood does not. Therefore there exists a phase angle in the current to voltage ratio that is only due to the myocardium. The phase angle or delay in the admittance signal is caused by the capacitive property of the myocardium. With constant current emission at 20 kHz and calculation of the magnitude and phase of instantaneous input current to output voltage ratio it is possible to estimate actual myocardial conductance and parallel conductance continuously and in real-time [25]. Although this method may be more compliant with catheter misalignment and more sensitive, it is still not thoroughly validated in most rodent models of cardiovascular disease [26].

To compute actual volumes from conductance readings according to Baan's equation, it is still necessary to determine blood resistivity. This can be done easily in large animals and humans since large blood volumes are available for direct determination. Care must be taken to maintain blood temperature constant because lower temperatures slightly increase blood resistivity. Also, if an experiment involves large fluctuations in the

Fig. 21.3 *Hemodynamic evaluation in rodents. Fundamental aspects of calibration* (**A**): (*1*) parallel conductance (G_p) or non-cavity conductance can be extrapolated by regressing end-diastolic (G_{ED}) and end-systolic (G_{ES}) conductances to the identity line after injecting a small volume of hypertonic saline which does not alter haemodynamic conditions or left ventricular (*LV*) pressure readings but artificially increases conductance (*G*), (*2*) in small rodents it is unfeasible to collect large blood samples therefore a final standard well calibration can substitute for blood resistivity measurement, nonetheless, the standard curve usually behaves non-linearly in the high volume range. *Practical tips during hemodynamic assessment* (**B**): (*1*) the weak conductance signal is prone to electrical interference which can be removed with a low-pass filter, (*2*) an end-systolic pressure peak can sometimes appear in the tracing particularly at low volumes and demands catheter repositioning, (*3*) recordings with arrhythmia should not be analysed altogether, excluding ectopic beats does not eliminate changes in contractility in the following beats, (*4*) avoid long inferior vena cava occlusions that jeopardize coronary perfusion and thus myocardial performance. *Aspects of pressure-volume loops analysis* (**C**): (*1*) the myocardium oscillates like a spring between maximal elastance (E_{max}) at end-systole, defining an end-systolic pressure-volume relationship (ESPVR), and minimal elastance at end-diastole, defining an end-diastolic pressure-volume relationship (EDPVR) according to the original conception of Suga & Sagawa, (*2*) the ESPVR (2a) can usually be analysed by linear fitting when the quadratic correction is dismal whereas the EDPVR (2b) due to the intrinsic properties of the myocardium should always be analysed by exponential fitting to avoid gross mistakes as the one illustrated, please note that the tracings in grey would have a steeper slope in a linear analysis while there was actually a downward shift in EDPVR by exponential analysis when compared with the tracing in black because the acquisitions were not performed at the same volume range hematocrit, resistivity must be measured at varying hematocrit levels because these have an important effect on resistivity. Resistivity usually ranges from 150 to 190 Ω.cm between 25 and 45 % of hematocrit, respectively, at 37 °C [27]. By approximating two additional electrode pairs to 0.2 mm of each other the catheter can measure resistivity continuously and in real time. Applying both dual-frequency excitation to evaluate parallel conductance and catheter measured resistivity it is even possible to perform telemetric monitoring of pressure-volume loops [28].

Nevertheless, other confounders contribute to underestimation of actual blood volume: the endocardial border is not smooth, trabeculae and papillary muscles contribute to field inhomogeneity, the placement of the catheter is frequently not central, and the electrodes cannot span all the long-axis range of the ventricle. After measuring blood resistivity and parallel conduction Baan et al. [20]. proposed another calibration factor, slope factor α, to account for these limitations.

$$V = (1/\alpha) * (G_t - G_p) * L^2 / \sigma$$

The term slope originates from the way it was originally derived as the slope of the linear regression between stroke volume as assessed by conductance and stroke volume assessed by either flow measurement or thermodilution during caval occlusion in a dog or in a set of human patients. Since conductance usually underestimated volume the slope (α) was lower than 1.

As for rodents, large volumes of blood (over 5 mL) are not easily collectable without at least major hemodynamic consequences. To circumvent this problem standardized wells of known dimensions can be used for catheter calibration with the animal's blood post mortem in order to perform a conductance – volume standard curve. These standard curves usually have a linear fitting over the small volume range and are enough for accurate volume determination in mice. For progressively higher volumes the fitting becomes exponential (Fig. 21.3A2). Non-linear fitting can be explained because the emitting electrodes are not plate electrodes but rather point electrodes and the electrical field is inhomogeneous. To solve this issue Wei et al. [29]. proposed an alternative to Baan's equation including an empirically determined non-linear calibration coefficient instead of slope factor α. Simpler approaches can be attained by selecting calibration values that precisely span the range of conductances recorded during the actual experiment. These are usually close to linear even in rats. Another possibility is just to correct the stroke volume assessed by conductance as the range from maximum to minimum (after excluding parallel conductance) by another method. Several methods can be used to measure cardiac output and stroke volume. In rodents, ECHO and flow probes are most common. Echocardiography cannot be performed continuously, is observer-dependent and usually overestimates cardiac output. Another important point is that stroke volume assessed by echocardiography before hemodynamic evaluation in a minimally sedated animal is of course much higher than stroke volume measured under anaesthesia and possibly even with open-chest. If the latter are corrected for the former a large overestimation of ventricular volumes is most likely. As for flow measurement currently the most viable option is transient time flow measurement. It provides a continuous real-time and observer-independent assessment of cardiac output and stroke volume without the need for estimating vessel cross-sectional area, which is prone to error in such small animals. Nonetheless it is not feasible in closed-chest preparations. For complete cardiac output measurement it should be placed in the ascending aorta, but some researchers prefer the descending aorta and then correct the signal for the proportion of non-measured cardiac output.

As grasped by the complexity and controversy surrounding volume analysis this technique should not be viewed as a straightforward and easily implementable technique. It is time-consuming and demands considerable know-how.

21.2.3.3 Practical Tips for a Good Acquisition and Analysis

Detailed experimental troubleshooting can be found elsewhere [19, 26]. We will go over some key points. Due to electrical interference conductance signal may show irregularities, particularly conspicuous during isovolumetric contraction and relaxation when pressure is rapidly changing and volume is constant, filtering with a low pass filter is usually enough to optimize signal without altering analysis (Fig. 21.3B1). Filtering with frequencies lower than 30–50 Hz may influence analysis and should be avoided.

The researcher will usually be able to obtain various conductance signals with a good morphology of the loops depending on the positioning of the catheter in the same preparation. As a general rule the best selection is the loop with the widest range. With experience the researcher will be familiarized with the expected conductance values for each animal species and model, and catheter making this choice easier. If the software used enables simultaneous acquisition and analysis, once hypertonic saline solution has been injected for calibration to parallel conduction an immediate analysis should be performed to gauge G_p values, these should never be negative or higher than total conductance. As stated for conductance with experience the researcher will be familiarized with expected values for each animal model.

Particularly for lower ventricular volumes, as during inferior vena cava occlusions an end-systolic peak may appear in the tracing (Fig. 21.3B2). This is usually due to direct contact of the pressure membrane with the myocardium and can only be solved by repositioning the catheter.

Inferior vena cava occlusions should be as transient as possible to prevent reflex or neuroendocrine mediated influences on performance. All recordings with arrhythmia should be excluded (Fig. 21.3B3) as well as those with significant variation of heart rate because frequency-dependent changes in myocardial performance last for many heartbeats. Also, a resting period between acquisitions should be safeguarded to avoid changes in performance due to previous load manipulations.

The drop in systolic pressure should not compromise myocardial perfusion. For lower pressures a notorious decrease in performance is clear (Fig. 21.3B4).

21.2.3.4 Hemodynamic Parameters Derived from Pressure-Volume Loops

Detailed reviews of derived parameters can be found in recent reviews [26, 30]. Volume analysis permits assessing preload by end-diastolic volume and ejection fraction. The pressure-volume loop analysis concept was originally laid out by Suga and Sagawa [21] who explored time varying-elastance (or pressure-volume ratio) as a means to measure pump function, by considering the ventricle a spring whose elastance increases during systole and decreases during diastole (Fig. 21.3C1) [21] according to the function:

$$E(t) = P(V,t) / \left[V(t) - V_0\right]$$

When both elastance and time are normalized this relationship is highly stable regardless of loading conditions or animal species [22] but it can be changed by drugs such as myosin activators that enhance effective myosin cross-bridge formation and duration and therefore lengthen systolic ejection time.

In ex situ perfused dog hearts Suga and Sagawa demonstrated the relative load-independence of maximum elastance (E_{max}) [31] that was thereafter taken as gold standard for myocardial contractility. In vivo with pressure-volume loops and acute preload reductions by vena cava occlusion a similar index can be derived, end-systolic elastance (E_{es}). It can be derived from linear regression of end-systolic points This index is also slightly load-dependent reflecting load influence on cross-bridge cycles and calcium sensitivity but since load conditions do not change markedly during experiments this is generally ignored. In a simple view E_{es} in units of mmHg.volume^{-1} is the slope of this regression and is proportional to inotropism. Nevertheless linear regression is characterized by both slope and intercept and as elegantly illustrated by Burkhoff [30] several combinations of slope and intercept variation can indeed indicate increased contractility. Accurate comparisons of inotropic state between experimental groups therefore require joint analysis of both parameters by either analysis of covariance or multiple regression with dummy variables [32]. Another aspect that complicates analysis is that the best fitting for end-systolic pressure-volume relationship is actually non-linear, particularly in rodents. A quadratic correction was proposed by Kass et al. [33] (Fig. 21.3C2a).

Non-linearity raises concerns when comparisons between groups of animals with distinct working pressure ranges are analysed as occurs in models of heart failure or arterial hypertension. In these cases preload reductions with caval occlusion may generate end-systolic pressure-volume relationships at distinct working ranges. If a linear analysis is performed differences in slope may simply be due to non-linearity. As a practical rule, when the quadratic correction is negligible over a wide range of pressure-volume variation encompassing a common working pressure, linear fitting can be used for comparisons between groups. This index is particularly well tailored to perform comparisons in the acute setting when there is no change in muscle mass or geometry, but in chronic disease changes in ventricular mass and geometry are important confounding factors. Values normalized for myocardial mass can be used but do not account for relative wall-thickness; therefore the most correct approach relies on estimation of stress-strain relationships by complementary methods such as sonomicrometers or ECHO [34]. Another approach that yields a less load-dependent index and accounts for slight cycle length changes between beats is time normalization of pressure-volume loops to obtain isophasical elastance and time-normalized E_{es} [35]. Other relatively load-independent indices of contractility have been proposed, such as the dP/dt_{max} to end-diastolic volume relationship, which is more sensitive to acute inotropic changes [36], or the preload recruitable stroke work, which is not dependent on chamber size or geometry and has units of mmHg [37]. This particular feature of preload recruitable stroke work makes it particularly useful since it is not influenced by chamber volume or geometry and can be applied reproducibly across animal species. Also as a rule of thumb in healthy animals values over 60 mmHg should be expected, while lower values suggest a poor experimental preparation.

Analysis of pressure-volume loops enables a more refined assessment of afterload. Sunagawa et al. [38] first coined the concept of effective arterial elastance (E_a) in isolated heart preparations [38], which was later documented in vivo [39]. E_a is a measurement of vascular load, can be derived from pressure-volume loops as the P_{ES} to stroke volume ratio and is customarily represented by a line that unites the end-systolic point and end-diastolic volume. Its fundamental determinants are heart rate and peripheral vascular resistance. By assessing the ratio between E_a and E_{es} derived from pressure-volume loops ventricular-arterial coupling can be assessed. Its healthy range is close to 1 (0.7–1.2) in the LV and deviations towards higher values have important pathophysiological consequences in the progression of heart failure [40].

Stroke work can easily be defined by the area encompassed by the pressure-volume loop and is the efficient or external mechanical output of the heart, but the total area circumscribed by time-varying elastance is higher, including a left side component of internal work [41]. Suga et al. explored, validated and recently reviewed this concept to the study of myocardial bioenergetics in isolated hearts with simultaneous measurement of oxygen consumption, but application to the in vivo and in situ heart is also possible [42].

As for diastolic function, myocardial stiffness can be assessed by the end-diastolic pressure-volume relationship obtained during inferior vena cava occlusions. Several fitting models have been used, but in contrast to the end-systolic pressure-volume relationship linear approaches are never accurate (Fig. 21.3C2b). In the lower pressure and volume range titin and intrinsic myofilament properties are more important, while collagen and extracelullar matrix components dominate in the higher pressure and volume range. Most researchers use an exponential model with a pressure offset (P_0) to account for non-zero pressures at zero volume (pericardial restraint, interventricular interaction, and intrathoracic pressure) and two constants, where β is chamber stiffness constant with units of volume^{-1}:

$$P_{ED} = \alpha * \left(e^{\beta * VED} - 1\right) + P_0$$

Several issues are important. Firstly the timing of end-diastole itself can be assessed either visually or automatically, ideally joint analysis of ECG and peak QRS detection is the most valuable time-point, if an ECG is not available percentage change in pressure can also be used to establish beginning of contraction. Secondly chamber size is important, particularly when dealing with experimental groups that have remarkably different weights. In this case, previous indexation of volumes to weight or body surface area may be useful [9] or, alternatively, indexes may be corrected to account for ventricular size and wall thickness or, ideally, using strain measures all of which require imaging methods [30]. Thirdly, if all fitting constants vary (α, β and P_0) group comparisons will require either analysis of covariance or multiple regression with dummy variables as previously mentioned for the end-systolic pressure-volume relationships.

Considerations on Right Ventricular Analysis

Although the right ventricle is a chamber with complex geometry, coarse trabeculations, somewhat triangular shaped loops which make end-systole determination more difficult, and with a potential for higher current loss to surrounding structures which makes precise determination of parallel conductance of paramount importance, the conductance methodology has been applied successfully to various animal species and disease models and load independent indexes derived from pressure-volume relationships originally validated for the LV have been extensively validated for right ventricular analysis as well [43]. In rodents simultaneous evaluation of both left ventricular and right ventricular volumes is currently unfeasible unless the conductance signal is alternately read from each ventricle due to the unresolved issue of interference in close electrical fields [44] but in larger animals and with multiple electrode catheters simultaneous recordings are possible [45].

21.3 Discussion and General Considerations

Beyond the evaluation of cardiac structure, telemetry, echocardiography and now also magnetic resonance imaging are increasingly substituting for more invasive approaches to cardiovascular function assessment such as hemodynamic evaluation. They have the advantage of enabling serial assessment with minimal sedation/anaesthesia. Precise evaluation of load-independent indices of contractility and relaxation however will mostly likely continue to depending on invasive hemodynamic function evaluation by pressure-volume loop analysis.

Conclusion

Assessing cardiac structure and function in rodent disease models is the cornerstone to basic and translational cardiovascular research. Throughout the chapter the grounding concepts of telemetry, echocardiography and hemodynamic evaluation in rodents were summarized. These are the essential tools for in vivo assessment of cardiovascular function that are closest to intact physiology but as emphasised are also time consuming and laborious techniques prone to many caveats and systemic biases. We have tried to review them and to share our hands-on experience with the reader. We hope it may have been useful for both newcomers to the cardiovascular research field and to the more experienced researcher.

References

1. Kramer K, Kinter LB. Evaluation and applications of radiotelemetry in small laboratory animals. Physiol Genomics. 2003;13:197–205.
2. Kaidi S, Brutel F, Van Deun F, Kramer K, Remie R, Dewe W, et al. Comparison of two methods (left carotid artery and abdominal aorta) for surgical implantation of radiotelemetry devices in CD-1 mice. Lab Anim. 2007;41:388–402.
3. Ram R, Mickelsen DM, Theodoropoulos C, Blaxall BC. New approaches in small animal echocardiography: imaging the sounds of silence. Am J Physiol Heart Circ Physiol. 2011;301:H1765–80.
4. Oyama MA. Advances in echocardiography. Vet Clin Small An. 2004;34:1083–104, v.
5. Schiller NB, Shah PM, Crawford M, DeMaria A, Devereux R, Feigenbaum H, et al. Recommendations for quantitation of the left ventricle by two-dimensional echocardiography. American Society of Echocardiography Committee on Standards, Subcommittee on Quantitation of Two-Dimensional Echocardiograms. J Am Soc Echocardiogr. 1989;2:358–67.
6. Citro R, Bossone E, Kuersten B, Gregorio G, Salustri A. Tissue Doppler and strain imaging: anything left in the echo-lab? Cardiovasc Ultrasound. 2008;6:54.

7. Collins KA, Korcarz CE, Lang RM. Use of echocardiography for the phenotypic assessment of genetically altered mice. Physiol Genomics. 2003;13:227–39.
8. Kanno S, Lerner DL, Schuessler RB, Betsuyaku T, Yamada KA, Saffitz JE, et al. Echocardiographic evaluation of ventricular remodeling in a mouse model of myocardial infarction. J Am Soc Echocardiogr. 2002; 15:601–9.
9. Hamdani N, Franssen C, Lourenco A, Falcao-Pires I, Fontoura D, Leite S, et al. Myocardial titin hypophosphorylation importantly contributes to heart failure with preserved ejection fraction in a rat metabolic risk model. Circ Heart Fail. 2013;6:1239–49.
10. Tei C, Nishimura RA, Seward JB, Tajik AJ. Noninvasive Doppler-derived myocardial performance index: correlation with simultaneous measurements of cardiac catheterization measurements. J Am Soc Echocardiogr. 1997;10:169–78.
11. Hardziyenka M, Campian ME, de Bruin-Bon HA, Michel MC, Tan HL. Sequence of echocardiographic changes during development of right ventricular failure in rat. J Am Soc Echocardiogr. 2006;19:1272–9.
12. Vogel M, Schmidt MR, Kristiansen SB, Cheung M, White PA, Sorensen K, et al. Validation of myocardial acceleration during isovolumic contraction as a novel noninvasive index of right ventricular contractility: comparison with ventricular pressure-volume relations in an animal model. Circulation. 2002;105:1693–9.
13. Paulus WJ, Tschope C, Sanderson JE, Rusconi C, Flachskampf FA, Rademakers FE, et al. How to diagnose diastolic heart failure: a consensus statement on the diagnosis of heart failure with normal left ventricular ejection fraction by the Heart Failure and Echocardiography Associations of the European Society of Cardiology. Eur Heart J. 2007;28:2539–50.
14. Urboniene D, Haber I, Fang YH, Thenappan T, Archer SL. Validation of high-resolution echocardiography and magnetic resonance imaging vs high-fidelity catheterization in experimental pulmonary hypertension. Am J Physiol Lung Cell Mol Physiol. 2010;299:L401–12.
15. Stypmann J, Engelen MA, Troatz C, Rothenburger M, Eckardt L, Tiemann K. Echocardiographic assessment of global left ventricular function in mice. Lab Anim. 2009;43:127–37.
16. Matsubara H, Takaki M, Yasuhara S, Araki J, Suga H. Logistic time constant of isovolumic relaxation pressure-time curve in the canine left ventricle. Better alternative to exponential time constant. Circulation. 1995;92:2318–26.
17. Leite-Moreira AF, Correia-Pinto J, Gillebert TC. Afterload induced changes in myocardial relaxation: a mechanism for diastolic dysfunction. Cardiovasc Res. 1999;43:344–53.
18. Leite-Moreira AF, Lourenco AP, Roncon-Albuquerque Jr R, Henriques-Coelho T, Amorim MJ, Almeida J, et al. Diastolic tolerance to systolic pressures closely reflects systolic performance in patients with coronary heart disease. Basic Res Cardiol. 2012;107:1–9.
19. Pacher P, Nagayama T, Mukhopadhyay P, Batkai S, Kass DA. Measurement of cardiac function using pressure-volume conductance catheter technique in mice and rats. Nat Protoc. 2008;3:1422–34.
20. Baan J, van der Velde ET, de Bruin HG, Smeenk GJ, Koops J, van Dijk AD, et al. Continuous measurement of left ventricular volume in animals and humans by conductance catheter. Circulation. 1984; 70:812–23.
21. Suga H, Sagawa K. Instantaneous pressure-volume relationships and their ratio in the excised, supported canine left ventricle. Circ Res. 1974;35:117–26.
22. Georgakopoulos D, Mitzner WA, Chen CH, Byrne BJ, Millar HD, Hare JM, et al. In vivo murine left ventricular pressure-volume relations by miniaturized conductance micromanometry. Am J Physiol. 1998; 274:H1416–22.
23. Georgakopoulos D, Kass DA. Estimation of parallel conductance by dual-frequency conductance catheter in mice. Am J Physiol Heart Circ Physiol. 2000;279: H443–50.
24. White PA, Brookes CI, Ravn HB, Stenbog EE, Christensen TD, Chaturvedi RR, et al. The effect of changing excitation frequency on parallel conductance in different sized hearts. Cardiovasc Res. 1998; 38:668–75.
25. Porterfield JE, Kottam AT, Raghavan K, Escobedo D, Jenkins JT, Larson ER, et al. Dynamic correction for parallel conductance, GP, and gain factor, alpha, in invasive murine left ventricular volume measurements. J Appl Physiol. 2009;107:1693–703.
26. Cingolani OH, Kass DA. Pressure-volume relation analysis of mouse ventricular function. Am J Physiol Heart Circ Physiol. 2011;301:H2198–206.
27. Tjin SC, Xie T, Lam YZ. Investigation into the effects of haematocrit and temperature on the resistivity of mammalian blood using a four-electrode probe. Med Biol Eng Comput. 1998;36:467–70.
28. Uemura K, Kawada T, Sugimachi M, Zheng C, Kashihara K, Sato T, et al. A self-calibrating telemetry system for measurement of ventricular pressure-volume relations in conscious, freely moving rats. Am J Physiol Heart Circ Physiol. 2004;287:H2906–13.
29. Wei CL, Valvano JW, Feldman MD, Pearce JA. Nonlinear conductance-volume relationship for murine conductance catheter measurement system. IEEE Trans Biomed Eng. 2005;52:1654–61.
30. Burkhoff D, Mirsky I, Suga H. Assessment of systolic and diastolic ventricular properties via pressure-volume analysis: a guide for clinical, translational, and basic researchers. Am J Physiol Heart Circ Physiol. 2005;289:H501–12.
31. Suga H, Sagawa K, Shoukas AA. Load independence of the instantaneous pressure-volume ratio of the canine left ventricle and effects of epinephrine and heart rate on the ratio. Circ Res. 1973;32:314–22.
32. Steendijk P, Baan Jr J, Van der Velde ET, Baan J. Effects of critical coronary stenosis on global systolic left ventricular function quantified by pressure-volume

relations during dobutamine stress in the canine heart. J Am Coll Cardiol. 1998;32:816–26.
33. Kass DA, Beyar R, Lankford E, Heard M, Maughan WL, Sagawa K. Influence of contractile state on curvilinearity of in situ end-systolic pressure-volume relations. Circulation. 1989;79:167–78.
34. Takaoka H, Esposito G, Mao L, Suga H, Rockman HA. Heart size-independent analysis of myocardial function in murine pressure overload hypertrophy. Am J Physiol Heart Circ Physiol. 2002;282:H2190–7.
35. Kind T, Westerhof N, Faes TJ, Lankhaar JW, Steendijk P, Vonk-Noordegraaf A. Cardiac phase-dependent time normalization reduces load dependence of time-varying elastance. Am J Physiol Heart Circ Physiol. 2009;296:H342–9.
36. Little WC. The left ventricular dP/dtmax-end-diastolic volume relation in closed-chest dogs. Circ Res. 1985; 56:808–15.
37. Glower DD, Spratt JA, Snow ND, Kabas JS, Davis JW, Olsen CO, et al. Linearity of the Frank-Starling relationship in the intact heart: the concept of preload recruitable stroke work. Circulation. 1985;71:994–1009.
38. Sunagawa K, Maughan WL, Sagawa K. Optimal arterial resistance for the maximal stroke work studied in isolated canine left ventricle. Circ Res. 1985; 56:586–95.
39. Kelly RP, Ting CT, Yang TM, Liu CP, Maughan WL, Chang MS, et al. Effective arterial elastance as index of arterial vascular load in humans. Circulation. 1992; 86:513–21.
40. Kass DA, Kelly RP. Ventriculo-arterial coupling: concepts, assumptions, and applications. Ann Biomed Eng. 1992;20:41–62.
41. Suga H. Cardiac energetics: from E(max) to pressure-volume area. Clin Exp Pharmacol Physiol. 2003;30: 580–5.
42. Takeshita D, Tanaka M, Mitsuyama S, Yoshikawa Y, Zhang GX, Obata K, et al. A new calpain inhibitor protects left ventricular dysfunction induced by mild ischemia-reperfusion in in situ rat hearts. J Physiol Sci. 2013;63:113–23.
43. White PA, Redington AN. Right ventricular volume measurement: can conductance do it better? Physiol Meas. 2000;21:R23–41.
44. Lourenco AP, Vasques-Novoa F, Oliveira-Pinto J, Fontoura D, Roncon-Albuquerque Jr R, Leite-Moreira AF. Haemodynamic and neuroendocrine effects of tezosentan in chronic experimental pulmonary hypertension. Intensive Care Med. 2012;38:1050–60.
45. Cardozo RL, de Vroomen M, van Bel F, Baan J, Steendijk P. Simultaneous measurement of right and left ventricular volume by the conductance catheter technique in the newborn lamb. Neth Heart J. 2003; 11:203–9.
46. Williams TD, Chambers JB, Henderson RP, Rashotte ME, Overton JM. Cardiovascular responses to caloric restriction and thermoneutrality in C57BL/6J mice. Am J Physiol Regul Integr Comp Physiol. 2002;282: R1459–67.
47. Obst M, Gross V, Luft FC. Systemic hemodynamics in non-anesthetized L-NAME- and DOCA-salt-treated mice. J Hypertens. 2004;22:1889–94.
48. Braga VA, Prabhakar NR. Refinement of telemetry for measuring blood pressure in conscious rats. J Am Assoc Lab Anim Sci. 2009;48:268–71.
49. Murphy DJ, Renninger JP, Schramek D. Respiratory inductive plethysmography as a method for measuring ventilatory parameters in conscious, non-restrained dogs. J Pharmacol Toxicol Methods. 2010;62: 47–53.
50. Garver J, Bermeo-Blanco OA, Gibson N, Bogie H, Grenwis J, Vela EM. Implantation and monitoring of a novel telemetry unit in the Syrian golden hamster model. J Invest Surg. 2012;25:186–96.
51. Cesarovic N, Jirkof P, Rettich A, Arras M. Implantation of radiotelemetry transmitters yielding data on ECG, heart rate, core body temperature and activity in free-moving laboratory mice. J Vis Exp. 2011;57.
52. Rey M, Weber EW, Hess PD. Simultaneous pulmonary and systemic blood pressure and ECG Interval measurement in conscious, freely moving rats. J Am Assoc Lab Anim Sci. 2012;51:231–8.

Non Invasive Imaging Modalities for Cardiovascular Translational Research-Technical Considerations

22

Anna N. Paschali, Stephan G. Nekolla, and Constantinos D. Anagnostopoulos

Abstract

Non-invasive imaging (PET, SPECT, MRI, CT, US, optical imaging and hybrid modalities) has contributed significantly to Cardiovascular Translational Research since it allows data to be obtained in the context of the whole living organism, often in a format suitable for quantification and performance of longitudinal studies both in animals and humans. During the last decade important developments have been achieved in the use of sophisticated imaging probes targeting key molecules and cells, thus creating a new multidisciplinary field, termed "molecular imaging." Amongst the various modalities, Single Photon Emission Computed Tomography (SPECT) and Positron Emission Tomography (PET) offer the greatest translational potential, because of the wide availability of existing clinical scanners, high imaging sensitivity, versatile radiochemistry options and the ongoing development of new imaging agents. Advances in nanoparticle probe development have made Magnetic Resonance Imaging (MRI) an emerging, radiation-free alternative technique, pending more demonstrations of clinical performance and safety for both gadolinium-based and iron oxide–based compounds. Optical imaging and molecular ultrasound (US) will probably require longer time for clinical translation, while computed tomography

A.N. Paschali, MD, MSc, PhD (✉)
Medical School and Centre for Clinical Research, University of Patras, Biomedical Research Foundation, Academy of Athens,
4 SoranouEphessiou Street, 11527 Athens, Greece
e-mail: apashali@upatras.gr

S.G. Nekolla, PhD, FESC
Multimodal Cardiac Imaging, NuklearmedizinischeKlinik und PoliklinikKlinikumrechts der Isar der Technischen Universitaet München,
Ismaningerstr. 22, D-81675 Munich, Germany
e-mail: stephan.nekolla@tum.de

C.D. Anagnostopoulos, MD, PhD, FRCP, FRCR, FESC
PET/CT unit, Centre for Experimental Surgery, Clinical and Translational Research, Biomedical Research Foundation, Academy of Athens,
4 SoranouEphessiou Street, 11527 Athens, Greece
e-mail: cdanagnostopoulos@bioacademy.gr; http://www.bioacademy.gr/lab/anagnostopoulos

D.V. Cokkinos (ed.), *Introduction to Translational Cardiovascular Research*,
DOI 10.1007/978-3-319-08798-6_22,

(CT) has low sensitivity to molecular targets and is currently the less explored modality. Combining different techniques in one system may compensate for some of the limitations that exist in all stand-alone imaging modalities while permitting sequential or even simultaneous recording of anatomy, function and molecular events for animals and humans.

Keywords
PET • SPECT • MRI • CT • US • Optical imaging • Hybrid modalities • Cardiovascular Translational Research

Abbreviations

ACE	Angiotensin converting enzyme
AT_1R	Angiotensin II type 1 receptor
BLI	Bioluminescence imaging
BMIPP	b-methyliodophenylpentadecanoic acid
BOLD	Blood oxygen level-dependent
CAD	Coronary artery disease
CCD	Charged coupled device
CEU	Contrast enhanced ultrasound
CT	Computed tomography
CTP	Computed tomography perfusion
CVD	Cardiovascular diseases
EBCT	Electron beam computed tomography
ECHO	Echocardiography
EPI	Epinephrine
FA	Fatty acids
FDA	Food and Drug Administration
FDG	Fluoro-deoxyglucose
FI	Fluorescence imaging
Gd	Gadolinium
HED	Hydroxyephedrine
LGE	Late gadolinium enhancement
LV	Left ventricle
MBF	Myocardial blood flow
MCP	Monocyte chemotactic protein
MDCT	Multidetector computed tomography
MI	Myocardial infarction
MIBG	Metaiodobenzylguanidine
MMP	Matrix metalloproteinase
MPI	Myocardial perfusion imaging
MPO	Myeloperoxidase
MRA	Magnetic resonance angiography
MRI	Magnetic resonance imaging
MRS	Magnetic resonance spectroscopy
NaF	Sodium fluoride
PET	Positron Emission Tomography
SPECT	Single Photon Emission Computed Tomography
US	Ultrasound

22.1 Introduction

Real world implementation of discoveries from "bench to bedside"—that has been termed "translational research"—has contributed significantly to prevention, diagnosis and therapy of cardiovascular diseases (CVD). Non- invasive imaging has played a pivotal role in this effort, because it allows data to be obtained in the context of the whole living organism, often in a format suitable for quantification, and performance of longitudinal studies both in animals and humans. During the last decade important developments have been made in the use of sophisticated imaging probes targeting key molecules and cells, thus creating, a new multidisciplinary field termed "molecular imaging". This has paved the way for new research opportunities well beyond the area of cardiovascular medicine and it is likely that in the near future, several molecular agents will be entering the clinical phase of development. Such probes need to have favourable pharmacokinetics and biodistribution, high binding efficacy and specificity combined with lack of toxicity and feasibility of synthesis and distribution, all of which require intense testing of numerous candidate agents and potentially high development costs. Performance of molecular imaging studies is based on identification of a target (intracellular or extracellular) and use of a pertinent probe along with an imaging system. Proteins are of most practical interest as a target, because of their abundance within a cell (0.01–1 million molecules compared with 1–2 DNA and 10–1,000 RNA), which contributes to the imaging sensitivity [1].

Amongst the various modalities, nuclear imaging in the form of Single Photon Emission Computed Tomography (SPECT) or Positron Emission Tomography (PET) has played a pivotal role due to the high detection sensitivity, but advances in nanoparticle probe development have made Magnetic Resonance Imaging (MRI) and ultrasound (US) emerging, radiation-free alternatives. The current trend in imaging technology is the development of hybrid multimodality scanners (PET/CT, SPECT/CT, PET/MRI) with improved characteristics by means of sensitivity and spatial resolution that permit sequential or even simultaneous recording of anatomy, function and molecular events for animals and humans. The intention of this chapter is not to provide a detailed description of non-invasive techniques but focus on a brief overview of the characteristics and performance of different non-invasive imaging modalities with an emphasis on *molecular probes* and aspects of imaging relevant to the pathological entities discussed in the next chapter. It will discuss in more detail techniques which have already entered into the clinical arena and the ones who are robust enough to undergo testing in the clinical setting, but only briefly those which are mostly confined to the experimental setting.

22.2 Non-invasive Imaging Techniques

22.2.1 Nuclear Imaging

Nuclear imaging is based on the injection of radionuclides in their native form or as a part of a chemical molecule following the tracer principle, which basically means that very minute amounts of active substances are used without disturbing vital biological processes. Thus, the body is imaged "from the inside out" using special devices which record the distribution of radioactivity from the intravenously administered radionuclides. Currently, PET and SPECT are the most translatable noninvasive molecular imaging platforms. The strengths of nuclear imaging are its high sensitivity, the continuously increasing number of clinical scanners installed and availability of a wide variety of targeted, radioactively labeled tracers in experimental and clinical applications.

22.2.1.1 PET/MicroPET Imaging

PET uses short-lived positron emitters such as oxygen-15 (^{15}O, $T_{1/2}$ = 2.1 min), nitrogen-13 (^{13}N, $T_{1/2}$ = 10 min), rubidium-82 (^{82}Rb, $T_{1/2}$ = 78 s), carbon-11 (^{11}C, $T_{1/2}$ = 20 min), gallium-68 (^{68}Ga, $T_{1/2}$ = 68 min) and fluorine-18 (^{18}F, $T_{1/2}$ = 110 min), for labelling of biomolecules in order to characterize in-vivo physiologic and biochemical processes. ^{15}O, ^{13}N, ^{11}C and ^{18}F are cyclotron produced while ^{82}Rb is produced from a strontium-82 (^{82}Sr) generator system and ^{68}Ga is produced from a Germanium-68 (^{68}Ge) generator system. The emitted positron travels a short distance in the order of millimeters (determined by its initial kinetic energy), before it meets an electron and undergoes the annihilation reaction. Upon annihilation, the mass of positron and electron is converted into two 511 keV photons that travel in approximately opposite directions. Coincidence detection of these annihilation photons followed by mathematical reconstruction of the images form the basis of PET imaging.

The advantages of PET imaging include high sensitivity and temporal resolution enabling dynamic imaging, use of radiolabeled probes with natural radioisotopes such as ^{11}C, that do not alter chemical behavior and absolute quantification of biological processes. List mode data acquisition provides an opportunity to correct for motion during cardiac and respiratory cycles [2]. The inherent resolution of PET system is technically limited by the size of the detection crystals and fundamentally limited by physical behavior of positron decay, associated with the significant movement of positron before annihilation, and deviation from exact 180° angular separation [3]. Current state-of-the-art clinical PET scanners have a spatial resolution of 3–5 mm. A major limitation for the widespread use of PET remains the high cost, reflecting the sophisticated imaging technology and the need of a cyclotron on-site, or in close proximity of production sites for short-lived tracers and availability of expensive generators. The development of fluorinated (^{18}F) tracers, which have a relatively long half-life, allows imaging to be performed even without access to an on-site-cyclotron.

For pre-clinical PET imaging, dedicated systems with small crystals and bore diameters between 10 and 20 cm are required to reach a reasonable spatial resolution. The first *microPET* scanner was developed at UCLA in 1996 and currently more than 80 preclinical PET systems are installed worldwide. Most animal PET and PET/CT scanners have a spatial resolution of 1–2 mm [1, 4].

Radiopharmaceuticals which have been applied for PET cardiac imaging in the clinical and preclinical setting are described below. In general, ^{18}F-labeled tracers are more likely to achieve broader clinical application from a logistical standpoint, while the clinical use of ^{11}C, ^{13}N, ^{15}O labeled tracers has been limited by the need of an on-site cyclotron.

Myocardial Perfusion Agents

A number of positron emitting radiopharmaceuticals can be used as tracers of myocardial perfusion. The most common are Nitrogen-13 ammonia (^{13}N-ammonia), Rubidium-82 (^{82}Rb), and Oxygen-15 labeled water (^{15}O-water). ^{13}N-ammonia enters the myocardial cells in proportion to blood flow by diffusion across the sarcolemma, followed by metabolic conversion to ^{13}N-glutamine by glutamine synthetase, becoming trapped within the cell. ^{82}Rb is potassium analog, actively taken up by myocytes in proportion to blood flow via the Na^+/K^+-ATPase. ^{15}O-water is a freely diffusible tracer and has been primarily utilized for absolute flow quantification research, but myocardial images are only obtained after application of kinetic modelling techniques (Table 22.1). At present, ^{13}N-ammonia and ^{82}Rb are the only Food and Drug Administration (FDA) approved PET tracers for the evaluation of individuals with suspected or known coronary artery disease (CAD). Myocardial perfusion PET imaging is accomplished using flow tracers ^{13}N-ammonia and ^{82}Rb at rest and during pharmacologic stress. For assessment of myocardial perfusion, PET is an excellent technique with sensitivity and specificity of about 90 % [5]. ^{18}F-flurpiridaz is a newly developed PET myocardial perfusion agent targeted to Mitochondrial Complex –I (MC-I) in the heart [6]. It has improved biological and imaging characteristics compared with currently available perfusion imaging agents, including rapid uptake in the myocardium, prolonged retention, and superior extraction versus flow profiles. A first in man study has established the safety and dosimetry of ^{18}F-flurpiridaz and confirmed high sustained cardiac uptake (Fig. 22.1). Subsequent studies performed in CAD patients established the dose and timing needed to detect perfusion deficits when the agent is administered under resting and stress conditions [7].

Myocardial Metabolism Agents

The primary tracer to image glucose metabolism is fluoro-deoxyglucose (FDG) labelled with fluorine-18 (^{18}F-FDG) (Table 22.1). ^{18}F-FDG is a glucose analog taken up by myocardial cells via two carriers, the glucose transporters 1 and 4 (GLUT1 and

Table 22.1 PET Radiopharmaceuticals for clinical cardiac imaging

Tracer	Biologic target
Blood flow	
^{13}N-ammonia	Perfusion
^{82}Rb	Perfusion
^{15}O-water	Perfusion
Metabolism	
^{18}F-FDG	Glucose transport, glucose metabolism
^{11}C-palmitate	Fatty acid metabolism
^{11}C-acetate	Oxidative metabolism (TCA cycle turnover)
Innervation	
^{11}C-hydroxyephedrine	Presynaptic catecholamine uptake
^{11}C-epinephrine	Presynaptic catecholamine uptake and storage
Receptors	
^{11}C-CGP12177	Beta-adrenergic receptor (nonselective)
^{11}C-MQNB	Muscarinic receptor

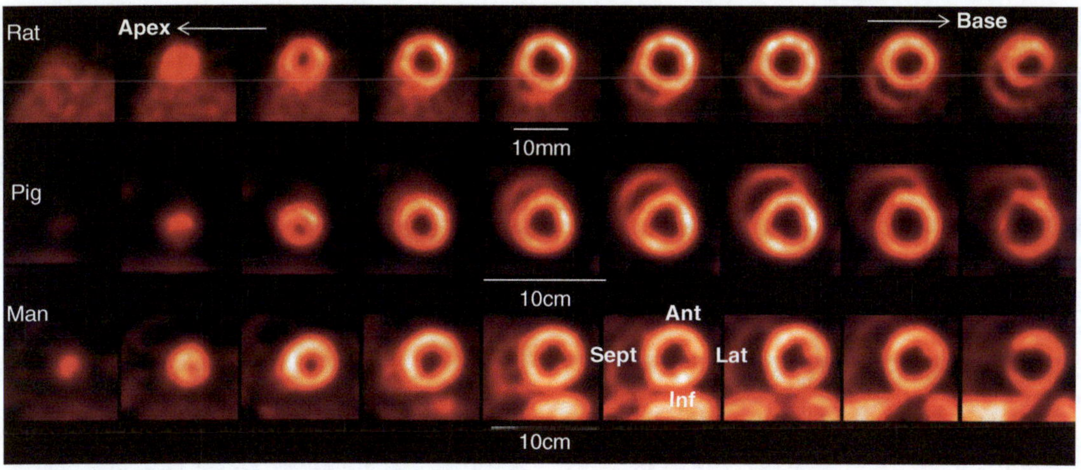

Fig. 22.1 Cardiac PET imaging of myocardial perfusion using F-18 labeled Flurpiridaz in rat, pig and man. The series of short axis images from apex to base were acquired in a dedicated animal PET/CT (rat) and a clinical PET/CT tomograph respectively. *Ant* anterior segment, *Lat* lateral segment, *Inf* inferior segment, *Sept* septum

GLUT 4). Similar to glucose, FDG is then phosphorylated by hexokinase to ^{18}F-FDG-6-phosphate but unlike glucose-6-phosphate, subsequent metabolism of ^{18}F-FDG-6-phosphate is minimal so that ^{18}F-FDG becomes essentially trapped in the myocardium. ^{18}F-FDG PET has been extensively used to assess myocardial viability and is still considered by some investigators as the gold standard for this assessment [8]. FDG is not a specific tracer, as it is also taken by activated macrophages and can be used to image inflammation.

Two tracers, palmitic acid and acetate have been labeled with ^{11}C. ^{11}C-palmitic acid can assess uptake and metabolism of long-chain fatty acids (FA). Their oxidation represents the major source of cardiac energy but complex kinetics and back-diffusion of the unmetabolized tracer by the myocytes allows only semi-quantitative measurements. ^{11}C-acetate, is a two-carbon-chain free FA which is extracted proportionally to myocardial blood flow, then rapidly enters the tricarboxylic acid cycle and is metabolized to carbon dioxide. It is considered a marker of overall oxidative metabolism without the complexity of substrate interaction between glucose and FA [9] (Table 22.1).

Myocardial Innervation Agents

The main tracers to image myocardial innervation are hydroxyephedrine (HED) and epinephrine (EPI) labeled with ^{11}C. HED is a false transmitter analog of norepinephrine and highly resistant to intraneuronal metabolic degradation. HED is considered a marker of uptake-1 mechanism, which is the reuptake for storage or catabolic disposal of norepinephrine into the presynaptic terminal by an energy dependent transporter. EPI is a true catecholamine that, in contrast to HED, is sensitive to metabolic degradation under normal conditions and has also gained interest as a potential neuronal imaging tracer (Fig. 22.2). ^{11}C-EPI labeled compounds are not FDA approved, and it is unlikely that they will not receive a broader clinical application due to their short half-life and need for an on-site cyclotron. New innervation tracers, such as LMI1195, a benzylguanidine derivative similar to metaiodobenzylguanidine (MIBG), but labeled with ^{18}F, are under investigation with the potential for a more widespread use from a logistical standpoint [10]. Post-synaptic receptor density can be assessed with a radiolabeled b-receptor antagonist CGP12177 and MQNB, a muscarinic receptor agonist, both labeled with ^{11}C (Table 22.1).

Further Molecular Probes

Beyond the tracers described above, a number of other agents have been tested mainly at a preclinical level and demonstrate potential for clinical translation. ^{18}F-galacto–arginine-glycine-aspartate

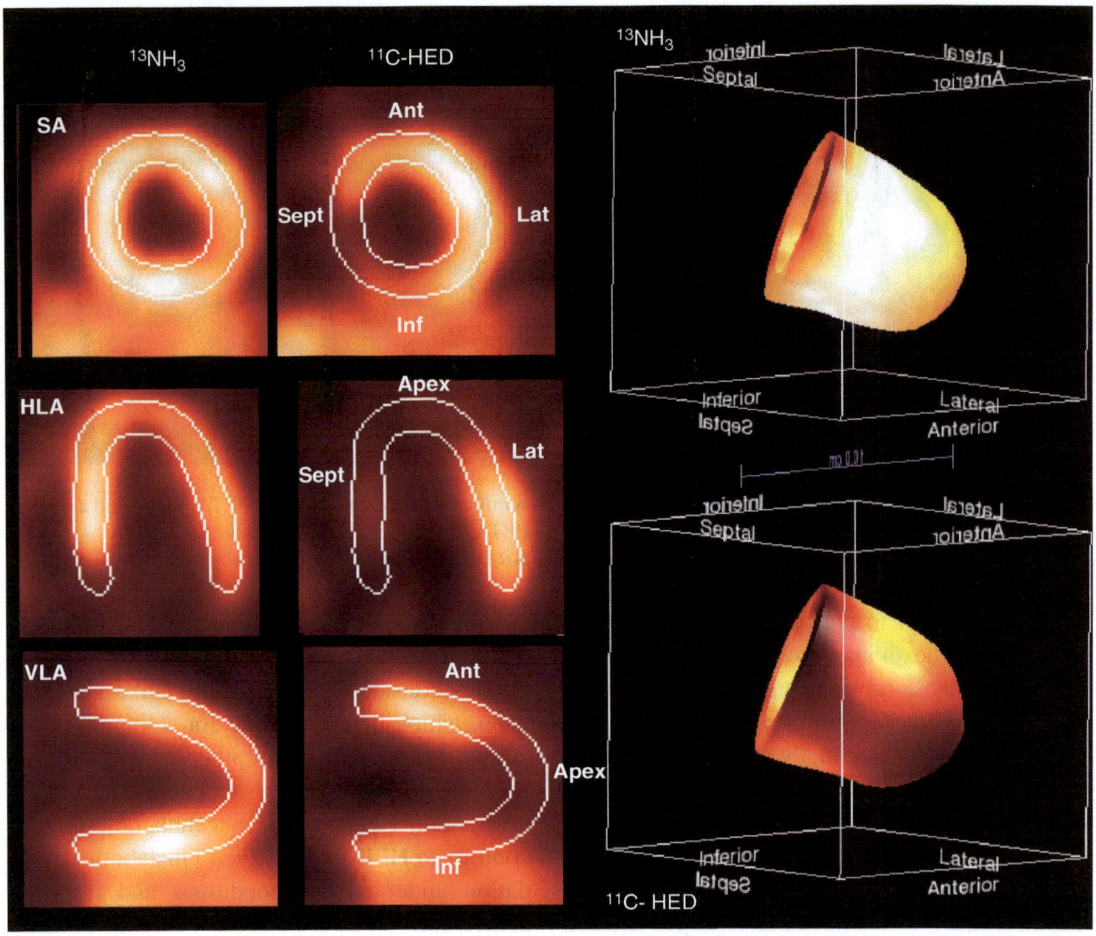

Fig. 22.2 Example of innervation imaging (performed with ^{11}C-HED) with demonstration of its relation to perfusion in a patient imaged after revascularization post MI. There is reduced ^{11}C-HED uptake in the anteroapical region as well as in the septum and most of the inferior wall indicating denervation in these areas. Perfusion as depicted by NH_3 uptake is normal in those areas and the rest of the LV myocardium. *SA* short axis, *VLA* vertical long axis, *HLA* horizontal axis, *Ant* anterior segment, *Lat* lateral segment, *Inf* inferior segment, *Sept* septum

(RGD) binds to $\alpha_v\beta_3$integrin receptors that are expressed on the endothelial surface during angiogenesis. Another option for angiogenesis imaging is to use the recently developed ^{68}Ga labelled RGD agent (^{68}Ga-NOTA-RGD) [11]. ^{68}Ga labeled tracers are highly appealing for imaging particularly for centers with no direct access to cyclotron, because ^{68}Ga is produced from a commercially available ^{68}Ge generator system. Annexin-V, a molecule which specifically binds to phosphatidylserine that is expressed on the surface of cells entering the apoptotic cascade, has been extensively tested in preclinical studies to image apoptosis. Radiolabeling of annexin-V for PET imaging has also been performed. Because annexin-V harbors numerous functional groups requiring protection and deprotection steps, its direct radiolabeling with ^{18}F is impractical. Recently, a set of novel small-molecule probes known as the Aposense compounds (a patented platform technology; Aposense Ltd.) has been designed to detect apoptotic membrane imprint [12]. Within this family, the PET tracer ^{18}F-ML-10 shows selective uptake by apoptotic cells, in correlation with the apoptotic hallmarks of breakdown of mitochondrial membrane potential, caspase activation, or apoptotic DNA fragmentation. Signal is lost on membrane rupture, and thus ^{18}F-ML-10 is capable of distinguishing between apoptotic and necrotic cells [12]. ^{18}F-ML-10 is the first PET tracer for apoptosis that has been advanced into clinical trials, with promising results to date in biodistribution and dosimetry profiles. For imaging necrosis, the tracer hypericin labeled with Iodine-124 (^{124}I), has shown a specific and high affinity, although the exact mechanism of action is still unknown [13]. The ^{11}C-labelled PET tracer PK11195, is a selective ligand of the translocator protein, known as peripheral benzodiazepine receptor (PBR) that is expressed in high density in circulating human phagocyte populations, particularly in monocytes and neutrophils [14]. Matrix metalloproteinase (MMP) imaging is also feasible through a newly developed MMP inhibitor labeled with ^{18}F [15]. Other probes targeting adhesion molecules (such as VCAM-1) labeled with ^{18}F are under investigation in experimental models. Recently, ^{18}F-sodium fluoride (^{18}F-NaF), a radiopharmaceutical used for skeletal imaging, was tested in patients with coronary atherosclerosis and symptomatic carotid disease and proved to provide relevant information regarding active micro-deposition of calcium in atherosclerotic plaques, a process that is associated with plaque instability [16].

Several angiotensin converting enzyme (ACE) inhibitors and angiotensin receptor 1 (AT_1R) antagonists have been radiolabeled for molecular imaging techniques. Initial attempts for developing specific ACE binding radiotracers were made by use of fluorine-18 labeled captopril (^{18}F–CAP), the first clinically available ACE inhibitor. ^{18}F–CAP, however, had a number of shortcomings that reduced its potential as a suitable tracer for examining ACE distribution. A new radiotracer, N-succinimidyl-4-[F-18]-fluorobenzoyllisinopril (^{18}F–FBL), was synthetized to bind more specifically to ACE. Multiple PET radiotracers for AT_1R have been developed labeled with ^{11}C, but major limitations in pharmakokinetics and biodistribution, rendered these tracers unsuitable for clinical use. Another probe labeled with ^{11}C (^{11}C-KR31173) was found to bind selectively to AT_1R in various tissues including the heart and first experimental studies in animals and first-in-man application (in four healthy volunteers) proved the feasibility and safety of imaging cardiac AT_1R expression [17]. These results provide a rationale for broader clinical testing of AT_1R -targeted molecular imaging.

22.2.1.2 SPECT/MicroSPECT Imaging

The detection system in conventional nuclear medicine is called Anger or γ-camera and typically has a sodium iodide (NaI) crystal. This camera permits planar and tomographic cardiac imaging (SPECT), if projections from different angles around the body are acquired. A new generation of cameras was recently introduced and uses cadmium zinc telluride (CZT) crystals. These systems show improved sensitivity and spatial resolution which allows for shorter acquisition times or reduction of injected tracer [18]. SPECT imaging probes are labeled with γ-emitting radionuclides, such as technetium-99 m (^{99m}Tc, $T_{1/2}$=6 h), thallium-201 (^{201}Tl, $T_{1/2}$=73 h), indium-111 (^{111}In, $T_{1/2}$=67 h), iodine-123 (^{123}I, $T_{1/2}$=13.2 h), and iodine-131 (^{131}I, $T_{1/2}$=8 days). Among these, ^{99m}Tc labeled tracers are the most readily available in everyday clinical practice from a commercially available molybdenum generator system, while the rest, are cyclotron produced. ^{99m}Tc has favorable physical and dosimetric features (it decays by isomeric transition and emits gamma rays at an energy level of 140 keV) and is the preferred isotope for SPECT imaging. The spatial resolution of clinical SPECT systems is 7–15 mm [1].

For pre-clinical research, a number of *micro-SPECT* systems are available commercially. MicroSPECT imaging offers several advantages in small animal models of CVD, such as the greater availability of radiotracers with a longer half-life compared to PET and the ability to image multiple tracers labeled with different isotopes simultaneously. The spatial resolution of microSPECT systems is 0.5–2 mm [1].

Currently available SPECT tracers used for myocardial perfusion imaging (MPI) are divided into two groups: ^{201}Tl and ^{99m}Tc labeled agents (Table 22.2). ^{201}Tl, an analog of potassium, is extracted actively by cell membrane Na^+/K^+ pumps on the first pass through the coronary vasculature and its uptake is proportional to regional perfusion over a wide range of flow rates. It has the highest myocardial extraction (85 % at the first passage of tracer from the myocytes) of the three available γ-emitting myocardial perfusion radiopharmaceuticals, with a peak myocardial concentration at 10 min after injection. ^{201}Tl is not sequestered permanently in the myocardial tissue, and it is continuously exchanged between the extracellular and intracellular spaces. ^{201}Tl decays by electron capture to mercury-201, and emits lower energy x-rays (75–80 keV) [19]. In contrast to ^{201}Tl, ^{99m}Tc must be bound to another compound so that can become suitable for assessing myocardial perfusion. ^{99m}Tc-sestamibi (methoxyisobutylisonitrile) and ^{99m}Tc tetrofosmin (1,2-bis[bis(2-ethoxyethyl)phosphino] ethane) are the two commercially available tracers. Both agents are lipophilic cations that passively diffuse into cardiomyocytes along an electropotential gradient and are actively trapped in mitochondria or in cytoplasma. The extraction of sestamibi and tetrofosmin by the myocytes is considerably lower than that of ^{201}Tl (65 and 54 % respectively). The intracellular passage of sestamibi and tetrofosmin is permanent, and redistribution is negligible, particularly with the tetrofosmin [19]. Myocardial uptake is proportional to myocardial blood flow in a specific range of flow rates, but lower than that of ^{201}Tl. The relationship between myocardial blood flow (MBF) and net myocardial uptake of various perfusion tracers (^{15}O-water, ^{13}N-ammonia, ^{82}Rb, ^{201}Tl, ^{99m}Tc-sestamibi and ^{99m}Tc tetrofosmin) is presented in Fig. 22.3.

SPECT MPI has a history of over 20 years in clinical practice. Such studies can be performed at rest or after physical exercise or pharmacological stress, with vasodilators (dipyridamole, adenosine, or regadenoson) or with the β-agonist dobutamine (Fig. 22.4). Perfusion studies can be coupled with electrocardiogram (ECG) gating (gated SPECT) allowing also assessment of ventricular function.

Beyond perfusion, other parameters can also be assessed such as FA metabolism and innervation by molecules labelled with ^{123}I (Table 22.2). ^{123}I emits predominantly γ photons with energies of 159 keV. 123-iodinated modified FA such as b-methyliodophenylpentadecanoic acid (BMIPP), have provided a sensitive SPECT marker of altered FA transport into the myocyte [20]. In contrast to straight long-chain FA that enter the mitochondria and are metabolized by b-oxidation immediately, BMIPP is not metabolized via b-oxidation because the methyl substitution precludes the formation of the ketoacyl coenzyme A intermediate. The prolonged retention of BMIPP in the cardiomyocyte is suitable for a longer acquisition time which is necessary for SPECT. Cardiac autonomic innervation imaging is also feasible by the use of a radiolabeled norepinephrine analog ^{123}I-MIBG. ^{123}I-MIBG, although similar to norepinephrine in terms of its storage, release, and reuptake in the presynaptic nerve terminal, it neither binds to the postsynaptic receptors nor undergoes presynaptic or postsynaptic metabolism. ^{123}I-MIBG undergoes avid uptake and storage in the cardiac nerve terminals through norepinephrine transporter-1. Myocardial retention of ^{123}I-MIBG depends mainly on the integrity of the presynaptic nerve terminal [21].

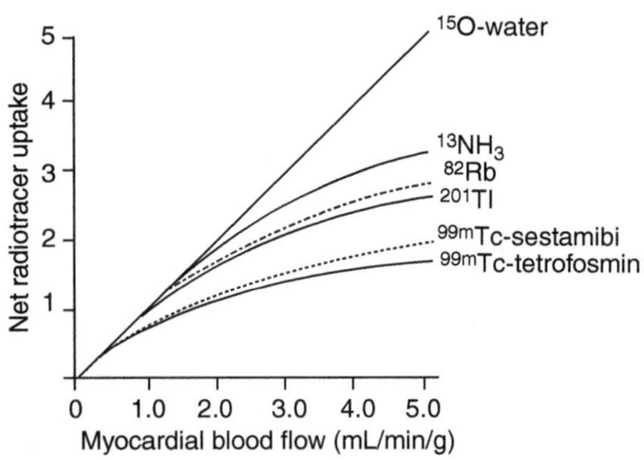

Fig. 22.3 Relation between net myocardial uptake of various perfusion tracers and MBF. With the exception of ^{15}O-water which exhibits a linear uptake-flow relation, the net uptake for all radiotracers increases non-linearly with higher flow rates. Please note that despite this limitation, ^{13}NH3 and ^{82}Rb demonstrate higher myocardial net uptake rates compared to SPECT perfusion tracers at higher flows (Reprinted, with permission from Bravo et al. *J Cardiovasc Transl Res*. 2011)

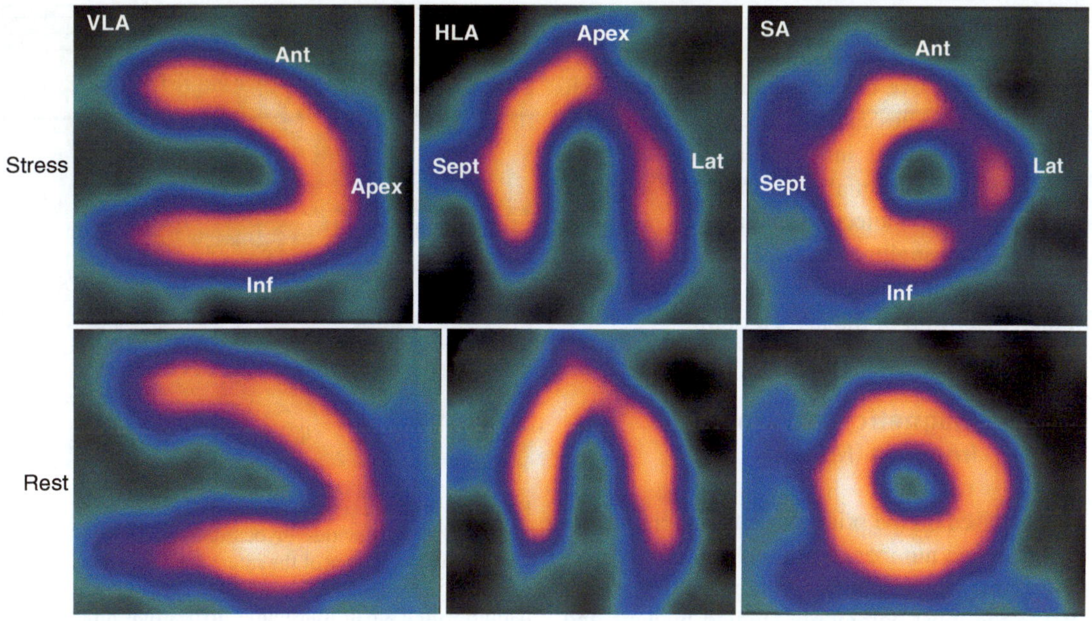

Fig. 22.4 SPECT myocardial perfusion imaging (MPI). *Top row* (stress study): there is reduced uptake of Thallium-201 in the lateral wall (HLA and SA views) following pharmacological stress with adenosine (140 μg/kg/min administered over a period of 6 min) but normal uptake elsewhere. *Bottom row* (resting study): the resting study is normal. Taken together, the stress and rest imaging data demonstrate an inducible perfusion abnormality in the lateral wall compatible with disease of the left circumflex artery. *SA* short axis, *VLA* vertical long axis, *HLA* horizontal long axis, *Ant* anterior segment, *Lat* lateral segment, *Inf* inferior segment, *Sept* septum

Table 22.2 SPECT radiopharmaceuticals for clinical cardiac imaging

Tracer	Biologic target
Blood flow	
^{201}Tl	Perfusion, viability
^{99m}Tc-sestamibi	Perfusion, viability
^{99m}Tc-tetrofosmin	Perfusion, viability
Metabolism	
^{123}I- BMIPP	Fatty acid metabolism
Innervation	
^{123}I-MIBG	Presynaptic catecholamine uptake

Imaging with ^{123}I-MIBG is in clinical use for many years. Semiquantitative measurement of ^{123}I-MIBG uptake is performed with early (10–20 min) or late (3–4 h) heart-to-mediastinum ratio (H/M) or washout rate of this tracer [22].

Further Molecular Probes

Beyond the aforementioned tracers which have been used in humans, there are additional agents that have been used mainly in experimental studies. ^{99m}Tc-labelled annexin-V has been used to image apoptosis as it shows selective, high-affinity binding to phosphatidyloserin on the surface of apoptotic cells. Since binding of annexin to phosphatidyloserin involves all four binding domains, there have been attempts to optimize target uptake and biodistribution characteristics in order to improve imaging of apoptosis. A new tracer ^{99m}Tc-HIS-AnxA5 has been developed for improved imaging of apoptosis [23]. For angiogenesis with SPECT imaging, radiolabeled RGD derivatives have been developed using radioisotopes such as ^{99m}Tc and ^{111}In. Other molecular probes under investigation include monocyte chemotactic protein (MCP) or macrophage's receptor LOX-1, labelled with ^{99m}Tc. Broad-spectrum inhibitors of active MMP have also been labeled with ^{99m}Tc (^{99m}Tc-RP805) and specifically bind to lesions that demonstrate significant MMP activity [24]. Recently, a ^{99m}Tc–labeled AT_1R ligand peptide (^{99m}Tc-labeled losartan) was developed and studied in a murine model of acute myocardial infarction (MI) [25].

From the above data it becomes evident that radioisotope studies can evaluate myocardial perfusion, metabolism, innervation and function, and have the potential to provide significant information on molecular parameters such as inflammation, angiogenesis, cell death (apoptosis or necrosis) and extracellular matrix alterations of the vessel wall or the myocardium.

22.2.2 Magnetic Resonance Imaging (MRI)

MRI is based on the principle that nuclei consisting of an odd number of protons and or neutrons have a magnetic moment or spin. Hydrogen-1 (^{1}H) is the most commonly studied nucleus and the most abundant in the body. When placed inside a strong magnetic field, the nuclei acquire a frequency directly proportional to the strength of the main magnetic field. Recovery of magnetization in the longitudinal and transverse directions is determined by the relaxation times T1 and T2 respectively, which is the basis of soft tissue contrast [26]. MRI pulse sequences that emphasize differences in T1 and T2 are commonly referred to as T1 and T2 weighted sequences. MRI is a cross-sectional technique but with the specific advantage of free selection of slice orientation and good three-dimensional capabilities which is very important for cardiac imaging. It has become the gold standard for assessing in detail cardiac structures and the derived functional parameters (volume curves, ejection fraction, wall thickness and thickening). All these functional parameters can also be acquired during pharmacologic (adenosine or dipiridamole) stress. Real-time cardiac MRI imaging with ECG gating is also feasible. Furthermore, MRI can provide precise information on tissue characterization by obtaining insights into the biological characteristics of the tissue of interest, such as scar delineation [late gadolinium enhancement (LGE) imaging] (Fig. 22.5), oedema and inflammation (T2-weighted sequences), identification of fat (T1-weighted black blood with fat suppression), water, and fibrous content. First-pass MRI perfusion imaging is another option and is clinically accurate under rest and pharmacologic stress [27]. In contrast to nuclear techniques, cardiac MRI with gadolinium (Gd) chelates does not image perfusion per se, but rather their distribution into the interstitial space. Constant improvements in MRI technology such as blood oxygen level-dependent (BOLD) or whole-heart coverage with dynamic 3D-cardiac imaging, allow performance of perfusion quantification [28], but this technique still needs to prove its diagnostic accuracy. MRI coronary angiography is feasible but there are still technical limitations that hamper the technique's routine clinical use. In contrast, magnetic resonance angiography (MRA) of larger vessels (e.g. carotids or aorta) is a well established technique with broad clinical use. Another interesting capability of MRI currently under investigation is magnetic resonance spectroscopy (MRS). MRS of the heart is a powerful research tool able to measure energy metabolism, intermediary metabolism, drug metabolism and ion homeostasis through analysis of nuclei, such as hydrogen (^{1}H), carbon (^{13}C), fluorine (^{19}F), sodium (^{23}Na), and phosphorus (^{31}P) [29]. However, the role of this

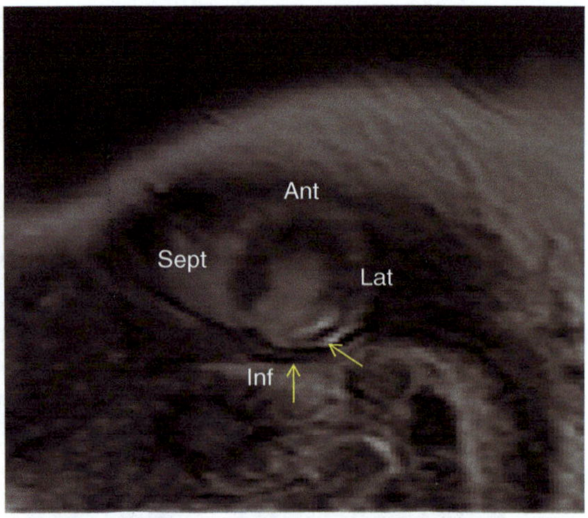

Fig. 22.5 Short axis view of a LGE MRI image from a patient with a previous myocardial infarction; there is LGE at the apical area of the inferior wall (*arrow*) and the adjacent part of the lateral wall (*arrow*), appearances compatible with a small transmural myocardial infarct. *LGE* late gadolinium enhancement, *Ant* anterior segment, *Lat* lateral segment, *Inf* inferior segment, *Sept* septum

approach in the clinical setting is yet to be determined considering the long acquisition times and low spatial resolution.

MRI has the advantages of providing very high temporal and spatial resolution (1.5–3 T, 0.5–1.5 mm), along with excellent soft tissue contrast [1]. micro-MRI scanners have a spatial resolution of 0.01–0.1 mm (>4.7 T) [1]. The major limitation of MRI in molecular imaging is its relatively lower sensitivity compared with nuclear imaging. While MRI does not involve ionizing radiation, the Gd contrast used is not without risk, and this is greater in patients with significantly impaired renal function. Although new and safe devices for MRI use have been engineered, at present MRI cannot be carried out in most patients with implanted pacemakers and implantable cardioverter-defibrillators.

For performance of molecular imaging, there is a need for the addition of contrast agents modulating the chemical environment inside an organism. There are two major classes of imaging agents based on gadolinium and iron. Gd-chelates are water soluble contrast agents that readily diffuse in all tissues, including the myocardial interstitium but do not enter intact cells. Gd-chelates conjugated to antibodies, peptides, or peptidomimetics, shorten the T1 relaxation time and thus lead to a contrast on T1 weighted images. Presently under investigation are macrophage, clot and apoptosis imaging probes. Macrophage imaging can be performed with Gd-containing immunomicelles [30] or lipid-based nanoparticles [31] that link to a macrophage-specific antibody. Also a Gd-based probe of myeloperoxidase (MPO) activity, an enzyme secreted by neutrophils and macrophages is under investigation. The probe becomes polymerized in the presence of MPO resulting in increased relaxivity, protein binding, and slow wash-out, all contributing to signal enhancement in areas of high MPO activity [32]. EP-2104R is a novel Gd-based fibrin-binding peptide that allows selective visualization of acute coronary, cardiac, and pulmonary thrombi [33]. Annexin-labelled magnetofluorescent nanoparticle (AnxCLIO-cy5.5) and a novel gadolinium chelate (Gd-DTPA-NBD), have also been developed for high-resolution MRI to image cardiomyocyte apoptosis and necrosis respectively [34].

Iron oxide based contrast agents lead to a signal reduction on T2 weighted images. Coated iron oxide particles [SPIO; 60–150 nm, including the ultrasmall (USPIO; 10–40 nm) and micron-sized (MPIO; 0.9–8 mm) versions] are engulfed by activated macrophages and, to a limited degree, by endothelial or smooth muscle cells within the inflamed plaques [35]. Oxide particles have already undergone extensive clinical evaluation that has not revealed safety problems. The major challenge facing USPIO imaging concerns the routine use of gradient recalled echo pulse sequences, which can lead to signal loss in areas of USPIO uptake. Newer MRI techniques that allow detection of USPIO as a positive contrast signal are under development and should help improve the diagnostic accuracy of the USPIO-enhanced MRI technique [36]. There have also been developed iron oxide nanoparticles to target specific molecular targets such as VCAM-1 targeted USPIO derivative (R832) and USPIO-R826 for apoptosis targeting [37]. Another novel approach uses perfluorocarbon nanoparticles carrying fluorine (^{19}F) that can be specifically detected by ^{19}F MRI [38]. This method detects signal that is distinct from any background signal and therefore quantifiable.

From the data already mentioned, it can be appreciated that MRI can assess the morphology, function, perfusion, viability and fibrosis of the cardiac tissue and also has the potential to provide significant information regarding inflammation, cell death (apoptosis or necrosis) and thrombus imaging.

22.2.3 Computed Tomography (CT)/ Micro-CT

CT imaging is based on the principle of attenuation of X-rays by tissues. The first electron beam CT (EBCT) system to scan the beating heart was introduced in 1979 and in 1989 the first use of an EBCT scanner in detection of coronary artery calcification was described. Nowadays multi-detector CT (MDCT) is widely used and technical improvements—including faster gantry rotation, increased number of detectors (64, 128, 256 and 320), decreased slice thickness, and use of dual x-ray sources—have considerably increased the temporal and the spatial resolution of MDCT. Current clinical CT scanners have a spatial resolution of 0.5–2 mm [1]. In patients investigated for CAD, MDCT coronary angiography has a high accuracy and, in particular, a very high negative predictive value (>98 %) [39]. Stress dynamic CT perfusion (CTP) imaging is a newly introduced non-invasive technique, and there are several approaches under investigation in experimental setting in pigs [40, 41] and in humans [42] to quantify myocardial perfusion, thereby providing information as to whether or not a coronary stenosis is flow limiting. Coronary calcium assessment can also be performed using MDCT. The main advantage of CT is rapid, non-invasive, cross sectional imaging of vessels to diagnose vascular occlusions and atherosclerotic calcified lesions. In addition, fast MDCT produces 3-dimensional volume data and allows acquisition of important information on pulmonary and cardiac arterial and venous systems prior to electrophysiology procedures, as well as evaluation of patients undergoing percutaneous procedures, such as transcatheter aortic valve replacement, resynchronization pacing and left atrial appendage closure. Unfortunately, CT has relatively low imaging sensitivity compared with nuclear imaging and exposes the patient to radiation and iodonized contrast agents which are often used during the procedure. *Small animal imaging* can be accomplished *by micro-CT scanners* which were developed in the early 1980s. Micro-CT as a standalone device or as a complement of micro-SPECT and PET provides high spatial resolution (0.02–0.3 mm) and micro-anatomic information [1]. Research efforts are evolving with CT molecular imaging using either iodinated [43] or gold nanoparticles [44].

22.2.4 Ultrasound Imaging

Echocardiography (ECHO) has seen a rapid evolution from single-crystal M mode to two-dimensional (2D) and three-dimensional (3D) ECHO. The recent introduction of real-time 3D echocardiographic imaging techniques permits images to be obtained in one beat with improved resolution and higher accuracy in quantification of left ventricle (LV) volumes. The addition of the fourth dimension (time) (4D), has become possible by recent advances in computer processing speed and memory, along with miniaturization of beam-formation hardware. Most contemporary clinical models provide a spatial resolution of 0.15–1 mm [1]. ECHO can assess the whole of the myocardium, valves and valve motion, chamber size, wall motion, and thickness from several projections so that one segment can be visualized from more than one view. A volumetric analysis can be performed manually or semi automatically using segmentation techniques. Doppler ECHO is another possibility that allows measurement of the differences between transmitted and returned wave produced when it hits moving blood cells (Fig. 22.6). It is used for determination of the direction and velocity of a moving blood volume as well as estimation of valvular gradients, and intracardiac pressures. Stress ECHO with the use of exercise or dobutamine can assess myocardial ischemia resulting from a coronary stenosis in the form of ischemia-induced regional wall motion abnormality. The combination of intravenous contrast injection (microbubbles) to assess perfusion during dobutamine stress ECHO, can increase the sensitivity without loss of specificity [45]. There are, however, some limitations yet to overcome when using this approach. The procedure remains highly operator dependent and there is a considerable learning curve both for image acquisition and interpretation. As for conventional transthoracic ECHO, the diagnostic yield depends greatly on image quality. What makes ECHO unique over other imaging modalities is the fact that it is a radiation free procedure and has the ability to provide significant myocardial anatomic and functional information at bedside.

High-frequency micro-US has been specifically developed for small animal research with frequencies ranging from 15 to 80 MHz compared with clinical US systems which range from 3 to

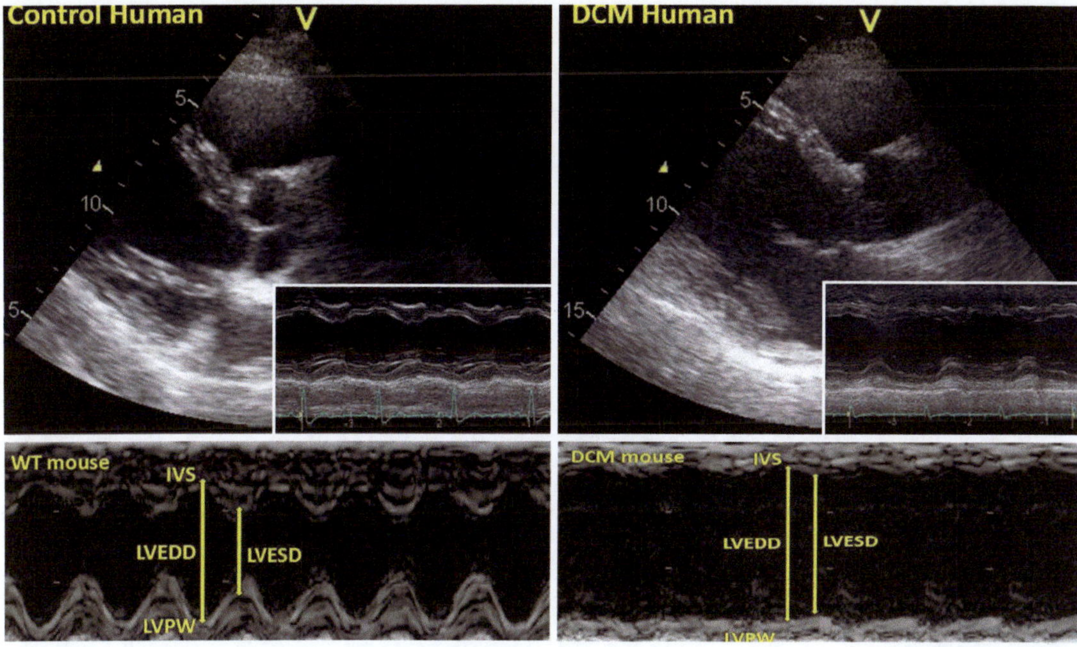

Fig. 22.6 *First panel*: two-dimensional (2D) echocardiographic images and 2D targeted M-mode recordings from the parasternal long axis view of a normal heart and a patient with dilated cardiomyopathy. *Second panel*: two-dimensional targeted M-mode recordings of the left ventricle (*LV*) at the level of the papillary muscles taken from a 6 months old wild type mouse and a mouse with dilated cardiomyopathy. The *yellow arrows* show left ventricular end diastolic (*LVEDD*) and end systolic dimension (*LVESD*), the intraventicular septum (*IVS*) and the left ventricular posterior wall in diastole

15 MHz. Current micro-US systems resolution is 0.04–0.1 mm [1]. Typically, micro-US can image tissue of around 3 cm below the skin, and this is more than sufficient for small animals such as mice. Recent advances have allowed imaging of molecular and cellular alterations of disease with targeted contrast enhanced ultrasound (CEU). Molecular US is performed with gas-containing microbubbles (2–5 μm in diameter) with nonlinear acoustic characteristics that have shells composed of protein, lipids, or biocompatible polymers. The basis for signal generation from these agents is thought to be largely from their different acoustic characteristics or the disruption with release of free highly echogenic gas of these particles [46]. Microbubbles are pure intravascular tracers that behave similarly to red cells in the microcirculation thereby limiting the selection of molecular targets to the endothelium. For the purposes of targeting, microbubbles can be retained in diseased tissue by virtue of ligands that are conjugated to the microbubble shell surface or, in a more simple fashion, by changing certain key chemical properties of the microbubble shell. Currently, molecular imaging with US has remained in the domain of preclinical research but there are efforts under way to develop agents for human use. This step will involve development of surface conjugation methods with a proven safety profile in humans and the intention to provide information that is useful and incremental in value to established diagnostic methods.

22.2.5 Optical Imaging

Optical imaging is divided into *fluorescence* and *bioluminescence* imaging. Fluorescence imaging (FI) works on the basis of fluorochromes inside the subject that are excited by an external light source, and which emit light of a different wavelength in response. Bioluminescence imaging (BLI), on the other hand, is based on light generated by chemiluminescent enzymatic reactions.

In both fluorescence and bioluminescence imaging, the light signals are captured by charged coupled device (CCD) cameras which are extremely light-sensitive and yield planar and tomographic images.

FI is typically performed by exogenous delivery of a fluorescent probe that interacts with the target or by direct imaging of an endogenously expressed fluorescent protein. A number of fluorescent imaging agents have been developed and are being scaled up for clinical testing [47]. Optical fluorescence imaging allows high-speed and high-sensitivity detection of multiple fluorescent tracers, complementing well other imaging modalities. Yet, the major limitation of tissue and organ-level optical imaging is its restricted depth of penetration, due to light absorption and scattering. Because light attenuation by tissue is wave-

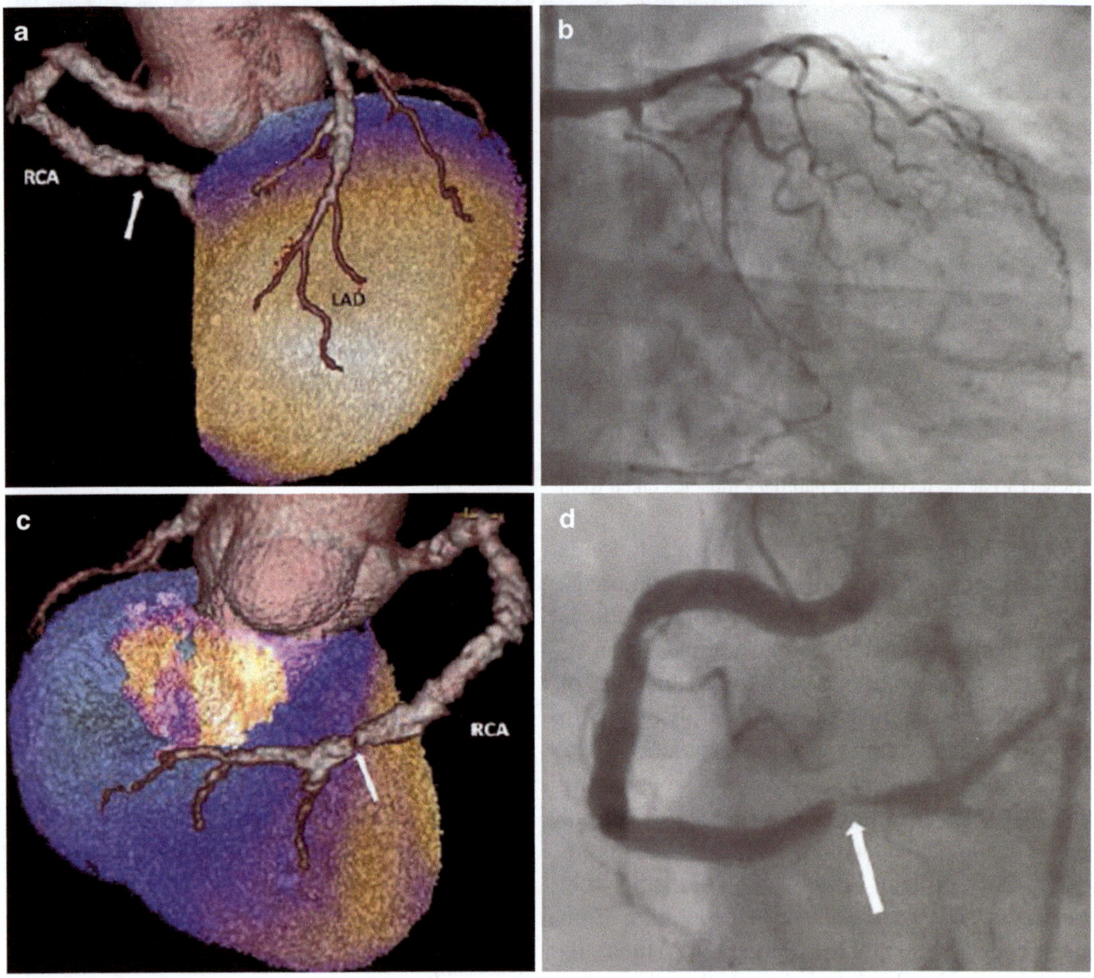

Fig. 22.7 An 80 year old man with exertion chest pain. Stress myocardial perfusion-CTA hybrid images corroborated with invasive angiography. (**a**) MPS-CTA hybrid image showing heavily calcified LAD and RCA. There is normal perfusion (*orange colouration*) to the LAD territory despite significant calcific coronary disease. There is a significant lesion in the mid/distal RCA (*white arrow*). (**b**) Angiography of the LAD shows no obstruction but the extensive calcification seen on CTA is not appreciated. There is a collateral vessel seen from the LCx to the RCA territory. (**c**) MPS-CTA hybrid image showing the inferior wall of the left ventricle and the extensively diseased RCA with obstructive lesion (*white arrow*). There is a moderate to severe reduction in perfusion of the inferior wall (purple and blue colouration). (**d**) Angiography of the RCA shows the obstructive lesion (*white arrow*) but the other extensive calcification is not fully appreciated. *CTA* computed tomography angiography, *MPS* myocardial perfusion scintigraphy, *LAD* left anterior descending, *RCA* right coronary artery, *LCx* left circumflex (Adapted and reproduced from Anagnostopoulos et al. [53]; Lang et al. [50] by permission)

length dependent, fluorescent probes or proteins with more red-shifted emission (near-infrared probes) have been developed to maximize imaging sensitivity and specificity. Optical imaging has inferior spatial resolution compared to other modalities, only reaching up to 1–10 mm. To overcome the problem of limited depth penetration of light in tissue, mostly catheter-based optical approaches have been used.

22.3 Hybrid and Multi-modality Imaging

Hybrid imaging modalities, introduced a decade ago, when the first PET/CT system was launched, are now indispensable, as they offer a combination of functional and anatomic information and correction of emission data, resulting in superior image quality required for quantification. The latest generation of both PET and SPECT clinical and pre-clinical scanners is equipped with ultrafast MDCT (PET/CT, microPET/CT, SPECT/CT, microSPECT/CT) making possible the evaluation of coronary calcification and coronary anatomy and atheromatous plaque morphology in the same setting with myocardial perfusion, viability, molecular targets and ventricular function [48] (Figs. 22.7 and 22.8). Some technical challenges do exist for quantitative cardiac PET/CT. Because CT is acquired during breathhold, misalignment with PET data, which reflect an average over the breathing cycle, can occur [2]. Studies addressing this issue, e.g. by respiratory gating, are currently underway and may provide the methodological

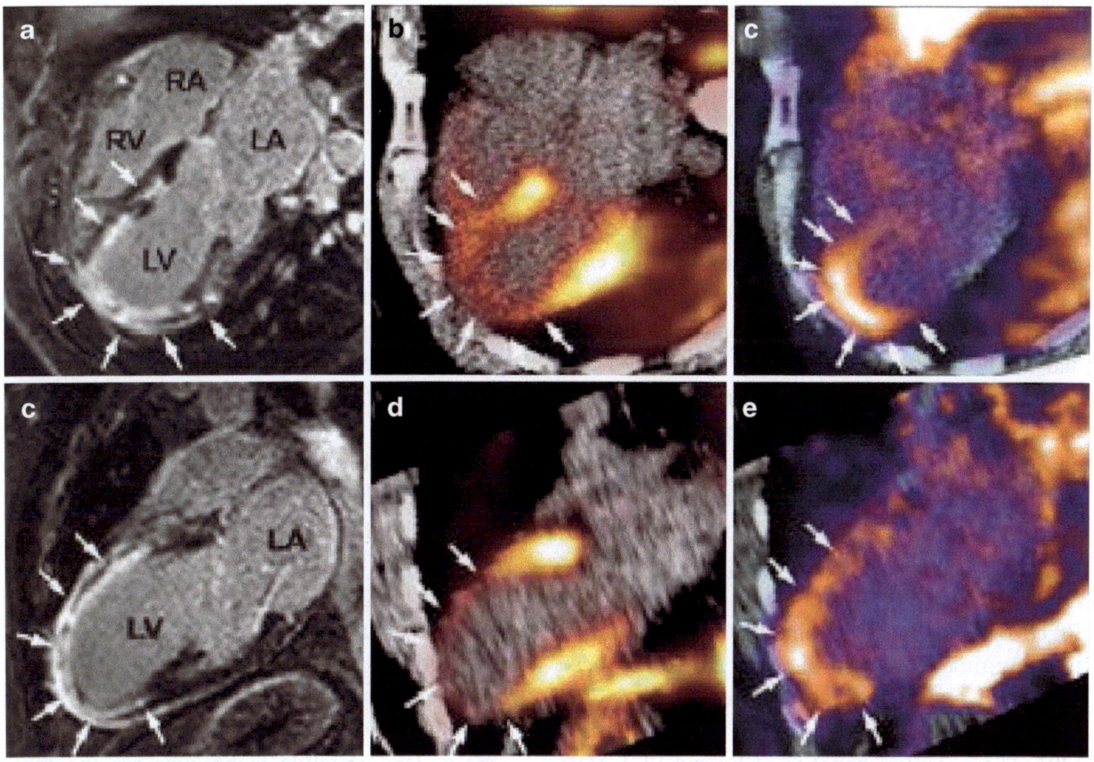

Fig. 22.8 *A* case study from a patient two weeks after MI and PCI who underwent MRI (LGE), ^{13}N ammonia PET/CT and ^{18}F-Galacto-RGD PET/CT. *Panel A and D;* Cardiac Magnetic Resonance with delayed enhancement (*arrows*) extending from the anterior wall to the apical region in the four- (*A*) and two-chamber (*D*) view. *Panel B and E;* Identically reproduced location and geometry with severely reduced myocardial blood flow using ^{13}N-ammonia, corresponding to the regions of delayed enhancement by Cardiac Magnetic Resonance (*arrows*). *Panel C and F;* Focal ^{18}F-RGD signal co-localized to the infarcted area. This signal may reflect angiogenesis within the healing area (*arrows*) (Adapted and reproduced from Makowski et al. [54]; Mulder et al. [51] by permission)

Table 22.3 Potential benefits of hybrid PET/MRI in cardiac imaging

Application	PET	MRI	PET/MRI
Myocardial perfusion imaging	Allows quantification of myocardial blood flow; accurate method to detect functionally significant coronary lesions.	A potential alternative for diagnosis of CAD and assessment of atheromatous plaques' morphology (in experienced centres)	MRI-based correction for attenuation, motion, and partial volume correction for improved quantification of myocardial blood flow?
Non-invasive coronary angiography	–	Presently inferior performance, but no radiation or contrast agents as in coronary CT angiography	Possibility to combine anatomy (plaque burden, luminal obstruction) with haemodynamic consequences (ischaemia) of CAD
Assessment of left ventricle function	Limited by low spatial resolution	Most accurate technique to determine left ventricle function and structure	Combination of left ventricle function with perfusion, metabolic or molecular imaging for improved stratification of heart failure
Assessment of infarction and viability	^{18}F-FDG uptake is a gold standard of viability.	High-resolution delineation of infarction by MRI LGE. Potential of magnetic resonance spectroscopy?	More detailed risk assessment by combining glucose uptake and LGE
Molecular imaging	Excellent sensitivity; tracers for many targets (inflammation, angiogenesis, sympathetic nervous function, therapeutic genes or cells etc.)	Lower sensitivity than PET; evolving tracers and imaging techniques for molecular targets	Exact anatomical localization and volume correction by MRI for detection and quantification of molecular targets by PET

background for future trials evaluating the clinical benefit of PET/CT imaging in patients with cardiac disease.

Hybrid PET/MRI scanners for small animals and humans have been recently introduced and have created high expectations, notably because of the potential for superior tissue contrast, inherent in the MRI modality, as well as the potential for multiparametric functional imaging in conjunction with PET. Access to co-registered, almost simultaneous anatomic, physiologic and molecular measurements have already made PET/MRI the most sophisticated quantitative imaging modality in cardiology. However, these combined approaches are in their infancy and their additive value has yet to be documented [49]. The potential benefits of hybrid PET/MRI in cardiac imaging are displayed in Table 22.3. Development of SPECT/MRI systems for small animals is also an active research area. Except from PET/CT, SPECT/CT and PET/MRI, the greater system flexibility provided by small animal imaging has resulted in the development of bimodal systems such as PET/optical and also of trimodal systems such as PET/SPECT/CT. In addition, attempts have been made to even co-register US images with other imaging modalities such as PET [50]. Accordingly, there is increasing interest in the development of nanoparticles suitable for more than one detection system in order to combine advantages of the different imaging modalities [51, 52].

Conclusions

The translatability of novel molecular imaging techniques depends on a combination of factors such as technological development, fitting animal disease models and probe development. Radionuclide techniques are the most translatable amongst the various non-invasive approaches because of the wide availability of existing scanners, high imaging sensitivity, versatile radiochemistry options and the ongoing development of new imaging agents. They provide superior sensitivity in the evaluation of different cardiovascular targets and pathways at cellular and subcellular level but they suffer from low spatial resolution, exposure to ionizing radiation, lack of anatomic information and there is a need for a generator/cyclotron for radionuclide production. Combining modalities (PET/CT, PET/MR, SPECT/CT and SPECT/MR) can compensate for some of the limitations that may exist in stand-alone imaging modalities while building on their respective strengths. In terms of the utilization of molecular imaging probes in the clinical arena, radionuclide techniques are the most capable for clinical use in the short-term. In the medium term, MRI molecular imaging techniques are certainly promising, pending more demonstrations of clinical performance and safety for both gd-based and iron oxide–based compounds [1]. Molecular US and optical imaging will probably take longer for clinical translation, while CT has low sensitivity to molecular targets and is currently the less explored modality.

References

1. Chen IY, Wu JC. Cardiovascular molecular imaging: focus on clinical translation. Circulation. 2011;123:425–43.
2. Martinez-Moller A, Zikic D, Botnar RM, Bundschuh RA, Howe W, Ziegler SI, et al. Dual cardiac-respiratory gated PET: implementation and results from a feasibility study. Eur J Nucl Med Mol Imaging. 2007;34:1447–54.
3. Phelps ME, Hoffman EJ, Huang S-C, Ter-Pogossian MM. Effect of positron range on spatial resolution. J Nucl Med. 1975;16:649–52.
4. Tai YC, Ruangma A, Rowland D, Siegel S, Newport DF, Chow PL, et al. Performance evaluation of the microPET-Focus: a third generation microPET scanner dedicated to animal imaging. J Nucl Med. 2005;46:455–63.
5. Mc Ardle BA, Dowsley TF, Dekemp RA, Wells GA, Beanlands RS. Does Rubidium-82 PET have superior accuracy to SPECT perfusion imaging for the diagnosis of obstructive coronary disease? A systematic review and meta-analysis. J Am Coll Cardiol. 2012;60:1828–37.
6. Nekolla SG, Reder S, Saraste A, Higuchi T, Dzewas G, Preissel A, et al. Evaluation of the novel myocardial perfusion positron-emission tomography tracer 18F-BMS-747158-02: comparison to 13N-ammonia and validation with microspheres in a pig model. Circulation. 2009;119:2333–42.
7. Berman DS, Maddahi J, Tamarappoo BK, Czernin J, Taillefer R, Udelson JE, et al. Phase II safety and clinical comparison with single-photon emission computed tomography myocardial perfusion imaging for detection of coronary artery disease: flurpiridaz F 18 positron emission tomography. J Am Coll Cardiol. 2013;6:469–77.
8. Ghosh N, Rimoldi OE, Beanlands RS, Camici PG. Assessment of myocardial ischaemia and viability: role of positron emission tomography. Eur Heart J. 2010;31:2984–95.
9. Schwaiger M, Hicks R. The clinical role of metabolic imaging of the heart by positron emission tomography. J Nucl Med. 1991;32:565–78.
10. Higuchi T, Yousefi BH, Kaiser F, Gärtner F, Rischpler C, Reder S, et al. Assessment of the 18F-labeled PET tracer LMI1195 for imaging norepinephrine handling in rat hearts. J Nucl Med. 2013;54:1142–6.
11. Jeong JM, Hong MK, Chang YS, Lee YS, Kim YJ, Cheon GJ, et al. Preparation of a promising angiogenesis PET imaging agent: 68Ga-labeled c(RGDyK)-isothiocyanatobenzyl-1,4,7-triazacyclononane-1,4,7-triacetic acid and feasibility studies in mice. J Nucl Med. 2008;49:830–6.
12. Cohen A, Shirvan A, Levin G, Grimberg H, Reshef A, Ziv I. From the Gla domain to a novel small-molecule detector of apoptosis. Cell Res. 2009;19:625–37.
13. De Saint-Hubert M, Bauwens M, Deckers N, Drummen M, Douma K, Granton P, et al. In vivo molecular imaging of apoptosis and necrosis in atherosclerotic plaques using microSPECT-CT and microPET-CT imaging. Mol Imaging Biol. 2014;16:246–54.
14. Veenman L, Gavish M. The peripheral-type benzodiazepine receptor and the cardiovascular system. Implications for drug development. Pharmacol Ther. 2006;110:503–24.
15. Wagner S, Faust A, Breyholz HJ, Schober O, Schäfers M, Kopka K. The MMP inhibitor (R)-2-(N-benzyl-4-(2-[18F]fluoroethoxy) phenylsulphonamido)-N-hydroxy-3-methylbutanamide: improved precursor synthesis and fully automated radiosynthesis. Appl RadiatIsot. 2011;69:862–8.
16. Joshi NV, Vesey AT, Williams MC, Shah AS, Calvert PA, Craighead FH, et al. 18F-fluoride positron emission tomography for identification of ruptured and high-risk coronary atherosclerotic plaques: a prospective clinical trial. Lancet. 2014;383:705–13.
17. Fukushima K, Bravo PE, Higuchi T, Schuleri KH, Lin X, Abraham MR, et al. Molecular hybrid positron emission tomography/computed tomography imaging of cardiac angiotensin II type 1 receptors. J Am Coll Cardiol. 2012;60:2527–34.
18. Bocher M, Blevis IM, Tsukerman L, Shrem Y, Kovalski G, Volokh L. A fast cardiac gamma camera with dynamic SPECT capabilities: design, system

validation and future potential. Eur J Nucl Med Mol Imaging. 2010;37:1887–902.
19. Baggish AL, Boucher CA. Radiopharmaceutical agents for myocardial perfusion imaging. Circulation. 2008;118:1668–74.
20. Tamaki N, Morita K, Kuge Y, Tsukamoto E. The role of fatty acids in cardiac imaging. J Nucl Med. 2000;41:1525–34.
21. Sisson JC, Wieland DM, Sherman P, Mangner TJ, Tobes MC, Jacques Jr S. Metaiodobenzylguanidine as an index of the adrenergic nervous system integrity and function. J Nucl Med. 1987;28:1620–4.
22. Flotats A, Carrió I, Agostini D, Le Guludec D, Marcassa C, Schäfers M, et al. Proposal for standardization of 123I-metaiodobenzylguanidine (MIBG) cardiac sympathetic imaging by the EANM Cardiovascular Committee and the European Council of Nuclear Cardiology. Eur J Nucl Med Mol Imaging. 2010;37:1802–12.
23. De Saint-Hubert M, Mottaghy FM, Vunckx K, Nuyts J, Fonge H, Prinsen K, et al. Site-specific labeling of 'second generation' annexin V with 99mTc(CO)3 for improved imaging of apoptosis in vivo. Bioorg Med Chem. 2010;18:1356–63.
24. Hartung D, Schäfers M, Fujimoto S, Levkau B, Narula N, Kopka K, et al. Targeting of matrix metalloproteinase activation for noninvasive detection of vulnerable atherosclerotic lesions. Eur J Nucl Med Mol Imaging. 2007;34 Suppl 1:1–8.
25. Verjans JW, Lovhaug D, Narula N, Petrov AD, Indrevoll B, Bjurgert E, et al. Noninvasive imaging of angiotensin receptors after myocardial infarction. JACC Cardiovasc Imaging. 2008;1:354–62.
26. Budinger TF, Lauterbur PC. Nuclear magnetic resonance technology for medical studies. Science. 1984;226:288–98.
27. Nandalur KR, Dwamena BA, Choudhri AF, Nandalur MR, Carlos RC. Diagnostic performance of stress cardiac magnetic resonance imaging in the detection of coronary artery disease: a meta-analysis. J Am Coll Cardiol. 2007;50:1343–53.
28. Gebker R, Jahnke C, Manka R, Frick M, Hucko T, Kozerke S, et al. High spatial resolution myocardial perfusion imaging during high dose dobutamine/atropine stress magnetic resonance using k–t SENSE. Int J Cardiol. 2012;158:411–6.
29. Hudsmith LE, Neubauer S. Magnetic resonance spectroscopy in myocardial disease. JACC Cardiovasc Imaging. 2009;2:87–96.
30. Lipinski MJ, Amirbekian V, Frias JC, Aguinaldo JG, Mani V, Briley-Saebo KC, et al. MRI to detect atherosclerosis with gadolinium-containing immunomicelles targeting the macrophage scavenger receptor. Magn Reson Med. 2006;56:601–10.
31. Lipinski MJ, Frias JC, Amirbekian V, Briley-Saebo KC, Mani V, Samber D, et al. Macrophage-specific lipid-based nanoparticles improve cardiac magnetic resonance detection and characterization of human atherosclerosis. JACC Cardiovasc Imaging. 2009;2:637–47.
32. Nahrendorf M, Sosnovik D, Chen JW, Panizzi P, Figueiredo JL, Aikawa E, et al. Activatable magnetic resonance imaging agent reports myeloperoxidase activity in healing infarcts and noninvasively detects the anti-inflammatory effects of atorvastatin on ischemia-reperfusion injury. Circulation. 2008;117:1153–60.
33. Spuentrup E, Fausten B, Kinzel S, Wiethoff AJ, Botnar RM, Graham PB, et al. Molecular magnetic resonance imaging of atrial clots in a swine model. Circulation. 2005;112:396–9.
34. Sosnovik DE, Nahrendorf M, Panizzi P, Matsui T, Aikawa E, Dai G, et al. Molecular MRI detects low levels of cardiomyocyte apoptosis in a transgenic model of chronic heart failure. Circ Cardiovasc Imaging. 2009;2:468–75.
35. Kooi ME, Cappendijk VC, Cleutjens KB, Kessels AG, Kitslaar PJ, Borgers M, et al. Accumulation of ultrasmall superparamagnetic particles of iron oxide in human atherosclerotic plaques can be detected by in vivo magnetic resonance imaging. Circulation. 2003;107:2453–8.
36. Howarth SP, Li ZY, Tang TY, Graves MJ, U-King-Im JM, Gillard JH. In vivo positive contrast IRON sequence and quantitative T(2)* measurement confirms inflammatory burden in a patient with asymptomatic carotid atheroma after USPIO-enhanced MR imaging. J Vasc Interv Radiol. 2008;19:446–8.
37. Burtea C, Ballet S, Laurent S, Rousseaux O, Dencausse A, Gonzalez W, et al. Development of a magnetic resonance imaging protocol for the characterization of atherosclerotic plaque by using vascular cell adhesion molecule-1 and apoptosis targeted ultrasmall superparamagnetic iron oxide derivatives. Arterioscler Thromb Vasc Biol. 2012;32:36–48.
38. Neubauer AM, Myerson J, Caruthers SD, Hockett FD, Winter PM, Chen J, et al. Gadolinium-modulated 19F signals from perfluorocarbon nanoparticles as a new strategy for molecular imaging. Magn Reson Med. 2008;60:1066–72.
39. Chang SM, Bhatti S, Nabi F. Coronary computed tomography angiography. Curr Opin Cardiol. 2011;26:392–402.
40. Rossi A, Uitterdijk A, Dijkshoorn M, Klotz E, Dharampal A, van Straten M, et al. Quantification of myocardial blood flow by adenosine-stress CT perfusion imaging in pigs during various degrees of stenosis correlates well with coronary artery blood flow and fractional flow reserve. Eur Heart J Cardiovasc Imaging. 2012;14:331–8.
41. So A, Hsieh J, Li JY, Hadway J, Kong HF, Lee TY. Quantitative myocardial perfusion measurement using CT perfusion: a validation study in a porcine model of reperfused acute myocardial infarction. Int J Cardiovasc Imaging. 2012;28:1237–48.
42. Rossi A, Dharampal A, Wragg A, Davies LC, van Geuns RJ, Anagnostopoulos C, et al. Diagnostic performance of hyperaemic myocardial blood flow index obtained by dynamic computed tomography: does it predict functionally significant coronary lesions? Eur Heart J Cardiovasc Imaging. 2014;15:85–94.

43. Hyafil F, Cornily JC, Rudd JH, Machac J, Feldman LJ, Fayad ZA. Quantification of inflammation within rabbit atherosclerotic plaques using the macrophage-specific CT contrast agent N1177: a comparison with 18F-FDG PET/CT and histology. J Nucl Med. 2009;50:959–65.
44. Cormode DP, Skajaa T, van Schooneveld MM, Koole R, Jarzyna P, Lobatto ME, et al. Nanocrystal core high-density lipoproteins: a multimodality contrast agent platform. Nano Lett. 2008;8:3715–23.
45. Dodla S, Xie F, Smith M, O'Leary E, Porter TR. Real-time perfusion echocardiography during treadmill exercise and dobutamine stress testing. Heart. 2010;96:220–5.
46. de Jong N, Bouakaz A, Frinking P. Basic acoustic properties of microbubbles. Echocardiography. 2002;19:229–40.
47. Jaffer FA, Libby P, Weissleder R. Optical and multimodality molecular imaging: insights into atherosclerosis. Arterioscler Thromb Vasc Biol. 2009;29:1017–24.
48. Blankstein R, Di Carli MF. Integration of coronary anatomy and myocardial perfusion imaging. Nat Rev Cardiol. 2010;7:226–36.
49. Rischpler C, Nekolla SG, Dregely I, Schwaiger M. Hybrid PET/MR imaging of the heart: potential initial experiences, and future prospects. J Nucl Med. 2013;5:402–15.
50. Lang N, Hermann S, Hold S, Mienkina M, Stegger L, Stypmann J, et al. Hybrid 3D Sono/PET in a mouse. Eur J Nucl Med Mol Imaging. 2007;34:1706–7.
51. Mulder WJ, Strijkers GJ, Briley-Saboe KC, Frias JC, Aguinaldo JG, Vucic E, et al. Molecular imaging of macrophages in atherosclerotic plaques using bimodal PEG-micelles. Magn Reson Med. 2007;58:1164–70.
52. Sosnovik DE, Schellenberger EA, Nahrendorf M, Novikov MS, Matsui T, Dai G, et al. Magnetic resonance imaging of cardiomyocyte apoptosis with a novel magneto-optical nanoparticle. Magn Reson Med. 2005;54:718–24.
53. Anagnostopoulos C, Neill J, Reyes E, Prvulovich E. Myocardial perfusion scintigraphy: technical innovations and evolving clinical applications. Heart. 2012;98:353–9.
54. Makowski MR, Ebersberger U, Nekolla S, Schwaiger M. In vivo molecular imaging of angiogenesis, targeting alphavbeta3 integrin expression, in a patient after acute myocardial infarction. Eur Heart J. 2008;29: 2201.

Cardiovascular Applications of Non-invasive Imaging in Cardiovascular Diseases: From Bench to Bedside

23

Constantinos D. Anagnostopoulos, Anna N. Paschali, and Stephan G. Nekolla

Abstract

Advances in basic cardiovascular sciences have enhanced our understanding of disease pathogenesis at the genomic, transcriptional and proteomic level. Translation of basic research into clinical practice has played a major role in prevention, diagnosis and therapy of cardiovascular diseases (CVD), and in this context, the contribution of non invasive imaging (PET, SPECT, MRI, CT, US, optical imaging and hybrid modalities) has been instrumental. In the years to come, evaluation of myocardial perfusion and ventricular function by non invasive techniques will remain important for diagnosis and management of patients investigated for CVD, but such information will be augmented by an understanding of the contribution of other parameters such as myocardial metabolism, innervation, inflammation, angiogenesis, apoptosis, thrombosis and extracellular matrix alterations of the vessel wall or the myocardium. Suitable imaging probes for those targets may provide tools for early identification of individuals who are at risk of cardiovascular events, refining prediction based on current risk scoring models and existing non invasive tools.

C.D. Anagnostopoulos, MD (✉)
Centre for Experimental Surgery, Clinical and Translational Research Biomedical Research Foundation, Academy of Athens,
4 Soranou Ephessiou Street, 11527 Athens, Greece
e-mail: cdanagnostopoulos@bioacademy.gr; http://www.bioacademy.gr/lab/anagnostopoulos

A.N. Paschali, MD, MSc, PhD
Medical School and Centre for Clinical Research, University of Patras, Biomedical Research Foundation, Academy of Athens,
4 Soranou Ephessiou Street, 11527 Athens, Greece
e-mail: apashali@upatras.gr

S.G. Nekolla, PhD
Multimodal Cardiac Imaging, Nuklearmedizinische Klinik und Poliklinik Klinikumrechts der Isar der Technischen Universitaet München,
Ismaningerstr. 22, D-81675 Munich, Germany
e-mail: stephan.nekolla@tum.de

D.V. Cokkinos (ed.), *Introduction to Translational Cardiovascular Research*,
DOI 10.1007/978-3-319-08798-6_23, © Springer International Publishing Switzerland 2015

Keywords
Cardiovascular Translational Research • Multimodality imaging • Atherosclerosis • Vulnerable plaque • Ischemic heart disease • LV remodeling • Heart failure

Abbreviations

ACS	Acute coronary syndromes
APO	Apoptosis
ATH	Atherosclerosis
AT_1R	Angiotensin II type 1 receptor
AVS	Aortic valve stenosis
bFGF	Basic fibroblast growth factor
BMCs	Bone marrow–derived stem cells
BMIPP	b-Methyliodophenylpentadecanoic acid
BNP	Blood natriuretic peptide
CAD	Coronary artery disease
CEUS	Contrast-enhanced ultrasonography
CRT	Cardiac resynchronisation therapy
CT	Computed tomography
CVD	Cardiovascular diseases
DSE	Dobutamine stress ECHO
EC	Endothelial cells
ECHO	Echocardiography
EPI	Epinephrine
FA	Fatty acids
FDG	Fluoro-deoxyglucose
FRS	Framingham risk score
Gd	Gadolinium
HED	Hydroxyephedrine
HF	Heart failure
HiB	Hibernation
HIPs	High-intensity plaques
ICAM-1	Intercellular adhesion molecule-1
IHD	Ischemic heart disease
INFL	Inflammation
LDL	Low density lipoprotein
LGE	Late gadolinium enhancement
LV	Left ventricle
MBF	Myocardial blood flow
MCP-1	Monocyte chemotactic protein-1
MDCT	Multidetector computed tomography
MI	Myocardial infarction
MIBG	Metaiodobenzylguanidine
MMPs	Matrix-metalloproteinases
MPI	Myocardial perfusion imaging
MPO	Myeloperoxidase
MPR	Myocardial perfusion reserve
MRA	Magnetic resonance angiography
MRI	Magnetic resonance imaging
MVO	Microvascular obstruction
N	Necrosis
NaF	Sodium fluoride
PBR	Peripheral benzodiazepine receptor
PCI	Percutaneous coronary intervention
PET	Positron Emission Tomography
RAAS	Renin Angiotensin-Aldosterone System
REM	Remodeling
SCA	Sudden cardiac arrest
SMCs	Smooth muscle cells
SPECT	Single Photon Emission Computed Tomography
SPIOs	Small iron-oxide nanoparticles
TCFA	Thin-cap fibroatheroma
TIA	Transient ischemic attack
US	Ultrasound
VCAM-1	Vascular cell adhesion molecule-1
VEGF	Vascular endothelial growth factor

23.1 Introduction

Cardiovascular research has enhanced our understanding of disease pathogenesis at the genomic, transcriptional and proteomic level. Translation of basic research into clinical practice has played a major role in prevention, diagnosis and therapy of cardiovascular diseases (CVD), and in this context, the contribution of non-invasive imaging has been instrumental. In this chapter we discuss the main directions of non invasive imaging in cardiovascular translational research. Novel molecular imaging approaches will be described in the context of investigation of different pathological entities with an emphasis on atherosclerosis (ATH) and its consequences to the vessel wall and the myocardium.

23.2 Pathological Entities

23.2.1 Atherosclerosis and the Vulnerable Plaque

ATH a leading cause of mortality in the developed world, is a chronic, progressive inflammatory and lipid deposition process in the arterial wall, with a long asymptomatic phase. The process starts at sites of endothelial injury resulting from a variety of factors, including hypertension, dyslipidemia and noxious substances in cigarette smoke among others. These factors downregulate endothelial cells (EC) production of nitric oxide, thereby impairing vasodilatory capacity and protective functions. As a result, low density lipoprotein (LDL) infiltrates the subendothelial space. Dysfunctional EC express a number of adhesion molecules (vascular cell adhesion molecule-1 ''VCAM-1'', intercellular adhesion molecule-1, ''ICAM-1'') and selectins (E-selectin and P-selectin) that promote the binding of circulating T-lymphocytes and monocytes to vascular EC. Chemokines such as monocyte chemotactic protein-1 (MCP-1) are also implicated in the recruitment process of leucocytes, predominantly monocytes to the vessel wall. In the vessel wall monocytes differentiate into macrophages that internalize oxidised LDL and evolve into foam cells. Over time, EC, macrophages, and smooth muscle cells (SMCs) die from apoptosis (APO) or necrosis (N), promoting the formation of a necrotic core and plaque expansion. Macrophages and T-lymphocytes via secreting proteolytic enzymes, such as matrix metalloproteinases (MMPs) and cathepsins, cytokines, growth factors and pro-inflammatory mediators create an inflammatory micro-environment. In this environment, SMCs travel from the media layer into the plaque, transform into fibroblasts and build a fibrotic tissue replacing the endothelium on top, forming the fibrous cap [1].

The predominant form of vulnerable plaque, termed thin-cap fibroatheroma (TCFA), has been shown by ex vivo histology of human cadavers to have a thin fibrous cap (<65 μm), a large necrotic lipid core (>10 % plaque area), a paucity of SMCs, and heavy infiltration of the fibrous cap by inflammatory cells (i.e., macrophages). The initiation of plaque rupture has been linked to macrophages that contribute to the digestion of the fibrous cap by upregulating MMPs. Also, high rate of macrophage and SMCs APO as well as intraplaque angiogenesis by proliferation of medial vasa vasorum and intraplaque haemorrhage have been implicated in plaque rupture [2].

At first, the vessel wall expands outwards rather than inwards, i.e. the whole cross sectional area of the vessel increases whilst the lumen does not change significantly (vascular remodeling). Due to outward remodeling (REM) of the atherosclerotic vessel wall which compensates the narrowing of the vessel lumen by the plaque, there is no significant luminal obstruction and patients remain asymptomatic. Therefore such plaques can be undetectable with the current morphological techniques (X-ray or CT angiography) and plaque rupture is unpredictable. However, as the plaque continues to enlarge, the lumen begins to be compromised and the changes which occur can be assessed by non invasive imaging. Conventional multidetector computed tomography (MDCT) and magnetic resonance angiography (MRA) are capable of non-invasively detecting plaques on the basis of their morphology or tissue composition but cannot distinguish the molecular signatures of rupture-prone (vulnerable) plaques from those of stable plaques. Molecular imaging can visualize the critical biological aspects that are otherwise undetected by conventional imaging methods. The major goal of imaging in this setting is to detect high-risk plaques, refine risk stratification and answer questions that guide treatment decisions, e.g. which lesion should be treated by mechanical intervention and which should be left alone.

In this section we describe the *non invasive imaging techniques* that have been tested in this field with emphasis in those which have evolved from the preclinical setting to the first in man application and then to clinical practice. They comprise a range of molecular imaging approaches based on the multifaceted pathophysiology of ATH progression, targeting EC activation, inflammation (INFL), APO, matrix REM, angiogenesis, lipid core and fibrous cup formation and thrombosis (Fig. 23.1, Table 23.1A). Invasive techniques such as intra-vascular ultrasound (IVUS and

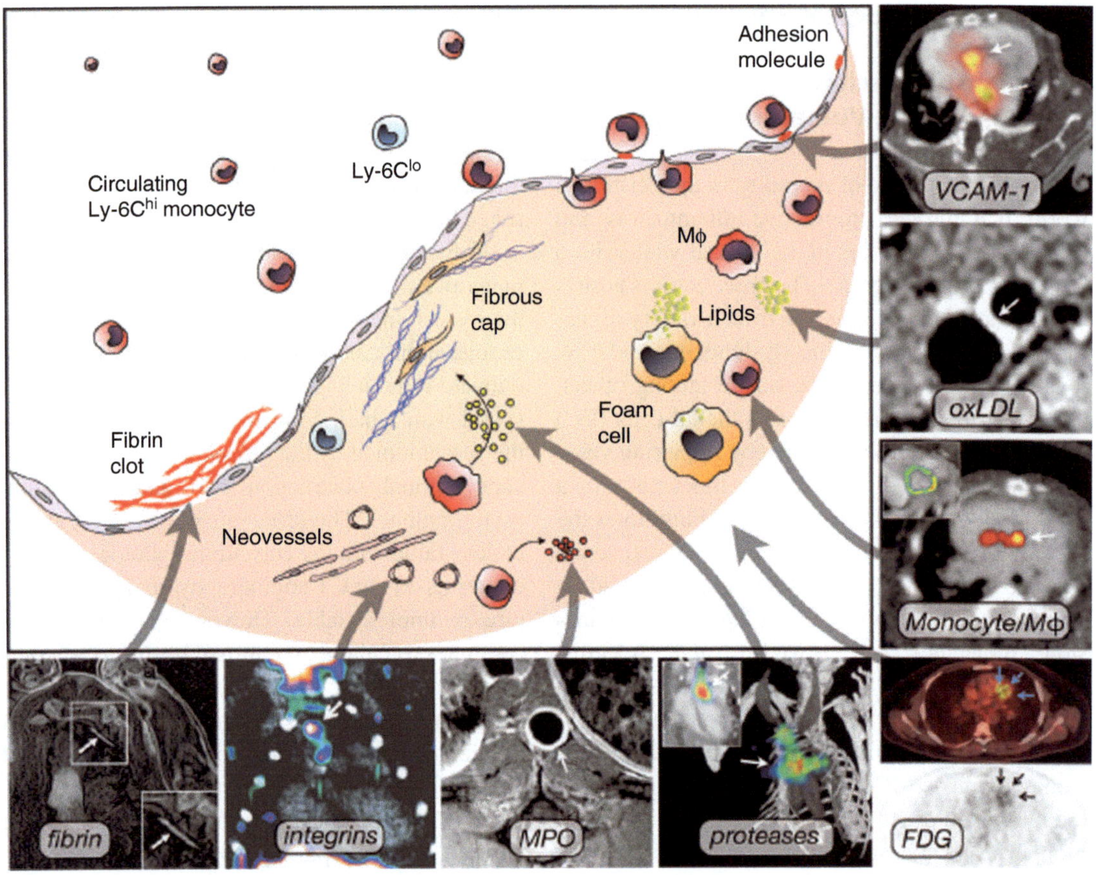

Fig. 23.1 Selected molecular imaging targets in atherosclerosis. (**a**) PET-CT imaging of adhesion molecule expression in apoE/mice with the ^{18}F -VCAM–1 ligand. (**b**) Gd-loaded microvesicles targeted to oxLDL macrophage receptor, result in increased T1 MRI contrast. (**c**) Macrophage quantitation in atherosclerotic plaque using iron oxide nanoparticles that increase T2* contrast on MRI. (**d**) FDG/PET-CT imaging of metabolic activity in a patient with coronary heart disease using the glucose analog ^{18}F-FDG. (**e**) Fluorescence Tomography-CT imaging of cathepsin protease activity in the root of apoE/mice. (**f**) MRI of myeloperoxidase activity in a rabbit model of atherosclerosis. (**g**) PET-CT imaging of integrins using ^{18}F-Galacto-RGD in LDLr/mice. (**h**) MRI of fibrin within coronary artery clots in a swine model (Adapted and reproduced from Leuschner and Nahrendorf [113], [3] by permission)

virtual histology IVUS) and intracoronary optical coherence tomography (OCT) which offer unique capabilities of superior resolution (100 μm for IVUS and 10–20 μm for OCT) for the detection of TCFA and for intravascular characterization of plaque architecture are by definition, outside the scope of this chapter.

23.2.1.1 Preclinical Molecular Imaging of Atherosclerosis and the Vulnerable Plaque

Endothelial dysfunction is one of the first changes occurring in patients with ATH. Imaging of EC activation has been accomplished targeting VCAM-1 in mice models with ATH, using microPET/CT imaging with the ^{18}F -VCAM–1 ligand or with small iron-oxide nanoparticles (SPIOs) [VCAM-1 targeted USPIO derivative (R832)] for microMRI imaging, offering also the possibility to add fluorescent dyes for optical verification in vivo [3]. Microbubbles that target VCAM-1, and P-selectin for molecular ultrasound (US) imaging have also been developed [4]. In addition, studies in rabbits have confirmed monocyte trafficking in atheroma using the monocyte chemotactic protein-1 (MCP-1)

Table 23.1 Non-invasive *molecular* imaging in cardiovascular translational research (from bench to bedside); *A. Atherosclerosis*, *B. Ischemic heart disease*, *C. Ischemic injury and post-infarction remodeling*, *D. Heart failure*

Imaging targets		Endothelial dysfunction/adhesion molecules (VCAM-1, selectins, MCP-1)	Inflammation/ activated macrophages	Spotty calcifications	Apoptosis (phosphatidylserine)	MMPs	Angiogenesis (integrin αvβ3)	Thrombus (fibrin, glycoprotein IIb/IIIa)
A. Atherosclerosis	Pre-clinical	PET, SPECT, MRI, optical imaging, ECHO.	PET, SPECT, MRI, CT	Optical imaging	SPECT, PET, MRI	SPECT, MRI, optical imaging	PET, MRI, optical imaging, ECHO	MRI, PET, ECHO
	Clinical	No	PET/FDG (clinical trials) MRI (studies)	PET/NaF (initial studies)	Limited data	No	Limited data	Fibrin-targeted MRI (clinical trials)

Imaging targets		Myocardial perfusion	Ischemic memory
B. Ischemic heart disease	Pre-clinical	SPECT and PET MPI, CE-MRI, ECHO, CT	SPECT/BMIPP, ECHO-microbubbles
	Clinical	SPECT and PET MPI, CE-MRI, ECHO, CT	SPECT/BMIPP

Imaging targets		Myocardial perfusion	Apoptosis/necrosis	Inflammation/activated macrophages	MMPs	RAAS	Angiogenesis/integrin αvβ3, VEGF
C. Ischemic injury and post-infarction remodeling	Pre-clinical	SPECT and PET MPI, CE-MRI, ECHO, CT	Dual-contrast MRI	PET/FDG, MRI, ECHO-microbubbles	SPECT, optical imaging	SPECT, PET	PET, SPECT, MRI, ECHO-microbubbles
	Clinical	SPECT and PET MPI, LGE-MRI, ECHO, CT	Limited data on apoptosis/necrosis	Limited data	No	Limited data	Limited data

Imaging targets		Myocardial perfusion	Myocardial viability	Myocardial innervation
D. Heart failure	Pre-clinical	SPECT and PET MPI, CE-MRI, ECHO, CT	Glucose metabolism (FDG PET) FA metabolism (SPECT, PET) Oxidative metabolism (PET) Cell membrane integrity (TL-SPECT) Intact mitochondria (Tc-SPECT) (Recruitment of) myocardial thickness/motion (ECHO, cine MRI, G-SPECT) LGE-MRI	PET (HED, EPI), SPECT (MIBG)
	Clinical	SPECT and PET MPI, CE-MRI	The same as in pre-clinical imaging	PET (HED), SPECT (MIBG)

CE-MRI contrast enhanced MRI, *CEUS* contrast enhanced ultrasound, *CT* computed tomography, *ECHO* echocardiography, *EPI* epinephrine, *FA* fatty acid, *G-SPECT* gated SPECT, *HED* hydroxyl-ephedrine, *LGE MRI* late gadolinium enhancement MRI, *MIBG* metaiodobenzylguanidine, *MPI* myocardial perfusion imaging, *MRI* magnetic resonance imaging, *NaF* sodium fluoride, *NP* nanoparticle, *PET* positron emission tomography, *RAAS* rennin angiotensin-aldosterone system, *SPECT* single photon emission computed tomography, *Tc* Technetium-99m, *TL* Thalium-201 labeled with ^{99m}Tc (microSPECT) [5]. All of these agents remain still in the preclinical level and further studies will be required to test their effectiveness towards clinical applications.

INFL is a key feature of plaque destabilization and therefore an attractive imaging target. A number of techniques and agents have been developed. Herein we describe these which have already been introduced in the clinical setting and those which have shown promising results at a preclinical level: Activated macrophages have been targeted with radionuclide methods based either on their increased glycolytic activity (by FDG PET) or by targeting specific receptors. The feasibility of plaque INFL imaging with ^{18}F-Fluoro-deoxyglucose (FDG) was established in animal (small and large) models of aortic ATH, with results showing a three- to fivefold greater ^{18}F-FDG uptake in atherosclerotic aortas than in normal aortas [6]. Several receptors upregulated in activated macrophages have been exploited in pre-clinical imaging of ATH, such as LOX-1 with the use of ^{99m}Tc anti-LOX-1 antibody for SPECT imaging [7] or peripheral benzodiazepine receptor (PBR) with the use of ^{11}C-PK11195 for PET imaging in mice and rabbits [8]. An MRI based approach has also been tested in animal models (rabbits) for imaging of vessel wall INFL using SPIOs [9] or alternatively with the Gd-containing immunomicelles [10] or lipid-based nanoparticles [11]. In addition, MDCT has been employed in imaging of INFL with the use of iodinated [12] or gold [13] nanoparticles that selectively accumulate into macrophages. Although promising, these results remain yet to be confirmed in clinical studies.

Arterial calcification is part of the development of ATH and is related to cardiovascular risk. *Active calcification* progressively increases given that the inflammatory cascade contributes to calcium deposition. Although large calcifications inside the plaque have been linked by some to plaque stability, *spotty calcifications*, especially inside the fibrous cap, are suggested to cause plaque rupture and thrombotic events, as it is assumed to be a product of osteogenic action by osteocytic- and chondrocytic-like cells inside the plaque [14]. In a mouse model of ATH, Aikawa et al. [15] were able to detect INFL and microcalcifications in early atherosclerotic plaques using a nanoparticle-based contrast agent to visualize macrophages and a bisphosphonate-derivatized near-infrared fluorescent imaging agent to detect calcifications. They showed that macrophage infiltration in early atherosclerotic plaques precedes calcification.

Another feature of plaque instability is the high rate of *macrophage APO*. It is a typical feature of fibrous caps of vulnerable and ruptured atherosclerotic plaques and it has also been an imaging target by a variety of non invasive techniques. In a pioneering study of molecular imaging of APO with ^{99m}Tc-labeled annexin-V (^{99m}Tc-anxA5) SPECT, Kolodgie et al. [16] demonstrated the feasibility to target APO in rabbit models of ATH. Further experimental studies in rabbits have demonstrated that novel therapies with caspase inhibitors suppress atherosclerotic plaque APO in vivo using ^{99m}Tc-anxA5 micro-SPECT/CT [17]. Moreover, in a recent study in mice models using novel radiotracers to image APO (^{99m}Tc-HIS-AnxA5) and N (^{124}I hypericin) with SPECT/CT and PET/CT respectively, De Saint-Hubert et al. [18] showed that APO and N imaging is feasible in principle, but there are still hurdles to overcome including further optimization in biodistribution probes characteristics that is essential before such findings are translated to humans. APO -targeted ultra small super paramagnetic iron oxide derivatives (USPIO-R826) have also been tested with MRI in mice models and seem to be highly promising tools for ATH imaging contributing to the detection of vulnerable plaques [3].

With vessel REM that occurs in ATH, there is activation of several proteases (e.g., MMPs or cathepsin G) that also have significant detrimental effects on cap thickness and therefore plaque stability. The advantage of imaging MMPs is the assessment of the activity of macrophages rather than their density in vulnerable plaques. Up to date, 23 MMPs have been identified. A large variety of synthetic MMPs ligands with high affinity has been developed in the past. These small molecules act as MMP inhibitors and were first tested as anticancer drugs. Different MMPs imaging approaches for SPECT, MRI and optical imaging have been successfully tested in various animal models of ATH. Recently the first GMP-conform MMP inhibitor labeled with ^{18}F suitable for PET imaging was described [19], paving the way for the first studies in humans in the near future.

An additional imaging target is *intraplaque angiogenesis* that is manifested by proliferation of medial vasa vasorum and has been implicated in rapid plaque growth, intraplaque haemorrhage, and plaque rupture. Integrin αvβ3 is a potential imaging target for plaque and vasa vasorum neovascularization. Winter et al. [20] showed in rabbits that in vivo imaging of neovascularization of atherosclerotic plaques using MRI targeting αvβ3 paramagnetic nanoparticles is feasible and might provide a method for defining the burden and evolution of ATH. More recently, cyclic peptides that contain the Arg-Gly-Asp (RGD) attachment site labeled for optical imaging or PET have demonstrated focally increased uptake in advanced, macrophage-rich atherosclerotic lesions of hypercholesterolaemic mice [21].

Thrombus formation may also be a useful target for identification of complicated atherosclerotic lesions as well as sources of thrombo-embolism. Inflamed endothelium and cells participating in the development of the necrotic core show high levels of fibrin and thrombin expression. Molecular MRI with the fibrin-targeted contrast-agent EP-2104R has been demonstrated in animal models allowing selective visualization of acute coronary, brachiocephalic artery, cardiac, and pulmonary thrombi [22]. MRI of thrombus has been otherwise achieved at high fields (9.4 T) in mouse models of carotid thrombosis by use of single-chain antibody-conjugated SPIOs targeted to the glycoprotein IIb/IIIa of activated platelets [23]. This approach represents a novel noninvasive technique allowing the detection and quantification of platelet-containing thrombi and could be further tested in humans. Whether it can also be applicable to assessing thrombosis in human coronary vessels where plaque assessment is challenging due to the small vessel size remains unknown at present. US microbubble targeting of the thrombus has also been investigated using an approach based on the surface conjugation of ligands that recognize the platelet glycoprotein IIb/IIIa, fibrin, and tissue factor. In terms of radionuclide imaging, a recently described tracer (^{99m}Tc-fucoidan) has demonstrated its use to image P-selectin overexpression in arterial thrombosis and EC activation in animal models [24]. Three new fibrin-targeted PET probes (FBP1, FBP2, FBP3) have been tested with micro-PET/MRI in rat models of carotid artery thrombosis with promising results, as identification of thrombi was confirmed in those experimental studies ex vivo by autoradiography [25].

23.2.1.2 Clinical Molecular Imaging of Atherosclerosis and the Vulnerable Plaque

A decade ago FDG uptake was for the first time described as an incidental finding in the vascular wall of large arteries in oncological patients. Yun et al. [26] reported that along all vascular beds (aorta, iliac, and femoral arteries), age and hypercholesterolemia were correlated with the degree of FDG uptake. The clinical feasibility of ^{18}F-FDG plaque imaging has been demonstrated in patients with carotid, aortic, femoral, and iliac ATH [27–29] with proven high reproducibility [27] (Fig. 23.2). Positive correlation has been observed between ^{18}F-FDG PET activity and CD68-immunostaining for macrophages in endarterectomy samples from carotid plaques [29], as well as between FDG and increased biomarkers of angiogenesis [vascular endothelial growth factor (VEGF)] [30]. Although quantification of FDG uptake is a highly reproducible measure, it does vary over time suggesting that INFL may be a transient feature of ATH which waxes and wanes as disease progresses [30].

Clinical FDG PET/CT studies have shown that vascular calcification (as assessed by CT) and vascular metabolic activity (assessed by PET) rarely overlap, whereas plaque calcification was inversely related to PET and histologic biomarkers of INFL, suggesting that these findings represent different stages in the evolution of atheroma [31]. INFL burden assessed by PET corresponds to high risk morphology plaques (positive REM

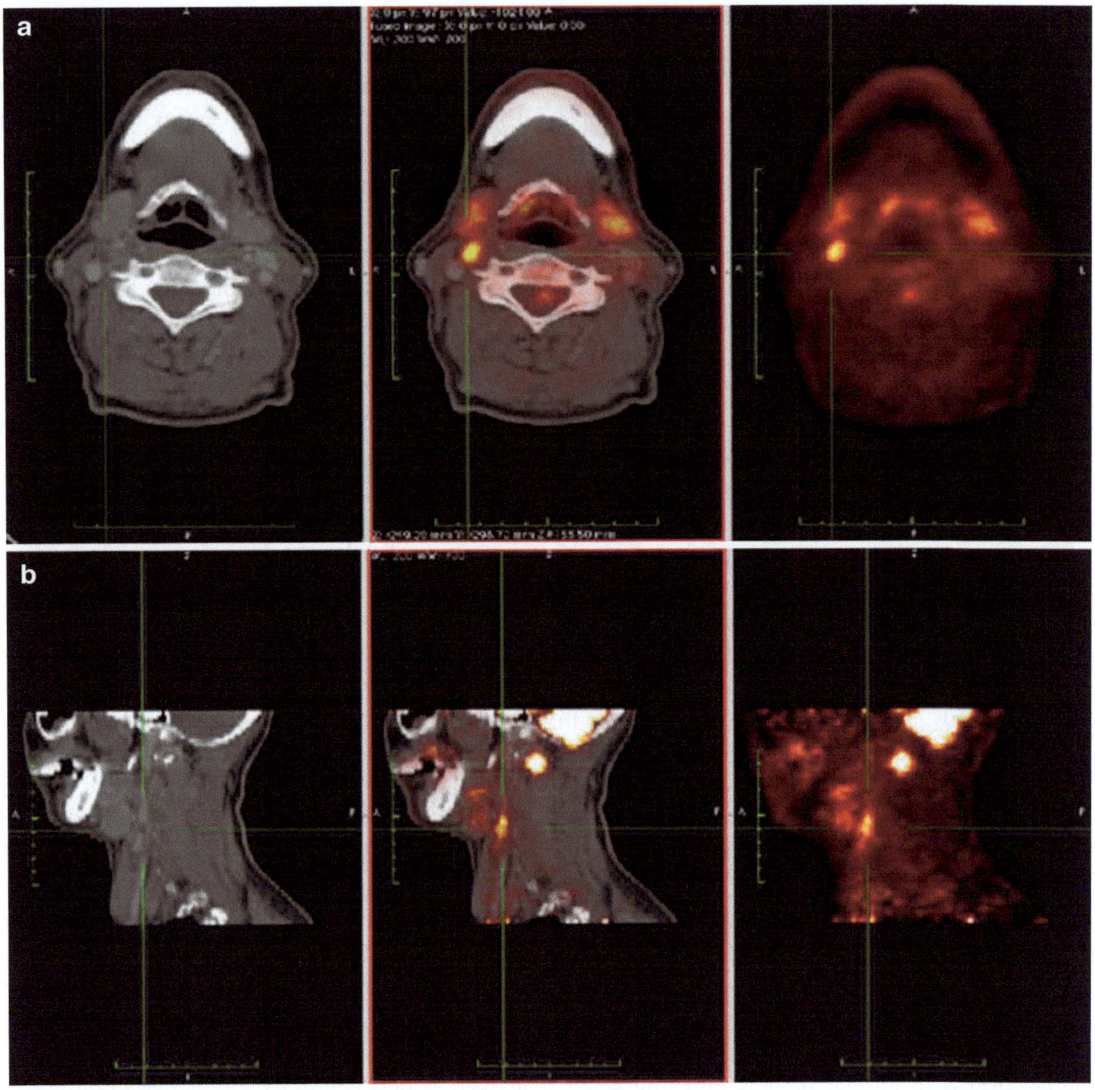

Fig. 23.2 Example of qualitative assessment of FDG uptake in right-side carotid artery plaque from a patient with high plaque uptake. (**a**) Transverse and (**b**) sagittal slice of same patient. Both CT (*left*), FDG-PET (*right*) and fused image (*middle*) are shown (Adapted and reproduced from Graebe et al. [114], [29] by permission)

and low attenuation), as assessed by CT [32]. The time interval between symptoms [transient ischaemic attack (TIA)/stroke] and a significantly positive ipsilateral FDG PET result in the culprit lesion was also investigated and found to be about 38 days [33]. The observation that PET imaging in close proximity to the time of the event (TIA or stroke) reveals higher lesional-to contralesional max SUV ratios in the culprit vessels compared to those with chronic stenosis was also confirmed more recently by a different research group [34]. Whether FDG PET could improve the clinical management of patients with carotid stenosis remains to be proven, but at the moment, FDG-PET can only complement conventional anatomic imaging (US, CT and MRA) towards risk assessment for future stroke [34]. The interrelationship of atherosclerotic disease across arterial beds has also been evaluated using FDG imaging. Rudd et al. [31] have demonstrated a positive relationship between uptake in adjacent territories and along paired left and right arterial beds.

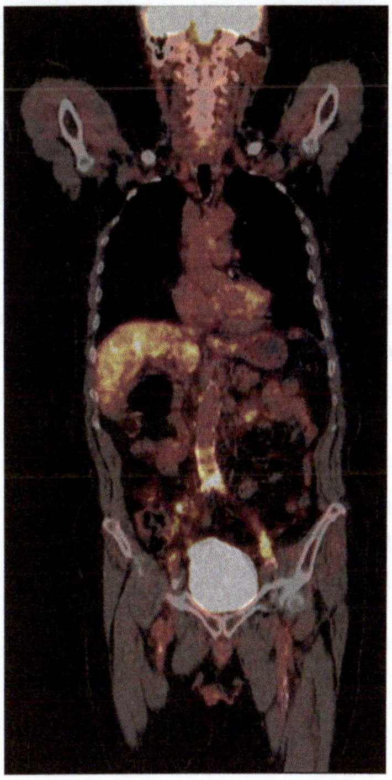

Fig. 23.3 Coronal ^{18}F PET/CT image of a patient depicting high uptake of tracer in the lower part of the abdominal aorta and the left common iliac artery suggestive of atherosclerosis

Multi-vascular evaluation of disease has been proposed, given that high FDG uptake across major vascular beds including the aorta, iliac, and carotid arteries is a predictor of future cardiovascular events [35] (Fig. 23.3).

Carotid FDG-PET/CT imaging has been employed for the first time in a phase 2b, double-blind, multicentre study (dal-PLAQUE), as a co-primary endpoint together with MRI-assessed indices to study the drug dalcetrapib that modulates cholesteryl ester transfer protein (CETP) activity to raise high-density lipoprotein (HDL) cholesterol. Total vessel area that was used to assess ATH burden by MRI was reduced in patients given dalcetrapib. However, PET/CT showed no evidence of change of vascular INFL assessed by FDG [36]. In a recent study, statin therapy (atorvastatin) produced significant rapid dose-dependent (10 versus 80 mg) reductions in FDG uptake within the artery wall, that may represent changes in atherosclerotic plaque INFL indicating a possible role of FDG PET in detecting early treatment effects in patients at risk or with established ATH [37].

Despite favorable results from a number of clinical studies, it should be noted that FDG signal is not only determined by inflammatory macrophages but other parameters; for instance, thrombus activity or SMCs function, which can also affect tracer uptake. More specific targets have also been tested clinically by Gaemperli et al. [38] demonstrating non-invasive detection and quantification of intraplaque INFL with peripheral benzodiazepine receptor PBR PET/CT imaging (^{11}C PK11195). Other surrogate markers of atheroma INFL have also been used in humans including ^{68}Ga-DOTATATE and ^{11}C-choline. ^{68}Ga-DOTATATE binds to somatostatin receptors subtype 2 that are expressed by macrophages [39]. ^{11}C-choline differs in that it is taken up by inflammatory cells—primarily macrophages, following which it undergoes phosphorylation and is metabolized into forming phosphatidylcholine that is eventually incorporated into the cellular membrane [40].

Beyond imaging of larger arterial beds, which has experienced rapid clinical translation, molecular imaging of coronary arterial plaques has also made progress recently (Fig. 23.4).^{18}F-FDG has been tested in this setting by various groups but with limited success, since physiological myocardial uptake of this tracer posses difficulties in identifying local INFL in coronary lesions in addition to those related to motion artifact, and partial volume effect. Employing a high-fat, low-carbohydrate diet before FDG-PET imaging to lower the physiological glucose uptake in the myocardium, studies have demonstrated the feasibility of FDG uptake in coronary plaques. Rogers et al. [41] studied FDG uptake in the left main coronary artery, as this is larger, more remote from myocardium, and less mobile. They found greater FDG uptake in left main artery in patients with acute coronary syndromes (ACS) compared to those with stable angina [41]. Dweck et al. [42] have employed PET/CT imaging with ^{18}F-sodium fluoride (^{18}F-NaF), a radiopharmaceutical used for skeletal imaging which provides relevant information regarding active micro-deposition of calcium in atherosclerotic plaques, a process that is associated with plaque instability. They found that ^{18}F-NaF uptake was higher in patients with coronary ATH versus control subjects and correlated with the calcium score, although 40 % of those with scores >1,000 displayed normal uptake [42]. Patients with increased coronary ^{18}F-NaF activity had higher rates of prior cardiovascular events and angina and higher Framingham risk scores [42] (Fig. 23.5). More recently, the same group have reported that ^{18}F-NaF localizes more avidly in plaques of patients with symptomatic carotid disease and in ruptured plaques of patients with acute MI compared to patients with stable coronary artery disease (CAD) [43]. This technique holds great promise for identifying high-risk and ruptured plaque however, further studies are needed to establish whether it can improve management of patients with CAD.

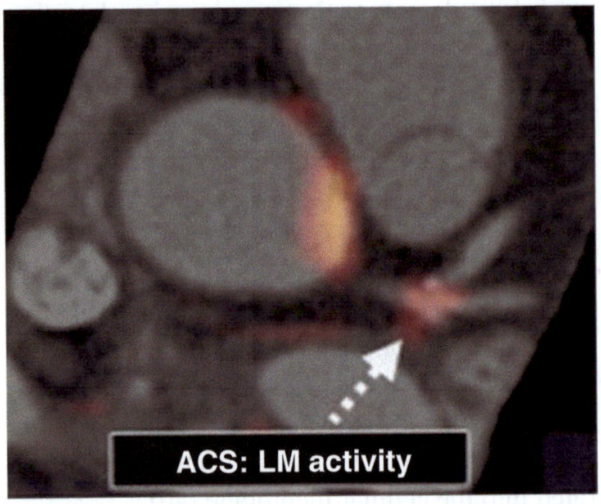

Fig. 23.4 Coregistered FDG PET/CT images showing FDG uptake at the trifurcation of the LM in a subject presenting with ACS. *ACS* acute coronary syndrome, *CT* computed tomography, *FDG* fluorodeoxyglucose, *LM* left main coronary artery, *PET* positron emission tomography (Adapted and reproduced from Rogers et al. [41], by permission)

Early studies involving symptomatic patients undergoing carotid endarterectomy found that up to a 24 % change in MRI signal could be observed for plaques 24 h after SPIOs delivery with histological proof of macrophage uptake [44]. The fast iron turnover renders repetitive imaging with this technique feasible and potentially useful to monitor treatment efficacy. Indeed, a recent prospective human study, ATHEROMA (Atorvastatin Therapy: Effects on Reduction of Macrophage Activity), showed the feasibility of using SPIOs with MRI to monitor serially the effect of atorvastatin on plaque INFL at 6-week intervals [45]. Reduction of SPIOs uptake was detected as early as 6 weeks after high-dose (80 mg) atorvastatin therapy, months to years earlier than changes in plaque morphology. These findings reaffirmed the advantage of molecular imaging over

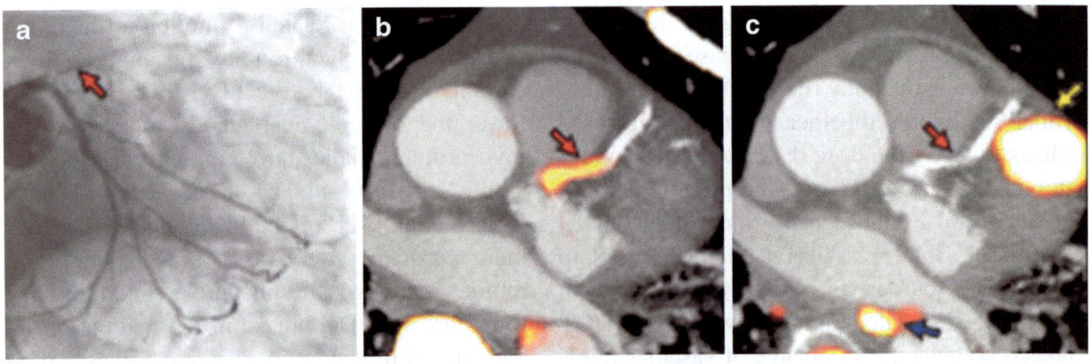

Fig. 23.5 Focal ^{18}F-NaF and ^{18}F-FDG uptake in patients with myocardial infarction and stable angina. Patient with acute ST-segment elevation myocardial infarction with (**a**) proximal occlusion (*red arrow*) of the left anterior descending artery on invasive coronary angiography and (**b**) intense focal ^{18}F-NaF uptake (*yellow-red*) at the site of the culprit plaque (*red arrow*) on the combined positron emission and computed tomogram (PET-CT). Corresponding *18F-FDG* PET-CT image (**c**) showing no uptake at the site of the culprit plaque. Note the significant myocardial uptake overlapping with the coronary artery (*yellow arrow*) and uptake within the oesophagus (*blue arrow*) (Adapted and reproduced from Joshi et al. [43], by permission)

morphometric imaging for assessment of the effectiveness of plaque-altering therapy.

Neovascularization in carotid plaques has been assessed semi-quantitatively by contrast-enhanced ultrasonography (CEUS) and it was shown that significant acoustic plaque enhancement is correlated both with histopathology and clinical presentation. This approach takes advantage of the fact that US contrast agents are pure intravascular tracers and hence, CEUS allows for the assessment of the amount of blood contained in the microvasculature within the region of interest. US molecular imaging, with specific ligands, such as for instance monoclonal antibodies, targeting integrins such as $\alpha_v\beta_3$, remain for the time being in the domain of preclinical research. Angiogenesis imaging with ^{18}F-Galacto-RGD PET/CT could be another option, with recent data from 10 patients with high-grade carotid artery stenosis scheduled for carotid endarterectomy, demonstrating specific tracer accumulation in atherosclerotic carotid plaques, which correlates with immunohistochemistry of avb3 expression [46].

Regarding APO imaging, ^{99m}Tc-anxA5 has been tested with SPECT in a small pilot study of four patients for its ability to detect cellular APO associated with unstable human carotid plaques [47]. Significant ^{99m}Tc-anxA5 uptake was found in the culprit lesions of patients with a recent history of transient ischemic attack, concordant to ex vivo histological confirmation after endarterectomy. Future prospective outcome studies in a larger group of patients will help determine its true discriminatory potential.

For *thrombus imaging* fibrin-targeted contrast agent EP-2104R has been used in a phase II clinical trial that included 11 patients with recent thrombosis (intracardiac, thoracic aorta, carotid artery) indicating that the agent provides strong enough signals for visualization of intracardiac, extracardiac arterial, and venous thrombi [48]. Black-blood MRI was performed 3.5 h after agent injection showing very good thrombus-to-adjacent soft tissue contrast and a sensitivity of 84 % for detection of known thrombi in the aforementioned vascular territories with this agent [48]. Ongoing efforts aim at increasing further its imaging sensitivity by optimizing the contrast dose and imaging parameters. Although the relatively long administration-to-imaging time possibly precludes widespread application of EP-2104R for acute arterial thrombosis syndromes, fibrin MRI may, at least conceptually, offer an alternative option to transesophageal echocardiography (ECHO) for left atrial thrombi. In addition, detection of subclinical thrombi on carotid atheroma could identify high risk patients.

In summary, significant progress has been made recently in the clinical setting towards identification of plaques which are prone to rupture. These first steps are important for the clinical community, as identification and appropriate treatment of these high-risk plaques can result in their stabilization and potentially reduce the incidence of stroke, acute MI and sudden cardiac death. It should be emphasized that we still need data on the natural history of these plaques, and at present, we lack outcome data (in terms of soft and hard cardiovascular events) from well designed prospective randomized trials upon which to develop treatment criteria for these plaques.

23.2.1.3 Imaging of Morphological Plaque Changes: Lipid Core and Fibrous Cup Formation

MDCT allows imaging of the vessel wall, potentially providing insights into the characteristics and extent of intramural ATH. Three parameters have been shown to be related to cardiovascular events: (1) CT density (<30 HU is an indicator of vulnerability); (2) lumen irregularities and (3) positive REM index. More recently, such parameters have been tested in a study aiming to assess their value for predicting ACS. Semiautomatic plaque quantification was employed (reporting plaque volume, burden area, noncalcified percentage, attenuation and positive REM). In this study, 1,650 patients were included and ROC analysis was performed comparing a model incorporating Framingham risk score (FRS) and conventional cardiac computed tomography angiography reading (consisting of calcium score, luminal stenosis, extent of CAD, and morphology assessment) with a model that also included semiautomated plaque quantification. The areas under the curve were 0.64 and 0.79 respectively, ($p < 0.05$), indicating an enhanced ability of CT to detect potentially vulnerable plaque by providing additional information beyond that obtained from conventional reading [49].

MRI has also been tested for assessing atheromatous plaque morphology particularly of large or "static" arteries, such as the carotid arteries. Lipid and fibrotic plaque components have been accurately quantified on T2-weighted images, in both animals and humans. T2-weighted images have also been used to measure the fibrous cap thickness and to identify fibrous cap rupture and intraplaque hemorrhage, features that are commonly found in symptomatic carotid ATH [50]. The main limitation of MRI in identifying vulnerable plaques is its relatively poor reproducibility. To overcome this limitation newer techniques have been developed and applied in patients. These include diffusion weighted, gado-fluorine enhanced and time of flight imaging which have the potential to identify lipid-rich necrotic core and fibrous cap as well as intra-plaque hemorrhage, an indicator of plaque rupture. Attempts have also been made for plaque assessment in coronary arteries. In a recent prospective study by Noguchi et al. [51], 568 patients with suspected or known CAD underwent non-contrast T1-weighted imaging to determine whether coronary high-intensity plaques (HIPs), which are associated with characteristics of vulnerability can predict future coronary events. The results showed that HIPs are significantly associated with coronary events, and may thus represent a novel predictive factor.

23.2.2 Ischemic Heart Disease

The most frequent cause of myocardial ischemia in man is coronary ATH. This can lead to chronic ischemic syndromes or to acute episodes of plaque instability that can be manifested as acute myocardial infarction (MI) or sudden death. In the clinical setting, non-invasive assessment of ischemic heart disease (IHD) focuses on functional and metabolic effects of coronary flow limitation related to stenotic plaques. The heart is metabolically a very active organ and requires a high level of oxygen delivery. Furthermore oxygen extraction from delivered blood is high even at rest. Any increase in oxygen demand therefore must be met by increasing coronary and microcirculatory blood flow, as there is little scope to increase oxygen extraction. The balance between myocardial oxygen requirements and oxygen delivery is central to understanding the mechanisms by which ischemia can occur. On a metabolic level, the myocardium uses a variety of substrates, but under physiological conditions in the fasting state most of the energy required comes from the oxidation of fatty acids (FA) and to a lesser degree from glucose. When glucose or insulin levels are high, such as after a meal, glucose oxidation increases and fatty acid use is suppressed. Myocardial ischemia results in a metabolic shift from FA to glucose, which results in 11 % more ATP produced per molecule of oxygen [52].

As myocardial oxygen demand increases or coronary blood flow falls, autoregulatory and metabolic regulatory mechanisms are activated towards maintaining myocardial perfusion at a normal level. When these compensatory changes (including autoregulation and metabolic regulation) become exhausted, ischemia finally results as myocardial blood flow falls. In patients with atherosclerotic heart disease, compensatory mechanisms to maintain myocardial perfusion in the face of significant epicardial stenoses are already active. Vasodilatation of the distal vascular bed occurs and pressure gradient across the stenosis increases. This exhaustion of compensatory mechanisms in patients with CAD is also compounded by abnormal endothelial function and impaired endothelium-derived vasodilator mechanisms. The first abnormality to become apparent during ischemia is therefore reduced perfusion to the affected territory. It is not until a diameter stenosis of around 80 % that resting perfusion is critically reduced, and as a rule of thumb, any stenosis less than 40 % diameter is unlikely to have any haemodynamic consequences even during maximum coronary dilatation. The pathophysiology of myocardial ischemia involves a series of progressive changes that have been described in terms of a 'cascade' from the cellular level through perfusion abnormalities, contractile dysfunction, electrocardiographic abnormalities and finally symptoms [53].

23.2.2.1 Functional and Metabolic Imaging in Ischemic Heart Disease

In patients with stenotic plaques but no reduction in flow at rest due to compensatory mechanisms, perfusion abnormalities can be induced by stressing the perfusion system (Table 23.1B). Rest and stress radionuclide myocardial perfusion imaging (MPI) is a well established technique for diagnosis and risk stratification. Comparison of tracer distribution at rest and exercise or pharmacological stress can describe the presence, severity, and extent of myocardial ischemia caused by flow-limiting coronary stenoses. There are alternative well validated techniques for non-invasive assessment of myocardial perfusion and these include ECHO and MRI, for an in depth review of the subject and comparisons of diagnostic accuracy that is beyond the scope of this chapter, the reader is referred to selected references [54, 55].

A different approach is to image the metabolic and molecular sequels of myocardial ischemia. This is termed "ischemic memory" and may reveal the ischemic origin of recent chest pain and define the extent of myocardium compromised by ischemia (Table 23.1B). There are experimental and clinical data demonstrating the feasibility and significance of metabolic radionuclide imaging in patients with stable disease but also in those with suspected ACS mostly using radiolabeled FA such as ^{123}I-BMIPP SPECT [56, 57]. However, despite encouraging results, a number of issues remain unsettled, including optimal imaging protocols, widespread tracer availability, utility of metabolic imaging in diabetic patients, incremental value for diagnosis and prognosis over and above that obtained by perfusion data and impact of radionuclide metabolic imaging on clinical management. Ischemic memory imaging with ECHO has also been achieved in mice models using microbubbles targeted to the EC adhesion molecule P-selectin, which is expressed in response to only a mild ischemic stimulus. P-selectin–targeted imaging has been shown to detect brief myocardial ischemic injury even after the ischemic insult has resolved and in the absence of MI [58] (Fig. 23.6). No clinical studies using this technique have been performed so far. For the initiation of clinical trials, several developments need to take place both for the contrast agents that are being used and the imaging technology for tracer detection.

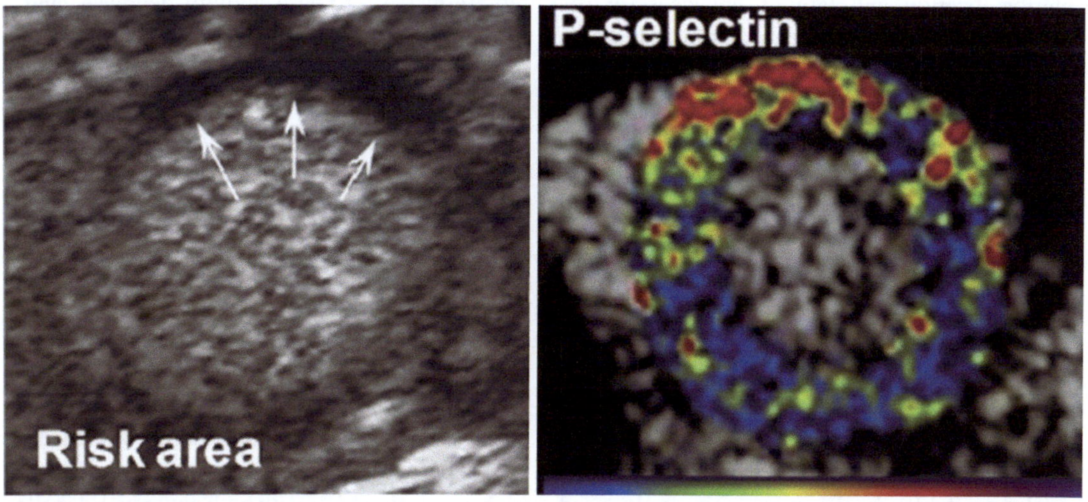

Fig. 23.6 Contrast echocardiographic imaging of recent myocardial ischemia with P-selectin–targeted microbubbles. Short-axis contrast echocardiographic images from a mouse illustrating hypoperfusion (*arrows*) of the anterior wall on perfusion imaging during brief occlusion of the left anterior descending (*left*) and enhancement within the previously ischemic anterior territory with P-selectin–targeted microbubbles injected intravenously 45 min after reflow. Color scale at *bottom* (Adapted and reproduced from Inaba and Lindner [115], [58] by permission)

23.2.2.2 Specific Issues Related to Ischemia-Reperfusion Injury and Post-infarction Remodeling

Acute MI is a common cause of REM of the left ventricle (LV). It is estimated that despite primary percutaneous coronary intervention (PCI) and standard current therapy, around 30 % of anterior MI will develop REM. The latter is a complex process by which mechanical, neurohormonal and genetic factors alter ventricular structure and function leading to reduced mechanical performance, electrical instability and sudden death. It is an important aspect of heart failure (HF) progression, characterized by dilation and change of the shape of the left LV and evolving alterations in the ventricular wall which include hypertrophy, loss of myocytes and increased interstitial fibrosis [59]. The three major biomechanical mechanisms contributing to the increase of LV volumes over time after MI are: (a) expansion of the infarct in the sub-acute phase, (b) subsequent non-ischemic infarct extension into the adjacent noninfarcted region, and (c) hypertrophy and dilation of non-infarcted myocardium in the chronic phase [59]. The main factors associated with REM are size of infarction, residual viability within the infarct territory, anterior location and late or unsuccessful (or absence of) reperfusion therapy both at the epicardial vessel level and at the microvasculature level (no reflow) [59].

Imaging techniques have been employed for prediction of LV REM. Non-invasive techniques in the form of ECHO, MRI, CT and radionuclide imaging have been utilized in this setting, as they are well suited for assessing parameters which either constitute phenotypic expressions of REM (e.g. alterations of heart size, shape and mass, end diastolic and end-systolic volumes and regional contractility) or are by themselves determinants of the REM process (e.g. myocardial perfusion, fibrosis and viability). ECHO which is widely available, is the most commonly used technique for prediction of LV REM, but MRI because of its high accuracy and reproducibility of measurements is currently the gold standard to assess the aforementioned parameters as well as microvascular obstruction, tissue oedema and infarct size at the early stage post-acute MI [60]. The later is a key determinant of long-term LV REM, however, microvascular obstruction, indexed by intramyocardial haemorrhage on T2-weighed images has also been found to be a powerful predictor of changes in global function and LV end-systolic volume [61]. Tomographic radionuclide imaging with ^{99m}Tc-labelled tracers (Sestamibi and Tetrofosmin) and ECG gating synchronisation (ECG-gated SPECT) is another option for predicting LV REM in the post primary PCI setting, as it offers the benefit of assessing both perfusion and function in the same myocardial segments as well as salvaged myocardium and final scar size, but it also allows accurate and highly reproducible measurements of global LV function and volumes [62].

However, there still exists a need for upstream imaging biomarkers that will allow timely and targeted intervention before disease has progressed beyond the point of no return. A key element to this, is knowledge of changes occurring at cellular or extracellular level that has been acquired over the last few years. It is now recognized that LV REM is characterized by a regression to the fetal pattern, i.e. increase of β-MHC, α-actin, ANP overexpression, sarcoendoplasmic reticulum Ca^{2+}-ATPase activity decrease, and a shift of myocardial metabolism towards glucose utilization [59]. In the following paragraphs, we discuss selected novel imaging strategies which could complement the more conventional techniques described above and may provide new possibilities for the management of post MI patients (Table 23.1C).

23.2.2.3 Molecular Imaging Targets in Ischemic Injury and Post-infarction Remodeling

APO is different from *N*, as it is a reversible process, and hence a therapeutic target, whereas N is not. The dual-contrast imaging technique for high-resolution MRI with both annexin-V labelled nanoparticle (AnxCLIO-cy5.5) to image APO and delayed-enhancement imaging with a novel gadolinium chelate (Gd-DTPA-NBD), to image N, has great potential for clinical translation as

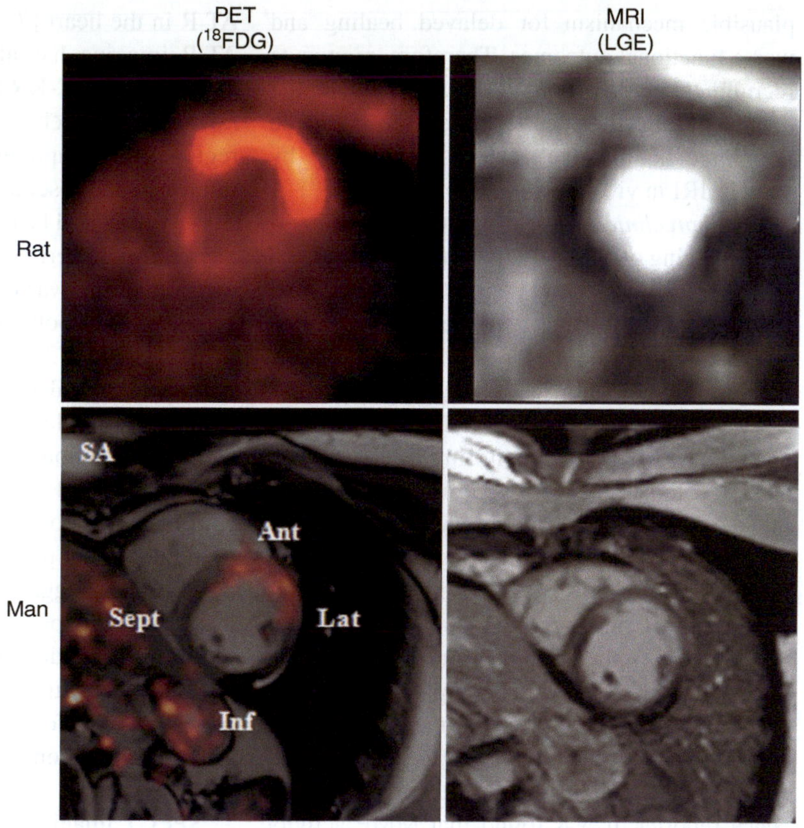

Fig. 23.7 FDG PET imaging in rat and man shortly after myocardial infarction and reperfusion corresponding to inflammation and/or a change in myocardial metabolism in the anterolateral region. The LGE MR images in the same area show a different volume of distribution for LGE pointing to local edema. For the rodent images, a preclinical PET and a clinical MRI was used. The human data were created on a fully integrated PET/MRI system. *LGE* late gadolinium enhancement, *SA* short axis, *Ant* anterior segment, *Lat* lateral segment, *Inf* inferior segment, *Sept* septum

demonstrated recently in a transgenic mouse model of myocardial ischaemia [63]. This method allowed the apoptotic cells to be differentiated from necrotic cells, which further helped to identify a group of apoptotic yet viable cells in the myocardium (4–6 h after ischemia reperfusion) that could benefit from antiapoptotic therapy. MRI agents that bind to exposed DNA are also under investigation in animal models [64].

Post-infarction INFL with FDG PET imaging has been assessed in mice models and in selected human case studies shortly after myocardial infarction and reperfusion in combination with LGE MRI [65, 66]. FDG uptake on PET, corresponding to matching LGE on MRI, shortly after myocardial infarction and reperfusion, indicates INFL and/or a change in myocardial metabolism (Fig. 23.7). Post-infarction INFL has also been attempted to be assessed more specifically in mice models with MRI and contrast microbubble ECHO to image monocytes/macrophages or myeloperoxidase (MPO) activity [67–70] providing considerable information regarding the progression of wound healing and scar formation in the LV after MI. In particular, in the recent study by Lee et al. [66], Gd-DTPA–enhanced infarcts showed high FDG uptake on day 5 after MI in a mouse model. Surprisingly, there was also considerable monocyte recruitment in the remote myocardium in parallel with a robust increase of recruiting adhesion molecules and chemokines, although levels were always lower compared to the infarct zone. In a very recent study by Ye et al. [71] spatiotemporal recruitment of monocytes was imaged with combined (^{19})F/(^{1})H magnetic resonance, in vivo in a rat model of reperfused MI. Blood monocytes were labeled by intravenous injection of ^{19}F-perfluorocarbon emulsion 1 day after MI. The distribution patterns of monocyte infiltration were correlated with the presence of microvascular obstruction (MVO) and intramyocardial hemorrhage assessed by MRI. Specifically, monocyte recruitment was highly reduced in MVO areas and that could be a plausible mechanism for delayed healing and worse functional outcomes. Therefore, monocyte recruitment in MI with MVO could be a potential diagnostic and therapeutic target that could be monitored noninvasively and longitudinally by $^{19}F/^{1}H$ MRI in vivo [71].

At a *preclinical* level, quantitative radionuclide imaging of MMPs activity that is correlated with extracellular matrix degradation is now feasible using radiolabeled molecules targeting MMPs. This can be performed at different time points in combination with radionuclide (ECG-gated MPI SPECT) or non-radionuclide based techniques (MRI) for monitoring both scar size and LV volumes changes over time thus introducing a molecular/mechanical imaging approach that could help to assess in a longitudinal fashion the relationship between enhanced MMPs activation after MI and altered regional myocardial deformation. In the aforementioned study of Lee et al. [66] in mice, which employed ^{18}F-FDG PET-MRI imaging for assessment of INFL, assessment of the activity of MMP-2 and MMP-9 was also performed using an activatable fluorescence reporter. It was found that MMP activity was significantly increased in non infarcted myocardium, suggesting that monocyte recruitment to the remote zone may contribute to post-MI dilation, although the precise cellular contribution of MMPs activity is unclear at this point.

Renin Angiotensin-Aldosterone System (RAAS) is another attractive imaging target due to its key role in various cardiac pathologies, including post-infarct LV REM. In a murine model of MI, investigators have used both a fluorescent angiotensin peptide analog and ^{99m}Tc-labeled losartan, an *angiotensin II type 1 receptor* (AT_1R) blocker. Uptake of the angiotensin-targeted fluorescent compound was seen in the infarct area at 1–12 weeks after MI using an open chest imaging preparation, with maximum uptake within the heart seen at approximately 3 weeks after infarction. Subsequent histopathologic analyses suggested specificity for myofibroblasts within the infarct region in the weeks after the infarction. The investigators also performed in vivo micro-SPECT/CT with ^{99m}Tc-labeled losartan, demonstrating the feasibility for in vivo imaging of AT_1R in the heart [72]. The potential of PET for AT_1R imaging has also been investigated. The novel ligand ^{11}C-KR31173 has been tested in a rat model of ischemia and reperfusion, where regional AT_1R upregulation was detected in the infarct area. Subsequent testing of the same PET tracer (^{11}C-KR31173) was performed in pigs 3–4 weeks after experimental MI [73] (Fig. 23.8). Ex vivo validation was carried out by immunohistochemistry and polymerase chain reaction. After MI, ^{11}C-KR31173 retention corrected for regional perfusion, revealed AT_1R up-regulation in the infarct area relative to remote myocardium, whereas retention was elevated in both regions when compared with myocardium of healthy controls. Postmortem analysis confirmed AT_1R up-regulation in remote and infarct tissue. These early studies suggest that accurate quantification of AT_1R overexpression by novel imaging techniques as mentioned above, if feasible, may become a helpful tool not only for identifying patients at risk for developing LV REM and HF after MI, but potentially for optimizing anti-RAS therapy.

SPECT imaging with the ^{99m}Tc-RGD peptide to target $\alpha_v\beta_3$ integrin, which is overexpressed on myofibroblasts has been used in mouse models with myocardial infarcts. Maximal tracer uptake was observed in the infarct area at 2 weeks, followed by 4 and 12 weeks compared with that in unmanipulated mice [74]. In another study measuring the efficacy of pharmacologic intervention in myocardial REM, ^{99m}Tc-RGD peptide was significantly reduced in mice treated with combination therapy (captopril, losartan and spironolactone) and correlated with echocardiographic parameters [75]. If proven clinically feasible, such a strategy could be useful for monitoring myocardial healing process and identifying post-MI patients likely to develop LV REM and HF. Angiogenesis probes in the form of radiolabelled or MRI nanoparticles and US microbubbles targeting up-regulation of vascular endothelial growth factor (VEGF) receptors [76] or $\alpha_v\beta_3$ integrin [77, 78] during neovessel formation in myocardial infract have also been tested in small animals. Experimental studies in rats subjected to transient left coronary artery occlusion followed

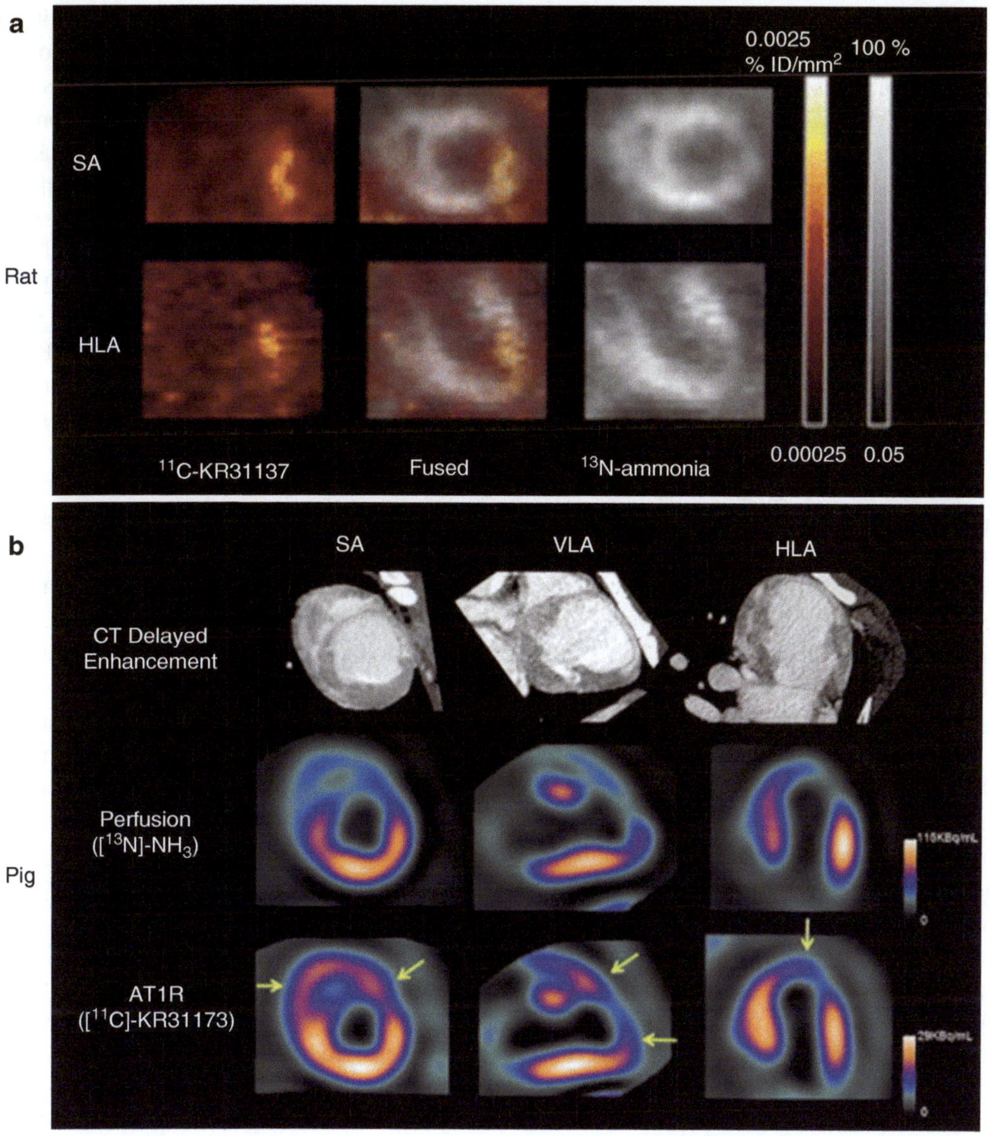

Fig. 23.8 ^{11}C-KR31137 and ^{13}N-ammonia PET studies in a rat (a) and in a pig (b) after myocardial infarction. (**a**) Short-axis (*SA*) view and horizontal-long-axis (*HLA*) views showing focal increased ^{11}C-KR31173 uptake in area of reduced myocardial perfusion by ^{13}N-ammonia. (**b**) CT delayed enhancement images, are shown, where the infarct region is visualized by a thin wall and mostly transmural contrast enhancement. Myocardial perfusion images using [^{13}N]-NH_3 show a defect that matches the area of delayed CT contrast enhancement. Images of AT1R, using [^{11}C]-KR31173 show a less pronounced reduction in the infarct region when compared with perfusion, and elevated binding in the right ventricular wall (*yellow arrows*). *CT* computed tomography, *HL* horizontal long axis, *LV* left ventricular, *SA* short axis, *VL* vertical long axis (Adapted and reproduced from Fukushima et al. [73] by permission)

by reperfusion showed an up-regulation of $\alpha_v\beta_3$ integrin expression (detected by ^{18}F-Galacto-RGD uptake), which peaks between 1 and 3 weeks post MI and remains detectable until 6 months after reperfusion suggesting a delayed but prolonged tissue response to a transient episode of coronary occlusion and reperfusion [78]. These are interesting observations, which, if clinically validated, may offer the means for monitoring therapeutic interventions in this setting. For instance, a treatment strategy targeting angiogenesis could be optimised with the help of imaging, as such approach may interfere with the healing process after MI. Basic fibroblast growth factor (bFGF) is one of the agents used in angiogenesis induction therapy (induces the expression of $\alpha_v\beta_3$ integrin in EC), which may reduce infract size, improve systolic function and increase collateral circulation. Another PET tracer has been tested recently: ^{68}Ga-NOTA-RGD was used to investigate imaging characteristics in a rat MI model and to monitor the efficacy of bFGF therapy, with promising results for assessment of pathophysiology or monitoring of therapeutic efficacy [79]. Feasibility of imaging VEGFRs with PET in the myocardium was also demonstrated in a rat model of MI. VEGFRs increased significantly after MI and remained elevated for 2 weeks, after which time it returned to baseline levels [76].

In the clinical setting although late gadolinium enhancement (LGE) MRI yields an excellent high-resolution image of myocyte loss and infarct size, it cannot differentiate between N and APO. SPECT with ^{99m}Tc-labeled annexin-V, although a promising technique to image APO in patients with acute coronary symptoms, was found to be limited by the high background signal within 12 h of probe administration, which made early detection of APO after ischemia difficult. Furthermore, this probe does not effectively differentiate APO from N, both of which expose the imaging target (phosphatidylserine) to annexin. Regarding novel radiopharmaceuticals such as radiolabelled RGD peptides there are only limited clinical data. Makowski et al. [77], studied a patient two weeks after MI and PCI who underwent MRI (LGE), ^{13}N ammonia PET/CT and ^{18}F-Galacto-RGD PET/CT. There was $\alpha_v\beta_3$ expression corresponding to the infarct area as defined by the extent of LGE MRI and severely reduced myocardial blood flow (perfusion defect with ^{13}N ammonia). This study demonstrated the feasibility of $\alpha_v\beta_3$ expression imaging in humans as an indicator of myocardial healing taking place within the infarcted area. Verjans et al. [80] used a ^{99m}Tc-labeled RGD imaging peptide to target integrins associated with collagen-producing myofibroblasts and neoangiogenesis in 10 patients with MI in conjunction with early SPECT MPI and LGE MRI. In this study, integrin SPECT signal at 3 and 8 weeks usually extended beyond the perfusion defects on SPECT MPI and colocalized with the infarct scar on follow-up MRI 1 year after the ischemic event. Further experimental and clinical research is underway focusing on the specificity of the new imaging probes for angiogenesis and their relationship to REM after MI. Regarding RAAS imaging, although the novel ligand ^{11}C-KR31173 has been tested in four healthy volunteers and was proved to be feasible and safe using clinical PET/CT technology (Fig. 23.9), it has not yet entered clinical trials to predict the risk for ventricular REM and to monitor the efficacy of anti-RAS drug therapy [73].

In concluding, there has been a remarkable progress in molecular imaging of infarct healing and remodelling in animals in the past decade, with the development of probes which target APO, N, INFL, angiogenesis, RAAS and MMPs. Translating this work to the bedside in a cost-effective and clinically beneficial manner remains a significant challenge [81].

23.2.3 Heart Failure

In HF several neurohormonal, immunological and biochemical mechanisms are common regardless of the underlying etiology and include (a) activation of molecular mechanisms, (b) structural changes in the heart and other organs such as the kidneys and lungs, and (c) systemic disturbances such as chronic INFL. In this multifaceted process, INFL, oxidative stress, extracellular matrix REM, neurohormonal activation (mainly involvement of the RAAS, and disturbance of the homeostasis of the sympathetic nervous system with overstimulation of the beta-adrenergic receptors) and myocyte injury/stress are the main contributors. Serum-based biomarkers associated with these processes are currently being investigated for their ability to stratify disease severity, predict mortality, guide therapy, and assess treatment efficacy, however, these are often non specific

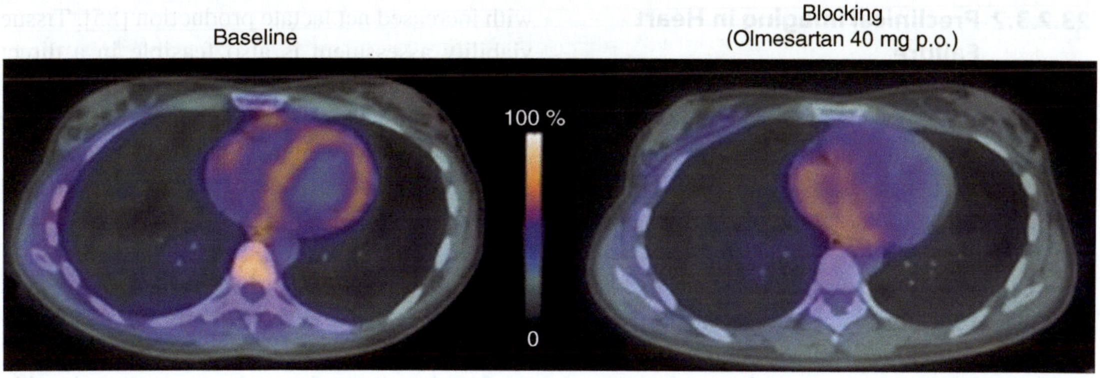

Fig. 23.9 PET/CT of myocardial AT1R in a healthy human subject. Transaxial fusion images are shown through the mid-cardiac region. Baseline images show regionally homogeneous uptake of the angiotensin II type 1 receptor (AT1R) ligand [^{11}C]-KR31173 in left ventricular myocardium (*left*). Repeat imaging 3 h after an oral (p.o.) dose of 40 mg olmesartan for specific blocking of AT1R shows complete absence of myocardial [^{11}C]-KR31173 uptake, confirming tracer specificity for the receptor (*right*). Tracer is only present in the blood pool of atria and ventricles (Adapted and reproduced from Fukushima K et al. [73] by permission)

and hence there is a need for developing molecular imaging approaches to assess those targets. Amongst the different causes of HF, IHD is the underlying etiology in around two thirds of cases. In those patients, distinction between reversible and irreversible causes of LV dysfunction leading to HF is important, as treatment strategies may be adapted accordingly. Reversible causes of LV dysfunction are two ischemic entities, which if treated, can lead to recovery of LV function and improvement of symptoms and prognosis. These are both forms of *viable* dysfunctional myocardium and termed "*stunning*" and "*hibernation*" (HiB). Non invasive imaging has been used extensively in this setting; the different techniques and derived signals of viability and HiB are discussed briefly below (Table 23.1D).

23.2.3.1 Specific Issues on Heart Failure of Ischemic Etiology: Imaging Myocardial Viability and Hibernation

Although the exact underlying phenomena in HiB remain to a significant degree unclear, alteration of structural proteins and metabolism, disorganisation of the cytoskeleton, loss of myofilaments, glycogen vacuoles and sarcomeric instability may all result from impairment of regional perfusion and lead to myocardial dysfunction. APO, patchy fibrosis, INFL, and depressed β-adrenergic control (for the latter see next section on innervation imaging) are present, underpinning the similarity of features of chronic myocardial HiB with those of HF regardless of its etiology (ischemic or non-ischemic). Non invasive imaging has contributed significantly to this area by increasing our understanding of the underlying concepts, and among the techniques, PET has played a pivotal role. The use of the latter is related to its ability to assess accurately myocardial perfusion at rest and stress and alterations of myocardial metabolism that occur following myocardial ischemia. Other non invasive imaging modalities (SPECT, ECHO and MRI) have also played an important role by targeting key pathophysiological parameters such as fibrosis and/or cellular viability, microcirculation and contractile reserve. The latter has been most frequently been evaluated by ECHO (or by MRI) using dobutamine stress. LGE MRI and ECHO can directly assess the presence of tissue fibrosis, or the consequences of fibrosis such as wall thickness/chamber size which are important determinants of the recovery of contractile function. Perfusion can be evaluated by PET or SPECT tracers, cell membrane integrity can be evaluated by ^{201}TL, intact mitochondria can be probed by ^{99m}Tc labeled tracers, glucose and free fatty acid metabolism can be assessed by FDG and radio-labeled fatty acids.

23.2.3.2 Preclinical Imaging in Heart Failure

A number of experimental studies focus on the quantitative relation of flow and function using models of acute (minutes), subacute (hours) and chronic (weeks) models of myocardial ischaemia. Pertinent to the setting of chronic LV dysfunction are the results of studies by Heusch et al. employing models of chronic stenosis which suggest that HiB probably represents a spectrum of changes, with *chronic repetitive stunning* showing normal or near normal resting perfusion and impaired myocardial perfusion reserve at one end (this condition has also been termed "functional HiB") and reduced resting perfusion at the other ("structural HiB"). At this advanced stage, there is also reduced myocardial oxygen consumption and lack of lactate extraction, even during inotropic stimulation with dobutamine [82]. Increased glucose utilization as assessed by PET with FDG is a consistent finding in animals with chronic stenosis (metabolic shift) and perfusion-contraction matching, but it has also been observed in chronic stunning characterized by perfusion-contraction mismatch [83]. In addition, it has been shown that clearance rates of ^{11}C-palmitate are reduced compared to control segments and that metabolic recovery after transient ischemia is slow and paralleled by the slow recovery of myocardial function [56]. Oxidative metabolism using ^{11}C-acetate, which reflects overall oxidative metabolism or myocardial oxygen consumption has also been assessed in experimental models of repetitive stunning [84]. It has been demonstrated that there is a prolonged yet reversible reduction in systolic function associated with a significant down-regulation of both glucose and oxidative metabolism (assessed by FDG and ^{11}C-acetate respectively) despite restoration of normal myocardial blood flow. Other experimental studies employing ECHO have shown that the hypoperfused viable myocardium retains its responsiveness to inotropic challenge with dobutamine. At higher doses, the inotropic response to dobutamine is blunted and thus overall, there is a biphasic response, with increased wall thickening at lower doses and contractile dysfunction at higher doses that is associated with increased net lactate production [85]. Tissue viability assessment is also feasible in a direct approach employing LGE MRI. A number of experimental studies have demonstrated that the technique can distinguish between myocardial scar, peri-infarction zone of edema, and normal myocardium [86, 87].

23.2.3.3 Clinical Imaging in Heart Failure-Hibernation

Numerous studies in patients with chronic LV dysfunction have focused on the relationship between regional perfusion and function. Taken together, the results of these studies are in agreement with those obtained from the experimental setting and demonstrate that in most cases, there is impairment of myocardial perfusion reserve (MPR), with the reduction of resting perfusion seen only in the most advanced cases of HiB (*perfusion-contraction matching*). The introduction of MRI for assessment of myocardial perfusion has been instrumental in depicting reduction of perfusion at the sub-endocardium in patients with hibernating myocardium that is also in agreement with preclinical studies. This has been eloquently demonstrated by Selvanayagam et al. [88] who have shown that perfusion is reduced at rest when compared to areas without significant coronary stenosis. Moreover, in the same patients, both subendocardial perfusion and LV function are normalized or improved, following revascularization. The relation between perfusion and metabolism has also been extensively investigated and is in agreement with studies from the preclinical setting. Higher FDG signal compared to perfusion (obtained by qualitative or quantitative analysis) in segments with reduced function is consistently predictive of functional recovery following reperfusion, thus determining prognosis [85] (Fig. 23.10). Other studies in patients with LV dysfunction using PET and ^{11}C-acetate have demonstrated that the rate constant of acetate clearance in areas with chronic HiB was reduced, largely in relation to the reduced myocardial perfusion [89].

As alluded above, although baseline contractile function is depressed, the viable hypoperfused myocardium retains its responsiveness to

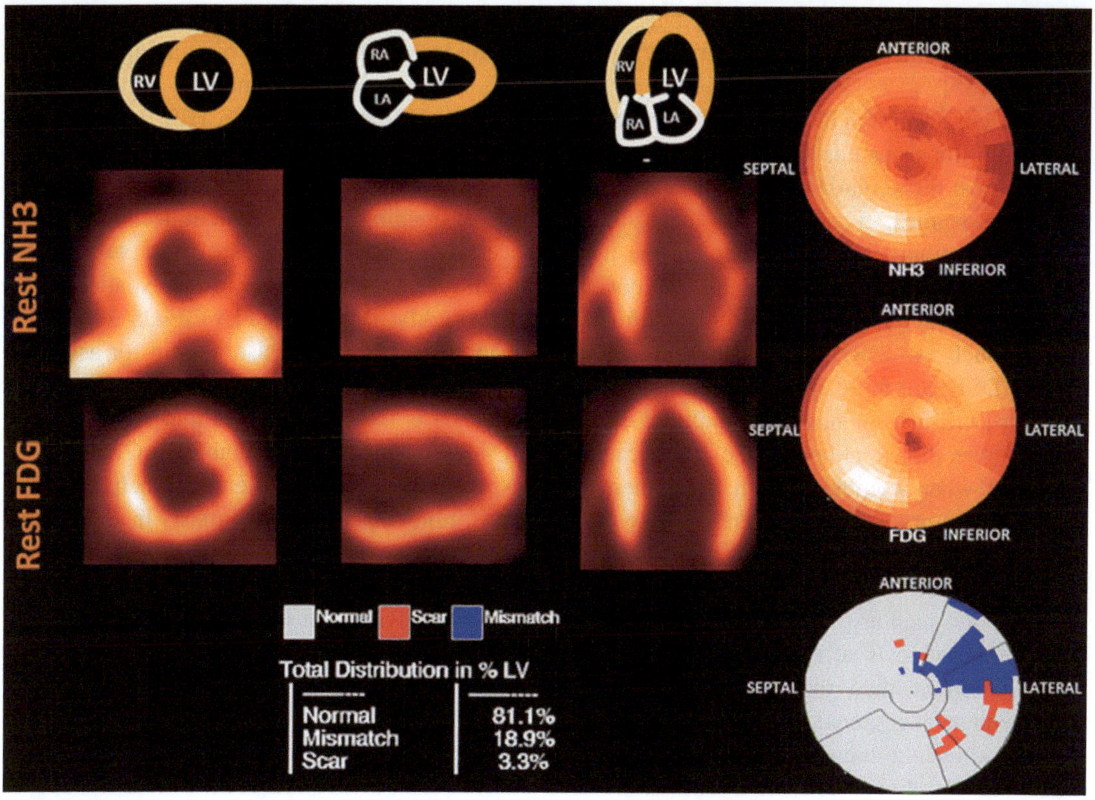

Fig. 23.10 Resting ^{13}N-ammonia and ^{18}F-FDG tomographic images and polar maps of a 68-year-old male with known CAD, previous myocardial infarctions, impaired LV function and multiple previous PCIs. He underwent a PET study for assessment of myocardial viability. Combined assessment of the resting 13N-ammonia and the ^{18}F-FDG images shows a large mismatch between perfusion and metabolism (19 % of the total myocardial mass) in the anterolateral region compatible with hibernating myocardium. There is an area with minor match inferolaterally (indicative of very limited myocardial damage involving only 3.1 % of the total myocardial mass) but otherwise well preserved perfusion and viability in the LV myocardium. *^{18}F-FDG* ^{18}F-Fluorodeoxyglucose, *CAD* coronary artery disease, *LV* left ventricle, *PCI* percutaneous coronary intervention, *PET* positron emission tomography, *RV* right ventricle, *RA* right atrium, *LA* left atrium (Adapted and reproduced from Anagnostopoulos et al. [91], [90] by permission)

an inotropic challenge but this depends upon the severity of MPR reduction. This is because the latter has a direct impact on the ability of viable myocardium to improve its contraction upon inotropic stimulation, as this requires augmentation of myocardial perfusion. As in preclinical studies, a biphasic pattern to dobutamine stimulation has also been observed in humans. The presence of a biphasic pattern is important to rule out other causes of regional dysfunction such as subendocardial scar or remodelled myocardium, as both of these conditions are characterized by preserved contractile reserve both at low and high levels of inotropic stimulation. There is a discrepancy between radionuclide techniques and those based on contractile reserve in about 20–25 % segments that are characterized as viable by the former but they do not improve functionally during stimulation with dobutamine. These segments usually have mild reduction of resting perfusion, avid uptake of FDG or SPECT tracers and almost completely exhausted MPR that prevents the segments from increasing their oxygen consumption upon inotropic stimulation and hence from increasing their contractile function. Apart from the exhaustion of MPR, other factors, such as the presence and severity of cardiomyocytic alterations or down-regulation of beta-adrenoreceptors, may also contribute to the lack of contractile reserve in apparently viable segments [85].

The accuracy of non invasive imaging tests for predicting improvement in regional or global function post revascularization has been tested in numerous studies. These studies consistently show that radionuclide techniques are the most sensitive for prediction of functional recovery, whereas techniques challenging contractile reserve such as MRI and dobutamine stress ECHO (DSE) are more specific [90]. MRI studies with LGE also demonstrate high sensitivity but low specificity, although the latter can be improved when combined with assessment of contractile reserve with dobutamine. The relatively low specificity of the radionuclide techniques however, is not a disadvantage because other factors, such as the improvement of symptoms and prognosis after revascularization are more important than the exact prediction of improvement of regional wall systolic function. Reperfusion of the hibernating myocardium stabilizes myocardial blood flow conditions by eliminating repetitive episodes of ischemia and protects the myocardium from REM, APO and cell death even when it does not lead to an improvement of LV function.

The role of non invasive imaging in the management of patients with LV dysfunction of ischemic etiology has been challenged recently by the results of the Surgical Treatment for Ischemic HF (STICH) trial [91]. According to this, the presence of viable myocardium was associated with an increased probability of survival but viability assessment failed to identify patients with a survival benefit from surgical revascularization as compared with medical therapy alone. This differs from the results from previous (mostly retrospective studies) and those from a post hoc analysis of the multi-centre randomized controlled trial "PET and Recovery Following Revascularization" (PARR-2) trial, which provide a reasonably good evidence for the impact of non invasive imaging on the identification of high-risk patients who may benefit from revascularization [92, 93]. Nevertheless, further randomized trials incorporating viability/HiB imaging as part of the work up for management of ischaemic HF are still required to assess the value of imaging in this setting. The Alternative Imaging Modalities in Ischemic HF (AIMI-IMAGE HF) Project is one such trial that is currently underway and is expected to address the issue around the role of cardiac imaging in management decisions and to ascertain which methods are most suitable for which types of patients, for instance patients with severely dilated hearts and LVEF <25 %.

Viability imaging is also helpful for assessing response to *cardiac resynchronisation therapy* (CRT). It is well documented that approximately 30 % of patients judged suitable for CRT will not respond. Viability assessment may help in identifying non-responders or assist in improving implantation to improve the likelihood of response. Extent of viability appears to be directly linked to improved CRT response as well as the presence of myocardial viability at the LV lead site, no matter whether measured by, SPECT, PET, ECHO or MRI [94]. Imaging studies are now focusing on the integration of dyssynchrony data with venous anatomy and myocardial scar in order to improve outcomes. A small study using MRI to guide the position of the LV lead to the latest activated LV segment, relative to the venous anatomy and away from areas of scar resulted in a 92 % response rate from 20 patients (reduction in LV end-systolic volume by >15 % on echo) [95]. Larger studies are underway in order to confirm the validity of multimodality imaging for assessing response to *cardiac resynchronisation therapy* (CRT).

23.2.3.4 Myocardial Innervation Imaging in Heart Failure

Human sympathetic neurons appear to be more susceptible than myocytes to ischemic injury. In ischemic HF, there is an activation of the sympathetic nervous system, in which an increased norepinephrine release from the cardiac sympathetic postganglionic nerve terminals causes desensitization of the postsynaptic b-adrenergic receptors, which leads to worsening of the LV systolic function. A decreased efficiency of norepinephrine reuptake through the presynaptic norepinephrine transporter-1 (uptake-1 mechanism) further contributes to norepinephrine spillover into the bloodstream in HF patients. The clinical significance of such neuropathic derangement is evidenced by the known benefit of β-blockade for reducing mortality. Noninvasive investigation of the myocardial adrenergic transmission in HF patients holds a great promise to predict their risk of lethal ventricular arrhythmia.

Preclinical Imaging

In pig hearts, hibernating myocardium was induced by chronic occlusion of the left anterior descending artery (LAD) in a study by Luisi et al. [96]. Physiologic studies (resting flow measurements) and ^{11}C-HED PET were performed 1–5 months later. After 3 months, anterior hypokinesis developed with reductions in resting flow and a critical reduction in subendocardial flow reserve. Extensive defects in hydroxyephedrine (HED) uptake were found for hibernating myocardium, with regional retention approximately 50 % lower than that in normally perfused remote myocardium. Relative HED uptake (left anterior descending coronary artery/remote) was lower in chronically instrumented animals than in control animals and animals studied 1 month after instrumentation. The regional reduction in sympathetic nerve function was persistent and unaltered for at least 2 months after the development of hibernating myocardium. The study showed that hibernating myocardium is associated with persistent reductions in regional uptake of norepinephrine by sympathetic nerves [96]. In another study by Sasano et al. [97] in pigs after an experimental myocardial infarct (in the mid LAD), PET of tissue perfusion, catecholamine uptake and storage was performed with ^{13}N-ammonia and ^{11}C-EPI respectively, 4–12 weeks later. MRI and invasive electrophysiology (electroanatomic mapping, basket catheter, ventricular tachycardia inducibility) were performed within 1 week of PET. The study showed that myocardial neuronal injury exceeded the perfusion defect size (perfusion/innervation mismatch) and these areas may be a substrate for post-infarct arrhythmias [97].

Clinical Imaging

In the ADMIRE-HF (AdreView Myocardial Imaging for Risk Evaluation in HF) study, a total of 961 subjects with New York Heart Association (NYHA) functional class II/III HF and left ventricular ejection fraction (LVEF) ≤35 % were included. Clinical assessment, as well as ^{123}I-MIBG and MPI was performed and blood natriuretic peptide (BNP) measurements were obtained in these patients who were then followed up for up to 2 years [98]. The ADMIRE-HF study demonstrated the capacity of quantitation of sympathetic innervation of the myocardium, measured by the late heart/mediastinum ratio (H/M) on ^{123}I-MIBG scintigraphy, for predicting prognosis for significant cardiac events in subjects with HF and significant left ventricular dysfunction. This is the population to which guidelines for use of implanted devices for management of HF and arrhythmic event risk usually apply. The ADMIRE-HF showed a highly significant relationship between time to HF-related events and the H/M quantification, which was independent of other commonly measured parameters such as LVEF and BNP, as well as demographic parameters such as age and renal function in a HF population on guidelines-based contemporary therapy. The study also showed a clear association between severity of myocardial sympathetic neuronal dysfunction and risk for subsequent cardiac death [98]. In the Prediction of ARrhythmic Events with Positron Emission Tomography (PAREPET) study, a total of 204 patients were followed up for 4.1 years using $^{11C\text{-}HED}$, perfusion (^{13}N-ammonia) and viability (FDG) imaging. The primary end-points of the study were sudden cardiac arrest (SCA) defined as arrhythmic death or ICD discharge for ventricular fibrillation or ventricular tachycardia >240 bpm [99]. The study showed that in ischemic cardiomyopathy, the volume of myocardium with reduced ^{11}C-HED accumulation and the area of ammonia/^{11}C HED mismatch were independently predictive of sudden cardiac death whilst LVEF and infarct volume were not [99]. These are important observations; however their implications are at present relevant only to centres in close proximity to a cyclotron. ^{18}F-labeled norepinephrine analogs, which have a longer half-life are currently under investigation. If the findings of the PAREPET study are confirmed by such tracers, they could facilitate broader application and provide an improved approach for the identification of patients most likely to benefit from an ICD.

23.3 Imaging in Other Cardiovascular Pathological Entities

23.3.1 Aortic Aneurysms

The evaluation of high risk features in the arterial wall of aneurysms, beyond simply measuring their size with U/S, CT and MRI, might predict those that are prone to rupture. Molecular imaging approaches are similar to those described in the ATH section (imaging of INFL, neovascularization, MMPs and cathepsins) [100].

23.3.1.1 Preclinical Imaging

In mice models, macrophage markers and MMPs tracers, were found to accumulate in progressing aneurysms [101]. Optical imaging of vascular endothelial growth factor (VEGF) expression as a function of aneurysm progression in a murine aneurysm model was also investigated [102].

23.3.1.2 Clinical Imaging

The clinical value of FDG PET seems to be unclear particularly in asymptomatic patients with abdominal aortic aneurysms whose diameter is close to surgical indication because of the marked decrease in SMCs density. Recently Courtois et al. [103] studied patients (mostly asymptomatic) with abdominal aortic aneurysms using FDG PET and biopsy samples that were analyzed by immunohistochemistry, quantitative real-time polymerase chain reaction, and zymography. They showed that positive ^{18}F-FDG uptake in the aneurysmal wall is associated with an active inflammatory process characterized by a dense infiltrate of proliferating leukocytes in the adventitia and an increased circulating C-reactive protein. Moreover, a loss of SMCs in the media and alterations of the expression of genes involved in the REM of adventitia and collagen degradation potentially participate in the weakening of the aneurysmal wall preceding rupture. Aortic wall INFL using SPIOs (MRI) has been proven feasible in patients. The use of quantitative T2 and T2* pulse sequences, also provides a quantitative method for assessing SPIOs uptake by the aortic wall [104].

23.3.2 Valvular Diseases

Aortic stenosis and mitral regurgitation are the two most common valvular heart diseases. Current imaging methods (Doppler ECHO, MDCT and MRI) which measure hemodynamic parameters, decreased leaflet mobility, calcification, and reduced valve area, only identify the disease at a relatively late stage. Detection of earlier molecular and functional abnormalities in aortic valves in vivo may predict the future risk of subclinical valvular lesions and identify targets for effective therapeutic strategies to prevent aortic valve stenosis. Certain aspects in the pathophysiology of degenerative aortic stenosis are similar to that of coronary ATH; adhesion molecules, macrophages/INFL, MMPs/cysteine proteases and calcific deposits.

23.3.2.1 Preclinical Imaging

In a study by Hamilton et al. [105], a cholesterol-fed rabbit model was used to test the efficacy of identifying macrophage infiltration in early stage of aortic valve stenosis (AVS) using SPIOs with MRI. Although SPIOs labeling of macrophage infiltration in AVS has the potential to detect the disease process early, the results were hampered by iron deposition within myofibroblasts from control and cholesterol-fed valves posing the need for a macrophage-specific iron compound rather than passive targeting. Advances in 3-dimensional micro–CT imaging, may prove to be useful for understanding the spatial distribution of calcium deposition during progression of calcific AVS.

23.3.2.2 Clinical Imaging

Recent studies in patients with aortic valve disease reported that PET/CT is a novel, feasible, and repeatable approach to detect and quantify valvular INFL (FDG uptake) and osteoblastic activity (NaF), which are two key mechanisms underlying the development and progression of calcific aortic valve disease. In two recent studies by Dweck et al. [106, 107] ^{18}F-NaF and ^{18}F-FDG activity was increased in patients with both aortic sclerosis and stenosis, displaying a progressive rise in uptake with increasing disease severity. However, calcification rather than INFL appears to be the predominant process affecting the valve, particularly in the latter stages of the disease, in which a more marked progression in ^{18}F-NaF activity was observed that was disproportionate to ^{18}F-FDG. Enhanced uptake of FDG in the region of the valve documented by PET/CT might also help to confirm the presence of endocarditis and prompt the initiation of therapy. Obviously, more research is necessary to further refine and validate clinical application of PET in valvular heart diseases.

Rapid development of transcatheter valve therapies has led to an increase in the use of multimodality imaging for assessment of parameters such as myocardial strain and fibrosis by ECHO and/or MRI to evaluate the impact of valve dysfunction on the myocardium and to improve planning and guiding of surgical/transcatheter valve procedures (with multimodality/3D/fusion imaging). Such imaging approaches have generated a growing interest for their implementation in this setting however, further prospective studies are needed to demonstrate their precise impact on clinical outcomes.

23.4 The Role of Non-invasive Imaging in Assessment of Novel Therapies

Cell therapy has been extensively studied as a potential treatment option for patients with impaired cardiac function due to cell death. Despite encouraging findings from early animal and initial small-scale human studies, a recent meta-analysis has shown only marginal benefits, mainly with the use of bone marrow–derived stem cells (BMCs) [108]. Monitoring of cell survival and differentiation has the potential to unravel the reasons for these non-favorable results. For this to happen, cell labeling is essential and it is performed by use of two general approaches, namely, direct cell labeling and reporter gene imaging. The former approach is accomplished by incubating cells with contrast agents that either bind to the cell surface or are imported into the cells via diffusion, endocytosis or active transport [e.g., ^{111}In-labelled oxine and ^{99m}Tc-exametazime (HMPAO) for SPECT imaging, ^{18}F-FDG for PET imaging or SPIOs for visualization by MRI] [109]. Reporter gene imaging by means of optical imaging is successful in small animal research, whereas scintigraphic techniques are more applicable to large animals and patients. Most studies label an enzyme or transporter (herpes simplex virus type I thymidine kinase) or the human iodide/symporter. The main advantage of the reporter gene approach is that the imaging signal becomes specific to only viable implanted cells capable of mediating reporter protein–probe interaction and becomes reflective of cell number if the reporter gene is integrated into the genome and replicates with cell division (Fig. 23.11). In contrast, with direct cell labeling, the contrast agent is diluted over time with cell division and may be engulfed by other cell types (eg, macrophages) on cell death, which leads to the signal either not being reflective of cell number or not being specific to the implanted cells [110].

Radionuclide direct cell labeling, although it does not permit to monitor cell viability beyond 4–5 days because of the half lives of the common isotopes used, it can be quickly translated into the clinical setting because similar cell-labeling/imaging techniques have been used clinically for years to monitor the trafficking of other cell populations (e.g., ^{111}In-oxine–labeled leukocytes for imaging infection) and their high imaging sensitivity allows the tracking of low numbers of cells. This is the main reason why only the radionuclide-based imaging techniques (PET, SPECT) with direct cell labeling have been used in human studies. Reporter gene imaging with PET has allowed longitudinal PET imaging of stem cells for at least 10 days in porcine animal models and greater than 2 weeks in murine models [111]. In

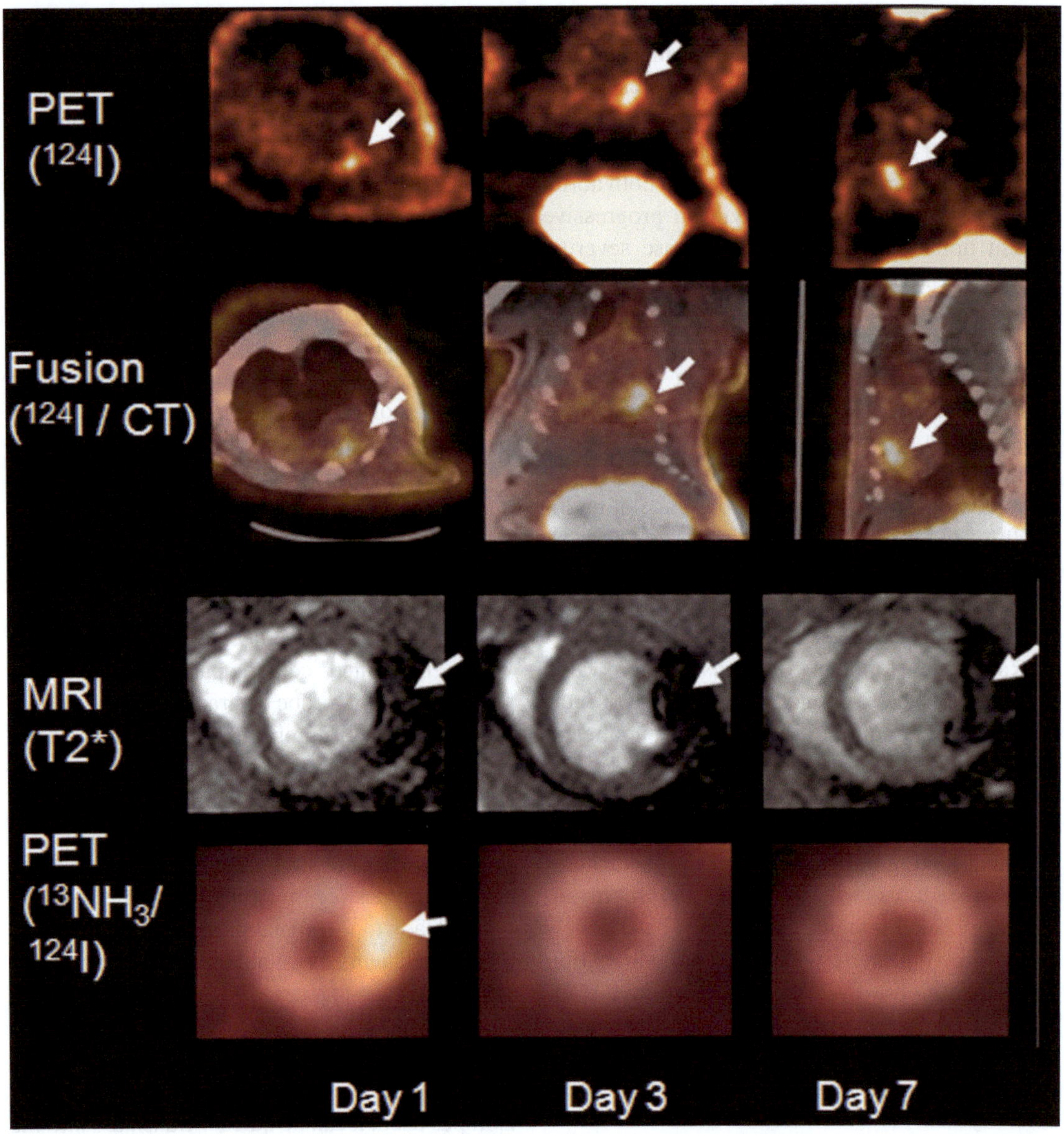

Fig. 23.11 Imaging of graft endothelial progenitor cells (*EPCs*) by multimodal reporter gene imaging in the rat heart. The *top panel* shows PET/CT 1 day after grafting the cells showing a clear signal from the viable cells. The *lower panel* depicts serial PET and MRI imaging revealing that the cells are dysfunctional at later time points and the persistent MR T2* signal only picks up the iron signal from the phagocytized cells (Modified with permission from Higuchi T, et al. Combined reporter gene PET and iron oxide MRI for monitoring survival and localization of transplanted cells in the rat heart. Higuchi TJ et al. [112] by permission)

a recent study by Higuchi et al. [112], combined reporter gene PET and SPIOs MRI were utilized for monitoring survival and localization of transplanted cells in the rat heart. Although iron labeling rapidly loses specificity for cell viability because of phagocytosis of iron particles released from dead cells, reporter gene expression provided specific information on the number of surviving cells (Fig. 23.11). This multimodality approach allowed complementary analysis of cell localization and viability, together with morphologic information about the heart. The application of these approaches to clinical research however, will require further documentation of suitability and safety to pass regulatory hurdles.

Conclusions

Beyond the areas of myocardial perfusion, ventricular function and tissue viability where imaging techniques have been available for many years, significant developments have been made recently in imaging fundamental processes such as angiogenesis, APO, MMPs expression etc., which are also of great interest to other disciplines beyond cardiovascular medicine; oncology is one such example. It is anticipated that in the near future, some of the molecular agents currently under investigation will enter the clinical phase of development and together with information from multiple other sources; e.g. genomic and proteomic technologies, can contribute to a patient–individualized risk assessment and treatment. For this to happen and overcome the challenges of the high costs which are involved, broad collaboration not only among different centers but between academia and industry is an essential component to success.

References

1. Ross R. Atherosclerosis: an inflammatory disease. N Engl J Med. 1999;340:115–26.
2. Virmani R, Kolodgie FD, Burke AP, Finn AV, Gold HK, Tulenko TN, et al. Atherosclerotic plaque progression and vulnerability to rupture: angiogenesis is a source of intraplaque hemorrhage. Arterioscler Thromb Vasc Biol. 2005;25:2054–61.
3. Burtea C, Ballet S, Laurent S, Rousseaux O, Dencausse A, Gonzalez W, et al. Development of a magnetic resonance imaging protocol for the characterization of atherosclerotic plaque by using vascular cell adhesion molecule-1 and apoptosis targeted ultrasmall superparamagnetic iron oxide derivatives. Arterioscler Thromb Vasc Biol. 2012;32:36–48.
4. Kaufmann BA, Sanders JM, Davis C, Xie A, Aldred P, Sarembock IJ, et al. Molecular imaging of inflammation in atherosclerosis with targeted ultrasound detection of vascular cell adhesion molecule-1. Circulation. 2007;116:276–84.
5. Kircher MF, Grimm J, Swirski FK, Libby P, Gerszten RE, Allport JR, et al. Noninvasive in vivo imaging of monocyte trafficking to atherosclerotic lesions. Circulation. 2008;117:388–95.
6. Aziz K, Berger K, Claycombe K, Huang R, Patel R, Abela GS. Noninvasive detection and localization of vulnerable plaque and arterial thrombosis with computed tomography angiography/positron emission tomography. Circulation. 2008;117:2061–70.
7. Li D, Patel AR, Klibanov AL, Kramer CM, Ruiz M, Kang BY, et al. Molecular imaging of atherosclerotic plaques targeted to oxidized LDL receptor LOX-1 by SPECT/CT and magnetic resonance. Circ Cardiovasc Imaging. 2010;3:464–72.
8. Laitinen I, Marjamäki P, Någren K, Laine VJ, Wilson I, Leppänen P, et al. Uptake of inflammatory cell marker [11C]PK11195 into mouse atherosclerotic plaques. Eur J Nucl Med Mol Imaging. 2009;36:73–80.
9. Hyafil F, Laissy JP, Mazighi M, Tchetche D, Louedec L, Adle-Biassette H, et al. Ferumoxtran-10-enhanced MRI of the hypercholesterolemic rabbit aorta: relationship between signal loss and macrophage infiltration. Arterioscler Thromb Vasc Biol. 2006;26:176–81.
10. Lipinski MJ, Amirbekian V, Frias JC, Aguinaldo JG, Mani V, Briley-Saebo KC, et al. MRI to detect atherosclerosis with gadolinium-containing immunomicelles targeting the macrophage scavenger receptor. Magn Reson Med. 2006;56:601–10.
11. Lipinski MJ, Frias JC, Amirbekian V, Briley-Saebo KC, Mani V, Samber D, et al. Macrophage-specific lipid-based nanoparticles improve cardiac magnetic resonance detection and characterization of human atherosclerosis. JACC Cardiovasc Imaging. 2009;2:637–47.
12. Hyafil F, Cornily JC, Rudd JH, Machac J, Feldman LJ, Fayad ZA. Quantification of inflammation within rabbit atherosclerotic plaques using the macrophage-specific CT contrast agent N1177: a comparison with 18F-FDG PET/CT and histology. J Nucl Med. 2009;50:959–65.
13. Cormode DP, Skajaa T, van Schooneveld MM, Koole R, Jarzyna P, Lobatto ME, et al. Nanocrystal core high-density lipoproteins: a multimodality contrast agent platform. Nano Lett. 2008;8:3715–23.
14. Ehara S, Kobayashi Y, Yoshiyama M, Shimada K, Shimada Y, Fukuda D, et al. Spotty calcification typifies the culprit plaque in patients with acute myocardial infarction: an intravascular ultrasound study. Circulation. 2004;110:3424–9.
15. Aikawa E, Nahrendorf M, Figueiredo JL, Swirski FK, Shtatland T, Kohler RH, et al. Osteogenesis associates with inflammation in early-stage atherosclerosis evaluated by molecular imaging in vivo. Circulation. 2007;116:2841–50.
16. Kolodgie FD, Petrov A, Virmani R, Narula N, Verjans JW, Weber DK, et al. Targeting of apoptotic macrophages and experimental atheroma with radiolabeled annexin V: a technique with potential for noninvasive imaging of vulnerable plaque. Circulation. 2003;108:3134–9.
17. Sarai M, Hartung D, Petrov A, Zhou J, Narula N, Hofstra L, et al. Broad and specific caspase

inhibitor induced acute repression of apoptosis in atherosclerotic lesions evaluated by radiolabeled annexin A5 imaging. J Am Coll Cardiol. 2007;50: 2305–12.
18. De Saint-Hubert M, Bauwens M, Deckers N, Drummen M, Douma K, Granton P, et al. In vivo molecular imaging of apoptosis and necrosis in atherosclerotic plaques using microSPECT-CT and microPET-CT imaging. Mol Imaging Biol. 2014;16:246–54.
19. Wagner S, Faust A, Breyholz HJ, Schober O, Schäfers M, Kopka K. The MMP inhibitor (R)-2-(N-benzyl-4-(2-[18F]fluoroethoxy) phenylsulphonamido)-N-hydroxy-3-methylbutanamide: improved precursor synthesis and fully automated radiosynthesis. Appl Radiat Isot. 2011;69:862–8.
20. Winter PM, Morawski AM, Caruthers SD, Fuhrhop RW, Zhang H, Williams TA, et al. Molecular imaging of angiogenesis in early-stage atherosclerosis with alpha(v)beta3-integrin-targeted nanoparticles. Circulation. 2003;108:2270–4.
21. Laitinen I, Saraste A, Weidl E, Poethko T, Weber AW, Nekolla SG, et al. Evaluation of alphavbeta3 integrin-targeted positron emission tomography tracer ^{18}F-galacto-RGD for imaging of vascular inflammation in atherosclerotic mice. Circ Cardiovasc Imaging. 2009;2:331–8.
22. Makowski MR, Forbes SC, Blume U, Warley A, Jansen CH, Schuster A, et al. In vivo assessment of intraplaque and endothelial fibrin in ApoE(−/−) mice by molecular MRI. Atherosclerosis. 2012;222: 43–9.
23. von zur Muhlen C, von Elverfeldt D, Moeller JA, Choudhury RP, Paul D, Hagemeyer CE, et al. Magnetic resonance imaging contrast agent targeted toward activated platelets allows in vivo detection of thrombosis and monitoring of thrombolysis. Circulation. 2008;118:258–67.
24. Rouzet F, Bachelet-Violette L, Alsac JM, Suzuki M, Meulemans A, Louedec L, et al. Radiolabeled fucoidan as a p-selectin targeting agent for in vivo imaging of platelet rich thrombus and endothelial activation. J Nucl Med. 2011;52:1433–40.
25. Ciesienski KL, Yang Y, Ay I, Chonde DB, Loving GS, Rietz TA, et al. Fibrin-targeted PET probes for the detection of thrombi. Mol Pharm. 2013;10: 1100–10.
26. Yun M, Jang S, Cucchiara A, Newberg AB, Alavi A. 18F FDG uptake in the large arteries: a correlation study with the atherogenic risk factors. Semin Nucl Med. 2002;32:70–6.
27. Rudd JH, Myers KS, Bansilal S, Machac J, Rafique A, Farkouh M, et al. (18)fluorodeoxyglucose positron emission tomography imaging of atherosclerotic plaque inflammation is highly reproducible: Implications for atherosclerosis therapy trials. J Am Coll Cardiol. 2007;50:892–6.
28. Rudd JH, Myers KS, Bansilal S, Machac J, Pinto CA, Tong C, et al. Atherosclerosis inflammation imaging with ^{18}F-FDG PET: carotid, iliac, and femoral uptake reproducibility, quantification methods, and recommendations. J Nucl Med. 2008;49:871–8.
29. Tawakol A, Migrino RQ, Bashian GG, Bedri S, Vermylen D, Cury RC, et al. In vivo ^{18}F-fluorodeoxyglucose positron emission tomography imaging provides a noninvasive measure of carotid plaque inflammation in patients. J Am Coll Cardiol. 2006;48:1818–24.
30. Menezes LJ, Kotze CW, Agu O, Richards T, Brookes J, Goh VJ, et al. Investigating vulnerable atheroma using combined ^{18}F-FDG PET/CT angiography of carotid plaque with immunohistochemical validation. J Nucl Med. 2011;52:1698–703.
31. Rudd JH, Myers KS, Bansilal S, Machac J, Woodward M, Fuster V, et al. Relationships among regional arterial inflammation, calcification, risk factors, and biomarkers: a prospective fluorodeoxyglucose positron-emission tomography/computed tomography imaging study. Circ Cardiovasc Imaging. 2009;2:107–15.
32. Figueroa AL, Subramanian SS, Cury RC, Truong QA, Gardecki JA, Tearney GJ, et al. Distribution of inflammation within carotid atherosclerotic plaques with high-risk morphological features: a comparison between positron emission tomography activity, plaque morphology, and histopathology. Circ Cardiovasc Imaging. 2012;5:69–77.
33. Kwee RM, Truijman MT, Mess WH, Teule GJ, ter Berg JW, Franke CL, et al. Potential of integrated [18F] fluorodeoxyglucose positron-emission tomography/CT in identifying vulnerable carotid plaques. AJNR Am J Neuroradiol. 2011;32:950–4.
34. Noh SM, Choi WJ, Kang BT, Jeong SW, Lee DK, Schellingerhout D, et al. Complementarity between 18F-FDG PET/CT and ultrasonography or angiography in carotid plaque characterization. J Clin Neurol. 2013;9:176–85.
35. Rominger A, Saam T, Wolpers S, Cyran CC, Schmidt M, Foerster S, et al. ^{18}F-FDG PET/CT identifies patients at risk for future vascular events in an otherwise asymptomatic cohort with neoplastic disease. J Nucl Med. 2009;50:1611–20.
36. Fayad ZA, Mani V, Woodward M, Kallend D, Abt M, Burgess T, et al. Safety and efficacy of dalcetrapib on atherosclerotic disease using novel non-invasive multimodality imaging (dal-PLAQUE): a randomised clinical trial. Lancet. 2011;378:1547–59.
37. Tawakol A, Fayad ZA, Mogg R, Alon A, Klimas MT, Dansky H, et al. Intensification of statin therapy results in a rapid reduction in atherosclerotic inflammation: results of a multi-center FDG-PET/CT feasibility study. J Am Coll Cardiol. 2013;62:909–17.
38. Gaemperli O, Shalhoub J, Owen DR, Lamare F, Johansson S, Fouladi N, et al. Imaging intraplaque inflammation in carotid atherosclerosis with ^{11}C-PK11195 positron emission tomography/computed tomography. Eur Heart J. 2012;33:1902–10.
39. Rominger A, Saam T, Vogl E, Ubleis C, la Fougere C, Forster S, et al. In vivo imaging of macrophage activity in the coronary arteries using 68Ga-DOTATATE

PET/CT: correlation with coronary calcium burden and risk factors. J Nucl Med. 2010;51:193–7.
40. Kato K, Schober O, Ikeda M, Schafers M, Ishigaki T, Kies P, et al. Evaluation and comparison of ^{11}C-choline uptake and calcification in aortic and common carotid arterial walls with combined PET/CT. Eur J Nucl Med Mol Imaging. 2009;36:1622–8.
41. Rogers IS, Nasir K, Figueroa AL, Cury RC, Hoffmann U, Vermylen DA, et al. Feasibility of FDG imaging of the coronary arteries: comparison between acute coronary syndrome and stable angina. J Am Coll Cardiol Img. 2010;3:388–97.
42. Dweck MR, Chow MW, Joshi NV, Williams MC, Jones C, Fletcher AM, et al. Coronary arterial ^{18}F-sodium fluoride uptake: a novel marker of plaque biology. J Am Coll Cardiol. 2012;59:1539–48.
43. Joshi NV, Vesey AT, Williams MC, Shah AS, Calvert PA, Craighead FH, et al. ^{18}F-fluoride positron emission tomography for identification of ruptured and high-risk coronary atherosclerotic plaques: a prospective clinical trial. Lancet. 2014;383:705–13.
44. Kooi ME, Cappendijk VC, Cleutjens KB, Kessels AG, Kitslaar PJ, Borgers M, et al. Accumulation of ultra small super paramagnetic particles of iron oxide in human atherosclerotic plaques can be detected by in vivo magnetic resonance imaging. Circulation. 2003;107:2453–8.
45. Tang TY, Howarth SP, Miller SR, Graves MJ, Patterson AJ, U-King-Im JM, et al. The ATHEROMA (Atorvastatin therapy: effects on reduction of macrophage activity) study: evaluation using ultrasmall superparamagnetic iron oxide-enhanced magnetic resonance imaging in carotid disease. J Am Coll Cardiol. 2009;53:2039–50.
46. Beer AJ, Pelisek J, Heider P, Saraste A, Reeps C, Metz S, et al. PET/CT imaging of integrin avb3 expression. J Am Coll Cardiol. 2014 (in press). http://dx.doi.org/10.1016/j.jcmg.2013.12.003.
47. Kietselaer BL, Reutelingsperger CP, Heidendal GA, Daemen MJ, Mess WH, Hofstra L, et al. Noninvasive detection of plaque instability with use of radiolabeled annexin A5 in patients with carotid-artery atherosclerosis. N Engl J Med. 2004;350:1472–3.
48. Vymazal J, Spuentrup E, Cardenas-Molina G, Wiethoff AJ, Hartmann MG, Caravan P, et al. Thrombus imaging with fibrin-specific gadolinium-based MR contrast agent EP-2104R: results of a phase II clinical study of feasibility. Invest Radiol. 2009;44:697–704.
49. Versteylen MO, Kietselaer BL, Dagnelie PC, Joosen IA, Dedic A, Raaijmakers RH, et al. Additive value of semiautomated quantification of coronary artery disease using cardiac computed tomographic angiography to predict future acute coronary syndromes. J Am Coll Cardiol. 2013;61:2296–305.
50. Cai J, Hatsukami TS, Ferguson MS, Kerwin WS, Saam T, Chu B, et al. In vivo quantitative measurement of intact fibrous cap and lipid-rich necrotic core size in atherosclerotic carotid plaque: comparison of high-resolution, contrast-enhanced magnetic resonance imaging and histology. Circulation. 2005;112:3437–44.
51. Noguchi T, Kawasaki T, Tanaka A, Yasuda S, Goto Y, Ishihara M, et al. High-intensity signals in coronary plaques on non-contrast T1-weighted magnetic resonance imaging as a novel determinant of coronary events. J Am Coll Cardiol. 2014 (Published online). doi:10.1016/j.jacc.2013.11.034.
52. Bolukoglu H, Goodwin GW, Guthrie PH, Carmical SG, Chen TM, Taegtmeyer H. Metabolic fate of glucose in reversible low-flow ischemia of the isolated working rat heart. Am J Physiol. 1996;270:817–26.
53. Gould KL, Lipscomb K. Effects of coronary stenoses on coronary flow reserve and resistance. Am J Cardiol. 1974;34:48–55.
54. Anagnostopoulos C, Neill J, Reyes E, Prvulovich E. Myocardial perfusion scintigraphy: technical innovations and evolving clinical applications. Heart. 2012;98:353–9.
55. Dowsley T, Al-Mallah M, Ananthasubramaniam K, Dwivedi G, McArdle B, Chow BJ. The role of noninvasive imaging in coronary artery disease detection, prognosis and clinical decision making. Can J Cardiol. 2013;29:285–96.
56. Schwaiger M, Schelbert HR, Ellison D, Hansen H, Yeatman L, Vinten-Johansen J, et al. Sustained regional abnormalities in cardiac metabolism after transient ischemia in the chronic dog model. J Am Coll Cardiol. 1985;6:336–47.
57. Dilsizian V. Metabolic imaging for identifying antecedent myocardial ischemia and acute coronary syndrome in the emergency department. Curr Cardiol Rep. 2011;13:96–9.
58. Villanueva FS, Lu E, Bowry S, Kilic S, Tom E, Wang J, et al. Myocardial ischemic memory imaging with molecular echocardiography. Circulation. 2007;115:345–52.
59. Cokkinos DV, Pantos C. Myocardial remodelling, an overview. Heart Fail Rev. 2011;16:1–4.
60. Nijveldt R, Beek AM, Hirsch A, Stoel MG, Hofman MB, Umans VA, et al. Functional recovery after acute myocardial infarction: comparison between angiography, electrocardiography, and cardiovascular magnetic resonance measures of microvascular injury. J Am Coll Cardiol. 2008;52:181–9.
61. Ørn S, Manhenke C, Greve OJ, Larsen AI, Bonarjee VV, Edvardsen T, et al. Microvascular obstruction is a major determinant of infarct healing and subsequent left ventricular remodelling following primary percutaneous coronary intervention. Eur Heart J. 2009;30:1978–85.
62. Berti V, Sciagrà R, Acampa W, Ricci F, Cerisano G, Gallicchio R, et al. Relationship between infarct size and severity measured by gated SPECT and long-term left ventricular remodelling after acute myocardial infarction. Eur J Nucl Med Mol Imaging. 2011;38:1124–31.
63. Sosnovik DE, Garanger E, Aikawa E, Nahrendorf M, Figuiredo JL, Dai G, et al. Molecular MRI of cardiomyocyte apoptosis with simultaneous delayed

enhancement MRI distinguishes apoptotic and necrotic myocytes in vivo: potential for midmyocardial salvage in acute ischemia. Circ Cardiovasc Imaging. 2009;2:460–7.
64. Garanger E, Hilderbrand SA, Blois JT, Sosnovik DE, Weissleder R, Josephson L. A DNA-binding Gd chelate for the detection of cell death by MRI. Chem Commun (Camb). 2009;29:4444–6.
65. Higuchi T, Nekolla SG, Jankaukas A, Weber AW, Huisman MC, Reder S, et al. Characterization of normal and infarcted rat myocardium using a combination of small-animal PET and clinical MR imaging. J Nucl Med. 2007;48:288–94.
66. Lee WW, Marinelli B, van der Laan AM, Sena BF, Gorbatov R, Leuschner F, et al. PET/MR of inflammation in myocardial infarction. J Am Coll Cardiol. 2012;59:153–63.
67. Panizzi P, Swirski FK, Figueiredo JL, Waterman P, Sosnovik DE, Aikawa E, et al. Impaired infarct healing in atherosclerotic mice with Ly-6C(hi) monocytosis. J Am Coll Cardiol. 2010;55:1629–38.
68. Flogel U, Ding Z, Hardung H, Jander S, Reichmann G, Jacoby C, et al. In vivo monitoring of inflammation after cardiac and cerebral ischemia by fluorine magnetic resonance imaging. Circulation. 2008;118:140–8.
69. Christiansen JP, Leong-Poi H, Klibanov AL, Kaul S, Lindner JR. Noninvasive imaging of myocardial reperfusion injury using leukocyte-targeted contrast echocardiography. Circulation. 2002;105:1764–7.
70. Nahrendorf M, Sosnovik D, Chen JW, Panizzi P, Figueiredo JL, Aikawa E, et al. Activatable magnetic resonance imaging agent reports myeloperoxidase activity in healing infarcts and noninvasively detects the anti-inflammatory effects of atorvastatin on ischemia-reperfusion injury. Circulation. 2008;117:1153–60.
71. Ye YX, Basse-Lüsebrink TC, Arias-Loza PA, Kocoski V, Kampf T, Gan Q, et al. Monitoring of monocyte recruitment in reperfused myocardial infarction with intramyocardial hemorrhage and microvascular obstruction by combined fluorine 19 and proton cardiac magnetic resonance imaging. Circulation. 2013;128:1878–88.
72. Verjans JW, Lovhaug D, Narula N, Petrov AD, Indrevoll B, Bjurgert E, et al. Noninvasive imaging of angiotensin receptors after myocardial infarction. J Am Coll Cardiol Img. 2008;1:354–62.
73. Fukushima K, Bravo PE, Higuchi T, Schuleri KH, Lin X, Abraham MR, et al. Molecular hybrid positron emission tomography/computed tomography imaging of cardiac angiotensin II type 1 receptors. J Am Coll Cardiol. 2012;60:2527–34.
74. van den Borne SWM, Isobe S, Verjans JW, Petrov A, Lovhaug D, Li P, et al. Molecular imaging of interstitial alterations in remodeling myocardium after myocardial infarction. J Am Coll Cardiol. 2008;52:2017–28.
75. van den Borne SWM, Isobe S, Zandbergen HR, Li P, Petrov A, Wong ND, et al. Molecular imaging for efficacy of pharmacologic intervention in myocardial remodeling. J Am Coll Cardiol Img. 2009;2:187–98.
76. Rodriguez-Porcel M, Cai W, Gheysens O, Willmann JK, Chen K, Wang H, et al. Imaging of VEGF receptor in a rat myocardial infarction model using PET. J Nucl Med. 2008;49:667–73.
77. Makowski MR, Ebersberger U, Nekolla S, Schwaiger M. In vivo molecular imaging of angiogenesis, targeting alphavbeta3 integrin expression, in a patient after acute myocardial infarction. Eur Heart J. 2008;29:2201.
78. Higuchi T, Bengel FM, Seidl S, Watzlowik P, Kessler H, Hegenloh R, et al. Assessment of alphavbeta3 integrin expression after myocardial infarction by positron emission tomography. Cardiovasc Res. 2008;78:395–403.
79. Eo JS, Paeng JC, Lee S, Lee YS, Jeong JM, Kang KW, et al. Angiogenesis imaging in myocardial infarction using 68Ga-NOTA-RGD PET: characterization and application to therapeutic efficacy monitoring in rats. Coron Artery Dis. 2013;24:303–11.
80. Verjans J, Wolters S, Laufer W, Schellings M, Lax M, Lovhaug D, et al. Early molecular imaging of interstitial changes in patients after myocardial infarction: comparison with delayed contrast-enhanced magnetic resonance imaging. J Nucl Cardiol. 2010;17:1065–72.
81. Jivraj N, Phinikaridou A, Shah AM, Botnar RM. Molecular imaging of myocardial infarction. Basic Res Cardiol. 2014;109:397.
82. Schulz R, Guth BD, Pieper K, Martin C, Heusch G. Recruitment of an inotropic reserve in moderately ischemic myocardium at the expense of metabolic recovery: a model of short-term hibernation. Circ Res. 1992;70:1282–95.
83. Fallavollita JA, Canty Jr JM. Differential ^{18}F-2-deoxyglucose uptake in viable dysfunctional myocardium with normal resting perfusion. Circulation. 1999;99:2798–805.
84. Di Carli MF, Prcevski P, Singh TP, Janisse J, Ager J, Muzik O, et al. Myocardial blood flow, function, and metabolism in repetitive stunning. J Nucl Med. 2000;41:1227–34.
85. Rahimtoola SH, Dilsizian V, Kramer CM, Marwick TH, Vanoverschelde JL. Chronic ischemic left ventricular dysfunction: from pathophysiology to imaging and its integration into clinical practice. J Am Coll Cardiol Img. 2008;1:536–55.
86. Witschey WR, Zsido GA, Koomalsingh K, Kondo N, Minakawa M, Shuto T, et al. In vivo chronic myocardial infarction characterization by spin locked cardiovascular magnetic resonance. J Cardiovasc Magn Reson. 2012;14:37.
87. Schuleri KH, Centola M, Evers KS, Zviman A, Evers R, Lima JA, Lardo AC. Cardiovascular magnetic resonance characterization of peri-infarct zone remodeling following myocardial infarction. J Cardiovasc Magn Reson. 2012;14:24.
88. Selvanayagam JB, Jerosch-Herold M, Porto I, Sheridan D, Cheng AS, Petersen SE, et al. Resting myocardial blood flow is impaired in hibernating myocardium: a magnetic resonance study of

quantitative perfusion assessment. Circulation. 2005;112:3289–96.
89. Hata T, Nohara R, Fujita M, Hosokawa R, Lee L, Kudo T, et al. Noninvasive assessment of myocardial viability by positron emission tomography with ^{11}C acetate in patients with old myocardial infarction. Usefulness of low-dose dobutamine infusion. Circulation. 1996;94:1834–41.
90. Anagnostopoulos C, Georgakopoulos A, Pianou N, Nekolla SG. Assessment of myocardial perfusion and viability by positron emission tomography. Int J Cardiol. 2013;167:1737–49.
91. Bonow RO, Maurer G, Lee KL, Holly TA, Binkley PF, Desvigne-Nickens P, et al. Myocardial viability and survival in ischemic left ventricular dysfunction. N Engl J Med. 2011;364:1617–25.
92. Beanlands RS, Nichol G, Huszti E, Humen D, Racine N, Freeman M, et al. F-18-fluorodeoxyglucose positron emission tomography imaging-assisted management of patients with severe left ventricular dysfunction and suspected coronary disease: a randomized controlled trial (PARR-2). J Am Coll Cardiol. 2007;50:2002–12.
93. D'Egidio G, Nichol G, Williams KA, Guo A, Garrard L, deKemp R, et al. Increasing benefit from revascularization is associated with increasing amounts of myocardial hibernation: a substudy of the PARR-2 trial. J Am Coll Cardiol Img. 2009;2:1060–8.
94. Becker M, Zwicker C, Kaminski M, Napp A, Altiok E, Ocklenburg C, et al. Dependency of cardiac resynchronization therapy on myocardial viability at the LV lead position. J Am Coll Cardiol Img. 2011;4:366–74.
95. Shetty AK, Duckett SG, Ginks MR, Ma Y, Sohal M, Bostock J, et al. Cardiac magnetic resonance-derived anatomy, scar, and dyssynchrony fused with fluoroscopy to guide LV lead placement in cardiac resynchronization therapy: a comparison with acute haemodynamic measures and echocardiographic reverse remodelling. Eur Heart J Cardiovasc Imaging. 2013;14:692–9.
96. Luisi Jr AJ, Suzuki G, Dekemp R, Haka MS, Toorongian SA, Canty Jr JM, et al. Regional ^{11}C-hydroxyephedrine retention in hibernating myocardium: chronic inhomogeneity of sympathetic innervation in the absence of infarction. J Nucl Med. 2005;46:1368–74.
97. Sasano T, Abraham MR, Chang KC, Ashikaga H, Mills KJ, Holt DP, et al. Abnormal sympathetic innervation of viable myocardium and the substrate of ventricular tachycardia after myocardial infarction. J Am Coll Cardiol. 2008;51:2266–75.
98. Jacobson AF, Senior R, Cerqueira MD, Wong ND, Lopez VA, Agostini D, et al. Myocardial iodine-123 metaiodobenzylguanidine imaging and cardiac events in heart failure: results of the prospective ADMIRE-HF (AdreView Myocardial Imaging for Risk Evaluation in Heart Failure) study. J Am Coll Cardiol. 2010;55:2212–21.
99. Fallavollita JA, Heavey BM, Luisi Jr AJ, Michalek SM, Baldwa S, Mashtare Jr TL, et al. Regional myocardial sympathetic denervation predicts the risk of sudden cardiac arrest in ischemic cardiomyopathy. J Am Coll Cardiol. 2014;63:141–9.
100. Osborn EA, Jaffer FA. The advancing clinical impact of molecular imaging in CVD. J Am Coll Cardiol Img. 2013;61:1327–41.
101. Nahrendorf M, Keliher E, Marinelli B, Leuschner F, Robbins CS, Gerszten RE, et al. Detection of macrophages in aortic aneurysms by nanoparticle positron emission tomography-computed tomography. Arterioscler Thromb Vasc Biol. 2011;31:750–7.
102. Tedesco MM, Terashima M, Blankenberg FG, Levashova Z, Spin JM, Backer MV, et al. Analysis of in situ and ex vivo vascular endothelial growth factor receptor expression during experimental aortic aneurysm progression. Arterioscler Thromb Vasc Biol. 2009;29:1452–7.
103. Courtois A, Nusgens BV, Hustinx R, Namur G, Gomez P, Somja J, et al. ^{18}F-FDG uptake assessed by PET/CT in abdominal aortic aneurysms is associated with cellular and molecular alterations prefacing wall deterioration and rupture. J Nucl Med. 2013;54:1740–7.
104. Sadat U, Taviani V, Patterson AJ, Young VE, Graves MJ, Teng Z, et al. Ultra small super paramagnetic iron oxide-enhanced magnetic resonance imaging of abdominal aortic aneurysms – a feasibility study. Eur J Vasc Endovasc Surg. 2011;41:167–74.
105. Hamilton AM, Rogers KA, Belisle AJ, Ronald JA, Rutt BK, Weissleder R, et al. Early identification of aortic valve sclerosis using iron oxide enhanced MRI. J Magn Reson Imaging. 2010;31:110–6.
106. Dweck MR, Jones C, Joshi NV, Fletcher AM, Richardson H, White A, et al. Assessment of valvular calcification and inflammation by positron emission tomography in patients with aortic stenosis. Circulation. 2012;125:76–86.
107. Dweck MR, Khaw HJ, Sng GK, Luo EL, Baird A, Williams MC, et al. Aortic stenosis, atherosclerosis, and skeletal bone: is there a common link with calcification and inflammation? Eur Heart J. 2013;34:1567–74.
108. Abdel-Latif A, Bolli R, Tleyjeh IM, Montori VM, Perin EC, Hornung CA, et al. Adult bone marrow derived cells for cardiac repair: a systematic review and meta-analysis. Arch Intern Med. 2007;167: 989–97.
109. Terrovitis J, Lautamäki R, Bonios M, Fox J, Engles JM, Yu J, et al. Noninvasive quantification and optimization of acute cell retention by in vivo positron emission tomography after intramyocardial cardiac-derived stem cell delivery. J Am Coll Cardiol. 2009;54:1619–26.
110. Chen IY, Wu JC. Cardiovascular molecular imaging: focus on clinical translation. Circulation. 2011;123: 425–43.
111. Gyongyosi M, Blanco J, Marian T, Tron L, Petnehazy O, Petrasi Z, et al. Serial noninvasive in vivo positron

emission tomographic tracking of percutaneously intramyocardially injected autologous porcine mesenchymal stem cells modified for transgene reporter gene expression. Circ Cardiovasc Imaging. 2008;1:94–103.
112. Higuchi T, Anton M, Dumler K, Seidl S, Pelisek J, Saraste A, et al. Combined reporter gene PET and iron oxide MRI for monitoring survival and localization of transplanted cells in the rat heart. J Nucl Med. 2009;50:1088–94.
113. Leuschner F, Nahrendorf M. Molecular imaging of coronary atherosclerosis and myocardial infarction: considerations for the bench and perspectives for the clinic. Circ Res. 2011;108:593–606.
114. Graebe M, Pedersen SF, Borgwardt L, Højgaard L, Sillesen H, Kjaer A. Molecular pathology in vulnerable carotid plaques: correlation with [18]-fluorodeoxyglucose positron emission tomography (FDG-PET). Eur J Vasc Endovasc Surg. 2009;37:714–21.
115. Inaba Y, Lindner JR. Molecular imaging of disease with targeted contrast ultrasound imaging. Transl Res. 2012;159:140–8.

Molecular Imaging of Inflammation Using Echocardiography. Advances with the Use of Microbubbles

24

James S.M. Yeh and Petros Nihoyannopoulos

Abstract

Ultrasound molecular imaging uses microbubbles conjugated with targeting ligands. When administered *intravenously* these 'targeting bubbles' attach to areas expressing the molecule of interest for ultrasound detection. The migration of this technology to human application has been limited by uncertainties regarding its safety and efficacy, including: (i) the lack of targeting bubbles that do not contain immunogenic (strept)avidin for ligand conjugation; (ii) the traditional use of high power ultrasound causing 'instantaneous' bubble destruction, raising concerns about biosafety and rendering it not a real-time imaging technique (limiting bedside interpretation); (iii) the absence of robust molecular quantification methods, diminishing its potential diagnostic power. Progress has been made in all three areas recently. An example is molecular imaging of E-selectin expression for detecting endothelial activation or inflammation in the heart. Inflammation underlies important cardiovascular diseases, such as coronary atheromatous heart disease, myocarditis and heart transplant rejection. Endothelial activation occurs early in inflammation and E-selectin is classically expressed only on activated endothelial cells. E-selectin targeting bubbles, based on maleimide-thiol conjugation chemistry, were successfully engineered. They allowed high resolution real-time and quantitative ultrasound molecular imaging of the heart in mice. Future directions in the field includes establishing 3-D ultrasound molecular imaging, and therapies using targeting bubbles as vehicles for

J.S.M. Yeh, MBChB, MRCP, PhD
National Heart and Lung Institute,
Imperial College London, London, UK

P. Nihoyannopoulos, MD, FRCP, FESC, FACC, FAHA (✉)
National Heart and Lung Institute,
Imperial College London, London, UK

Hammersmith Hospital,
Du Cane Road, London W12 0NN, UK
e-mail: petros@imperial.ac.uk

D.V. Cokkinos (ed.), *Introduction to Translational Cardiovascular Research*,
DOI 10.1007/978-3-319-08798-6_24, © Springer International Publishing Switzerland 2015

targeted delivery of therapeutic agents such as drugs or genetic materials. All these help gather the financial and research momentum required to establish the technology in humans.

Keywords
Molecular imaging • Ultrasound molecular imaging • Microbubbles • Targeted-microbubbles • Contrast echocardiography • Contrast ultrasonography • Real-time imaging • Time signal intensity curve • Quantification • E-selectin • Inflammation

Abbreviations

KO	Knock-out
LV	Left ventricle, left ventricular
mAb	Monoclonal antibody
MCU	Microbubble contrast enhanced ultrasound/ultrasonography
MI	Mechanical index
PEG	Polyethylene glycol
RES	Reticuloendothelial system
TIC	Time signal intensity curve
WT	Wild-type

24.1 Introduction

Inflammation underlies important cardiovascular diseases such as coronary heart disease, myocarditis and heart transplant rejection. Endothelial activation is an early inflammatory event, characterised by up-regulated expression of endothelial adhesion molecules, including E-selectin, P-selectin, ICAM-1 and VCAM-1. Quantitative molecular imaging of endothelial adhesion molecule(s) potentially allows the detection and characterisation of inflammation for early diagnosis, monitoring of response to treatment and possibly prediction of prognosis in these patients.

Echocardiography or ultrasonography is a common imaging modality that is non-invasive and relatively inexpensive compared to other imaging modalities such as nuclear imaging, computed tomography (CT), positron emission tomography (PET) and magnetic resonance imaging (MRI). Importantly, it does not involve ionising radiation, can be performed quickly, and has high temporal and spatial resolutions. Uniquely, it can be performed by the bedside, a clear advantage in severely ill or unstable patients. Ultrasound molecular imaging is therefore a potentially elegant and powerful diagnostic tool.

The strategy for ultrasound molecular imaging involves the use of targeting microbubbles as ultrasound contrast enhancement agents. Phospholipid-based targeting bubbles are gas encapsulated within a phospholipid shell containing targeting ligands (e.g. antibodies or peptides) on the shell's outer surface. They average ≈1 to 5 μm in diameter with similar rheology to that of the red blood cells. In an acoustic field, the bubbles may undergo non-linear oscillation generating strong back scattered signals. Following their *intravenous* (*iv*) administration, they circulate and accumulate in tissues by attaching to the molecules of interest for subsequent ultrasound detection – localising and defining the spatial extent and intensity of the targeted molecule expression. Such imaging technique is here termed 'targeted microbubble contrast enhanced ultrasonography' (targeted MCU). It has been described for ultrasound molecular imaging of various pathophysiological processes, including inflammation, angiogenesis and thrombosis in animal models of human diseases [1].

Limiting factors for the clinical translation of ultrasound molecular imaging include: (a) the traditional use of biotin-(strept)avidin conjugation chemistry for attaching targeting ligands to the bubble-shell surface, which made the targeting bubbles immunogenic and should best be avoided in humans (streptavidin or avidin is a bacterium *Streptomyces avidinii* protein or egg white protein, respectively); (b) the historical use of high ultrasound power bubble destructive imaging technique, which raised safety concerns regarding the bioeffects of the high power bubble destruction; it also made acquisition of complete cardiac cycles and bedside interpretations difficult (ie, it was not a real-time imaging method and extensive off-line image subtraction analysis was required to isolate the retained bubble signals from that of the circulating bubbles, in order to visualise the targeted molecules); and (c) the technique's ability to quantitatively measure the level of molecular expression has not been established. Favourable demonstrations of the technique's safety, effectiveness and breadth of potential clinical applications would help gather the financial and research momentum required to establish it for human applications.

24.1.1 Inflammation and Endothelial Adhesion Molecules

Inflammation is a common pathogenic pathway in major human diseases. These include cardiovascular diseases such as atherosclerosis involving the coronary arteries (and its sequelae of acute coronary syndrome or ischaemia-reperfusion injury), the aorta, carotid and renal arteries; myocarditis; congestive heart failure or dilated cardiomyopathy; and heart transplant rejection. Non cardiovascular diseases include connective tissue diseases (such as rheumatoid arthritis), vasculitis, glomerulonephritis, inflammatory bowel disease, inflammatory skin conditions, acute lung injury and organ transplant rejection [2–10].

Endothelial activation occurs early in inflammation, one characteristic being the up-regulated expression of endothelial adhesion molecules, such as E-selectin, P-selectin, ICAM-1 and VCAM-1 (Table 24.1). The endothelial adhesion molecules are involved in recruiting circulating leukocytes to the sites of inflammation, through the leukocyte adhesion cascade [7]. They also participate in immunological processes [17], as well as angiogenesis e.g., in tumour formation and ischaemia-led vasculogenesis. The leukocyte adhesion cascade consists of a sequence of events. First, leukocytes roll along the vessel wall through low-affinity adhesive interactions with E-selectin and P-selectin. This results in activation and firm adhesion of the leukocytes to the endothelium through ICAM-1 and VCAM-1. Adherent leukocytes then transmigrate through the vascular wall into tissues, mediated by chemo-attractants.

Stimuli for the up-regulated expression of endothelial adhesion molecules include tumour necrosis factor, interleukin-1β, γ-interferon, substance P and bacterial endotoxin lipopolysaccharide [18]. Maximal endothelial adhesion molecule expression is generally noted between 3 and 6 h following exposure to the stimulus [7].

Transcription factors such as NF-κB and AP-1 have been shown to regulate the expression of endothelial adhesion molecules. NF-κB also leads to further production of inflammatory mediators, such as tumour necrosis factor, by the recruited leukocytes. Thus a vicious cycle occurs at the site of inflammation with inflammatory mediator induced endothelial adhesion molecule expression, leading to leukocyte recruitment, leading to further production of inflammatory mediators from the recruited leukocytes, leading to further endothelial adhesion molecule expression and leukocyte recruitment [7, 19].

There are species [20] and tissue [16] differences in endothelial adhesion molecule expression. More recently, genetic polymorphisms of endothelial adhesion molecules have been associated with their altered expressions in inflammatory conditions, such as atherosclerosis, rheumatoid arthritis, other connective tissues diseases, vasculitis and diabetes mellitus [20].

The up-regulated expression of endothelial adhesion molecules may be used as molecular markers of endothelial activation or inflammatory activity in a number of important cardiovascular and non-cardiovascular diseases [1, 31–33]. Furthermore, imaging of a series of endothelial adhesion molecules may be relevant because the expression profile (combination and level) of individual adhesion molecules may differ in different types and/or stages of diseases e.g., acute *vs* chronic *vs* resolving inflammation. For example, there is evidence that E- and P-selectin are involved in the selective recruitment of T-helper

Table 24.1 Characteristics of endothelial adhesion molecules

Adhesion molecule	Alternative designation	Localisation	Ligand	Function	Basal expression
Selectin family					
P-selectin	CD62P	Endothelial cell	L-selectin	Rolling	Yes
	PADGEM	Platelet	PSGL-1		
	GMP-140		120 kD PSL		
E-selectin	CD62E	Endothelial cell	L-selectin	Rolling	No[a]
	ELAM-1		CLA, SSEA-1		
			250 kD ESL-1		
Ig-supergene family					
ICAM-1	CD54a	Endothelial cell	CD11a/CD18	Adherence/transmigration	Yes
		Leukocyte (myocyte, haematopoietic cell, fibroblast) [13]	CD11b/CD18		
VCAM-1	CD106	Endothelial cell (myocyte, fibroblast, follicular dendritic cell) [14]	CD49d/CD29	Adherence	No/very low
PECAM-1	CD31	Endothelial cell	PECAM-1	Adherence/transmigration	Yes
		Leukocytes			
		Platelet			
MAdCAM-1		Endothelial cell	L-selectin	Adherence/transmigration	Yes
		(Intestine)	CD49d/β_7		

Adapted from Krieglstein et al. [7]

CLA cutaneous lymphocyte antigen, *ELAM-1* endothelial leukocyte adhesion molecule-1, *ESL-1* E-selectin Ligand-1, *GMP-140* granule membrane protein-140, *ICAM-1* intercellular adhesion molecule-1, *MAdCAM-1* mucosal address in cell adhesion molecule-1, *PADGEM* platelet activation-dependent granule external membrane protein, *PECAM-1* platelet endothelial cell adhesion molecule-1, *PSGL-1* P-selectin glycoprotein ligand-1, *SSEA-1* sialyl stage-specific embryonic antigen-1, *VCAM-1* vascular endothelial cell adhesion molecule-1

[a]Basal expression of E-selectin in resting endothelial cells, where present, is very low or undetectable. However, detectable low levels of constitutive E-selectin expression has been reported in some vascular beds of certain animals in the absence of overt inflammation [15, 16]

1 cells [22, 23]. In myocarditis, T-helper 1-dominated responses are associated with the induction of myocarditis, whilst T-helper 2-dominated responses are associated with enhanced recovery [21]. Thus it may be possible to determine the status of myocarditis without tissue biopsy, by non-invasively imaging the endothelial adhesion molecule expression profile using quantitative ultrasound molecular imaging.

24.1.1.1 E-Selectin

Classically, E-selectin is expressed only on activated endothelial cells in the post-capillary venules. Its basal expression in resting endothelial cells, where present, is very low or undetectable. However, detectable low levels of constitutive E-selectin expression has been reported in some vascular beds of certain animals in the absence of overt inflammation [15, 16]. In addition to the post-capillary venules (the classical site of E-selectin expression), E-selectin expression has also been found in inflamed myocardial microvasculature [24], renal glomeruli [10] and the aorta [25, 26], in mouse models of Coxsackievirus B3 myocarditis [24], glomerulonephritis [10], and atherosclerosis [25], respectively.

E-selectin interacts with N- and O-glycans that contain the sialyl Lewis x tetrasaccharide or its isomers, such as the glycoprotein L-selectin (in man, not mice), E-selectin ligand-1 (ESL-1) and P-selectin glycoprotein ligand-1 (PSGL-1). These E-selectin ligands are present on neutrophils, monocytes, lymphocytes, myeloid cells, dendritic cells, and eosinophils [15].

E-selectin on the endothelial cell surface may be cleaved, releasing soluble E-selectin that lacks the intact cytoplasmic domain. The normal blood level of soluble E-selectin has been reported to be in the range of 0.1–3 ng/ml [12]. Cell-surface E-selectin may also be internalised into the endothelial cell by endocytosis [27].

E-selectin has been detected in human tissues of cardiac transplant rejection [28], myocarditis [29], dilated cardiomyopathy [29], coronary atheromatous heart disease [30], rheumatoid arthritis [31], inflammatory bowel disease [8], chronic inflammatory disease of the skin [9], cytomegalovirus infection [11] and sepsis [12].

E-selectin's mono cell type expression and specificity for endothelial activation/inflammation made it an attractive prototype molecule for developmental work in quantitative real-time ultrasound molecular imaging Yeh et al. 2008 [1, 34].

24.1.2 Microbubbles as Ultrasound Contrast Enhancement Agents

24.1.2.1 Ultrasound Imaging for Microbubble Detection

Microbubbles are strong scatterers of ultrasound, readily detectable at typical clinical ultrasound frequencies of 2–13 MHz, despite being <6–10 um in diameter which is significantly smaller than the resolution of ultrasound. The echogenicity of the bubbles is dependent on the bubble size (size distribution), compressibility of the bubbles or gas, shell thickness/elasticity/viscosity, bubble scattering: attenuation ratio, insonating ultrasound frequency and power.

Microbubbles are compressible and may undergo non-linear radial oscillation in an acoustic field generating strong backscattered signals that can be differentiated from tissue signals using special non-linear ultrasound imaging modes (e.g., pulse inversion, Contrast Pulse Sequencing, Power Modulation).

In the acoustic field, microbubbles have different responses depending on the insonating acoustic power (peak negative pressure or mechanical index (MI)). At very low acoustic powers (e.g., <0.1 MPa or MI <0.1), bubbles oscillate linearly (contraction and expansion are similar in amplitude). At low-moderate powers (e.g., 0.1–1 MPa or MI 0.1–1), bubble expansion is larger than contraction (non-linear oscillation), and produces signals whose frequencies are multiples (harmonics) of the incident ultrasound wave. At high powers (e.g., >1 MPa or MI >1), the bubbles are destroyed rapidly, producing a brief non-linear response and harmonic signal of high amplitudes.

Non-linear imaging methods allow sensitive and specific detection of bubbles by evaluating the frequency components due to nonlinear response of the bubbles and suppressing those due to linear response of the tissues. Methods include high or low acoustic power (MI) settings (see below). High acoustic power settings are usually >1 MPa (MI >1), while the low power settings are usually 0.1–0.25 MPa (MI 0.1–0.25). The MI used for contrast ultrasound studies in clinical practice ranges 0.05–1.9.

The high acoustic power imaging modes (0.8–2.5 MPa or MI >0.8) are based on harmonic B-mode, harmonic Doppler or Power Doppler techniques. They cause rapid bubble destruction, associated with a brief emission of intense nonlinear bubble signals, giving high bubble sensitivity. These bubble destructive imaging modes exhibit a higher signal-to-noise ratio, better bubble-to-tissue contrast and lesser nonlinear signal propagation in tissues compared with fundamental B-mode or Doppler imaging. However only intermittent single-frame contrast ultrasound images can be acquired, due to the rapid bubble destruction. This precludes continuous real-time imaging/assessment.

The low acoustic power imaging modes (0.05–0.5 MPa or MI 0.05–0.5) are based on pulse inversion (harmonic or Doppler), multi-pulse or coded excitation techniques. They cause minimal bubble destruction, allowing continuous real-time imaging. However, the lower acoustic power used has higher attenuation and lower bubble backscatter signal intensity, which reduces bubble detection sensitivity compared with the high acoustic power techniques. In harmonic mode, the attenuation is higher for returning harmonics than for the incident pulse. This effect cannot be compensated for by a higher amplitude of the incident pulse because it would give rise to: (a) nonlinear signal propagation in tissues, reducing signal-to-noise ratio and bubble-to-tissue contrast; (b) increased bubble destruction. Newer imaging modes based on multi-pulse sequence or coded excitation have increased signal-to-noise ratio and bubble-to-tissue contrast, allowing highly sensitive and specific bubble imaging at low acoustic powers. E.g., Contrast Pulse Sequencing [74] and Power Modulation imaging [75].

In practice, the relationship between the backscatter signal intensity and bubble concentration is exponential, with an approximately linear-range at low bubble concentrations [1, 76, 77]. At higher bubble concentrations, the increase in signal intensity plateaus; and at even higher concentrations, the signal intensity decreases because of: (a) signal saturation due to the limited dynamic range of the ultrasound system; and (b) signal attenuation due to multiple scattering effect [78], absorption, other ultrasound energy dissipating mechanisms such as viscous loss and thermal damping [79].

24.1.2.2 Microbubble Stability

Bubbles decay by dissolution (gas deflation), resulting in a decrease in size and number, and contrast ultrasound signal intensity. Factors influencing the stability of bubbles include the bubble size, characteristics of the bubble gas (low solubility, high molecular weight, low Ostwald coefficient, high saturated vapour pressure or low lipophilicity gives more stable bubbles), diffusivity of the gas across the shell, the shell thickness, surface tension, and solubility (bubbles with water soluble galactose shell last for shorter periods than those with relatively insoluble albumin- or phospholipid-shell), shell stability against mechanical perturbation, and the presence/absence of mechanical perturbation such as ultrasound insonation, shear force and systemic pressures *in vivo* [1, 36–39].

24.1.2.3 Biodistribution and Elimination of Microbubbles *In Vivo*

Microbubbles are considered as flow tracers which remain within the intravascular space and have rheology similar to that of the red blood cells [35]. The lungs and reticuloendothelial system (RES) are their major routes of elimination. They differ from iodinated or other contrast agents commonly used in scintigraphy, CT, MRI or PET imaging, which diffuse into the interstitium or cells, with often the kidneys as one of the major routes of elimination.

Following *iv* administration, the bubbles first reach the right heart, then the pulmonary circulation in the lungs, then return to the left heart and onwards to the systemic circulation. They continuously decay (decreasing in size and number) in the blood stream by gaseous deflation, the rate of which is influenced by the surrounding milieu for gaseous diffusion, such as the diffusion gradient and changes in the ambient pressure (such as in the ventricle, lungs or acoustic field) [36–39].

Iv administered bubbles undergo first-pass elimination in the lungs by size filtration, whereby those larger than the capillaries (e.g., >6–10 μm diameter) are mechanically trapped in the pulmonary microcirculation. The gas is exhaled out of the lungs unmetabolised. There is no significant sequestration of the bubbles in the lungs [40], presumably because the large trapped bubbles deflate rapidly. This first pass lung extraction has been shown to occur within 20–60 s [41, 42] in man following *iv* injection, and may decrease the total bubble gas volume by 30–50 %, depending on the size distribution of the bubbles administered. The bubbles are continuously removed from the circulation by RES uptake – primarily in the liver and spleen – involving phagocytosis by Kupffer cells or splenic macrophages, respectively [40, 43–48]. This is similar to other macromolecular contrast agents such as liposomes [49], supramagnetic iron oxide particles [50] and quantum dots [51]. The bubble shells are metabolised through pathways dictated by its component composition. Bubble elimination approximated to first-order kinetics (reviewed in Yeh et al. 2010 [1]).

In the pig, a significant proportion of microbubbles are removed by the pulmonary intravascular macrophages lining the lung capillaries [46, 52]. Pulmonary intravascular macrophages are only found in certain species such as cats and some mammals of the order *Artiodactyla*, which includes pigs, sheep, goats, and cattle. They are absent or negligible in rodents, rabbits, chickens, monkeys or man [53, 54]. The uptake of bubbles by the pulmonary macrophages causes powerful pulmonary vasoconstriction – apparently mediated by thromboxane [55]. An important implication of this is that experiments using certain animals (e.g., pigs) would require pre-treatment with steroids or non steroidal anti-inflammatory drugs, in order to prevent adverse effects from pulmonary vasoconstriction induced by the bubbles. The experiments would need to be designed such that the critical region of the hypothesis being tested will not be affected by these variables.

The biodistribution or elimination of targeting microbubbles are seldom described, however they are expected to be similar to that of the non-targeting bubbles, with the exception that targeting bubbles accumulate additionally at site(s) of their targeted molecule expression [44, 45]. Unlike circulating bubbles, retained bubbles at target sites are eliminated primarily by passive and/or ultrasound mediated gaseous deflation [39]; RES-uptake or rapid gaseous deflation in the lungs do not occur unless the bubbles targeted molecules expressed in the RES or lungs, respectively. Retained bubbles in non-RES tissues may be phagocytosed and degraded by leukocytes [56], but this is not universal [1] and likely dependent on the bubble property (e.g., chemical composition, physico-chemical and biological properties), the biology of the targeted molecule, the targeted cell, tissue or disease process. The elimination of targeting bubbles approximates to first-order kinetics [1]. The half-life of retained bubbles is longer the greater its initial (maximum) concentration [1]. This may be due to a bubble-to-bubble protection phenomenon recently described *in vitro* [57] and *in vivo* [1]–as the distance between adjacent bubbles shortens at higher concentrations, there is: (i) increased acoustical interactions between adjacent bubbles causing mechanical responses such that the net diffusion of gas out of the bubble population is reduced; and/or (ii) reduced concentration gradient for gas diffusion out of the bubbles, due to increased gas saturation in the micro-environment surrounding them. Such phenomenon highlights an important pitfall of conventional acoustic quantification methods (see Sect. 24.2.1).

24.1.2.4 Composition and Preparation of Microbubbles

The chemical composition and processing condition of the microbubbles influence their physical chemistry and mechanical properties, thus affecting their stability, yield, charge, size distribution, acoustic response, degree of non-specific adherence/retention in tissues, elimination and toxicity *in vivo*. Some of these variables are interrelated [1, 58–63].

Non-targeting and targeting microbubbles, produced by the pharmaceutical industry and others, which demonstrated ultrasound imaging *in vivo* are shown in Table 24.2. Detailed information on the composition and processing conditions required for making them is generally lacking in the public domain. For phospholipid-based microbubbles, the phospholipids can be dispersed along with surfactant polyethylene glycol (PEG) stearate

Table 24.2 Examples of microbubbles used in humans (albumin-, phospholipid- or other-shelled bubbles)

Microbubble	Composition	Gas	Net charge/ zeta potential	Mean size or cumulative size distribution (μm)	Conc (x10⁹/ ml)	Application	Clinical trial status	Approval status	Developer
BY963	Phospholipid shell: contains DSPG	Air				LVO	Phase III (Europe)		Byk Gulden
						Doppler (cerebral, central and peripheral vessels)	Phase III		
Definity (Perflutren, Aerosomes, MRX 115, DMP 115)	Phospholipid shell (8 nm thick): DPPA: DPPC: MPEG5000DPPE in 10:82:8 molar ratio	C_3F_8	Neg	1.1–3.3 98 % <10 μm	1–1.5	LVO	FDA-filed (USA and Europe), Phase III (Japan)	Licensed	Bristol-Myers Squibb (ImaRx Pharmaceuticals?)
						MP	Phase II/III		
						Hepatic and renal masses	FDA-filed (USA and Europe), Phase III (liver, Japan)		
						Breast masses	Phase II		
Imagent (Imavist, AFO-150)	Phospholipid shell: contains DMPC	C_6F_{14}	Neut	5 99.8 % <10 μm	0.5	LVO	FDA-filed (USA)	Licensed	Alliance Pharmaceutical Corporation + Schering AG
						MP	Phase II completed		
						Stress echo (pharmacological stress)	Phase II		
						Lesions and blood flow abnormalities	Phase II		
						Prostate and breast	Phase II		
Sonazoid (NC100100)	Phospholipid shell	C_4F_{10}	Neg	3	1	LVO	FDA-submitted (USA)	Not approved	Nycomed Imaging
						MP	Phase II		
						Visualisation of liver lesions	Phase II completed		
SonoVue (BR1)	Phospholipid shell: contains DSPC, DPPG, palmitic acid, PEG4000	SF_6	Neg	2.5 >90 % <8 μm	0.1–0.5	LVO	FDA-filed (USA and Europe)	Licensed	Bracco Diagnostics
						Macrovasculature	FDA-filed (USA and Europe)	Licensed	
						MP	Phase II		

BR55 (VEGFR2 targeting bubble)	Phospholipid shell: contains DSPE-PEG(2000), DSPE-PEG(2000)-peptide	$C_4F_{10}+N_2$		1.5±0.1(SD), range 1–3 μm	2	Prostate cancer imaging	Phase 0 (results awaited)		Bracco Diagnostics
Echovist (SH U454)	Galactose-based shell	Air		99 %<12 μm, 95 %<8 μm				Licensed	Schering AG
Levovist (SHU 508A)	Galactose-based shell: 99.9 % galactose, 0.1 % palmitic acid	Air	Neg	95 %<10 μm		LVO Doppler and CFI; vascular	Marketed in Europe, etc. Phase III completed in USA and Japan	Licensed (EU, Japan, Canada)	Schering AG
Albunex (ABX)	Albumin shell (15 nm thick): 5 % human serum albumin	Air	−3 mV	4±2 (SD)	0.5–0.8			Withdrawn	Mallinckrodt
Optison (FS069)	Albumin shell: albumin N-acetyltryptophan, caprylic acid	C_3F_8	Slight neg	2–4.5 93 % <10 μm	0.5–0.8	LVO MP Stress echo Liver imaging TCD and kidney	Marketed in USA and Europe Phase II/III Phase II Phase II/III	Withdrawn	Molecular Biosystems
Quantison	Albumin: Human serum albumin (recombinant)	Air		3.2	1.5	MP	Phase II (suspended)	Not approved/ withdrawn	Andaris Ltd
Cardiosphere (PB 127)	Bilayer polylactide/ albumin shell	N_2	Slight neg			MP	Phase III completed		POINT Biomedical
Sonovist (Sonavist, SHU 563A)	Polycyanoacrylate shell	Air				Liver, kidney, MP	Phase II		Schering AG
Acusphere (Imagify, AI 700)	Poly(lactic-co-glycolic acid) based shell	C_4F_{10}	Neg			MP	Phase III		Acusphere Inc

(continued)

Table 24.2 (continued)

Microbubble	Composition	Gas	Net charge/zeta potential	Mean size or cumulative size distribution (μm)	Conc (10^9/ml)	Application	Clinical trial status	Approval status	Developer
EchoGen[a] (QW3600)	Charged surfactant (liquid droplet without shell):	DDFP	Neg	3–10	3–5	LVO	Approved for marketing in Europe	Withdrawn	Sonus Pharmaceuticals
	2 % DDFP emulsion containing surfactant (PEG Telomer B) + sucrose					MP	Phase II		
						Stress echo (exercise and pharmacological stress)	Phase III completed		
						Chest pain in ER	Phase II		
						3D echocardiography	Phase III		
						Prostate	completed		

Adapted and modified from Yeh et al. [1]

Microbubbles produced in the industry not reaching beyond Phase I clinical trial are omitted (e.g., BR14, Myomap (AIP 201), SonoGen (QW7437), SHU 616A), except BR55 (the only targeting microbubble tested in humans, Phase 0)

Abbreviations: *CFI* colour flow imaging, *Conc* concentration, *DDFP* dodecafluoropentane, *DPPA* dipalmitoylphosphatidic acid, *DPPC* dipalmitoylphosphatidylcholine, *DPPE* dipalmitoylphosphatidalethanolamine, *DPPE-MPEG5000* N-(methoxypolyethylene glycol 5000 carbamoyl)-DPPE, *DPPG* dipalmitoylphosphatidylglycerol, *DSPC* distearoylphosphatidylcholine, *DSPG-Na* 3-sn-phosphatidyl-1-DL-glycero-distearyl sodium derivative of phospholipid isolated from soybeans, *LVO* left ventricular opacification, also known as endocardial border delineation (EBD)), *MP* myocardial perfusion, *PEG4000* macrogol 4000, *TCD* transcranial Doppler

[a]Echogen is a liquid-in-liquid fluorocarbon emulsion containing surfactant (PEG Telomer B), where DDFP microdroplets phase shift to bubbles after physical activation *in vivo* (hypobaric activation by body temperature, NB. boiling point = 29.3 °C) [73]

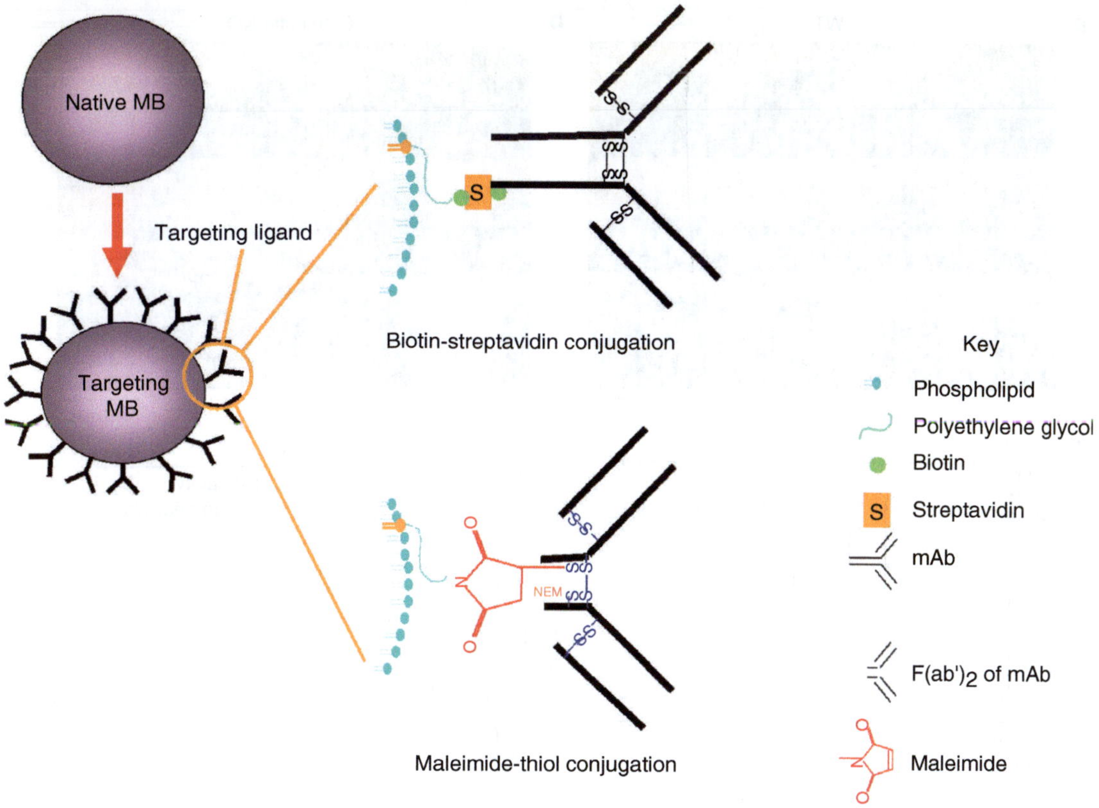

Fig. 24.1 Strategy for converting native (non-targeting) microbubbles to targeting microbubbles for ultrasound molecular imaging. Native bubbles containing biotin or maleimide on its shell surface are conjugated with targeting ligands (e.g., mAb or its $F(ab')_2$ fragment). *Top*: traditional biotin-streptavidin conjugation where biotinylated mAb is linked to bubbles containing biotin on its surface, via streptavidin. *Bottom*: maleimide-thiol conjugation where reduced $F(ab')_2$ containing thiol (thiol produced from the reduction of interchain disulfide bond) is linked to bubbles containing maleimide on its surface. Abbreviations: *mAb* monoclonal antibody, *NEM* N-ethylmaleimide

in an organic solvent. The solvent is evaporated and replaced with an aqueous buffer. Bubbles are then formed using shear mixing approaches [58], where the mixture is sonicated or agitated vigorously in the presence of the filling-gas. For making targeting bubbles, targeting ligands can be conjugated to bubbles after the bubble formation (Fig. 24.1); or they can be conjugated to one of the shell components (e.g., a phospholipid species) prior to bubble formation [60].

Conjugation chemistries used in making targeting bubbles include non-covalent biotin-(strept)avidin and covalent maleimide-thiol [1, 64], pyridyldithio-thiol [102], carbodiimide [65], benzotriazole-amine [66], succinate-amine [103] or amine-succinimidyl [67] conjugations. To date, the biotin-(strept)avidin conjugation chemistry is the most commonly used, it being simple, robust, efficient, and forms very strong stable bonds. Although attractive for early developmental work, it is not suitable for human use because streptavidin or avidin is a bacterium *Streptomyces avidinii* protein or egg white protein, respectively, both known to produce unwanted immunogenic side effects [68]. An alternative maleimide-thiol conjugation chemistry has the advantage of low potential immunogenicity. Conjugate products containing maleimide have been tested in humans without significant immunogenic or toxic side-effects attributable to maleimide *per se* [69, 70]. This includes the maleimide-PEG-hemoglobin conjugate, Hemospan®, which has completed Phase III clinical trial [70]. The thioether bond formation

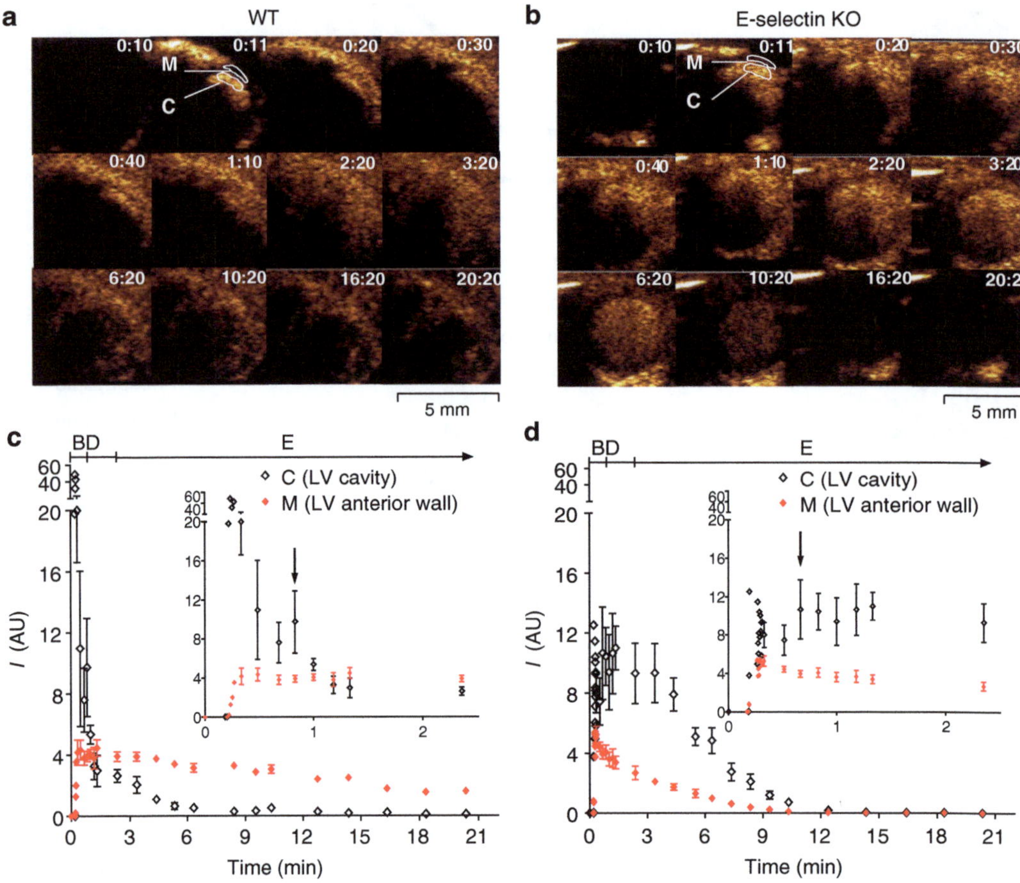

Fig. 24.2 Ultrasound molecular imaging of E-selectin expression in the mouse heart. Sequential Images (**a**, **b**). E-selectin targeting microbubbles were administered as a rapid *iv* bolus via the tail vein at 10s (0:10) to anaesthetised WT (**a**) and E-selectin KO (**b**) mice, both pretreated with lipopolysaccharide to induce systemic inflammation involving the heart. Shown are sequential 14 MHz low MI Contrast Pulse Sequencing (**a** bubble-specific imaging mode) images of the heart in end-diastole, in parasternal short axis view of the LV. Bubble signal intensities are shown in a heated object scale (*orange colour*), tissue signals are not displayed. Results: Signals in the LV cavity and myocardium peaked within a few heart beats (<1 s). Signal attenuation in the LV cavity and myocardium decreased with time (e.g., frame 0:30 *vs* 6:20) as bubble concentrations decreased. Signal in the LV cavity (representing the concentration of free flowing bubbles in the blood pool) decreased more rapidly in the WT than the E-selectin KO mouse. Signal in the myocardium persisted after clearance of bubbles from the blood pool in the WT but not the KO mouse, indicating retention of the E-selectin targeting bubbles by E-selectin expressed in the WT myocardium. Time intensity curves of the LV cavity and myocardium in the WT (**c**) and E-selectin KO (**d**) mice. Plotted are the background subtracted mean acoustic units (*AU*) ± SD for the LV cavity (region of interest (ROI) C) and myocardium (ROI M). Suggested bolus (*B*), distribution (*D*) and elimination phases (*E*) of the bubbles are shown. A second lower peak signal intensity ≈ 40–50s post bubble administration could be observed in most animals (*arrow*, *inset*) as ultrasound signal attenuation reduced with decreased bubble concentration in the distribution phase

between the maleimide on the bubble-shell and thiol on the targeting-ligand is strong and rapid at near neutral pH (bond strength in the order of nano newtons; second-order rate constant 0.8–$1.2 \times 10^4\ M^{-1}\ s^{-1}$) [71]. The near neutral pH is advantageous in avoiding negative impact on the ligands and bubbles during the conjugation reaction, and in preventing dissociation of the ligands from the bubble-shell *in vivo*. In 2008, Yeh et al. reported E-selectin targeting bubbles, based on maleimide-thiol conjugation chemistry, that were effective for ultrasound molecular imaging *in vivo* (Figs. 24.2 and 24.3). These bubbles were stable, echogenic, specific to the targeted molecule and effective for real-time and quantitative ultrasound molecular imaging *in vivo*.

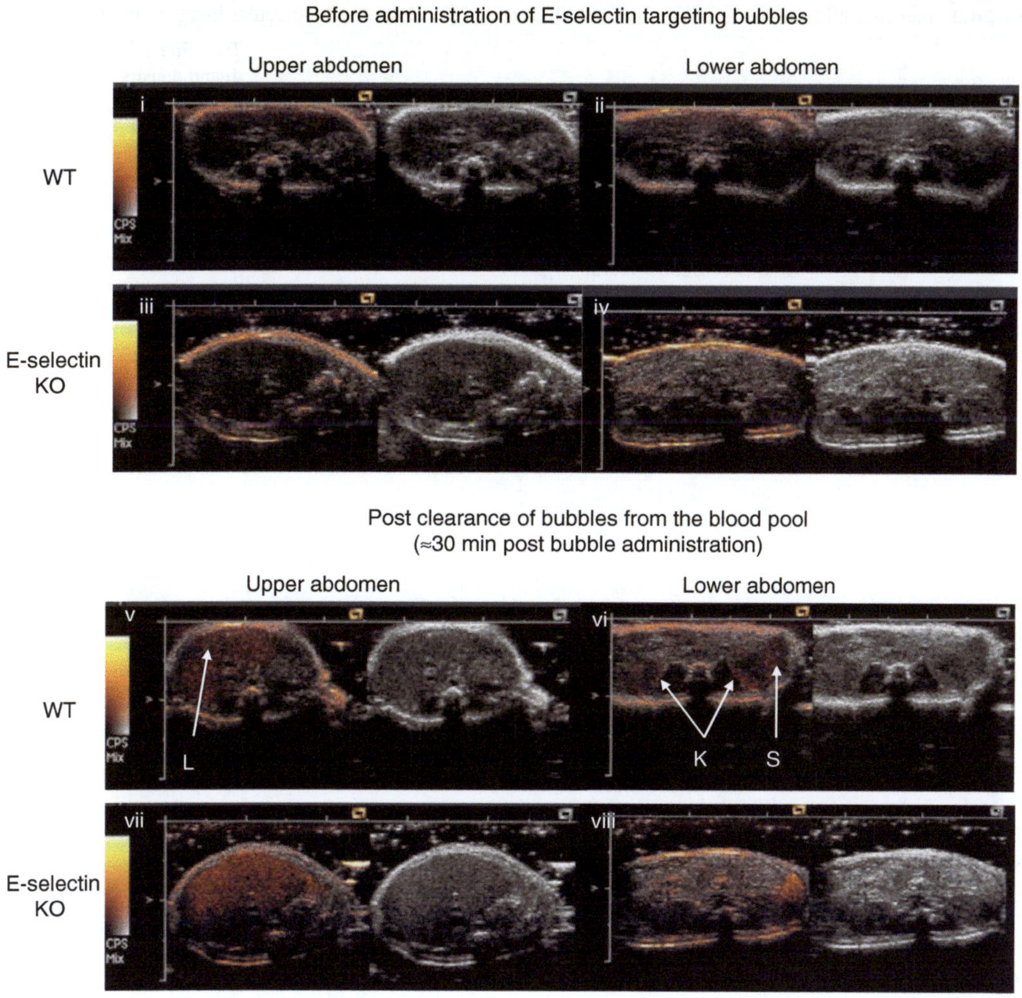

Fig. 24.3 Ultrasound molecular imaging of E-selectin expression in the mouse kidneys. WT and E-selectin KO mice were both pre-treated with lipopolysaccharide to induce systemic inflammation involving the kidneys. Baseline transverse images of the abdomen were obtained by scanning in a cranial-caudal direction, before *iv* bolus administration of E-selectin targeting microbubbles (i–iv). Imaging of the abdomen was resumed at ~30min post bubble administration (v–viii). Shown are 14 MHz low MI Contrast Pulse Sequence images of the upper abdomen encompassing the liver (i, iii, v, vii) and lower abdomen encompassing the kidneys (*K*) and spleen (*S*) (ii, iv, vi, viii). Bubble signal intensities are displayed in a heated object scale (*orange colour*) superimposed with tissue signals in grey scale. Results: The elimination of the circulating bubbles by RES-uptake could be inferred from the persistence of bubble signals in the liver and spleen, in both the WT and E-selectin KO mice, following the clearance of circulating bubbles from the blood pool. Specific targeting of the bubbles to E-selectin in the kidneys was observed in the WT, shown as the persistence of bubble signals in the kidneys after clearance of the circulating bubbles from the blood pool, which occurred in the WT but not E-selectin KO mice. The targeted bubble signal for E-selectin was located predominantly in the renal cortex, as expected (E-selectin was expressed predominantly on the endothelial cells of the renal glomeruli, which are concentrated in the renal cortex)

Non-specific retention in non-RES tissues and adverse effects were minimal following *iv* administration [1, 34, 64]. Elsewhere, an amine-succinimidyl conjugation chemistry has been used in BR55 (a VEGFR2 targeting microbubble) [67], the only targeting bubble tested in humans so far – the results of its Phase 0 clinical trial are still awaited [72].

The number of targeting ligands per bubble ranged 0.3–80 × 10^4 (0.6–300 × 10^3 ligands/μm^2), most in the order of 1–10 × 10^4/bubble (1–10 x 10^3 ligands/μm^2) Table 24.3.

Table 24.3 Phospholipid-shelled targeting microbubbles tested for ultrasound molecular imaging *in vivo*

Origin (bubble ID, where available)	Conjugation chemistry	Bubble shell composition	Bubble gas	Targeting ligand	Targeting ligand density on bubble *(conjugation reaction ratio)*	Bubble diameter (μm)
UVA	Biotin-streptavidin	DSPC (83 mol %) PEG40-stearate (16 mol %) DSPE-PEG2000- biotin (1 mol %) ±DiI, DiO or rhodamine DHPE (small unspecified amount)	C_4F_{10}	mAb Peptide Protein	2–165 k/μm^2 60–300 k/ bubble	Mean: 1.9–3.4 Range: 94–97 % are <5

Targeted molecules	Disease model	Tissues imaged	Host & bubble dose (number of bubbles)	Application[a]	References
α_5-integrins α_v-integrins β_1-and β_3-integrins CX3CR-1 H-2Kk (mouse MHC class I H-2Kk protein) on transfected bone-marrow derived endothelial progenitor cell ICAM-1 VCAM-1 MAdCAM-1 P-selectin Platelet glycoprotein-1bα Selectins (not discriminating amongst E-, P-, and L-selectin) vWF (A1-domain)	Angiogenesis (chronic ischemia, stem cell therapy, tumor) Coronary thrombosis & angioplasty Inflammation (atherosclerosis, cardiac transplant rejection, Crohn's disease (small bowel), ischemia-reperfusion injury)	Aorta Bowel Heart Kidney Skeletal muscle Tumor (implanted in brain or flanks) Matrigel plug (implanted in abdomen)	Mouse: 1–10 × 10^6 Rat: 2.5–100 × 10^6 Dog: 10^8	RT SQ	Lindner JR et al., *Circulation* 2001;104:2107 Ellegala DB et al., *Circulation* 2003;108:336 Leong-Poi H et al., *Circulation* 2003;107:455; *Circulation* 2005;111:3248 Weller GE et al., *Circulation* 2003;108:218; *Cancer Res* 2005;65:533 Sakuma T et al., *Cardiovasc Res* 2005;66:552 Bachmann C et al., *Gastroenterology* 2006;130:8 Villanueva FS et al., *Circulation* 2007;115:345 Kaufmann BA et al., *Circulation* 2007;116:276; *Eur Heart J* 2007;28:2011; *J Am Soc Echocardiogr* 2010;23:79; *Arterioscler Thromb Vasc Biol* 2010;30:54 Behm CZ et al., *Circulation* 2008;117:2902 Kuliszewski MA et al., *Cardiovasc Res* 2009;83:653 McCarty OJ et al., *JACC Cardiovasc Imaging* 2010;3:947 Carr CL et al., *Arterioscler Thromb Vasc Biol* 2011;31:2526 Davidson BP et al., *J Am Coll Cardiol* 2012;60:1690 Khanicheh E et al., *Arterioscler Thromb Vasc Biol* 2013;33:2187 Liu Y et al., *Circ Cardiovasc Imaging* 2013;6:74 Ryu JC et al., *Circulation* 2013;127:710

(continued)

Table 24.3 (continued)

Origin (bubble ID, where available)	Conjugation chemistry	Bubble shell composition	Bubble gas	Targeting ligand	Targeting ligand density on bubble *(conjugation reaction ratio)*	Bubble diameter (μm)
UVA	Biotin-streptavidin	DSPC (83 mol %) PEG40-stearate (16 mol %) DSPE-PEG3400- biotin (1 mol %)	C_4F_{10}	mAb Protein Peptide	NA	Mean: 3.2
UVA (bubbles loaded with plasmid DNA)	Biotin-streptavidin	DSPC (70 mol %) PEG40-stearate (13 mol %) DSPE-PEG2000- biotin (1 mol %) DSTAP (16 mol %) cDNA (plasmid containing firefly luciferase gene): 0.04 pg loaded per bubble ±DiI or DiO	C_4F_{10}	mAb	NA	Mean: 2.5–3.1
Targeson (TargeStar-series)	Biotin-streptavidin	TargeStar/TargeStar-B Biotin coated bubbles Component details not disclosed TargeStar-SA Streptavidin coated bubbles, containing 2.7 k streptavidin/μm^2 (streptavidin on distal tip of PEG) Component details not disclosed	Perfluorocarbon (not specified)	mAb Peptide scFvs	*(Reaction ratio: ligands at >20x excess necessary to saturate streptavidin binding sites)*	Mean: 1.9–2.5 Range: 1–8; >98 % are <8
Targeson (TS-02-008, bubbles loaded with plasmid DNA)	Biotin-streptavidin	DSPC PEG40-stearate DSPE-PEG40- biotin (1 %) DSTAP (2 mol %) cDNA (plasmid containing firefly luciferase gene): 0.04 pg loaded bubble	C_4F_{10}	mAb	200 k/bubble (not actually measured) *(Reaction ratio: 5 μg mAb/107 bubbles)*	Mean: 1.8

Targeted molecules	Disease model	Tissues imaged	Host & bubble dose (number of bubbles)	Application[a]	References
Selectins (not discriminating between E- and P-selectin) VCAM-1 VEGFR2	Angiogenesis (inflammation, tumor) Atherosclerosis	Aorta Tumor (implanted in hind limb)	Mouse: $1–10 \times 10^6$	Not RT	van Wamel A et al., *Proc IEEE Ultrason Symp* 2007;961 (abstract) Khanicheh E et al., *PLos One* 2013;8:e58761
P-selectin	Microbubble targeted gene delivery in ischemia (ischemia-reperfusion)	Skeletal muscle	Mouse: 2×10^8	Not RT	Xie A et al., *J Am Coll Cardiol Img* 2012;5:1253
$\alpha_v\beta_3$-integrin $\alpha_{IIb}\beta_3$ (GPIIb/IIIa) CD147[b] EGFR[b] P-selectin VEGFR2	Angiogenesis (tumor) Thrombosis Tumorigenesis	Artery (carotid) Tumor (prostate) Tumor (implanted in flank, hind limb or mammary fat pad)	Mouse: $0.84–100 \times 10^6$	RT SQ	Rychak JJ et al., *Mol Imaging* 2007;6:289 Xuan JW et al., *Mol Imaging* 2009;8:209 Hu X et al., *Invest Radiol* 2012;47:398 Sorace AG et al., *J Ultrasound Med* 2012;31:1543 Knowles JA et al., *Arch Otolaryngol Head Neck Surg* 2012;138:662 Wang X et al., *Circulation* 2012;125:3117
MAdCAM-1 VCAM-1	Microbubble targeted gene delivery in Crohn's disease	Bowel	Mouse: 10^7	RT	Tlaxca JL et al., *J Control Release* 2013;165:216

(continued)

Table 24.3 (continued)

Origin (bubble ID, where available)	Conjugation chemistry	Bubble shell composition	Bubble gas	Targeting ligand	Targeting ligand density on bubble *(conjugation reaction ratio)*	Bubble diameter (μm)
Visual-Sonics, Bracco (Micro Marker Target Ready Contrast Agent)	Biotin-streptavidin	Streptavidin coated bubbles (streptavidin on distal tip of PEG) No further details disclosed	$C_4F_{10}+N_2$	mAb Peptide	6–8 k/μm^2 40–54 k/1.5 μm bubble	Mean: 1–3
SMU	Biotin- avidin	ND	ND	mAb	NA	NA
SMU	Biotin-streptavidin	Unspecified modification of bubbles from UVA	C_3F_8	mAb	NA	Mean: 2.4
SMU[c]	Biotin-streptavidin	DPPC (55 mol %) PEG40 stearate (20 mol %) DSPE-PEG2000- biotin (4 mol %) ±DiI (21 mol %)	C_3F_8	mAb	(*Reaction ratio: streptavidin: mAb:bubble ≈ 10^5:3x10^5:1 or 10^6 mAb/ bubble*)	Mean: 2.3 IQR: 1.7–3.6

Targeted molecules	Disease model	Tissues imaged	Host & bubble dose (number of bubbles)	Application[a]	References
$\alpha_v\beta_3$-integrin Human CD276 on transfected mouse vascular endothelial cell DEspR Endogolin ICAM-1 P-selectin Thy1 VCAM-1 VEGFR2	Angiogenesis (atherosclerosis, tumor) Inflammation (atherosclerosis, ischemia-reperfusion injury, TNFα -induced) Mural haemorrhage	Artery (carotid, femoral) Bowel Hind limb Kidney Tumor (thyroid, pancreas) Tumor (implanted in flank, hind limb, mammary fat pad, pancreas or prostate) Vasa vasorum neovessel (carotid)	Mouse: $3.8–7 \times 10^7$ Rat: 3.1 (1.3×10^8/kg)–40×10^7 Rabbit Monkey: 10^8	RT SQ	Bettinger T et al., *Proceedings of the 12th European Symposium on Ultrasound Contrast Imaging* 2007;81 (Rottedam) (abstract) Lyschik A et al., *J Ultrasound Med* 2007;26:1575 Lee DJ et al., *J Ultrasound Med* 2008;27:855 Willmann JK et al., *Radiology* 2008;246:508, *Radiology* 2008;248:936, *J Nuc Med* 2010;51:433 Andonian S et al., *J Endourol* 2009;23:373 Lee SC et al., *JACC Cardiovasc Imaging* 2010;3:1265 Tardy I et al., *Invest Radiol* 2010;45:573 Decano JL et al., *Mol Imaging Biol* 2011;13:1096 Deshpande N et al., *Radiology* 2011;258:804; *Radiology* 2012;262:172 Foygel K et al., *Gastroenterology* 2013;145:885 Mancini M et al., *BMC Medical Imaging* 2013;13:31 Lutz AM et al., *Clin Cancer Res* 2014;20:1313 Chadderdon SM et al., *Circ* 2014;129:471
P-selectin	Ischemia-reperfusion injury	Kidney	Mouse	RT(NS) Q	Bin JP et al., *Eur Heart J* 2008;29(Suppl 1):21 (abstract)
α_v-integrin ICAM-1	Angiogenesis (ischemia) Ischemia-reperfusion injury	Heart Hind limb	Mouse: $5–10 \times 10^6$	RT SQ	Yan Y et al., *Cardiovasc Res* 2011;89:175 Xie J et al., *Cardiovasc Res* 2011;92:256
VCAM-1	Atherosclerosis	Artery (abdominal aorta)	Mouse: 10^6	RT SQ	Wu J et al., *Radiology* 2011;260:463

(continued)

Table 24.3 (continued)

Origin (bubble ID, where available)	Conjugation chemistry	Bubble shell composition	Bubble gas	Targeting ligand	Targeting ligand density on bubble *(conjugation reaction ratio)*	Bubble diameter (μm)
UCA Davis	Biotin-streptavidin	DSPC (90 mol %) DSPE-PEG2000 (5 mol %) DSPE-PEG2000- biotin (5 mol %)	C_4F_{10}	Peptide	0.6 k/μm² 3 or 7 k/1.3 or 1.8 μm bubble, respectively	Mode: 1.8, 4.5, 7.5 Median: 1.3
UCA Davis	Biotin- avidin	ND	ND	Peptide	NA	Mean: ≈2
WKU	Biotin- avidin	DSPC (77 mol %) PEG40-stearate (15 mol %) DSPE-PEG2000- biotin (8 mol %)	C_4F_{10}	Peptide	NA	Mean: 3.2[d]
TMMU	Biotin-streptavidin	DPPG DSPC DSPE-PEG2000- biotin PEG4000	C_3F_8	mAb	NA	NA
NTHU (bubbles loaded with drug)	Biotin- avidin	DPPC (66 mol %) DSPE-PEG2000 (17 mol %) DSPE-PEG2000- biotin (17 mol %) BCNU (2.8 mg)[e]	C_3F_8	mAb	9 k/μm² 92 k/1.8 μm bubble	Mean: 1.8
Bracco (BG0470)	Maleimide -thiol	DPPE-MPB (5 mol %) Other components not disclosed	ND	Avidin[f]	NA	NA
Bracco	Maleimide -thiol	Phospholipid (which?) -MPB Other components not disclosed	ND	Fab	2 k/μm² 17 k/bubble	Mean: 1.5–2.8 Range: >95 % are <8
Bracco	Maleimide –thiol-streptavidin-biotin	DSPC Palmitic acid DSPE-PEG2000-maleimide (5 mol %)	$C_4F_{10}+N_2$ (35:65 v/v)	mAb Peptide Protein (YSPSL)	3 k–86 k/μm² 21–608 k/1.5 μm bubble	NA
	Maleimide –thiol	DSPC Palmitic acid DSPE-PEG2000-maleimide (5 mol %)	$C_4F_{10}+N_2$ (35:65 v/v)	Protein (YSPSL)	3 k/μm² 21 k/1.5 μm bubble	Mean: 1.5 Range: 1–2

Targeted molecules	Disease model	Tissues imaged	Host & bubble dose (number of bubbles)	Application[a]	References
β_1-and β_3-integrins	Angiogenesis	Matrigel plug (implanted in groin)	Rat: 4×10^8	RT	Stieger SM et al., *Contrast Media Mol Imaging* 2008;3:9
$\alpha_v\beta_3$-integrin	Angiogenesis (tumor)	Tumor (implanted in mammary fat pad)	Mouse: 10^8	RT	Hu X et al., *Invest Radiol* 2012;47:398
$\alpha_v\beta_3$-integrin	Angiogenesis (tumor)	Tumor (implanted in inguinal area)	Mouse: 10^9/kg (2.25×10^7)	RT	Jun HY et al., *Acad Radiol* 2010;17:54
VEGFR2	Atherosclerosis (neovascularisation)	Artery (abdominal aorta)	Rabbit	RT(NS) SQ	Liu H et al., *J Clin Ultrasound* 2011;39:83
VEGFR2	Angiogenesis (tumor)	Tumor (implanted in brain)	Rat: 6.1×10^9	RT(NS)	Fan CH et al., *Biomaterials* 2013;34:2142
αIIbβ3 (GPIIb/IIIa)	Thrombosis	Artery (abdominal artery thrombus)	Rabbit	RT	Tardy I et al., *Acad Radiol* 2002;9(Suppl 2):S294
αIIbβ3 (GPIIb/IIIa)	Thrombosis	Artery (human blood in rat carotid)[g]	Rat	RT	Alonso A et al., *Stroke* 2007;38:1508
E-selectin P-selectin Selectins (not discriminating between E- and P-selectin)	Inflammation (ischemia-reperfusion injury, LPS-induced)	Heart Skeletal muscle (hind-limb)	Rat: 1–5×10^8/kg (3.3–15×10^7)	RT	Bettinger T et al., *Invest Radiol* 2012;47:516 Hyvelin JM et al., *Invest Radiol* 2014;49:224
Selectins (not discriminating between E- and P-selectin)	Inflammation (acute colitis, ischemia-reperfusion injury)	Heart Large bowel	Mouse: 5×10^7 Rat: 2.6×10^8/kg (8.7×10^7) Monkey: 2×10^8	RT	Wang H et al., *Radiology* 2013;267:818 Hyvelin JM et al., *Invest Radiol* 2014;49:224 Davidson BP et al., *J Am Soc Echocardiogr* 2014;27:786

(continued)

Table 24.3 (continued)

Origin (bubble ID, where available)	Conjugation chemistry	Bubble shell composition	Bubble gas	Targeting ligand	Targeting ligand density on bubble *(conjugation reaction ratio)*	Bubble diameter (μm)
Imperial College London	Maleimide -thiol	DSPC (75 mol %) PEG40-stearate (14 mol %) DSPE-PEG2000-maleimide (9 mol %) DiI (2 mol %)	C_3F_8	$F(ab')_2$ (each reduced $F(ab')_2$ contained 2 thiol groups for maleimide conjugation)	(*Reaction ratio ≈ 4,000 k F(ab') 2/bubble; F(ab')2: maleimide ≥10:1*)	Mean: 2.2 Range: 98.6 % are <6; 100 % are <10
UVA/ Targeson	Maleimide -thiol	PC (which?) PEG40-stearate DSPE-PEG2000-maleimide	C_4F_{10}	Peptide	6 k/μm² 120 k/bubble	Mean: 2.5 Range: >99 % are <8
SMU	Maleimide –thiol (of lipid- peptide before bubble formation)	DPPC (97.2 mol %) Poloxamer-188 (1.8 mol %) DSPE-PEG3400-maleimide-peptide (1 mol %)	C_3F_8	Peptide	5–7 k/um² 110 k/bubble	Mean: 2.3–2.5
Borden	Maleimide -thiol	DSPC (90 mol %) DSPE-PEG2000 (5 mol %) DSPE-PEG2000-maleimide (5 mol %)	C_4F_{10}	Peptide	(*Reaction ratio: 30 peptide/ maleimide*)	Size selected to 4–5 μm (actual measurements not given)
Borden	Maleimide -thiol	DSPC (90 mol %) DSPE-PEG5000 (5 mol %) DSPE-PEG2000-maleimide (5 mol %)	C_4F_{10}	Peptide	(*Reaction ratio: 30 peptide/ maleimide*)	Size selected to 4–5 μm (actual measurements not given)
UT (bubbles loaded with plasmid DNA)	Maleimide -thiol	HSPC (96 mol %) DOTMA (6 mol %) DSPE-PEG2000-maleimide (2 mol %) pcDNA3 plasmids containing either the firefly luciferase or mouse Timp3 gene (0.20 mg/kg body weight incubated with 0.10 mL bubbles)	C_3F_8?	mAb	ND	Mean: 2.1
ImaRx therapeutics (MRX-408)	Succinate-amine reaction forming carboxamide linkage (of lipid- peptide before bubble formation)	DPPG-PEG- peptide in aerosome (MRX-113, ImaRx) lipid mixture No further details disclosed	C_4F_{10}	Peptide	NA	Mean: 2–2.5

Targeted molecules	Disease model	Tissues imaged	Host & bubble dose (number of bubbles)	Application[a]	References
E-selectin	Inflammation (LPS-induced)	Heart Kidney	Mouse: 10^8	RT Q	Yeh JSM et al., *J Am Coll Cardiol* 2008;51(Suppl): A124-5 (abstract) Yeh JSM et al., *Heart* 2008; 94(Suppl II);A21 (abstract) Yeh JSM et al., *Eur Heart J* 2008;29(Suppl 1):21 (abstract) Current manuscript
VEGFR2	Angiogenesis (tumor)	Tumor (implanted in hind limb)	Mouse: 2×10^7	RT	Anderson CR et al., *Invest Radiol* 2010;45:579
$\alpha_{IIb}\beta_3$ (GPIIb/IIIa)	Thrombosis	Artery (thrombus in abdominal aorta or carotid)	Mouse: 10^6 Rat: 10^6	RT	Hu G et al., *Thromb Haemost* 2012;107:172 Wu W et al., *Invest Radiol* 2013;48:803
$\alpha_v\beta_3$-integrin	Angiogenesis (tumor)	Tumor (implanted in kidney or hind limb)	Mouse: 2.5×10^7 Rat: 5×10^6	RT	Sirsi SR et al., *Ultrasound Med Biol* 2012;38:1019 Borden MA et al., *Mol Imaging* 2013;12:357
$\alpha_v\beta_3$-integrin	Angiogenesis (tumor)	Tumor (implanted in hind limb)	Rat: 5×10^6	RT	Borden MA et al., *Mol Imaging* 2013;12:357
MMP2 (extravascular target)[h]	Microbubble targeted gene delivery in myocardial infarction (ischemia –reperfusion)	Heart	Rat: 0.2 ml (imaging) 0.1 ml (therapy) Bubble concentration not disclosed	RT?	Yan P et al., *Biomaterials* 2014;35:1063
αIIbβ3 (GPIIb/IIIa)	Thrombosis	Vein (inferior vena cava or left atrial appendage thrombus)	Dog: 6×10^7/min	Not RT	Takeuchi M et al., *J Am Soc Echocardiog* 1999;12:1015

(continued)

Table 24.3 (continued)

Origin (bubble ID, where available)	Conjugation chemistry	Bubble shell composition	Bubble gas	Targeting ligand	Targeting ligand density on bubble *(conjugation reaction ratio)*	Bubble diameter (μm)
Bracco (BG0024)	Undisclosed covalent conjugation chemistry (of lipid- peptide before bubble formation)	Lipid (which?) -peptide Other components not disclosed	ND	Peptide	NA	NA
Bracco (BR55)	Amine-succinimidyl linkage[i] (of lipid- peptide before bubble formation)	DSPE-PEG2000 & DSPE-PEG2000 -peptide (at 15:1 mol:mol?) Other components not disclosed	$C_4F_{10}+N_2$	Peptide	34 ± 1 k, range 32–37 k or 57 k/μm^2 240 k/1.5 μm bubble or 400 k/bubble	Mean: 1.5 Range: 1–3, or 97 % are <4
XJU	Benzotriazole-amine reaction forming carbamate linkage (of lipid- peptide before bubble formation)	DPPG (73 wt %) DSPE-PEG-BTC (21 wt %) DPPG:DSPE-PEG- BTC-peptide (6 wt %)	SF_6	Peptide	1,644 k/μm^2 100,000 k/4.4 μm bubble	Mean: ≈4.4 Range: >90 % are 1–10

Targeted molecules	Disease model	Tissues imaged	Host & bubble dose (number of bubbles)	Application[a]	References
$\alpha_{IIb}\beta_3$ (GPIIb/IIIa)	Thrombosis	Artery (abdominal artery thrombus)	Rabbit	RT	Tardy I et al., *Acad Radiol* 2002;9(Suppl 2):S294
VEGFR2	Angiogenesis (tumor)	Tumor (breast, liver or prostate) Tumor (implant in hind limb, mammary fat pad or prostate)	Mouse: $0.5–10 \times 10^7$ Rat: $0.94–3.7 \times 10^7$; 0.1 ml/kg (1.6 μL bubble volume/kg) Man (phase-0 clinical trial)	RT Q	Pochon S et al., *Invest Radiol* 2010;45:89 Tardy I et al., *Invest Radiol* 2010;45:573 Fischer T et al., *Invest Radiol* 2010;45:675 Pillai R et al., *Bioconj Chem* 2010;21:556 Pysz MA et al., *Radiology* 2010;256:519, *Quant Imaging Med Surg* 2012;2:68 Bzyl J et al., *Eur Radiol* 2011;21:1988, *Eur Radiol* 2013;23:468 Frinking PJ et al., *Ultrasound Med Biol* 2012;38:1460 Bachawal SV et al., *Cancer Res* 2013;73:1689 Grouls C et al., *Radiology* 2013;267:487 Wijkstra H et al., *Proceedings of the 18th European Symposium on Ultrasound Contrast Imaging* 2013 (Rotterdam) ClinicalTrials.gov, National Institutes of Health, NCT01253213, 2010–2012
$\alpha_{IIb}\beta_3$ (GPIIb/IIIa)	Thrombosis	Vein (femoral vein thrombus)	Dog	Not RT	Wang B et al., *Acad Radiol* 2006;13:428

(continued)

Table 24.3 (continued)

Origin (bubble ID, where available)	Conjugation chemistry	Bubble shell composition	Bubble gas	Targeting ligand	Targeting ligand density on bubble *(conjugation reaction ratio)*	Bubble diameter (μm)
UNC	Undisclosed covalent conjugation chemistry (of lipid- peptide before bubble formation)	DSPC (90 mol %) DSPE-PEG2000 (5 mol %) DSPE-PEG2000- peptide (5 mol %)	ND	Peptide	NA	NA
Targeson (Visistar-Integrin®)	Pyridyldithio -thiol	DSPC PEG40-stearate DSPE-PEG-PDP ±DiI (2 mol %)	C_4F_{10}	Peptide	35 k/μm² 820 ± 160 k/bubble	Mean: 2.75 Range: >98 % are <8
UCA La Jolla/UC[j]	DNA-DNA linkage (non-covalent)	DPPC 18 mg + DPPA 2 mg (mixture at 1 mg/mL) DSPE-PEG5000 (0.075 mg/mL) DSPE-PAA-DNA (mean 3.3 DNA strands per DSPE-PAA molecule) (0.3 mg/mL)	C_4F_{10}	Aptamer (TACS)	*(TACS added to bubbles at molar ratio 1.5:1 relative to the available number of DNA sites)*	Mean: 1.6

Modified and updated from Yeh et al. 2010 [1]

Targeting microbubbles based on phospholipid-shell and published in the English language upto July 2014

Targeting ligands are conjugated to the microbubbles after they are formed, unless indicated otherwise

Abbreviations: *abstr* abstract, *BCNU* 1,3-bis(2-chloroethyl)-1-nitrosourea, also known as Carmustine – an anti-neoplastic agent against eg malignant glioma, *Conc* concentration, *DEspR* dual endothelin-1/vascular endothelial growth factor-signal peptide receptor, *DHPE* dihexadecanoyl phosphoethanolamine, *DiI* 1,1'-dioctadecyl-3,3,3',3'-tetramethylindocarbocyanine perchlorate, *DiO* 3,3'-dioctadecyloxacarbocyanine perchlorate, *DOTMA* 1,2-di-O-octadecenyl-3-trimethylammonium propane, *DPPC* 1,2-dipalmitoyl-*sn*-glycero-3-phosphatidylcholine, *DPPE-MPB* 1,2-dipalmitoyl-*sn*-glycero-3-phosphoethanolamine-4(p-maleimidophenyl) butyramide, *DPPG* 1,2-dipalmitoyl-*sn*-glycero-3-phospho-(1'-*rac*-glycerol), *DSPC* 1,2-distearoyl-*sn*-glycero-3-phosphocholine, *DSPE* 1,2-distearoyl-*sn*-glycero-3-phosphoethanolamine, *DSPE-PAA-DNA* poly(acrylic acid) (PAA) is coupled to DSPE via carbodiimide-mediated amidation, two amine terminated DNA strands (5'H_2N-CCAACCACAAAA, 5' AAAACAACCCCA-NH_2) are then attached to the carboxyl groups of PAA, on average there are 3.3 DNA strands per DSPE-PAA molecule, *DSPE-PEG-BTC* distearoylphosphatidylethanolamine-polyethylene glycol-benzotriazole carbonate, *DSPE-PEG2000* 1,2-distearoyl-*sn*-glycero-3-phosphoethanolmine-N-methoxy(polyethylene glycol)-2000, *DSPE-PEG2000-Biotin* 1,2-distearoyl-*sn*-glycero-3-phosphoethanolamine-N-(biotinyl (polyethylene glycol)-2000), *DSPE-PEG3400-Biotin* 1,2-distearoyl-*sn*-glycero-3-phosphoethanolamine-N-(biotinyl (polyethylene glycol)-3400), *DSPE-PEG2000-Maleimide* 1,2-distearoyl-*sn*-glycero-3-phosphoethanolamine-N-(maleimide(polyethylene glycol)-2000), *DSPE-PEG3400-Maleimide-peptide* distearoylphosphatidylethanolamine-polyethylene glycol (3400)-Maleimide-peptide, *DSPE-PEG-PDP* distearoylphosphatidylethanolamine-PEG 2000-pyridyldithio propionate, *DSTAP* 1,2-distearoyl-3-trimethylammoniumpropane; provides positive charge, *HSPC* hydrogenated soy L-α-phosphatidylcholine, *ID* identification, *IQR* inter quartile range, *GPIIb/IIIa* glycoprotein IIb/IIIa receptor on activated platelets, *LPS* lipopolysaccharide, *mol* mole, *mol %* mole %, *mAb* monoclonal antibody, *MPB* maleimido-4(p-phenylbutyrate), *NA* not available/applicable, *ND* not disclosed, *NRT* non real-time imaging, *NTHU* National Tsing Hua University, Taiwan, *PEG* polyethylene glycol, *PEG4000* polyethylene glycol-4000, *PEG40-Stearate* mono-stearate poly(ethylene)glycol-40, *Q* quantitative imaging, *RT* real-time imaging, *RT(NS)* real-time non bubble specific mode imaging, *scFvs* single-chain antibody, *SMU* Southern Medical University, Guangzhou, China, *SQ* semi-quantitative imaging, *TACS* thrombin aptamer crosslinking sequence: a complementary DNA strand GGTTGGTGTGGTTGGTGTTTTTTTTTGTGG TTGGTGTGGTTGG, it cross-links DNA (of DSPE-PAA-DNA) on the bubble surface, but subsequent interaction with thrombin results in its displacement from the DNA cross-links, making the bubble shell less rigid,

Targeted molecules	Disease model	Tissues imaged	Host & bubble dose (number of bubbles)	Application[a]	References
$\alpha_v\beta_3$-integrin	Angiogenesis (tumor)	Tumor (implanted in flank)	Rat: 1.4×10^8	RT	Streeter JE et al., *Mol Imaging* 2010;9:87, *Mol Imaging* 2011;10:460, *Technol Cancer Res Treat* 2013;12:311 Gessner RC et al., *Ultrasound Med Biol* 2012;38:651
$\alpha_v\beta_3$-integrin	Angiogenesis (tumor)	Tumor (implanted in mammary fat pad)	Mouse: $5–10 \times 10^7$	RT	Anderson CR et al., *Invest Radiol* 2011:46:215 Hu X et al., *Am J Nucl Med Mol Imaging* 2013;3:336
Thrombin	Thrombosis (active clotting)	Vein (vena cava thrombus)	Rabbit: 10^7	RT	Nakatsuka MA et al., *Biomaterials* 2013;34:9559

and hence more echogenic, *Thy1* thymocyte differentiation antigen 1 – a specific biomarker of pancreatic ductal adenocarcinoma neovasculature, *TMMU* Third Military Medical University, Chongqing, China, *UC* University of Colorado, USA, *UCA Davis* University of California, Davis, USA, *UCA La Jolla* University of California, La Jolla, USA, *UNC* University of North Carolina, USA, *UT* University of Toronto, Canada, *UVA* University of Virginia, USA, *v/v* volume/volume, *WKU* Wonkwang University, Iksan, Jeonbuk, South Korea, *XJU* Xi'an Jiaotong University, Xi'an Shaanxi, China, *YSPSL* P-selectin glycoprotein ligand 1 fused to a human fragment crystallizable (Fc) domain (rPSGL-Ig)

Keys

[a]Quantitative or semi-quantitative imaging is achieved when acoustic quantification of the targeted molecule correlates with that using an independent (non-acoustic) quantification method which is quantitative or semi-quantitative in nature, respectively

[b]On tumor derived endothelial cells

[c]Superparamagnetic microbeads coated (via streptavidin) phospholipid bubbles

[d]By microscopy, which tends to give larger size and smaller concentration measurements compared with electrozone sensing

[e]BCNU is attached to the phospholipid shell by electrostatic and hydrophobic interactions. BCNU encapsulated in the bubbles = 1.02 ± 0.37 mg/mL (bubble concentration = $12.29 \pm 0.25 \times 10^9$ bubbles/mL)

[f]Avidin on the bubbles target biotinylated anti-glycoprotein IIb/IIIa receptor mAb administered *iv* 30 min prior to *iv* administration of the bubbles

[g]The clot was incubated with targeting bubbles *ex-vivo* then implanted into the carotid artery for ultrasound imaging, therefore the bubbles' *in vivo* targeting specificity (including absence of non-specific adherence to non-RES tissues), absence of adverse effects, stability for transpulmonary passage were not demonstrated. The same investigators also reported using the same bubbles for ultrasound-mediated clot thrombolysis in rats(99). Although the bubbles were administered *intravenously*, no imaging was performed to exclude non-specific bubble retention in non-RES issues

[h]In order for the targeting bubbles (confined to the intravascular space) to target MMP2, microvascular permeability was transiently increased by triggered myocardial contrast echocardiography

[i]Disuccinimidyl glutarate linking amine on targeting peptide with amine on DSPE-PEG2000, producing (DSPE-PEG2000)-disuccinimidyl glutarate-(peptide). This conjugation strategy introduces glutaric acid linker between the phospholipid-PEG and peptide

[j]Microbubble shell outer surface contains a network of single-stranded oligonucleotides (DNA from DSPE-PAA-DNA) which are cross-linked by TACS (a complementary DNA strand). This increases the rigidity of the bubble shell, reducing its echogenicity. In the presence of clinically-relevant, elevated amounts of thrombin, TACS preferentially binds to free thrombin, thus displaced from the DNA cross-links. This decreases the rigidity of the bubble shell, increasing its echogenicity

A complete recipe suitable for making targeting microbubbles (based on maleimide-thiol conjugation chemistry) against molecules of choice and shown to be effective for quantitative and real-time ultrasound molecular imaging *in vivo* can be found in Yeh et al. 2010 [1]. Microbubbles are unstable, its size distribution and concentration may change significantly within hours at 4C. For long term storage, they can be snap frozen in liquid nitrogen and kept at −80 °C. Alternatively, they can be lyophilized and stored in septum sealed vials containing the bubble gas; bubbles can then be reconstituted by adding aqueous solution (e.g., normal saline) and shaking.

24.2 Techniques for Ultrasound Molecular Imaging

Targeted MCU traditionally revolved around the use of high ultrasound-power (high MI) causing 'instantaneous' bubble destruction, originally proposed by Lindner et al. in 2000 [80, 81]. Although the high power bubble destructive imaging technique allows detection of lower bubble concentrations, conferring higher imaging sensitivity, it has the following disadvantages:

(a) The bioeffects of high acoustic power bubble destruction, raising safety concerns [82–85].
(b) Non real-time nature of the imaging technique. The instantaneous bubble destruction precludes continuous contrast imaging. Thus whole cardiac cycle(s) cannot be examined in real-time. Visual appreciation of molecular expressions at the time of scanning by the bedside is difficult – extensive off-line image subtraction analysis is required to isolate the retained bubble signals from that of the circulating bubbles, in order to visualise the targeted molecule expression [80, 81].
(c) The reliance on a single image frame (bubbles are destroyed 'instantaneously') containing the targeted bubble signal for image subtraction analysis makes it prone to noise and motion artefact errors. It precludes the use of frame averaging for noise reduction, or selection of image frames to exclude those with significant motion artefact.

Low MI non-bubble specific imaging modes can be used for real-time contrast enhanced imaging (e.g., low MI fundamental B-mode imaging). However, they are not specific for bubble signals and require off-line image processing to remove causing tissue signals for the display of the bubble signals. Thus they are not real-time molecular imaging modes.

Real-time molecular imaging requires the use of bubble-specific imaging modes at low acoustic power that minimise bubble destruction, e.g., Contrast Pulse Sequencing or Power Modulation imaging at low MI. Around 2002/3, these imaging modes had just become available on some clinical ultrasound scanners for contrast imaging using non-targeting microbubbles. They were not yet tested for molecular imaging using targeting microbubbles. In 2008, Yeh et al. reported high resolution real-time ultrasound molecular imaging of E-selectin expression in the mouse heart, using low MI CPS mode imaging at 14 MHz (spatial resolution $\approx$0.2 mm [64]. This showed that bedside visualisation of molecular targets is feasible. Figures 24.2 and 24.3 show examples of real-time imaging of E-selectin expression in the mouse heart and kidneys. The non bubble destructive nature of the imaging technique potentially allows 3-D volume scanning for 3-D molecular imaging in the near future.

The ability of targeted MCU to detect a particular molecule of interest depends on several factors, including the abundance of the targeted molecule, targeting ligand density on the bubble surface, targeting ligand-molecule binding characteristics, bubble dose, echogenicity of the targeting bubbles, the sensitivity of the imaging mode and settings used for bubble detection, and the imaging protocol employed [1].

Currently, there is no gold standard in bubble dosing for ultrasound molecular imaging. Reported dosages range 4×10^7–4×10^9 bubbles/kg body weight (*iv* bolus), with the vast majority in the low and mid levels of this range (Table 24.3). It seems logical that for molecular quantifications based on the retained bubble signal intensity, saturation of the molecular targets by the bubbles is required for robust quantification of the molecules. For example, five bubbles may only detect molecule expressions of up to five molecules. The optimal bubble dose is the minimum required for detecting the clinical range of molecular expression that is safe.

24.2.1 Quantification of Molecular Expressions Using Ultrasound

The spatial and temporal expression of targeted molecules may vary according to the types and stages of disease/disease process (e.g., acute *vs* chronic *vs* resolving inflammation). Therefore the ability of ultrasound molecular imaging to quantify the level of molecular expression would be important in the diagnosis, prediction of prognosis and monitoring response to therapy of diseases. However, the imaging technique's ability to quantify the level of molecular expression remains unestablished.

Acoustic quantifications have often been assessed against independent (non-acoustic) methods which were semi-quantitative in nature, demonstrating at best the semi-quantitative capability of the imaging technique. Only a handful of studies used highly quantitative independent assays to assess the acoustic quantifications [1, 86–90]. These showed that the correlation between the acoustic and non-acoustic quantifications varied from moderate to strong [1, 88–90], or was not calculated [86, 87]. Corresponding scatter plots that would allow examination of the correlations claimed were not available [86–89], except in Yeh et al. monitoring response to therapy of diseases [1, 34].

It is likely that different quantification algorithms have different levels of sensitivity and accuracy [1]. Yeh et al. (2010) reported acoustic quantification of E-selectin expression in the mouse heart, by analysing the time signal intensity curve (TIC) from the bubble elimination perspective [1]. This consisted of curve-fitting the bi-exponential equation, $I_{\text{tissue}}(t) = A_f e^{-\lambda_f t} + A_r e^{-\lambda_r t}$ (derived using first-order elimination kinetics and linear acoustics theory), to the elimination-phase of the tissue (myocardium) TIC. I_{tissue} (t) is the bubble signal intensity in the tissue at time t; A_r or A_f is the maximum signal intensity (concentration) of the retained or freely circulating bubbles in the tissue, respectively; λ_r or λ_f is the elimination rate constant of the retained or circulating bubbles in the tissue, respectively. Acoustic half-life of the retained or circulating bubbles in the tissue may be calculated as $\frac{\ln 2}{\lambda}$, where $\lambda = \lambda_r$ or λ_f, respectively. A_r correlated strongly with the level of E-selectin expression ($|r| > 0.8$). By comparison, a conventional quantification method based on the retained bubble signal intensity at a single late time-point post bubble administration (e.g., 25min) also allowed acoustic quantification of E-selectin expression ($|r| = 0.8$) [34]. However, scatter plots showed that the TIC-method (A_r) had a greater dynamic range and was more sensitive and able to quantify lower levels of E-selectin expression than the conventional method. A further advantage of the TIC-method was that other useful characteristics could be quantified simultaneously, such as the retained or circulating microbubble half-life [1].

A 'bubble-to-bubble protection' phenomenon (see Sect. 24.1.2.3) likely contributed to the lower sensitivity and accuracy of the conventional quantification method, ie, by the time of signal sampling, the retained bubbles would have decreased by a different number of half-lives amongst subjects with different levels of molecular expression – leading to under-estimation or even missed detection of the targeted molecules in subjects with lower expression levels (lower maximum retained bubble concentrations), because the retained bubble half-life is shorter the lower the maximum retained bubble concentration. In contrast, the TIC-method takes into account the retained bubble half-life, allowing a more sensitive and accurate quantification of the targeted molecule expression. This is important because the expression levels of targeted molecules may vary and be relatively low in natural/human disease states.

Other TIC-based quantification methods have been described [91–96]. However, unlike that of Yeh et al. (2010), their performance for molecular quantification have not been tested [91, 92, 94–96], or only tested against independent (non-acoustic) assays semi-quantitatively [93]. Importantly, they all require curve-fitting the entire TIC, which makes them prone to errors due to signal saturations/attenuations in the early time points of the TIC where bubble concentrations are high. Low bubble dosages would be required when using these methods, risking under-estimation of the targeted molecules due to non-saturation of the targets by the bubbles. In contrast, the method by Yeh et al. (2010) requires curve-fitting only part of the elimination-phase TIC (the curve is fitted and extrapolated from the linear acoustic region of the elimination-phase) – thus attenuated/saturated signals are not curve-fitted. Overall, the method is simpler, quicker, likely more quantitative, and allows higher bubble dosages to be used [1]. Nonetheless, the method remains to be tested in other tissues and disease processes, and for other molecular targets.

As with all ultrasound quantifications, the retained bubble signal intensities used to relate to the targeted molecule concentration will vary with the imaging depth, ultrasound setting, type of tissue and bubbles. These variables are likely to vary in clinical practice. Here, calibration of the bubble signal intensity (e.g., against bubble concentration) in the region(s) of interest will be necessary for molecular quantification, and for inter-/intra- subject comparisons [1].

24.3 *In Vivo* Applications of Ultrasound Molecular Imaging

Ultrasound molecular imaging using targeted MCU was first described in the kidneys in 2000-1 [80, 81]. The technique is currently mainly limited to the imaging of intravascular molecular targets (including the vasa vasorum) [97], as the circulation of *iv* administered targeting bubbles is confined to the intravascular space. However, interstitially (subcutaneous, submucosal, parenchyma) administered microbubbles may reach the lymphatic drainage system and sentinel lymph nodes [98], allowing imaging of intra-lymphatic molecular targets in the future, relevant for assessing tumour and other diseases. Also in the future, exit of bubbles from the intravascular space by their small size (targeting 'nanobubbles'), or endocytosis/phagocytosis following attachment to cell surface may allow imaging of molecular events outside the intravascular space.

To date, targeted MCU has been reported for the *in vivo* detection of various intravascular molecules/cells in various pathophysiological processes of different diseases in animals, including (reviewed in Yeh 2010 [1], see also Table 24.3):

(i) E-selectin, P-selectin, selectins (E-, P-, and L-selectins non-selectively), ICAM-1, VCAM-1, MAdCAM-1, β_1, β_3–containing integrin (e.g., $\alpha_5\beta_1$, $\alpha_v\beta_3$, $\alpha_{IIb}\beta_3$ (GPIIb/IIIa receptor)), platelet glycoprotein Ibα, or activated von Willebrand factor (A1-domain) in the inflammatory processes of atherosclerosis, ischaemia-reperfusion injury, acute myocardial infarction and primary angioplasty, chronic ischaemia, heart transplant rejection, encephalomyelitis, inflammatory bowel disease, endotoxaemia, mural haemorrhage, prothrombotic atherosclerosis, or tumour irradiation, in tissues such as the aorta, heart, skeletal muscle, kidney, brain, bowel or prostate cancer (hind limb implant), in mice, rats or dogs.

(ii) VEGFR2, β_1,β_3– or α_v- containing integrins (e.g., $\alpha_5\beta_1$, $\alpha_v\beta_3$), endogolin, dual endothelin-1/vascular endothelial growth factor-signal peptide receptor, P-selectin, or thymocyte differentiation antigen 1 (a specific biomarker of pancreatic ductal adenocarcinoma) in the angiogenesis of: (a) tumour (breast, prostate, ovarian, colon, pancreatic, thyroid, liver cancer, melanoma, angiosarcoma, fibrosarcoma, glioma, neuroblastoma, or Ewing tumour) located in the brain, pancreas, thyroid, liver, kidney, mammary fat pad, hind limb, flanks, or inguinal area of mice or rats; (b) chronic ischaemia (hind limb skeletal muscle) in mice or rats; (c) matrigel plug angiogenesis model implanted in the groin and abdomen of mice or rats; and (d) atherosclerosis in the aorta or carotids in rats or rabbits.

(iii) $\alpha_{IIb}\beta_3$ (GPIIb/IIIa receptor) in thrombosis (blood clots) in the carotid artery, left atrial appendage, inferior vena cava, aorta or abdominal artery in animal models of stroke or thrombo-embolic disease, in mouse, rats, rabbits or dogs.

(iv) P-selectin for detecting activated endothelium and fractalkine receptor (CX3CR-1), for detecting pro-angiogenic monocytes stimulated by progenitor cell therapy in hind limb ischaemia in mice.

(v) L-selectin ligand expressed on the endothelial cells of post capillary high endothelial venules for molecular imaging of peripheral lymph nodes in dogs (using targeting bubbles administered *iv*).

(vi) EGFR and CD147 on tumour derived endothelial cells of squamous cell carcinoma (SCC-1) implanted in the flanks of mice.

(vii) Matrix metalloproteinase-2 in ischaemia-reperfusion remodeling of the heart in rats.

(viii) Reporter molecules (MHC class I H 2Kk protein) on transfected bone-marrow derived endothelial progenitor cells, in endothelial progenitor cell therapy in rats.

(ix) Tumour angiogenic endothelium in prostate cancer implanted in the flanks of mice (using targeting bubbles conjugated with cyclic RRL peptide – the molecular target of cyclic RRL peptide is unknown).

(x) Activated leukocytes in ischaemia-reperfusion injury, acute myocardial infarction and primary angioplasty, or heart transplant rejection in the heart or kidneys, in mice, rats, rabbits or dogs (using non-conjugated bubbles containing phosphatidyl serine or Sonovue – the mechanism for the binding of these bubbles to activated leukocytes include charge interaction and binding through complement).

24.4 Clinical Translations

24.4.1 Microbubble Contrast Enhanced Ultrasonography

Current clinical applications of MCU basically use non-targeting microbubbles as flow tracers confined to the intravascular space, or for enhancing Doppler signals in Doppler-based imaging techniques. Clinically licensed microbubbles include Definity, Imagent, Sonazoid, Sonovue, Echovist and Levovist. Albunex, Optison and EchoGen have been withdrawn (Table 24.2).

Well established clinical applications include:

(i) The delineation of endomyocardial border for assessing left ventricular (LV) wall motion with/without stress (left ventricular opacification).

(ii) Macrovascular assessment of the central, cerebral and peripheral vessels.

(iii) Characterisation of lesions in the liver and kidney by their vascular pattern or contrast enhancement characteristics.

(iv) Assessment of myocardial perfusion.

(v) Identification of intra- and extra-cardiac shunts, e.g., atrial septal defect, patent foramen ovale, ventricular septal defect, and pulmonary-venous shunting.

(vi) Identification of ventricular thrombus or non-compaction.

Less well established clinical applications include:

(i) Characterisation of breast, prostate and splenic lesions by their vascular pattern or contrast enhancement characteristics.

(ii) Identification of residual defect, patch or endovascular leak following cardiac or vascular surgery.

(iii) Functional assessment of heart valve regurgitation or stenosis.

(iv) Identification of extra-cardiac thrombus.

Not so well established clinical applications include:

(i) Assessment of lymph nodes, pancreatic pathology, intestinal pathology (tumour, inflammatory bowel disease and its complications), ovarian tumour, uterine fibroids and synovial vascularisation in rheumatic joint disease, by their vascular pattern reflected in their contrast enhancement characteristics (angiogenesis is involved in inflammatory diseases (e.g., rheumatoid arthritis, psoriasis) as well as tumour growth).

(ii) Assessment of intra-cardiac mass.

Clinical applications using extra-vascular administration of microbubbles for contrast enhanced ultrasonography include:

(i) Evaluation of fallopian tube patency – hysterosalpingo contrast sonography (bubbles introduced into the fallopian tube via the uterine cavity with a transcervical intrauterine balloon catheter for trans-vaginal ultrasound).

(ii) Identification and assessment of vesicoureteral reflux – contrast-enhanced voiding sonocystography (bubbles introduced into the bladder for imaging before and after voiding).

24.4.2 Ultrasound Molecular Imaging

To date, BR55, a VEGFR2 targeting microbubble for cancer detection, is the only targeting bubble tested in humans – the results of its Phase-0 clinical trial for prostate cancer imaging (completed in December 2012) are still awaited [72]. Notably, BR55 has been found to have moderate degrees of non-specific retention in the healthy tissue (albeit this was in the rat prostate) [99].

The translation of ultrasound molecular imaging using targeting microbubbles into clinical use has been slow, partly because of uncertainties regarding its safety and efficacy, and partly because of FDA concerns and regulatory issues. Favourable demonstrations of the technique's safety, effectiveness and breadth of potential clinical applications would help gather the financial and research momentum required to establish it for human use.

24.5 Conclusion – Future Directions

Currently direct information on specific molecular events that take place in man is largely limited to histological study of pathological specimens, often obtained relatively late in the course of the disease. Ultrasound molecular imaging allows temporal follow up of molecular events in real-time non-invasively, and can be combined with anatomical and other functional imaging (e.g., tissue structure, ventricular function, perfusion). This potentially allows: (1) earlier diagnosis before gross structural or functional abnormalities causing symptoms or signs occur; (2) monitoring of response to therapeutic interventions; and (3) more accurate prediction of prognosis. This chapter shows how ultrasound imaging can identify and quantify molecular events, such as inflammation in the heart, through the use of targeting microbubbles as ultrasound contrast enhancement agents. The technique can potentially image any molecules accessible to the intravascular microbubble, in any tissues amenable to ultrasonography. Recent advances in targeting bubble engineering, ultrasound imaging and quantification algorithms help to strengthen the potential of ultrasound molecular imaging as a clinical diagnostic tool. Future directions for development in the field includes establishing 3-D ultrasound molecular imaging and therapies using targeting bubbles as vehicles for targeted delivery of therapeutic agents such as drugs or genetic materials [100, 101]. It has recently been shown that the efficiency of gene transfection can be augmented using targeted bubbles (*vs* non-targeted bubbles) [100].

References

1. Yeh JSM. Molecular imaging of inflammation using echocardiography. PhD thesis. London: University of London; 2010.
2. Ross R. Atherosclerosis – an inflammatory disease. N Engl J Med. 1999;340:115–26.
3. Bevilacqua MP, Nelson RM, Mannori G, Cecconi O. Endothelial-leukocyte adhesion molecules in human disease. Annu Rev Med. 1994;45:361–78.
4. Martino TA, Liu P, Petric M, Sole M. Enteroviral myocarditis and dilated cardiomyopathy: a review of clinical and experimental studies. In: Rotbard H, editor. Human enterovirus infections. Washington, DC: ASM Press; 1995. p. 291–351.
5. Mann DL. Inflammatory mediators and the failing heart: past, present, and the foreseeable future. Circ Res. 2002;91:988–98.
6. Devaux B, Scholz D, Hirche A, Klovekorn WP, Schaper J. Upregulation of cell adhesion molecules and the presence of low grade inflammation in human chronic heart failure. Eur Heart J. 1997;18:470–9.
7. Krieglstein CF, Granger DN. Adhesion molecules and their role in vascular disease. Am J Hypertens. 2001;14(6 Pt 2):S44–54.
8. Bhatti M, Chapman P, Peters M, Haskard D, Hodgson HJ. Visualising E-selectin in the detection and evaluation of inflammatory bowel disease. Gut. 1998;43:40–7.
9. Chu W, Presky DH, Swerlick RA, Burns DK. Alternatively processed human E-selectin transcripts linked to chronic expression of E-selectin *in vivo*. J Immunol. 1994;153:4179–89.
10. Timoshanko JR, Sedgwick JD, Holdsworth SR, Tipping PG. Intrinsic renal cells are the major source of tumor necrosis factor contributing to renal injury in murine crescentic glomerulonephritis. J Am Soc Nephrol. 2003;14:1785–93.

11. Allen MD, King C, MacDonald TO, Himes V. VCAM-1 and E-selectin expression during cytomegalovirus infection in post-transplant myocardial biopsies. Clin Transplant. 1996;10:528–37.
12. Newman W, Beall LD, Carson CW, Hunder GG, Graben N, Randhawa ZI, et al. Soluble E-selectin is found in supernatants of activated endothelial cells and is elevated in the serum of patients with septic shock. J Immunol. 1993;150:644–54.
13. Seko Y, Matsuda H, Kato K, Hashimoto Y, Yagita H, Okumura K, et al. Expression of intercellular adhesion molecule-1 in murine hearts with acute myocarditis caused by coxsackievirus B3. J Clin Invest. 1993;91:1327–36.
14. Seko Y, Yagita H, Okumura K, Yazaki Y. Expression of vascular cell adhesion molecule-1 in murine hearts with acute myocarditis caused by coxsackievirus B3. J Pathol. 1996;180:450–4.
15. Lowe JB. Glycosylation in the control of selectin counter-receptor structure and function. Immunol Rev. 2002;186:19–36.
16. Eppihimer MJ, Wolitzky B, Anderson DC, Labow MA, Granger DN. Heterogeneity of expression of E- and P-selectins *in vivo*. Circ Res. 1996;79:560–9.
17. Springer TA. Adhesion receptors of the immune system. Nature. 1990;346(6283):425–34.
18. Kansas G. Selectins and their ligands in inflammation. In: Ley K, editor. Physiology of inflammation. Oxford: Oxford University Press; 2001. p. 222–41.
19. Collins T, Read MA, Neish AS, Whitley MZ, Thanos D, Maniatis T. Transcriptional regulation of endothelial cell adhesion molecules: NF-kappa B and cytokine-inducible enhancers. Faseb J. 1995;9:899–909.
20. Marshall D, Haskard DO. Clinical overview of leukocyte adhesion and migration: where are we now? Semin Immunol. 2002;14:133–40.
21. Goldsby RA, Kindt TJ, Osborne BA, Kuby J. Autoimmunity. In: Goldsby RA, Kindt TJ, Osborne BA, Kuby J, editors. Immunology. 5th ed. New York: W. H. Freeman and Company; 2003. p. 460–78.
22. Austrup F, Vestweber D, Borges E, Lohning M, Brauer R, Herz U, et al. P- and E-selectin mediate recruitment of T-helper-1 but not T-helper-2 cells into inflammed tissues. Nature. 1997;385(6611):81–3.
23. Xie H, Lim YC, Luscinskas FW, Lichtman AH. Acquisition of selectin binding and peripheral homing properties by CD4(+) and CD8(+) T cells. J Exp Med. 1999;189:1765–76.
24. Yeh JSM, Tracy S, Drescher KM, Sunde J, Kono K, Chapman N, et al. E-selectin is expressed in coxsackievirus B3 myocarditis. J Am Coll Cardiol. 2005;45 Suppl 1:142A.
25. Hajra L, Evans AI, Chen M, Hyduk SJ, Collins T, Cybulsky MI. The NF-kappa B signal transduction pathway in aortic endothelial cells is primed for activation in regions predisposed to atherosclerotic lesion formation. Proc Natl Acad Sci U S A. 2000;97:9052–7.
26. Eriksson EE, Werr J, Guo Y, Thoren P, Lindbom L. Direct observations *in vivo* on the role of endothelial selectins and alpha(4) integrin in cytokine-induced leukocyte-endothelium interactions in the mouse aorta. Circ Res. 2000;86:526–33.
27. Kuijpers TW, Raleigh M, Kavanagh T, Janssen H, Calafat J, Roos D, et al. Cytokine-activated endothelial cells internalize E-selectin into a lysosomal compartment of vesiculotubular shape. A tubulin-driven process. J Immunol. 1994;152:5060–9.
28. Allen MD, McDonald TO, Himes VE, Fishbein DP, Aziz S, Reichenbach DD. E-selectin expression in human cardiac grafts with cellular rejection. Circulation. 1993;88:II243–7.
29. Kuhl U, Noutsias M, Seeberg B, Schultheiss HP. Immunohistological evidence for a chronic intramyocardial inflammatory process in dilated cardiomyopathy. Heart. 1996;75:295–300.
30. Semaan HB, Gurbel PA, Anderson JL, Muhlestein JB, Carlquist JF, Horne BD, et al. Soluble VCAM-1 and E-selectin, but not ICAM-1 discriminate endothelial injury in patients with documented coronary artery disease. Cardiology. 2000;93:7–10.
31. Jamar F, Houssiau FA, Devogelaer JP, Chapman PT, Haskard DO, Beaujean V, et al. Scintigraphy using a technetium 99m-labelled anti-E-selectin Fab fragment in rheumatoid arthritis. Rheumatology. 2002;41:53–61.
32. Reynolds PR, Larkman DJ, Haskard DO, Hajnal JV, Kennea NL, George AJ, et al. Detection of vascular expression of E-selectin *in vivo* with MR imaging. Radiology. 2006;241:469–76.
33. Yeh JSM, Sennoga C, McConnell E, Eckersley J, Tang M, Dawson D, et al. Echo identification and quantification of inflammatory molecules in the heart. Heart. 2008;94(Suppl II):A21–2.
34. Yeh JSM, Sennoga C, McConnell E, Eckersley R, Tang M, Hill R, et al. Molecular imaging of the heart using contrast ultrasound: acoustic quantification of molecular expressions. Eur Heart J. 2008;29 Suppl 1:21.
35. Jayaweera AR, Edwards N, Glasheen WP, Villanueva FS, Abbott RD, Kaul S. *In vivo* myocardial kinetics of air-filled albumin microbubbles during myocardial contrast echocardiography. Comparison with radiolabeled red blood cells. Circ Res. 1994;74:1157–65.
36. Vuille C, Nidorf M, Morrissey RL, Newell JB, Weyman AE, Picard MH. Effect of static pressure on the disappearance rate of specific echocardiographic contrast agents. J Am Soc Echocardiogr. 1994;7:347–54.
37. Kabalnov A, Klein D, Pelura T, Schutt E, Weers J. Dissolution of multicomponent microbubbles in the bloodstream: 1. Theory. Ultrasound Med Biol. 1998;24:739–49.
38. Kabalnov A, Bradley J, Flaim S, Klein D, Pelura T, Peters B, et al. Dissolution of multicomponent microbubbles in the bloodstream: 2. Experiment. Ultrasound Med Biol. 1998;24:751–60.
39. Chomas JE, Dayton P, Allen J, Morgan K, Ferrara KW. Mechanisms of contrast agent destruction.

IEEE Trans Ultrasoun Ferroelectr Freq Control. 2001;48:232–48.
40. Killam AL, Mehlhaff PM, Zavorskas PA, Greener Y, McFerran BA, Miller JJ, et al. Tissue distribution of ^{125}I-labeled albumin in rats, and whole blood and exhaled elimination kinetics of octafluoropropane in anesthetized canines, following intravenous administration of OPTISON R (FS069). Int J Toxicol. 1999;18:49–63.
41. Hutter JC, Luu HM, Mehlhaff PM, Killam AL, Dittrich HC. Physiologically based pharmacokinetic model for fluorocarbon elimination after the administration of an octafluoropropane-albumin microsphere sonographic contrast agent. J Ultrasound Med. 1999;18:1–11.
42. Morel DR, Schwieger I, Hohn L, Terrettaz J, Llull JB, Cornioley YA, et al. Human pharmacokinetics and safety evaluation of SonoVue, a new contrast agent for ultrasound imaging. Invest Radiol. 2000;35:80–5.
43. Perkins AC, Frier M, Hindle AJ, Blackshaw PE, Bailey SE, Hebden JM, et al. Human biodistribution of an ultrasound contrast agent (Quantison) by radiolabelling and gamma scintigraphy. Br J Radiol. 1997;70:603–11.
44. Willmann JK, Cheng Z, Davis C, Lutz AM, Schipper ML, Nielsen CH, et al. Targeted microbubbles for imaging tumor angiogenesis: assessment of whole-body biodistribution with dynamic micro-PET in mice. Radiology. 2008;249:212–9.
45. Palmowski M, Morgenstern B, Hauff P, Reinhardt M, Huppert J, Maurer M, et al. Pharmacodynamics of streptavidin-coated cyanoacrylate microbubbles designed for molecular ultrasound imaging. Invest Radiol. 2008;43:162–9.
46. Walday P, Tolleshaug H, Gjoen T, Kindberg GM, Berg T, Skotland T, et al. Biodistributions of air-filled albumin microspheres in rats and pigs. Biochem J. 1994;299:437–43.
47. Tartis MS, Kruse DE, Zheng H, Zhang H, Kheirolomoom A, Marik J, et al. Dynamic microPET imaging of ultrasound contrast agents and lipid delivery. J Control Release. 2008;131:160–6.
48. Toft KG, Hustvedt SO, Hals PA, Oulie I, Uran S, Landmark K, et al. Disposition of perfluorobutane in rats after intravenous injection of Sonazoid. Ultrasound Med Biol. 2006;32:107–14.
49. Ishida T, Harashima H, Kiwada H. Liposome clearance. Biosci Rep. 2002;22:197–224.
50. Thorek DL, Chen AK, Czupryna J, Tsourkas A. Superparamagnetic iron oxide nanoparticle probes for molecular imaging. Ann Biomed Eng. 2006;34:23–38.
51. Schipper ML, Cheng Z, Lee SW, Bentolila LA, Iyer G, Rao J, et al. microPET-based biodistribution of quantum dots in living mice. J Nucl Med. 2007;48:1511–8.
52. Walday P, Ostensen J, Tolleshaug H, Holtz E. Albunex–a new ultrasound contrast agent. Effects on hemodynamics, contrast, and biodistribution in different species. Invest Radiol. 1994;29 Suppl 2:S142–4.
53. Brain JD, Molina RM, DeCamp MM, Warner AE. Pulmonary intravascular macrophages: their contribution to the mononuclear phagocyte system in 13 species. Am J Physiol. 1999;276(1 Pt 1):L146–54.
54. Winkler GC. Review of the significance of pulmonary intravascular macrophages with respect to animal species and age. Exp Cell Biol. 1989;57:281–6.
55. Ostensen J, Hede R, Myreng Y, Ege T, Holtz E. Intravenous injection of Albunex microspheres causes thromboxane mediated pulmonary hypertension in pigs, but not in monkeys or rabbits. Acta Physiol Scand. 1992;144:307–15.
56. Lindner JR, Dayton PA, Coggins MP, Ley K, Song J, Ferrara K, et al. Noninvasive imaging of inflammation by ultrasound detection of phagocytosed microbubbles. Circulation. 2000;102:531–8.
57. Klibanov AL, Ferrara KW, Hughes MS, Wible Jr JH, Wojdyla JK, Dayton PA, et al. Direct video-microscopic observation of the dynamic effects of medical ultrasound on ultrasound contrast microspheres. Invest Radiol. 1998;33:863–70.
58. Klibanov AL. Ultrasound contrast agents: development of the field and current status. Topics Curr Chem. 2002;222:73–106.
59. Ferrara KW, Borden MA, Zhang H. Lipid-shelled vehicles: engineering for ultrasound molecular imaging and drug delivery. Acc Chem Res. 2009;42:881–92.
60. Myrset AH, Fjerdingstad HB, Bendiksen R, Arbo BE, Bjerke RM, Johansen JH, et al. Design and characterization of targeted ultrasound microbubbles for diagnostic use. Ultrasound Med Biol. 2011;37:136–50.
61. Leong-Poi H, Song J, Rim SJ, Christiansen J, Kaul S, Lindner JR. Influence of microbubble shell properties on ultrasound signal: implications for low-power perfusion imaging. J Am Soc Echocardiogr. 2002;15(10 Pt 2):1269–76.
62. Lindner JR, Wei K. Contrast echocardiography. Curr Probl Cardiol. 2002;27:454–519.
63. Seidel G, Beller KD, Aaslid R, Hummel RP, Thibaut U, Vidal-Langwasser M, et al. The influence of different gases on acoustic properties of a spherosome-based ultrasound contrast agent (BY963). A transcranial Dopplersonography study. J Neuroimaging. 1998;8:83–7.
64. Yeh JSM, Sennoga CA, McConnell E, Scheiermann C, Li Y, Dawson D, et al. Real-time molecular imaging using targeted microbubble ultrasound for early detection of disease: a step closer towards application in humans. J Am Coll Cardiol. 2008;51(Suppl):A124–5.
65. Villanueva FS, Jankowski RJ, Klibanov S, Pina ML, Alber SM, Watkins SC, et al. Microbubbles targeted to intercellular adhesion molecule-1 bind to activated coronary artery endothelial cells. Circulation. 1998;98:1–5.
66. Wang B, Zang WJ, Wang M, Ai H, Wang YW, Li YP, et al. Prolonging the ultrasound signal

enhancement from thrombi using targeted microbubbles based on sulfur-hexafluoride-filled gas. Acad Radiol. 2006;13:428–33.
67. Pochon S, Tardy I, Bussat P, Bettinger T, Brochot J, von Wronski M, et al. BR55: a lipopeptide-based VEGFR2-targeted ultrasound contrast agent for molecular imaging of angiogenesis. Invest Radiol. 2010;45:89–95.
68. Chinol M, Casalini P, Maggiolo M, Canevari S, Omodeo ES, Caliceti P, et al. Biochemical modifications of avidin improve pharmacokinetics and biodistribution, and reduce immunogenicity. Br J Cancer. 1998;78:189–97.
69. French RR, Bell AJ, Hamblin TJ, Tutt AL, Glennie MJ. Response of B-cell lymphoma to a combination of bispecific antibodies and saporin. Leuk Res. 1996;20:607–17.
70. Vandegriff KD, Winslow RM. Hemospan: design principles for a new class of oxygen therapeutic. Artif Organs. 2009;33:133–8.
71. Knight CG, Green NM. The accessibility of protein-bound dinitrophenyl groups to univalent fragments of anti-dinitrophenyl antibody. Biochem J. 1976; 159:323–33.
72. ClinicalTrials.gov NIoH. BR55 in prostate cancer: an exploratory clinical trial (NCT01253213). 2010–2012.
73. Correas JM, Quay SD. EchoGen emulsion: a new ultrasound contrast agent based on phase shift colloids. Clin Radiol. 1996;51 Suppl 1:11–4.
74. Phillips P, Gardner E. Contrast-agent detection and quantification. Eur Radiol Suppl. 2004;14 Suppl 8:P4–10.
75. Mor-Avi V, Caiani EG, Collins KA, Korcarz CE, Bednarz JE, Lang RM. Combined assessment of myocardial perfusion and regional left ventricular function by analysis of contrast-enhanced power modulation images. Circulation. 2001;104: 352–7.
76. Skyba DM, Jayaweera AR, Goodman NC, Ismail S, Camarano G, Kaul S. Quantification of myocardial perfusion with myocardial contrast echocardiography during left atrial injection of contrast. Implications for venous injection. Circulation. 1994;90:1513–21.
77. Lankford M, Behm CZ, Yeh J, Klibanov AL, Robinson P, Lindner JR. Effect of microbubble ligation to cells on ultrasound signal enhancement: implications for targeted imaging. Invest Radiol. 2006;41:721–8.
78. de Jong N, Hoff L, Skotland T, Bom N. Absorption and scatter of encapsulated gas filled microspheres: theoretical considerations and some measurements. Ultrasonics. 1992;30:95–103.
79. de Jong N. Acoustic properties of ultrasound contrast agents. PhD thesis . Rotterdam: Erasmus University; 1993.
80. Lindner JR, Song J, Xu F, Klibanov AL, Singbartl K, Ley K, et al. Noninvasive ultrasound imaging of inflammation using microbubbles targeted to activated leukocytes. Circulation. 2000;102:2745–50.
81. Lindner JR, Song J, Christiansen J, Klibanov AL, Xu F, Ley K. Ultrasound assessment of inflammation and renal tissue injury with microbubbles targeted to P-selectin. Circulation. 2001;104: 2107–12.
82. Skyba DM, Price RJ, Linka AZ, Skalak TC, Kaul S. Direct *in vivo* visualization of intravascular destruction of microbubbles by ultrasound and its local effects on tissue. Circulation. 1998;98:290–3.
83. Miller DL, Averkiou MA, Brayman AA, Everbach EC, Holland CK, Wible Jr JH, et al. Bioeffects considerations for diagnostic ultrasound contrast agents. J Ultrasound Med. 2008;27:611–32.
84. Fowlkes JB. American Institute of Ultrasound in Medicine consensus report on potential bioeffects of diagnostic ultrasound: executive summary. J Ultrasound Med. 2008;27:503–15.
85. Blomley M, Claudon M, Cosgrove D. WFUMB safety symposium on ultrasound contrast agents: clinical applications and safety concerns. Ultrasound Med Biol. 2007;33:180–6.
86. Korpanty G, Carbon JG, Grayburn PA, Fleming JB, Brekken RA. Monitoring response to anticancer therapy by targeting microbubbles to tumor vasculature. Clin Cancer Res. 2007;13:323–30.
87. Lyshchik A, Fleischer AC, Huamani J, Hallahan DE, Brissova M, Gore JC. Molecular imaging of vascular endothelial growth factor receptor 2 expression using targeted contrast-enhanced high-frequency ultrasonography. J Ultrasound Med. 2007;26: 1575–86.
88. Deshpande N, Ren Y, Foygel K, Rosenberg J, Willmann JK. Tumor angiogenic marker expression levels during tumor growth: longitudinal assessment with molecularly targeted microbubbles and US imaging. Radiology. 2011;258:804–11.
89. Bachawal SV, Jensen KC, Lutz AM, Gambhir SS, Tranquart F, Tian L, et al. Earlier detection of breast cancer with ultrasound molecular imaging in a transgenic mouse model. Cancer Res. 2013;73: 1689–98.
90. Yeh JSM, Sennoga C, McConnell E, Eckersley RJ, Tang M, Seddon JM, et al. Quantification of E-selectin expression in the mouse heart using targeted microbubble contrast enhanced echocardiography. In: Ten Cate FJ, de Jong N, Albrecht T, editors. Proceedings of the thirteenth European symposium on ultrasound contrast imaging. Rotterdam; 2008. p. 91–2.
91. Lindner JR, Ismail S, Spotnitz WD, Skyba DM, Jayaweera AR, Kaul S. Albumin microbubble persistence during myocardial contrast echocardiography is associated with microvascular endothelial glycocalyx damage. Circulation. 1998;98:2187–94.
92. Fisher NG, Christiansen JP, Leong-Poi H, Jayaweera AR, Lindner JR, Kaul S. Myocardial and microcirculatory kinetics of BR14, a novel third-generation

intravenous ultrasound contrast agent. J Am Coll Cardiol. 2002;39:530–7.
93. Behm CZ, Kaufmann BA, Carr C, Lankford M, Sanders JM, Rose CE, et al. Molecular imaging of endothelial vascular cell adhesion molecule-1 expression and inflammatory cell recruitment during vasculogenesis and ischemia-mediated arteriogenesis. Circulation. 2008;117:2902–11.
94. Carr CL, Qi Y, Davidson B, Chadderdon S, Jayaweera AR, Belcik JT, et al. Dysregulated selectin expression and monocyte recruitment during ischemia-related vascular remodeling in diabetes mellitus. Arterioscler Thromb Vasc Biol. 2011;31:2526–33.
95. Sirsi SR, Hernandez SL, Zielinski L, Blomback H, Koubaa A, Synder M, et al. Polyplex-microbubble hybrids for ultrasound-guided plasmid DNA delivery to solid tumors. J Control Release. 2012;157(2):224–34. PubMed PMID: 21945680.
96. Chen CC, Sirsi SR, Homma S, Borden MA. Effect of surface architecture on *in vivo* ultrasound contrast persistence of targeted size-selected microbubbles. Ultrasound Med Biol. 2012;38:492–503.
97. Decano JL, Moran AM, Ruiz-Opazo N, Herrera VL. Molecular imaging of vasa vasorum neovascularization via DEspR-targeted contrast-enhanced ultrasound micro-imaging in transgenic atherosclerosis rat model. Mol Imaging Biol. 2011;13: 1096–106.
98. Goldberg BB, Merton DA, Liu JB, Murphy G, Forsberg F. Contrast-enhanced sonographic imaging of lymphatic channels and sentinel lymph nodes. J Ultrasound Med. 2005;24:953–65.
99. Frinking PJ, Tardy I, Theraulaz M, Arditi M, Powers J, Pochon S, et al. Effects of acoustic radiation force on the binding efficiency of BR55, a VEGFR2-specific ultrasound contrast agent. Ultrasound Med Biol. 2012;38:1460–9.
100. Xie A, Belcik T, Qi Y, Morgan TK, Champaneri SA, Taylor S, et al. Ultrasound-mediated vascular gene transfection by cavitation of endothelial-targeted cationic microbubbles. JACC Cardiovasc Imaging. 2012;5:1253–62.
101. Tlaxca JL, Rychak JJ, Ernst PB, Konkalmatt PR, Shevchenko TI, Pizarro TT, et al. Ultrasound-based molecular imaging and specific gene delivery to mesenteric vasculature by endothelial adhesion molecule targeted microbubbles in a mouse model of Crohn's disease. J Control Release. 2013;165:216–25.
102. Anderson CR et al. Ultrasound molecular imaging of tumor angiogenesis with an integrin targeted microbubble contrast agent. Invest Radiol. 2011:46:215.
103. Takeuchi M et al. Enhanced visualization of intravascular and left atrial appendage thrombus with the use of a thrombus-targeting ultrasonographic contrast agent (MRX-408A1): In vivo experimental echocardiographic studies. J Am Soc Echocardiog. 1999;12:1015.

Clinical Aspects and Genetics of Cardiomyopathies

25

Aris Anastasakis

Abstract

Cardiomyopathies (CMP) are myocardial disorders that are not explained by abnormal loading conditions and coronary artery disease. They are classified into a number of morphological and functional phenotypes that can be caused by genetic and non-genetic mechanisms. Despite considerable heterogeneity within the categories of hypertrophic, dilated, restrictive, arrhythmogenic right ventricular, and other types of CMP, these diagnostic classifications can predict major complications and delineate treatment options for each group. Recently, we face the development of more sophisticated methods, including the genetic evaluation, for predicting adverse clinical events.

Keywords

Cardiomyopathy • Sudden death • Genetics • Heart failure • Stroke • Arrhythmias

Abbreviations

AAD	Antiarrhythmic Drugs
ACM	Arrhythmogenic cardiomyopathy
AF	Atrial fibrillation
ALVC	Arrhythmogenic left ventricular cardiomyopathy
ARVC	Arrhythmogenic right ventricular cardiomyopathy
CMP	Cardiomyopathy
DCM	Dilated cardiomyopathy
ECG	Electrocardiographic
HCM	Hypertrophic cardiomyopathy
HD	Heart disease
HF	Heart failure
ICD	Implantable cardioverter defibrillator
LA	Left Atrium
LBBB	Left branch bundle block
LDAC	Left Dominant Arrhythmogenic Cardiomyopathy
LMNA	Lamin A (Laminopathies)
LV/RV	Left/Right ventricular/ventricle
LVH	Left Ventricular Hypertrophy

A. Anastasakis, MD, PhD
Unit of Inherited Cardiovascular Diseases, 1st Department of Cardiology, University of Athens, 2, Michalakopoulou str, Athens 11527, Greece
e-mail: anastasakisaris@gmail.com

D.V. Cokkinos (ed.), *Introduction to Translational Cardiovascular Research*,
DOI 10.1007/978-3-319-08798-6_25, © Springer International Publishing Switzerland 2015

LVOTO	Left ventricular outflow obstruction
NSVT	Non-Sustained Ventricular tachycardia
PVS	Programmed ventricular stimulation
RBBB	Right branch bundle block
RV	Right ventricle
SCD	Sudden Cardiac Death
VT	Ventricular Tachycardia
EKKAN	Heart center for the young and athletes

25.1 Introduction

Cardiomyopathies (CMP) are a clinically heterogeneous group of heart muscle disorders. They are defined by the presence of abnormal myocardial structure and/or function in the absence of ischemic heart disease (HD) or abnormal loading conditions [1–3].

Familial CMP are a major cause of heart disease in all age groups, often with an onset in adolescence or early adult life. Not only the patients but also their families can be severely burdened by these illnesses. The current classifications of CMP continue to be based on phenotype defined by clinical evaluation of affected individuals, incorporating genotype when possible [2, 4, 5]. Despite considerable heterogeneity within the categories of hypertrophic, dilated, restrictive, arrhythmogenic right ventricular, and other types of CMP, these diagnostic classifications can predict major complications and delineate treatment options for each group (Figs. 25.1 and 25.2) [3].

25.1.1 Incomplete Penetrance and Variable Expressivity

Inherited CMPs show marked phenotypic variability, even within families [1–4]. Penetrance, the proportion of mutation carriers with clinically detectable disease increases with age but remains less than 100 %. In most persons with hypertrophic CMP, hypertrophy is manifested in adolescence, whereas the age at onset in patients with sarcomeric dilated CMP is bimodal, with a peak during childhood and mid-adulthood [5]. The disease is gradually progressive in patients with dilated CMP due to laminopathy (LMNA) [1, 2]. It is uncommon to find numerous persons with clinically apparent arrhythmogenic right ventricular cardiomyopathy (ARVC) in a single pedigree, which indicates a low level of penetrance [1, 2]. Early reports of all CMPs

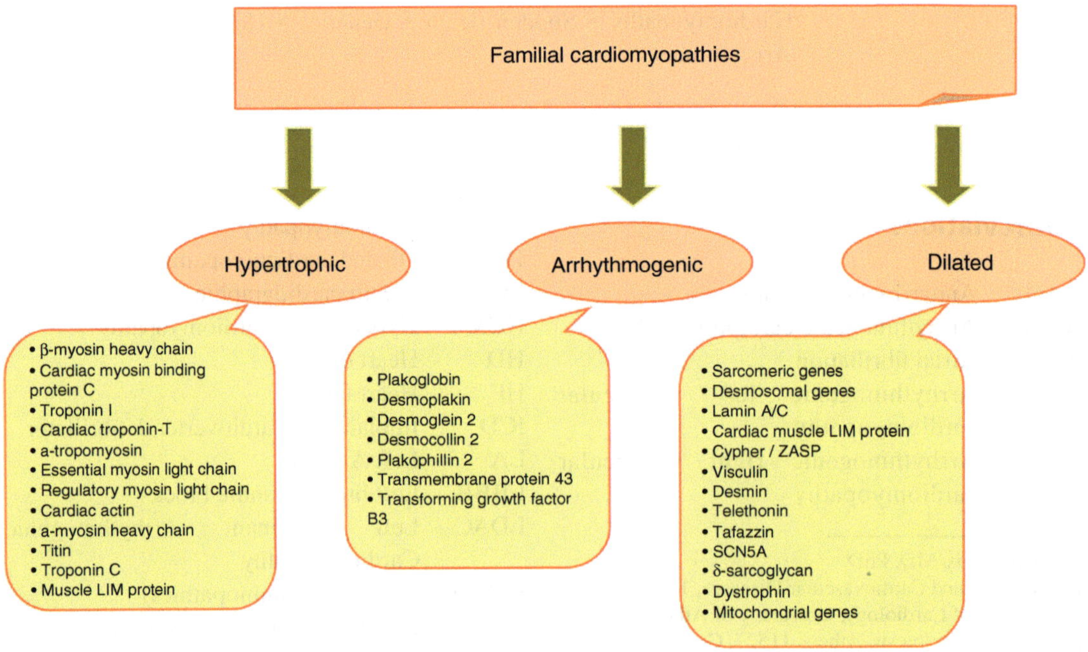

Fig. 25.1 Familial Cardiomyopathies and genetic substrate (Image modified from original image courtesy of EKKAN)

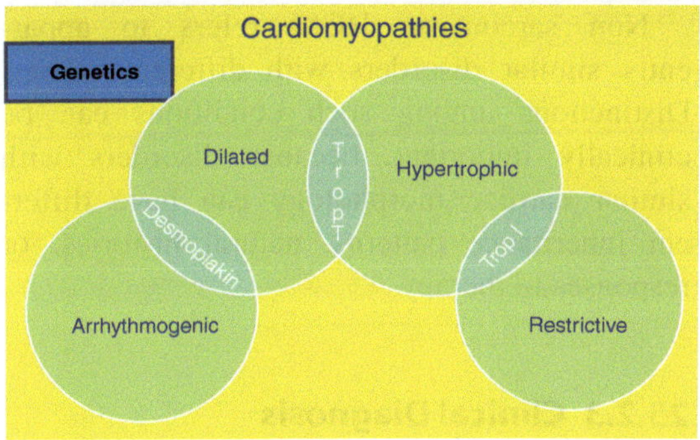

Fig. 25.2 Cardiomyopathies and overlapping in genetic substrates (Image reproduced courtesy of EKKAN)

described, as expected, patients with severe forms of the disease. Subsequent studies, however, have shown that most of the affected persons have mild, sometimes atypical forms of the disease; as a result, the number of cases in a given family, and thus the proportion of familial cases, is greater than originally suspected. Only a minority of patients with hypertrophic CMP have the classic feature of outflow obstruction at rest, and up to half the cases of idiopathic dilated CMP are familial [1–8]. It has also become apparent that ARVC often goes unrecognized and is more common than was first thought [1, 2]. Incomplete penetrance requires diagnostic criteria of less than the usual stringency for first-degree relatives; clinicians caring for families at risk now use complex diagnostic algorithms to interpret minor abnormalities [1, 2]. The corollary is that, in the general population, patients with subtle features of inherited CMP are difficult to recognize. Thus, population screening is generally ineffective; instead, cascade screening (sequential identification of related family members, increasingly guided by genetic testing) is the key.

25.1.2 Genetic Heterogeneity and Genotype–Phenotype Correlations

Hypertrophic and dilated CMP can be allelic, each caused by specific missense mutations in the same genes encoding sarcomeric proteins [2]. Since these diseases arise from mutations with opposing biophysical consequences [2], a variant "breeds true" within each family; there has been no reliable documentation of families in which a single sarcomere mutation causes hypertrophic CMP in some members and dilated CMP in others. However, other aspects of the CMP phenotype can vary within families, indicating the absence of a precise relationship between the mutation and its biophysical consequences [1, 2]. For example, familial restrictive CMP is part of the spectrum of sarcomeric hypertrophic CMP, with a loose relationship between certain mutations and this variant of the phenotype [1, 2, 5, 8].

In certain circumstances, knowledge of the gene underlying the CMP may alter patient care. One example is forms of hypertrophic CMP with different inheritance patterns and natural histories [8–12]. Another example is the susceptibility to disturbances of the conduction system of patients with dilated CMP due to LMNA mutations; when this is sufficient to warrant pacemaker insertion, use of an implantable cardioverter – defibrillator should be considered [1, 2]. However, for most CMPs, correlation between the disease gene and the phenotype are currently of limited utility for managing the care of individual patients [4, 8]; some quantitative differences exist, but there is substantial overlap between disease-gene groups, and exceptions are common [1, 2]. Additional complexities include the presence of two or more variants, as either compound or double heterozygosity (some families may have more than one causative mutation). The proportion of genotyped persons with more than one variant is higher in diseases with low penetrance — notably, ARVC. The presence of multiple variants complicates genetic testing in families [1, 2, 4, 8].

25.2 Hypertrophic Cardiomyopathy

25.2.1 Definition and Epidemiology

Hypertrophic cardiomyopathy (HCM) is defined as left ventricular (LV) hypertrophy in the absence of abnormal loading conditions sufficient to explain the degree of hypertrophy. HCM is a complex but relatively common form of genetic heart muscle disease that occurs in 1 out of 500 people, but often goes undiagnosed in the community. HCM is the most common cause of heart-related sudden death (SD) in people under 20 years of age, and it can also be responsible for exercise disability at almost any age. HCM occurs equally in both sexes and has been reported in many races (Fig. 25.3) [8–21].

25.2.2 Genetics

HCM is a familial disease in approximately half of the cases. It is inherited mainly as an autosomal dominant trait caused by mutations in genes that encodes proteins of the cardiac sarcomere. The commonest are β-myosin heavy chain, cardiac troponin T, cardiac troponin I, α-tropomyosin, cardiac myosin binding protein C, the essential and regulatory myosin light chains, and cardiac actin. Other genes, such as those encoding α-myosin, titin, and proteins of the Z-disc, account for less than 1 % of cases (Table 25.1).

Non sarcomeric HCM refers to apparently similar disorders with different causes. Distinctions among such conditions can be clinically important, because disorders with similar cardiac morphology can have different inheritance patterns, natural histories, or responses to therapy.

25.2.3 Clinical Diagnosis

Most patients with HCM are asymptomatic. Some experience chest pain, breathlessness, fatigue, and palpitations, often with day-to-day variation. Syncope is also common and can be caused by many mechanisms including left ventricular outflow obstruction (LVOTO), hypotension secondary to abnormal vascular responses, and arrhythmias. Changes in LV loading conditions during exercise, heavy meals, and dehydration often precipitate symptoms. The cardiovascular examination in most patients is normal. On auscultation, LVOTO causes a harsh ejection systolic murmur at the left sternal edge, which increases in intensity during the strain phase of the Valsalva, or when standing from the squatting position.

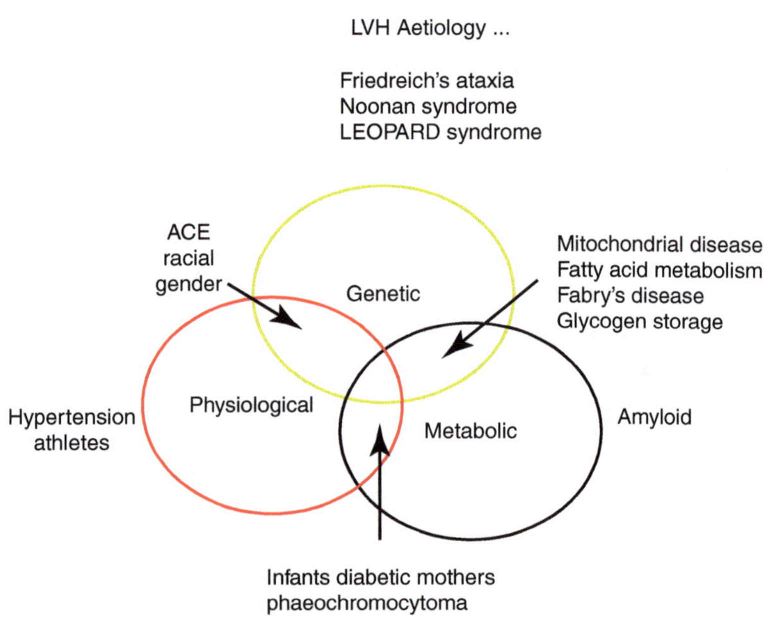

Fig. 25.3 LVH Aetiology

Table 25.1 Classification and causes of HCM

Familial	Nonfamilial
Familial, unknown gene	Obesity Infants of diabetic mothers
Sarcomeric protein disease	Athletic training
β-Myosin heavy chain	Amyloid (AL/prealbumin)
Cardiac myosin binding protein C	See Fig. 25.3
Cardiac troponin I	
Troponin T	
α-Tropomyosin	
Essential myosin light chain	
Regulatory myosin light chain	
Cardiac actin	
α-Myosin heavy chain	
Titin	
Troponin C	
Muscle LIM protein	
Glycogen storage disease	
e.g., GSD II (Pompe disease); GSD III (Forbes disease); AMP kinase (WPW, HCM, conduction disease)	
Danon disease	
Lysosomal storage diseases	
e.g., Anderson-Fabry disease, Hurler syndrome	
Disorders of fatty acid metabolism	
Carnitine deficiency	
Phosphorylase B kinase deficiency	
Mitochondrial cytopathies	
e.g., MELAS, MERRF, LHON	
Syndromic HCM	
Noonan syndrome	
LEOPARD syndrome	
Friedreich ataxia	
Beckwith-Wiedermann syndrome	
Swyer syndrome (pure gonadal dysgenesis)	
Costello syndrome	
Other	
Phospholamban promoter	
Familial amyloid	

Table reproduced courtesy of EKKAN

Most patients with LVOTO also have mitral regurgitation, caused by abnormal coaptation of the mitral valve leaflets during systole.

The resting 12-lead ECG is abnormal in 95 % of patients with HCM. Atrioventricular conduction abnormalities (including first-degree block) are rare, except in particular subtypes of HCM (e.g., PRKAG2 mutations, mitochondrial disease, Danon or Fabry disease) where they are more frequent (Fig. 25.3) [7, 9, 11].

25.2.3.1 Imaging

In patients with HCM, absolute left-ventricular wall thickness ranges widely from mild (13–15 mm) to massive (>50 mm) [4, 8, 15–19]. The diagnosis of HCM relies on the presence of a maximal LV wall thickness of more than 2 standard deviations from the normal (typically ≥13 mm in an adult). Hypertrophy is typically asymmetric, involving the interventricular septum in more than other segments, but any pattern of

LV hypertrophy, including concentric, eccentric, distal, and apical, is consistent with the diagnosis of HCM. In resting conditions, 25 % of patients have obstruction of the LV outflow tract. As many as 70 % of symptomatic patients may have latent or provocable LV systolic function. A proportion of adults with HCM develop progressive myocardial thinning, global LV systolic impairment, and cavity dilatation. Characteristically, patients with HCM have diastolic LV impairment shown by reduced early diastolic (Ea) velocities in the mitral annulus and septum and reversal of the ratio of early/late diastolic velocities (Ea/Aa) (Fig. 25.4). Cardiac magnetic resonance imaging provides a detailed assessment of cardiac morphology as well as an accurate assessment of systolic function. It also permits tissue characterization, particularly detection of myocardial scarring by the assessment of delayed gadolinium enhancement. Studies suggest that the extent of gadolinium enhancement correlates with risk factors for sudden death and with progressive LV remodeling [4, 8, 16, 20].

25.2.3.2 Further Investigation

Symptom limited exercise testing is safe in HCM [50, 51] and provides a quantitative assessment of a patient's exercise tolerance, particularly when combined with metabolic functional testing. An abnormal blood pressure response to exercise is associated with an increased risk of SD in young adults. Ambulatory electrocardiographic monitoring is important in the assessment of symptoms and in the prediction of arrhythmic risk [21–48]. Nonsustained ventricular tachycardia occurs in 20 % of adults with HCM. Paroxysmal supraventricular arrhythmias occur in 30–50 % of patients; sustained atrial fibrillation (AF) is present in 5 % of patients at diagnosis, and develops in a further 10 % in the subsequent 5 years. The main indications for coronary angiography are exclusion of coronary artery disease and, much less commonly, assessment of cardiac output, filling pressures, and intraventricular pressure gradients in patients with severe symptoms. Endomyocardial biopsy is occasionally indicated when an infiltrative or metabolic disease, such as amyloidosis or Anderson-Fabry disease, is suspected [52–54].

25.2.4 Natural History

HCM can present at any age. Many patients follow a stable and benign course, with a low risk of adverse events, but a minority experience progressive symptoms caused by slow deterioration in diastolic and sometimes in LV systolic function. A proportion of individuals die suddenly, whereas others may die from progressive heart failure, thromboembolism, and, rarely, infective endocarditis [55].

25.2.4.1 Sudden Cardiac Death

Overall, HCM is a relatively benign disease but at the same time is one of the commonest causes of SCD in the young. Most contemporary studies report an annual incidence of SCD in HCM populations of 0.5–1 % per year, rising to 2 % or higher in certain groups. The mechanism of SCD is rarely documented but factors that contribute to a propensity to ventricular arrhythmias include dispersion of repolarization, which increases susceptibility to triggered arrhythmias; myocyte disarray and areas of conduction block that predispose to reentry arrhythmias. Other morphologic and physiologic factors influence the vulnerability of the underlying substrate, such as myocardial ischemia, LVOTO, and diastolic dysfunction [4, 8, 38–61].

25.2.4.2 End Stage HCM, Stroke and Infective Endocarditis

End-stage HCM develops at all ages but, in most patients, the time from onset of heart failure (HF) symptoms to diagnosis of severe systolic impairment is about 10–15 years. The development of severe systolic HF is associated with a poor prognosis, with rapid progression to death or transplantation and an overall mortality of up to 11 % per year. The prevalence of severe systolic impairment in HCM using conventional echocardiographic criteria ranges from 2 % to nearly 10 %, with an annual incidence of less than 1 %. The annual incidence of stroke varies from 0.56 to 0.8 %/y, rising to 1.9 % in patients more than 60 years old. The major cause is atrial fibrillation [AF], which affects about a quarter of patients with HCM, with an incidence of 2 % per annum. Risk factors for AF

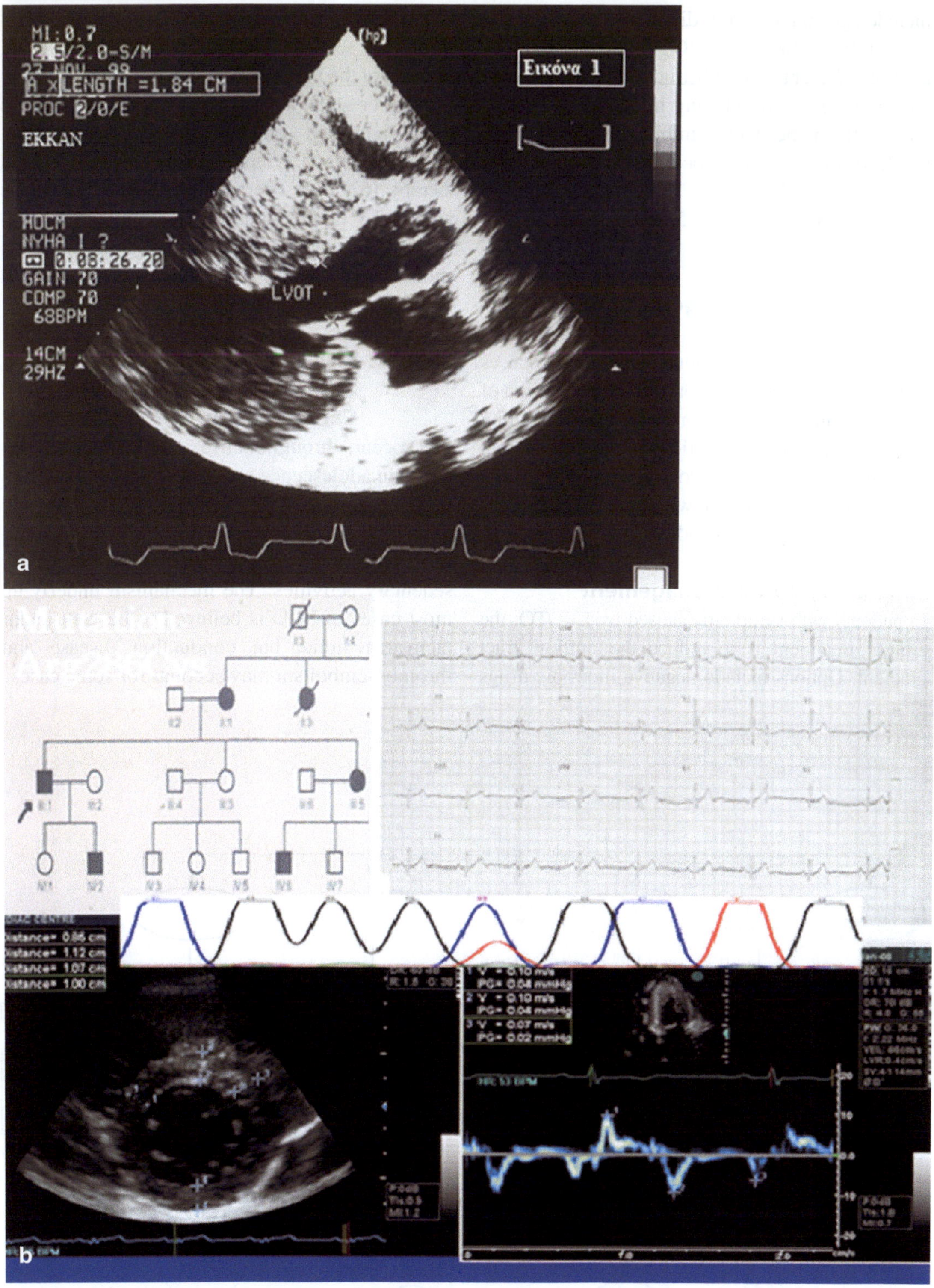

Fig. 25.4 Hypertrophic cardiomyopathy: (**a**) Typical form (**b**) Subclinical form (Image reproduced courtesy of EKKAN)

include age and left atrial dilation (a consequence of diastolic dysfunction, LVOTO, and mitral regurgitation). Patients with obstructive HCM have an increased risk of developing infective endocarditis, usually on the anterior mitral valve leaflet. The incidence of infective endocarditis is 1.4 per 1,000 person-year and 3.8 per 1,000 person-year in patients with obstruction [55, 56].

25.2.5 Clinical Management of HCM

The treatment of most patients with HCM focuses on the management of symptoms, the prevention of disease-related complications and the counseling of family members. Exceptions include lysosomal storage diseases, such as Pompe, Anderson-Fabry disease or amyloidosis, for which specific therapies are available (Figs. 25.3 and 25.5).

25.2.5.1 Symptom Management

In patients with symptoms caused by LVOTO, the aim of treatment is to reduce the outflow tract gradient. Options include negative inotropic drugs (β-blockers, disopyramide, and verapamil), atrioventricular sequential pacing, percutaneous alcohol ablation of the interventricular septum, and surgery. Surgery or septal ablation is considered in patients with significant outflow obstruction (gradient >50 mmHg) and symptoms refractory to medical therapy [62, 63]. Therapeutic options in patients without LV outflow gradients are limited predominantly to pharmacologic therapy. Anticoagulation should be considered in all patients with sustained or paroxysmal AF [58, 59].

25.2.5.2 Risk Stratification and Prevention of Sudden Cardiac Death

SCD occurs throughout life, with a maximal incidence in adolescence and young adulthood, often without warning signs or symptoms. Although there is an excess of deaths during or after strenuous exertion, most occur during mild exertion or sedentary activities. The mechanism underlying most cases of SCD is believed to be ventricular tachyarrhythmia, but conduction disease and thrombo-embolism may account for some cases.

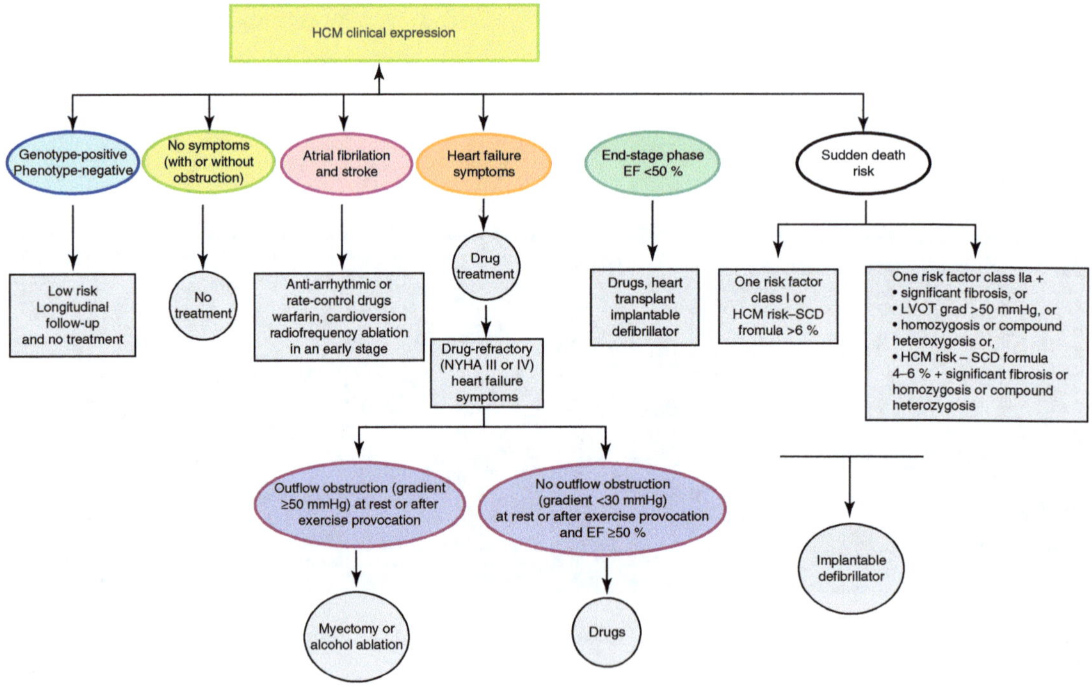

Fig. 25.5 Natural history and management of Hypertrophic Cardiomyopathy (Image reproduced courtesy of EKKAN). *LVOT* Left ventricular outflow track, *EF* Ejectiar fraction, *NYHA* New york heart association

In general, the presence of one or more conventional clinical risk factors should prompt consideration of an implantable cardioverter defibrillator (ICD). Patients with two or more risk factors have a 4–5 % annual risk of SCD. More problematic are patients who have only a single risk factor (up to 25 % of patients). When assessing the need for ICDs in this group, age, symptoms, and the presence of so-called minor risk factors should be taken into account and balanced against the risk of complications of ICD therapy, particularly in young people. Patients with HCM should refrain from intense exercise. This restriction has significant implications for all patients, underlining the importance of accurate diagnosis [42–48].

25.2.5.3 Clinical Risk Stratification in HCM

The Following Data are Being Used

1. **Conventional primary prevention risk markers**
   Family history of sudden death due to hypertrophic cardiomyopathy
   Unexplained recent syncope
   Multiple repetitive non-sustained ventricular tachycardia (on ambulatory ECG)
   Hypotensive or attenuated blood pressure response to exercise
   Massive left-ventricular hypertrophy (thickness, ≥30 mm)
2. **Potential high-risk subsets for primary prevention**
   End-stage phase (ejection fraction <50 %)
   Left-ventricular apical aneurysm and scarring
3. **Potential arbitrators for primary prevention**[1]
   Substantial left-ventricular outflow gradient at rest
   Multiple sarcomere mutations
   Extensive and diffuse late gadolinium enhancement
   Modifiable
   - Intense competitive sports
   - Coronary artery disease

[1] *A number of disease features can be regarded as arbitrators when the level of risk based on conventional markers is ambiguous. They may be useful in resolving otherwise uncertain ICD decisions on a case-by-case basis. Routine use of electrophysiology testing is not recommended.*

Recently a more sophisticated model (HCM Risk-SCD) was published for predicting SCD in HCM. This is the first validated SCD risk prediction model for patients with HCM. The model provides accurate individualized estimates for the probability of SCD using readily collected clinical parameters such as LVH, LVOT gradient at rest, NSVT in Holter, familial SCD, LA size and age [47].

Pregnancy

Serious complications during pregnancy in women with HCM occur in less than 2 % of pregnancies. Maternal mortality seems to be confined to women with high risk profiles [4, 8, 63].

25.2.5.4 Clinical Value of Genetic Testing

A genetic diagnosis is obtainable in 70 % of consecutive patients with familial HCM, though the yield is lower (30 %) when sporadic disease is considered [4, 8]. Those with special characteristics such as conduction disorders, pre-excitation, or systemic disease may represent phenocopies of sarcomere-associated HCM and focused genetic testing may be helpful with diagnosis and treatment (e.g. Danon's disease, Fabry disease). The greatest benefit of genetic testing in HCM derives from cascade screening with the ability to identify which individuals in a family are, or are not, at risk of disease development [1, 2, 4, 5, 8, 32, 60, 63, 64].

25.2.6 Evaluation of Families and Genetic Counselling

Current guidelines recommend screening with a 12-lead ECG and echocardiogram for family members of HCM patients [4, 5, 8, 63].

At age <12 years
Screening optional unless:
- Either a malignant family history of premature death from hypertrophic cardiomyopathy is known or other adverse complications are present
- Child is a competitive athlete in an intensive training programme

- Onset of symptoms
- Other clinical suspicion of early left-ventricular hypertrophy has been noted

At age 12–21 years

- Screening should be performing every 12–18 months

At older than 21 years

- Imaging should be performed either at onset of symptoms or possibly at 5-year intervals (at least through mid-life); more frequent intervals are appropriate in families with a malignant clinical course or history of late-onset hypertrophic cardiomyopathy

Thus at the present time hypertrophic cardiomyopathy has been transformed from a rare and largely untreatable disorder to a common genetic disease with effective management strategies.

25.3 Arrhythmogenic (ARVC/ALVC) Cardiomyopathy

25.3.1 Definition-Epidemiology

Arrhythmogenic right ventricular cardiomyopathy (ARVC) is a genetically determined heart muscle disease that predominantly affects the right ventricle (RV). The disease is characterized by fibrofatty replacement of the right and/or the left ventricular myocardium, segmental dysfunction of the RV or/and LV and arrhythmias. ARVC is mainly a desmosomal disease resulting from defective cell adhesion proteins. The estimated prevalence of ARVC in the general population ranges from 1 in 2,000 to 1 in 5,000. A familial background has been demonstrated in about 50 % of ARVC cases (Fig. 25.6). The disease becomes clinically overt most often in the third or fourth decade of life. Clinical diagnosis of ARVC is often difficult because of the nonspecific nature of the disease and the broad spectrum of phenotypic manifestation, ranging from severe to concealed forms. In 2010, the International Task Force proposed revised criteria for the clinical diagnosis of ARVC (Table 25.2) [65].

25.3.2 Genetics

The disease is familial, and typically autosomal dominant, in about half the cases. Mutations in five genes that encode desmosomal proteins (desmoplakin, plakoglobin, plakophilin 2, desmoglein 2, and desmocollin 2) have been found in ARVC. The same holds true for two related autosomal recessive disorders: (1) Naxos disease (ARVC accompanied by woolly hair and palmoplantar keratoderma) and, (2) The Carvajal syndrome (which has a similar dermatologic phenotype but in which left ventricular involvement is predominant). Mutant desmosomes may therefore compromise cell-to-cell adhesion at intercalated disks, lessening the ability of myocytes to withstand mechanical forces during the cardiac cycle. Damage to the cell surfaces, causing cell detachment and cell death, probably ensues [65, 66].

The majority of causative mutations are insertions or deletions or nonsense mutations that result in premature truncation of the encoded proteins. Two other, nondesmosomal genes have been implicated in ARVC: one for the transforming growth factor β3 (TGF-β3) and the other for the transmembrane protein 43 (TMEM43). Experimental data indicating that mutant desmosomes also cause remodeling of gap junctions 63 explain how electrocardiographic changes and ventricular arrhythmias can develop before the loss of myocytes and dysfunction of the RV become apparent (the concealed phase of the disease) [65–71].

25.3.2.1 Morphologic Types of ACM

The spectrum of RV alterations ranges from global RV dilatation/dysfunction to regional wall motion abnormalities or "bulges" typically localized in the triangle of dysplasia, (i.e., subtricuspid, apical, and infundibular regions). The LV and the septum are usually involved to a lesser extent; whereas, biventricular or left dominant variants of disease have been reported [71–76].

The extent of LV involvement and variations in the perceptible timing has allowed recognition of three distinct patterns of disease expression:

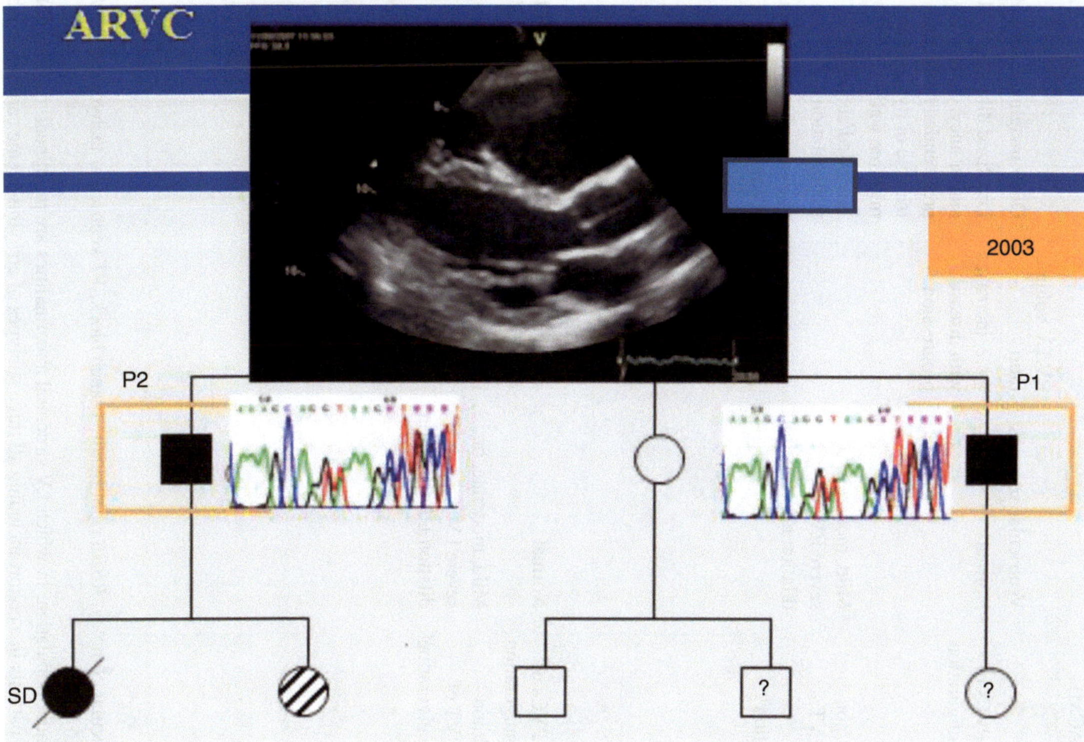

Fig. 25.6 ARVC is a familial cardiomyopathy (Image reproduced courtesy of EKKAN)

1. **Classic (right dominant)**. The early stages of the disease are characterized by isolated RV involvement, evolving from localized to diffuse. LV involvement may arise after the onset of global RV dysfunction.
2. **Left dominant**, characterized by early prominent LV involvement; the LV is consistently more severely affected than the right.
3. **Biventricular**, characterized by parallel bilateral involvement with no apparent proclivity to either ventricle.

Left-dominant arrhythmogenic cardiomyopathy (LDAC) is characterized pathologically by fibroadipose replacement of the LV. In classic right dominant disease, LV involvement is frequently confined to the inferolateral and inferior walls, sparing the septum. LDAC, in contrast, affects the septum in more than 50 % of cases. Cardiovascular magnetic resonance commonly shows late gadolinium enhancement in a subepicardial or midmyocardial distribution, consistent with that observed in pathology [74].

25.3.3 Clinical Diagnosis

25.3.3.1 Original and Modified Task Force Criteria

The 1994 Task Force Criteria were initially designed to guarantee an adequate specificity for ARVC among index cases with overt clinical manifestations. However, the 1994 Criteria lack sensitivity for identification of early/minor phenotypes, particularly in the setting of familial ARVC. Accordingly, diagnostics criteria have been recently revised with the aim of improving diagnostic sensitivity [65]. Comparison of dignostic criteria of ARVC versus ALVC [LDAC] is presented in Table 25.2. The approach of classifying structural, histopathologic, electrocardiographic (ECG), arrhythmic, and genetic features of the disease as major and minor criteria has been maintained. As far as ECG and arrhythmic features are concerned, in the revised Task Force Criteria T-wave inversion in V1 to V3 as well as VT with left bundle branch block (LBBB) morphology with superior/indeterminate QRS axis,

Table 25.2 Clinical diagnostic criteria for right versus left arrhythmogenic cardiomyopathy (ACM)

Diagnosis ACM	12-Lead ECG	Signal-averaged ECG	Arrhythmia		Ventricular volumes	RV/LV volume ratio	Other imagine abnormalities
Classic right dominant ARVC	Normal	Late potentials	Both supraventricular tachycardia and atrial fibrillation/flutter are observed but are not contributory to diagnosis	Frequent PVCs of LBBB configuration	Normal	≥1.2, increases with disease progression	Localized dilation, WMA, and/or aneyrysms in RV, preferentially affecting triangle of dyplasia and mid-free wall
	Poor R-wave progression[a] IVCD in V1-3 Incomplete RBBB RBBB Epsilon waves in V1-3 Inverted/flat T-waves in V1-3, extending to V4-6 with LV involvement ST elevation in V1-3			Sustained/non-sustained VT of LBBB configuration[b]	Mild, moderate, or severe RV dilation ± dysfunction		Increased/abnormal trabeculation Fat/late enhancement in RV myocardium
Left dominant ALVC	Normal	–		Frequent PVCs of RBBB configuration	Normal	<1, diminishes with disease progression	Localized dilation, WMA, and/or aneyrysms in LV
	Leftward QRS axis (–30°< QRS axis <0) or left-axis deviation (QRS axis <–30°)			Sustained/non-sustained VT of RBBB configuration[c]	Mild, moderate, or severe LV dilation ± dysfunction		Non-compacted appearance
	Early transition LBBB Epsilon waves in inferior (II, III, aVF) and/or lateral leads (V5-V6±V4, I, aVL) Inverted/flat T-waves in (infero) lateral leads, extending to V1-3 with RV involvement						Late enhancement in LV myocardium in subepicardial/midwall distribution

Data compiled from Marcus et al. [65] and Sen-Chowdhry et al. [76]

IVCD intraventricular conduction delay, *LBBB* left bundle branch block, *PVC* premature ventricular complex, *RBBB* right bundle branch block, *VT* ventricular tachycardia, *WMA* wall motion abnormality

[a]PoorR-wave progression is the primary ECG abnormality observed in the Newfoundland founder population, in which LV structural abnormalities are prominent, but the subtype of arrhythmogenic cardiomyopahty is still being elucidated. It has also been reported in ~10 % of patients in a cohort including all three subtypes of arrhythmogenic cardiomyopahty

[b]Non-sustained VT is defined as three or more consecutive beats at a rate of >120 bpm; sustained VT has a duration of >30 s

either sustained or non-sustained, have become major criteria. The following findings have been included among minor criteria: (1) T-wave inversion in V1 and V2 in the absence of right bundle block (RBBB) and from V1 to V4 in the presence of complete RBBB; (2) Positivity of any one of the three signal-averaged ECG (SAECG) parameters for late potentials; and (3) premature ventricular beats more frequent than 500 per 24 h on the Holter monitoring. Moreover, revised guidelines provide quantitative cutoff values in imaging and histopathological criteria. Finally, the identification of a pathogenetic gene mutation in a first-degree relative has become a major criterion for ARVC diagnosis [65, 71, 74, 76].

25.3.4 Clinical Genetics in Arrhythmogenic Cardiomyopathy

A familial background has been identified in 50 % of patients with ARVC. Once a proband is diagnosed with the disease, family genetic screening is indicated for the detection of affected family members, before their clinical symptoms become evident. The first ARVC-causing gene (i.e., the plakoglobin gene [JUP]) was identified in patients with Naxos disease, a syndrome characterized by palmoplantar keratosis, woolly hair, and ARVC with an autosomal recessive pattern of inheritance. Plakoglobin protein is a component of desmosomes, which are specialized intercellular structures providing mechanical attachment of myocytes.

A cardio-cutaneous syndrome, similar clinical profile to Naxos disease, mainly involving the LV has also been reported (so-called Carvajal disease). The cause of Carvajal syndrome is a defective desmoplakin gene (DSP). Dominant forms of ARVC caused by DPS gene mutations in plakophilin-2 (PKP-2) have been reported in almost one-third of unrelated probands from three different cohorts of subject with ARVC across the world. Subsequently, desmoglein-2 (DSG2) and desmocollin –2 (DSC2) were detected as rare disease-causing desmosomal genes [65, 71, 74, 76–82].

Other gene mutations unrelated to cell adhesion complex were also identified. Data demonstrate the importance of multiple variants in clinically significant ARVC and indicate that sequencing of all five desmosomal genes is required when genetic evaluation of an ARVC/ACM proband and family is undertaken. In cases where clinical diagnosis in the proband is certain or highly probable, genetic testing is reasonable if cascade screening is desired by the family members [1, 2].

Arrhythmic SCD might occur in a preclinical stage of ARVC before diagnostic histopathologic features become evident at post mortem. Therefore, diagnosis of the cause of death may depend on molecular genetic testing with identification of a pathogenetic gene defect [67–69, 72, 73, 77–79].

25.3.5 Clinical Management

The current evidence suggests that asymptomatic individuals should be included in a follow-up program with noninvasive evaluation on a regular basis for early identification of warning symptoms and demonstration of disease progression or ventricular arrhythmias. Whether prophylactic use of β-blockers, anti-arrhythmic drugs (AADs), and angiotensin-converting enzyme (ACE) inhibitors/angiotensin receptor blocker may reduce arrhythmic complications and disease progression in asymptomatic patients or gene carriers, remains to be proven. AAD therapy is the first-line treatment for patients with well-tolerated and non-life threatening ventricular arrhythmias. Sotalol has been frequently used for prevention of ventricular arrhythmia or the reduction of ICD intervention. Amiodarone alone or in combination with β-blockers has been reported as an alternative approach, although potentially dangerous cardiac and noncardiac side effects should be taken into account. In patients with biventricular heart failure, classical treatment of HF seems adequate. The main mechanism of ventricular tachycardia

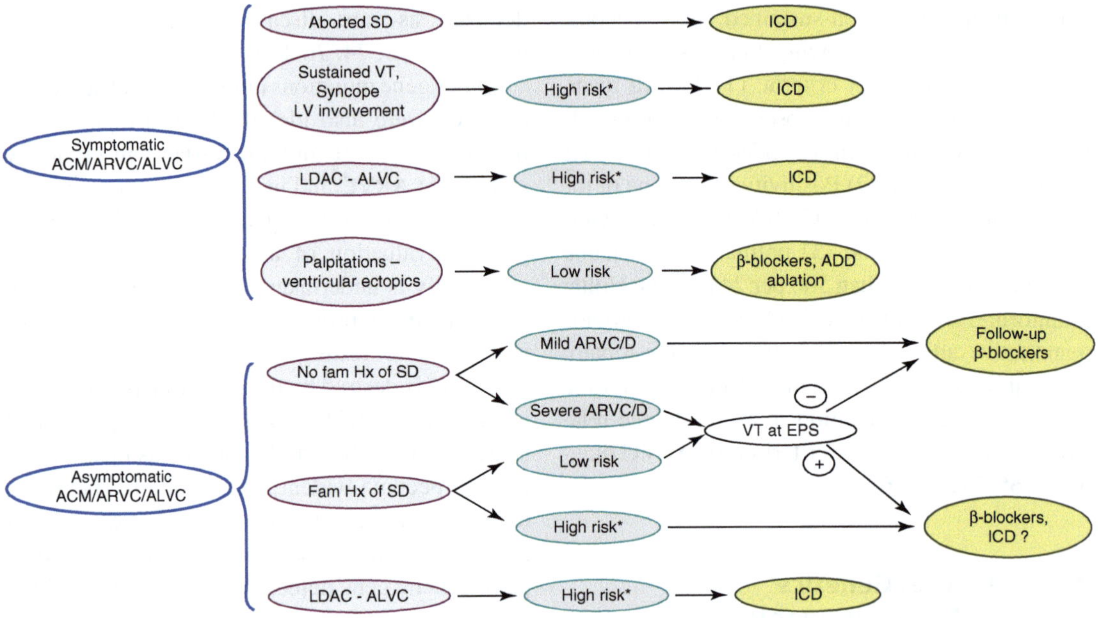

Fig. 25.7 Risk stratification and management in ARVC/ACM. * Risk factors: history of syncope, severe RV dysfunction, LV involvement, hemodynamically unstable VT/VF, QRS dispersion ≥40 ms, epsilon waves, family history of premature SCD, *fam HX* family history of SC; *ICD* implantable cardioverter/defibrillator, *EPS* electrophysiological study; *SD* sudden death, *VT* ventricular tachycardia (Image reproduced courtesy of EKKAN)

(VT) in ARVC is scar-related reentry. Three-dimensional (3D) electroanatomical mapping by CARTO system offers the possibility to delineate electroanatomical scar, which corresponds to areas of low amplitude and fractionated intracardiac electrograms [70–72, 75, 77–82].

25.3.5.1 Risk Stratification

Mortality rate of patients with ARVC/ACM on medical therapy is estimated to be around 1 % per year. Most of the deaths are related to arrhythmias, which can occur at any time during the disease course. Patients with prior cardiac arrest and those with hemodynamically unstable VT carry the highest risk of SCD and benefit of ICD implantation (secondary prevention).

ICD implantation for primary prevention seems problematic The available data based on autopsy series or retrospective clinical studies suggest that young age, fast and poorly tolerated VT, syncope, severe RV dysfunction, LV involvement with HF and, perhaps, familial occurrence of juvenile SD are potential predictors of SCD and worse outcome [79]. Progressive ventricular dysfunction leading to HF and embolic stroke may cause death in a small proportion of patients. There are conflicting data on the prognostic values of electrophysiologic study (EPS) with programmed ventricular stimulation (PVS) in ARVC. Further studies in larger subject populations over a longer follow-up are needed to conclusively determine the value of PVS for risk stratification of patients with ARVC [70, 71, 79, 80].

In conclusion, ARVC/ACM shows an autosomal dominant pattern of inheritance with incomplete penetrance and variable clinical expression, although an autosomal recessive mode has been identified. Molecular genetic analysis is a powerful tool for preclinical diagnosis of ARVC/ACM in asympomatic family members of gene-positive probands and may contribute to risk stratification and clinical management. The most important therapeutic objective in ARVC/ACM is to prevent arrhythmic SD (Fig. 25.7).

25.4 Dilated Cardiomyopathy (DCM)

DCM is characterized by left ventricular dilatation and systolic dysfunction in the absence of hypertension, coronary artery disease, valve disease, congenital heart disease, and other overloading conditions. Analysis of asymptomatic relatives of affected patients indicates that familial disease accounts for one-third to one-half of cases [40, 41].

DCM is the most common cardiomyopathy worldwide and accounts for 25 % of HF cases in the US. Prevalence in adults is 1:2,500. This disorder develops at any age, and in either sex, but more commonly in men than in women [85].

25.4.1 Genetics

25.4.1.1 Familial and Genetic

At presentation, a family history and screening of first-degree relatives (for ventricular dilation, conduction disturbances and skeletal myopathy) should be considered. More than 40 disease-causing genes have been identified in DCM, most of which encode proteins of the sarcolemma, cytoskeleton, sarcomere, nuclear envelope (e.g. Lamin), and mitochondrion. The structural and functional consequences of DCM mutations include impairment of myocardial force generation, force transmission, and cell survival. DCM is inherited as an autosomal dominant trait in 90 % of families. This mode of transmission is often associated with reduced and age-related penetrance, although onset by the fourth decade of life is typical. Expression is also variable and frequently incomplete: although symptomatic disease may not be present, cardiac evaluation may reveal unexplained electrocardiographic ECG or echocardiographic abnormalities [84, 85].

Autosomal dominant forms of DCM may be associated with conduction disease or skeletal myopathy. Other modes of inheritance include autosomal recessive, X-linked recessive, and mitochondrial. In autosomal recessive DCM, patients usually present at a younger age than those with the dominant form. The disease course is characterized by more rapid progression to death or cardiac transplantation. X-linked inheritance is characterized by the absence of male-to-male transmission. Women may be affected but usually express a milder form of disease expression with onset later in life. Affected patients usually have an increase in creatine-kinase (CK) – MM isoform level (e.g. Mutations in dystrophin that also cause Duchenne and Becker muscular dystrophy).

Matrilineal inheritance is usually associated with signs of mitochondrial-related phenotype, such as lactacidemia, hypoacusia, palpebral ptosis, myopathy with ragged red fibers, ophthalmoplegia, encephalopathy, or retinitis pigmentosa. In this form of inheritance the mother, son, or daughter may be affected, but the affected men do not transmit the disease to their offspring.

Causative genes in DCM seem to predominantly encode cytoskeletal and sarcomeric proteins with subsequent defects of force generation and transmission. Metabolic abnormalities and disturbed calcium homeostasis are additional mechanisms. In DCM, mutations in the genes encoding contractile proteins result in functional changes that are the opposite of the changes caused by mutations in the same contractile genes that cause HCM [84–86].

A large number of mutations have been identified in **LMNA**, the gene encoding lamins A and C, which is 12 exons in length and located on the long arm of chromosome 1 (1q21.2-q21.3). Phenotypic manifestations are diverse, including an array of rare but dominantly transmitted diseases affecting cardiac and skeletal muscle (laminopathies): Emery-Dreifuss muscular dystrophy, Dunnigan-type familial partial lipodystrophy (a rare degenerative disorder of the adipose tissue), limb girdle muscular dystrophy 1B, and dilated cardiomyopathy with conduction system disease. Lamin mutations may cause disruption of nuclear function, resulting in cell death. Mice lacking the LMNA gene have been shown to develop rapidly progressive DCM with conduction defects (slow heart rates, prolonged PR and QRS intervals) [85–92].

Finally, although LDAC (desmosomal disease) is now accepted as a variant of ARVC, it can be clinically mistaken for DCM or myocarditis owing to its early and predominant left ventricular involvement [76, 85].

25.4.2 Clinical Diagnosis

25.4.2.1 Patients with the Disease

In index cases, DCM is diagnosed in the presence of depressed fractional shortening (<25 %) of reduced left ventricular ejection fraction (LVEF) (<45 %), and a dilated LV (end-diastolic diameter >117 % of the predicted value corrected for age and body surface area) [83, 85]. DCM patients present with shortness of breath and fatigue or signs of overt HF. Physical examination may be unremarkable or reveal the signs of HF.

Normal ECG is not unusual in the early phase. No ECG abnormalities are specific for DCM. First or second degree AV block, intraventricular block, ST-T wave changes, Q waves, atrial fibrillation, or ventricular arrhythmias may be seen. New ventricular arrhythmias or second or third degree heart block in patients with apparently chronic DCM suggest sarcoidosis.

In echocardiography the LV is dilated, and more spherical than usual with increased wall stress and depressed systolic function with or without mitral regurgitation. Usually contractility is globally reduced with or without segmental abnormalities. Additionally, pericardial effusion (especially in myocarditis) and signs of right HF may be present. Magnetic resonance imaging provides the most accurate estimate of ventricular structure and function and allows detection of inflammation and scarring [83, 85].

Endomyocardial biopsy is controversial. It can be used to distinguish between disease processes that need alternative treatment strategies, such as storage diseases, sarcoidosis, and haemochromatosis. It is reasonable to implement it in patients with new-onset CMP and fulminant HF, who may benefit from an early diagnosis. Usually however, microscopic examination reveals areas of interstitial and perivascular fibrosis, and sometimes areas of necrosis and cellular infiltrate. Additionally, testing for secondary or specific causes that mimic DCM is suggested with clinical suspicion of haemochromatosis, sleep-apnea, HIV infection, rheumatological disease, storage diseases, or pheochromocytom may be warranted [85].

25.4.2.2 Relatives

Incomplete phenotypic expression is common among relatives, contributing to underrecognition of familial disease. Nevertheless, nearly a third of asymptomatic relatives of patients with DCM have echocardiographic abnormalities on screening (e.g., depressed fractional shortening, LV enlargement), and more than a quarter of these patients develop overt DCM. Furthermore, cardiac-specific autoantibodies were present in more than 30 % of asymptomatic relatives of patients with DCM, and are weak independent predictors of DCM development at 5-year follow-up [5, 83, 85].

Familial DCM is diagnosed in the presence of at least two affected individuals in the same family, or a history of unexplained SD before the age of 35 years in a first-degree relative Data compiled from Mestroni L et al. [83].

25.4.3 Risk of Sudden Death

The prognosis of DCM is highly variable. Earlier studies reported 5-year mortality rates of 50 %, which have declined to 20 % in more recent reports. This improvement in survival reflects both advances in HF therapy and early disease detection. An important unsolved challenge in the management of DCM is individual assessment of the lifetime risk of SD [84, 85].

Few parameters, such as LVEF and syncope, have been identified as good predictors of SD in DCM. Scant data exist on the natural history associated with specific genetic mutations and

Table 25.3 Definition of the clinical status of members of families with familial dilated cardiomyopathy compiled from [83]

Major criteria	Minor criteria
1. The presence of two or more affected individuals in a single family; or 2. The presence of a first-degree relative of a dilated cardiomyo-pathy patient, with well documented unexplained sudden death at <35 years of age.	1. Unexplained supraventricular (atrial fibrillation or sustained arrhythmias) or ventricular arrhythmias, frequent (>1,000/24 h) or repetitive (three or more beats with >120 bpm) before the age of 50 2. Left ventricular dilatation >112 % of the predicted value 3. Left ventricular dysfunction: ejection fraction <50 % or fractional shortening <28 % 4. Unexplained conduction disease: II or III atrioventricular conduction defects, complete left-ventricular bundle branch block, sinus nodal dysfunction 5. Unexplained sudden death or stroke before 50 years of age 6. Segmental wall motion abnormalities (<1 segment, or 1 if not previously present) in the absence of intraventricular conduction defect or ischaemic heart disease.

Assessment of the clinical status

Affected	Unknown	Unaffected
Presence of:	Presence of one or two minor criteria	Individuals with normal hearts
The major criteria (left ventricular dilatation and systolic dysfunction)		
Or left ventricular dilatation (>117 %)+one minor criterion		The presence of other causes of myocardial disease
Or three minor criteria		

predisposition to arrhythmia. However, recent studies have shown that arrhythmogenic risk is higher in certain subtypes of DCM, such as the laminopathies and desmosomal disease of the left ventricle (LDAC/ACM) [85–92].

25.4.3.1 Mild DCM with Severe Arrythmogenicity and Indications for Genetic Testing

Current data support the view that LMNA mutations are among the most common defects in familial DCM, accounting for 5–8 % of all DCM cases, and up to 70 % of cases of DCM with conduction defects and/or muscle contractures.

Although initial reports have emphasized that patients with DCM from lamin A/C (LMNA) mutation often have a conduction defect or AF prior to the development of HF, it is increasingly apparent that SD from ventricular arrhythmia is a major prognostic determinant, and often occurs before the onset of severe LV dysfunction. Because as reliable risk stratification in LMNA disease remains an unsolved challenge, consideration should be given to prophylactic ICD implantation in all patients who have a probable disease-causing mutation, particularly in the presence of a family history of premature SD [88, 89, 91, 92].

Additionally, LDAC/ACM is now accepted as a variant of ARVC and it can be clinically mistaken for DCM or myocarditis owing to its early and predominant LV involvement.

LDAC/ACM should be suspected in patients of any age with unexplained arrhythmia of LV origin, (infero) lateral T wave inversion, apparent DCM with arrhythmic presentation or myocarditis. The significant risk of SD in patients with LDAC justifies mutation screening for desmosomal genes in apparent DCM and warrants a low threshold for ICD placement if the diagnosis is confirmed. As noted, DCM with conduction disease and/or arrhythmia represents a special subset of familial DCM in which focused testing for LMNA, desmosomal, and to a lesser degree for SCN5A mutations, may have a substantial clinical impact. When there is a strong family history of important ventricular arrhythmias, heart block, or SD, practitioners may consider recommending early prophylactic ICD implantation for genotype-positive relatives, even in the presence of mild or no phenotype [85, 88–97].

Thus, unexpected sustained VT or SD in the absence of significant LV dysfunction should raise suspicion of either LMNA or a desmosomal mutation as the cause of the CMP and should prompt familial and genetic evaluation (Fig. 25.7).

Conclusions

The identification of the most clinically relevant genes underlying inherited CMP and demonstration of clinical relevance of genotype phenotype correlation require that cardiologists are aware of the possibilities and limitations of genetic testing, to squeeze out the maximum possible benefit. During the past two decades, numerous disease-causing genes for different CMP have been identified. These discoveries have led to better understanding of disease pathogenesis and are the initial steps in the clinical application of mutation analysis in the evaluation of the patients and their families.

References

1. Watkins H, Astrafian H, Redwood C. Inherited cardiomyopathies. N Engl J Med. 2011;364:1643.
2. Jacoby D, McKenna WJ. Genetics of inherited cardiomyopathy. Eur Heart J. 2012;33:296–304.
3. Elliott P, Anderson B, Arbustini E, Bilinska Z, Cecchi F, Charron P, et al. Classification of cardiomyopathies: a position statement from the European Working Group on Myocardial and Pericardial Diseases. Eur Heart J. 2008;29:270–6.
4. Elliott P, McKenna W. Hypertrophic cardiomyopathy. Lancet. 2004;363:1881–91.
5. Charron P, Arad M, Arbustini E, Basso C, Bilinska Z, Elliott P, et al. Genetic counselling and testing in cardiomyopathies: a position statement of the European Society of Cardiology Working Group on Myocardial and Pericardial Diseases. Eur Heart J. 2010;31:2715–26.
6. Anastasakis A, Sevdalis E, Papatheodorou E, Stefanadis C. Anderson-Fabry disease: a cardiomyopathy that can be cured. Hellenic J Cardiol. 2011;52:316–26.
7. Elliott P, Baker R, Pasquale F, Quarta G, Ebrahim H, Mehta AB, Hughes DA, ACES study group. Prevalence of Anderson-Fabry disease in patients with hypertrophic cardiomyopathy: the European Anderson-Fabry Disease survey. Heart. 2011;97:1957–60.
8. Maron BJ, Maron MS. Hypertrophic cardiomyopathy. Lancet. 2013;381(9862):242–55.
9. Anastasakis A, Papatheodorou E, Steriotis AK. Fabry disease and cardiovascular involvement. Curr Pharm Des. 2013;19:5997–6008.
10. Seidman CE, Seidman JG. Identifying sarcomere gene mutations in hypertrophic cardiomyopathy: a personal history. Circ Res. 2011;108:743–50.
11. Sabourdy F, Michelakakis H, Anastasakis A, Garcia V, Mavridou I, Nieto M, et al. Danon disease: further clinical and molecular heterogeneity. Muscle Nerve. 2009;39:837–44.
12. Theopistou A, Anastasakis A, Miliou A, Rigopoulos A, Toutouzas P, Stefanadis C. Clinical features of hypertrophic cardiomyopathy caused by an Arg278Cys missense mutation in the cardiac troponin T gene. Am J Cardiol. 2004;94:246–9.
13. Anastasakis A, Karandreas N, Stathis P, Rigopoulos A, Theopistou A, Sepp R, et al. Subclinical skeletal muscle abnormalities in patients with hypertrophic cardiomyopathy and their relation to clinical characteristics. Int J Cardiol. 2003;89:249–56.
14. Landstrom AP, Ackerman MJ. Mutation type is not clinically useful in predicting prognosis in hypertrophic cardiomyopathy. Circulation. 2010;122:2441–9.
15. Maron MS, Maron BJ, Harrigan C, Buros J, Gibson CM, Olivotto I, et al. Hypertrophic cardiomyopathy phenotype revisited after 50 years with cardiovascular magnetic resonance. J Am Coll Cardiol. 2009;54:220–8.
16. Moon JC, Fisher NG, McKenna WJ, Pennell DJ. Detection of apical hypertrophic cardiomyopathy by cardiovascular magnetic resonance in patients with non-diagnostic echocardiography. Heart. 2004;90:645–9.
17. Valeti US, Nishimura RA, Holmes DR, Araoz PA, Glockner JF, Breen JF, et al. Comparison of surgical septal myectomy and alcohol septal ablation with cardiac magnetic resonance imaging in patients with hypertrophic obstructive cardiomyopathy. J Am Coll Cardiol. 2007;49:350–7.
18. Maron BJ, Maron MS, Wigle ED, Braunwald E. The 50-year history, controversy, and clinical implications of left ventricular outflow tract obstruction in hypertrophic cardiomyopathy: from idiopathic hypertrophic subaortic stenosis to hypertrophic cardiomyopathy. J Am Coll Cardiol. 2009;54:191–200.
19. Elliott PM, Gimeno Blanes JR, Mahon NG, Poloniecki JD, McKenna WJ. Relation between severity of left-ventricular hypertrophy and prognosis in patients with hypertrophic cardiomyopathy. Lancet. 2001;357:420–4.
20. Ho CY. Genetics and clinical destiny: improving care in hypertrophic cardiomyopathy. Circulation. 2010;122:2430–40.
21. Maron BJ, Gardin JM, Flack JM, Gidding SS, Kurosaki TT, Bild DE. Prevalence of hypertrophic cardiomyopathy in a general population of young adults: echocardiographic analysis of 4111 subjects in the CARDIA Study. Circulation. 1995;92:785–9.
22. Cecchi F, Olivotto I, Gistri R, Lorenzoni R, Chiriatti G, Camici PG. Coronary microvascular dysfunction and prognosis in hypertrophic cardiomyopathy. N Engl J Med. 2003;349:1027–35.
23. Harris KM, Spirito P, Maron MS, Zenovich AG, Formisano F, Lesser JR, et al. Prevalence, clinical pro-

file, and significance of left ventricular remodeling in the end-stage phase of hypertrophic cardiomyopathy. Circulation. 2006;114:216–25.
24. Maron BJ, Maron MS, Semsarian C. Genetics of hypertrophic cardiomyopathy after 20 years: clinical perspectives. J Am Coll Cardiol. 2012.
25. Watkins H. Sudden death in hypertrophic cardiomyopathy. N Engl J Med. 2000;342:422–4.
26. Kelly M, Semsarian C. Multiple mutations in genetic cardiovascular disease: a marker of disease severity? Circ Cardiovasc Genet. 2009;2:182–90.
27. Kubo T, Gimeno JR, Bahl A, Steffensen U, Steffensen M, Osman E, et al. Prevalence, clinical significance, and genetic basis of hypertrophic cardiomyopathy with restrictive phenotype. J Am Coll Cardiol. 2007; 49:2419–26.
28. Corrado D, Basso C, Schiavon M, Thiene G. Screening for hypertrophic cardiomyopathy in young athletes. N Engl J Med. 1998;339:364–9.
29. Spirito P, Bellone P, Harris KM, Bernabo P, Bruzzi P, Maron BJ. Magnitude of left ventricular hypertrophy and risk of sudden death in hypertrophic cardiomyopathy. N Engl J Med. 2000;342:1778–85.
30. McLeod CJ, Ackerman MJ, Nishimura RA, Tajik AJ, Gersh BJ, Ommen SR. Outcome of patients with hypertrophic cardiomyopathy and a normal electrocardiogram. J Am Coll Cardiol. 2009;54:229–33.
31. Ho CY, Sweitzer NK, McDonough B, Maron BJ, Casey SA, Seidman JG, et al. Assessment of diastolic function with Doppler tissue imaging to predict genotype in preclinical hypertrophic cardiomyopathy. Circulation. 2002;105:2992–7.
32. Maron BJ, Yeates L, Semsarian C. Clinical challenges of genotype positive (+)-phenotype negative (—) family members in hypertrophic cardiomyopathy. Am J Cardiol. 2011;107:604–8.
33. Rowin EJ, Maron MS, Lesser JR, Maron BJ. CMR with late gadolinium enhancement in genotype positive-phenotype negative hypertrophic cardiomyopathy. JACC Cardiovasc Imaging. 2012;5:119–22.
34. Ho CY, López B, Coelho-Filho OR, Lakdawala NK, Cirino AL, Jarolim P, et al. Myocardial fibrosis as an early manifestation of hypertrophic cardiomyopathy. N Engl J Med. 2010;363:552–63.
35. Maron BJ, Casey SA, Hauser RG, Aeppli DM. Clinical course of hypertrophic cardiomyopathy with survival to advanced age. J Am Coll Cardiol. 2003;42:882–8.
36. Morita H, Rehm HL, Menesses A, McDonough B, Roberts AE, Kucherlapati R, et al. Shared genetic causes of cardiac hypertrophy in children and adults. N Engl J Med. 2008;358:1899–908.
37. Maron BJ, Shen WK, Link MS, Epstein AE, Almquist AK, Daubert JP, et al. Efficacy of implantable cardioverter-defibrillators for the prevention of sudden death in patients with hypertrophic cardiomyopathy. N Engl J Med. 2000;342:365–73.
38. McKenna WJ, Deanfield JE. Hypertrophic cardiomyopathy: an important cause of sudden death. Arch Dis Child. 1984;59:971–5.
39. Spirito P, Seidman CE, McKenna WJ, Maron BJ. The management of hypertrophic cardiomyopathy. N Engl J Med. 1997;336:775–85.
40. Olivotto I, Cecchi F, Casey SA, Dolara A, Traverse JH, Maron BJ. Impact of atrial fibrillation on the clinical course of hypertrophic cardiomyopathy. Circulation. 2001;104:2517–24.
41. Guttmann OP, Rahman MS, O' Mahony C, Anastasakis A, Elliott PM. Atrial fibrillation and thromboembolism in patients with hypertrophic cardiomyopathy: systematic review. Heart. 2014;100:465–72.
42. Elliott PM, Poloniecki J, Dickie S, Sharma S, Monserrat L, Varnava A, et al. Sudden death in hypertrophic cardiomyopathy: identification of high risk patients. J Am Coll Cardiol. 2000;36:2212–8.
43. Spirito P, Autore C, Rapezzi C, Bernabò P, Badagliacca R, Maron MS, et al. Syncope and risk of sudden death in hypertrophic cardiomyopathy. Circulation. 2009;119:1703–10.
44. Monserrat L, Elliott PM, Gimeno JR, Sharma S, Penas-Lado M, McKenna WJ. Non-sustained ventricular tachycardia in hypertrophic cardiomyopathy: an independent marker of sudden death risk in young patients. J Am Coll Cardiol. 2003;42:873–9.
45. Elliott PM, Gimeno JR, Tomé MT, Shah J, Ward D, Thaman R, et al. Left ventricular outflow tract obstruction and sudden death risk in patients with hypertrophic cardiomyopathy. Eur Heart J. 2006;27:1933–41.
46. Anastasakis A, Theopistou A, Rigopoulos A, Kotsiopoulou C, Georgopoulos S, Fragakis K, et al. Sudden cardiac death: investigation of the classical risk factors in a community-based hypertrophic cardiomyopathy cohort. Hellenic J Cardiol. 2013;54:281–8.
47. O'Mahony C, Jichi F, Pavlou M, Monserrat L, Anastasakis A, Rapezzi C, et al., for the Hypertrophic Cardiomyopathy Outcomes Investigators. A novel clinical risk prediction model for sudden cardiac death in hypertrophic cardiomyopathy (HCM Risk-SCD). Eur Heart J. 2014;35(30):2010–20.
48. Maron BJ, Spirito P, Ackerman MJ, Casey SA, Semsarian C, Estes 3rd NA, et al. Prevention of sudden cardiac death with implantable cardioverter-defibrillators in children and adolescents with hypertrophic cardiomyopathy. J Am Coll Cardiol. 2013;61:1527–35.
49. Sorajja P, Ommen SR, Nishimura RA, Gersh BJ, Berger PB, Tajik AJ. Adverse prognosis of patients with hypertrophic cardiomyopathy who have epicardial coronary artery disease. Circulation. 2003;108:2342–8.
50. Pelliccia A, Fagard R, Bjørnstad HH, Anastassakis A, Arbustini E, Assanelli D, et al. Recommendations for competitive sports participation in athletes with cardiovascular disease: a consensus document from the Study Group of Sports Cardiology of the Working Group of Cardiac Rehabilitation and Exercise Physiology and the Working Group of Myocardial and Pericardial Diseases of the European Society of Cardiology. Eur Heart J. 2005;26:1422–45.
51. Anastasakis A, Kotsiopoulou C, Rigopoulos A, Theopistou A, Protonotarios N, Panagiotakos D, et al. Similarities in the profile of cardiopulmonary exercise

testing between patients with hypertrophic cardiomyopathy and strength athletes. Heart. 2005;91:1477–8.
52. Melacini P, Basso C, Angelini A, Calore C, Bobbo F, Tokajuk B, et al. Clinicopathological profiles of progressive heart failure in hypertrophic cardiomyopathy. Eur Heart J. 2010;31:2111–23.
53. Nagueh SF, Ommen SR, Lakkis NM, Killip D, Zoghbi WA, Schaff HV, et al. Comparison of ethanol septal reduction therapy with surgical myectomy for the treatment of hypertrophic obstructive cardiomyopathy. J Am Coll Cardiol. 2001;38:1701–6.
54. Toutouzas K, Karanasos A, Anastasakis A, Vavuranakis M, Seggewiss H, Stefanadis C, et al. Optimal branch selection in alcohol septal ablation. Int J Cardiol. 2011;147:143–4.
55. Maron BJ, Lever H. In defense of antimicrobial prophylaxis for prevention of infective endocarditis in patients with hypertrophic cardiomyopathy. J Am Coll Cardiol. 2009;54:2339–40.
56. Spirito P, Rapezzi C, Bellone P, Betocchi S, Autore C, Conte MR, et al. Infective endocarditis in hypertrophic cardiomyopathy: prevalence, incidence, and indications for antibiotic prophylaxis. Circulation. 1999;99:2132–7.
57. Olivotto I, Maron BJ, Appelbaum E, Harrigan CJ, Salton C, Gibson CM, et al. Spectrum and clinical significance of systolic function and myocardial fibrosis assessed by cardiovascular magnetic resonance in hypertrophic cardiomyopathy. Am J Cardiol. 2010;106:261–7.
58. Fang MC, Go AS, Chang Y, Borowsky L, Pomernacki NK, Singer DE for the ATRIA study group. Comparison of risk stratification schemes to predict thromboembolism in people with nonvalvular atrial fibrillation. J Am Coll Cardiol. 2008;51:810–5.
59. Di Donna P, Olivotto I, Delcrè SD, Caponi D, Scaglione M, Nault I, et al. Efficacy of catheter ablation for atrial fibrillation in hypertrophic cardiomyopathy: impact of age, atrial remodelling, and disease progression. Europace. 2010;12:347–55.
60. Marian AJ. Hypertrophic cardiomyopathy: from genetics to treatment. Eur J Clin Invest. 2010;40:360–9.
61. Fifer MA, Vlahakes GJ. Management of symptoms in hypertrophic cardiomyopathy. Circulation. 2008;117:429–39.
62. Maron BJ, Nishimura RA, McKenna WJ, Rakowski H, Josephson ME, Kieval RS. Assessment of permanent dual-chamber pacing as a treatment for drug-refractory symptomatic patients with obstructive hypertrophic cardiomyopathy. A randomized, double-blind, crossover study (M-PATHY). Circulation. 1999;99:2927–33.
63. Gersh BJ, Maron BJ, Bonow RO, Dearani JA, Fifer MA, Link MS, et al. 2011 ACCF/AHA guideline for the diagnosis and treatment of hypertrophic cardiomyopathy: executive summary: a report of the American College of Cardiology Foundation/American Heart Association Task Force on Practice Guidelines. J Am Coll Cardiol. 2011;58:2703–38.
64. Maron BJ, Roberts WC, Arad M, Haas TS, Spirito P, Wright GB, et al. Clinical outcome and phenotypic expression in LAMP2 cardiomyopathy. JAMA. 2009;301:1253–9.
65. Marcus FI, McKenna WJ, Sherrill D, Basso C, Bauce B, Bluemke DA, et al. Diagnosis of arrhythmogenic right ventricular cardiomyopathy/dysplasia: proposed modification of the Task Force Criteria. Eur Heart J. 2010;31:806–14.
66. McKoy G, Protonotarios N, Crosby A, Tsatsopoulou A, Anastasakis A, Coonar A, et al. Identification of a deletion in plakoglobin in arrhythmogenic right ventricular cardiomyopathy with palmoplantar keratoderma and woolly hair (Naxos disease). Lancet. 2000;355:2119–24.
67. Kaplan SR, Gard JJ, Protonotarios N, Tsatsopoulou A, Spiliopoulou C, Anastasakis A, et al. Remodelling of myocyte gap junctions in arrhythmogenic right ventricular cardiomyopathy due to a deletion in plakoglobin (Naxos disease). Heart Rhythm. 2004;1:3–11.
68. Protonotarios N, Tsatsopoulou A, Anastasakis A, Sevdalis E, McKoy G, Stratos K, et al. Genotype-phenotype assessment in autosomal recessive arrhythmogenic right ventricular cardiomyopathy (Naxos disease) caused by a deletion in plakoglobin. J Am Coll Cardiol. 2001;38:1477–84.
69. Antoniades L, Tsatsopoulou A, Anastasakis A, Syrris P, Asimaki A, Panagiotakos D, et al. Arrhythmogenic right ventricular cardiomyopathy caused by deletions in plakophilin-2 and plakoglobin (Naxos disease) in families from Greece and Cyprus: genotype-phenotype relations, diagnostic features and prognosis. Eur Heart J. 2006;27:2208–16.
70. Lazaros G, Anastasakis A, Tsiachris D, Dilaveris P, Protonotarios N, Stefanadis C. Naxos disease presenting with ventricular tachycardia and troponin elevation. Heart Vessels. 2009;24:63–5.
71. Basso C, Corrado D, Marcus FI, Nava A, Thiene G. Arrhythmogenic right ventricular cardiomyopathy. Lancet. 2009;373:1289–300.
72. Protonotarios N, Anastasakis A, Antoniades L, Chlouverakis G, Syrris P, Basso C, et al. Arrhythmogenic right ventricular cardiomyopathy/dysplasia on the basis of the revised diagnostic criteria in affected families with desmosomal mutations. Eur Heart J. 2011;32:1097–104.
73. Gehmlich K, Syrris P, Peskett E, Evans A, Ehler E, Asimaki A, et al. Mechanistic insights into arrhythmogenic right ventricular cardiomyopathy caused by desmocollin-2 mutations. Cardiovasc Res. 2011;90:77–87.
74. McKenna WJ, Thiene G, Nava A, Fontaliran F, Blomstrom-Lundqvist C, Fontaine G, et al. Task Force of the Working Group Myocardial and Pericardial Disease of the European Society of Cardiology and of the Scientific Council on Cardiomyopathies of the International Society and Federation of Cardiology. Diagnosis of arrhythmogenic right ventricular dysplasia/cardiomyopathy. Br Heart J. 1994;71:215–8.
75. Marcus FI, Zareba W, Calkins H, Towbin JA, Basso C, Bluemke DA, et al. Arrhythmogenic right ventricular cardiomyopathy/dysplasia clinical presentation and diagnostic evaluation: results from the North American Multidisciplinary Study. Heart Rhythm. 2009;6:984–92.

76. Sen-Chowdhry S, Syrris P, Prasad SK, Hughes SE, Merrifield R, Ward D, et al. Left-dominant arrhythmogenic cardiomyopathy: an under-recognized clinical entity. J Am Coll Cardiol. 2008;52:2175–87.
77. Corrado D, Basso C, Leoni L, Tokajuk B, Turrini P, Bauce B, et al. Three-dimensional electroanatomical voltage mapping and histologic evaluation of myocardial substrate in right ventricular outflow tract tachycardia. J Am Coll Cardiol. 2008;51:731–9.
78. Asimaki A, Tandri H, Huang H, et al. A new diagnostic test for arrhythmogenic right ventricular cardiomyopathy. N Engl J Med. 2009;360:1075–84.
79. Corrado D, Calkins H, Link MS, Leoni L, Favale S, Bevilacqua M, et al. Prophylactic implantable defibrillator in patients with arrhythmogenic right ventricular cardiomyopathy/dysplasia and no prior ventricular fibrillation or sustained ventricular tachycardia. Circulation. 2010;122:1144–52.
80. Marcus GM, Glidden DV, Polonsky B, Zareba W, Smith LM, Cannom DS, et al.; Multidisciplinary Study of Right Ventricular Dysplasia Investigators. Efficacy of antiarrhythmic drugs in arrhythmogenic right ventricular cardiomyopathy: a report from the North American ARVC Registry. J Am Coll Cardiol. 2009;54:609–15.
81. Corrado D, Basso C, Pilichou K, Thiene G. Molecular biology and the clinical management of arrhythmogenic right ventricular cardiomyopathy/dysplasia. Heart. 2011;97:530–9.
82. Anastasakis A, Vouliotis AI, Protonotarios N, Stefanadis C. Arrhythmogenic right ventricular cardiomyopathy: the challenge of genetic interpretation in clinically suspected cases. Cardiology. 2012;123:190–4.
83. Mestroni L, Maisch B, McKenna WJ, Schwartz K, Charron P, Rocco C, et al. Guidelines for the study of familial dilated cardiomyopathies. Collaborative Research Group of the European Human and Capital Mobility Project on Familial Dilated Cardiomyopathy. Eur Heart J. 1999;20:93–102.
84. Lehnart SE, Ackerman MJ, Benson Jr DW, Brugada R, Clancy CE, Donahue JK, et al. Inherited arrhythmias: a National Heart, Lung, and Blood Institute and Office of Rare Diseases workshop consensus report about the diagnosis, phenotyping, molecular mechanisms, and therapeutic approaches for primary cardiomyopathies of gene mutations affecting ion channel function. Circulation. 2007;116:2325–45.
85. Jefferies JL, Towbin JA. Dilated cardiomyopathy. Lancet. 2010;375:752–62.
86. Hershberger RE, Morales A, Siegfried JD. Clinical and genetic issues in dilated cardiomyopathy: a review for genetics professionals. Genet Med. 2010;12:655–67.
87. Burkett EL, Hershberger RE. Clinical and genetic issues in familial dilated cardiomyopathy. J Am Coll Cardiol. 2005;45:969–81.
88. Taylor MR, Fain PR, Sinagra G, Robinson ML, Robertson AD, Carniel E, et al.; Familial dilated cardiomyopathy Registry Research Group. Natural history of dilated cardiomyopathy due to lamin A/C gene mutations. J Am Coll Cardiol. 2003;41:771–780.
89. Olson TM, Michels VV, Ballew JD, Reyna SP, Karst ML, Herron KJ, et al. Sodium channel mutations and susceptibility to heart failure and atrial fibrillation. JAMA. 2005;293:447–54.
90. Caforio AL, Mahon NG, Baig MK, Tona F, Murphy RT, Elliott PM, et al. Prospective familial assessment in dilated cardiomyopathy: cardiac autoantibodies predict disease development in asymptomatic relatives. Circulation. 2007;115:76–83.
91. Antoniades L, Eftychiou C, Kyriakides T, Christodoulou K, Katritsis DG. Malignant mutation in the lamin A/C gene causing progressive conduction system disease and early sudden death in a family with mild form of limb-girdle muscular dystrophy. J Interv Card Electrophysiol. 2007;19:1–7.
92. Kourgiannidis G, Anastasakis A, Lampropoulos K, Iliopoulos T. A patient with ventricular tachycardia due to a novel mutation of the lamin A/C gene: case presentation and mini review. Hellenic J Cardiol. 2013;54:326–30.
93. Mavrogeni S, Anastasakis A, Sfendouraki E, Gialafos E, Aggeli C, Stefanadis C. Ventricular tachycardia in patients with family history of sudden cardiac death, normal coronaries and normal ventricular function. Can cardiac magnetic resonance add to diagnosis? Int J Cardiol. 2013;168:1532–3.
94. Kotta CM, Anastasakis A, Stefanadis C. Effects of mutations and genetic overlap in inherited long-QT and Brugada arrhythmia syndromes. Hellenic J Cardiol. 2012;53:439–46.
95. Felker GM, Thompson RE, Hare JM, Hruban RH, Clemetson DE, Howard DL, et al. Underlying causes and long-term survival in patients with initially unexplained cardiomyopathy. N Engl J Med. 2000;342:1077–84.
96. Frustaci A, Russo MA, Chimenti C. Randomized study on the efficacy of immunosuppressive therapy in patients with virus-negative inflammatory cardiomyopathy: the TIMIC study. Eur Heart J. 2009;30:1995–2002.
97. Anastasakis A, McKenna W, Stefanadis C. Prevention of sudden cardiac death in the young: targeted evaluation of those at risk. Hellenic J Cardiol. 2006;47:251–4.

Cardiorenal Syndrome: What Basic Research Can Contribute

26

Aristidis S. Charonis

Abstract

Cardiorenal syndrome is defined as the coexistence of heart failure and renal failure. Under this term, several syndromes with distinct etiology and pathophysiology can be discriminated. This short review focuses on what we have learned from basic research approaches, using animal models. The use of animal models, albeit useful, should always be followed with reservations about extrapolation of results. Two models are presented in detail, one where heart dysfunction is caused by ligation of the left anterior descending artery and another where renal dysfunction is caused by subtotal nephrectomy; in both cases, anatomical and functional alterations in the other organ are presented. Next, future directions in this field are proposed, focused mainly on the need to use system biology approaches for gaining a more holistic understanding and on the promise that interventions on histone deacetylases holds for generating specific and effective pharmaceuticals.

Keywords

Cardiorenal syndrome • Heart failure • Renal failure • Myocardial infarction • Indoxyl sulfate

Abbreviations

ANP	Atrial Natriuretic Peptide
αSMA	Alpha Smooth Muscle Actin
BiP	Binding immunoglobulin Protein
βMHC	Beta-Myosin Heavy Chain
CKD	Chronic Kidney Disease
GFR	Glomerular Filtration Rate
GRP78	Glucose Responsive Protein 78
IL-6	Interleukine-6
IS	Indoxyl Sulfate
KIM-1	Kidney Injury Molecule-1
MAPK	Mitogen-Activated Protein Kinase
MI	Myocardial Infarction
NFκB	Nuclear Factor κB
NGAL	Neutrophil Gelatinase Associated Lipocalin
RAAS	Rennin-Angiotensin-Aldosterone System

A.S. Charonis, MD, PhD
Center of Clinical, Experimental Surgery and Translational Research, Biomedical Research Foundation of the Academy of Athens, Athens, Greece
e-mail: acharonis@bioacademy.gr

D.V. Cokkinos (ed.), *Introduction to Translational Cardiovascular Research*,
DOI 10.1007/978-3-319-08798-6_26, © Springer International Publishing Switzerland 2015

SMAD Similar to Mothers Against Decapentaplegic protein
STN Subtotal Nephrectomy
TGF-β Transforming Growth Factor-beta
UPR Unfolded Protein Response

26.1 Introduction

The cardiorenal syndrome could be defined in simple terms as the coexistence of heart failure and renal failure. This coexistence reflects the tight functional coupling of heart and kidneys. Indeed, current views appreciate the fact that although heart is the pump and kidneys are the filters, both organs are involved in the regulation of vital functions such as blood pressure, vascular tone, diuresis, fluid volume, tissue oxygenation, secretion of hormones [1]. Clinical observations have provided strong evidence for such a functional coupling, since about 1/5 of hospitalized patients with acute myocardial infarction exhibit compromised renal function [2] and death from heart-related causes is increased by a factor of at least ten in patients in dialysis compared to the general population [3].

Recently, it has been proposed that the term "cardiorenal syndrome" may describe a situation where different syndromes, distinct as regards their initiating cause and possibly for the operating pathohysiological mechanisms are clustered together. Therefore, a need to discriminate between them led to the proposal for a classification of "cardio-renal syndrome" in five different categories, based on the primary source of the dysfunction, as follows [1, 4]:

Type 1: starting with acute heart failure
Type 2: starting with chronic heart failure
Type 3: starting with acute renal failure
Type 4: starting with chronic renal failure
Type 5: starting with other systemic disease

This chapter will concentrate on the contributions of basic research for our understanding of the mechanisms underlying the cardio-renal syndrome, and the factors involved. As can be seen from Fig. 26.1, the field of cardio-renal research has witnessed an impressive growth in related publications; however, very few of them (less than 7 %) have used animal models and basic research tools to improve our understanding. Such an improvement should be considered of utmost importance, in order to develop in the future novel and specifically targeted therapeutic approaches.

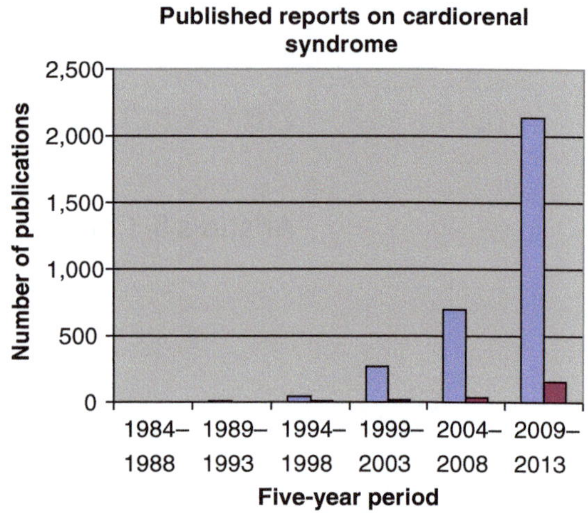

Fig. 26.1 With *blue* color all reports, with *red* color reports using animal models

26.2 What Has Been Done

The most frequently used animal models for studying cardiorenal syndrome are rodent models. The studies can be classified in

(a) those focusing on cardiac alterations in models of chronic kidney disease usually caused by subtotal nephrectomy,
(b) those focusing on renal alterations in models of heart failure usually caused by left anterior descending coronary artery ligation and
(c) those (actually very few and largely inconclusive) focusing on combined cardiac and renal damage.

These studies and their cumulative results can be found tabulated in a recent excellent review by Bongarts et al. [5].

From these studies, we would like to review in detail two from the group of H. Krum, quite representative of the status of the field.

26.2.1 The Acute Heart Failure Model

In order to assess the role of myocardial infarction (MI) on renal anatomy and function (the type 1 cardiorenal syndrome according to the already presented classification), Lekawanvijit and colleagues [6] have used a rat model where the left anterior descending artery was ligated [7]; this method leads to an overall mortality rate of about 30 %. Animals (operated, sham-operated and controls) were sacrificed at several time intervals post-infarction, ranging from 1 to 16 weeks. Assessment of cardiac function demonstrated that animals with MI had a lower ejection fraction compared to the other groups; blood pressure was unchanged, except for the early (1 week) interval in the animals with MI. Systolic and diastolic dysfunction was documented for all time intervals in the infarct group.

Renal function was evaluated by measurement of Glomerular Filtration Rate (GFR) and albuminuria. GFR was decreased at early time points (1 and 4 weeks) but tended to reach normal levels in subsequent time intervals. Albumin in 24 h urine was normal till the 4-week interval and showed an increase at later time points, reaching statistical significance at 16 weeks. Half of the infarct animals exhibited focal tubulointerstitial scarring at 16 weeks; they all showed peritubular fibrosis in the cortex in a time-dependant fashion. The interstitial space of those animals also exhibited macrophage infiltration at the 1-week interval only; along the same lines, IL-6 mRNA was upregulated at the 1 week interval. The TGF-β mRNA, the protein itself and downstream effector phospho-SMAD-2 (a crucial for signaling transcription factor) were upregulated with different kinetics. Study of acute kidney injury biomarkers showed no change in NGAL (Neutrophil Gelatinase Associated Lipocalin) but a biphasic increase in KIM-1 (Kidney Injured Molecule 1) positive tubules.

The authors postulate that there may be a biphasic effect of myocardial infarction on renal structure and function: At an early phase, the decrease in ejection fraction and hypotension may lead to reduction in blood flow through the kidneys and reduction of GFR, resulting in hypoxic/ischemic injury. Following this phase and as a result of these early changes, profibrotic cytokines such as IL-6 and TGF-β are responsible for a gradual development of fibrosis in the renal parenchyma, leading to long-term anatomical changes and renal dysfunction. Contributors to this second phase may not be limited to the TGF-β pathways; although experimental evidence is lacking, it is possible that the rennin-angiotensin-aldosterone system and the endothelin system may be involved as well [8].

26.2.2 The Chronic Renal Failure Model

In order to evaluate the role of chronic kidney disease on cardiac function (the type 4 cardiorenal syndrome according to the proposed classification) Lekawanvijit and colleagues [9] have used the rat model of subtotal nephrectomy (STN). In this model, one kidney is removed and two-thirds of the blood supply of the other kidney are blocked. These interventions are followed by a substantial reduction of the functional renal mass, leading to fibrosis and chronic kidney disease. At different time intervals (4, 8 and 12 weeks), experimental and control animals were studied for the levels of the uremic toxin indoxyl sulfate, renal function, cardiac function, cardiac anatomy/fibrosis and for macromolecules with possible involvement in the alterations observed. Indoxyl Sulfate (Fig. 26.2) is a protein-bound, poorly dialyzable toxin; it is a derivative of tryptophan (tryptophan absorbed at the intestine is metabolized to indole and indole in the liver is metabolize to indoxyl sylfate). Indoxyl

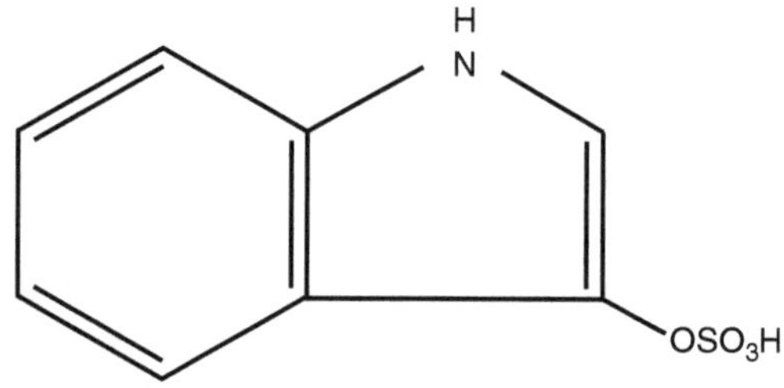

Fig. 26.2 Chemical formula of Indoxyl Sulfate

sulfate is normally excreted in the urine, but in CKD elevated serum levels are observed [10]. The reason for focusing on indoxyl sulfate was that previous findings in vitro have indicated that indoxyl sulfate exerts pro-inflammatory, pro-fibrotic and pro-hypertrophic effects on cardiac fibroblasts and cardiomyocytes [11].

A consistent decrease in body weight, in the range of 10 % was observed in animals with STN. A significant increase in systolic blood pressure, in the range of 50 % was recorded at all time intervals. As expected, animals with STN had increased serum creatinine and urine total protein concentrations and reduced GFR. Also, regarding indoxyl sulfate, animals with STN had almost four times higher concentrations in serum and reduced concentrations in urine. Administration of an oral charcoal absorbent of indoxyl sulfate, kremezin (AST-120), had no effect on blood pressure or body weight, but could improve serum creatinine and urine total protein. The heart weight, the left ventricular weight and the lung weight, all adjusted to body weight, were increased in animals with STN; echocardiography established early diastolic dysfunction and cardiac hypertrophy. Cardiac tissue findings relate to inflammation, fibrosis and hypertrophy. The pro-inflammatory cytokines IL-6 and TNF-α were examined at the mRNA level and no difference was detected between sham-operated and STN animals. Cardiac fibrosis was studied both morphologically and biochemically. Extracellular matrix evaluation with Sirius Red staining demonstrated an extensive fibrosis, which was reduced 50 % in animals taking kremezin. Examination of genes and pathways related to fibrosis indicated that TGF-β was increased at the mRNA and the protein level in STN animals and signaling pathways involving NFκB, p38 and p44/42 MAKPs were activated; some of these phenomena were partly reversed by the use of kremezin. Regarding hypertrophy, it was observed that cardiomyocyte cross-sectional area was significantly increased in STN animals and pro-hypertrophic genes such as ANP, βMHC and αSMA were also upregulated; none of these phenomena was affected by administration of kremezin.

Based on these results it can be concluded that CKD-generated uremic toxin IS contributes to uremic cardiomyopathy by inducing cardiac fibrosis. Despite signaling defects in cardiomyocytes, detected with high levels of IS, the study did not clearly document a functional impairment in the heart. These findings, combined with previous studies using the IS absorbent kremezin, imply a beneficial effect of reducing this specific uremic toxin. However, the contributions of the rennin-angiotensin-aldosterone system should be also examined in this model, as acknowledged by the authors.

Based on the studies presented above as well as others reviewed by Bongartz et al. [5], it can be concluded that so far, there is evidence for cardiac pathology and dysfunction as a result of compromised renal function, but there is not strong evidence for the reverse. We can propose as a working hypothesis for cardiorenal syndrome type 4 the following sequence of events, shown also in Fig. 26.3:

At the beginning, renal dysfunction causes a gradual increase in circulating blood volume, rise in blood pressure, and increase in the concentration of toxic metabolites in the circulation.

As a next step, consequences of the above changes are the activation of known pathways involving oxidative stress, inflammatory reactions and the activation of the RAAS system.

Next, activation of these systems exerts major negative effects on the myocardium. More specifically, it leads to alterations of cardiomyocytes, including hypertrophy and dysfunction; alterations in the heart interstitium, leading to gradual development of fibrotic tissue; and alterations in the heart microvasculature, a decrease in density and finally, in conjunction with wall thickening, less efficient exchange of nutrients and gases.

Finally, these changes in the myocardium cause diastolic and systolic dysfunction, leading to heart failure and in cases where fibrosis is prominent, to sudden death.

A word of caution is necessary in evaluating the results from animal models. First, it is well established that differences exist between any of

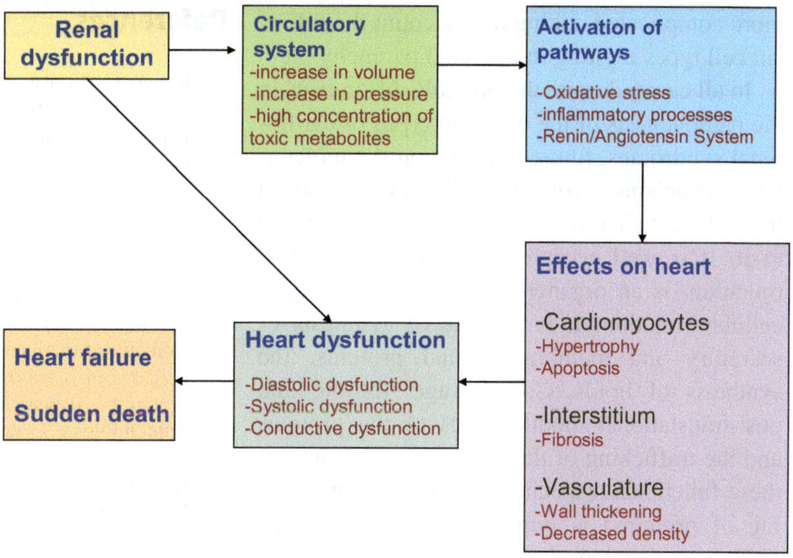

Fig. 26.3 Pathophysiological sequence of events in cardiorenal syndrome (type 4)

these models and the human situation. In addition, especially for type 2 and type 4 cardiorenal syndrome, it should be noted that all models used are far from mimicking conditions in the human, since the models used exert a sudden insult to either organ and do not simulate the gradual decline in function most frequently seen in patients with type 2 and type 4 cardiorenal syndrome. However, these models are closer to the human situation when type 1 and type 3 cardiorenal syndromes are considered, since the abrupt changes of the animal models (acute decline in heart and renal function) simulate the initiating pathology in the case of humans.

26.3 What Needs to Be Done

Cardiorenal syndrome involves the cross-talk between these two organs, which may be mediated by hemodynamic factors and by humoral factors in various combinations. The complexity of the process clearly necessitates System Biology approaches, using a combination of transcriptomics, proteomics and metabolomics and strong bioinformatic analysis. Results from such approaches are not reported yet in any detail. However, a glimpse of data from such approaches is given in a recent review by Ben-Shoshan et al. [12]. The authors have performed a gene chip array analysis of cardiac tissue during renal failure, using animal models. They claim to have identified that "cardiorenal syndrome-specific genetic alterations are highly related to the regulation of liquid surface tension, coagulation homeostasis and extracellular matrix metabolism". Bioinformatic analysis of their data indicated that even at early stages of renal failure cardiac tissue hypertrophy is initiated and the molecular pathways involved are distinct from those activated in hypertrophy due to infarction. It is mentioned that endoplasmic reticulum stress may be a key player in these early phenomena.

Although this information is not published yet in full detail, it is tempting to speculate that it would be very useful to explore the effect of hemodynamic factors and toxins (even at low concentrations) on the phenotype of cardiomyocytes, focusing on endoplasmic reticulum stress. In this respect, it is imperative to generate in the near future a more detailed analysis of the circulating toxins in the serum that are related to a reduced function of the kidneys and also of the toxins that are related to dialysis.

A similar approach could be suggested for the study of cardiorenal syndromes types 1 and 2, where hemodynamic factors and humoral factors should be examined for their effect on different renal cell phenotypes, although this approach is more complicated, taking into account the different cell types existing in the renal parenchyma.

In all cases, despite the possible differences in the pathogenesis of the different types of cardiorenal syndromes, future research on the molecular mechanisms involved should concentrate on the endoplasmic reticulum and the stress imposed to it. It is well accepted that the endoplasmic reticulum is an organelle with a central role in cellular function. It is the site of synthesis of secretory and membrane-bound proteins, the synthesis of lipids, Ca^{2+} storage, folding and post-translational modifications of the proteins and the trafficking of the proteins in it. If any of these functions, (especially the appropriate folding of proteins) is impaired, the endoplasmic reticulum is endowed with mechanisms that try to correct the problem, collectively known as the Unfolded Protein Response (UPR). At least three distinct signaling pathways participate in this response, having as common starting macromolecule the GRP78 protein (also known as BiP) which resides in the lumen of the endoplasmic reticulum [13]. These pathways are activated in order to overcome the problem and restore the normal function of the endoplasmic reticulum; their failure to do so leads to cell death [14]. Therefore detailed understanding at the molecular level of the specific pathways that are activated in cases of cardiorenal syndrome in the specific cell types involved, holds the promise to allow the design of targeted and more effective therapeutic interventions [15].

Regarding future therapeutic interventions, an interesting field where more works should be anticipated is the field of inhibition of protein deacetylation. This process is thought to be involved in the pathogenesis of both heart and kidney failure. Inhibitors of histone deacetylation have given encouraging data on cardiac and renal dysfunction in animal models, possibly because they affect a constellation of cell types and pathways [16]. In this respect, a lot needs to be learned about their specific targets (both histone and non-histone proteins) and even more importantly the specific isoforms of histone deacetylases involved, in order to improve the efficacy and specificity of future therapeutic regiments.

References

1. Ronco C, House AA, Haapio M. Cardiorenal syndrome: refining the definition of a complex symbiosis gone wrong. Intensive Care Med. 2008;34:957–62.
2. Parikh CR, Coca SG, Wang Y, Masudi FA, Krumholz HM. Long-term prognosis of acute kidney injury after acute myocardial infarction. Arch Intern Med. 2008;168:987–95.
3. Sarnak MJ, Levey AS, Schoolwerth AC, Coresh J, Culleton B, et al. Kidney disease as a risk factor for development of cardiovascular disease: a statement from the American Heart Association Councils on Kidney in cardiovascular Disease, High Blood Pressure Research, Clinical Cardiology and Epidemiology and Prevention. Circulation. 2003;108:2154–69.
4. Ronco C. Cardiorenal Syndromes: Definition and Classification. In: Ronco C, Costanzo MR, Bellomo R, Maisel AS, editors. Fluid overload: diagnosis and management, vol. 64. Basel: Karger; 2010. p. 33–8.
5. Bongartz LG, Braam B, Gaillard CA, Cramer MJ, Goldschmeding R, Verhaar MC, et al. Target organ cross talk in cardiorenal syndrome: animal models. Am J Physiol Renal Physiol. 2012;303:F1253–63.
6. Lekawanvijit S, Kompa AR, Zang Y, Wang BH, Kelly DJ, Krum H. Myocardial infarction impairs renal function, induces renal interstitial fibrosis, and increases renal KIM-1 expression: implications for cardiorenal syndrome. Am J Physiol Heart Circ Physiol. 2012;302:H1884–93.
7. Tzanidis A, Lim S, Hannan RD, See F, Ugoni AM, Krum H. Combined angiotensin and endothelin receptor blockade attenuates adverse cardiac remodeling post-myocardial infarction in the rat: possible role of transforming growth factor beta. J Mol Cell Cardiol. 2001;33:969–81.
8. Wolf G. Renal injury due to rennin-angiotensin-aldosterone system activation of the transforming growth factor-beta pathway. Kidney Int. 2006;70:1914–9.
9. Lekawanvijit S, Kompa AR, Manabe M, Wang BH, Langham RG, Nishijima F, et al. Chronic kidney disease-induced cardiac fibrosis is ameliorated by reducing circulating levels of a non-dialysable uremic toxin, indoxyl sulfate. PLoS One. 2012;7:e41281.
10. Niwa T. Uremic toxicity of indoxyl sulfate. Nagoya J Med Sci. 2010;72:1–11.
11. Lekawanvijit S, Adrahtas A, Kelly DJ, Kompa AR, Wang BH, Krum H. Does indoxyl sulfate, a uraemic toxin, have direct effects on cardiac fibroblasts and myocytes? Eur Heart J. 2010;31:1771–9.
12. Ben-Shoshan J, Entin-Meer M, Guzner-Gur H, Keren G. The cardiorenal syndrome: a mutual approach to concomitant cardiac and renal failure. Isr Med Assoc J. 2012;14:570–6.
13. Xu C, Bailly-Maitre B, Reed JC. Endoplasmic reticulum stress: cell life and death decisions. J Clin Invest. 2005;115:2656–64.

14. Kim I, Xu W, Reed JC. Cell death and endoplasmic reticulum stress: diseases relevance and therapeutic opportunities. Nat Rev Drug Discov. 2008;7:1013–30.
15. Dickhout JG, Carlisle RE, Austin RC. Interrelationship between cardiac hypertrophy, heart failure and chronic kidney disease. Endoplasmic reticulum stress as a mediator of pathogenesis. Circ Res. 2011;106:629–42.
16. Bush EW, McKinsey TA. Protein acetylation in the cardiorenal axis: the promise of histone deacetylase inhibitors. Circ Res. 2010;106:272–84.

27 Clinical Aspects of Cardiorenal Syndrome: Consequences of Therapy with the Renin-Angiotensin System Inhibitors

Demetrios V. Vlahakos

Abstract

The term "cardiorenal syndrome" has been introduced in an effort to describe problems of various kinds related to the simultaneous existence of heart and renal insufficiency. Synergism between two epidemiologic trends may support the construct of this syndrome, namely the population ageing and the epidemics of obesity and diabetes. Most studies indicate that the prevalence of anemia is increased in heart failure populations with co-morbid kidney disease, and therefore the term cardiorenal anemia syndrome has often been used. While rennin-angiotensin system inhibition improves morbidity and mortality in patients with congestive heart failure, it can further deteriorate renal function and increase incident anemia in patients with the cardiorenal syndrome. The mechanism is not yet fully understood, but angiotensin II, the active octapeptide of RAS, regulates intraglomerular filtration pressure and has been proven capable to both stimulate erythropoietin secretion and act as a direct growth factor on erythroid progenitors. Thus, RAS inhibition in patients with CRS may somehow diminish the beneficial effect anticipated from the studies in patients with CHF. Careful dose titration and frequent assessment of hemoglobin and hematocrit levels, estimated glomerular filtration rate, creatinine, sodium and potassium concentrations at the introduction of therapy is necessary to prevent this occurrence.

Keywords

Congestive cardiac failure(CHF) • Chronic renal failure • Syndrome Overweight • Obesity • Nephropathy • Diabetes • NT-proBNP • BNP Rennin angiotensin system (RAS) • Angiotensin converting enzyme (ACE) • Angiotensin receptor blockers (ARB) • Angiotensin II • Oxygen tension • Hypoxia inducible factor-1 (HIF-1) • Erythropoietin • Anemia

D.V. Vlahakos
Renal Unit, B' Department of Medicine,
Attikon University Hospital, Haidari, Athens, Greece
e-mail: vlahakos@otenet.gr

D.V. Cokkinos (ed.), *Introduction to Translational Cardiovascular Research*,
DOI 10.1007/978-3-319-08798-6_27, © Springer International Publishing Switzerland 2015

Abbreviations

ACE	Angiotensin converting enzyme
ACEi	Angiotensin converting enzyme inhibitor
ARB	Angiotensin receptor blocker
CHF	Congestive heart failure
CKD	Chronic kidney disease
CRAS	Cardiorenal anemia syndrome
CRS	Cardiorenal syndrome
Egfr	Estimated glomerular filtration rate
GFR	Glomerular filtration rate
HIF-1, LVEF	Left ventricular ejection fraction
HIF-1	Hypoxia inducible factor-1
NHANES	National Health and Nutrition Examination Survey
NYHA	New York Heart Association
RAS	Renin-angiotensin system.

27.1 Introduction

The incidence of congestive cardiac failure (CHF) and chronic renal failure has been increasing simultaneously in Western type societies over the past 30 years [1]. It has now become clear that these two problems co-exist in a substantial subset of the affected population and carry and extremely bad prognosis. For example, 46 % of patients with CHF have Chronic kidney disease (CKD) with glomerular filtration rate (GFR) <60 ml/min/1.73 m^2, while about 1/3 of patients with CHF stage III or IV according to New York Heart Association (NYHA) criteria have severe renal insufficiency (GFR <30 ml/min/1.73 m^2) [2, 3]. In recent years, the term cardiorenal syndrome CRS was introduced in an effort to describe problems of various kinds related to the simultaneous existence of heart and renal insufficiency. Despite lack of an accepted definition for the CRS and the controversies regarding its precise clinical or pathophysiologic foundation, reminiscent of the problems emerged with the proposition of the "metabolic syndrome", the term CRS has been increasingly used over the past 10 years (Fig. 27.1) [4, 5].

The term syndrome derives from the Greek συνδρομή (*sundromē*) that means "concurrence of symptoms, concourse" and reflects the presence of various common disorders. Although no genetic factors that encompass all traits of the syndrome have been identified, synergism between two epidemiologic trends may support the construct of the CRS, namely the population ageing and the epidemics of obesity and diabetes.

In the entirety of recorded human history, the world has never seen as aged a population as currently exists globally, and the UN predicts that the rate of population aging in the twenty-first century will exceed that in the 20th. Population aging has profound implications for many facets of human life affecting simultaneously the

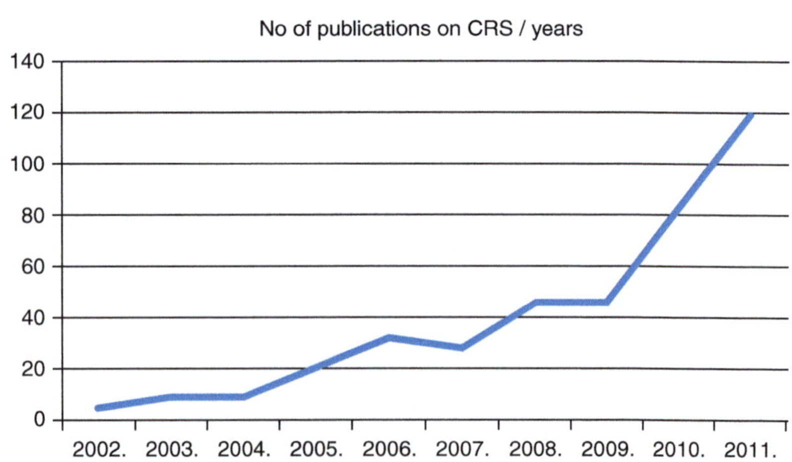

Fig. 27.1 Increasing number of publications in PUBMED regarding cardiorenal syndrome

cardiac and renal function. Elderly individuals have the highest incidence of coronary heart disease and hypertension, which constitute the two most powerful risk factors for heart failure. The prevalence of CKD also rises dramatically with age. Based on the results of the NHANES 1999–2004, more than one-third of those aged 70 or older have moderate or severe CKD defined as an eGFR <60 ml/min/1.73 m^2. Thus, parallel aging of the cardiovascular system and the kidney is at least in part the common soil for CRS in our time.

In addition, overweight and obesity have grown to pandemic proportions in industrialized countries during the past 50 years. For example, from 1960–1962 to 2005–2006, the prevalence of obesity increased from 13.4 to 35.1 % in U.S. adult age 20–74. Obesity increases the likelihood of type 2 diabetes, whose incidence is increasing in correlation with the rise in obesity. The American Diabetes Association estimates that about 21 million people have diabetes, with another 54 million people diagnosed with prediabetes. Diabetic patients carry an increased risk of coronary heart disease, hypertension, heart failure and nephropathy, in other words components of the CRS [6, 7].

Despite inconsistencies in the definition of anemia cases, most studies indicate that the prevalence of anemia is increased in CHF populations with co-existing kidney disease, advanced age, hypertension and more severe symptoms (range, 30–61 %) when compared with less symptomatic ambulatory populations (range, 4–23 %). Of note, even in patients with CHF and preserved ejection fraction, who represent the most common form of heart failure in westernized cultures anemia is also highly prevalent.

Since obesity and diabetes seem to be the driving force behind the development of heart disease and CKD, conditions with high prevalence of anemia, the term CRS has been enriched by many researchers to encompass anemia (cardiorenal anemia syndrome, CRAS) and metabolic syndrome (cardiorenal metabolic syndrome), in an effort to improve the practical utility, as a diagnostic and management tool among cardiologists, endocrinologists, nephrologists, hematologists and intensivists [8, 9].

Various pathophysiological pathways link cardiac and renal function and mediate clinical outcomes in CRS, including sympathetic and the renin-angiotensin aldosterone axis activation, vasopressin oversecretion, nitric oxide bioavailability, inflammation and overproduction of reactive oxygen species [10]. This very complex interaction of various processes is reflected in the great diversity of biomarkers used for detection of the concurrent kidney injury and heart failure by Palazzuoli et al. [11]:

NT-proBNP. BNP: Hemodynamic overload, neurohormonal activity. Troponins: Myocardial injury, hemodynamic overloads KIM-1, NGAL: Ischemia and nephrotoxins. NHE 3: Ischemia, pre-and post renal acute kidney injury. Cytokines (IL-6, 8, 18): Delayed graft function inflammatory activity. Actin, actin depolymerizing factor: Ischemia and delayed graft function. Cystatin-C: proximal tubule injury.

Among various therapeutic modalities introduced to interrupt those pathways and modulate morbidity and mortality, inactivation of rennin angiotensin system (RAS) has emerged, as the cornerstone treatment decision introduced by major guideline developers in cardiovascular, renal and endocrine medicine. An almost unexplored idea is that RAS inhibition, although benefiting heart failure, further deteriorates renal function and anemia in patients with CRS. If we accept this basic idea then wide use of RAS inhibition in large subsets of patients may be considered an iatrogenic cause of CRS with anemia.

27.2 RAS Inhibition May Further Deteriorate Renal Function in the Cardiorenal Syndrome

RAS inhibition has provided a major improvement in the management of CHF, resulting in both amelioration of symptoms and an increase in survival. In addition, angiotensin converting enzyme (ACE) inhibitors (ACEi) or angiotensin receptor blockers (ARB) are recommended for primary prevention of HF in patients with coronary artery disease, peripheral vascular disease, stroke, and diabetes with another major risk factor, such as smoking or microalbuminuria. RAS inhibition is also recommended for patients with reduced LVEF, regardless of symptoms.

RAS inhibition has been shown to be effective in slowing the progressive decay of GFR in diabetic nephropathy in both diabetes mellitus type 1 and type 2, as well as in non-diabetic individuals with CKD and proteinuria >1,000 mg/day. Intense RAS blockade in subjects with cardiovascular disease and relatively preserved renal function by a combination of high-dose ACE inhibitor and ARB therapy worsened GFR despite improving proteinuria in the ONTARGET study [11]. A high burden of renal vascular atherosclerosis, preexisting CKD not revealed by serum creatinine or both may have contributed to these outcomes. Of note, RAS inhibition in patients with CRS has not been established as yet to be renoprotective. On the contrary, RAS inhibition could further deteriorate renal function in CRS and somehow diminish the beneficial effect anticipated from the studies in patients with CHF.

Animal studies by several laboratories, most notably that of B. Brenner, have revealed that the glomerular capillary pressure and proteinuria depends on arterial perfusion pressure and the constriction of efferent arteriole, the dominant site of angiotensin II action. Consequently, RAS inhibition exerts its renoprotective effect by reducing arterial pressure and relaxing the efferent arteriole. These effects of RAS inhibition on renal hemodynamics vary widely depending on the preexisting physiologic and pathologic state of the kidneys. RAS inhibition is usually well tolerated in patients with normal cardiac function or mild heart failure and preserved renal perfusion. However, in cardiac patients with moderate-to-severe heart failure or systemic hypotension and sodium and fluid depletion due to high dose diuretic therapy, renal perfusion pressures may already be at or near the autoregulatory breakpoint and GFR could be maintained due to angiotensin II-mediated selective vasoconstriction of the efferent arteriole of the glomerulus. Complete or sustained RAS inhibition with the longer-acting agents regularly administered in our days in cardiac patients may be detrimental to renal function, especially if coexisting renal impairment exists, in other words in patients with CRS [12, 13].

Although ACEi and ARBs are not nephrotoxic drugs per se, they must be used with extreme caution because severe hyperkalemia and acute deterioration of renal function may occur in patients with CRS. In the management of such patients, especially if the eGFR is less than 30–40 mL/min/1.73 m^2, it is of paramount significance to commence these agents with the smallest dose and carefully and slowly titrate the dose to the highest dose tolerated. However, many physicians still rely on serum creatinine, as an index of renal function, and not on the considerably more precise estimates of the GFR and therefore, tend to underestimate the severity of renal dysfunction, particularly in elderly women, who may have severely compromised renal function despite a serum creatinine concentration within the normal range. Those physicians usually prescribe ACE inhibitors or ARBs in the "recommended" dosage. As a result, a vicious cycle begins to operate because the higher the RAS inhibition, the worse the deterioration of the renal function, leading to even higher accumulation of the ACEi or ARBs administered [14].

27.3 RAS Inhibition May Increase Incidence of Anemia in Cardiorenal Syndrome

The discovery of ACEi and ARB's at the beginning of 80s and 90s, respectively, and the finding that RAS inhibition reduces morbidity and mortality in patients with CHF, created the basis for most authorities worldwide to develop guidelines introducing this type of therapy, as the cornerstone therapy in CHF. Despite the inconsistencies in the definition of anemia cases, most studies indicate that the prevalence of anemia is increased in CHF populations with co-existing kidney disease, the so called CRS, advanced age, and more severe symptoms (range, 30–61 %) when compared with less symptomatic ambulatory populations (range, 4–23 %). Anemia is more common in CHF than could be accounted for by age or the degree of renal dysfunction. The few published reports in patients with CHF and preserved ejection fraction indicate that anemia is also highly prevalent. In most cases of anemia in heart failure no specific etiology can be found [15–17].

The RAS is historically known as a major regulator of blood pressure and plasma volume. Angiotensin II receptors are, however, also found on erythroid progenitors, indicating that beyond blood pressure and salt and water homeostasis, RAS may also have a role in the regulation of red blood cell mass [18]. This is supported by observations of genetically manipulated animals. Thus, transgenic mice that carried both the human renin and angiotensinogen genes developed persistently increased hematocrits, which remained normal when the two transgenes were introduced into the AT1-receptor null background, an observation that highlights the pivotal role of the AT1 receptor. Moreover, knockout mice for the ACE gene developed substantial and highly reproducible anemia, which was corrected almost fully by infusion of Ang II for 2 weeks [19].

Although there may of course exist a host of causative or contributory factors operative in CRS that can cause anemia, RAS inactivation may be implicated in the majority of mechanisms involved with anemia development in such patients. For example, bone marrow can be suppressed by uremic toxin accumulation due to the original renal disease, which maybe further deteriorated by the concomitant therapy with ACEi or ARBs, as previously described. Increased angiotensin II signaling in the kidney alters peritubular oxygen tension, a key regulatory factor for erythropoietin secretion [20]. Reduced oxygen tension in the peritubular fibroblasts of the renal cortex is associated with increased intracellular concentrations of reactive oxygen species, which, in turn, increases activation of hypoxia inducible factor-1 (HIF-1) and erythropoietin gene expression [21]. Angiotensin II, therefore, may increase erythropoietin secretion by reducing renal blood flow and increasing proximal tubular reabsorption. Erythropoietin levels are modestly increased in patients with CHF in proportion to measures of activation of the RAS. Inhibition of the RAS with either ACE inhibitors or angiotensin receptor blockers is associated with decreased erythropoietin production and reduced hemoglobin levels. In addition, ACEi therapy may reduce hemoglobin concentrations via increased levels of the tetra-peptide, N-acetyl-serylaspartyl-lysyl-proline, which is an inhibitor of hematopoiesis and a substrate for the ACE [22]. On the other hand, angiotensin II acts as a direct growth factor of erythroid progenitors by activating specific AT1 receptors located on them. Subsequently, angiotensin II receptor blockers or ACE inhibitors block the direct growth effect of angiotensin in erythroid progenitors and decrease RBC mass.

Anemia is frequently associated with clinical signs and symptoms of congestion, a finding that suggests that plasma volume expansion may contribute to anemia in CHF by a process of hemodilution. In 37 ambulatory nonedematous anemic patients with CHF, a radiolabeled albumin technique for direct measurement of plasma volume demonstrated that 46 % of the patients with low hematocrit values had a normal red blood cell volume; therefore the anemia could be considered entirely attributable to expanded plasma volume and consequent hemodilution. Thus, the combination of a true decrease in RBC mass and plasma volume expansion might be the critical feature that determines susceptibility to anemia in patients with CRS.

Conclusions

The term "cardiorenal syndrome" has been introduced in an effort to describe problems of various kinds related to the simultaneous existence of heart and renal insufficiency. Synergism between two epidemiologic trends may support the construct of the CRS, namely the population ageing and the epidemics of obesity and diabetes. Most studies indicate that the prevalence of anemia is increased in CHF populations with co-morbid kidney disease, advanced age, hypertension and more severe symptoms. Inactivation of the RAS has emerged as the cornerstone treatment decision introduced by major guideline developers in cardiovascular, renal and endocrine disease. While RAS inhibition improves morbidity

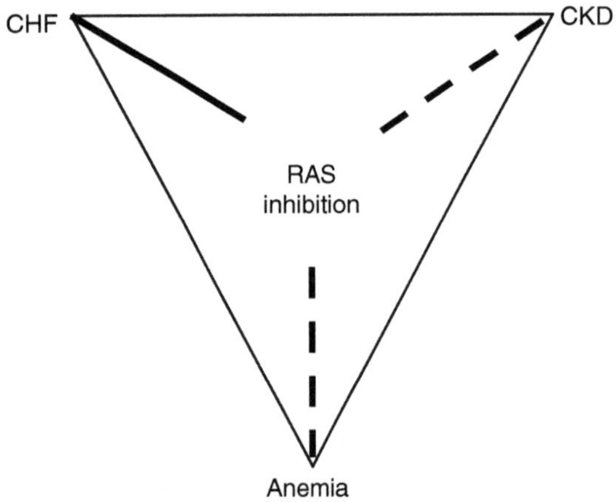

Fig. 27.2 The Cardiorenal Anemia Syndrome and Renin-Angiotensin-System (*RAS*) inhibition. While RAS inhibition improves morbidity and mortality in patients with congestive heart failure (*solid line*), it can further deteriorate renal function and increase incident anemia (*dashed lines*)

and mortality in patients with congestive heart failure, it can further deteriorate renal function and increase incident anemia. Thus, RAS inhibition in patients with CRS may somehow diminish the beneficial effect anticipated from the studies in patients with CHF. Careful dose titration and frequent assessment of hemoglobin and hematocrit levels, estimated GFR, creatinine, sodium and potassium concentrations at the introduction of therapy is necessary to prevent this occurrence (Fig. 27.2).

References

1. Triposkiadis F, Starling RC, Boudoulas H, Giamouzis G, Butler J. The cardiorenal syndrome in heart failure: cardiac? renal? syndrome? Heart Fail Rev. 2012;17:355–66.
2. Sarnak MJ, Levey AS, Schoolwerth AC, Coresh J, Culleton B, Hamm LL, et al. Kidney disease as a risk factor for development of cardiovascular disease: a statement from the American Heart Association Councils on Kidney in Cardiovascular Disease, High Blood Pressure Research, Clinical Cardiology and Epidemiology and Prevention. Circulation. 2003;108:2154–69.
3. Bock JS, Gottlieb SS. Cardiorenal syndrome: new perspectives. Circulation. 2010;121:2592–600.
4. Silverberg DS, Wexler D, Sheps D, Blum M, Keren G, Baruch R, et al. The effect of correction of mild anemia in severe, resistant congestive heart failure using subcutaneous erythropoietin and intravenous iron: a randomized controlled study. J Am Coll Cardiol. 2001; 37:1775–80.
5. Ronco C, Haapio M, House AA, Anavekar N, Bellomo R. Cardiorenal syndrome. J Am Coll Cardiol. 2008;52:1527–39.
6. Bakris G, Vassalotti J, Ritz E, Wanner C, Stergiou G, Molitch M, et al.; CKD Consensus Working Group. National Kidney Foundation consensus conference on cardiovascular and kidney diseases and diabetes risk: an integrated therapeutic approach to reduce events. Kidney Int. 2010;78:726–36.
7. Hsu CY, McCulloch CE, Iribarren C, Darbinian J, Go AS. Body mass index and the risk for end-stage renal disease. Ann Intern Med. 2006;144:21–8.
8. Ezekowitz JA, McAlister FA, Armstrong PW. Anemia is common in heart failure and is associated with poor outcomes. Insights from a cohort of 12,065 patients with new-onset heart failure. Circulation. 2003;107: 223–5.
9. Felker GM, Shaw LK, Stough WG, O'Connor CM. Anemia in patients with heart failure and preserved systolic function. Am Heart J. 2006;151:457–62.
10. Dec GW. Anemia in heart failure: time to rethink its etiology and treatment? J Am Coll Cardiol. 2006;48: 2490–2.
11. Palazzuoli A, Masson S, Ronco C, Maisel A. Clinical relevance of biomarkers in heart failure and cardiorenal syndrome: the role of natriuretic peptides and troponin. Heart Fail Rev. 2014;19:267–84.
12. Mann JF, Anderson C, Gao P, Gerstein HC, Boehm M, Rydén L, et al. Dual inhibition of the renin-angiotensin system in high-risk diabetes and risk for stroke and other outcomes: results of the ONTARGET trial. J Hypertens. 2013;31:414–21.
13. Abdi R, Brenner BM. Impact of renin angiotensin system blockade on renal function in health and disease: an end or a beginning? Semin Nephrol. 2004;24: 141–6.
14. Shlipak MG, Fried LF, Stehman-Breen C, Siscovick D, Newman AB. Chronic renal insufficiency and cardiovascular events in the elderly: findings from the Cardiovascular Health Study. Am J Geriatr Cardiol. 2004;13:81–90.
15. McClellan WM, Flanders WD, Langston RD, Jurkovitz C, Presley R. Anemia and renal insufficiency are independent risk factors for death among patients with congestive heart failure admitted to community hospitals: a population-based study. J Am Soc Nephrol. 2002;13:1928–36.
16. Mozaffarian D, Nye R, Levy WC. Anemia predicts mortality in severe heart failure: the prospective randomized amlodipine survival evaluation (PRAISE). J Am Coll Cardiol. 2003;41:1933–9.
17. Al-Ahmad A, Rand WM, Manjunath G, Konstam MA, Salem DN, Levey AS, Sarnak MJ. Reduced kidney function and anemia as risk factors for motality in patients with left ventricular dysfunction. J Am Coll Cardiol. 2001;38:955–62.
18. Gupta M, Miller BA, Ahsan N, Ulsh PJ, Zhang MY, Cheung JY, Yang HC. Expression of angiotensin II

type I receptor on erythroid progenitors of patients with post transplant erythrocytosis. Transplantation. 2000;70:1188–94.
19. Vlahakos DV, Marathias KP, Madias NE. The role of the renin-angiotensin system in the regulation of erythropoiesis. Am J Kidney Dis. 2010;56: 558–65.
20. Nangaku M, Inagi R, Miyata T, Fujita T.Angiotensin-induced hypoxia in the kidney: functional and structural changes of the renal circulation. Adv Exp Med Biol. 2007;618:85–99.
21. Jelkmann W. Regulation of erythropoietin production. J Physiol. 2011;589:1251–8.
22. van der Meer P, Lipsic E, Westenbrink BD, van de Wal RM, Schoemaker RG, Vellenga E, et al. Levels of hematopoiesis inhibitor N-acetyl-seryl-aspartyl-lysyl-proline partially explain the occurrence of anemia in heart failure. Circulation. 2005;112:1743–7.

Part V

Therapeutic Aspects

Pre- Peri- Post-Conditioning the Ischemic Myocardium: Challenges, Confounders and Expectations

28

Efstathios K. Iliodromitis, Ioanna Andreadou, Nikolaos Dagres, and Dimitrios T. Kremastinos

Abstract

The heart is afforded with endogenous mechanisms of protection against ischemic-reperfusion injury. Both preconditioning with short-lived periods of ischemia-reperfusion prior to a prolonged ischemia and postconditioning with very brief episodes of ischemia-reperfusion immediately after an index ischemia confer effective protection. Initial experimental studies investigated the natural history, the signal transduction pathways and the pharmaceutical agents that are involved in myocardial protection. Clinical studies that followed verified the laboratory findings transferring the acquired knowledge into clinical practice. Autacoids like adenosine, bradykinin and opioids are some of the experimentally and clinically most used agents that trigger the mechanism of protection by up-regulation of several kinases and of mediators, which prevent the opening of mitochondrial permeability pores. Clinical studies may be categorized as observational, reproducible and pharmacological. The remote form of myocardial conditioning by application of ischemia in a distal vascular territory, e.g. by blood pressure cuff inflation at the time of an evolving myocardial infarction, has shown promising results and may be used as an adjunctive to clinical methods of flow restoration and in parallel to the other treatment modalities. Although there are chances, there are also some confounders, which render the reproducibility of conditioning more difficult in clinical reality.

Keywords

Preconditioning • Postconditioning • Myocardial protection

E.K. Iliodromitis (✉) • N. Dagres
D.T. Kremastinos
Second Department of Cardiology,
University of Athens Medical School,
Attikon University Hospital, Athens, Greece
e-mail: iliodromitis@yahoo.gr

I. Andreadou
Department of Pharmaceutical Chemistry,
University of Athens School of Pharmacy,
Athens, Greece

D.V. Cokkinos (ed.), *Introduction to Translational Cardiovascular Research*,
DOI 10.1007/978-3-319-08798-6_28, © Springer International Publishing Switzerland 2015

Abbreviations

AR	Adenosine receptors
IPC	Ischemic preconditioning
mPTP	Mitochondrial permeability transition pores
PKC	Protein kinase C
PostC	Postconditioning
ROS	Reactive oxygen species
SAFE	Survival activating factor Enhancement

28.1 Introduction

Total coronary occlusion without development of collateral vessels results in myocardial infarction with a wave-front of necrosis, which spreads from the subendocardial to subepicardial layers. The early restoration of coronary flow by mechanical or pharmaceuticals means is the cornerstone of therapy in clinical practice. Despite the enormous value of reperfusion as the principal method of therapy, it also carries a series of side effects, which are summarized by the term of reperfusion injury. Among the more severe expressions of reperfusion injury are the extension of myocardial necrosis, apoptosis, the appearance of severe and potentially lethal arrhythmias, stunning and endothelial dysfunction [1].

28.1.1 Preconditioning

Almost 30 years ago, a group of investigators analyzing the effects of brief coronary artery occlusions with prolonged arterial occlusion on ATP depletion and necrosis, found a significant reduction of the final infarct size when brief periods of ischemia-reperfusion preceded a more sustained period of ischemia. This very important finding, called ischemic preconditioning (IPC) [2], was afterwards verified in every species studied, including human, and independently of the presence of collateral vessels [1].

Initial studies described the natural history of this phenomenon in terms of number and duration of each short ischemic insult, presence and duration of the short intervening reperfusion intervals, duration of the prolonged ischemic insult and finally the territory of brief ischemic applications [2–4].

28.1.2 Postconditioning

In 2003, the Vinten-Johansen's group using a dog model found that the application of a series of very short periods of ischemia-reperfusion immediately upon reperfusion after index ischemia reduces the final infarct size [5]. This phenomenon is called postconditioning (PostC) and has been verified in a large number of experimental models and in humans [6]. Although PostC consists of staccato ischemic-reperfusion intervals, earlier studies had already described that gentle or gradual reperfusion is a more preferable method for restoration of the coronary flow compared to the abrupt reperfusion [7, 8]. The initial studies of PostC also described the natural history of the effective interventions in terms of the number and the duration of the brief periods of ischemia-reperfusion and of the time of the first application of short-lived ischemia. Several studies suggest that IPC and PostC are equally effective in infarct size reduction although other studies have found that the protection provided by PostC is weaker compared to that conferred by IPC [9–11].

28.2 Natural History

28.2.1 Number and Duration of Short Ischemic-Reperfusion Intervals

One or more short-lived ischemic insults of 5 min ischemia separated by 5–10 min of reperfusion each, seems to be the more appropriate cardioprotective strategy. However, there is a controversy regarding the "frequency-dependency" of preconditioning with some studies suggesting that one cycle is as efficacious as multiple cycles, others suggesting that more cycles provide greater protection and others indicating that repetitive cycles exhaust the protective effect of IPC [3, 4]. Currently, a 5-min ischemic period is considered the preferable duration for an effective stimulus of protection, although a shorter duration seems also to be effective in some species and a longer duration of brief ischemia has been also applied.

28.2.2 Reperfusion Interval Prior to the Index Ischemia

After the application of the short ischemic insult(s), two periods of protection follow. The first one, called first window of protection, lasts approximately 60 min and confers the stronger protection to the myocardium reducing the final infarct size by approximately 70 %. After this period and for approximately 12 h, any protection ceases and the preconditioned myocardium behaves as a naïve organ comparable to controls [12]. However, the lost protection can be recaptured after appropriate interventions during the periods where protection is fade. Interestingly, there is a delayed form of protection, called second window of protection, starting 24 h later without any additional intervention and lasting up to in 72–96 h [13]. The delayed form of protection is therefore longer albeit weaker compared to the protection afforded by the first one. Although the algorithms of effective preconditioning regarding the duration and the number of stimuli have been mostly elucidated, there have been major concerns regarding the effectiveness of various algorithms of postconditioning. Of note, the same algorithms may be either effective or ineffective in limiting the infarct size with their effectiveness depending on the animal species and the experimental conditions [11, 14].

28.2.3 Duration of Index Ischemia

After total coronary occlusion, a wave-front of necrosis moves from the sub-endocardium to the sub-epicardium. Any early intervention that may restore the normal flow by mechanical or by pharmaceutical means or even spontaneous resolution of thrombus that blocks normal flow, interrupts the mechanism of necrosis and rescues the ischemic myocardial tissue.

Protection provided by preconditioning is not perpetual, fades and is eventually lost if the duration of the index ischemia extends beyond a period of approximately 3 h. Therefore, any form of conditioning rather delays the ensuing myocardial necrosis and "buys" some time from ischemia instead of entirely protecting the heart from this.

However, shorter periods of ischemia cause substantially reduced infarct size compared to longer ones [11]. Thus, the total ischemic burden seems to be responsible for the final infarct size regardless of the way of its application. In other words, conditioning may not be effective in limiting the infarct size when the myocardium is not exposed to a sustained or a heavy burden of ischemia [15].

28.3 Mechanisms Involved in Protection

After initial studies describing the physical history of the protective mechanisms, research focused on the recognition of the mechanisms that make the heart tolerant against ischemic-reperfusion injury. In the first few years after the discovery of preconditioning, the most prominent hypothesis was that IPC protects by improving the metabolic balance during the ischemic insult. Several studies examined the metabolic and ionic effects of IPC on hearts and it was found that after application of an IPC protocol, the myocardium has a smaller adenine nucleotide pool, a creatine phosphate overshoot, excess intracellular glucose, and a contractile deficit termed stunning [16, 17]. During these early years, an effect on reperfusion injury was not seriously considered as most investigators were convinced that the protection conferred by IPC occurs during ischemia. However, after the first initial studies, most of the evidence suggests that IPC exerts its protection in the first minutes of reperfusion. That was first demonstrated when the blockade of the PI3 kinase or ERK in the first minutes of reperfusion abrogated the IPC protection in rat [18] and rabbit hearts [19].

Both interventions, pre- and postconditioning, decrease the infarct size because they are capable of eliminating reperfusion injury sharing some common intracellular pathways [20]. Adenosine, opioids and bradykinin are critical ligands that occupy specific cell surface receptors and initiate numerous signaling pathways that activate-phosphorylate a series of intracellular mediators and the final targets [21]. Multiple adenosine receptor subtypes are involved in the initial cascade of events [22]. Some of the receptor subtypes are critical in some species while others are more important in other species [23, 24]. However, except for consistent data on cardioprotection mediated by A_{2B} stimulation, which seems to play a crucial role in infarct limitation [25], there are conflicting results regarding the role of adenosine receptors (ARs) in ischemic postconditioning and the involvement of AR subtypes in cardioprotection.

Nevertheless, adenosine receptors are coupled to inhibitory G protein and activate protein kinase C (PKC), which has a significant contribution to myocardial protection [26]. More specifically, PKC plays a role in both IPC phases. The first response to the preconditioning stimulus, the so-called "preconditioning phase" takes place during the preconditioning stimulus. This phase includes activation of PI3K/Akt and members of the MAPK kinase family (MEK1/2, ERK1/2) via G protein- related mechanisms, convergence of both the pathways on mitochondria, generation of reactive oxygen species (ROS) with subsequent activation of PKC-e, and opening of K_{ATP} channels. The second phase takes place during reperfusion and results in decreasing reperfusion injury. During this phase, a quick burst in ROS generation can activate PKC with further phosphorylation of the participants of the RISK (Reperfusion Injury Salvage kinase) cascade, which in turn activate mitochondrial K_{ATP} channels and lead to closure of the mitochondrial permeability transition pore [18, 27]. There are different PKC isoforms, which are either involved in the protection, such as PKCε, or in the abrogation of the entire mechanism, such as PKCδ [26].

Contrary to adenosine, the other two ligands, namely opioids and bradykinin, activate directly the mitochondrial K_{ATP} channels, which then produce free radicals that activate PKC [28]. Bradykinin is elevated during and after an ischemic insult [29]. Two bradykinin receptors exist in cardiomyocytes, a constitutive B2 receptor and a B1 receptor that is induced after stress [30]. IPC-induced cardioprotection is abolished in B2 receptor knockout mice [31]. The results of studies with knockout of the B1 receptor in female mice suggest that B1 receptors have no effect on the remodeling after a myocardial infarction, however, the cardioprotective role of the B1 receptor is unknown [32]. Myocardial ischemia results in the synthesis and release of endogenous opioid peptides [33]. Morphine is cardioprotective when administered either just prior to reperfusion or prior to ischemia in rats [34] and many data suggest that opioids elicit or mimic IPC in rat hearts [35, 36]. The pathway that intervenes between opioid or bradykinin receptors and the mitochondrial K_{ATP} channels is complex and a series of different kinases or mediators are activated. In fact, ERK1/2, PI3, Akt, eNOS, cyclic GMP, PKG are appropriately activated before the opening of the KATP channels, which then produce free radicals (ROS) leading to upregulation of PKC [37]. The opening of mitochondrial K_{ATP} channels, with subsequent generation of reactive oxygen species (ROS), is considered to be a pivotal step in the mechanism of preconditioning [38].

Oxygen-derived free radicals are involved in the protective mechanism of ischemic preconditioning in rabbits [39] and rats [40] and it has been shown that diazoxide, a mito K_{ATP} channel opener, triggers the protective mechanism of the IPC via free radical production, while the administration of free radical scavengers negates this protective effect in isolated rabbit and rat hearts [41, 42]. Nevertheless, there is a controversy regarding the role of exogenously administered free radical scavengers in the attenuation of the effect of ischemic preconditioning in vivo. Our group has previously shown in vivo that the abrogation or not of the infarct size limiting effect of IPC by antioxidants depends of the antioxidant administered. Thus, melatonin and acetyl-cysteine do not prevent the protection of IPC in vivo, although they protect from oxidative damage during ischemia and reperfusion [43]. Acute administration of vitamin E triggers preconditioning via K_{ATP} channels and cyclic-GMP without inhibiting lipid peroxidation [44], whereas acute administration of vitamin C abrogates the effect of ischemic preconditioning in rabbits by decreasing blood and tissue levels of lipid peroxidation products [45]. Independently of whether PKC is activated after adenosine, opioids, bradykinin or other ligands, there is a common pathway that follows afterwards. Free radicals are very important for the protection in preconditioning. It should be noted that ROS have been recognized as part of the trigger pathway that preconditions the heart prior to the onset of the index ischemia [46]. One could summarize: no ROS no protection. Thus, preconditioning is mediated in part by elaboration of ROS, possibly from mitochondria via signaling cascades that involve PKC and postconditioning may lead directly or indirectly to a reduction in ROS and more gradual restoration in pH [6].

28.3.1 Reperfusion Injury

Although free radicals are necessary for myocardial protection provided by preconditioning, they are entirely detrimental at the time of reperfusion, having double facets as God Janus. Free radicals and calcium overload as well as acute pH changes occurring immediately after flow restoration contribute to reperfusion injury and cell death. Free radicals are generated upon reperfusion and destroy all membranes increasing their permeability for various agents [47]. The calcium paradox is the phenomenon where additional calcium enters into the cell despite the fact that its intracellular levels are already increased as a result of the ischemic period [48]. Abrupt pH normalization is also detrimental contributing to the increase of the infarct size [49]. All these changes are responsible for the mitochondrial permeability transition pore (mPTP) opening at the beginning of reperfusion, which allows any agent smaller than 1.5 kD to enter inside the mitochondrion and to cause swelling, disruption and finally necrosis of the cell [50]. In order to target the apoptotic component of reperfusion- induced cell death, the activation of existing innate cellular anti-apoptotic pathways of survival, may provide an opportunity for protecting the heart against lethal reperfusion- induced injury. Ischaemia–reperfusion has been shown to activate the pro-survival kinase signalling cascades, (RISK) phosphatidylinositol-3-OH kinase (PI3K)–Akt and p42/p44 extra-cellular signal-regulated kinases (Erk 1/2), both of which have been implicated in cellular survival, through their recruitment of anti-apoptotic pathways of protection [51]. In IPC and PostC, the final activation of A2b receptors upregulates the RISK pathway, which prevent mPTP opening and thus mitochondrial and cell death. Furthermore, various agents such as insulin, statins, erythropoietin and others can pharmacologically increase the level of RISK kinases [18], while cyclosporine directly prevents mPTP opening [52]. All these agents have been extensively used in different experiments as well as in clinical practice.

Another pathway that is involved in the mechanism of postconditioning is called SAFE (Survival Activating Factor Enhancement) and has been proposed as an alternative cascade that plays a significant role in postconditioning. Cytokines like IL-6 and TNFα increase the kinase

JAK, which then phosphorylates the transcription of factors that act as end-effectors conferring cardioprotection [53].

28.3.2 Remote Interventions

Local mechanical interventions in the same artery where the index ischemia occurs, has been extensively investigated both in the preconditioning and in the postconditioning era with very strong evidence. Apart from this, remote ischemia and reperfusion of another vascular territory was initially described as a preconditioning analogue in 1993, called remote preconditioning [54]. Later studies investigated the mechanism by which ischemia and reperfusion of another artery or another distal organ can confer protection to the heart [55]. Indeed, it was found that systemic response, humoral factors or neural pathways target the distal tissue or the distal organ [56, 57]. Remote protection affects not only the heart but also other organs such as kidneys [58], brain [59] and liver [60] providing promising expectations for applicability in clinical practice [61].

Extending the existing knowledge of remote preconditioning, several investigators tested the possibility that remote postconditioning could be also effective. In fact, the application of ischemia at a distal artery immediately upon reperfusion of the index organ, or at the time of the index ischemia or both during index ischemia and reperfusion was found to be an effective and attractive intervention limiting the final infarct size [62]. Remote postconditioning seems to be at least equally effective with local postconditioning [63, 64]. Since the remote short-lived episodes of ischemia/reperfusion are applied while the target organ is already exposed to sustained ischemia, this intervention is called *perconditioning* and not *remote postconditioning* [65].

28.4 Clinical Studies

Knowledge acquired from the natural history and from the mechanism of preconditioning, postconditioning and their forms of delayed protection or remote application has been transferred from the experimental conditions into clinical practice.

Clinical studies in this field may be categorized into observational, reproducible and pharmacological studies. For ethical or practical reasons, a number of clinical studies have used surrogate endpoints instead of more hard endpoints. Such surrogate endpoints have been the resolution of ST elevation or the level of ST deviation, the intensity of chest pain, the left ventricular wall motion score index, the endothelial function and others. Hard endpoints used in many clinical trials are the final infarct size, survival and elimination of lethal arrhythmias.

28.4.1 Observational Studies

Numerous clinical studies have described the outcome of patients with pre infarction angina, which acts as a preconditioning stimulus before the index ischemia leading to the myocardial infarction [66–70]. Several end points such as short-term or long-term mortality, duration of hospital stay, development of lethal arrhythmias, cardiogenic shock or preservation of viable myocardium have been examined. Most of these clinical studies were positive corroborating the beneficial effect of preconditioning and the potential role in everyday practice. However, negative findings were also reported due to the lack of strict time limitations as well as of stable experimental conditions in clinical reality [71, 72]. These are the reasons why some studies were not able to demonstrate the expected benefit in patients who are potentially in a preconditioning state.

Another explanation for the divergent results in clinical studies is that many patients are already in medical treatment with drugs, which may enhance or attenuate any benefit from conditioning [73]. Finally co-morbidities such as diabetes mellitus [74], hypercholesterolemia [75] or hypertension [76] increase the threshold of protection as shown previously and may thus blunt any benefit provided by preconditioning. These explanations fit to all forms of myocardial protection, i.e. delayed preconditioning [77], postconditioning [78–80] and remote preconditioning as well as to the other types of clinical studies that will be described below [81].

28.4.2 Reproducible Studies

Coronary angioplasty and treadmill exercise tests are some of the clinical forms that may reproduce ischemic preconditioning. Balloon inflation may cause larger initial ST elevation followed by less pronounced ST elevation during the subsequent balloon inflations because the first ischemia acts as preconditioning stimulus, which expresses its protective effect in the following. Similarly, consequent exercise treadmill tests may show an attenuation of the ischemic findings because the initial test acts as preconditioning stimulus to the second one [82]. There is a decline of the afforded protection when the intervening reperfusion intervals are extended to the periods where protection fades and finally lasts. It is of interest that the delayed protection is feasible because the second window of protection can be also reproduced as shown in clinical studies with treadmill test or scintigraphy [83].

Postconditioning is more relevant than preconditioning in clinical practice because the associated intervention(s) is/are applied not prior to the sustained ischemia, which naturally cannot be predicted, but immediately upon reperfusion. Furthermore, remote interventions could be also applied either at the time of the index ischemia in an evolving myocardial infarction or at the beginning of reperfusion. Based on the experimental findings, clinical studies have shown that additional short-lived episodes of ischemia-reperfusion by balloon inflation at the time of stenting in acute coronary syndromes provide benefit to the (post) ischemic myocardium reducing the infarct size by approximately one-third [84, 85]. These findings were verified in further clinical studies of acute coronary syndromes with or without ST elevation. However, due to the lack of strict experimental conditions in the protocols and for the other reasons that were previously mentioned, several clinical studies failed to demonstrate the effectiveness of postconditioning [86–88].

Remote conditioning is a safer and more easily applicable intervention that may evoke protection. It is safer because there is no reason to perform additional manipulations by inflating the balloon in an artery that was recently opened and more easily applicable because remote ischemia can be obtained by the simple inflation of a blood pressure cuff [89]. Of note, blood pressure cuff inflation in the ambulance, during transportation of patients with evolving myocardial infarction, were shown to increase the salvaged index and to reduce the size of myocardial infarction in large areas at risk [89]. Similar findings were also described in clinical studies with patients who underwent Coronary Aortocoronary Bypass Grafting and released lower troponin levels as a result of such interventions [90]. Once again, divergent results from similar studies by other investigators also appear in the literature [91].

It is of interest that remote conditioning does not protect only the heart but any organ exposed to ischemia reperfusion and this intervention seems to be promising for organs such as brain, kidneys, liver, or pancreas conferring, for instance, better preservation of the organs and possible transplantation under better conditions.

28.4.3 Pharmacological Studies

The identification of surface receptors and their ligands as well as the elucidation of the intracellular mediators that make the cell tolerant against ischemia/reperfusion injury resulted in the use of pharmacological agents that may trigger or mimic the protective mechanism(s) of conditioning. Adenosine, opioids and bradykinin, which occupy the specific receptors, have been used in human tissue studies, in elective coronary angioplasty and in other clinical circumstances as conditioning mimetics [92–95]. Nicorandil, which activates mitochondrial K_{ATP} channels [96, 97] insulin, statins and erythropoietin which indirectly prevent mitochondrial PTP opening by the activation of RISK kinases, and cyclosporine, which directly prevents mitochondrial PTP opening, have been extensively used in many clinical studies [98–102]. More specifically, adenosine and its analogues have been used as an adjunctive therapy to thrombolysis in patients with acute myocardial infarction with positive findings in those who had large areas at risk [103, 104]. These agents have been also used in patients undergoing CABG [105]. Nicorandil has been also used in patients with coronary artery disease [106] while cyclosporine provides promising results as an adjunctive therapy at the time of flow restoration [102].

As already noted, we must always take into account that there are co morbidities in most of the patients suffering from coronary artery disease and that many patients are already treated with drugs that may facilitate (statins, opioids, ACE inhibitors) or attenuate (glibenclamide) the protective effect of conditioning.

In conclusion, there are promising findings that local or remote conditioning is effective in limiting the final infarct size and these interventions can be additionally applied as adjunctive to conventional therapies in humans, at the time of evolving myocardial infarction.

References

1. Yellon DM, Hausenloy DJ. Myocardial reperfusion injury. N Engl J Med. 2007;357:1121–35.
2. Murry CE, Jennings RB, Reimer KA. Preconditioning with ischemia: a delay of lethal cell injury in ischemic myocardium. Circulation. 1986;74:1124–36.
3. Iliodromitis EK, Kremastinos DT, Katritsis DG, Papadopoulos CC, Hearse DJ. Multiple cycles of preconditioning cause loss of protection in open-chest rabbits. J Mol Cell Cardiol. 1997;29:915–20.
4. Sandhu R, Diaz RJ, Mao GD, Wilson GJ. Ischemic preconditioning. Differences in protection and susceptibility to blockade with single-cycle versus multicycle transient ischemia. Circulation. 1997;96:984–95.
5. Zhao ZQ, Corvera JS, Halkos ME, Kerendi F, Wang NP, Guyton RA, et al. Inhibition of myocardial injury by ischemic postconditioning during reperfusion: comparison with ischemic preconditioning. Am J Physiol Heart Circ Physiol. 2003;285:H579–88.
6. Vinten-Johansen J. Postconditioning: a mechanical maneuver that triggers biological and molecular cardioprotective responses to reperfusion. Heart Fail Rev. 2007;12:235–44.
7. Okamoto F, Allen BS, Buckberg GD, Bugyi H, Leaf J. Reperfusion conditions: importance of ensuring gentle versus sudden reperfusion during relief of coronary occlusion. J Thorac Cardiovasc Surg. 1986;92:613–20.
8. Na HS, Kim YI, Yoon YW, Han HC, Nahm SH, Hong SK. Ventricular premature beat-driven intermittent restoration of coronary blood flow reduces the incidence of reperfusion-induced ventricular fibrillation in a cat model of regional ischemia. Am Heart J. 1996;132:78–83.
9. Kin H, Zatta AJ, Lofye MT, Amerson BS, Halkos ME, Kerendi F, et al. Postconditioning reduces infarct size via adenosine receptor activation by endogenous adenosine. Cardiovasc Res. 2005;67:124–33.
10. Downey JM, Cohen MV. Why do we still not have cardioprotective drugs? Circ J. 2009;73:1171–7.
11. Skyschally A, van Caster P, Iliodromitis EK, Schulz R, Kremastinos DT, Heusch G. Ischemic postconditioning: experimental models and protocol algorithms. Basic Res Cardiol. 2009;104:469–83.
12. Pagliaro P, Gattullo D, Rastaldo R, Losano G. Ischemic preconditioning: from the first to the second window of protection. Life Sci. 2001;69:1–15.
13. Yamashita N, Hoshida S, Taniguchi N, Kuzuya T, Hori M. A "second window of protection" occurs 24 h after ischemic preconditioning in the rat heart. J Mol Cell Cardiol. 1998;30:1181–9.
14. Iliodromitis EK, Downey JM, Heusch G, Kremastinos DT. What is the optimal postconditioning algorithm? J Cardiovasc Pharmacol Ther. 2009;14:269–73.
15. Iliodromitis K, Farmakis D, Andreadou I, Zoga A, Bibli SI, Manolaki T, et al. Various models of cardiac conditioning in single or sequential periods of ischemia: comparative effects on infarct size and intracellular signaling. Int J Cardiol. 2013;168:1336–41.
16. Murry CE, Richard VJ, Jennings RB, Reimer KA. Myocardial protection is lost before contractile function recovers from ischemic preconditioning. Am J Physiol. 1991;260:H796–804.
17. Jennings RB, Sebbag L, Schwartz LM, Crago MS, Reimer KA. Metabolism of preconditioned myocardium: effect of loss and reinstatement of cardioprotection. J Mol Cell Cardiol. 2001;33:1571–88.
18. Hausenloy DJ, Yellon DM. New directions for protecting the heart against ischaemia-reperfusion injury: targeting the Reperfusion Injury Salvage Kinase (RISK)-pathway. Cardiovasc Res. 2004;61:448–60.
19. Solenkova NV, Solodushko V, Cohen MV, Downey JM. Endogenous adenosine protects preconditioned heart during early minutes of reperfusion by activating Akt. Am J Physiol. 2006;290:H441–9.
20. Andreadou I, Iliodromitis EK, Koufaki M, Farmakis D, Tsotinis A, Kremastinos DT. Alternative pharmacological interventions that limit myocardial infarction. Curr Med Chem. 2008;15:1304–13.
21. Xin W, Yang X, Rich TC, Krieg T, Barrington R, Cohen MV, et al. All preconditioning-related G protein-coupled receptors can be demonstrated in the rabbit cardiomyocyte. J Cardiovasc Pharmacol Ther. 2012;17:190–8.
22. Kin H, Zhao ZQ, Sun HY, Wang NP, Corvera JS, Halkos ME, et al. Postconditioning attenuates myocardial ischemia-reperfusion injury by inhibiting events in the early minutes of reperfusion. Cardiovasc Res. 2004;62:74–85.

23. Methner C, Schmidt K, Cohen MV, Downey JM, Krieg T. Both A2A and A2B adenosine receptors at reperfusion are necessary to reduce infarct size in mouse hearts. Am J Physiol Heart Circ Physiol. 2010;299:H1262–4.
24. Philipp S, Yang XM, Cui L, Davis AM, Downey JM, Cohen MV. Postconditioning protects rabbit hearts through a protein kinase C-adenosine A2B receptor cascade. Cardiovasc Res. 2006;70:308–14.
25. Liu Y, Yang X, Yang XM, Walker S, Förster K, Cohen MV, et al. AMP579 is revealed to be a potent A2B-adenosine receptor agonist in human 293 cells and rabbit hearts. Basic Res Cardiol. 2010;105:129–37.
26. Simkhovich BZ, Przyklenk K, Kloner RA. Role of protein kinase C in ischemic "conditioning": from first evidence to current perspectives. J Cardiovasc Pharmacol Ther. 2013;18:525–32.
27. Hausenloy DJ, Tsang A, Mocanu MM, Yellon DM. Ischemic preconditioning protects by activating prosurvival kinases at reperfusion. Am J Physiol. 2004;288: H971–6.
28. Gross ER, Gross GJ. Ligand triggers of classical preconditioning and postconditioning. Cardiovasc Res. 2006;70:212–21.
29. Baumgarten CR, Linz W, Kunkel G, Scholkens BA, Wiemer G. Ramiprilat increases bradykinin outflow from isolated hearts of rat. Br J Pharmacol. 1993;108:293–5.
30. Marceau F, Hess JF, Bachvarov DR. The B1 receptors for kinins. Pharmacol Rev. 1998;50:357–86.
31. Yang XP, Liu YH, Scicli GM, Webb CR, Carretero OA. Role of kinins in the cardioprotective effect of preconditioning: study of myocardial ischemia/reperfusion injury in B2 kinin receptor knockout mice and kininogen-deficient rats. Hypertension. 1997;30:735–40.
32. Xu J, Carretero OA, Sun Y, Shesely EG, Rhaleb NE, Liu YH, et al. Role of the B1 kinin receptor in the regulation of cardiac function and remodeling after myocardial infarction. Hypertension. 2005;45:747–53.
33. Romano MA, Seymour EM, Berry JA, McNish RA, Bolling SF. Relative contribution of endogenous opioids to myocardial ischemic tolerance. J Surg Res. 2004;118:32–7.
34. Gross ER, Hsu AK, Gross GJ. Opioid-induced cardioprotection occurs via glycogen synthase kinase beta inhibition during reperfusion in intact rat hearts. Circ Res. 2004;94:960–6.
35. Gross ER, Hsu AK, Gross GJ. Acute aspirin treatment abolishes, whereas acute ibuprofen treatment enhances morphine-induced cardioprotection: role of 12-lipoxygenase. J Pharmacol Exp Ther. 2004;310:185–91.
36. Gross ER, Peart JN, Hsu AK, Auchampach JA, Gross GJ. Extending the cardioprotective window using a novel delta-opioid agonist fentanyl isothiocyanate via the PI3-kinase pathway. Am J Physiol Heart Circ Physiol. 2005;288:H2744–9.
37. Oldenburg O, Qin Q, Krieg T, Yang XM, Philipp S, Critz SD, et al. Bradykinin induces mitochondrial ROS generation via NO, cGMP, PKG, and mitoKATP channel opening and leads to cardioprotection. Am J Physiol Heart Circ Physiol. 2004;286:H468–76.
38. Schulz R, Cohen MV, Behrends M, Downey JM, Heusch G. Signal transduction of ischemic preconditioning. Cardiovasc Res. 2001;52:181–98.
39. Skyschally A, Schulz R, Gres P, Korth H, Heusch G. Attenuation of ischemic preconditioning in pigs by scavenging of free oxyradicals with ascorbic acid. Am J Physiol Heart Circ Physiol. 2003;284:H698–703.
40. Steeves G, Singh N, Singal PK. Preconditioning and antioxidant defense against reperfusion injury. Ann N Y Acad Sci. 1994;723:116–27.
41. Pain T, Yang XM, Critz SD, Yue Y, Nakano A, Liu GS, et al. Opening of mitochondrial K_{ATP} channels triggers the preconditioned state by generating free radicals. Circ Res. 2000;15:460–6.
42. Forbes A, Steenbergen C, Murphy E. The protective effect of diazoxide is blocked by antioxidants. Circulation. 1999;100(Suppl I):I342.
43. Andreadou I, Iliodromitis EK, Mikros E, Bofilis E, Zoga A, Constantinou M, et al. Melatonin does not prevent the protection of ischemic preconditioning in vivo despite its antioxidant effect against oxidative stress. Free Radic Biol Med. 2004;37:500–10.
44. Andreadou I, Iliodromitis EK, Tsovolas K, Aggeli IK, Zoga A, Gaitanaki C, et al. Acute administration of vitamin E triggers preconditioning via K(ATP) channels and cyclic-GMP without inhibiting lipid peroxidation. Free Radic Biol Med. 2006;41:1092–9.
45. Tsovolas K, Iliodromitis EK, Andreadou I, Zoga A, Demopoulou M, Iliodromitis KE, et al. Acute administration of vitamin C abrogates protection from ischemic preconditioning in rabbits. Pharmacol Res. 2008; 57:283–9.
46. Andreadou I, Iliodromitis EK, Farmakis D, Kremastinos DT. To prevent, protect and save the ischemic heart: antioxidants revisited. Expert Opin Ther Targets. 2009;13:945–56.
47. Penna C, Mancardi D, Rastaldo R, Pagliaro P. Cardioprotection: a radical view Free radicals in pre and postconditioning. Biochim Biophys Acta. 2009;1787:781–93.
48. Kawabata KI, Netticadan T, Osada M, Tamura K, Dhalla NS. Mechanisms of ischemic preconditioning effects on Ca(2+) paradox-induced changes in heart. Am J Physiol Heart Circ Physiol. 2000;278:H1008–15.
49. Inserte J, Barba I, Hernando V, Abellán A, Ruiz-Meana M, Rodríguez-Sinovas A, et al. Effect of acidic reperfusion on prolongation of intracellular acidosis and myocardial salvage. Cardiovasc Res. 2008;77: 782–90.
50. Javadov S, Karmazyn M. Mitochondrial permeability transition pore opening as an endpoint to initiate cell death and as a putative target for cardioprotection. Cell Physiol Biochem. 2007;20:1–22.
51. Cross TG, Scheel-Toellner D, Henriquez NV, Deacon E, Salmon M, Lord JM. Serine/threonine protein kinases and apoptosis. Exp Cell Res. 2000;256:34–41.
52. Halestrap AP, Clarke SJ, Javadov SA. Mitochondrial permeability transition pore opening during myocardial reperfusion–a target for cardioprotection. Cardiovasc Res. 2004;61:372–85.

53. Ovize M, Baxter GF, Di Lisa F, Ferdinandy P, Garcia-Dorado D, Hausenloy DJ, et al. Postconditioning and protection from reperfusion injury: where do we stand? Cardiovasc Res. 2010;87:406–23.
54. Przyklenk K, Bauer B, Ovize M, Kloner RA, Whittaker P. Regional ischemic 'preconditioning' protects remote virgin myocardium from subsequent sustained coronary occlusion. Circulation. 1993;87:893–9.
55. Wolfrum S, Schneider K, Heidbreder M, Nienstedt J, Dominiak P, Dendorfer A. Remote preconditioning protects the heart by activating myocardial PKCepsilon-isoform. Cardiovasc Res. 2002;55:583–9.
56. Opie LH. Cardioprotection at a distance - remote conditioning takes the stage. Exp Physiol. 2012;97:905.
57. Weinbrenner C, Nelles M, Herzog N, Sarvary L, Strasser RH. Remote preconditioning by infrarenal occlusion of the aorta protects the heart from infarction: a newly identified non-neuronal but PKC-dependent pathway. Cardiovasc Res. 2002;55:590–601.
58. Kerendi F, Kin H, Halkos ME, Jiang R, Zatta AJ, Zhao ZQ, et al. Remote postconditioning. Brief renal ischemia and reperfusion applied before coronary artery reperfusion reduces myocardial infarct size via endogenous activation of adenosine receptors. Basic Res Cardiol. 2005;100:404–12.
59. Koch S, Gonzalez N. Preconditioning the human brain: proving the principle in subarachnoid hemorrhage. Stroke. 2013;44:1748–53.
60. Huerta L, Rancan L, Simón C, Isea J, Vidaurre E, Vara E, et al. Ischaemic preconditioning prevents the liver inflammatory response to lung ischaemia/reperfusion in a swine lung autotransplant model. Eur J Cardiothorac Surg. 2013;43:1194–201.
61. Rentoukas I, Giannopoulos G, Kaoukis A, Kossyvakis C, Raisakis K, Driva M, et al. Cardioprotective role of remote ischemic periconditioning in primary percutaneous coronary intervention: enhancement by opioid action. JACC Cardiovasc Interv. 2010;3:49–55.
62. Hausenloy DJ, Yellon DM. Remote ischaemic preconditioning: underlying mechanisms and clinical application. Cardiovasc Res. 2008;79:377–86.
63. Hausenloy DJ, Iliodromitis EK, Andreadou I, Papalois A, Gritsopoulos G, Anastasiou-Nana M, et al. Investigating the signal transduction pathways underlying remote ischemic conditioning in the porcine heart. Cardiovasc Drugs Ther. 2012;26:87–93.
64. Gritsopoulos G, Iliodromitis EK, Zoga A, Farmakis D, Demerouti E, Papalois A, et al. Remote postconditioning is more potent than classic postconditioning in reducing the infarct size in anesthetized rabbits. Cardiovasc Drugs Ther. 2009;23:193–8.
65. Schmidt MR, Smerup M, Konstantinov IE, Shimizu M, Li J, Cheung M, et al. Intermittent peripheral tissue ischemia during coronary ischemia reduces myocardial infarction through a KATP-dependent mechanism: first demonstration of remote ischemic preconditioning. Am J Physiol Heart Circ Physiol. 2007;292:H1883–90.
66. Andreotti F, Pasceri V, Hackett DR, Davies GJ, Haider AW, Maseri A. Preinfarction angina as a predictor of more rapid coronary thrombolysis in patients with acute myocardial infarction. N Engl J Med. 1996;334:7–12.
67. Ishihara M, Sato H, Tateishi H, Kawagoe T, Shimatani Y, Kurisu S, et al. Implications of prodromal angina pectoris in anterior wall acute myocardial infarction: acute angiographic findings and long-term prognosis. J Am Coll Cardiol. 1997;30:970–5.
68. Kloner RA, Shook T, Antman EM, Cannon CP, Przyklenk K, Yoo K, et al. Prospective temporal analysis of the onset of preinfarction angina versus outcome: an ancillary study in TIMI-9B. Circulation. 1998;97:1042–5.
69. Gheeraert PJ, Henriques JP, De Buyzere ML, De Pauw M, Taeymans Y, Zijlstra F. Preinfarction angina protects against out-of-hospital ventricular fibrillation in patients with acute occlusion of the left coronary artery. J Am Coll Cardiol. 2001;38:1369–74.
70. Solomon SD, Anavekar NS, Greaves S, Rouleau JL, Hennekens C, Pfeffer MA, HEART Investigators. Angina pectoris prior to myocardial infarction protects against subsequent left ventricular remodeling. J Am Coll Cardiol. 2004;43:1511–4.
71. van den Munckhof I, Riksen N, Seeger JP, Schreuder TH, Borm GF, Eijsvogels TM, et al. Aging attenuates the protective effect of ischemic preconditioning against endothelial ischemia-reperfusion injury in humans. Am J Physiol Heart Circ Physiol. 2013;304:H1727–32.
72. Pêgo-Fernandes PM, Jatene FB, Kwasnicka K, Hueb AC, Moreira LF, Gentil AF, et al. Ischemic preconditioning in myocardial revascularization with intermittent aortic cross-clamping. J Card Surg. 2000;15:333–8.
73. Yang XM, Liu Y, Cui L, Yang X, Liu Y, Tandon N, et al. Platelet P2Y12 blockers confer direct postconditioning-like protection in reperfused rabbit hearts. J Cardiovasc Pharmacol Ther. 2013;18:251–62.
74. Fullmer TM, Pei S, Zhu Y, Sloan C, Manzanares R, Henrie B, et al. Insulin suppresses ischemic preconditioning-mediated cardioprotection through Akt-dependent mechanisms. J Mol Cell Cardiol. 2013;64:20–9.
75. D'Annunzio V, Donato M, Buchholz B, Pérez V, Miksztowicz V, Berg G, et al. High cholesterol diet effects on ischemia-reperfusion injury of the heart. Can J Physiol Pharmacol. 2012;90:1185–96.
76. Takeuchi T, Ishii Y, Kikuchi K, Hasebe N. Ischemic preconditioning effect of prodromal angina is attenuated in acute myocardial infarction patients with hypertensive left ventricular hypertrophy. Circ J. 2011;75:1192–9.
77. Zhang FJ, Ma LL, Wang WN, Qian LB, Yang MJ, Yu J, et al. Hypercholesterolemia abrogates sevoflurane-induced delayed preconditioning against myocardial infarct in rats by alteration of nitric oxide synthase signaling. Shock. 2012;37:485–91.
78. Iliodromitis EK, Zoga A, Vrettou A, Andreadou I, Paraskevaidis IA, Kaklamanis L, et al. The effectiveness of postconditioning and preconditioning on infarct size in hypercholesterolemic and normal anesthetized rabbits. Atherosclerosis. 2006;188:356–62.

79. Iliodromitis EK, Andreadou I, Prokovas E, Zoga A, Farmakis D, Fotopoulou T, et al. Simvastatin in contrast to postconditioning reduces infarct size in hyperlipidemic rabbits: possible role of oxidative/nitrosative stress. Basic Res Cardiol. 2010;105:193–203.
80. Andreadou I, Farmakis D, Prokovas E, Sigala F, Zoga A, Spyridaki K, et al. Short-term statin administration in hypercholesterolemic rabbits resistant to postconditioning: effects on infarct size, endothelial nitric oxide synthase and nitro-oxidative stress. Cardiovasc Res. 2012;94:501–9.
81. Heusch G. Cardioprotection: chances and challenges of its translation to the clinic. Lancet. 2013;381: 166–75.
82. Edwards RJ, Redwood SR, Lambiase PD, Tomset E, Rakhit RD, Marber MS. Antiarrhythmic and anti-ischaemic effects of angina in patients with and without coronary collaterals. Heart. 2002;88:604–10.
83. Iliodromitis EK, Koutelou M, Paraskevaidis IA, Theodorakos A, Farmakis D, Tsoutsanis J, et al. Treadmill exercise test with dual isotope scintigraphy documents the second window of preconditioning in humans. Atherosclerosis. 2008;198:122–8.
84. Iliodromitis EK, Paraskevaidis IA, Fountoulaki K, Farmakis D, Andreadou I, Antoniadis A, et al. Staccato reperfusion prevents reperfusion injury in patients undergoing coronary angioplasty: a 1-year follow-up pilot study. Atherosclerosis. 2009;204:497–502.
85. Xue F, Yang X, Zhang B, Zhao C, Song J, Jiang T, et al. Postconditioning the human heart in percutaneous coronary intervention. Clin Cardiol. 2010;33:439–44.
86. Freixa X, Bellera N, Ortiz-Pérez JT, Jiménez M, Paré C, Bosch X, et al. Ischaemic postconditioning revisited: lack of effects on infarct size following primary percutaneous coronary intervention. Eur Heart J. 2012;33:103–12.
87. Tarantini G, Favaretto E, Marra MP, Frigo AC, Napodano M, Cacciavillani L, et al. Postconditioning during coronary angioplasty in acute myocardial infarction: the POST-AMI trial. Int J Cardiol. 2012;162: 33–8.
88. Hahn J-Y, Song YB, Kim EK, Yu CW, Bae J-W, Chung W-Y, et al. Ischemic postconditioning during primary percutaneous coronary intervention: POST randomized trial. Circulation. 2013;128:1889–94.
89. Botker HE, Kharbanda R, Schmidt MR, Bøttcher M, Kaltoft AK, Terkelsen CJ, et al. Remote ischaemic conditioning before hospital admission, as a complement to angioplasty, and effect on myocardial salvage in patients with acute myocardial infarction: a randomized trial. Lancet. 2010;375:727–34.
90. Ali N, Rizwi F, Iqbal A, Rashid A. Induced remote ischemic pre-conditioning on ischemia-reperfusion injury in patients undergoing coronary artery bypass. J Coll Physicians Surg Pak. 2010;20:427–31.
91. Yetgin T, Manintveld OC, Boersma E, Kappetein AP, van Geuns RJ, Zijlstra F, et al. Remote ischemic conditioning in percutaneous coronary intervention and coronary artery bypass grafting. Circ J. 2012;76: 2392–404.
92. Kopecky SL, Aviles RJ, Bell MR, Lobl JK, Tipping D, Frommell G, et al. A randomized, double-blinded, placebo-controlled, dose-ranging study measuring the effect of an adenosine agonist on infarct size reduction in patients undergoing primary percutaneous transluminal coronary angioplasty: the ADMIRE (AmP579 Delivery for Myocardial Infarction REduction) study. Am Heart J. 2003;146: 146–52.
93. Cleveland Jr JC, Meldrum DR, Rowland RT, Banerjee A, Harken AH. Adenosine preconditioning of human myocardium is dependent upon the ATP-sensitive K+ channel. J Mol Cell Cardiol. 1997;29: 175–82.
94. Wong GT, Huang Z, Ji S, Irwin MG. Remifentanil reduces the release of biochemical markers of myocardial damage after coronary artery bypass surgery: a randomized trial. J Cardiothorac Vasc Anesth. 2010;24:790–6.
95. Liuba P, Batra S, Pesonen E, Werner O. Bradykinin preconditions postischemic arterial endothelial function in humans. J Card Surg. 2005;20:420–4.
96. Patel DJ, Purcell HJ, Fox KM. Cardioprotection by opening of the K(ATP) channel in unstable angina. Is this a clinical manifestation of myocardial preconditioning? Results of a randomized study with nicorandil. CESAR 2 investigation. Clinical European studies in angina and revascularization. Eur Heart J. 1999;20:51–7.
97. Kato T, Yoshimoto N. Ischaemic preconditioning and outcomes after angioplasty: effects of drug therapy. Drugs. 2003;63:33–8.
98. Pache J, Kastrati A, Mehilli J, Bollwein H, Ndrepepa G, Schühlen H, et al. A randomized evaluation of the effects of glucose-insulin-potassium infusion on myocardial salvage in patients with acute myocardial infarction treated with reperfusion therapy. Am Heart J. 2004;148:e3.
99. Paraskevaidis IA, Iliodromitis EK, Ikonomidis I, Rallidis L, Hamodraka E, Parissis J, et al. The effect of acute administration of statins on coronary microcirculation during the pre-revascularization period in patients with myocardial infarction. Atherosclerosis. 2012;223:184–9.
100. Furlani D, Klopsch C, Gäbel R, Ugurlucan M, Pittermann E, Klee D, et al. Intracardiac erythropoietin injection reveals antiinflammatory potential and improved cardiac functions detected by Forced Swim Test. Transplant Proc. 2008;40:962–6.
101. Gerczuk PZ, Kloner RA. An update on cardioprotection: a review of the latest adjunctive therapies to limit myocardial infarction size in clinical trials. J Am Coll Cardiol. 2012;59:969–78.
102. Piot C, Croisille P, Staat P, Thibault H, Rioufol G, Mewton N, et al. Effect of cyclosporine on reperfusion injury in acute myocardial infarction. N Engl J Med. 2008;359:473–81.
103. Mahaffey KW, Puma JA, Barbagelata NA, DiCarli MF, Leesar MA, Browne KF, et al. Adenosine as an adjunct to thrombolytic therapy for acute myocardial

infarction: results of a multicenter, randomized, placebo-controlled trial: the Acute Myocardial Infarction STudy of ADenosine (AMISTAD) trial. J Am Coll Cardiol. 1999;34:1711–20.

104. Ross AM, Gibbons RJ, Stone GW, Kloner RA, Alexander RW, AMISTAD-II Investigators. A randomized, double-blinded, placebo-controlled multicenter trial of adenosine as an adjunct to reperfusion in the treatment of acute myocardial infarction (AMISTAD-II). J Am Coll Cardiol. 2005;45: 1775–80.

105. Lee HT, LaFaro RJ, Reed GE. Pretreatment of human myocardium with adenosine during open heart surgery. J Card Surg. 1995;10:665–76.

106. IONA Study Group. Effect of nicorandil on coronary events in patients with stable angina: the Impact Of Nicorandil in Angina (IONA) randomised trial. Lancet. 2002;359:1269–75.

Gene Therapy for the Heart

29

Eleni Papanikolaou and Nicholas P. Anagnou

Abstract

Gene therapy refers to the use of DNA or of any other type of nucleic acid, as a pharmaceutical agent to treat a disease. This therapeutic approach was initially designed to treat several monogenic diseases, and is especially suited for the treatment of blood diseases such as hemoglobinopathies or immunodeficiencies. However, the advances in understanding the molecular basis of myocardial dysfunction, the identification and characterization of the properties and plasticity of several subpopulations of cardiac cells, combined with the development of increasingly efficient gene transfer technologies, has rendered heart failure another excellent candidate for gene-based therapies. Moreover, there is still a critical need to further explore novel therapeutic approaches in heart failure, and thus, gene therapy has emerged as a realistic alternative. Particularly, cardiovascular gene therapy has benefitted from recent advancements in vector technology and delivery modalities, and stem cell biology. This chapter reviews the available gene transfer technologies and the molecular features that constitute the main targets in the field of cardiac gene therapy, it presents the current status of gene therapy for the heart, and discusses how the knowledge gained from the initial clinical trials can be used to develop a safer and more efficient gene transfer approach. Since the first demonstration of the *in vivo* gene transfer into myocardium, there have been a series of advancements that have transformed gene therapy from an experimental tool to the threshold of becoming a viable clinical option.

E. Papanikolaou • N.P. Anagnou, MD, PhD (✉)
Laboratory of Cell and Gene Therapy,
Biomedical Research Foundation
of the Academy of Athens (IIBEAA),
4 Soranou Ephessiou Street, Athens 115 27, Greece

Laboratory of Biology,
University of Athens School of Medicine,
75 Mikras Asias Street, Athens 11527, Greece
e-mail: anagnou@med.uoa.gr

D.V. Cokkinos (ed.), *Introduction to Translational Cardiovascular Research*,
DOI 10.1007/978-3-319-08798-6_29,

Keywords
Gene therapy • Lentiviral vector • Retroviral integration • Insertional mutagenesis • Hematopoietic stem cells (HSCs) • Cardiac stem cells (CSCs) • β-adrenergic system • Calcium cycling proteins • Heart failure

Abbreviations

AAV	Adeno-Associated Virus
ADA	Adenosine Deaminase
ADCY6	Adenylate Cyclase type 6
AdV	Adenovirus
β-AR	β-Adrenergic Receptor
CAR	Coxsackie-Adenovirus Receptor
CHF	Congestive Heart Failure
CMV	Cytomegalovirus
DRPs	DNase Resistant Particles
GRK	G protein-coupled Receptor Kinase
GTh	Gene Therapy
HIV	Human Immunodeficiency Virus
LTR	Long Terminal Repeat
LVAD	Left Ventricular Assist Device
MAR	Matrix Attachment Region elements
miRNAs	Micro Interfering RNAs
MLV	Murine Leukemia Virus
PAA	Polyamidoamine
PEI	Polyethylenimines
PIC	Pre-Integration Complex
PLN	Phospholamban
PP1	Protein Phosphatase 1
RNAi	RNA interfering
RSV	Rous Sarcoma Virus
SDF1	Stromal cell-Derived Factor-1
SERCA	Sarcoplasmic Reticulum Ca^{2+} ATPase
SIN	Self-inactivating
VSV	Vesicular Stomatitis Virus
VSV-G	Vesicular Stomatitis Virus envelope glycoprotein G
X-SCID	X-linked Severe Combined Immunodeficiency

29.1 Introduction

Gene therapy (GTh) refers to the use of DNA or of any other type of nucleic acid, as a pharmaceutical agent to treat a disease. The name derives from the idea that primarily DNA can be used to either substitute a deficient gene or replace a mutated gene within an individual's cells. Thus, in gene therapy protocols, DNA encoding a therapeutic protein is packaged within a vector which is used to facilitate the entrance of DNA into the cells. Once inside the cell, in most types of viral vectors, the DNA integrates into the host genome and is expressed for life by the cell machinery, resulting in the production of the therapeutic protein, which eventually leads to the treatment of the disease.

Therapy by gene transfer in general, is not suitable for the treatment of complex disease phenotypes associated with multiple affected genes or for the multiple genetic variations that underlie complex disorders. Rather, gene therapy, with the exception of cancer and several other multifactorial disorders, is mostly applicable for monogenic disorders, such as the hereditary disorders caused by mutations in more than 1,800 gene loci [1]. Thus, it is conceivable that if sufficient correction or compensation can be achieved with gene transfer, monogenic disorders could be prevented and/or treated [1]. Therefore, this therapeutic approach was initially designed to treat several monogenic diseases and is especially suited for treatment of blood diseases such as hemoglobinopathies or immunodeficiencies.

However, the advances in understanding the molecular basis of myocardial dysfunction, the identification and characterization of the properties and plasticity of several subpopulations of cardiac cells, combined with the development of increasingly efficient gene transfer technologies, has rendered heart failure (HF) another excellent candidate for gene-based therapy.

The most important issue to resolve in a gene therapy trial is the adequate correction of the phenotype of the disease, by constructing the most efficient vector in terms of (a) gene delivery,

(b) stability, (c) appropriate and tissue-specific transgene expression and (d) safety. Furthermore, the type of cell to be selected for correction, is of critical importance, and generally depends on the type of organ(s) and/or tissues that manifest the abnormal phenotype.

Three main types of gene therapy approaches are currently being employed:

(a) *In situ* gene therapy in which the vector carrying the therapeutic genetic material is directly administered to the affected tissue, such as by an injection into a tumor nodule or organ [2]. This type of therapy applies for gene transfer to the heart.
(b) *Ex vivo* gene therapy during which the patients' cells are harvested and co-cultured in the laboratory in the presence of the therapeutic vector. The "corrected" cells with the new genetic material are then transplanted back to the patient from whom they were originally derived [2].
(c) *In vivo* gene therapy is defined as the administration of the vector carrying the therapeutic genetic material directly to a live animal. The vector can be delivered by a variety of methods, such as intravenous injection or by other physical means of administration such as hypodermic injection, aerosol, or employing other routes [2].

29.2 Gene Therapy Vectors

Vectors constitute the vehicles or carriers that contain the therapeutic gene for delivery to the cells. Especially for the heart, the design must account for the tissue-specific and spatial patterns of the cardiovascular pathophysiological process, depending on whether it is a global process such as HF or a focal process such as nodal dysfunction. Therefore, the optimal vector format in HF must be able to effectively deliver and drive sustained transgene expression to guarantee long term improvement, as well as broad transduction efficiency to the majority of cardiomyocytes to ensure significant impact on ventricular function. In all cases, the designed vector should not induce cytotoxic effects and should be rescuable after injection in order to maximize the safety of the whole gene/cell therapy approach.

Gene delivery systems derive either from genetically engineered viruses or from non-viral formulations such as those manufactured by the use of nanotechnology [3]. Non-viral vectors include: (a) naked plasmid DNA, (b) liposomes, (c) DNA polymer-carrying particles and (d) oligonucleotides [4].

Several types of recombinant viruses are used as vehicles of the therapeutic genes in cardiac gene therapy. These include:

- Retroviruses belonging to the subfamily of *Oncoretroviridae* e.g. Murine Leukemia Virus (MLV) or *Lentiviridae* e.g. Human Immunodeficiency Virus (HIV)
- Adeno-Associated viruses
- Adenoviruses

Each vector delivery system provides different specificity, exhibits different tropism and displays a distinct expression pattern at the molecular level. The appropriate choice of a delivery system will ensure a successful therapy. Moreover, the selection of the appropriate vector delivery method is critical for the proper implementation of the therapeutic strategy and for efficient transgene expression in the myocardium. Especially for cardiovascular disease, both the invasiveness of vector delivery method and the patient safety need to be critically assessed prior to initiating gene therapy trials. There are three ways of delivering the vectors to the myocardium and include (a) coronary artery and venous infusion, (b) direct intramyocardial injection and (c) pericardial delivery [4].

29.2.1 Retroviruses

29.2.1.1 Oncoretroviruses or Gamma-Retroviruses

Retroviruses are widely used as efficient tools for genetic manipulation of stem cells, mainly because of their ability to integrate into the host cell's genome through the reverse transcription process during which the viral single-stranded (ss) RNA is converted to double-stranded (ds) DNA. Integration of the retroviral DNA genome into the host cell DNA is an essential step in the retrovirus replication cycle, permitting viral genomes to become permanently fixed as proviruses into the DNA of the host. During this process, the retroviral DNA is associated within a large complex with a subset of retroviral proteins known as the pre-integration complex (PIC). For oncoretroviruses, such as the murine leukemia virus (MLV), uncoating, DNA synthesis, and formation of the PIC occur at the same rate, both in non-dividing cells as well as in dividing cells, but integration fails to occur. However, during mitosis, the nuclear membrane disassembles, rendering the chromosomes accessible to the virus, suggesting that successful infection by oncoretroviruses such as MLV requires cell division [5].

Oncoretroviruses consist of an enveloped capsid that contains a plus (+) strand RNA genome ranging from 7 to 10 kb. Their tropism often includes hematopoietic stem cells. Oncoretroviral vectors present several advantages as they exhibit (a) efficient and stable gene transfer, transduction rates of up to 40 % of hematopoietic stem cells in non-human primates and (b) high fidelity gene transfer due to intact integration and absence of chromosomal rearrangements. However, their use in the clinic has been hampered by the development of T-cell acute lymphoblastic leukemia, due to integration of the viral genome in the second intron of the LMO-2 proto-oncogene in several patients during the gene therapy clinical trial for X-linked severe combined immunodeficiency (X-SCID) conducted in France [6]. Moreover, utilization of a gamma-retroviral vector led to genomic instability and myelodysplasia subsequent to EVI1 activation after gene therapy for chronic granulomatous disease [7]. It is therefore anticipated that oncoretroviral vectors will be gradually displaced in the field of hemopoietic gene therapy [8]. However, no studies have been conducted to date in the context of cardiac stem cells and/or cardiomyocytes and therefore, this field represents another challenge, due to the fact that there are basic issues that remain to be fully addressed regarding the level of myocyte regeneration.

29.2.1.2 Lentiviruses

Lentiviruses, display one major advantage compared to gamma-retroviruses as they do not require dissociation of the nuclear envelope in order to integrate their genome into the host's genome, as it has been extensively documented, and therefore they can efficiently infect both dividing and non-dividing cells [9]. HIV in particular, has the capacity to cross the nuclear membrane of interphasic cells because the pre-integration complex contains a nuclear localization signal that allows transport through the nuclear pore complexes [10]. This represents a crucial aspect for genetically modifying tissues, especially those considered as the main potential cell targets of gene therapy, such as the brain, muscle, liver and the hematopoietic system, as they can transduce even non-dividing cells residing in the G_0 phase of the cell cycle.

Lentiviruses also consist of an enveloped capsid that contains a plus (+) strand RNA genome of approximately 10 kb. Wild-type HIV naturally infects cells of the hematopoietic system and specifically $CD4^+$ T-cells. However, in the gene therapy context, HIV-based vectors are pseudotyped by alternative envelope glycoproteins such as the glycoprotein derived from vesicular stomatitis virus (VSV), namely the VSV-G envelope glycoprotein that confers significant tropism for many cells, including stem cells of the hematopoietic and the cardiac system. Pseudotyping with VSV-G presents an additional advantage, as it allows for the vector formulates to be concentrated by ultracentrifugation and therefore can lead to increased vector titers. Several human clinical trials utilizing lentiviral vectors have shown promise for various disorders including ADA-deficient SCID [11], β-thalassemia [12], Wiskott-Aldrich syndrome [13] and metachromatic leukodystrophy [14]. It is therefore clear that lentiviral vectors have outperformed oncoretroviral vectors in terms of safety and efficiency and represent an effective agent of gene transfer that can be also employed in the cardiac gene therapy field. However, although successful lentiviral transduction has been documented in cardiac micro-vascular endothelial cells [15], cardiomyocytes [16], cardiac stem cells and progenitors [17, 18], it seems that utilization of lentiviral vectors in the cardiac gene therapy field, is still far from reaching the clinic.

Despite the therapeutic effect that retroviruses have demonstrated, there is always the risk for insertional mutagenesis, i.e. activation of proto-oncogenes or down-regulation of tumour suppressor genes upon viral integration. While the possibility of insertional mutagenesis using replication-defective vectors has been discussed as theoretically possible [19], such risks had been originally estimated to be extremely low [20], based on the assumption that proviral integration into the genome was random [21].

29.2.1.3 Additional Safety Data on Retroviruses and Lentiviruses

With the readily accessible human genome sequence data, mapping studies of retroviral integration sites in cell lines, have uncovered non-random integration patterns, using wild-type HIV, HIV-derived, or murine leukemia virus (MLV)-derived vectors [22–26], while it was extensively documented that retroviral integration is actually not such a random process and that each virus presents a unique pattern of integration. Thus, MLV integrants are located predominantly around transcription start sites, while HIV integrants strongly favour transcription units and gene-dense regions of the genome. The basis for these preferences is unknown, and conceivably they may reflect interaction of the pre-integration complex with specific proteins or with specific DNA sequences or structures that are associated with transcription.

In order to make gene therapy based on retroviral vectors safer, the use of specific DNA elements called insulators, exhibiting the capacity to block enhancer activity and maintain the chromatin status of distinct chromosomal regions, was eventually introduced in the construction of vectors in order to (a) diminish variable expression and silencing of the transgene and (b) reduce the risk of insertional mutagenesis [27, 28]. This strategy combined with the deletion of the U3 region of the LTR in the self-inactivating (SIN) configuration of lentiviruses, has rendered over the past decade, lentiviral vectors as powerful tools in the fields of neuroscience, hematology, developmental biology, stem cell biology and transgenesis.

29.2.2 Adeno-Associated Viruses

Adeno-associated viruses (AAV) are members of the family Parvoviridae, and constitute non-pathogenic, non-enveloped viruses containing a 4.7 kb single-stranded DNA genome that encodes the structural proteins of the viral capsid, encoded by the *cap* gene and the non-structural proteins necessary for viral replication and assembly, encoded by the *rep* gene, flanked by short inverted terminal repeats. Their life cycle involves two phases, the replicative and the latent phase. In the productive phase, it co-infects the host cell only when a helper virus is present [29]. In the absence of a helper virus, AAV usually enters the latent phase, integrating into the human genome, commonly within a specific region of chromosome 19, although this has been observed only in cell lines. Its principal advantage for gene therapy is the poor inflammatory response to infected cells. As a therapeutic vector, AAV consists only of the inverted terminal repeats which are necessary for replication, packaging, and integration, while the viral coding sequences are entirely removed, rendering AAV vectors replication-deficient. The resulting recombinant vectors can efficiently deliver a transgene and safely mediate long-term gene expression in dividing and non-dividing cells of numerous tissues. AAV has the potential to facilitate long-term transgene expression in the absence of destructive T-cell responses, and such vectors have been generally proven safe. However, naturally occurring AAV variants are typically inefficient in infecting a number of stem cell types, particularly human embryonic stem cells [29].

There are 13 reported serotypes of AAV that display different tissue tropism, depending on the structure of the capsid protein. Serotypes AAV-1, 6, 8 and 9 have been shown to be the most cardiotropic. However, significant transduction in non-target tissues such as liver, skeletal muscle and lung has been documented [4]. In order to improve AAV cardiotropism, several methods have been introduced and novel viral capsid AAV libraries were constructed through DNA shuffling and chimeric strain production. This strategy simultaneously enhances tissue tropism and also helps AAV-based vectors to evade naturally occurring neutralizing antibodies [30–34]. Neutralizing antibodies to various AAV serotypes are present in approximately 20–80 % of the population, severely limiting the potential therapeutic use of AAV. Thus, the presence of such antibodies constitutes a major exclusion criterion in many AAV-based clinical trials [35]. There are numerous publications describing the efficient transduction of cardiac cells by AAV vectors [36, 37], and it appears that the AAVs constitute the most effective way for gene transfer in cardiac cells to date. Moreover, there are ongoing gene therapy clinical trials for HF in which gene transfer is mediated by AAV vectors.

Specifically, the first clinical trial of gene therapy was launched in the United States in 2007 [35, 38] and was based on gene delivery of the SERCA2 cDNA via a recombinant AAV1 (AAV1.SERCA2a) for calcium up-regulation in patients with advanced heart failure (CUPID). The study was a two-part, Phase 1/2 multicenter trial designed to evaluate the safety and the biological effects of gene transfer of the SERCA2a cDNA via the recombinant AAV1. In part 1, participants were administered a single intracoronary infusion of AAV1.SERCA2a in an open-label approach. A 12-month follow-up of these patients documented an acceptable safety pattern; moreover, improvement of cardiac function was detected in several patients. Overall, the results of the specific study suggested that gene transfer of AAV1.SERCA2a confers quantitative biological benefit. During the second part of the trial, 39 patients with advanced HF, received the AAV1-mediated SERCA2a transgene in one or three doses of DNase resistant particles (DRPs), i.e. low dose (6×10^{11} DRPs), middle dose (3×10^{12} DRPs), and high dose (1×10^{13} DRPs), or placebo [39]. Over a 1-year period, the cumulative recurrent cardiovascular events such as death, heart failure admission, left ventricular assist device (LVAD) insertion, cardiac transplantation, and myocardial infarction, increased in the placebo group but not in the low and middle-dose AAV1.SERCA2a groups which exhibited diminished recurrent cardiovascular events for the first 6 months. However, from months 6 to 12, these groups demonstrated events that were similar to placebo. The high-dose AAV1.SERCA2a group, continued to do significantly better than all groups at 12 months without any increase in adverse events, laboratory abnormalities, or arrhythmias [39]. Furthermore, the CUPID 2 Phase 2b trial (NCT01643330) is underway, designed to evaluate whether increasing SERCA2a activity via gene therapy improves clinical outcome [40]. Available data so far, indicate that calcium up-regulation by AAV1/SERCA2a gene therapy is safe and of potential benefit in advanced HF [40]. The promising results of the CUPID clinical trial, have prompted researchers to conduct two other clinical trials targeting SERCA2a, that will be enrolling patients soon. The first trial, which is conducted in the United Kingdom, includes patients with advanced heart failure who received LVAD at least 1 month prior to treatment. These patients will be treated either with AAV1.SERCA2a or saline. Simultaneously, a Phase 2, single-center, double-blind, randomized, placebo-controlled, parallel-group study will be conducted at the Institute de Cardiologie Pitié-Salpêtrière in Paris, France, with the primary objective of investigating the impact of AAV1.SERCA2a on cardiac remodelling parameters in patients with severe HF [4].

29.2.3 Adenoviruses

Human adenoviruses constitute another viral family used in gene therapy approaches, which are classified into 51 immunologically distinct serotypes divided into six subgroups, namely subgroups A–F. Adenoviruses are non-enveloped, double-stranded (ds) DNA viruses and contain large protein complexes that bind to CD46 or to coxsackie-adenovirus receptor (CAR), depending on the serotype for viral binding and cellular entry. Upon cellular entry via clathrin-mediated endocytosis, the dsDNA is transported to the nucleus across nuclear pores, allowing efficient transduction of both mitotic and non-mitotic cells. Their genome size ranges from approximately 30 to 35 kb and contains five segments that encode early gene products (E1a, E1b, E2a, E2b, E3, and E4), and five segments that encode late gene products (L1–L5). The E1, E2, and E4 gene products regulate transcription and translation of the late genes and therefore, are indispensable for viral replication [41]. Adenoviral vectors are among the most promising gene transfer vehicles for the *in vivo* treatment of a range of human diseases, e.g. cystic fibrosis and haemophilia, because of their ability to infect a wide spectrum of cell types, including quiescent cells. Adenoviral vectors present the following advantages: (a) they provide high efficiency of gene transfer because they are able to deliver many genome copies per target cell that typically translates into very high expression, (b) they can deliver relatively large therapeutic genes of approximately 25–30 kb in size especially with the latest generation vectors, and (c) they confer high fidelity of gene transfer because the vector genomes are genetically stable. However, although replication-deficient vectors based on adenoviruses can be produced easily and at high titres, two main disadvantages occur, i.e. (a) the transgene's expression is transient and typically lasts 1–2 months in non-dividing cells, while is much shorter in dividing cells and (b) there is a significant induction of both cellular and humoral host immune response. First-generation adenoviral vectors may be applied where short-term expression and single dosing is desirable, such as cancer vaccine therapies. Initial enthusiasm toward the use of first-generation adenoviral vectors in gene replacement therapy has diminished, because not only they did fail to achieve sustained gene transfer, but also resulted in significant toxicity and death of an individual [41]. Furthermore, the pre-existing immunity against adenoviruses in patients, may result in low levels of transgene delivery and expression. Third-generation gutless or helper-dependent adenoviral vectors have attenuated immunogenic potential, but still a significant risk remains. Finally, CAR receptors are particularly prevalent in liver tissue, thus limiting adenoviral tissue specificity. Due to the aforementioned limiting factors, adenoviral mediated strategies are limited in cardiovascular gene therapy trials [42].

At present, adenoviral vector delivery is being utilized in an ongoing clinical trial. This research study is designed to determine (a) whether gene transfer using the adenovirus 5- encoding human adenylate cyclase type 6 (Ad5.hAC6) can be safely administered to patients with congestive heart failure (CHF) and (b) whether this agent may be of benefit in heart failure. In initial extensive animal experiments, it was found that increased amounts of ADCY6 protein in heart cells appear to make the heart pump more vigorously [43]. In the specific study, adenovirus-encoding human ADCY6 will be delivered through intracoronary injection with dose escalation to patients with CHF.

29.2.4 Non-viral Vectors

In general, non-viral vectors are based on a DNA construct, usually a plasmid that typically includes a constitutive promoter sequence such as the cytomegalovirus (CMV) or Rous sarcoma virus (RSV) promoters, as well as enhancer sequences that provide tissue specificity of the therapeutic gene. Plasmids are double stranded circular DNA molecules of approximately 2–12 kb in size, bearing several characteristics such as an origin of replication to ensure replication in bacteria and in certain cases eukaryotic cells and an antibiotic resistance gene. Plasmid DNA vector-based systems have several advantages, as they are extremely easy to manufacture, are low cost and present a reduced risk of systemic immunological responses. Plasmids can be readily delivered in *in vitro* cultured cells by several means of transfection such as lipofection, electroporation and calcium phosphate precipitation. In fact, plasmid transfection is being globally employed in cell lines during the course of lentiviral, AAV and adenoviral vector production. However, delivery of naked plasmids to tissues has been shown to be inefficient and challenging for several reasons. Plasmids are rapidly and systematically degraded within the cell and moreover, they exhibit poor cellular entry, followed by intracellular compartmentalization leading to short-term expression. Moreover, transient expression can also be the result of *de novo* methylation, histone modification and heterochromatin formation. All these features limit the utilization of plasmids as efficient DNA delivery tools.

In order to overcome these issues, one approach combines incorporation of the recently identified matrix attachment region (MAR) elements that have been shown to prevent transgene silencing by partly inhibiting DNA methylation [44] and/or by effectively insulating the transgene and creating independent euchromatin domains. Another strategy that confers greater plasmid stability is being addressed through the use of carrier molecules including liposomal and polymer systems. This approach provides stability of the plasmid DNA in the systemic circulation because it shields the DNA within liposome-DNA complexes. Polymer based DNA complexes involving polyethylenimines (PEI) and polyamidoamine complexes (PAA) have improved gene transfer through enhanced uptake, with reduced cytotoxicity and protection from endosomal degradation. However, even by this method, the DNA is cleared quickly and the main expression is located predominantly in the lungs [45].

Currently, an ongoing clinical trial examines the effects of injecting stromal cell-derived factor-1 (SDF1) directly into the myocardium of patients with ischemic heart disease [46]. In this open-label trial, the safety of a single escalating dose of SDF1-naked plasmid DNA by an endomyocardial injection at multiple sites will be evaluated. Preliminary efficacy will be evaluated by measuring the impact on cardiac function via standard echocardiography measurements, cardiac perfusion via SPECT imaging, and improvement according to the NYHA classification.

29.3 Molecular Targets

Over the past 20 years, extensive insights have been provided regarding our understanding of the pathophysiology and the molecular and cellular dimensions of HF. These advancements, paved the way towards the generation of novel therapeutic strategies based on gene-transfer technology. Currently, the molecular events that constitute the main targets in the field of cardiac gene therapy can be classified in two main categories: (a) molecular targets of the β-adrenergic system and (b) molecular targets of calcium cycling proteins. For these targets to be validated, it is extremely important to first prove that they can rescue cardiac function in animal models of established HF, that this rescue is not associated with arrhythmogenesis, and that a gene-dose effect can be established.

29.3.1 The β-Adrenergic System

Heart failure provokes multiple changes in the β-adrenergic signalling that essentially lead to β-adrenergic receptor (β-AR) down-regulation and desensitization. Therefore, a rationale based on gene transfer to treat HF, includes overexpression of β-AR as a simple way to overcome β-AR down-regulation. It has been demonstrated that transgenic mice overexpressing the human β_1-ARs suffered from severe cardiomyopathy [47], but in contrast, mice with cardiac overexpression of β_2-AR demonstrated increased basal myocardial adenylate cyclase activity with increased left ventricular (LV) function [48]. Consequently, direct and intracoronary myocardial delivery of adenovirus containing the human β_2-AR transgene resulted in enhanced cardiac function in rodents and mammalian models [48, 49].

Another molecular target for potential gene transfer is GRK2 that constitutes a G protein-coupled receptor kinase (GRK2), is the most abundantly expressed GRK in the heart and has been implicated in the pathogenesis of dysfunctional cardiac β-AR signalling. GRKs phosphorylate the agonist-occupied receptors, resulting in functional uncoupling. In mice, selective GRK2 ablation after HF induced by myocardial infarction, resulted in increased survival, halted ventricular remodelling, and enhanced cardiac contractile performance [50]. Finally, βARKct, a peptide that inhibits GRK2-mediated β-AR desensitization, has been evaluated *in vivo* in animals. Intracoronary administration of adenovirus-mediated βARKct transgene to rabbits three weeks after induced myocardial infarction, demonstrated a marked reversal of ventricular dysfunction [51].

The last target of the β-adrenergic system is adenylate cyclase 6 (ADCY6), is an enzyme used to catalyse the formation of cAMP by ATP. Overexpression of ADCY6 in transgenic mice resulted in improved cardiac function in response to adrenergic stimulation combined with increased cAMP production in isolated cardiomyocytes. Importantly, upregulation of ADCY6 had a neutral effect on basal cardiac function and was not associated with structural heart abnormalities [52]. Moreover, intracoronary administration of adenovirus encoding ADCY6 in a pacing model of HF in pigs, resulted in improved LV function and remodeling, associated with increased cAMP-generating capacity [53]. These promising effects of upregulation of ADCY6 in preclinical studies, are currently under investigation for initiation of clinical trials in patients with HF [43].

29.3.2 Calcium Cycling Proteins

Gwathmey et al. [54], were the first to report that calcium cycling is abnormal in human heart failure regardless of the etiology, partially due to decreased sarcoplasmic reticulum Ca^{2+} ATPase 2a (SERCA2a) activity [4]. Consequently, gene transfer of SERCA2a led to improvement in cardiac contractility in a large number of experimental models of heart failure [55, 56]. Apparently, gene transfer of SERCA2a has proven to provide additional advantages that include (a) restoration of the normal state of cardiac energetics [57], (b) decrease in ventricular arrhythmias [58], and (c) enhancement of coronary flow through activation of eNOS in endothelial cells [59]. Therefore, it is not surprising that SERCA2a has been utilized as the first molecular target for gene transfer in the context of heart failure gene therapy. A further validation of this strategy was recently documented by the identification of a series of miRNAs that suppress intracellular calcium handling in heart muscle, by interacting with mRNA encoding SERCA2a [60]. Particularly, *miR-25* potently delayed calcium uptake kinetics in cardiomyocytes *in vitro* and was upregulated in heart failure, both in mice and humans. Adeno-associated virus 9 (AAV9)-mediated overexpression of *miR-25* *in vivo*, resulted in a significant loss of contractile function, while injection of an antisense oligonucleotide against *miR-25*, markedly halted established heart failure in a mouse model, improving cardiac function and survival compared to control. These data reveal that endogenous *miR-25* contributes to declining cardiac function during heart failure and suggest that it might be targeted therapeutically to restore function.

Several other molecules have served as candidates for the treatment of heart failure through gene transfer. These include the inhibition of phospholamban (PLN) through RNAi technology [61], the inhibition of protein phosphatase 1 (PP1) by direct gene addition of the protein phosphatase-1 inhibitor-1 [62], and finally the upregulation of S100. The latter, is part of a family of Ca^{2+}-modulated proteins that are implicated in intracellular regulatory activities. It promotes cardiac contractile and relaxation function by enhancing the activity of both ryanodine receptors (RYRs) and SERCA2a. More recently, AAV9 gene transfer of S100A1 in a preclinical model of ischemic cardiomyopathy induced dramatic improvements in contractile function, suggesting that a clinical trial of S100A1 gene therapy for human HF appears in the horizon [4].

29.3.3 Other Targets

Recently, the ability of the SDF1/CXCR4 complex to promote the homing of stem cells to infarcted myocardium has promoted their use as therapeutic targets in ischemic heart failure [63]. Furthermore, as previously mentioned, a clinical trial is underway to investigate the therapeutic benefit of SDF1 overexpression in ischemic cardiomyopathy [46] by gene transfer of SDF1 incorporated in a naked plasmid.

Conclusions

Novel insights about the molecular mechanisms associated with heart failure combined with the identification and development of vectors with the best cardiotropic properties, have made gene therapy a realistic adjunctive treatment to mechanical, and pharmacological therapies for heart failure. Furthermore, the ongoing parallel approaches world-wide to validate the therapeutic effects of cell-based regenerative medicine in heart failure, will immensely contribute to the advancement of rational therapies targeting cardiovascular disease [64]. In the future, extensive research for the identification of novel targets as well as for the improvement of vector systems, will undoubtedly lead to safer and more effective clinical trials in gene therapy.

Acknowledgements This study was supported by a Grant No. 11E-RARE-09-155 by the European Research Projects on Rare Diseases (ERA-Net) of the European Union to N.P. A.

References

1. O'Connor TP, Crystal RG. Genetic medicines: treatment strategies for hereditary disorders. Nat Rev Genet. 2006;7:261–76.
2. American Society of Cell and Gene Therapy. Educational Resources. Gene Therapy and Cell Therapy Defined. 2014. http://www.asgct.org/general-public/educational-resources/gene-therap--nd-cell-therapy-defined. Accessed 23 Mar 2014.
3. Yang F, Green JJ, Dinio T, Keung L, Cho SW, Park H, et al. Gene delivery to human adult and embryonic cell-derived stem cells using biodegradable nanoparticulate polymeric vectors. Gene Ther. 2009;16:533–46.
4. Hajjar RJ. Potential of gene therapy as a treatment for heart failure. J Clin Invest. 2013;123:53–61.
5. Miller DG, Adam MA, Miller AD. Gene transfer by retrovirus vectors occurs only in cells that are actively replicating at the time of infection. Mol Cell Biol. 1990;10:4239–42.
6. Hacein-Bey-Abina S, von Kalle C, Schmidt M, Le Deist F, Wulffraat N, McIntyre E, et al. A serious adverse event after successful gene therapy for X-linked severe combined immunodeficiency. N Engl J Med. 2003;348:255–6.
7. Stein S, Ott MG, Schultze-Strasser S, Jauch A, Burwinkel B, Kinner A, et al. Genomic instability and myelodysplasia with monosomy 7 consequent to EVI1 activation after gene therapy for chronic granulomatous disease. Nat Med. 2010;16:198–204.
8. Ariga T. A possible turning point in the hematopoietic stem cell gene therapy for primary immunodeficiency diseases? Lentiviral vectors could take the place of retroviral vectors. Expert Rev Clin Immunol. 2013;11:1015–8.
9. Naldini L. Lentiviruses as gene transfer agents for delivery to nondividing cells. Curr Opin Biotechnol. 1998;9:457–63.
10. Vodicka MA. Determinants for lentiviral infection of non-dividing cells. Somat Cell Mol Genet. 2001;26:35–49.
11. Hassan A, Booth C, Brightwell A, Allwood Z, Veys P, Rao K, et al. Outcome of hematopoietic stem cell transplantation for adenosine deaminase-deficient severe combined immunodeficiency. Blood. 2012;120:3615–24.
12. Cavazzana-Calvo M, Payen E, Negre O, Wang G, Hehir K, Fusil F, et al. Transfusion independence and HMGA2 activation after gene therapy of human β-thalassaemia. Nature. 2010;467:318–22.
13. Aiuti A, Biasco L, Scaramuzza S, Ferrua F, Cicalese MP, Baricordi C, et al. Lentiviral hematopoietic stem cell gene therapy in patients with Wiskott-Aldrich syndrome. Science. 2013;341:1233151.
14. Biffi A, Montini E, Lorioli L, Cesani M, Fumagalli F, Plati T, et al. Lentiviral hematopoietic stem cell gene therapy benefits metachromatic leukodystrophy. Science. 2013;341:1233158.
15. Kuang L, Feng J, He G, Jing T. Knockdown of Nrf2 inhibits the angiogenesis of rat cardiac micro-vascular endothelial cells under hypoxic conditions. Int J Biol Sci. 2013;7:656–65.
16. Du Y, Zhu H, Li D, Wang L, Zhang L, Luo Y, et al. Lentiviral-mediated overexpression of Akt1 reduces anoxia-reoxygenation injury in cardiomyocytes. Cell Biol Int. 2014;38:488–96.
17. Zanetti BF, Gomes WJ, Han SW. Identification, selection, and enrichment of cardiomyocyte precursors. Biomed Res Int. 2013;2013:390789.
18. Barth AS, Kizana E, Smith RR, Terrovitis J, Dong P, Leppo MK, et al. Lentiviral vectors bearing the cardiac promoter of the Na+–Ca2+ exchanger report cardiogenic differentiation in stem cells. Mol Ther. 2008;5:957–64.
19. Cornetta K, Morgan RA, Anderson WF. Safety issues related to retroviral mediated gene transfer to humans. Hum Gene Ther. 1991;2:5–14.
20. Moolten FL, Cupples LA. A model for predicting the risk of cancer consequent to retroviral gene therapy. Hum Gene Ther. 1992;3:479–86.
21. Coffin JM, Hughes SH, Varmus HE. Retroviruses. Plainview/New York: Cold Spring Harbor Laboratory Press; 1997.
22. Elleder D, Pavlicek A, Paces J, Hejnar J. Preferential integration of human immunodeficiency virus type 1 into genes, cytogenetic R bands and GC-rich DNA regions: insight from the human genome sequence. FEBS Lett. 2002;517:285–6.
23. Schroder AR, Shinn P, Chen H, Berry C, Ecker JR, Bushman F. HIV-1 integration in the human genome favors active genes and local hotspots. Cell. 2002;110:521–9.
24. Laufs S, Gentner B, Nagy KZ, Jauch A, Benner A, Naundorf S, et al. Retroviral vector integration occurs

in preferred genomic targets of human bone marrow repopulating cells. Blood. 2003;101:2191–8.
25. Mitchell RS, Beitzel BF, Schroder AR, Shinn P, Chen H, Berry CC, et al. Retroviral DNA integration: ASLV, HIV, and MLV show distinct target site preferences. PLoS Biol. 2004;2:e234.
26. Wu X, Li Y, Crise B, Burgess SM. Transcription start regions in the human genome are favored targets for MLV integration. Science. 2003;300:1749–51.
27. Papanikolaou E, Georgomanoli M, Stamateris E, Panetsos F, Karagiorga M, Tsaftaridis P, et al. The new SIN-lentiviral vector for thalassemia gene therapy combining two HPFH activating elements corrects human thalassemic hematopoietic stem cells. Hum Gene Ther. 2012;23:15–31.
28. Hanawa H, Yamamoto M, Zhao H, Shimada T, Persons DA. Optimized lentiviral vector design improves titer and transgene expression of vectors containing the chicken β-globin locus HS4 insulator element. Mol Ther. 2009;17:667–74.
29. Mays LE, Wilson JM. The complex and evolving story of T cell activation to AAV vector-encoded transgene products. Mol Ther. 2011;19:16–27.
30. Asokan A, Conway JC, Phillips JL, Li C, Hegge J, Sinnott R, et al. Re-engineering a receptor footprint of adeno-associated virus enables selective and systemic gene transfer to muscle. Nat Biotechnol. 2010;28: 79–82.
31. Wang J, Faust SM, Rabinowitz JE. The next step in gene delivery: molecular engineering of adeno-associated virus serotypes. J Mol Cell Cardiol. 2011; 50:793–802.
32. Mitchell AM, Nicolson SC, Warischalk JK, Samulski RJ. AAV's anatomy: roadmap for optimizing vectors for translational success. Curr Gene Ther. 2010;10:319–40.
33. Li W, Asokan A, Wu Z, Van Dyke T, DiPrimio N, Johnson JS, et al. Engineering and selection of shuffled AAV genomes: a new strategy for producing targeted biological nanoparticles. Mol Ther. 2008;16: 1252–60.
34. Ying Y, Müller OJ, Goehringer C, Leuchs B, Trepel M, Katus HA, et al. Heart-targeted adeno-associated viral vectors selected by in vivo biopanning of a random viral display peptide library. Gene Ther. 2010;17:980–90.
35. Jaski BE, Jessup ML, Mancini DM, Cappola TP, Pauly DF, Greenberg B, et al. Calcium upregulation by percutaneous administration of gene therapy in cardiac disease (CUPID Trial), a first-in-human phase 1/2 clinical trial. J Card Fail. 2009;15:171–81.
36. Wang D, Zhong L, Nahid MA, Gao G. The potential of adeno-associated viral vectors for gene delivery to muscle tissue. Expert Opin Drug Deliv. 2014;11:345–64.
37. Asokan A, Samulski RJ. An emerging adeno-associated viral vector pipeline for cardiac gene therapy. Hum Gene Ther. 2013;24:906–13.
38. Hajjar RJ, Zsebo K, Deckelbaum L, Thompson C, Rudy J, Yaroshinsky A, et al. Design of a phase 1/2 trial of intracoronary administration of AAV1/ SERCA2a in patients with heart failure. J Card Fail. 2008;14:355–67.
39. Jessup M, Greenberg B, Mancini D, Cappola T, Pauly DF, Jaski B, et al. Calcium upregulation by percutaneous administration of gene therapy in cardiac disease (CUPID): a phase 2 trial of intracoronary gene therapy of sarcoplasmic reticulum Ca2+-ATPase in patients with advanced heart failure. Circulation. 2011;124:304–13.
40. Greenberg B, Yaroshinski A, Zsebo KM, Butler J, Felker GM, Voors AA, et al. Design of a phase 2b trial of intracoronary administration of AAV1/SERCA2a in patients with advanced heart failure. JACC Heart Fail. 2014;2:84–92.
41. Lasaro MO, Ertl HCJ. New insights on adenovirus as vaccine vectors. Mol Ther. 2009;17:1333–9.
42. Naim C, Yerevanian A, Hajjar RJ. Gene therapy for heart failure: where do we stand? Curr Cardiol Rep. 2013;15:333.
43. Hammond HK. Adenylyl cyclase gene transfer in heart failure. Ann N Y Acad Sci. 2006;1080:426–36.
44. Argyros O, Wong SP, Harbottle RP. Non-viral episomal modification of cells using S/MAR elements. Expert Opin Biol Ther. 2011;11:1177–91.
45. Yockman JW, Kastenmeier A, Erickson HM, Brumbach JG, Whitten MG, Albanil A, et al. Novel polymer carriers and gene constructs for treatment of myocardial ischemia and infarction. J Control Release. 2008;132:260–6.
46. Kawase Y, Ladage D, Hajjar RJ. Rescuing the failing heart by targeted gene transfer. J Am Coll Cardiol. 2011;57:1169–80.
47. Milano CA, Allen LF, Rockman HA, Dolber PC, McMinn TR, Chien KR, et al. Enhanced myocardial function in transgenic mice overexpressing the beta 2-adrenergic receptor. Science. 1994;264:582–6.
48. Maurice JP, Hata JA, Shah AS, White DC, McDonald PH, Dolber PC, et al. Enhancement of cardiac function after adenoviral-mediated in vivo intracoronary beta2-adrenergic receptor gene delivery. J Clin Invest. 1999;104:21–9.
49. Shah AS, Lilly RE, Kypson AP, Tai O, Hata JA, Pippen A, et al. Intracoronary adenovirus-mediated delivery and overexpression of the beta(2)-adrenergic receptor in the heart: prospects for molecular ventricular assistance. Circulation. 2000;101:408–14.
50. Raake PW, Vinge LE, Gao E, Boucher M, Rengo G, Chen X, et al. G protein-coupled receptor kinase 2 ablation in cardiac myocytes before or after myocardial infarction prevents heart failure. Circ Res. 2008;103:413–22.
51. Shah AS, White DC, Emani S, Kypson AP, Lilly RE, Wilson K, et al. In vivo ventricular gene delivery of a beta-adrenergic receptor kinase inhibitor to the failing heart reverses cardiac dysfunction. Circulation. 2001;103:1311–6.
52. Gao MH, Lai NC, Roth DM, Zhou J, Zhu J, Anzai T, et al. Adenylylcyclase increases responsiveness to catecholamine stimulation in transgenic mice. Circulation. 1999;99:1618–22.
53. Lai NC, Roth DM, Gao MH, Tang T, Dalton N, Lai YY, et al. Intracoronary adenovirus encoding adenylyl

cyclase VI increases left ventricular function in heart failure. Circulation. 2004;110:330–6.
54. Gwathmey JK, Copelas L, MacKinnon R, Schoen FJ, Feldman MD, Grossman W, et al. Abnormal intracellular calcium handling in myocardium from patients with end-stage heart failure. Circ Res. 1987;61:70–6.
55. Miyamoto MI, del Monte F, Schmidt U, DiSalvo TS, Kang ZB, Matsui T, et al. Adenoviral gene transfer of SERCA2a improves left-ventricular function in aortic-banded rats in transition to heart failure. Proc Natl Acad Sci U S A. 2000;97:793–8.
56. del Monte F, Harding SE, Schmidt U, Matsui T, Kang ZB, Dec GW, et al. Restoration of contractile function in isolated cardiomyocytes from failing human hearts by gene transfer of SERCA2a. Circulation. 1999;100:2308–11.
57. Sakata S, Lebeche D, Sakata N, Sakata Y, Chemaly ER, Liang LF, et al. Restoration of mechanical and energetic function in failing aortic-banded rat hearts by gene transfer of calcium cycling proteins. J Mol Cell Cardiol. 2007;42:852–61.
58. Lyon AR, Bannister ML, Collins T, Pearce E, Sepehripour AH, Dubb SS, et al. SERCA2a gene transfer decreases sarcoplasmic reticulum calcium leak and reduces ventricular arrhythmias in a model of chronic heart failure. Circ Arrhythm Electrophysiol. 2011;4:362–72.
59. Hadri L, Bobe R, Kawase Y, Ladage D, Ishikawa K, Atassi F, et al. SERCA2a gene transfer enhances eNOS expression and activity in endothelial cells. Mol Ther. 2010;18:1284–92.
60. Wahlquist C, Jeong D, Rojas-Muñoz A, Kho C, Lee A, Mitsuyama S, et al. Inhibition of *miR-25* improves cardiac contractility in the failing heart. Nature. 2014. doi:10.1038/nature13073.
61. Suckau L, Fechner H, Chemaly E, Krohn S, Hadri L, Kockskämper J, et al. Long-term cardiac-targeted RNA interference for the treatment of heart failure restores cardiac function and reduces pathological hypertrophy. Circulation. 2009;119:1241–52.
62. Nicolaou P, Rodriguez P, Ren X, Zhou X, Qian J, Sadayappan S, et al. Inducible expression of active protein phosphatase-1 inhibitor-1 enhances basal cardiac function and protects against ischemia/reperfusion injury. Circ Res. 2009;104:1012–20.
63. Ghadge SK, Muhlstedt S, Ozcelik C, Bader M. SDF-1alpha as a therapeutic stem cell homing factor in myocardial infarction. Pharmacol Ther. 2011;129:97–108.
64. Behfar A, Crespo-Diaz R, Terzic A, Gersh BJ. Cell therapy for cardiac repair –lessons from clinical trials. Nat Rev Cardiol. 2014;11:232–46.

Cell Therapy in Cardiac Diseases

30

Vasileios Sousonis, Konstantinos Malliaras, John Terrovitis†, and John Nanas

Abstract

The mammalian heart is nowadays viewed as a dynamic organ, capable of endogenous regeneration. However, the intrinsic rate of cardiomyocyte renewal is low and cannot make up for the extensive loss of cardiomyocytes occurring after a major heart injury, such as a myocardial infarction. Multiple cell types (including skeletal myoblasts, bone marrow-derived cells, heart-derived progenitor cells, embryonic stem cells and induced pluripotent stem cells) have been used in preclinical animal models and in clinical trials to repair or regenerate the injured heart, either directly (through formation of new transplanted tissue) or indirectly (through paracrine stimulation of endogenous regeneration). Herein, we provide a critical assessment of the various cell types used for heart repair and regeneration, discuss the insights arising from the first decade of clinical trials, and touch upon future directions of cell therapy for heart disease.

Keywords

Heart regeneration • Cell therapy • Progenitor cells • Myocardial infarction • Cardiosphere-derived cells

Abbreviations

BMMNCs	Bone marrow mononuclear cells
CABG	Coronary bypass grafting
CDCs	Cardiosphere-derived cells
CPCs	Cardiac progenitor cells
CSps	Cardiospheres
EF	Ejection fraction
EPCs	Endothelial progenitor cells
ESCs	Embryonic stem cells
GCSF	Granulocyte colony stimulating factor
HSCs	Hematopoietic stem cells
iPSCs	Induced pluripotent stem cells
LV	Left ventricle
MI	Myocardial infarction
MRI	Magnetic resonance imaging
MSCs	Mesenchymal stromal cells
SKMs	Skeletal myoblasts

†This Chapter is dedicated to the memory of John Terrovitis

V. Sousonis, MD • K. Malliaras, MD (✉)
J. Terrovitis†, MD • J. Nanas, MD, PhD
3rd Department of Cardiology, University of Athens, 67th Mikras Asias str, Athens 11527, Greece
e-mail: malliaras@gmail.com

D.V. Cokkinos (ed.), *Introduction to Translational Cardiovascular Research*,
DOI 10.1007/978-3-319-08798-6_30, © Springer International Publishing Switzerland 2015

30.1 Heart Regeneration and Cell Therapy

Heart disease is, and is predicted to remain (at least until 2030), the single leading cause of death globally [1]. Cardiomyocyte deficiency underlies most types of heart disease. The human left ventricle (LV) contains ~4 billion myocytes, and a myocardial infarction (MI) can instantly wipe out up to 40 % of these. Cardiac pressure and/or volume overload (e.g. due to hypertension or valvular heart disease) result in gradual slow myocyte death over long periods of time, while normal ageing is associated with the loss of ~20 million myocytes per year [2]. While conventional therapies aim to limit myocardial injury and to block maladaptive pathways, the "holy grail" of therapy for heart disease is to achieve myocardial regeneration (i.e. regrow healthy working heart muscle).

Endogenous heart regeneration has been a controversial issue for decades. The human heart was traditionally viewed as a terminally differentiated organ, incapable of postnatal cardiomyogenesis (i.e. generation of new cardiomyocytes); the potential for cardiac regeneration was only recognized in lower vertebrate species, like newts and zebrafish [2]. Nowadays, the concept of the adult mammalian heart as a dynamic organ capable of endogenous regeneration has been convincingly established [3]. However, the rate of new cardiomyocyte formation is clearly low [3] and inadequate to replenish the substantial losses of cells occurring after major cardiac injuries.

During the last 13 years, cell therapy has emerged as a potentially useful approach to achieve therapeutic regeneration of the diseased heart [4]. Multiple cell types with progenitor properties (including skeletal myoblasts, bone marrow-derived cells, heart-derived cells, embryonic stem cells and induced pluripotent stem cells) have been used in preclinical animal models and in clinical trials to repair or regenerate the injured heart, either directly (through formation of new transplanted tissue) or indirectly (through paracrine stimulation of endogenous regeneration). Although no consensus has yet emerged, the ideal cell type for the treatment of heart disease [4], from a theoretic standpoint, should:

(a) be safe, i.e. not be tumorigenic or arrhythmiogenic;
(b) improve heart function and structure (attenuate or reverse adverse cardiac remodeling);
(c) generate (directly or indirectly) functional cardiac muscle and vasculature, structurally and functionally integrated into the host tissue;
(d) be easily harvested using routine clinical methods, readily grown in large numbers, and amenable to delivery by minimally invasive approaches;
(e) be available as a standardized "off the shelf" product that can be readily administered in the clinical setting;
(f) be tolerated by the immune system;
(g) not raise ethical concerns.

At present, the "perfect" cell for the treatment of heart disease remains elusive; however, it is apparent that some cell types are more promising than others.

Herein, we critically assess the various cell types used in efforts to achieve heart regeneration (focusing on large scale randomized controlled clinical trials, where available), discuss the insights arising from the first decade of clinical trials, and touch upon future directions of cell therapy for heart disease.

30.2 The Road to Clinical Application

Figure 30.1 depicts the ideal "pathway to clinical application" of cell therapy for heart disease, and how far along this path each candidate cell type has progressed [5]. The pathway begins with preclinical small- and large-animal studies, before moving on to human subjects. The goal of small-animal studies is to investigate cell product safety and efficacy, and provide insight into mechanisms of action. Subsequently, experiments in large animals should be performed to optimize the cell product's clinical formulation, dose, and delivery method, as well as to test safety and efficacy in clinically relevant

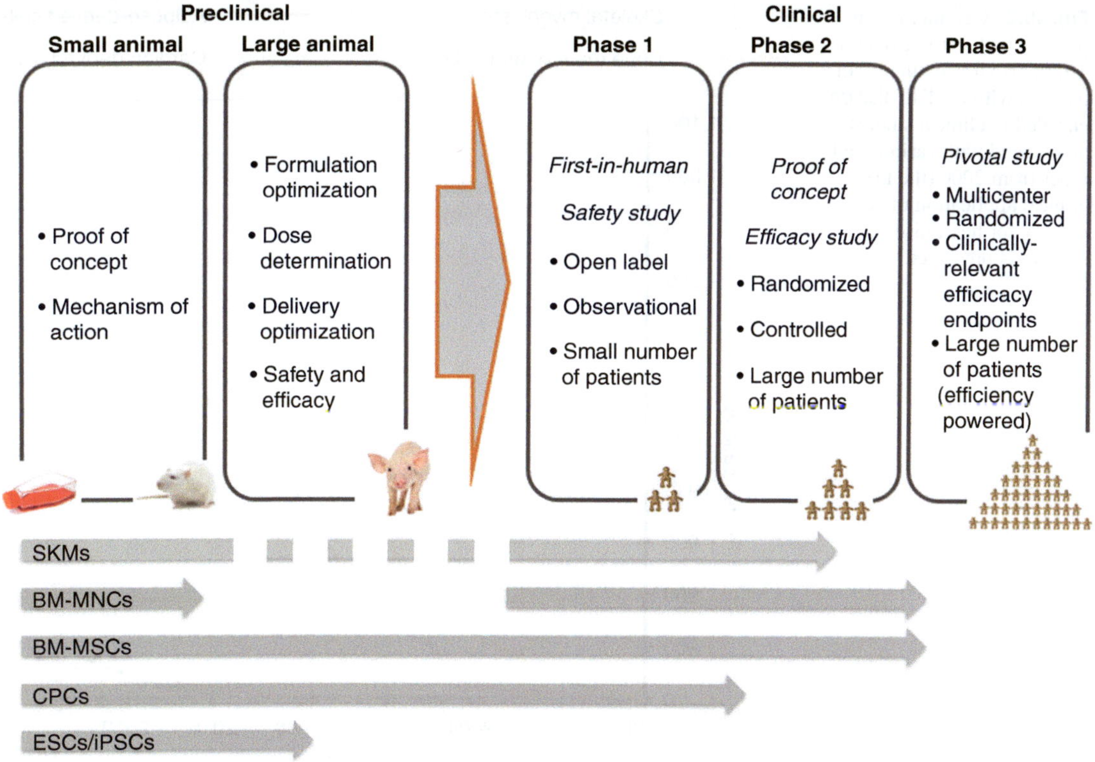

Fig. 30.1 The pathway to clinical translation. Vital steps along the path involve small-animal studies (proof-of-concept studies and studies to investigate the mechanism of action) and large-animal studies (to optimize dosage, formulation, and delivery as well as to test safety and efficacy in clinically relevant models), before moving on to human subjects. Skeletal myoblasts (*SKMs*) followed a fairly convincing preclinical developmental program (without systematic testing in large animals) before moving on to humans; they are currently being tested in phase 2 trials. On the other hand, bone marrow mononuclear cells (*BM-MNCs*) entered the clinical arena immediately after the first reports of rodent studies; currently large-scale phase 3 outcome trials are about to commence. In the case of bone marrow mesenchymal stromal cells (*BM-MSCs*) and heart-derived cells, a more logical and systematic approach for clinical translation has been employed; BM-MSCs are now entering phase 3 trials while heart-derived cells are currently being tested in phase 2 trials. Embryonic stem cells (ESCs) and induced pluripotent stem cells (iPSCs) are currently being tested in large animals. The *arrows* represent the progression of the discussed cell types along the path to clinical translation

models before moving into first-in-human clinical trials. Figure 30.2 depicts the approximate number of patients with cardiac disease enrolled in clinical studies and treated with various cell types from 2000 (the first clinical application of cell therapy for heart disease) to 2013. Such clinical studies begin with safety (phase 1) to determine whether the cell product is tolerated in humans, often with a dose-ranging protocol. If no significant safety concerns are raised, an efficacy signal is sought in phase II trials, which enroll a larger patient population. Phases 1 and 2 can be combined in a way that a relatively small study yields both preliminary safety and efficacy data; such phase 1/2 trials need to be prospective, randomized, controlled, with pre-specified exploratory efficacy endpoints and blinded data analysis. The goal in phase 2 is to determine the efficacy readout for a larger phase 3 trial, which is powered for efficacy and for rare safety events that may have been missed in earlier phases. The primary endpoint of phase 3 trials should reflect clinically relevant effects (morbidity and/or mortality) and the goal is to prove the efficacy of the new therapy over the current standard of care.

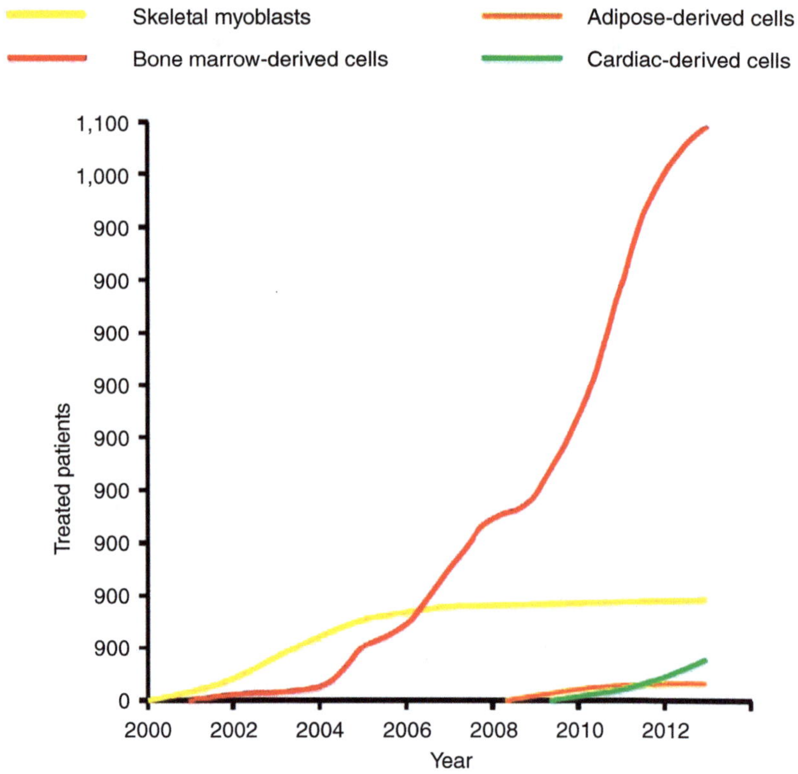

Fig. 30.2 Cell therapy in patients with cardiac disease. The approximate number of patients with cardiac disease enrolled in clinical studies and treated with various cell types from 2000 (the first clinical application of cell therapy for heart disease) to 2013 is presented

Within this framework, we now consider and critically assess each of the major cell types that has been tested (or is planned to be tested in the case of embryonic stem cells/induced pluripotent stem cells) in patients.

30.3 Skeletal Myoblasts

Skeletal myoblasts (SKMs), mononucleated cells located between the basal lamina and the sarcolemma of skeletal myofibers, are activated, proliferate, differentiate and fuse to form new skeletal muscle fibers (myotubes) in response to injury. They are resistant to ischemia, and can be easily harvested in abundant numbers and expanded for autologous transplantation. These features, along with their myogenic phenotype, have made SKMs an attractive population for cardiac repair and regeneration.

Preclinical experimental studies suggested that administration of autologous SKMs improves LV function and attenuates remodeling in animal models of ischemic heart disease [6, 7]. In recipient myocardium, SKMs differentiate into multinucleated myotubes (not cardiomyocytes) that lack expression of connexin-43 and gap junctions, forming islands of conduction block that slow conduction velocity and create the substrate for reentrant arrhythmias [8].

After a decade of experimental studies [6, 7] SKMs were the first cell type to enter the clinical arena for heart regeneration. In June 2000 autologous SKMs, isolated and expanded from a thigh muscle biopsy, were intramyocardially injected in a patient with severe ischemic heart failure as an adjunct to coronary bypass grafting (CABG) surgery [9]. Several small non-randomized phase I studies ensued demonstrating functional benefit in treated patients, albeit with a high incidence of ventricular arrhythmias, confirming the concerns raised by preclinical research [10, 11]. The first phase II SKM trial, MAGIC, enrolled patients with chronic ischemic cardiomyopathy randomized to receive direct intramyocardial injections (as an adjunct to CABG surgery) of autologous myoblasts or placebo solution. The MAGIC trial failed to demonstrate efficacy and was discontinued prematurely, while a trend towards more ventricular arrhythmias in the treated groups was observed, despite the prophylactic use of amiodarone [12]. Increased incidence of ventricular arrhythmias in treated patients was also observed in the pilot MARVEL-1 study, a randomized, placebo-controlled trial of catheter-guided SKM transplantation in patients with ischemic heart failure that was also discontinued prematurely (due to financial reasons) [13]. On the other hand, the SEISMIC trial demonstrated a more favorable safety profile of catheter-guided SKM administration in patients with ischemic heart failure, along with a trend towards increased exercise tolerance in treated patients; nevertheless, no significant effect on LV ejection fraction (EF) was observed [14]. Taken together, the trajectory of SKMs is instructive and argues against premature enthusiasm solely on the basis of preclinical studies.

30.4 Bone Marrow-Derived Cells

The bone marrow is a highly heterogeneous tissue, containing several different cell populations with progenitor-like properties. These progenitor cells can be roughly divided into the following three categories: (a) hematopoietic stem cells (HSCs) that can give rise to all types of mature blood cells; (b) endothelial progenitor cells (EPCs), a subset of hematopoietic cells that promote neovascularization either directly (differentiation into endothelial cells) or indirectly (secretion of pro-angiogenic cytokines); and (c) mesenchymal stromal cells (MSCs) that can differentiate into osteoblasts, chondroblasts and adipocytes.

In the clinical field, bone-marrow derived cells have been administered in the following forms: (a) autologous bone marrow mononuclear cells (BMMNCs) either unfractionated or after purification for a progenitor cell marker (CD34 or CD133); and (b) autologous or allogeneic MSCs. These cellular products are considered individually below.

30.4.1 Bone Marrow Mononuclear Cells

Unlike SKMs, BMMNCs moved into patients without the benefit of a convincing preclinical development program; the first report of clinical application of BMMNCs for heart regeneration [15] surfaced within 4 months of the publication of a rodent study reporting extensive engraftment and cardiogenic differentiation of bone marrow-derived cells in mice [16]. Clinical application was catalyzed by the relative accessibility of bone marrow, the large numbers of unfractionated autologous cells that can be obtained without ex vivo expansion, and the extensive clinical experience with bone marrow transplantation. Ironically, the initial report of extensive transdifferentiation of bone marrow-derived cells into cardiomyocytes has proven to be controversial; several laboratories have been unable to reproduce the findings [17, 18]. Nevertheless, clinical studies have continued apace. It should be noted that BMMNCs, isolated by density centrifugation of bone marrow aspirates, actually contain very few progenitor cells (~2–4 % HSCs/EPCs and ~0.01 % MSCs); the vast majority of BMMNCs comprise committed hematopoietic cells at various stages of maturation [19].

In the clinical setting, autologous BMMNCs are by far the most frequently administered cell type for treatment of heart disease and have been used primarily in the setting of acute MI. To date >1,000 patients have been treated with BMMNCs in numerous clinical trials worldwide. As with SKMs, early small and uncontrolled pilot studies of BMMNC delivery after acute MI demonstrated consistently positive results [20, 21]. However, the results of later large randomized studies of intracoronary infusion of BMMNCs in acute MI have been conflicting. The first large-scale randomized but not placebo-controlled study (BOOST) demonstrated a transient functional benefit (increase in EF) at 6 months after BMMNC infusion [22] that was not sustained at 18 months or 5 years after therapy [23]. Two subsequent placebo-controlled studies yielded varied results: REPAIR-AMI showed a significant improvement in EF at 4 months [24], whereas a study by Jannsens et al. [25] (in which BMMNCs were infused within 24 h after reperfusion, earlier than in the other studies) showed no improvement in EF at 4 months but a more profound decrease in scar size in cell-treated patients. In contrast to the previous studies, results of the randomized but not placebo-controlled ASTAMI trial were resoundingly negative [26]. The results of subsequent large randomized studies have also been conflicting, ranging from: (a) positive: the FINCELL trial [27], the first study of BMMNC infusion in patients treated with thrombolysis, showed improvement of EF at 6 months; (b) marginally positive: in the REGENT study [28], EF improved in the cell-treated patients but not in controls at 6 months; however, no difference was observed when the treatment effect was compared among groups; (c) mixed: in the BONAMI trial no difference in EF but an increase in myocardial viability was observed after BMMNC therapy [29]; or (d) resoundingly negative: in the HEBE trial [30], SCAMI trial [31], TIME trial [32], LateTIME trial [33], and SWISS-AMI trial [34] no benefits of BMMNC infusion in patients with acute MI were observed. The reasons for the inconsistent outcomes of the aforementioned clinical trials are unclear but may be attributed to differences in cell isolation and preparation protocols [35]. Nevertheless, a recent meta-analysis (including 811 patients participating in 13 randomized trials) showed modest but significant benefit following BMMNC therapy: EF increased by ~3 %, end-systolic volume decreased by ~5 ml and scar size decreased by ~3.5 % in the cell-treated groups compared with controls [36].

Critically reviewing the accumulated data of BMMNC therapy in the acute MI setting, a number of conclusions can be drawn:

(i) Intracoronary infusion of autologous BMMNCs through a recently reopened infarct-related coronary artery is feasible and safe. Infusion is not associated with additional ischemic myocardial damage [22], increased incidence of arrhythmias [27] or increased in-stent/culprit vessel restenosis [27, 36];
(ii) Sustained functional benefits after BMMNC therapy in acute MI remain in doubt;
(iii) The patient population enrolled in BMMNC trials was not very ill at baseline (first MI population receiving prompt reperfusion, with a median EF of ~50 % pre-therapy) leaving little room for improvement.

The legacy of the studies of BMMNC therapy in acute MI has left the field puzzled. The next (and possibly definitive) chapter for BMMNCs will be the BAMI study (NCT01569178), a large phase 3 trial to be conducted in Europe with all-cause mortality as the primary endpoint. 3,000 patients with acute MI and EF <45 % will be randomized to either conventional therapy or intracoronary infusion of autologous BMMNCs. The BAMI study is powered to detect a 25 % relative decrease in 2-year all-cause mortality after cell therapy (11.5 % vs. 8.6 %). This highly anticipated study will hopefully answer, once and for all, whether BMMNCs are a useful adjunctive therapy in acute MI.

BMMNCs have also been used for the treatment of refractory angina. To date, four randomized controlled studies have been published. The study by van Ramhorst et al. showed that catheter-guided injection of BMMNCs resulted in improvements in myocardial perfusion as assessed by single photon emission computed tomography and EF at 3 months after therapy [37]; such improvements were not observed, however, in the PROTECT-CAD trial and the study by Losordo et al. (catheter-guided injection of BMMNCs and granulocyte colony stimulating factor [GCSF]–mobilized CD34+ cells, respectively) [38, 39]. A subsequent placebo-controlled phase 2 trial by the Losordo group, in which patients with refractory angina were randomized to receive catheter-guided transendocardial injections of GCSF-mobilized autologous CD34+ cells (collected from the peripheral blood via leukapheresis) or placebo, revealed significant improvements in symptoms (reduced angina frequency) and functional capacity (increased exercise tolerance) in cell-treated patients. However, cell-mobilization and collection procedures were associated with cardiac enzyme elevations in 4.6 % of patients [40]. CD34+ cells for the treatment of refractory angina are currently entering phase 3 trials (RENEW study, NCT01508910). In RENEW (which is currently recruiting participants) 444 patients with refractory angina will be randomized in a 2:1:1 fashion to cell therapy (transendocardial injection of GCSF-mobilized autologous CD34+ cells collected from the peripheral blood via leukapheresis), active control (GCSF-mediated stem cell mobilization, apheresis, and intramyocardial placebo injection), or open-label standard of care. The primary efficacy endpoint of RENEW is change in exercise treadmill time (the study has 90 % power to detect a 60-s difference in exercise time between cell-treated and active control patients) [41].

Finally, BMMNCs have also been investigated in the setting of chronic ischemic cardiomyopathy and heart failure, albeit on a much smaller scale compared with acute MI (or to a lesser extent refractory angina). Early, small clinical studies have shown some hints of efficacy [42–44]. However, the FOCUS trial (a multicenter phase II, randomized, placebo-controlled trial investigating the efficacy of transendocardial injection of BMMNCs in patients with chronic ischemic cardiomyopathy and heart failure) was resoundingly negative and failed to meet any of its pre-specified efficacy endpoints (no change in end-systolic left ventricular volumes, maximal oxygen consumption or myocardial perfusion) [45].

With regard to mechanism of action, well designed studies employing genetic labeling techniques have convincingly demonstrated that bone marrow-derived cells cannot readily transdifferentiate into cardiomyocytes. Thus, the prevailing concept of bone marrow-derived cell bioactivity has shifted towards the 'paracrine hypothesis', according to which the transplanted cells are proposed to produce soluble factors that are beneficial to the infarcted heart. With regard to the latter, studies in rodents have shown that exogenously administered bone marrow-derived cells can indirectly (in a paracrine manner) protect resident cardiomyocytes from apoptosis, stimulate angiogenesis and upregulate recruitment of endogenous cardiac progenitors in the infarcted heart [46].

30.4.2 Bone Marrow Mesenchymal Stromal Cells

MSCs reside in the bone marrow and their physiologic role is to create/function as a stromal network supporting the differentiation of HSCs into blood lineages. MSCs are self-renewing cells characterized by: (1) adherence to plastic in culture; (2) surface expression of CD105, CD90, and CD73; (3) lack of expression of hematopoietic markers; and (4) the capacity to differentiate into osteoblasts, adipocytes, and chondroblasts under specific in vitro conditions. While the ability of MSCs to undergo true cardiomyogenic transdifferentiation remains highly controversial [47, 48], MSCs are known to secrete a broad variety of cytokines, chemokines and growth factors involved in cardiac repair. To that end, preclinical animal studies have shown that MSCs can indirectly (in a paracrine manner) protect resident cardiomyocytes from apoptosis [49], promote angiogenesis [50], stimulate proliferation of endogenous cardiac progenitors and amplify resident cardiomyocyte cell-cycle re-entry in the infarcted heart [51]. These indirect mechanisms seem to underlie the reduction in infarct size, attenuation of LV remodeling and improvement in cardiac function observed in large animal models of MI and chronic ischemic cardiomyopathy [52, 53].

In the clinical field, MSCs have been primarily used in the setting of chronic ischemic cardiomyopathy. The Hare group performed a head-to-head comparison of autologous bone marrow-derived MSCs versus autologous BMMNCs (delivered by catheter-guided transendocardial injections) in patients with chronic ischemic cardiomyopathy (randomized-controlled TAC-HFT study) [54]. While both MSCs and BMMNCs did not raise significant safety concerns and improved quality of life, only MSCs (but not BMMNCs) decreased scar size, improved regional contractility and increased 6-min walk distance. However, chamber volumes and EF did not improve with either cell population.

The benefit of autologous MSC therapy may be enhanced by exposing cells in vitro to a "cardiogenic cocktail", a combination of cytokines that promotes adoption of a cardiopoietic phenotype (as indicated by expression of cardiac transcription factors in bone marrow-derived MSCs) [55]. In a rodent study by the Terzic group, infarcted animals treated with "cardiopoietic" bone marrow-derived MSCs derived greater functional benefit compared to animals treated with naïve MSCs [55]. The first clinical trial of "cardiopoietic" bone marrow-derived MSCs (delivered by catheter-guided transendocardial injections) for the treatment of ischemic heart failure, the randomized controlled C-CURE trial, demonstrated the safety and feasibility of this approach. C-CURE also revealed intriguing hints of efficacy: treatment with "cardiopoietic" MSCs improved systolic function, reduced LV end-systolic volume and improved 6-min walk distance compared to standard of care [56]. Following this initial study, a larger phase 3 trial powered to evaluate efficacy in ischemic heart failure patients has been approved and is currently recruiting participants (the CHART-1 study, with a composite primary endpoint comprising mortality, worsening of heart failure, quality of life, exercise capacity, cardiac volumes and EF [NCT01768702]).

Bone marrow-derived MSCs lack major histocompatibility complex class II receptors and costimulatory molecules, and possess immunomodulatory/immunosuppressive properties; these characteristics have made them attractive for allogeneic transplantation (without immunosuppression). A randomized, placebo-controlled trial of intravenous infusion of proprietary allogeneic bone marrow-derived MSCs (Prochymal, Osiris) in patients with acute MI did not raise any significant safety concerns and revealed hints of efficacy (improved EF) [57]. The latter is somewhat paradoxical, taking into account that preclinical studies have demonstrated that intravenous infusion is hampered by trapping of cells in the lungs, resulting in acute cardiac retention rates of <1 % [58]. With regard to chronic ischemic cardiomyopathy, the Hare group recently performed a head-to-head comparison between autologous and allogeneic bone marrow-derived MSCs, delivered by catheter-guided transendocardial injections. The major finding of POSEIDON is that therapy with allogeneic MSCs (without immunosuppression) appears to be safe and at least as effective as therapy with autologous MSCs (both allogeneic and autologous MSCs reduced infarct size and LV sphericity index but did not increase EF) [59]. The results of POSEIDON are encouraging, particularly with regard to the safety of allogeneic MSCs, but the small sample size and the lack of a proper control group (receiving standard of care without cell therapy) should prompt some caution regarding claims of efficacy [35]. With regard to heart failure, catheter-guided transendocardial injection of allogeneic proprietary stro-3+ bone marrow-derived MSCs (Revascor, Mesoblast) in 60 patients with ischemic and non-ischemic heart failure was not associated with a clinically significant immune response and resulted in a significant reduction of major adverse cardiac event rate. A phase III study of catheter-guided transendocardial injection of allogeneic stro-3+ bone marrow-derived MSCs is currently in preparation and plans to enroll 1,700 heart failure patients (Mesoblast). The primary efficacy endpoint of the trial is a time-to-first event analysis of heart failure-related major adverse cardiac events (defined as a composite of cardiac related death and decompensated heart failure events).

Bone marrow aside, subcutaneous adipose tissue is an alternative source of MSCs. Like bone marrow-derived MSCs, adipose-derived MSCs produce cytokines that promote angiogenesis, improve cardiac function and attenuate adverse remodeling in animal models of acute MI [60]. Importantly, autologous adipose-derived MSCs can be easily harvested in abundant numbers from lipoaspirates (with no need for ex vivo expansion, in contrast to bone marrow-derived MSCs); this enables therapeutic administration of an autologous cell product early in the course of an acute MI. In the clinical field, the randomized, placebo-controlled APOLLO trial demonstrated the feasibility and safety of intracoronary infusion of autologous adipose-derived MSCs in the setting of acute MI [61]. In addition, cell infusion in the APOLLO trial resulted in significant reductions in myocardial perfusion defect and scar size; however, the very small size of the control group (n=4) precludes any efficacy-related conclusions. The efficacy of intracoronary infusion of autologous adipose-derived MSCs in the setting of acute MI is currently being investigated in the phase 2 ADVANCE trial (NCT01216995). In addition, ongoing clinical studies are assessing a potential role of adipose-derived MSCs in ischemic heart failure and refractory angina.

30.5 Heart-Derived Progenitor Cells

During the past decade several studies supported the notion that the adult mammalian heart contains its own reservoir of progenitor cells. Numerous populations of putative adult endogenous cardiac progenitor cells (CPCs) have been proposed, largely based on expression of surface markers or functional properties that have been used to mark progenitors in other organs. Putative adult CPCs include: c-kit$^+$ (CD117$^+$, the receptor for stem cell antigen) cells [62], cardiosphere-forming cells (CSps, three-dimensional structures of CPCs and supportive cells) [63], cardiosphere-derived cells (CDCs) [64], sca-1$^+$ cells (stem cell antigen-1$^+$ cells) [65], cardiac side population cells [66], and SSEA-1$^+$ (stage-specific embryonic antigen-1$^+$) cells [67]. The high number of distinct populations of putative endogenous CPCs is difficult to reconcile with the limited regenerative capacity of the adult mammalian heart. Importantly, while all of the aforementioned cell types have been shown to express cardiac proteins *in vitro* or after delivery into recipient hearts following *ex vivo* expansion, their physiologic importance and contribution to cardiomyocyte replenishment in the normal or injured adult heart remains a topic of intense debate. Nevertheless, most studies suggest that endogenous CPCs (the identity of which still remains elusive) may generate new myocytes in the adult heart. While the role of endogenous CPCs in postnatal cardiomyogenesis during normal ageing appears to be limited (as most studies concur that myocyte turnover in the healthy aging heart most likely occurs through proliferation of pre-existing myocytes [68, 69]), multiple studies indicate CPC-mediated cardiomyocyte renewal occurs following myocardial injury [68–70]. From a therapeutic perspective, since CPCs may presumably be endogenously programmed to replenish heart muscle, their isolation and ex vivo expansion for the treatment of heart diseases seems a logical (yet challenging) strategy. So far, only c-kit$^+$ cells and CDCs have proceeded into human studies; these cellular products are considered individually below.

30.5.1 C-kit$^+$ Cells

C-kit$^+$ cells are self-renewing, clonogenic and can differentiate in vitro and in vivo into endothelial cells, smooth muscle cells and (possibly) cardiomyocytes [62]. Delivery of c-kit$^+$ cells in small and large animal models of MI and ischemic cardiomyopathy results in improved systolic performance and attenuation of LV remodeling purportedly through generation of newly-formed cardiomyocytes and vessels by transplanted cells [62, 71, 72]. However, the ability of c-kit$^+$ cells to readily differentiate into cardiomyocytes has been disputed by several studies reporting that adult c-kit$^+$ cells have only angiogenic but not cardiomyogenic potential [73]. With regard to clinical translation, intracoronary infusion of autologous c-kit$^+$ cells (isolated from right atrial appendages discarded during CABG surgery) in surgically revascularized patients with chronic ischemic heart failure is currently being investigated in the phase 1 SCIPIO trial. An interim analysis of the still-ongoing SCIPIO trial revealed that administration of c-kit$^+$ cells resulted in striking improvement in EF (measured by echo), that was not observed in control patients [74]. MRI (which was only performed in a subset of treated patients but not in controls) revealed a significant reduction in scar mass and a significant increase in viable myocardium after cell therapy [75]. While SCIPIO demonstrated that isolation and intracoronary infusion of c-kit cells is feasible and does not raise significant safety concerns, claims of efficacy are undermined by methodological concerns (poor randomization scheme, lack of MRI in control patients, and confounding effect of CABG surgery which can by itself result in gradual natural improvement of heart function) [76].

30.5.2 Cardiosphere Derived Cells

CDCs are a naturally heterogeneous cell population of intrinsic cardiac origin. CDCs are uniformly positive for CD105, while a subset of CDCs (~25 %) is positive for CD90 (a marker of MSCs) and a small fraction (~3–10 %) is positive for c-kit (a putative marker of endogenous CPCs [as explained above]) [64]. CDCs can be readily grown in clinically relevant numbers from percutaneous endomyocardial biopsy specimens [64], and exhibit clonogenicity, self-renewal capacity and multipotentiality [77]. Several preclinical animal studies have demonstrated that CDCs can improve cardiac function, decrease scar size and increase viable myocardium post-MI in mice [64, 78], rats [79–81] and pigs [82, 83]. Importantly, the salutary effects of CDC transplantation cannot be explained by direct cardiomyogenic differentiation of transplanted cells (such events represent "needle in haystack" incidents [78, 81]) and should be attributed instead to indirect (paracrine) mechanisms of action. To that end, CDCs are potent secretors of cytokines that indirectly stimulate endogenous repair and regeneration [78, 81, 84], by promoting angiogenesis, recruitment of resident cardiac progenitor cells, and proliferation of preexisting cardiomyocytes in the infarct border zone [69, 78, 81]. This indirect mechanism of action (without the need for long-term engraftment of transplanted cells) rationalizes the efficacy of allogeneic CDCs; it has been shown that allogeneic CDCs are just as effective as syngeneic CDCs in a rat model of MI and in a pig model of ischemic cardiomyopathy [81, 83, 85]. With regard to clinical translation, a phase 1/2 clinical study of autologous CDCs—the CADUCEUS study, has been recently completed. In CADUCEUS, human subjects with convalescent MI (1.5–3 months post-MI) LV dysfunction (EF: 25–45 %) were randomized to receive intracoronary infusion of autologous CDCs (harvested from endomyocardial biopsies), or conventional treatment, by prospective randomized assignment. Intracoronary infusion of autologous CDCs did not raise significant safety concerns in CADUCEUS. Analysis of exploratory efficacy endpoints revealed a decrease in scar size, an increase in viable myocardium and improved regional function of infarcted myocardium (but not global function) in CDC-treated patients compared to controls [86, 87]. These intriguing hints of efficacy (which are consistent with therapeutic regeneration) need to be confirmed in future larger clinical trials. The safety and efficacy of allogeneic CDCs in human subjects with LV dysfunction post-MI is currently being tested in the phase 1/2 multicenter, randomized, placebo-controlled ALLSTAR trial (NCT01458405).

30.6 Embryonic Stem Cells and Induced Pluripotent Stem Cells

Embryonic stem cells (ESCs), derived from the inner mass of the developing embryo in the blastocyst stage, are the prototypical stem cells. They have the capacity of self-renewal, can be clonally expanded and are capable of differentiating into any cell type in the body, including atrial, ventricular and nodal cardiomyocytes. However, significant obstacles need to be overcome before ESCs can be used clinically for heart regeneration. First, the unlimited differentiation potential of ESCs is a double-edged sword: when ESCs are transplanted in their primitive undifferentiated state, they form teratomas in recipient hearts [88]. The risk of oncogenicity greatly diminishes after cardiomyogenic differentiation of ESCs in vitro prior to administration; the feasibility and safety of this approach has so far been demonstrated in small animal MI models [89]. Second, ESC-derived cardiac grafts could plausibly contribute to arrhythmogenesis through automaticity and triggered activity, while their irregular graft geometry/architecture (abnormal alignment of ESC-derived cardiomyocytes with host myocardium, smaller size of ESC-derived cardiomyocytes, abnormal distribution of connexins) could promote reentry [90]. Third, due to their allogeneic origin, ESCs carry the risk of immune rejection; there is now clear evidence that the differentiated progeny of ESCs are rejected by the host immune system [88]. Since ESCs regenerate the heart directly (through cardiomyogenic differentiation of exogenously administered cells), sustained benefits would presumably require permanent engraftment of transplanted ESCs, rendering the use of long-term immunosuppression in the clinical setting mandatory. Finally, ESCs are ethically problematic since they are created from early human embryos (discarded after in vitro fertilization).

In the past 6 years, induced pluripotent stem cells (iPSCs) from somatic (adult) cells have been generated through ectopic expression of selected transcription factors via viruses, plasmids, or bioengineered proteins [91]. The resultant iPSCs closely resemble ESCs and can be subsequently guided to differentiate into desired specific cell types (including cardiomyocytes) using specific protocols developed for ESC differentiation. These techniques make patient-specific (autologous) pluripotent stem cells an imaginable reality and provide an alternative source for cardiogenic cell lines; functional cardiomyocytes have been successfully derived from both mouse [92] and human iPSCs [93]. Nevertheless, significant roadblocks preclude near-term clinical applicability for heart regeneration, including the risk of oncogenicity associated with the pluripotent state, risk of arrhythmiogenicity, insertional mutagenesis due to integrating vectors, low efficiency of successful nuclear reprogramming and of subsequent cardiogenic differentiation, genetic abnormalities, potential immunogenicity despite the autologous origin, and high cost. Methods to expedite the generation of cardiomyocytes from noncontractile somatic cells, without transit through a pluripotent state, are intriguing [94]. Nevertheless, the use of genetically modified cells that have undergone nuclear reprogramming will most likely face significant regulatory hurdles before clinical applications commence.

Currently, both ESCs and iPSCs are being tested for cardiac applications in large animals. Rigorous safety studies (focusing primarily on arrhythmiogenicity and oncogenicity) are essential before these pluripotent cells can enter the arena of clinical investigation.

30.7 Future Directions

Going forward (and regardless of investigated cell type), the pursuit of improved methods for cell delivery, means to boost cardiac cell retention, more potent and better-standardized "off the shelf" cellular products, and more apt patient populations is certainly merited [4, 5]. These points are considered individually below.

30.7.1 The Challenge of Low Cell Retention After Cardiac Delivery

Low cell retention after delivery to the heart is a persistent obstacle to successful myocardial regeneration [79, 95]. Numerous studies have investigated short-term cell retention both in experimental animals [96] and in humans [97] and the results have been overwhelmingly disappointing; acute cell retention (i.e., within 24 h of delivery) in the heart is generally <10 %, regardless of the cell type or delivery route. Cells acutely lost from the heart are washed out via the coronary venous system or mechanically ejected via the injection site, while retention rates in beating hearts are markedly lower than in non-beating hearts [79]. Taking into account that studies of bone marrow-derived and heart-derived cells [65, 79, 98] reveal a strong correlation between acute cell retention and long-term functional benefit, there is good reason to believe that: (a) the development of more effective delivery methods, combined with (b) successful means of boosting transplanted cell retention (ensuring that once cells are delivered, they will biologically bond with the host tissue and survive), would significantly enhance the utility of cell therapy.

With regard to delivery methods, cellular products for heart repair have so far been delivered clinically via three routes: systemic intravenous infusion, intracoronary infusion, and intramyocardial injection (either by direct open-chest injections as an adjunct to CABG surgery or by transendocardial catheter-based injections), while retrograde coronary venous, transvenous intramyocardial and intrapericardial approaches have been used mostly in preclinical studies.

Intravenous infusion, albeit simple in execution, is hampered by trapping of cells in the lungs, resulting in acute retention rates of <1 % [58]. Intracoronary delivery of cells into a recanalized infarct-related artery is safe and convenient (can be performed with standard balloon catheters) and has the inherent advantage that cells are homogeneously infused into myocardial regions with preserved oxygen and nutrient supply.

However, retention of cells is suboptimal (most cells are washed away before they can migrate into the surrounding tissue), unperfused regions of the myocardium are inaccessible, and the high dependence on endogenous homing signals makes this approach more attractive for use relatively early after acute MI, when such signals are highly expressed. In addition, safety concerns are raised during infusion of larger cells because of potential capillary plugging and microinfarction; this problem, if recognized, can be overcome by appropriate cell dosing and optimization of the infusate [82]. It should be noted, however, that in the vast majority of preclinical and clinical studies to date dosing has, by and large, been arbitrary, guided more by feasibility and accessibility than by systematic dosage optimization; a remarkable 6,700-fold range in cell dose is observed in human bone marrow-derived cell trials [99]. All things considered, the intracoronary delivery route seems to be best suited for the treatment of acute MI. With regard to heart failure, intracoronary infusion into multiple coronary vessels, allowing for delivery of higher total cell doses (compared with infusion into one artery only) and greater myocardial coverage (also targeting remote uninfarcted remodeled myocardium), may be potentially useful [100].

On the other hand, intramyocardial delivery (either open chest or catheter-based) results in better cardiac retention of cells (and less washout to off-target organs) compared to intracoronary [96] or systemic approaches [58]. In addition, it can access unperfused myocardial regions and can allow for delivery of high number of cells (up to one billion cells [56]) that would be microembolic if delivered intracoronarily. However, intramyocardial delivery is invasive and results in highly localized cell distribution around the injection sites [101]. Since freshly infarcted myocardium might engender a higher risk of perforation, intramyocardial delivery may probably be more suitable for patients with chronic ischemic cardiomyopathy and for patients with refractory ischemia lacking options for revascularization.

Delivery optimization should be combined with strategies to increase cell retention. Multiple lines of evidence indicate that strategies that effectively boost acute retention translate into greater functional benefit downstream [79, 80]. Several methods have been used, including: (a) priming of host tissue to increase homing, (b) preconditioning of transplanted cells with cytokines, prosurvival factors and physical stimuli, (c) genetic engineering of cells, (d) use of biomaterial scaffolds, and (e) delivery of three-dimensional cellular aggregates [95]. While much work has focused on improving transplanted cell quality and creating a more hospitable host environment, most cells are mechanically ejected via the injection site or washed away too quickly to be effective. Physical approaches (capping the injection site with fibrin glue to prevent back-flux of injected cells [79] and magnetic targeting of iron-loaded cells [80] to retain cells in the diseased tissue long enough to enable biologic bonding) may boost treatment efficacy and would be synergistic with efforts to improve cell quality or environmental receptiveness.

30.7.2 Use of Allogeneic Cells

In the first decade of cell therapy for human heart regeneration, most clinical trials have been conducted using autologous cells. Autologous sources are attractive because immunologic rejection is avoided by default. Nevertheless, autologous therapy is associated with serious limitations that complicate widespread clinical application. Specifically, autologous therapy necessitates patient-specific tissue harvesting, cell processing, and quality control, which pose significant logistic, economic, and timing constraints, thus limiting the scalability of cell therapy for heart diseases. In addition, progenitor cell growth properties and plasticity may be hampered by age and comorbidities [102], resulting in interpatient variability in cell potency. The use of allogeneic cells, if safe and effective, would obviate such limitations, enabling the generation of highly-standardized "off the shelf" cellular products and thus opening up a new treatment paradigm. Progenitor cells could be grown in large numbers from allogeneic tissue sources in a central facility under strict quality control and banked for future use, enabling safe and effective myocardial repair and regeneration in a timely, cost-efficient manner. The obvious disadvantage of allogeneic therapy is the risk of immune rejection, which may limit effectiveness (whether or not it poses safety hazards) and potential development of immune memory.

To that end, bone marrow-derived MSCs and heart-derived CDCs (both of which have been shown to be hypoimmunogenic cells lacking major histocompatibility complex class II receptors and costimulatory molecules) have attracted interest as therapeutic allogeneic agents. In the POSEIDON trial a head-to-head comparison between autologous and allogeneic MSCs was performed in patients with chronic ischemic cardiomyopathy. The major finding of POSEIDON is that therapy with allogeneic MSCs (without immunosuppression) appears to be safe and at least as effective as therapy with autologous MSCs [59], even though the small sample size and the lack of a proper control group (receiving standard of care without cell therapy) preclude definite conclusions [35]. Importantly, the theoretical risk of allosensitization appears to be low; only 1 of 15 patients in POSEIDON developed donor-specific antibodies, even without immunosuppression. A low risk of allosensitization was also observed in the MESOBLAST trial, in which only 2 of 45 patients developed persisting donor-specific antibodies after catheter-guided transendocardial injection of allogeneic MSCs (without immunosuppression). With regard to CDCs, their safety and efficacy as allogeneic agents has been validated in preclinical small- [81, 85] and large-animal [83] models. Allogeneic CDCs are now undergoing phase 1/2 clinical testing in the placebo-controlled ALLSTAR study of 270 patients with LV dysfunction post-MI (NCT01458405).

It should be noted that, without immunosuppression or HLA matching, most allogeneic cells (even MSCs or CDCs) will eventually be rejected after in vivo transplantation [81, 83, 103]. Nevertheless, since the vast majority of the observed functional benefit after therapy with adult progenitor cells is attributable to indirect pathways, rejection of allogeneic cells may not be an issue if it is delayed long enough to allow them to exert their protective and regenerative paracrine effects, resulting in sustained benefit without the requirement for stable engraftment of transplanted cells. On the other hand, ESCs (which are by default allogeneic) and iPSCs (if used in a "universal donor" paradigm) can regenerate the heart directly (through formation of new transplanted tissue by the exogenously administered cells). Thus, long-term immunosuppression (or HLA matching in the case of induced pluripotent stem cells) would be required for clinical applications.

30.7.3 Targeting a Sicker Patient Population

The majority of cell therapy trials to date have been performed in the setting of acute or convalescent MI and have enrolled patients who were not very sick (first-infarct population with minimal LV dysfunction [EF of ≈50 %] receiving aggressive, prompt reperfusion and optimal drug- and device-based therapies), leaving little room for improvement. However, data from various different trials suggest that patients with more severe ischemic damage (the ones with the worse prognosis) benefit most from cell therapy. In the REPAIR-AMI study, patients with a lower baseline EF (<48.9 %) showed a significant, threefold higher recovery in EF than seen in the converse group [104]. In addition, the beneficial effect on clinical endpoints was also preferentially observed in those patients with a lower baseline EF after myocardial infarction [24]. In the REGENT study, significant functional benefit was observed only in cell-treated patients who had baseline EF <37 % [28]. In the BOOST trial, sustained functional improvement was observed only in patients with greater infarct transmurality [23], and in the study by Janssens et al. [25], BMMNC administration led to enhanced recovery of regional function only in the most severely infarcted myocardial segments (characterized by the greatest infarct transmurality). In the CADUCEUS trial, infusion of CDCs resulted in greater absolute reduction of scar size in patients with larger infarcts (i.e. patients with higher baseline scar size) [87]. Taken together, the results indicate that the greatest benefits of cell therapy may occur in patients with the greatest infarct-induced myocardial damage. This finding has major implications for the design of future clinical studies: cell therapy may maximize its potential for successful myocardial repair and regeneration possibly by targeting a sicker patient population [105].

30.8 Closing Remarks

Cell therapy for heart disease began clinically more than a decade ago and the results so far have been mixed. The experience with skeletal myoblasts has been resoundingly negative, due to their arrhythmiogenicity. Bone marrow-derived cells (now entering phase 3 trials) have an established, excellent safety profile, but efficacy has been inconsistent and, overall, modest. Cautious optimism prevails for heart-derived cells (now entering phase 2 trials), which have yielded promising results, consistent with therapeutic regeneration of infarcted myocardium, in early phase 1 studies; however, these results need to be reproduced in larger trials. ESCs and iPSCs are currently being tested for cardiac applications in large animals. Rigorous safety studies (with a focus on arrhythmiogenicity and oncogenicity) are essential before these pluripotent cells can be administered in human subjects. Going forward (and regardless of cell type), the pursuit of improved methods for cell delivery, means to boost cardiac cell retention, more potent and better-standardized cellular products, and more apt patient populations is certainly merited.

References

1. Mathers CD, Lopez AD, Murray CJL. The burden of disease and mortality by condition: data, methods, and results for 2001. In: Lopez AD, Mathers CD, Ezzati M, Jamison DT, Murray CJL, editors. Global burden of disease and risk factors. Washington, DC: World Bank; 2006. p. 45–93.
2. Laflamme MA, Murry CE. Heart regeneration. Nature. 2011;473:326–35.
3. Bergmann O, Bhardwaj RD, Bernard S, Zdunek S, Barnabé-Heider F, Walsh S, et al. Evidence for cardiomyocyte renewal in humans. Science. 2009;324:98–102.
4. Malliaras K, Marbán E. Cardiac cell therapy: where we've been, where we are, and where we should be headed. Br Med Bull. 2011;98:161–85.
5. Malliaras K, Kreke M, Marbán E. The stuttering progress of cell therapy for heart disease. Clin Pharmacol Ther. 2011;90:532–41.
6. Jain M, DerSimonian H, Brenner DA, Ngov S, Teller P, Edge AS, et al. Cell therapy attenuates deleterious ventricular remodeling and improves cardiac performance after myocardial infarction. Circulation. 2001;103:1920–7.
7. He KL, Yi GH, Sherman W, Zhou H, Zhang GP, Gu A, et al. Autologous skeletal myoblast transplantation improved hemodynamics and left ventricular function in chronic heart failure dogs. J Heart Lung Transplant. 2005;24:1940–9.
8. Abraham MR, Henrikson CA, Tung L, Chang MG, Aon M, Xue T, et al. Antiarrhythmic engineering of skeletal myoblasts for cardiac transplantation. Circ Res. 2005;97:159–67.
9. Menasché P, Hagège AA, Scorsin M, Pouzet B, Desnos M, Duboc D, et al. Myoblast transplantation for heart failure. Lancet. 2001;357:279–80.
10. Siminiak T, Kalawski R, Fiszer D, Jerzykowska O, Rzeźniczak J, Rozwadowska N, et al. Autologous skeletal myoblast transplantation for the treatment of postinfarction myocardial injury: phase I clinical study with 12 months of follow-up. Am Heart J. 2004;148:531–7.
11. Hagège AA, Marolleau JP, Vilguin JT, Alhéritière A, Peyrard S, Duboc D, et al. Skeletal myoblast transplantation in ischemic heart failure: long-term follow-up of the first phase I cohort of patients. Circulation. 2006;114 Suppl 1:I108–13.
12. Menasché P, Alfieri O, Janssens S, McKenna W, Reichenspurner H, Tringuart L, et al. The myoblast autologous grafting in ischemic cardiomyopathy (MAGIC) trial: first randomized placebo-controlled study of myoblast transplantation. Circulation. 2008;117:1189–200.
13. Povsic TJ, O'Connor CM, Henry T, Taussig A, Kereiakes DJ, Fortuin FD, et al. A double-blind, randomized, controlled, multicenter study to assess the safety and cardiovascular effects of skeletal myoblast implantation by catheter delivery in patients with chronic heart failure after myocardial infarction. Am Heart J. 2011;162:654–62.
14. Duckers HJ, Houtgraaf J, Hehrlein C, Schofer J, Waltenberger J, Gershlick A, et al. Final results of a phase IIa, randomised, open-label trial to evaluate the percutaneous intramyocardial transplantation of autologous skeletal myoblasts in congestive heart failure patients: the SEISMIC trial. EuroIntervention. 2011;6:805–12.

15. Strauer BE, Brehm M, Zeus T, Gattermann N, Hernandez A, Sorg RV, et al. Intracoronary, human autologous stem cell transplantation for myocardial regeneration following myocardial infarction. Dtsch Med Wochenschr. 2001;126:932–8.
16. Orlic D, Kajstura J, Chimenti S, Jakoniuk I, Anderson SM, Li B, et al. Bone marrow cells regenerate infracted myocardium. Nature. 2001;410:701–5.
17. Murry CE, Soonpaa MH, Reinecke H, Nakajima H, Nakajima HO, Rubart M, et al. Haematopoietic stem cells do not transdifferentiate into cardiac myocytes in myocardial infarcts. Nature. 2004;428:664–8.
18. Balsam LB, Wagers AJ, Christensen JL, Kofidis T, Weissman IL, Robbins RC. Haematopoietic stem cells adopt mature haematopoietic fates in ischaemic myocardium. Nature. 2004;428:668–73.
19. Dimmeler S, Zeiher AM. Cell therapy of acute myocardial infarction: open questions. Cardiology. 2009; 113:155–60.
20. Fernández-Avilés F, San Román JA, Garcia-Frade J, Fernández ME, Peñarrubia MJ, de la Fuente L, et al. Experimental and clinical regenerative capability of human bone marrow cells after myocardial infarction. Circ Res. 2004;95:742–8.
21. Bartunek J, Vanderheyden M, Vandekerckhove B, Mansour S, De Bruyne B, De Bondt P, et al. Intracoronary injection of CD133-positive enriched bone marrow progenitor cells promotes cardiac recovery after recent myocardial infarction: feasibility and safety. Circulation. 2005;112 Suppl 9:I178–83.
22. Wollert KC, Meyer GP, Lotz J, Ringes-Lichtenberg S, Lippolt P, Breidenbach C, et al. Intracoronary autologous bone-marrow cell transfer after myocardial infarction: the BOOST randomised controlled clinical trial. Lancet. 2004;364:141–8.
23. Meyer GP, Wollert KC, Lotz J, Pirr J, Rager U, Lippolt P, et al. Intracoronary bone marrow cell transfer after myocardial infarction: 5-year follow-up from the randomized-controlled BOOST trial. Eur Heart J. 2009;30:2978–84.
24. Schächinger V, Erbs S, Elsässer A, Haberbosch W, Hambrecht R, Hölschermann H, et al. Improved clinical outcome after intracoronary administration of bone-marrow-derived progenitor cells in acute myocardial infarction: final 1-year results of the REPAIR-AMI trial. Eur Heart J. 2006;27:2775–83.
25. Janssens S, Dubois C, Bogaert J, Theunissen K, Deroose C, Desmet W, et al. Autologous bone marrow-derived stem-cell transfer in patients with ST-segment elevation myocardial infarction: double-blind, randomised controlled trial. Lancet. 2006;367:113–21.
26. Lunde K, Solheim S, Aakhus S, Arnesen H, Abdelnoor M, Egeland T, et al. Intracoronary injection of mononuclear bone marrow cells in acute myocardial infarction. N Engl J Med. 2006;355:1199–209.
27. Huikuri HV, Kervinen K, Niemelä M, Ylitalo K, Säilv M, Koistinen P, et al. Effects of intracoronary injection of mononuclear bone marrow cells on left ventricular function, arrhythmia risk profile, and restenosis after thrombolytic therapy of acute myocardial infarction. Eur Heart J. 2008;29:2723–32.
28. Tendera M, Wojakowski W, Ruzyllo W, Chojnowska L, Kepka C, Tracz W, et al. Intracoronary infusion of bone marrow-derived selected CD34+CXCR4+ cells and non-selected mononuclear cells in patients with acute STEMI and reduced left ventricular ejection fraction: results of randomized, multicentre Myocardial Regeneration by Intracoronary Infusion of Selected Population of Stem Cells in Acute Myocardial Infarction (REGENT) Trial. Eur Heart J. 2009;30:1313–21.
29. Roncalli J, Mouquet F, Piot C, Trochu JN, Le Corvoisier P, Neuder Y, et al. Intracoronary autologous mononucleated bone marrow cell infusion for acute myocardial infarction: results of the randomized multicenter BONAMI trial. Eur Heart J. 2011;32: 1748–57.
30. Hirsch A, Nijveldt R, van der Vleuten PA, Tijssen JG, van der Giessen WJ, Tio RA, et al. Intracoronary infusion of mononuclear cells from bone marrow or peripheral blood compared with standard therapy in patients after acute myocardial infarction treated by primary percutaneous coronary intervention: results of the randomized controlled HEBE trial. Eur Heart J. 2011;32:1736–47.
31. Wöhrle J, Merkle N, Mailänder V, Nusser T, Schauwecker P, von Scheidt F, et al. Results of intracoronary stem cell therapy after acute myocardial infarction. Am J Cardiol. 2010;105:804–12.
32. Traverse JH, Henry TD, Pepine CJ, Willerson JT, Zhao DX, Ellis SG, et al. Effect of the use and timing of bone marrow mononuclear cell delivery on left ventricular function after acute myocardial infarction: the TIME randomized trial. JAMA. 2012;308:2380–9.
33. Traverse JH, Henry TD, Ellis SG, Pepine CJ, Willerson JT, Zhao DX, et al. Effect of intracoronary delivery of autologous bone marrow mononuclear cells 2 to 3 weeks following acute myocardial infarction on left ventricular function: the Late TIME randomized trial. JAMA. 2011;306:2110–9.
34. Sürder D, Manka R, Lo Cicero V, Moccetti T, Rufibach K, Soncin S, et al. Intracoronary injection of bone marrow-derived mononuclear cells early or late after acute myocardial infarction: effects on global left ventricular function. Circulation. 2013;127:1968–79.
35. Marbán E, Malliaras K. Mixed results for bone marrow-derived cell therapy for ischemic heart disease. JAMA. 2012;308:2405–6.
36. Martin-Rendon E, Brunskill SJ, Hyde CJ, Stanworth SJ, Mathur A, Watt SM. Autologous bone marrow stem cells to treat acute myocardial infarction: a systematic review. Eur Heart J. 2008;29:1807–18.
37. van Ramshorst J, Bax JJ, Beeres SL, Dibbets-Schneider P, Roes SD, Stokkel MP, et al. Intramyocardial bone marrow cell injection for chronic myocardial ischemia: a randomized controlled trial. JAMA. 2009;301:1997–2004.
38. Tse HF, Thambar S, Kwong YL, Rowlings P, Bellamy G, McCrohon J, et al. Prospective

randomized trial of direct endmyocardial implantation of bone marrow cells for treatment of severe coronary diseases (PROTECT-CAD trial). Eur Heart J. 2007;28:2998–3005.
39. Losordo DW, Schatz RA, White CJ, Udelson JE, Veereshwarayya V, Durgin M, et al. Intramyocardial transplantation of autologous CD34+ stem cells for intractable angina: a phase I/Iia double-blind, randomized controlled trial. Circulation. 2007;115:3165–72.
40. Losordo DW, Henry TD, Davidson C, Sup Lee J, Costa MA, Bass T, et al. Intramyocardial, autologous CD34+ cell therapy for refractory angina. Circ Res. 2011;109:428–36.
41. Povsic TJ, Junge C, Nada A, Schatz RA, Harrington RA, Davidson CJ, et al. A phase 3, randomized, double-blind, active-controlled, unpublished standard of care study assessing the efficacy and safety of intramyocardial autologous CD34+ cell administration in patients with refractory angina: design of the RENEW study. Am Heart J. 2013;165:854–61.
42. Hendrikx M, Hensen K, Clijsters C, Jongen H, Koninckx R, Bijnens E, et al. Recovery of regional but not global contractile function by the direct intramyocardial autologous bone marrow transplantation: results from a randomized controlled clinical trial. Circulation. 2006;114 Suppl 1:I101–7.
43. Stamm C, Kleine HD, Choi YH, Dunkelmann S, Lauffs JA, Lorenzen B, et al. Intramyocardial delivery of CD133+ bone marrow cells and coronary artery bypass grafting for chronic ischemic heart disease: safety and efficacy studies. J Thorac Cardiovasc Surg. 2007;133:717–25.
44. Pokushalov E, Romanov A, Chernyavsky A, Larionov P, Terekhov I, Artyomenko S, et al. Efficiency of intramyocardial injections of autologous bone marrow mononuclear cells in patients with ischemic heart failure: a randomized study. J Cardiovasc Transl Res. 2010;3:160–8.
45. Perin EC, Willerson JT, Pepine CJ, Henry TD, Ellis SG, Zhao DX, et al. Effect of transendocardial delivery of autologous bone marrow mononuclear cells on functional capacity, left ventricular function, and perfusion in chronic heart failure: the FOCUS-CCTRN trial. JAMA. 2012;307:1717–26.
46. Takehashi M, Li TS, Suzuki R, Kobayashi T, Ito H, Ikeda Y, et al. Cytokines produced by bone marrow cells can contribute to functional improvement of the infarcted heart by protecting cardiomyocytes from ischemic injury. Am J Physiol Heart Circ Physiol. 2006;291:H886–93.
47. Pijnappels DA, Schalij MJ, Ramkisoensing AA, van Tuyn J, de Vries AA, van der Laarse A, et al. Forced alignment of mesenchymal stem cells undergoing cardiomyogenic differentiation affects functional integration with cardiomyocyte cultures. Circ Res. 2008;103:167–76.
48. Rose RA, Jiang H, Wang X, Helke S, Tsoporis JN, Gong N, et al. Bone marrow-derived mesenchymal stromal cells express cardiac-specific markers, retain the stromal phenotype, and do not become functional cardiomyocytes in vitro. Stem Cells. 2008;26:2884–92.
49. Gnecchi M, He H, Liang OD, Melo LG, Morello F, Mu H, et al. Paracrine action accounts for marked protection of ischemic heart by Akt-modified mesenchymal stem cells. Nat Med. 2005;11:367–8.
50. Kinnaird T, Stabile E, Burnett MS, Lee CW, Barr S, Fuchs S, et al. Marrow-derived stromal cells express genes encoding a broad spectrum of arteriogenic cytokines and promote in vitro and in vivo arteriogenesis through paracrine mechanisms. Circ Res. 2004;94: 678–85.
51. Hatzistergos KE, Quevedo H, Oskouei BN, Hu Q, Feigenbaum GS, Margitich IS, et al. Bone marrow mesenchymal stem cells stimulate cardiac stem cell proliferation and differentiation. Circ Res. 2010;107:913–22.
52. Amado LC, Saliaris AP, Schuleri KH, St John M, Xie JS, Cattaneo S, et al. Cardiac repair with intramyocardial injection of allogeneic mesenchymal stem cells after myocardial infarction. Proc Natl Acad Sci U S A. 2005;102:11474–9.
53. Schuleri KH, Feigenbaum GS, Centola M, Weiss ES, Zimmet JM, Tuerney J, et al. Autologous mesenchymal stem cells produce reverse remodeling in chronic ischaemic cardiomyopathy. Eur Heart J. 2009;30:2722–32.
54. Heldman AW, Difede DL, Fishman JE, Zambrano JP, Trachtenberg BH, et al. Transendocardial mesenchymal stem cells and mononuclear bone marrow cells for ischemic cardiomyopathy: the TAC-HFT randomized trial. JAMA. 2013. doi:10.1001/jama.2013.282909.
55. Behfar A, Yamada S, Crespo-Diaz R, Nesbitt JJ, Rowe LA, Perez-Terzic C, et al. Guided cardiopoiesis enhances therapeutic benefit of bone marrow human mesenchymal stem cells in chronic myocardial infarction. J Am Coll Cardiol. 2010;56:721–34.
56. Bartunek J, Behfar A, Dolatabadi D, Vanderheyden M, Ostojic M, Dens J, et al. Cardiopoietic stem cell therapy in heart failure: the C-CURE (Cardiopoietic stem Cell therapy in heart failURE) multicenter randomized trial with lineage-specified biologics. J Am Coll Cardiol. 2013;61:2329–38.
57. Hare JM, Traverse JH, Henry TD, Dib N, Strumpf RK, Schulman SP, et al. A randomized, double-blind, placebo-controlled, dose-escalation study of intravenous adult human mesenchymal stem cells (prohymal) after acute myocardial infarction. J Am Coll Cardiol. 2009;54:2277–86.
58. Freyman T, Polin G, Osman H, Crary J, Lu M, Cheng L, et al. A quantitative, randomized study evaluating three methods of mesenchymal stem cell delivery following myocardial infarction. Eur Heart J. 2006;27:1114–22.
59. Hare JM, Fishman JE, Gerstenblith G, DiFede Velazquez DL, Zambrano JP, Suncion VY, et al. Comparison of allogeneic vs autologous bone marrow-derived mesenchymal stem cells delivered by transendovardial injection in patients with ischemic cardiomyopathy: the POSEIDON randomized trial. JAMA. 2012;308:2369–79.

60. Valina C, Pinkernell K, Song YH, Bai X, Sadat S, Campeau RJ, et al. Intracoronary administration of autologous adipose tissue-derived stem cells improves left ventricular function, perfusion, and remodeling after acute myocardial infarction. Eur Heart J. 2007; 28:2667–77.
61. Houtgraaf JH, den Dekker WK, van Dalen BM, Springeling T, de Jong R, van Geuns RJ, et al. First experience in humans using adipose tissue-derived regenerative cells in the treatment of patients with ST-segment elevation myocardial infarction. J Am Coll Cardiol. 2012;59:539–40.
62. Beltrami AP, Barlucchi L, Torella D, Baker M, Limana F, Chimenti S, et al. Adult cardiac stem cells are pluripotent and support myocardial regeneration. Cell. 2003;114:763–6.
63. Messina E, De Angelis L, Frati G, Morrone S, Chimenti S, Fiordaliso F, et al. Isolation and expansion of adult cardiac stem cells from human and murine heart. Circ Res. 2004;95:911–21.
64. Smith RR, Barile L, Cho HC, Leppo MK, Hare JM, Messina E, et al. Regenerative potential of cardiosphere-derived cells expanded from percutaneous endomyocardial biopsy specimens. Circulation. 2007;115:896–908.
65. Oh H, Bradfute SB, Gallardo TD, Nakamura T, Gaussin V, Mishina Y, et al. Cardiac progenitor cells from adult myocardium: homing, differentiation, and fusion after infarction. Proc Natl Acad Sci U S A. 2003;100:12313–8.
66. Martin CM, Meeson AP, Robertson SM, Hawke TJ, Richardson JA, Bates S, et al. Persistent expression of the ATP-binding cassette transporter, Abcg2, identifies cardiac SP cells in the developing and adult heart. Dev Biol. 2004;265:262–75.
67. Ott HC, Matthiesen TS, Brechtken J, Grindle S, Goh SK, Nelson W, et al. The adult human heart as a source for stem cells: repair strategies with embryonic-like progenitor cells. Nat Clin Pract Cardiovasc Med. 2007;4 Suppl 1:S27–39.
68. Hsieh PC, Segers VF, Davis ME, MacGillivray C, Gannon J, Molkentin JD, et al. Evidence from a genetic fate-mapping study that stem cells refresh adult mammalian cardiomyocytes after injury. Nat Med. 2007;13:970–4.
69. Malliaras K, Zhang Y, Seinfeld J, Galang G, Tseliou E, Cheng K, et al. Cardiomyocyte proliferation and progenitor cell recruitment underlie therapeutic regeneration after myocardial infarction in the adult mouse heart. EMBO Mol Med. 2013;5:191–209.
70. Tamura Y, Matsumura K, Sano M, Tabata H, Kimura K, Ieda M, et al. Neural crest-derived stem cells migrate and differentiate into cardiomyocytes after myocardial infarction. Arterioscler Thromb Vasc Biol. 2011;31:582–9.
71. Dawn B, Stein AB, Urbanek K, Rota M, Whang B, Rastaldo R, et al. Cardiac stem cells delivered intravascularly traverse the vessel barrier, regenerate infarcted myocardium, and improve cardiac function. Proc Natl Acad Sci U S A. 2005;102:3766–71.
72. Bolli R, Tang XL, Sanganalmath SK, Rimoldi O, Mosna F, Abdel-Latif A, et al. Intracoronary delivery of autologous cardiac stem cells improves cardiac function in a porcine model of chronic ischemic cardiomyopathy. Circulation. 2013;128:122–31.
73. Zaruba MM, Soonpaa M, Reuter S, Field LJ. Cardiomyogenic potential of C-kit(+)-expressing cells derived from neonatal and adult mouse hearts. Circulation. 2010;121:1992–2000.
74. Bolli R, Chugh AR, D'Amario D, Loughran JH, Stoddard MF, Ikram S, et al. Cardiac stem cells in patients with ischaemic cardiomyopathy (SCIPIO): initial results of a randomized phase 1 trial. Lancet. 2011;378:1847–57.
75. Chugh AR, Beache GM, Loughran JH, Mewton N, Elmore JB, Kajstura J, et al. Administration of cardiac stem cells in patient with ischemic cardiomyopathy: the SCIPIO trial: surgical aspects and interim analysis of myocardial function and viability by magnetic resonance. Circulation. 2012;126 Suppl 1:S54–64.
76. Kreke M, Smith RR, Marbán L, Marbán E. Cardiospheres and cardiosphere-derived cells as therapeutic agents following myocardial infarction. Expert Rev Cardiovasc Ther. 2012;10:1158–94.
77. Davis DR, Zhang Y, Smith RR, Cheng K, Terrovitis J, Malliaras K, et al. Validation of the cardiosphere method to culture progenitor cells from myocardial tissue. PLoS One. 2009;4:e7195.
78. Chimenti I, Smith RR, Li TS, Gerstenblith G, Messina E, Giacomello A, et al. Relative roles of direct regeneration versus paracrine effects of human cardiosphere-derived cells transplanted into infarcted mice. Circ Res. 2010;106:971–80.
79. Terrovitis J, Lautamäki R, Bonios M, Fox J, Engles JM, Yu J, et al. Noninvasive quantification and optimization of acute cell retention by in vivo positron emission tomography after intramyocardial cardiac-derived stem cell therapy. J Am Coll Cardiol. 2009;54: 1619–26.
80. Cheng K, Li TS, Malliaras K, Davis DR, Zhang Y, Marbán E. Magnetic targeting enhances engraftment and functional benefit of iron-labeled cardiosphere-derived cells in myocardial infarction. Circ Res. 2010;106:1570–81.
81. Malliaras K, Li TS, Luthringer D, Terrovitis J, Cheng K, Chakravarty T, et al. Safety and efficacy of allogeneic cell therapy in infarcted rats transplanted with mismatched cardiosphere-derived cells. Circulation. 2012; 125:100–12.
82. Johnston PV, Sasano T, Mills K, Evers R, Lee ST, Smith RR, et al. Engraftment, differentiation, and functional benefits of autologous cardiosphere-derived cells in porcine ischemic cardiomyopathy. Circulation. 2009;120:1075–83.
83. Malliaras K, Smith R, Kanazawa H, Yee K, Seinfeld J, Tseliou E, et al. Validation of contrast-enhanced MRI to monitor regenerative efficacy after cell therapy in a porcine model of convalescent myocardial infarction. Circulation. 2013;128:2764–75.

84. Li TS, Cheng K, Malliaras K, Smith RR, Zhang Y, Sun B, et al. Direct comparison of different stem cell types and subpopulations reveals superior paracrine potency and myocardial repair efficacy with cardiosphere-derived cells. J Am Coll Cardiol. 2012;59:942–53.
85. Tseliou E, Pollan S, Malliaras K, Terrovitis J, Sun B, Galang G, et al. Allogeneic cardiospheres safely boost cardiac function and attenuate adverse remodeling post-myocardial infarction in immunologically-mismatched rat strains. J Am Coll Cardiol. 2013;61:1108–19.
86. Makkar RR, Smith RR, Cheng K, Malliaras K, Thomson LE, Berman D, et al. Intracoronary cardiosphere-derived cells for heart regeneration after myocardial infarction (CADUCEUS): a prospective, randomised phase 1 trial. Lancet. 2012;379:895–904.
87. Malliaras K, Makkar RR, Smith RR, Cheng K, Wu E, Bonow RO, et al. Intracoronary cardiosphere-derived cells after myocardial infarction: evidence for therapeutic regeneration in the final 1-year results of the CADUCEUS trial. J Am Coll Cardiol. 2014;63:110–22.
88. Nussbaum J, Minami E, Laflamme MA, Virag JA, Ware CB, Masino A, et al. Transplantation of undifferentiated murine embryonic stem cells in the heart: teratoma formation and immune response. FASEB J. 2007;21:1345–57.
89. Shiba Y, Fernandes S, Zhu WZ, Filice D, Muskheli V, Kim J, et al. Human ES-cell-derived cardiomyocytes electrically couple and suppress arrhythmias in injured hearts. Nature. 2012;489:322–5.
90. Chen MQ, Yu J, Whittington RH, Wu JC, Kovacs GT, Giovangrandi L. Modeling conduction in host-graft interactions between stem cell grafts and cardiomyocytes. Conf Proc IEEE Eng Med Biol Soc. 2009;2009:6014–7.
91. Nelson TJ, Martinez-Fernandez A, Terzic A. Induced pluripotent stem cells: developmental biology to regenerative medicine. Nat Rev Cardiol. 2010;7:700–10.
92. Nazaraki G, Uosaki H, Teranishi M, Okita K, Kim B, Matsuoka S, et al. Directed and systematic differentiation of cardiovascular cells from mouse induced pluripotent stem cells. Circulation. 2008;118:498–506.
93. Zhang J, Wilson GF, Soerens AG, Koonce CH, Yu J, Palecek SP, et al. Functional cardiomyocytes derived from human induced pluripotent stem cells. Circ Res. 2009;104:e30–41.
94. Ieda M, Fu JD, Delgado-Olguin P, Vedantham V, Hayashi Y, Bruneau BG, et al. Direct reprogramming of fibroblasts into functional cardiomyocytes by defined factors. Cell. 2010;142:375–86.
95. Terrovitis JV, Smith RR, Marbán E. Assessment and optimization of cell engraftment after transplantation into the heart. Circ Res. 2010;106: 479–94.
96. Hou D, Youssef EA, Brinton TJ, Zhang P, Rogers P, Price ET, et al. Radiolabeled cell distribution after intramyocardial, intracoronary, and interstitial retrograde coronary venous delivery: implications for current clinical trials. Circulation. 2005;112 Suppl 9:I150–6.
97. Hofmann M, Wollert KC, Meyer GP, Menke A, Arseniev L, Hertenstein B, et al. Monitoring of bone marrow cell homing into the infarcted human myocardium. Circulation. 2005;111:2198–202.
98. Vrtovec B, Poglajen G, Lezaic L, Sever M, Socan A, Domanovic D, et al. Comparison of transendocardial and intracoronary CD34+ cell transplantation in patients with nonischemic dilated cardiomyopathy. Circulation. 2013;128 Suppl 1:S42–9.
99. Murry CE, Field LJ, Menasché P. Cell-based cardiac repair: reflections at the 10-year point. Circulation. 2005;112:3174–83.
100. Suzuki G, Iyer V, Lee TC, Canty Jr JM. Autologous mesenchymal stem cells mobilize cKit+ and CD133+ bone marrow progenitor cells and improve regional function in hibernating myocardium. Circ Res. 2011;109:1044–54.
101. Li Q, Guo Y, Ou Q, Chen N, Wu WJ, Yuan F, et al. Intracoronary administration of cardiac stem cells in mice: a new, improved technique for cell therapy in murine models. Basic Res Cardiol. 2011;106: 849–64.
102. Dimmeler S, Leri A. Aging and disease as modifiers of efficacy of cell therapy. Circ Res. 2008;102: 1319–30.
103. Zangi L, Margalit R, Reich-Zeliger S, Bachar-Lustig E, Beilhack A, Negrin R, et al. Direct imaging of immune rejection and memory induction by allogeneic mesenchymal stromal cells. Stem Cells. 2009;27:2865–74.
104. Schächinger V, Erbs S, Elsässer A, Haberbosch W, Hambrecht R, Hölschermann H, et al. Intracoronary bone marrow-derived progenitor cells in acute myocardial infarction. N Engl J Med. 2006;355: 1210–21.
105. Malliaras K, Marbán E. Moving beyond surrogate endpoints in cell therapy trials for heart disease. Stem Cells Transl Med. 2014;3:2–6.

Moving Towards a Novel Paradigm in Drug Development for Worsening Heart Failure: The T1 Model (Mechanistic Translational Phase)

31

Sadiya S. Khan, Mihai Gheorghiade, and Gerasimos Filippatos

Abstract

Hospitalization for worsening heart failure (WHF) represents a clinical entity with high burden of global disease, unacceptable postdischarge mortality and rehospitalization rates reaching 45 % within 60–90 days, and enormous economic expenditures worldwide. Despite the use of evidence-based therapies and implementation of policy measures on the governmental level, there has been minimal impact on the event rate following hospitalization for worsening heart failure over the past decade. In addition, the aging population and improved survival post-myocardial infarction will continue to fuel the growing population of patients with heart failure. There exists a substantial unmet need for novel therapeutic strategies that will improve outcomes in patients hospitalized with WHF. The current paradigm of sequentially conducting trials from phase I to III has not resulted in successful identification of therapies that improve outcomes and a different approach is needed. Herein we describe potential reasons for the failure of current phase III clinical trails, lessons learned, and outline the T1 or translational phase model as a novel paradigm to move forward to successfully develop drug development in patients hospitalized with WHF.

Keywords

Heart failure • Worsening heart failure • Clinical trials • Translational phase models

S.S. Khan, MD • M. Gheorghiade, MD
Division of Cardiology, Department of Medicine, Center for Cardiovascular Innovation, Northwestern University Feinberg School of Medicine, Chicago, IL, USA

G. Filippatos, MD, FESC, FACC (✉)
Department of Cardiology, Athens University Hospital Attikon,
1 Rimini St. Haidari, Athens 12461, Greece
e-mail: geros@oetenet.gr

D.V. Cokkinos (ed.), *Introduction to Translational Cardiovascular Research*,
DOI 10.1007/978-3-319-08798-6_31, © Springer International Publishing Switzerland 2015

Abbreviations

BNP	Brain natriuretic peptide
CAD	Coronary artery disease
CMRI	Cardiac magnetic resonance imaging
HF	Heart failure
LV	Left ventricular dysfunction
N	Terminal pro-B type natriuretic peptide
NT	proBNP
T1	Translational phase model
WHF	Worsening heart failure

31.1 Introduction: The Global Health Burden of Heart Failure

Heart failure (HF) poses a significant clinical, economic, and public health challenge affecting an estimated 26 million people globally. In the United States alone, the prevalence is almost six million with an additional 15 million patients with HF in the countries represented by the European Society of Cardiology [1–4]. Hospitalization for worsening heart failure (WHF) is the leading cause of hospitalization in both the United States and Europe representing over two million admissions as a primary diagnosis accounting for the majority of the US $39 billion spent on HF care, with similar numbers in Europe [1, 5]. Heart failure is associated with significant morbidity and was listed on 1 in 9 death certificates (279,098 deaths) in the United States in 2010. Furthermore, patients who are hospitalized for worsening HF (WHF) are amongst the highest risk subset of patients with an unacceptably high post-discharge mortality and readmission rate [6, 7].

Incredibly, despite the advances in evidence-based drug and device therapies and policy measures to augment implementation of guideline based recommendations, there has not been a significant impact in the post-discharge event rate over the past two decades and rates of death or recurrent hospitalization remain dismal at 6 months approaching 50 % [8, 9]. Current projections based on epidemiological trends suggest that the prevalence of hospitalization for HF will continue to increase as a result of the aging population, improved survival after myocardial infarction, and reduction in sudden death with defibrillator implantation. In fact, despite international attention focused on this critical problem, clinical trails have failed to successfully identify novel therapies for patients hospitalized with WHF. It is imperative that we identify the reasons why phase II trials have not translated into successful phase III trials and shift our approach towards a novel paradigm in drug development and clinical trial design: the T1 or translational phase model.

31.2 Challenges of Conducting Clinical Trials in Hospitalized Patients with Worsening Heart Failure

There exists a clear discrepancy between the promise of basic science and the improvement of human health. Many possible etiologies have been cited for the negative trial results to date, which include, the drug itself, the patient selection protocol, the end points, and/or trial execution (Table 31.1). Any single one or a combination of these possibilities may be the reason that clinical benefits observed in phase II trials have not been reproduced in phase III trials for patients with WHF (Table 31.2). These disappointing results over a decade of efforts and hundreds of millions of research dollars spent stress the importance of identifying the reasons why benefits observed during phase II did not translate into benefits in phase III trials.

The International Working Group on Acute Heart Failure Syndromes has conducted a series of meetings at the United States Food and Drug Administration over the past 5 years, and we believe that we are now better equipped to conduct future studies with improved trial design as a result of the group's dialogue, which included representatives from academia, industry and regulatory authorities from both the United States and Europe [10, 11]. The group's consensus on the leading cause of failure to convincingly demonstrate safety and efficacy of agents in patients hospitalized with WHF was identified as the lack of in-depth understanding of the

Table 31.1 Contributors to lack of success in phase III AHFS trials

Pathophysiology and epidemiology	1. Poor understanding of the pathophysiology in AHFS 2. Heterogeneous patient population in terms of pathophysiology, etiology, and clinical presentation 3. Uncertain relationship between hemodynamics and neurohormonal changes and outcomes 4. Clinical course (particularly soon after discharge) of AHFS has not been well studied
The therapy (experimental drug or device)	5. Cardiac and noncardiac comorbid conditions influence the outcome and interaction with therapy 6. The transition from animal studies to clinical studies has occurred without comprehensive understanding of the mechanistic properties of the drug in specific patient subgroups. Not "knowing" the drug 7. Not having the correct dose 8. Possible variation of efficacy and safety with time given significant fluctuations in symptoms, hemodynamics, neurohormones, renal function, and myocardial injury during the course of hospitalization and postdischarge, the efficacy and/or safety of the drug may be dependent on the time of the intervention 9. The majority of drugs tested thus far reduce systemic BP, which may potentially decrease coronary perfusion, thereby contributing to myocardial and/or kidney injury
The protocol	10. Patient selection 11. Surrogate end points and clinical outcomes in phase II do not predict the results of a phase III trial 12. Choice of end points 13. Because most patients' signs and symptoms improve with standard therapy, it is difficult to prove that novel therapies are producing further and substantial improvements
Study execution	14. Selection of incorrect patients and/or less than ideal follow-up

Adapted and reproduced from Gheorghiade et al. [21] by permission

Table 31.2 Summary of failed phase III studies

Phase III studies	Primary end point(s)	Phase III primary end point reached?	Contributors to lack of success per Table 31.1
Tolvaptan			4,6,7,8,11
EVEREST (n=4,133)	Long term	No	
	1. All-cause mortality (superiority and non-inferiority) 2. Cardiovascular death or hospitalization for HF (superiority only) Short-term Composite of global clinical status and body weight reduction	Yes (driven by body weight reduction)	
Tezosentan			2,3,4,5,7,8,9,10,13
VERITAS (n=1,448)	1. Change in dyspnea (visual analog scale) over 24 h (in the individual trials) 2. Death or worsening HF at 7 days (in both trials combined)	No	
Levosimendan			3, 5,6,7,9,11

(continued)

Table 31.2 (continued)

Phase III studies	Primary end point(s)	Phase III primary end point reached?	Contributors to lack of success per Table 31.1
REVIVE-2 (n=600)	Composite of clinical signs/symptoms of HF and 1. Patient reported moderately or markedly improve at 6 h, 24 h, and 5 days (and no criteria for worsening) 2. Worsening (death, patient reported moderate or severe deterioration at any time point) or worsening symptoms at any time or persistent severe symptoms after 24 h requiring rescue therapy (ie intravenous diuretic, vasodilator or inotropic agents) 3. Unchanged	Yes—excess hypotension and arrhythmia with trends towards early mortality with levosimendan	
SURVIVE (n=1,327)	All-cause mortality at 180 days	No	
PROTECT (n=2,033)	Trichotomous classification of patients 1. Success: Improvement in dyspnea (Likert scale-moderately or markedly better) at 24 and 48 h or day of discharge, and not meeting criteria for treatment failure 2. Failure: death, HF readmission within 7 days, worsening HF (by physician assessment by day 7), or persistent renal impairment 3. Unchanged: neither criteria for success or failure	No	
Nesiritide			3,4,7,8,9,12,13
ASCEND-HF	1. Composite of all-cause mortality+HF rehospitalization at 30 days 2. Dyspnea at 6 and 24 h	No	

Adapted and reproduced from Gheorghiade et al. [21] by permission

molecules before pivotal multi-center international trials were conducted. This is not a problem simply in drug development in patients with WHF, but rather a systematic problem spanning different disease syndromes.

In the current paradigm of drug development, the successful completion of animal model studies is followed by phase I trials, which are focused on the investigation of the safety of novel agents in healthy subjects. This is followed by phase II studies to further understand the mechanistic properties, dose selection, and broad safety assessment in the context of a hypothesis-drive study in the desired target population. In a heterogeneous condition such HF, selection of the right patient population to target in a small phase II trial can be difficult and is critical for both efficacy and safety. This then culminates in a pivotal large-scale phase III trial (Fig. 31.1). Unfortunately, under this schema, every large trial conducted to date in patients hospitalized with WHF has failed to produce positive results in terms of efficacy and/or safety [12–19].

As described in Chap. 1, the Clinical Research Roundtable at the Institute of Medicine outlined 2 main obstacles limiting the transfer of discovery of disease mechanisms at the "bench" from being implemented at the "bedside" as novel methods for diagnosis, therapy, and prevention in the biomedical sciences [20]. These are defined as the T1 Block, translation from basic sciences to human studies, while the T2 block focuses on translation of new knowledge into everyday clinical practice and health care decision-making.

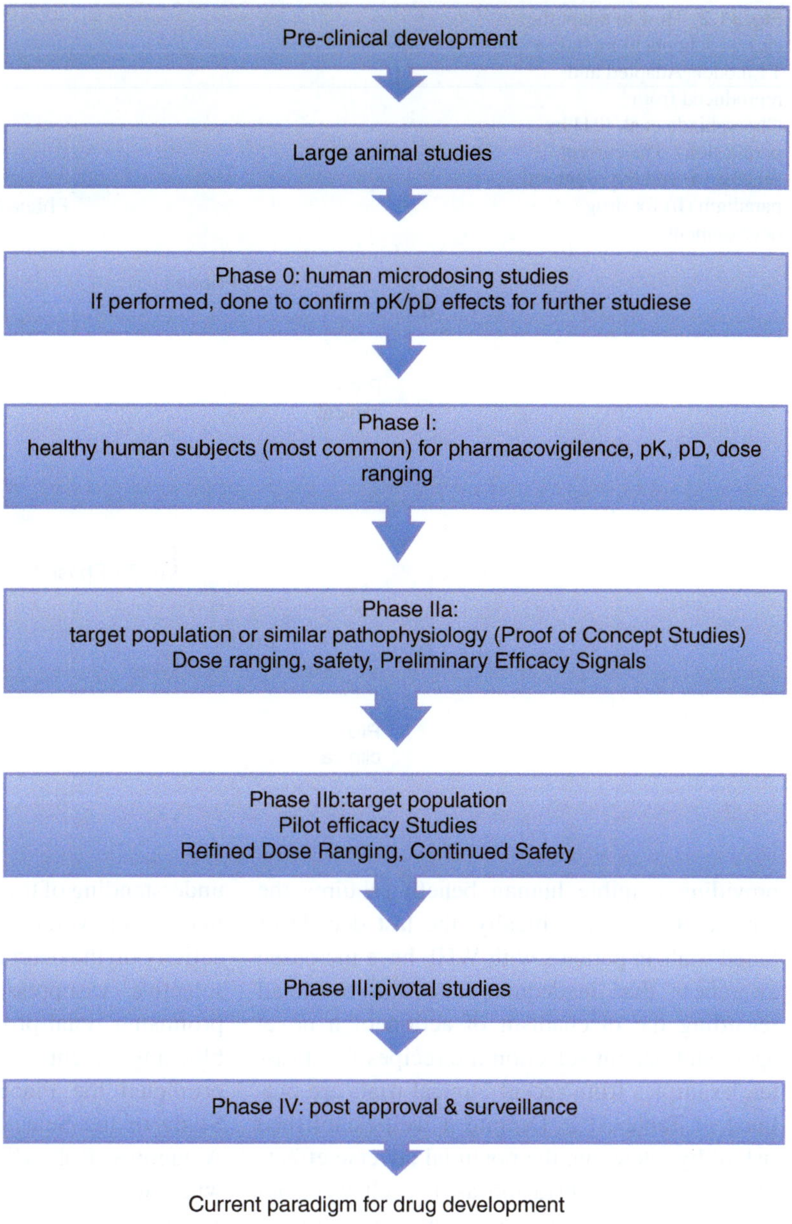

Fig. 31.1 Current Paradigm for Drug Development (Adapted and reproduced from Gheorghiade et al. [21] by permission)

Based on the group's prior experiences in clinical trial design, the main obstacle to overcome in patients hospitalized with WHF was identified as the T1 block. Therefore, we propose a novel paradigm of the T1 model to focus on investigation of the mechanistic effects of experimental agents prior to phase II studies prior to pivotal large-scale testing. We anticipate that this novel paradigm will improve the likelihood of successful translation of the beneficial effects of experimental agents observed in animal models into patients (Fig. 31.2) [21].

31.2.1 T1: Translational Mechanistic Phase of Research

The transition from preclinical studies to clinical trials in the quest for a novel agent developed at the "bench" to be administered at the "bedside"

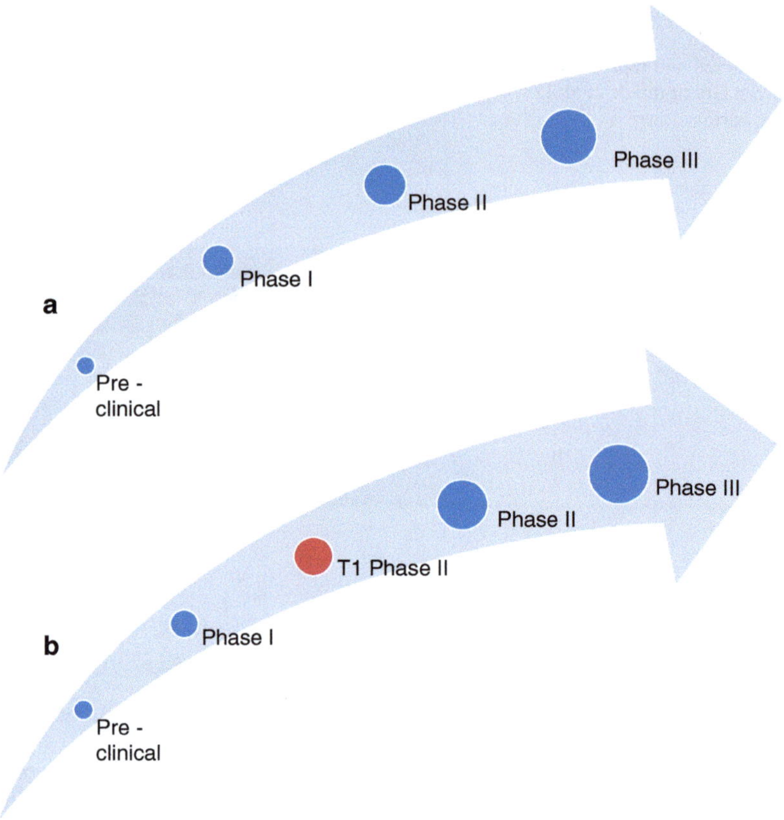

Fig. 31.2 How to adapt the current schema to include a T1 model (Adapted and reproduced from Gheorghiade et al. [21] by permission). The current schema (**a**) and the proposed paradigm (**b**) for drug development

providing tangible human benefit requires the utmost of care. Specifically, the last decade of failed trials in patients with WHF have increased awareness that inadequate attention to detail regarding the mechanism of action of a novel agent and patient selection are recipes for disaster. Examples from recent clinical trials are outlined in Table 31.2. Despite a well-established risk of hypotension, the potential adverse effects of coronary hypoperfusion as a result were not well studied in Levosimendan, especially in patients with concomitant coronary artery disease (CAD) [22]. The negative result in the Value of Endothelin Receptor Inhibition with Tezosentan in Acute Heart Failure Studies [15], while disappointing, was not unexpected as the hemodynamic and mechanistic effects of tezosentan were not previously tested in-depth at the lower dose in phase II trials prior to escalation to a multi-center international phase III trial [15, 23]. Tolvaptan, an oral vasopressin 2 receptor antagonist was developed without complete understanding of the physiologic response, which may be unfavorable, to unopposed vasopressin 1 activity on the heart and vasculature as a result of selective vasopressin 2 inhibition [24]. The promising renal-protective effects of adenosine blocking agents in small early-phase trials prompted the Placebo-Controlled Randomized Study of the Selective A1 Adenosine Receptor Antagonist Rolofylline for Patients Hospitalized with Acute Decompensated Heart Failure and Volume Overload to Assess Treatment Effect on Congestion and Renal Function (PROTECT) without an intermediate study assessing the impact of improved renal function on mortality and morbidity [25]. It was only after a decade of investigation and nearly $1 billion dollars that the Acute Study of Clinical Effectiveness of Nesiritide in Decompensated Heart Failure (ASCEND-HF) demonstrated lack of clinical efficacy, either in short-term improvement of dyspnea, or 30-days mortality or rehospitalization for heart failure [26].

T1 phase studies will be designed to occur after initial human studies in phase 0 and 1 studies, which will have demonstrated safety to proceed with further drug development and investigation in human subjects. This proposed schema would promote a seamless transition from animal studies to phase II investigations. T1 studies will be designed similar to animal studies with relatively small numbers of homogenous patients to allow for initial hypothesis testing. As we will explore later, the heart failure population is quite heterogeneous and clinical conditions, such as variable background therapy cannot be controlled in a clinical trial, and this may significantly affect results of small early phase studies. Therefore, patients entered into a T1 study will have a common etiology for WHF, a narrow range of age, ejection fraction, background therapy, and kidney function, as these are critical regulators of prognosis and may result in differential responses to novel therapies. This emphasis on homogeneity will be an obstacle in recruitment, however, the relatively small sample size required for the T1 studies will be expected to mitigate the difficulty. Further, investigation of multiple small homogenous groups will allow the ability to best capture which subgroup may benefit the most and should be considered as the initial target population in larger studies.

T1 studies will focus on mechanistic investigation of the novel therapeutic agent in the pre-specified patient population. These studies will focus on clearly defined end-points (e.g. changes in pulmonary capillary wedge pressure, renal function), but not on outcomes, as the small sample size would be prohibitive. This will allow for comprehensive initial investigation targeting the new drug's effect specifically on the heart. The advances in the past decade in biomarkers and cardiac imaging, such as 3-D echocardiography and cardiac magnetic resonance imaging (CMRI) make this phase possible today by allowing us the ability to assess, not only the left ventricular gross function, but also the myocyte, the interstitium, and the metabolism of the heart. This sets the stage for a novel characterization of HF patients to assist in enrollment of a more homogenous patient population. Experts in these imaging areas as well as electrophysiology, angiography, nephrology, and clinical trialists, will need to be identified up-front for successful trial design and execution. A small consortium of experienced centers is currently being created to conduct these trials with experience and expertise in these fields, especially in novel echocardiography techniques (tissue Doppler imaging, strain rate analysis, three-dimensional image acquisition), novel imaging modalities with cardiac magnetic resonance imaging and spectroscopy to evaluate myocardial metabolism, and invasive hemodynamics with right heart catheterization. In addition to standardization and optimization of the quality of hemodynamic assessment and image acquisition and interpretation, the use of concomitant "standard" background therapy has significant variability in large clinical trials as it is often left up to the discretion of the individual investigator or treating physician. The use of select T1 centers with a pre-specified protocol for initiation and up-titration of "standard" evidence-based background therapy will be critical to minimize variability in this regard. Furthermore, this may help attenuate the continental differences that were observed in the EVEREST Tolvaptan trial [27].

The T1 schema highlights the need to focus on patient selection to optimize homogeneity in the investigation of novel therapies. Identification of the patients who are most likely to respond to an experimental agent as well as exclusion of the patients who are most likely to experience adverse events will lay the groundwork and establish a foundation upon which to build later phases of drug development and phase II and phase III trials. This will essentially strengthen the "signal to noise" ratio and reduce the rate of both false positive and false negative results in small early-phase studies. This is especially important as promising novel therapeutics may be prematurely halted when a negative signal is identified in a small but heterogeneous sample size overshadows the positive effects. Conversely, a false positive signal may promote aggressive escalation of drug development, which fails to pan out in a large population in a phase III trial.

It is clear that patients with differing substrates will have a differential response to therapies for WHF. For example, patients with chronic ischemia and hibernating myocardium may respond differently to an inotrope compared with patients with primary cardiomyopathy. Similarly, patients with myocardial scarring may respond entirely differently. These critical differences in the myocardial substrate need to be identified and drug response on each substrate needs to be investigated in a thorough and comprehensive manner in a dedicated mechanistic phase of development, T1 phase. This highlights the need for a continued emphasis on defining and targeting the appropriate study population based on the mechanism of the proposed agent. The heterogeneity of the patient population with WHF is a significant challenge and has been a major limitation of prior clinical trials. A "one size fits all" approach is no longer appropriate.

One under recognized comorbid condition in patients with WHF is the presence of coronary artery disease (CAD). In OPTIME-CHF, patients had a differential effect in response to milrinone, with potentially beneficial effects in patients with nonischemic cardiomyopathy as well as clear evidence of harm in those patients with CAD [17]. In addition, reduction in coronary perfusion may be a key mechanism for progressive left ventricular (LV) dysfunction in patients with obstructive CAD. Further, in patients with ischemic myocardium that may be hibernating but viable, therapies that cause increases in oxygen demand and/or lead to myocardial injury may be particularly associated with adverse outcomes in these patients with a "vulnerable" myocardium. This highlights the need to return to the heart as a target and understand the pathophysiology for drug development.

Another high-risk subset of patients with WHF includes those with renal dysfunction at presentation or development during hospitalization as both of these groups experience a very high post-discharge event rate. In the Efficacy of Vasopressin Antagonism in Heart Failure Outcome Study with Tolvaptan [28], of the 2021 patients in the placebo group, renal dysfunction defined as estimated glomerular filtration rate <60.0 mL/min/1.73 m^2 was highly prevalent at baseline (53 %) as was worsening renal function defined as increase in serum creatinine of ≥0.3 mg/dL during hospitalization (14 %) and post-discharge (12 %), and was predictive of cardiovascular mortality and HF hospitalization [28]. The varying etiology of renal dysfunction adds another level of heterogeneity in this patient population, which includes comorbid diabetes, hypertension, and arteriosclerosis. Despite the association of renal dysfunction at baseline as well as worsening renal function during hospitalization or post-discharge follow-up with morbidity and mortality, the PROTECT trial highlights that improvement in renal function alone can not be used as a surrogate, as Rolofylline did not translate into improvement in symptoms or clinical outcomes [29].

Novel biomarkers may be a unique method to select a patient population for a small T1 study to highlight a higher risk subset, such as brain natriuretic peptide (BNP) or N-terminal pro-B-type natriuretic peptide (NT pro-BNP) or troponin as these have been identified with poorer prognosis in large registries and clinical trials of WHF [30]. Further, more the use of BNP to guide intensity of drug treatment in ambulatory patients with HF reduced total cardiovascular events [31]. In addition, mildly elevated troponin may reflect ongoing cardiac damage in the patient with WHF. Troponin elevation is not uncommon, and was present in 50 % of patients in the ASCEND-HF trial at baseline and was associated with worse prognosis [32]. Serial assessment of troponin performed in the PROTECT study demonstrated an increase in troponin during hospitalization in 21 % of patients, which was associated with worse outcomes at 60-days [33].

Dose investigation during T1 studies should focus on at minimum three distinct doses with a clear pharmacologic rationale for why the dosing was chosen. While the "correct" dose may not lead to a positive result, the "wrong" dose may lead to a negative result or a neutral study despite a "good" drug and a "good" target.

The timing of therapy initiation is as critical for success as the utilization of the "right" therapy in the "right" patient population. One proposed system divides the evaluation of the patient

Table 31.3 A proposal for a mechanistic translational phrase

T1 concept
1. A more thorough understanding of all of a molecule's effects on the heart (effects on viable but noncontractile myocardium, coronary perfusion, diastolic function, etc) is important
2. Reproduce the results obtained in large animal HF models in homogeneous groups of patients taking into account systolic and diastolic dysfunction, extent and severity of CAD, viable but dysfunctional myocardium, etc.
3. These in-depth evaluations should take advantage of recent progress made in noninvasive methods of assessment of cardiac function and structure (echocardiography, MRI spectroscopy, etc)
4. These studies would also expand our understanding of the pharmacokinetic and pharmacodynamic properties of novel molecules because, unlike animal models to date, patients with HF are commonly on background therapy for HF and have substantial comorbid conditions that might influence safety, efficacy, and outcomes
5. These studies should be conducted in dedicated centers that have the patient population, technology, and expertise to conduct such technically challenging studies

Adapted and reproduced from Gheorghiade et al. [21] by permission

presenting with WHF in the following phases: (1) the initial or emergency department phase, (2) the hospitalization phase, and (3) the pre-discharge phase. The management goals at each of these stages of phases of evaluation differ and require different therapies with different targets [34]. The T1 phase will allow mechanistic studies to investigate the drug's effects at the various phases to improve timing of selection and administration of experimental agent.

While a more methodological approach as described here with the T1 paradigm is necessary, it is important to note that a successful investigative approach also requires clarity, teamwork, consensus, and ever-present focus on execution (Table 31.3). We acknowledge that this "additional" phase may add time in an already lengthy drug development process, however, we strongly believe this additional time would be offset by the substantial benefits that the knowledge obtained from the mechanistic studies will provide, at a fraction of the overall cost of a large phase III trial.

31.3 Conclusions and Next Steps

Innovation in trial design and drug development for patients hospitalized with WHF remains a high priority given the unacceptably high post-discharge mortality and rehospitalization rate despite the available therapies. Identification of the current challenges is the first critical step prior to discussion of potential solutions for moving forward. We outline and describe the use of the T1 model or a translational phase to achieve a comprehensive mechanistic understanding of experimental agents to improve successful transition from the "bench" to the "bedside" for novel therapies in patients hospitalized with WHF. In addition, it is imperative that we focus on improved standardization in clinical classification, inclusion–exclusion criteria, and clinical endpoints as we design future clinical trials in hospitalized WHF patients to facilitate identification of the "right" patient population at the "right" time for administration of the "right" therapy. To continue to achieve progress in this field, we will need ongoing cooperation and collaboration from the scientific community, industry, and regulatory agencies to promote the incorporation of the T1 phase followed by carefully and well-executed phase II and III trials.

References

1. Hunt SA, Abraham WT, Chin MH, Feldman AM, Francis GS, Ganiats TG, et al. ACC/AHA 2005 Guideline Update for the Diagnosis and Management of Chronic Heart Failure in the Adult: a report of the American College of Cardiology/American Heart Association Task Force on Practice Guidelines (Writing Committee to Update the 2001 Guidelines for the Evaluation and Management of Heart Failure): developed in collaboration with the American College of Chest Physicians and the International Society for Heart and Lung Transplantation: endorsed by the Heart Rhythm Society. Circulation. 2005;112:e154–235.

2. Go AS, Mozaffarian D, Roger VL, Benjamin EJ, Berry JD, Blaha MJ, et al. Heart disease and stroke statistics–2014 update: a report from the American Heart Association. Circulation. 2014;129:e28–292.
3. Gheorghiade M, Zannad F, Sopko G, Klein L, Pina IL, Konstam MA, et al. Acute heart failure syndromes: current state and framework for future research. Circulation. 2005;112:3958–68.
4. Dickstein K, Cohen-Solal A, Filippatos G, McMurray JJ, Ponikowski P, Poole-Wilson PA, et al. ESC guidelines for the diagnosis and treatment of acute and chronic heart failure 2008: the Task Force for the diagnosis and treatment of acute and chronic heart failure 2008 of the European Society of Cardiology. Developed in collaboration with the Heart Failure Association of the ESC (HFA) and endorsed by the European Society of Intensive Care Medicine (ESICM). Eur J Heart Fail. 2008;10:933–89.
5. Fang J, Mensah GA, Croft JB, Keenan NL. Heart failure-related hospitalization in the U.S., 1979 to 2004. J Am Coll Cardiol. 2008;52:428–34.
6. Bueno H, Ross JS, Wang Y, Chen J, Vidan MT, Normand SL, et al. Trends in length of stay and short-term outcomes among Medicare patients hospitalized for heart failure, 1993–2006. JAMA. 2010;303:2141–7.
7. Jencks SF, Williams MV, Coleman EA. Rehospitalizations among patients in the Medicare fee-for-service program. N Engl J Med. 2009;360:1418–28.
8. Felker GM, Leimberger JD, Califf RM, Cuffe MS, Massie BM, Adams Jr KF, et al. Risk stratification after hospitalization for decompensated heart failure. J Card Fail. 2004;10:460–6.
9. Fonarow GC, Abraham WT, Albert NM, Stough WG, Gheorghiade M, Greenberg BH, et al. Factors identified as precipitating hospital admissions for heart failure and clinical outcomes: findings from OPTIMIZE-HF. Arch Intern Med. 2008;168:847–54.
10. Gheorghiade M, Adams KF, Cleland JG, Cotter G, Felker GM, Filippatos GS, et al. Phase III clinical trial end points in acute heart failure syndromes: a virtual roundtable with the Acute Heart Failure Syndromes International Working Group. Am Heart J. 2009;157:957–70.
11. Felker GM, Pang PS, Adams KF, Cleland JG, Cotter G, Dickstein K, et al. Clinical trials of pharmacological therapies in acute heart failure syndromes: lessons learned and directions forward. Circ Heart Fail. 2010;3:314–25.
12. Cuffe MS, Califf RM, Adams Jr KF, Benza R, Bourge R, Colucci WS, et al. Short-term intravenous milrinone for acute exacerbation of chronic heart failure: a randomized controlled trial. JAMA. 2002;287:1541–7.
13. Gheorghiade M, Konstam MA, Burnett Jr JC, Grinfeld L, Maggioni AP, Swedberg K, et al. Short-term clinical effects of tolvaptan, an oral vasopressin antagonist, in patients hospitalized for heart failure: the EVEREST Clinical Status Trials. JAMA. 2007;297:1332–43.
14. Konstam MA, Gheorghiade M, Burnett Jr JC, Grinfeld L, Maggioni AP, Swedberg K, et al. Effects of oral tolvaptan in patients hospitalized for worsening heart failure: the EVEREST Outcome Trial. JAMA. 2007;297:1319–31.
15. McMurray JJ, Teerlink JR, Cotter G, Bourge RC, Cleland JG, Jondeau G, et al. Effects of tezosentan on symptoms and clinical outcomes in patients with acute heart failure: the VERITAS randomized controlled trials. JAMA. 2007;298:2009–19.
16. Mebazaa A, Nieminen MS, Packer M, Cohen-Solal A, Kleber FX, Pocock SJ, et al. Levosimendan vs dobutamine for patients with acute decompensated heart failure: the SURVIVE Randomized Trial. JAMA. 2007;297:1883–91.
17. Sackner-Bernstein JD, Kowalski M, Fox M, Aaronson K. Short-term risk of death after treatment with nesiritide for decompensated heart failure: a pooled analysis of randomized controlled trials. JAMA. 2005;293:1900–5.
18. Sackner-Bernstein JD, Skopicki HA, Aaronson KD. Risk of worsening renal function with nesiritide in patients with acutely decompensated heart failure. Circulation. 2005;111:1487–91.
19. Publication Committee for the VI. Intravenous nesiritide vs nitroglycerin for treatment of decompensated congestive heart failure: a randomized controlled trial. JAMA. 2002;287:1531–40.
20. Sung NS, Crowley Jr WF, Genel M, Salber P, Sandy L, Sherwood LM, et al. Central challenges facing the national clinical research enterprise. JAMA. 2003;289:1278–87.
21. Gheorghiade M, Pang PS, O'Connor CM, Prasad K, McMurray J, Teerlink JR, et al. Clinical development of pharmacologic agents for acute heart failure syndromes: a proposal for a mechanistic translational phase. Am Heart J. 2011;161:224–32.
22. Cleland JG, Freemantle N, Coletta AP, Clark AL. Clinical trials update from the American Heart Association: REPAIR-AMI, ASTAMI, JELIS, MEGA, REVIVE-II, SURVIVE, and PROACTIVE. Eur J Heart Fail. 2006;8:105–10.
23. Louis A, Cleland JG, Crabbe S, Ford S, Thackray S, Houghton T, et al. Clinical Trials Update: CAPRICORN, COPERNICUS, MIRACLE, STAF, RITZ-2, RECOVER and RENAISSANCE and cachexia and cholesterol in heart failure. Highlights of the Scientific Sessions of the American College of Cardiology, 2001. Eur J Heart Fail. 2001;3:381–7.
24. Finley JJ, Konstam MA, Udelson JE. Arginine vasopressin antagonists for the treatment of heart failure and hyponatremia. Circulation. 2008;118:410–21.
25. Massie BM, O'Connor CM, Metra M, Ponikowski P, Teerlink JR, Cotter G, et al. Rolofylline, an adenosine A1-receptor antagonist, in acute heart failure. N Engl J Med. 2010;363:1419–28.
26. Cleland JG, Coletta AP, Buga L, Antony R, Pellicori P, Freemantle N, et al. Clinical trials update from the American Heart Association meeting 2010:

EMPHASIS-HF, RAFT, TIM-HF, Tele-HF, ASCEND-HF, ROCKET-AF, and PROTECT. Eur J Heart Fail. 2011;13:460–5.

27. Blair JE, Zannad F, Konstam MA, Cook T, Traver B, Burnett Jr JC, et al. Continental differences in clinical characteristics, management, and outcomes in patients hospitalized with worsening heart failure results from the EVEREST (Efficacy of Vasopressin Antagonism in Heart Failure: Outcome Study with Tolvaptan) program. J Am Coll Cardiol. 2008;52:1640–8.
28. Blair JE, Pang PS, Schrier RW, Metra M, Traver B, Cook T, et al. Changes in renal function during hospitalization and soon after discharge in patients admitted for worsening heart failure in the placebo group of the EVEREST trial. Eur Heart J. 2011;32:2563–72.
29. Weatherley BD, Cotter G, Dittrich HC, DeLucca P, Mansoor GA, Bloomfield DM, et al. Design and rationale of the PROTECT study: a placebo-controlled randomized study of the selective A1 adenosine receptor antagonist rolofylline for patients hospitalized with acute decompensated heart failure and volume overload to assess treatment effect on congestion and renal function. J Card Fail. 2010;16:25–35.
30. Anand IS, Fisher LD, Chiang YT, Latini R, Masson S, Maggioni AP, et al. Changes in brain natriuretic peptide and norepinephrine over time and mortality and morbidity in the Valsartan Heart Failure Trial (Val-HeFT). Circulation. 2003;107:1278–83.
31. Troughton RW, Frampton CM, Yandle TG, Espiner EA, Nicholls MG, Richards AM. Treatment of heart failure guided by plasma aminoterminal brain natriuretic peptide (N-BNP) concentrations. Lancet. 2000;355:1126–30.
32. Felker GM, Hasselblad V, Tang WH, Hernandez AF, Armstrong PW, Fonarow GC, et al. Troponin I in acute decompensated heart failure: insights from the ASCEND-HF study. Eur J Heart Fail. 2012;14:1257–64.
33. O'Connor CM, Fiuzat M, Lombardi C, Fujita K, Jia G, Davison BA, et al. Impact of serial troponin release on outcomes in patients with acute heart failure: analysis from the PROTECT pilot study. Circ Heart Fail. 2011;4:724–32.
34. Weintraub NL, Collins SP, Pang PS, Levy PD, Anderson AS, Arslanian-Engoren C, et al. Acute heart failure syndromes: emergency department presentation, treatment, and disposition: current approaches and future aims: a scientific statement from the American Heart Association. Circulation. 2010;122:1975–96.

Index

D.V. Cokkinos (ed.), *Introduction to Translational Cardiovascular Research*,
DOI 10.1007/978-3-319-08798-6, © Springer International Publishing Switzerland 2015

I

N